MAYO CLINIC BODY MRI CASE REVIEW

Mayo Clinic Scientific Press

Mayo Clinic Atlas of Regional Anesthesia and Ultrasound-Guided Nerve Blockade
Edited by James R. Hebl, MD, and Robert L. Lennon, DO

Mayo Clinic Preventive Medicine and Public Health Board Review
Edited by Prathibha Varkey, MBBS, MPH, MHPE

Mayo Clinic Challenging Images for Pulmonary Board Review
Edited by Edward C. Rosenow III, MD

Mayo Clinic Gastroenterology and Hepatology Board Review, Fourth Edition
Edited by Stephen C. Hauser, MD

Mayo Clinic Infectious Diseases Board Review
Edited by Zelalem Temesgen, MD

Mayo Clinic Antimicrobial Handbook: Quick Guide, Second Edition
Edited by John W. Wilson, MD, and Lynn L. Estes, PharmD

Just Enough Physiology
By James R. Munis, MD, PhD

Mayo Clinic Cardiology: Concise Textbook, Fourth Edition
Edited by Joseph G. Murphy, MD, and Margaret A. Lloyd, MD

Mayo Clinic Internal Medicine Board Review, Tenth Edition
Edited by Robert D. Ficalora, MD

Mayo Clinic Internal Medicine Board Review: Questions and Answers
Edited by Robert D. Ficalora, MD

Mayo Clinic Electrophysiology Manual
Edited by Samuel J. Asirvatham, MD

Mayo Clinic Gastrointestinal Imaging Review, Second Edition
By C. Daniel Johnson, MD

Arrhythmias in Women: Diagnosis and Management
Edited by Yong-Mei Cha, MD, Margaret A. Lloyd, MD, and Ulrika M. Birgersdotter-Green, MD

MAYO CLINIC BODY MRI CASE REVIEW

Christine U. Lee, MD, PhD

CONSULTANT, DEPARTMENT OF RADIOLOGY

MAYO CLINIC, ROCHESTER, MINNESOTA

ASSISTANT PROFESSOR OF RADIOLOGY

MAYO CLINIC COLLEGE OF MEDICINE

James F. Glockner, MD, PhD

CONSULTANT, DEPARTMENT OF RADIOLOGY

MAYO CLINIC, ROCHESTER, MINNESOTA

ASSISTANT PROFESSOR OF RADIOLOGY

MAYO CLINIC COLLEGE OF MEDICINE

MAYO CLINIC SCIENTIFIC PRESS

OXFORD UNIVERSITY PRESS

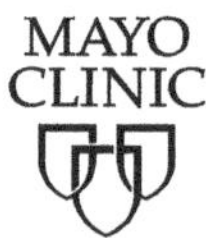

OXFORD
UNIVERSITY PRESS

Oxford University Press is a department of the University of Oxford. It furthers the University's objective of excellence in research, scholarship, and education by publishing worldwide.

Oxford New York
Auckland Cape Town Dar es Salaam Hong Kong Karachi
Kuala Lumpur Madrid Melbourne Mexico City Nairobi
New Delhi Shanghai Taipei Toronto

With offices in
Argentina Austria Brazil Chile Czech Republic France Greece
Guatemala Hungary Italy Japan Poland Portugal Singapore
South Korea Switzerland Thailand Turkey Ukraine Vietnam

Published in the United States of America by
Oxford University Press
198 Madison Avenue, New York, NY 10016
www.oup.com

Library of Congress Cataloging-in-Publication Data
Lee, Christine U., author.
Mayo Clinic body MRI case review / Christine U. Lee, James F. Glockner.
p. ; cm. — (Mayo Clinic scientific press)
ISBN 978-0-19-991570-5 (alk. paper)
I. Glockner, James F., author. II. Title. III. Series: Mayo Clinic scientific press (Series).
[DNLM: 1. Magnetic Resonance Imaging—methods—Case Reports. 2. Whole Body Imaging—methods—Case Reports. 3. Image Interpretation, Computer-Assisted—Case Reports. WN 185]
RC386.6.M34
616.07′548—dc23
2014001272

DEDICATION

We would like to dedicate this book to our parents,

Dr W. Yee and Agnes Lee and Warren and Mary Glockner.

PREFACE

Body MRI was once considered the weak stepsister of neurologic MRI (and probably still is by many neuroradiologists). This was reflected in the MR schedule during our training, when body MRI cases were relatively few and far between, and the job of the MR or abdominal fellow was to arrive at 6 AM for the 2 early cases and then wait for all the neurologic MRI examinations to be completed during the prime hours from 8 AM to 3 PM, after which any remaining body MRI cases could then be scanned.

The development of body MRI was hindered by problems of motion, whether breathing, cardiac pulsation, or anxious patients, and also by oddly shaped anatomy that couldn't be accommodated by a single coil. Nevertheless, many of the early pioneers persisted, and now body MRI is well established, widely accepted as a valuable imaging technique, and experiencing rapid growth in many areas.

Despite the increasingly prominent role of body MRI, training remains somewhat haphazard—there are relatively few dedicated body MRI fellowships, and exposure of residents and fellows to body MRI in the various subspecialty rotations is often limited to interpretation of images generated remotely using a standard protocol, without much reflection on how the images are obtained, which pulse sequences are optimal for a given clinical situation, and what can be done to fix the problems that inevitably arise. While protocol standardization does have the advantage of establishing a baseline level of examination quality, it remains surprisingly easy to generate truly horrible images, particularly when technologists and radiologists forget (or never learned) how to adapt an individual examination to accommodate the wide variety of sizes, breath-hold abilities, and temperaments of patients.

In our opinion, the opportunity for the technologist or radiologist to have a real impact on the quality of an examination is one of the most rewarding elements of body MRI, and we try to encourage our residents and fellows (with varying degrees of success) to learn enough of the nuts and bolts of scanning so that they can recognize when they are being fed substandard images and can even occasionally suggest possible solutions. We have tried to incorporate that philosophy into this book, particularly in the chapter on image artifacts, and have included several tangential but relatively brief discussions related to practical MR physics or optimization of protocols throughout the text.

While there are several excellent texts covering the fundamentals of body MRI, the teaching file format appeals to us because it represents the natural unit of radiologic analysis: Working radiologists examine a series of cases every day, and residents and fellows are continually forced to expose their knowledge (or lack thereof) in the semipublic forum of case conferences. The texts that we remember most fondly from our training (and, for the most part, the ones that we actually read all the way through) were teaching files, which exposed us to pathologies not prevalent at our institution and provided us with perspectives and analytical approaches that were occasionally different from those of our staff, all in an easily digestible format that could be incorporated into the occasional short breaks in the daily schedule.

The body MRI practice at Mayo Clinic has been large and fairly robust for many years, and we have accumulated a sizable collection of interesting cases encompassing a wide range of pathologies, organ systems, and imaging techniques. The chapters in this book are arranged primarily by organ systems, and we have attempted to include many examples of standard pathology as well as the occasional unusual and interesting cases that were missed by us (and a few others) either justifiably, because no one had ever heard of the diagnosis before, or less justifiably, because we hadn't heard of it but probably should have, or because we overlooked or misinterpreted some relevant findings. Our combined expertise (such as it is) encompasses the abdominal and pelvic chapters, while as individuals we participate in cardiac and vascular (J.F.G.) and breast and thoracic (C.U.L.) MRI practices. The musculoskeletal chapter is something of an anomaly since neither of us has read orthopedic MRI for many years; however, nearly all the examples in the chapter are cases that, for one reason or another, were scheduled for abdominal MRI. It is true, however, that all body MRI examinations include musculoskeletal anatomy, and we have attempted to provide a framework from the abdominal imager's perspective for handling the inevitable musculoskeletal-related abnormalities.

We have tried to make the text opinionated, readable, and at least somewhat entertaining, and we have eliminated references for the individual cases (we can count on 1 hand with several fingers left over the number of references looked up from texts we read during our training). The unwary reader should remember that our opinions are not universally shared and that, in fact, many aspects of body MRI remain extremely contentious. Most of all, we hope that this book will communicate our enthusiasm for the subject and stimulate a similar interest in trainees and even practicing radiologists.

We would like to acknowledge Benjamin H. Lee for his effort in creating the illustrations in Chapters 4 and 12—time which could otherwise have been devoted to his primary hobby of creating aliens.

TABLE OF CONTENTS

1.

LIVER: FOCAL MASSES

CASE 1.1

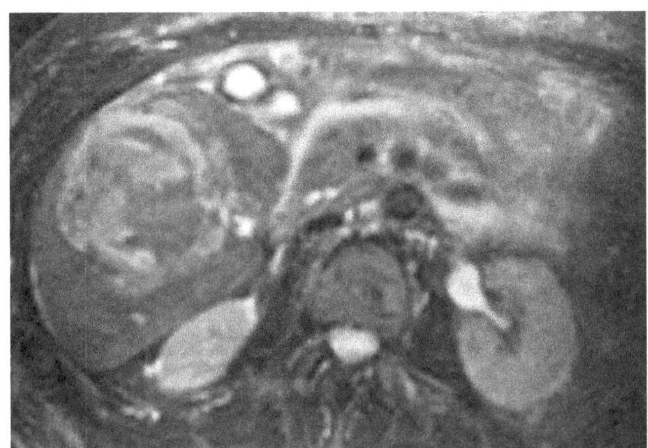

Figure 1.1.1

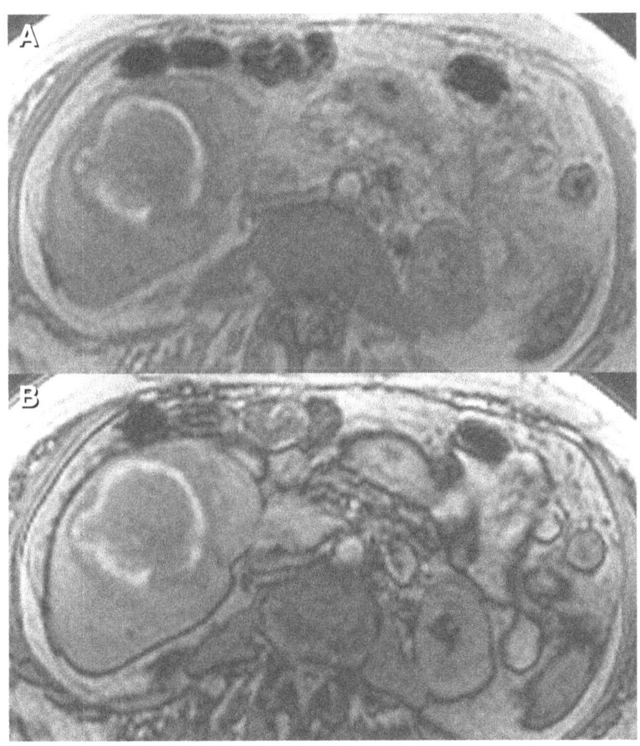

Figure 1.1.2

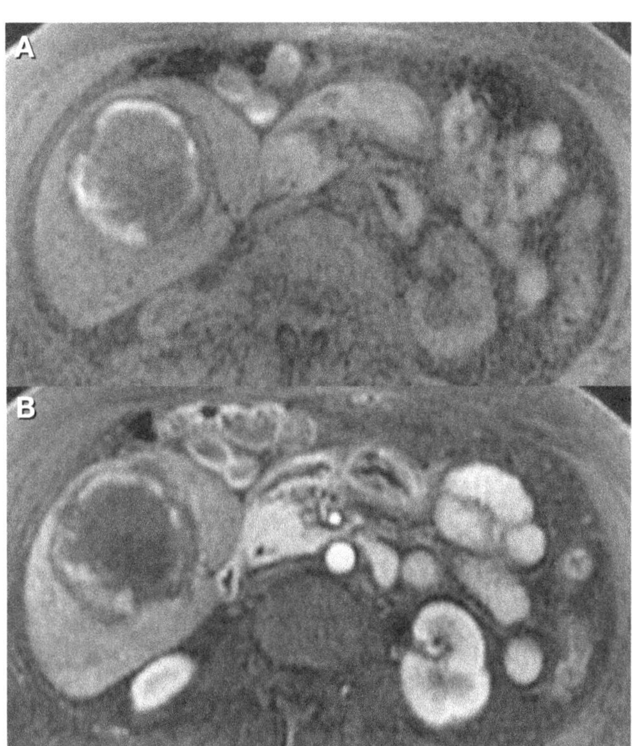

Figure 1.1.3

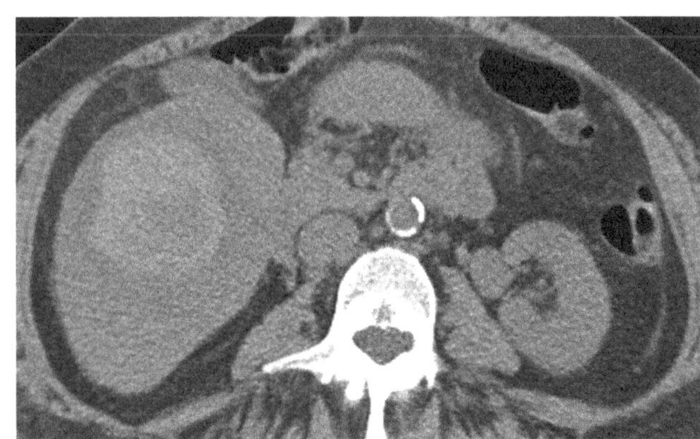

Figure 1.1.4

HISTORY: 71-year-old woman hospitalized for cholestasis and lymphadenopathy; history of recent aortic valve replacement

IMAGING FINDINGS: Axial fat-suppressed T2-weighted FSE (Figure 1.1.1), and axial IP and OP T1-weighted 2D SPGR (Figure 1.1.2) images demonstrate a large right hepatic lobe mass with a hyperintense peripheral rim and hypointense center. Pre- and postgadolinium arterial phase 3D SPGR images (Figure 1.1.3) reveal no enhancement of the mass. A CT scan performed later the same day (Figure 1.1.4) showed high attenuation in the mass, most consistent with hemorrhagic blood products.

DIAGNOSIS: Hepatic hematoma

COMMENT: Spontaneous nontraumatic hepatic hematomas that don't originate in a preexisting mass are relatively uncommon and generally occur in patients with a bleeding diathesis or patients who are anticoagulated. Hematomas seen in body MRI are most frequently the subacute type and often have a peripheral rim of high T1-signal intensity, representing intracellular methemoglobin. As the hematoma ages, methemoglobin may be converted to hemosiderin, with low signal intensity on both T1- and T2-weighted images.

The appearance of a subacute hematoma is distinctive, and the diagnosis can be made easily in most cases. The main concern, however, is whether the hematoma was caused by an underlying lesion. Dynamic gadolinium-enhanced 3D SPGR images are critical for answering this question since hematomas don't enhance (except for peripheral granulation tissue at the margins), whereas nearly every solid mass shows some degree of enhancement. Because hematomas are often complex, heterogeneous lesions containing large amounts of material with high signal intensity on precontrast T1-weighted acquisitions, subtraction images (ie, postcontrast minus precontrast) are often helpful to demonstrate the presence or absence of focal enhancement. Subtraction images should never be taken at face value, of course, without inspection of the unadulterated source images, since motion and misregistration artifacts can occasionally generate very convincing pseudolesions.

In this case, the radiologist indicated that the MRI findings could not entirely exclude the possibility of an underlying mass, so the clinician ordered a CT scan, which resulted in the same conclusions. It turned out that the patient had undergone a liver biopsy while still taking anticoagulation medication (for the aortic valve)—information that provides a plausible explanation for a hepatic hematoma without an underlying lesion.

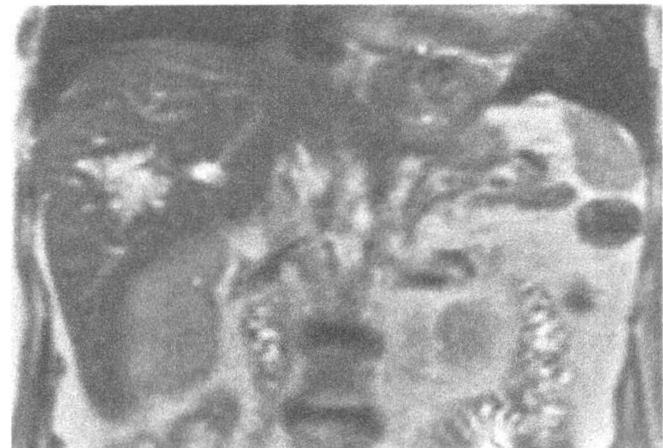

Figure 1.2.1

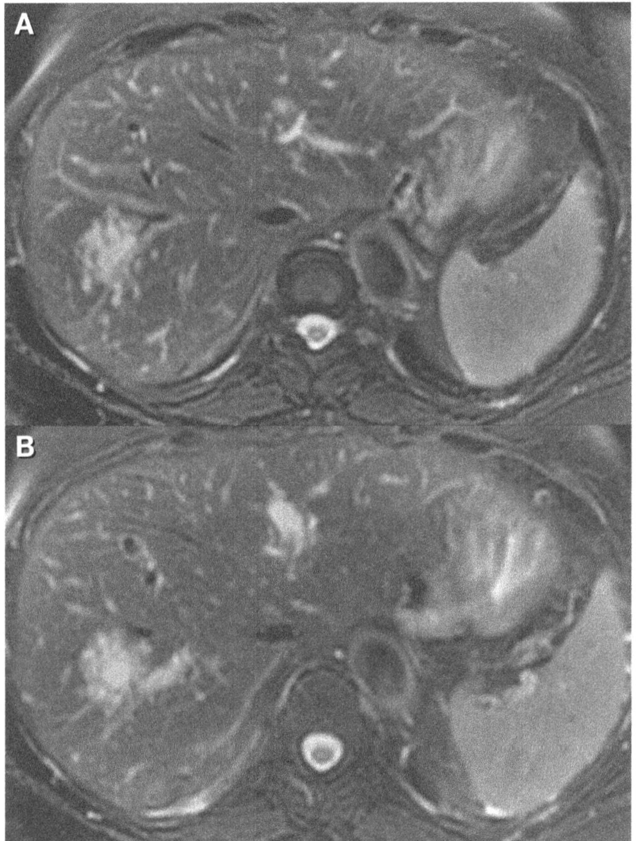

Figure 1.2.2

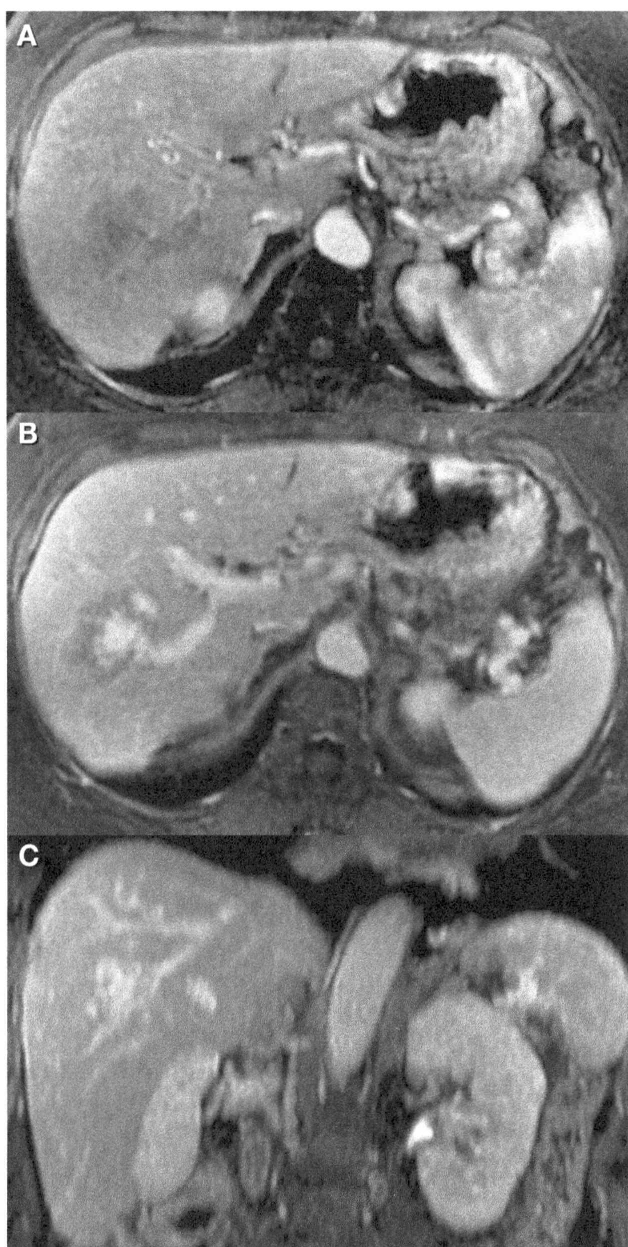

Figure 1.2.3

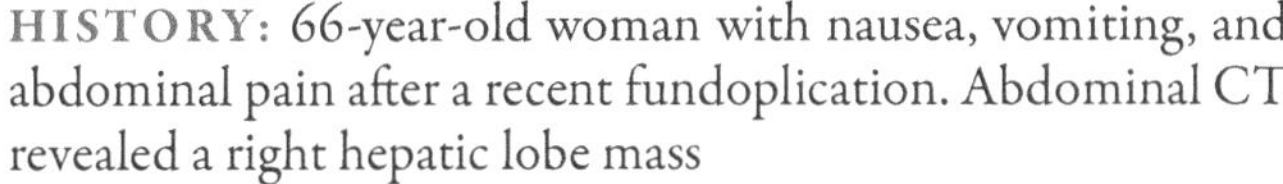

HISTORY: 66-year-old woman with nausea, vomiting, and abdominal pain after a recent fundoplication. Abdominal CT revealed a right hepatic lobe mass

IMAGING FINDINGS: Coronal SSFSE (Figure 1.2.1) and axial fat-suppressed FSE T2-weighted (Figure 1.2.2) images demonstrate a lobulated mass with high signal intensity in the right hepatic lobe. Axial arterial phase, portal venous phase, and coronal oblique reformatted equilibrium phase post-gadolinium 3D SPGR images (Figure 1.2.3) reveal no arterial phase enhancement of the lesion and prominent central enhancement on the portal phase image, as well as a mildly dilated portal vein extending to the lesion. The equilibrium phase coronal oblique reformatted image shows progressive enhancement of the mass, as well as continuity of the lesion with a mildly prominent right hepatic vein.

DIAGNOSIS: Hepatic vascular malformation

COMMENT: Hepatic vascular malformations are rarely discussed outside the context of congenital pediatric vascular lesions or hereditary hemorrhagic telangiectasia. Vascular malformations are uncommon in the liver but do occur occasionally in patients without a systemic vascular disorder or previous traumatic history. They can be classified on the basis of their feeding and draining vessels and into high-flow and slow-flow lesions.

In most cases, the diagnosis can be made with a reasonable degree of confidence. This patient, for example, had a lobulated lesion that is markedly hyperintense on T2-weighted images, resembling a hemangioma. On the dynamic postgadolinium images, however, it doesn't have enhancement characteristics consistent with a hemangioma since the initial enhancement is central rather than peripheral. There is a prominent feeding portal vein, an arguable draining hepatic vein, and persistent enhancement of the lesion to the level of the blood pool, all of which suggest that this is a vascular lesion.

This lesion can be classified as an intrahepatic portosystemic shunt but is small enough that it probably has no clinical implications.

The main differential diagnostic consideration is a hypervascular mass (see Case 1.18). The absence of any clearly defined solid component is reassuring, and diffusion-weighted images (not performed for this case) can be particularly helpful since a vascular malformation, even a slow-flow lesion such as this one, should appear as a flow void without a prominent high-signal-intensity focal mass. High-flow arterioportal fistulas or arteriovenous malformations also show flow voids on diffusion-weighted images and often on FSE acquisitions as well.

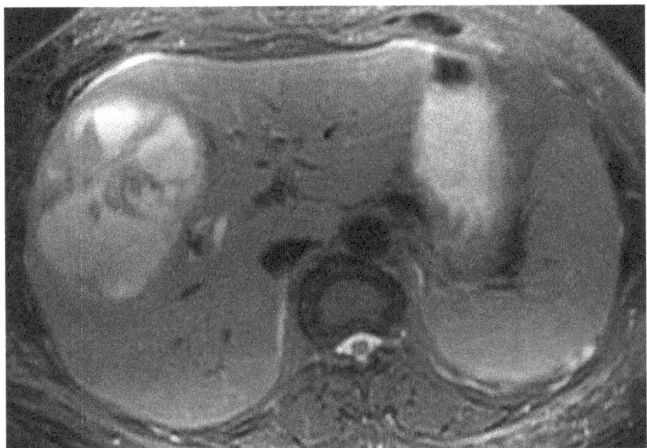

Figure 1.3.1

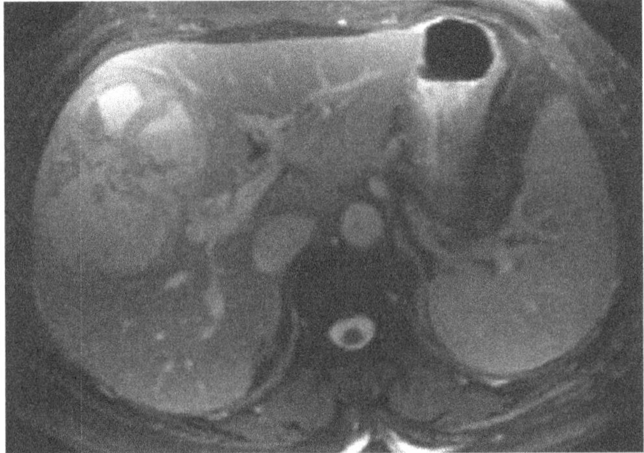

Figure 1.3.2

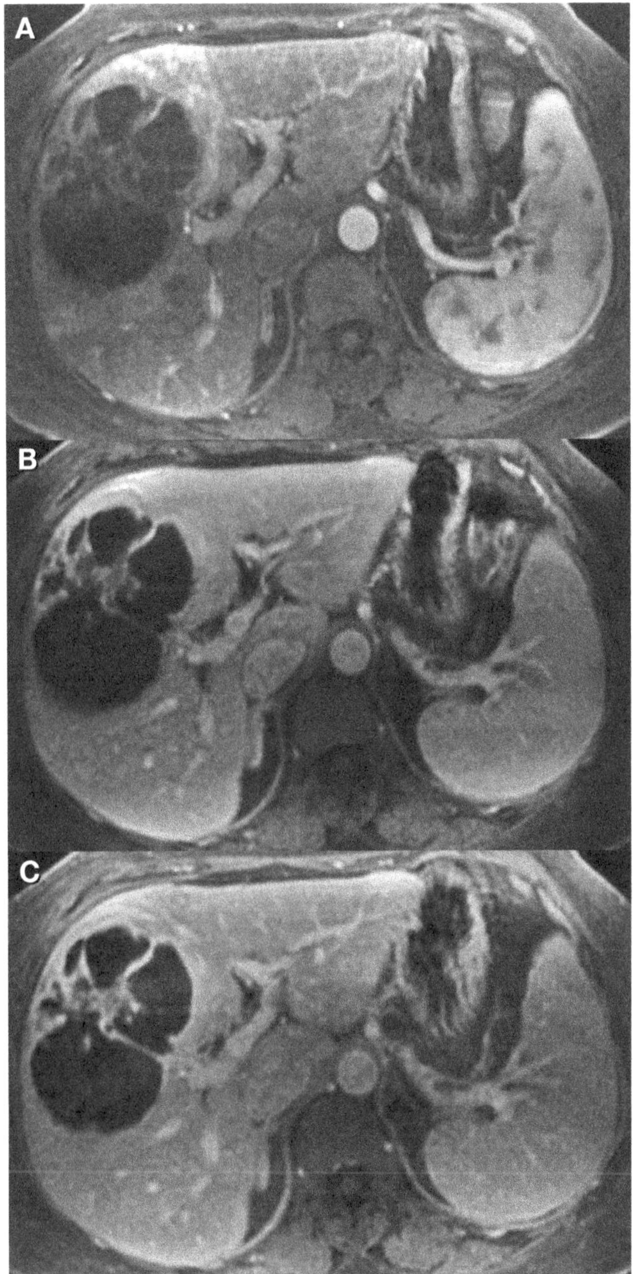

Figure 1.3.3

HISTORY: 70-year-old woman with nausea and weakness, elevated liver function tests, and elevated white blood cell count

IMAGING FINDINGS: Axial fat-saturated FSE (Figure 1.3.1) and SSFP (Figure 1.3.2) images demonstrate a large heterogeneous, predominantly cystic lesion in the right hepatic lobe containing multiple thick septations. Note the internal fluid-fluid levels, better seen on the SSFP image. Axial postgadolinium arterial, portal venous, and equilibrium phase images (Figure 1.3.3) show mild enhancement of the rim and septations. Notice also the adjacent parenchymal enhancement on the arterial phase image, suggestive of inflammation.

DIAGNOSIS: Hepatic abscess

COMMENT: A complex rim-enhancing cystic lesion in a patient with leukocytosis should be sufficient to suggest the diagnosis, although other causes such as a necrotic primary or metastatic neoplasm should also be considered.

Pyogenic liver abscesses are most often caused by biliary obstruction and ascending cholangitis or by hematogenous spread from an intestinal infection such as diverticulitis.

Common causative organisms include *Escherichia coli* and *Klebsiella pneumoniae*, with polymicrobial infections accounting for more than half of all cases. A small but increasing percentage of hepatic abscesses result from various interventional procedures, including transarterial chemoembolization and percutaneous radiofrequency ablation. Although most hepatic abscesses in the developed world are pyogenic, it is worth remembering that worldwide, the leading cause is parasitic infection from *Entamoeba histolytica*. Fungal infections, particularly candidiasis, are common in immunocompromised patients.

The appearance of abscesses on MRI is variable. Most lesions have low T1- and high T2-signal intensity, with early rim enhancement after gadolinium administration. Perilesional edema on T2-weighted images (and perilesional early enhancement) is more typical of abscesses than neoplasms, but this is not a particularly specific sign. Gas within an abscess is a helpful finding, appearing as a signal void and usually best seen on gradient echo pulse sequences.

Atypical abscesses can have an appearance more suggestive of a solid mass. Occasionally, atypical signal intensity on T1- and T2-weighted images may reflect the presence of proteinaceous debris, hemorrhage, or fibrosis.

A few studies have investigated the ability of DWI to distinguish abscesses from cysts, hemangiomas, and cystic or necrotic neoplasms. The general idea is that the center of an abscess has restricted diffusion in comparison to simple fluid in cysts, blood in hemangiomas, or necrotic fluid within a neoplasm, and therefore diffusion-weighted images obtained with a relatively high b value to minimize T2 shine-through will demonstrate higher signal intensity within an abscess. The corresponding ADC parametric image will show lower signal intensity (ie, lower ADC values) in the abscess compared to normal liver, and the other lesions will have higher ADC values. This sign is not universally true, but it is occasionally helpful, particularly in situations where gadolinium cannot be administered.

Pyogenic hepatic abscesses have an associated mortality rate estimated at 3% to 10%, although this rate has declined with earlier detection and more aggressive therapy. Standard treatment includes antibiotics with or without percutaneous aspiration, drainage, or surgery.

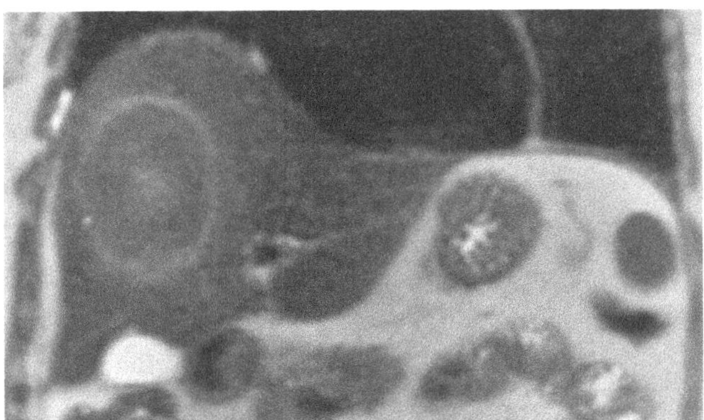

Figure 1.4.1

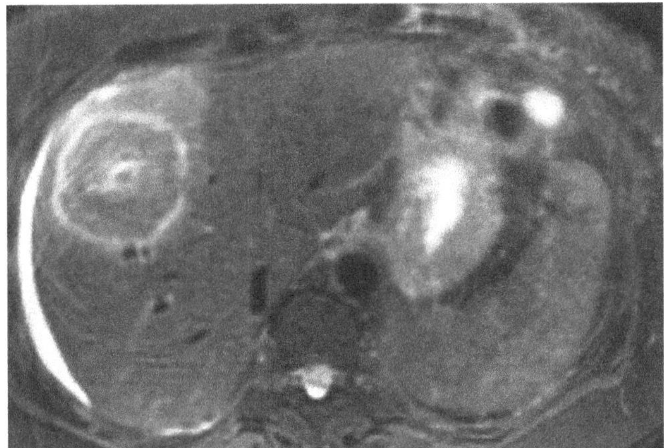

Figure 1.4.2

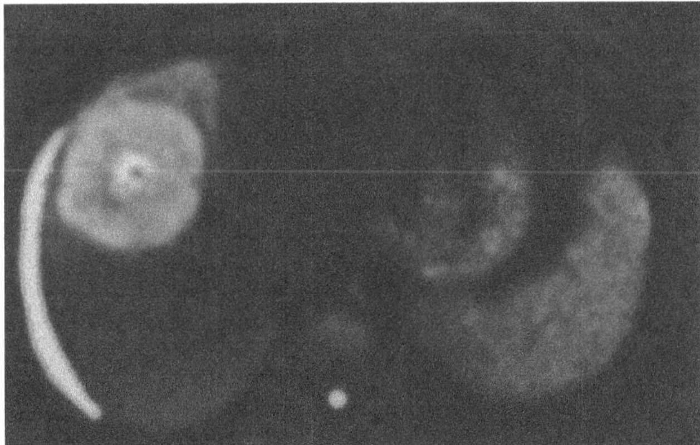

Figure 1.4.3

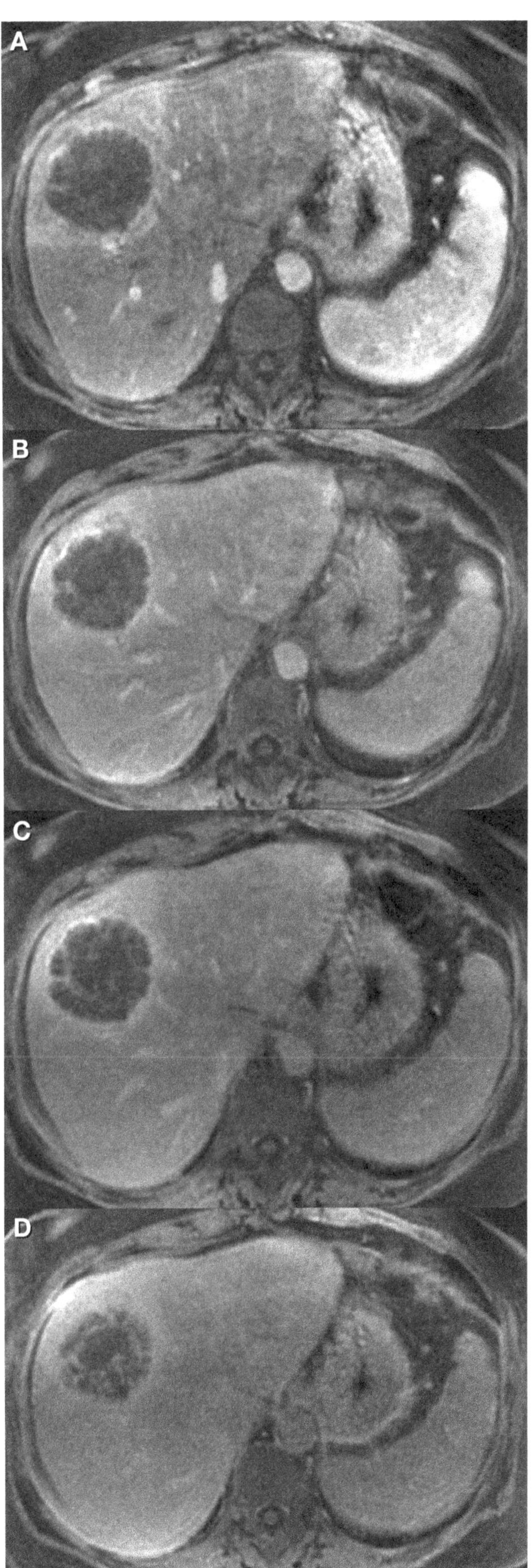

Figure 1.4.4

HISTORY: 67-year-old woman status post fundoplication 2 months ago, with development of fever and nonproductive cough shortly afterward; laboratory tests revealed normal liver function and an increased neutrophil count

IMAGING FINDINGS: Coronal SSFSE image (Figure 1.4.1) and axial fat-suppressed T2-weighted FSE image (Figure 1.4.2) demonstrate a slightly lobulated lesion with mildly increased signal intensity compared to normal liver and a prominent hyperintense rim. Notice the mildly increased signal intensity in the adjacent hepatic parenchyma, as well as a small amount of perihepatic ascites. Axial diffusion-weighted image (b=600 s/mm^2) (Figure 1.4.3) shows similar findings, with prominent high signal intensity centrally. Axial arterial, portal venous, equilibrium, and delayed phase postgadolinium 3D SPGR images (Figure 1.4.4) demonstrate mild rim enhancement on the arterial phase image and gradual, heterogeneous internal enhancement best appreciated on equilibrium and delayed phase images. Notice also the segmental parenchymal hyperenhancement adjacent to the lesion.

DIAGNOSIS: Organizing hepatic abscess

COMMENT: This case represents a less typical appearance of a pyogenic hepatic abscess, with unusually low T2-signal intensity and prominent gradual internal enhancement (ie, it's not predominantly cystic). The perilesional edema in the adjacent liver seen on the T2-weighted and postgadolinium images is suggestive of an abscess but is not a particularly compelling sign since large neoplasms often compress or encase vessels, leading to associated perfusion abnormalities.

The initial report was appropriately vague and favored metastatic disease over abscess. This led to a series of biopsies, all of which were inadequate or indeterminate, until the final successful biopsy yielded a diagnosis of an organizing abscess.

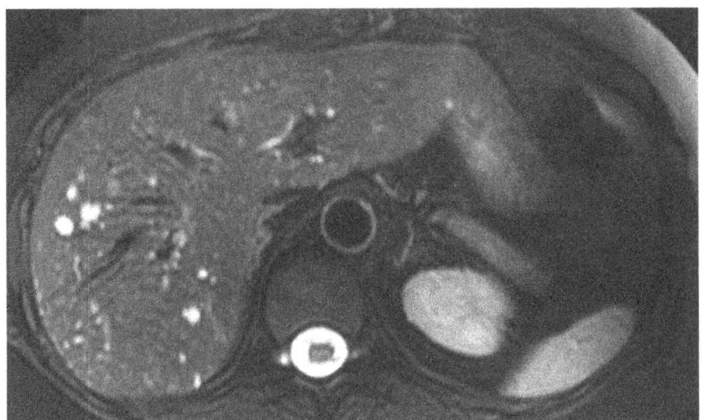

Figure 1.5.1

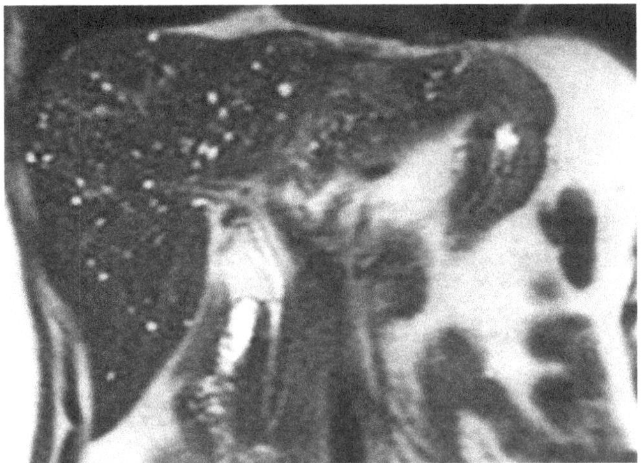

Figure 1.5.2

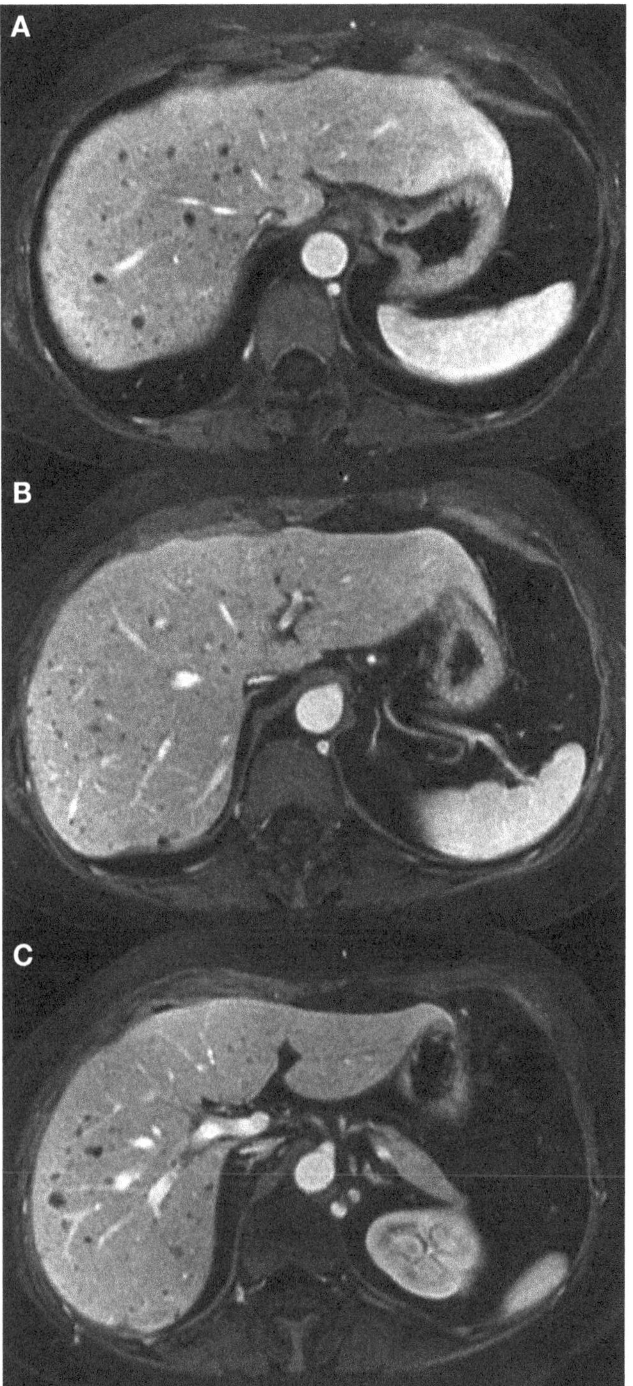

Figure 1.5.3

HISTORY: 33-year-old woman with multiple liver lesions on CT performed elsewhere

IMAGING FINDINGS: Axial fat-suppressed FSE T2-weighted (Figure 1.5.1), coronal SSFSE (Figure 1.5.2), and axial postgadolinium 3D SPGR (Figure 1.5.3) images demonstrate multiple, very small, nonenhancing cystic lesions

DIAGNOSIS: Biliary hamartomas

COMMENT: Biliary hamartomas, also called *von Meyenburg complexes*, belong to a spectrum of ductal plate anomalies that include polycystic liver disease and Caroli disease. Although it is relatively straightforward to distinguish biliary hamartomas and hepatic cysts from Caroli disease, the same cannot be said for biliary hamartomas vs hepatic cysts. By definition, Caroli disease represents saccular, dilated intrahepatic ducts, while neither biliary hamartomas nor hepatic cysts communicate with the biliary system. (So, injecting a hepatobiliary contrast agent and waiting for gadolinium to appear in the cystic cavity of a biliary hamartoma is a fruitless proposition.)

Distinction between biliary hamartomas and hepatic cysts is often difficult or impossible, but fortunately it is not particularly important since both are benign entities that should be left alone. There are a few imaging findings that may help suggest the diagnosis of biliary hamartoma. In general, biliary hamartomas are smaller (<1.5 cm) than most hepatic cysts and may follow a peribiliary distribution, which can be better appreciated in a second example, shown in Figures 1.5.4, 1.5.5, and 1.5.6.

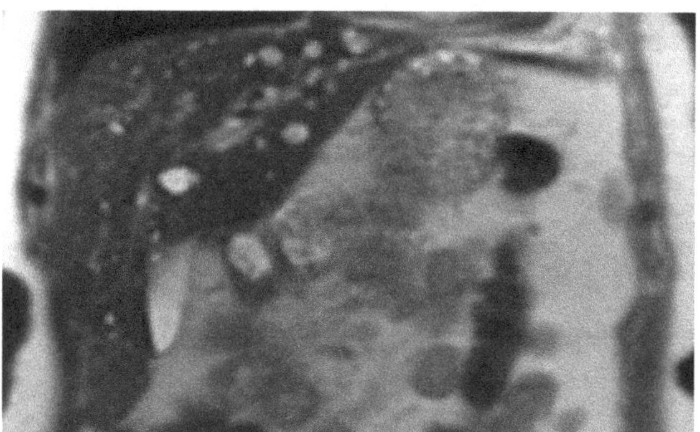

Figure 1.5.4

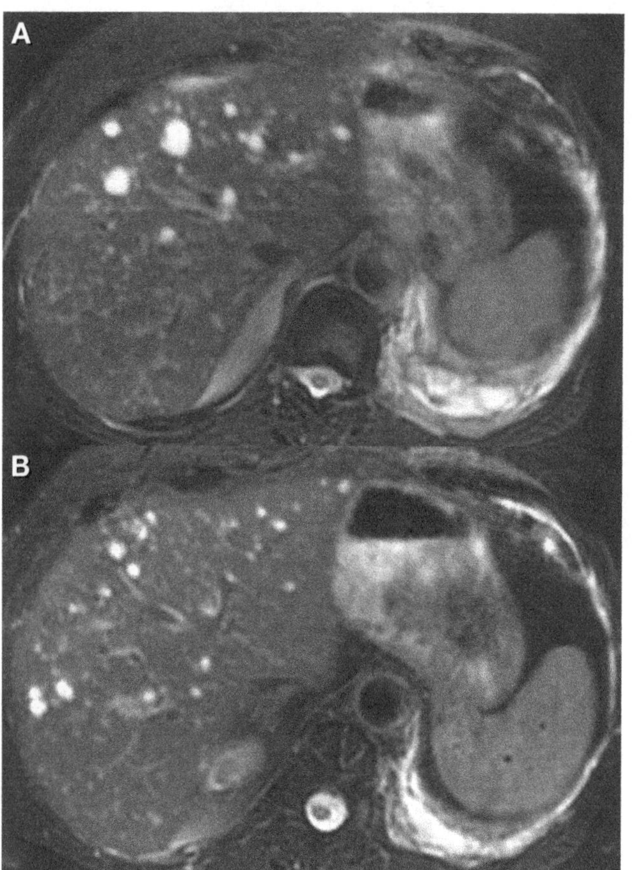

Figure 1.5.5

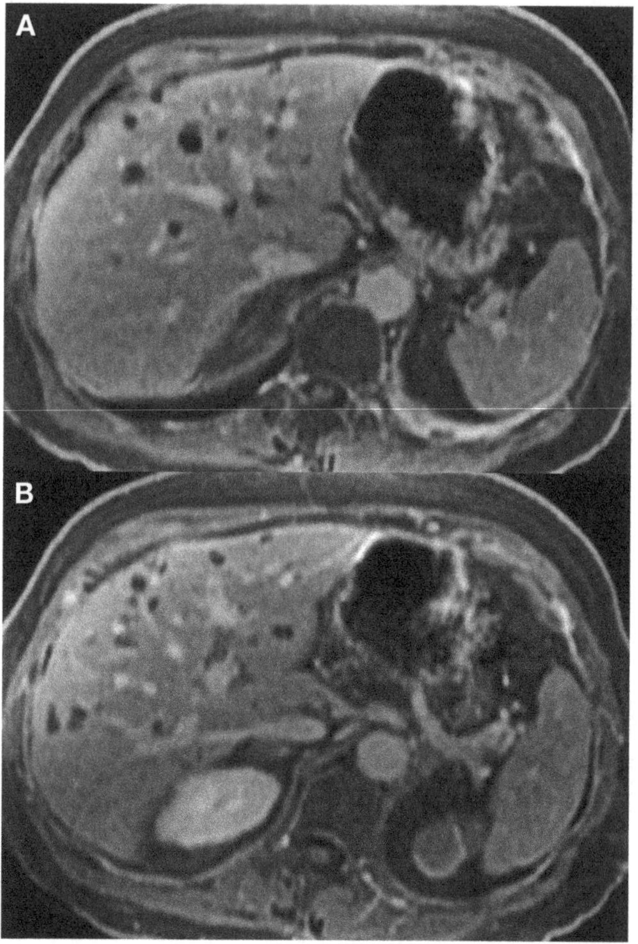

Figure 1.5.6

Coronal SSFSE (Figure 1.5.4), axial fat-suppressed FSE T2-weighted (Figure 1.5.5), and axial portal venous phase postgadolinium 3D SPGR (Figure 1.5.6) images demonstrate multiple small, nonenhancing cystic lesions in a segmental distribution.

Biliary hamartomas may have perceptible, slightly irregular walls that occasionally show mild enhancement; hepatic cysts have imperceptible walls without enhancement (unless it's a complex cyst). Another clue to distinguishing biliary hamartomas from hepatic cysts is simply one of likelihood. Biliary hamartomas are much less common than hepatic cysts, and so if you favor cysts in your differential diagnosis of these lesions, you'll be right most of the time.

The only important differential diagnosis (ie, one that would make a difference clinically) is a pathologic cystic lesion, such as an abscess or cystic metastasis. Usually, the distinction is obvious since both of these entities should have thicker walls with much greater enhancement—this is probably borne out by the fact that all of our pathologically proven cases of biliary hamartomas come either from lobectomies performed to resect another lesion that also happened to contain biliary hamartomas or from blind biopsies to assess for diffuse parenchymal disease.

CASE 1.6

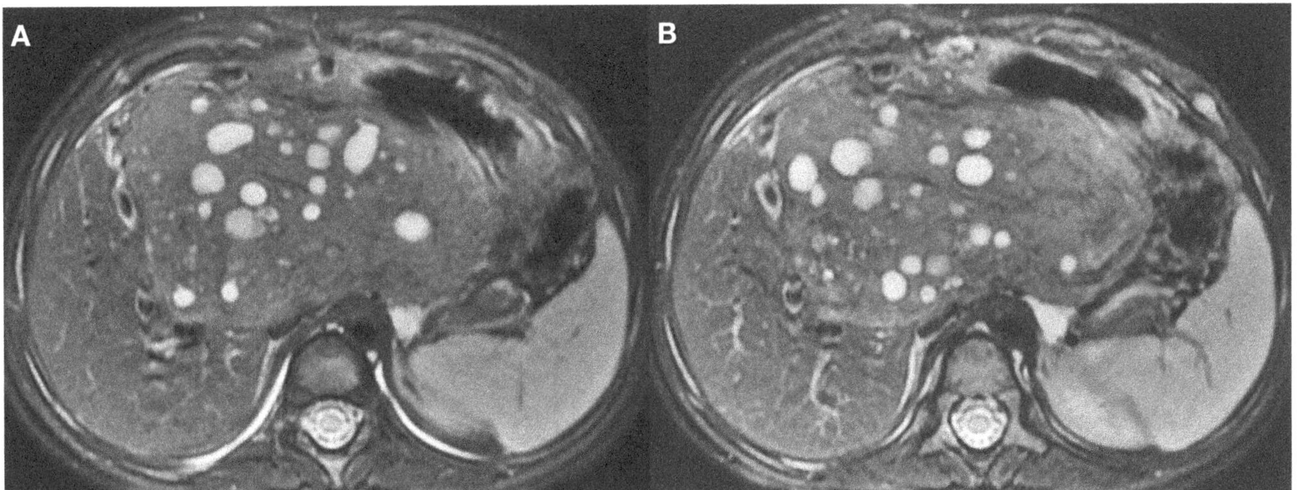

Figure 1.6.1

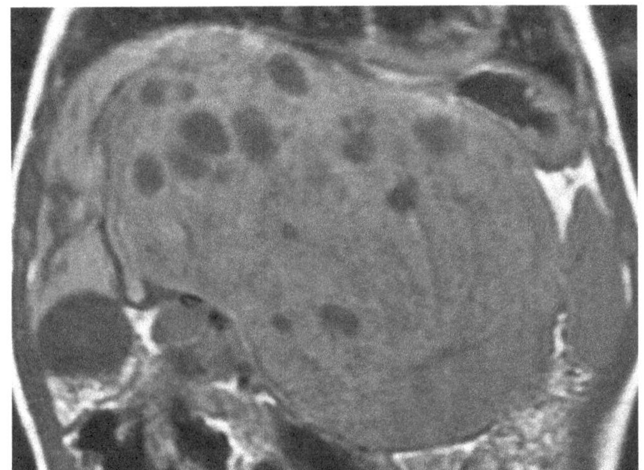

Figure 1.6.2

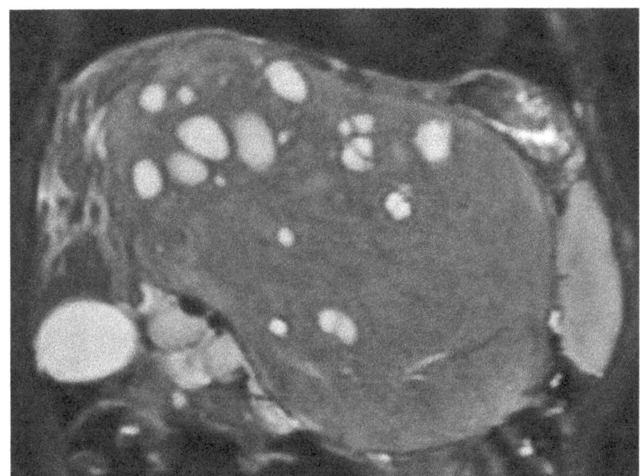

Figure 1.6.3

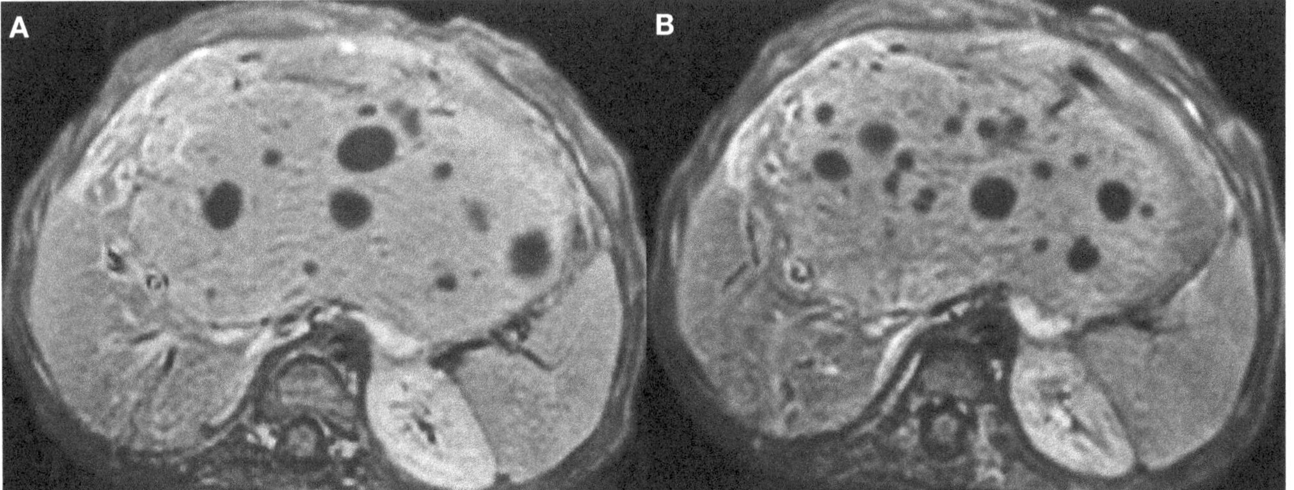

Figure 1.6.4

HISTORY: 3-year-old girl with an enlarging abdomen

IMAGING FINDINGS: Axial fat-suppressed FSE T2-weighted (Figure 1.6.1) and coronal T1-weighted (Figure 1.6.2) and T2-weighted (Figure 1.6.3) images demonstrate a large, well-circumscribed mixed solid and cystic mass occupying the entire left hepatic lobe. Axial postgadolinium 2D SPGR images (Figure 1.6.4) reveal mild hyperenhancement of the solid component of the mass relative to normal liver and no enhancement of the cystic components.

DIAGNOSIS: Mesenchymal hamartoma

COMMENT: Mesenchymal hamartoma is a rare lesion but is nevertheless the second most common benign liver mass in children, after infantile hemangioendothelioma. Mesenchymal hamartomas are typically discovered in children younger than 2 years (nearly all lesions are detected before 5 years of age) who present with a painless abdominal mass. Laboratory markers are generally unrevealing, although serum AFP levels are occasionally mildly elevated.

Mesenchymal hamartoma favors the right hepatic lobe and appears as a disordered proliferation of mesenchymal tissue containing variably sized cysts, bile ducts, and hepatocyte cords. The cystic components have no discrete endothelial lining and are thought to develop as a result of cystic degeneration of mesenchymal tissue and resultant accumulation of fluid from lymphatic and biliary duct obstruction.

Mesenchymal hamartoma has generally been considered a congenital lesion rather than a true neoplasm. However, recent cytogenic analysis has detected chromosomal translocations and aneuploidy, suggesting that a neoplastic cause may be more likely.

The imaging appearance of mesenchymal hamartoma is determined by the relative preponderance of cystic and solid components; 80% have macroscopic cysts and usually appear as multiloculated cystic masses with a variable amount of solid tissue.

Differential diagnosis includes other pediatric hepatic masses. Hepatoblastoma occurs in a similar age-group but is generally a solid lesion (Case 1.19), often associated with markedly elevated serum AFP levels. Infantile hemangioendothelioma may contain myxoid or cystic components, but the predominant vascular nature of these lesions is usually easily appreciated. Undifferentiated embryonal sarcoma (Cases 1.20 and 1.21) can have an appearance similar to mesenchymal hamartoma and, in fact, shares many cytogenic features, but it occurs in an older age-group and is typically more heterogeneous and aggressive in appearance. For predominantly cystic mesenchymal hamartomas, the differential diagnosis also includes simple cyst, hydatid disease, choledochal cyst, and lymphangioma.

The definitive treatment of mesenchymal hamartoma is surgical resection, with an excellent prognosis: Long-term survival is greater than 90%, even for patients with incomplete resection.

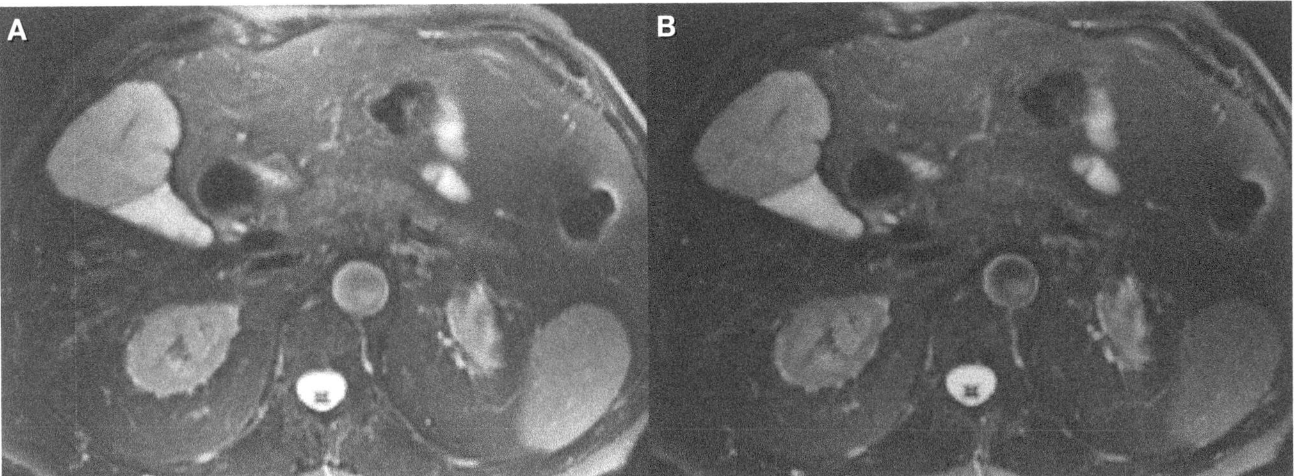

Figure 1.7.1

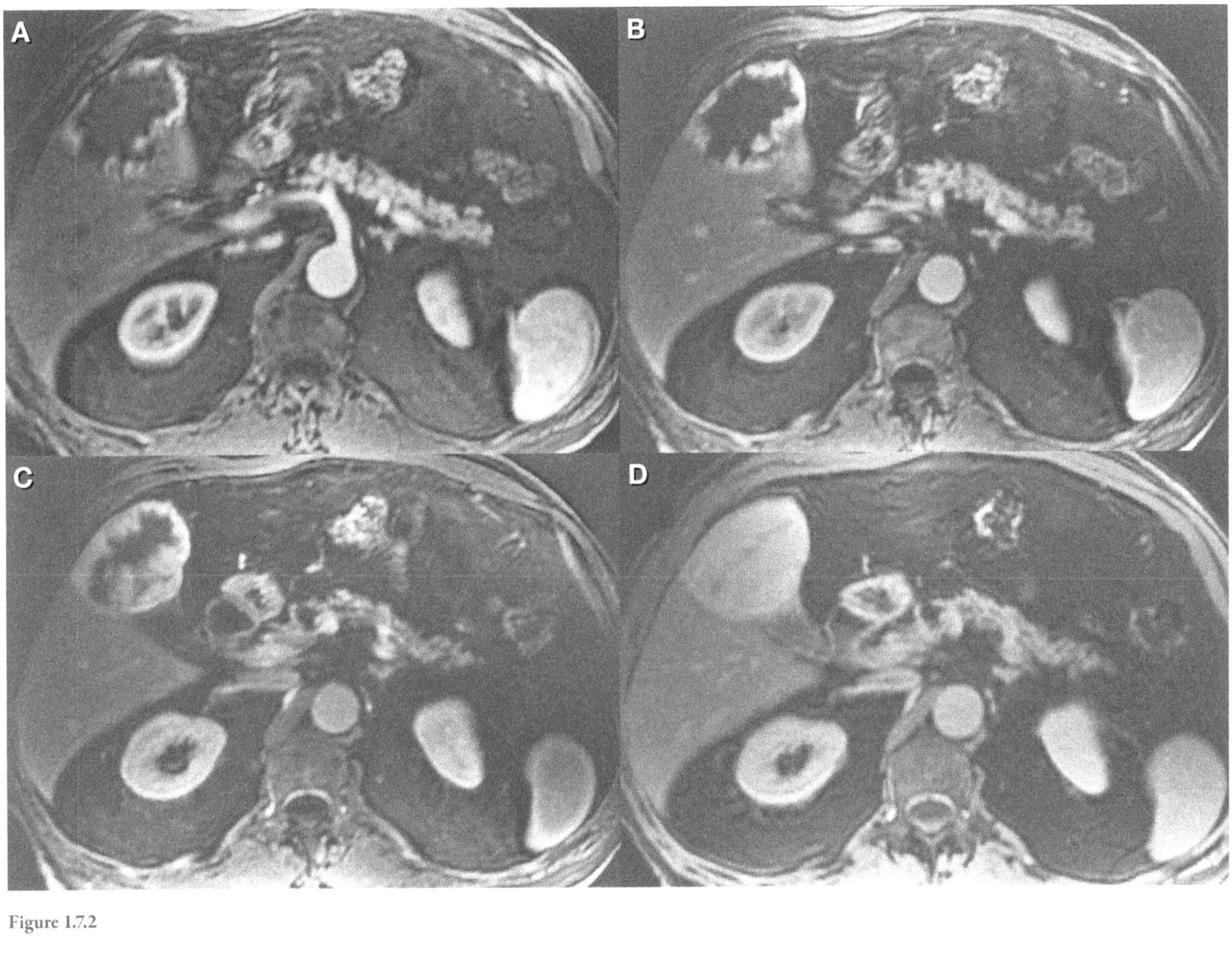

Figure 1.7.2

HISTORY: 75-year-old man with right upper quadrant pain

IMAGING FINDINGS: Axial fat-suppressed dual echo FSE T2-weighted images (Figure 1.7.1) reveal a lobulated mass in the right hepatic lobe with diffuse high signal intensity. Note that on the dual echo images, there is little signal loss between the first (TE, 80 ms) and second (TE, 160 ms) echoes. Axial arterial, portal venous, equilibrium, and 5-minute delayed phase postgadolinium 3D SPGR images (Figure 1.7.2) demonstrate early globular peripheral enhancement of the lesion, with gradual filling on subsequent images.

DIAGNOSIS: Hemangioma

COMMENT: Hemangiomas are benign masses consisting of vascular spaces of variable sizes lined with endothelial cells and interspersed fibrous or myxoid stroma. They are the most common hepatic mass (excluding cysts), with autopsy studies reporting an incidence of 1% to 20%, and are often found incidentally because the vast majority of patients with hemangioma are asymptomatic. Hemangiomas are much more common in women, who account for 75% of lesions, and are solitary in 70% to 90% of cases.

Three classic (or 1 classic and 2 somewhat problematic) appearances have been described on dynamic contrast-enhanced CT or MRI. Hemangiomas demonstrate early peripheral globular enhancement on arterial phase postgadolinium images, followed by gradual centripetal filling on portal venous and equilibrium phase images. Diffuse enhancement of the lesion is seen on delayed images with signal intensity similar to the blood pool (the inferior vena cava is a handy reference). This pattern is seen in 75% to 80% of lesions. A small percentage of hemangiomas, usually small lesions less than 1.5 cm in diameter, may show immediate diffuse enhancement on arterial phase images, again with persistent enhancement on portal venous and equilibrium phase images similar to blood pool. A third pattern, seen most commonly in larger lesions, is peripheral globular enhancement with centripetal filling but with persistent hypoenhancement in the center of the lesion.

This third pattern is becoming more common in our practice as more and more examinations are completed without anyone checking the images before the patient is dismissed, thereby losing the opportunity to obtain delayed images demonstrating complete enhancement of the lesion. Usually this isn't a tragedy, but the finding of persistent late enhancement equivalent to the blood pool is a very helpful sign in atypical lesions.

On T2-weighted imaging, hemangiomas are typically markedly hyperintense, similar to cerebrospinal fluid, and in our minds these represent the true "light bulb" lesions rather than pheochromocytomas. Our rule of thumb is that when a hepatic lesion is bright and easily visualized on SSFSE images or when it's nearly as bright as cerebrospinal fluid on standard FSE images, then it's a cyst or hemangioma. This is usually true, and the occasional exceptions can be diagnosed on dynamic postgadolinium images in most cases. In the dark ages of MRI before dynamic contrast-enhanced images could reliably be obtained (and illustrated by this case from the early years of 3D dynamic imaging), we often performed a dual echo FSE acquisition with 2 TEs, one at 80 ms with typical T2 weighting and a second longer TE of about 160 ms. The main reason for doing this was to distinguish cysts and hemangiomas from solid lesions; while all lesions might be at least somewhat bright on the first echo, only lesions that were mostly fluid had T2s long enough to be very bright on the second echo. We still occasionally see a dual echo FSE acquisition on examinations performed elsewhere that are submitted for review, but for the most part, this is a deservedly archaic technique. The vast majority of cysts and hemangiomas are much brighter than solid lesions on standard T2-weighted images, and the small amount of added confidence provided by the second echo does not justify the extra 3 to 4 minutes spent acquiring it.

Hemangiomas are usually hyperintense relative to liver on diffusion-weighted images performed with the typical b values used in abdominal imaging (ie, 50-800 s/mm^2), because of T2 shine-through rather than restricted diffusion. The ADC values of hemangiomas are consistently lower than for most solid lesions, and many of the early diffusion studies seeking to distinguish benign lesions from malignant ones on this basis inflated their statistics by comparing cysts and hemangiomas to solid cancers (on the other hand, there are not reliable differences in ADC values between solid benign and solid malignant lesions in the liver). A lesion that loses a significant amount of signal intensity between a low b-value and a high b-value acquisition is likely a cyst or hemangioma; similarly, one that has an ADC value higher than adjacent normal liver is also likely a cyst or hemangioma.

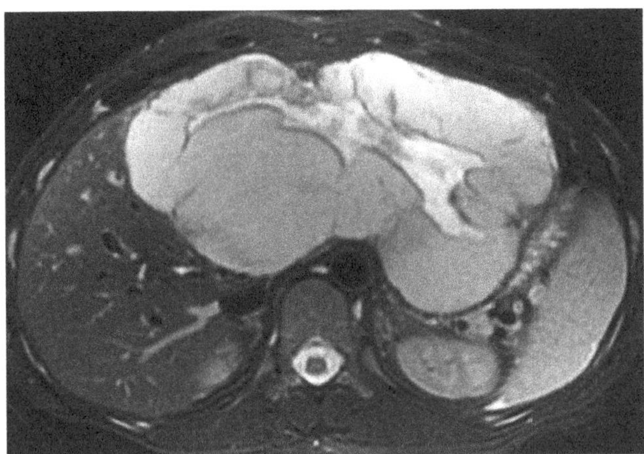

Figure 1.8.1

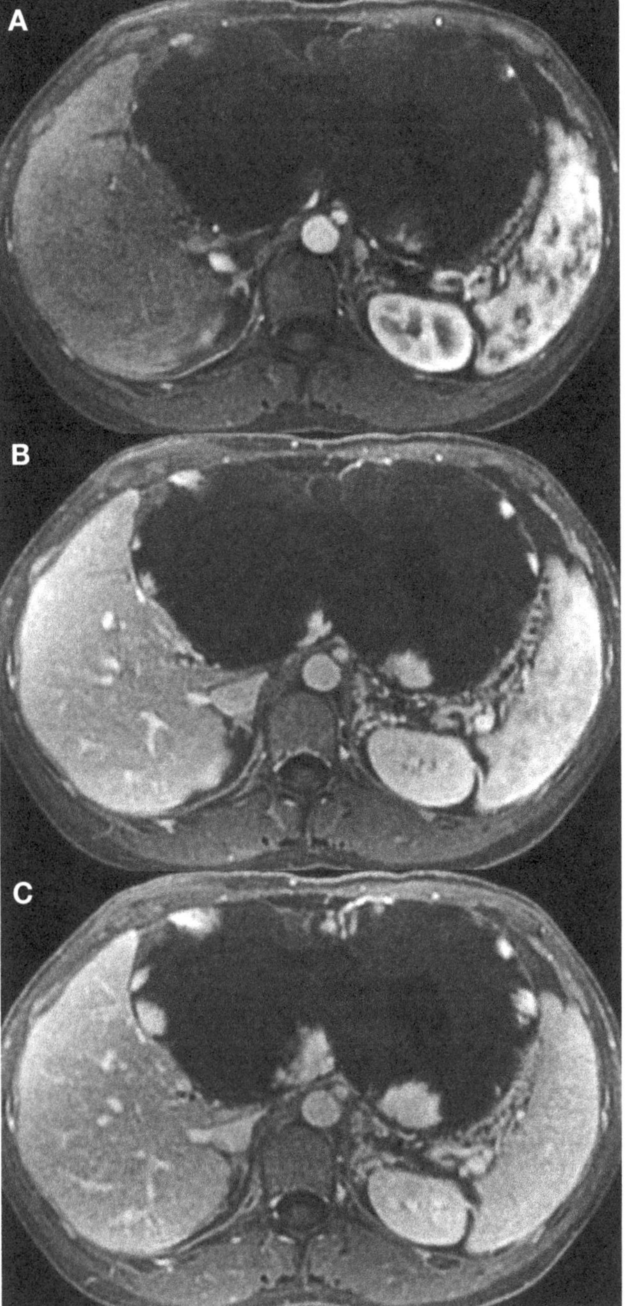

Figure 1.8.2

HISTORY: 36-year-old woman with early satiety and abdominal discomfort

IMAGING FINDINGS: Axial fat-suppressed FSE T2-weighted image (Figure 1.8.1) demonstrates a large mass in the left hepatic lobe with high signal intensity, greatest in the center of the lesion. Axial arterial, portal venous, and equilibrium phase postgadolinium 3D SPGR images (Figure 1.8.2) reveal gradually increasing globular peripheral enhancement.

DIAGNOSIS: Giant cavernous hemangioma

COMMENT: As noted in Case 1.7, early peripheral globular enhancement that continues to fill in on portal venous, equilibrium, and delayed phase postgadolinium 3D SPGR images is a radiologic "Aunt Minnie" for benign cavernous hemangiomas. Giant hemangiomas sometimes confuse our residents on the basis of sheer size and the somewhat heterogeneous appearance on T2-weighted images. They're reluctant to dismiss these lesions as clearly benign, but the characteristic appearance on dynamic postgadolinium 3D SPGR images is usually evident and the diagnosis straightforward. Central hyperintensity on T2-weighted images is a very common feature of giant hemangiomas, in our experience, and likely represents a central fibrotic core. The few exceptions to this generalization occur in patients with central thrombosis and calcification.

Giant cavernous hemangioma is defined as a hemangioma larger than 4 cm. They rarely rupture or cause other catastrophic problems (patients with giant hemangiomas have been cleared for parachute jumping, according to the literature), and indications for surgical resection are primarily based on clinical symptoms, such as progressive abdominal pain with hemangiomas larger than 5 cm.

The patient in this case underwent left and caudate lobectomies. Pathologic evaluation demonstrated a cavernous hemangioma forming a 19.6×14.5×6.4-cm mass, as well as a focus of FNH (0.9 cm) involving the caudate lobe. Even in retrospect, this small FNH was not well appreciated; it likely blended into the peripherally enhancing nodules of the giant hemangioma.

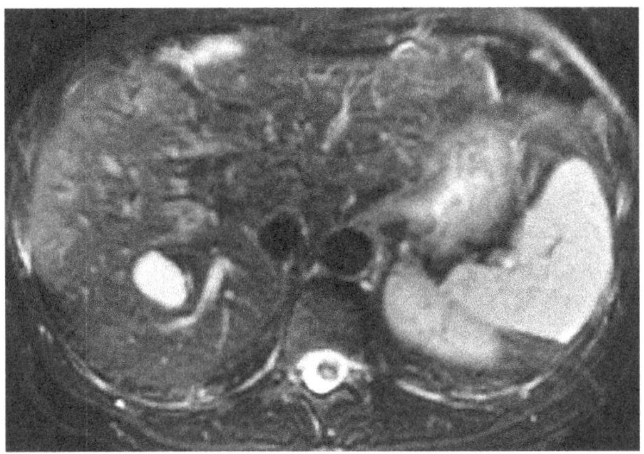

Figure 1.9.1

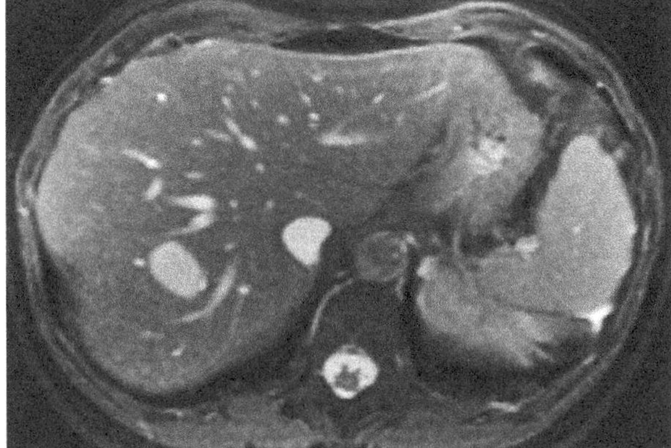

Figure 1.9.2

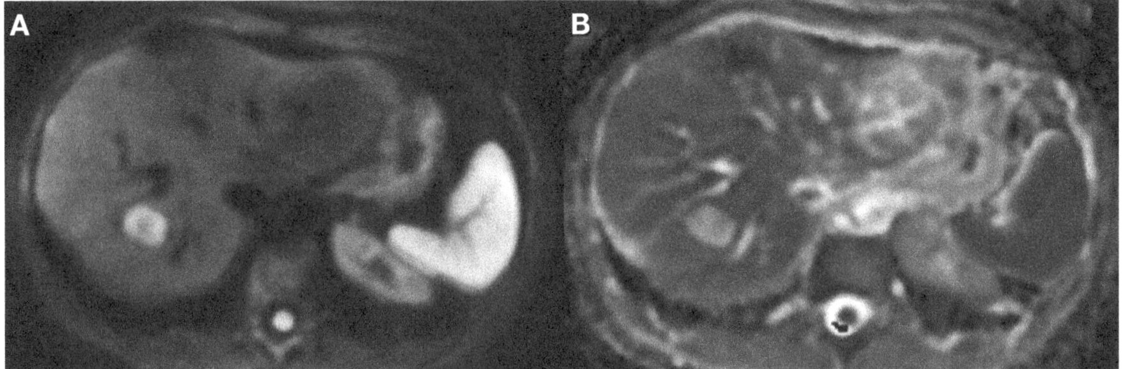

Figure 1.9.3

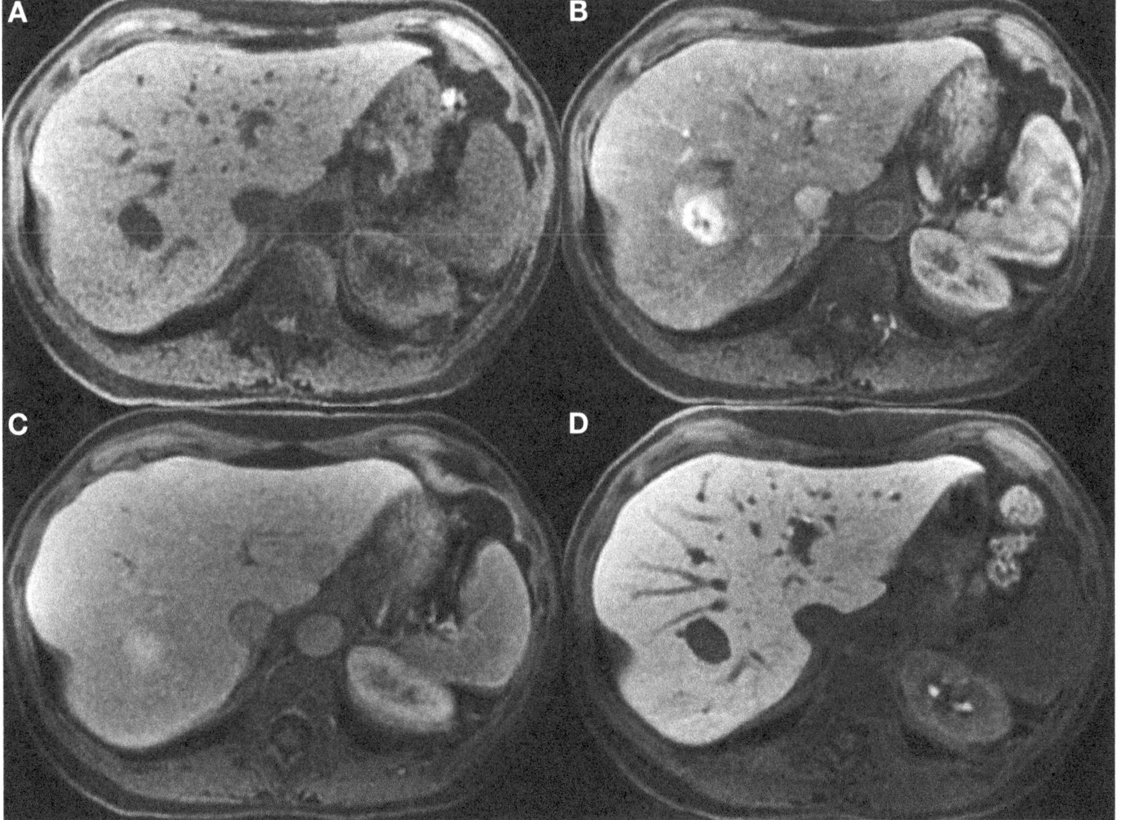

Figure 1.9.4

HISTORY: 63-year-old female potential kidney donor with an indeterminate liver mass

IMAGING FINDINGS: Axial fat-suppressed FSE T2-weighted (Figure 1.9.1) and SSFP (Figure 1.9.2) images demonstrate a focal lesion with high signal intensity in the right hepatic lobe. Diffusion-weighted image (b=600 s/mm^2) and corresponding ADC map (Figure 1.9.3) show high signal intensity within the lesion and a high ADC relative to liver. Axial precontrast, arterial phase, portal venous phase, and 20-minute delayed 3D SPGR images (Figure 1.9.4) before and after administration of a hepatobiliary-specific contrast agent (gadoxetate disodium; Eovist) reveal slightly globular peripheral enhancement during the arterial phase, with mild diffuse enhancement on the portal venous phase image, and no contrast retention on the hepatobiliary phase image.

DIAGNOSIS: Hemangioma (with Eovist)

COMMENT: Hepatobiliary-specific gadolinium-based contrast agents can be very helpful in distinguishing between FNH and adenomas, but they may occasionally be problematic in the setting of hemangiomas, as in this case. These agents are taken up by the hepatocytes and, in varying degrees, are excreted into the bile ducts. They include gadobenate dimeglumine (Multihance) and gadoxetic acid (or gadoxetate disodium) (Eovist in the United States and Primovist in the European Union and Australia). Another agent, mangafodipir trisodium (Teslascan), from which much experience has been gained, is no longer available for clinical use in the United States. Multihance and Eovist are comparable in T1 relaxivity, although a smaller volume for the same dose is used for Eovist in comparison to Multihance. With Multihance, there is approximately 3% to 5% biliary excretion compared with 50% biliary excretion with Eovist. Perhaps the most noticeable difference is that it takes much less time for Eovist (10-20 minutes) to reach the hepatobiliary phase than Multihance (60-90 minutes), which minimizes the logistical difficulties involved in obtaining hepatobiliary phase images.

Eovist is somewhat problematic for depicting the classic peripheral nodular enhancement and centripetal filling of hemangiomas because the small dose makes timing of the arterial phase somewhat more difficult. In addition, the rapid uptake of the agent by hepatocytes means that the portal venous phase is often suboptimal and that there is no real equilibrium phase, so that persistent hyperenhancement cannot be documented. This case is a nice illustration of such challenges; the arterial phase images are reasonably good but probably slightly later than ideal, and the nodular enhancement is more imagined than real. The portal phase image shows mild hyperenhancement and the 3-minute image shows hypoenhancement. Hepatobiliary phase images are not helpful for hemangiomas since the lesions contain no hepatocytes and do not retain the contrast agent. If the arterial phase characteristics are not absolutely classic, then it is difficult to be confident in your diagnosis on the basis of postgadolinium images alone (this case, for example, could also represent a hypervascular metastasis). This argument is not valid for Multihance, which has much lower hepatobiliary excretion and essentially normal portal venous and equilibrium phase images. If the clinical question is FNH vs hemangioma, then Multihance is probably the better choice, even though you may have to bring the patient back for delayed images.

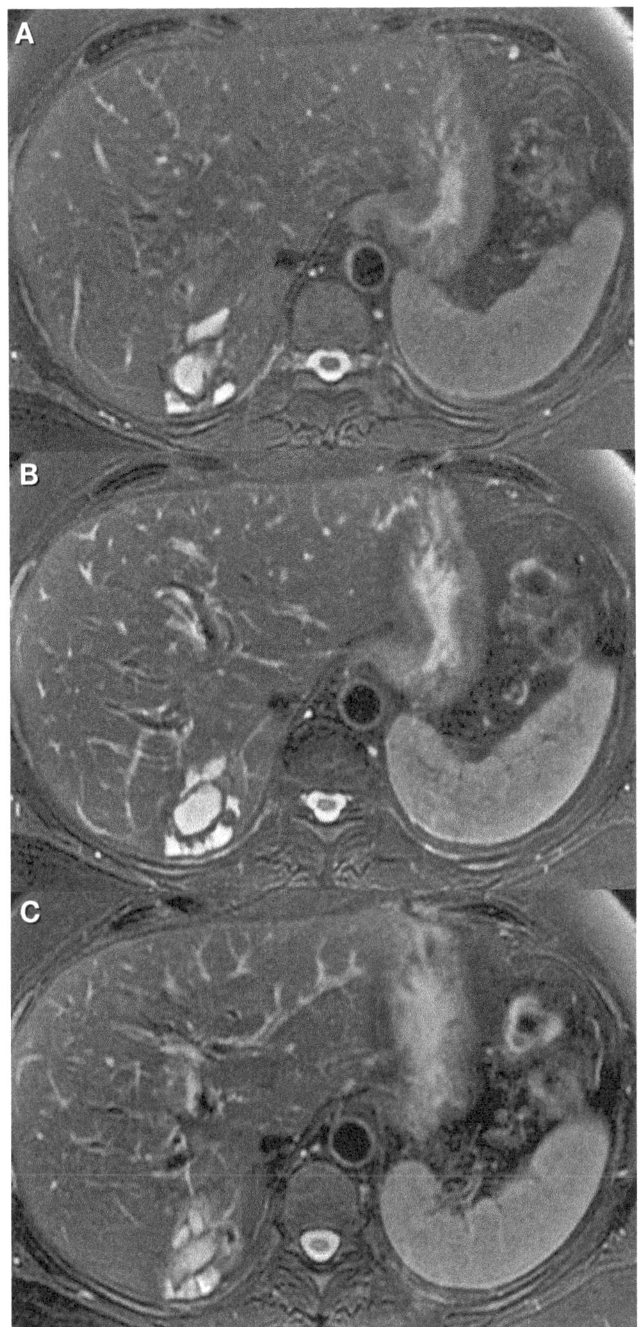

Figure 1.10.1

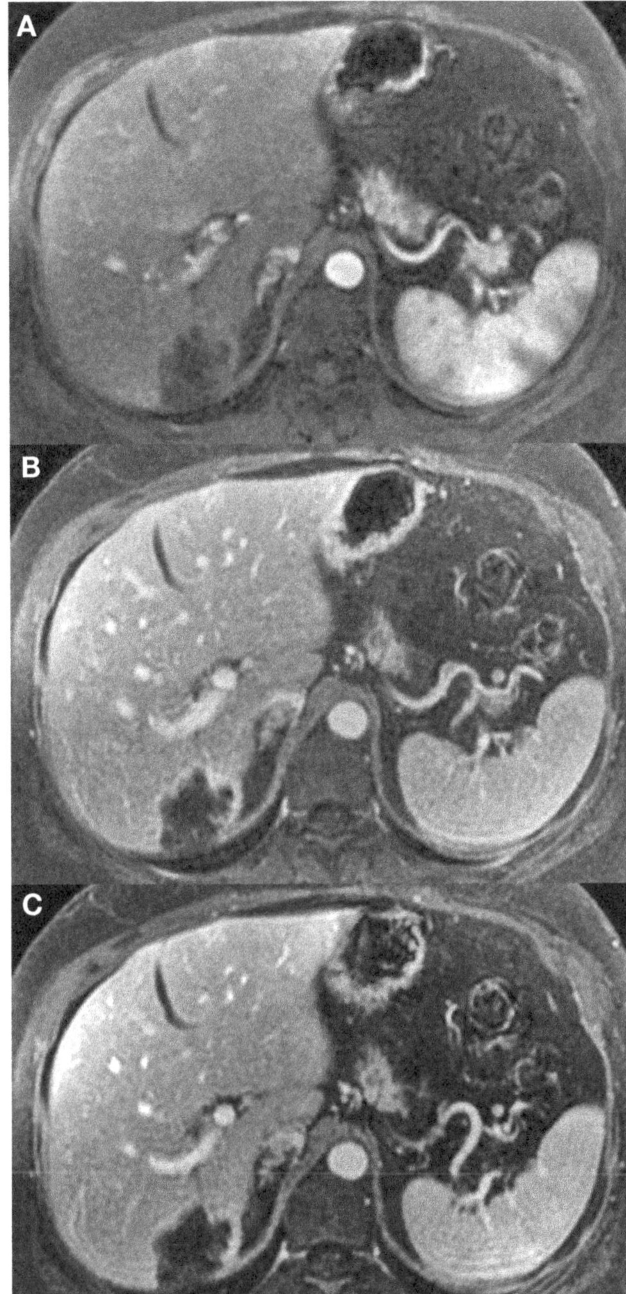

Figure 1.10.2

HISTORY: 59-year-old woman who presents for a second opinion of well-differentiated HCC that was biopsy proven elsewhere

IMAGING FINDINGS: Axial fat-suppressed FSE T2-weighted images (Figure 1.10.1) demonstrate a lesion in the posterior right hepatic lobe with central hyperintensity surrounded by smaller foci of similar high signal intensity. Axial arterial, portal venous, and equilibrium phase post-gadolinium 3D SPGR images (Figure 1.10.2) show a lobulated mass with mild peripheral progressive enhancement.

DIAGNOSIS: Sclerosed or sclerosing hemangioma

COMMENT: Cavernous hemangiomas occasionally undergo a benign sclerosing-thrombosing-hyalinizing process that begins centrally and gradually effaces the vascular spaces as it extends to the periphery. Although there are no pathognomonic imaging features for sclerosing hemangiomas, some clues that help to distinguish these from cancers include their very high T2-signal intensity, occasional geographic morphology, and contracture on follow-up imaging. Capsular retraction has been described in association with these lesions but isn't a particularly helpful feature because this sign is more commonly associated with cholangiocarcinoma—often a major consideration in the differential diagnosis. The typical peripheral globular enhancement of cavernous hemangiomas is less often seen, and instead patchy or uniform rim enhancement with absent central enhancement is the more typical appearance. DWI can also be problematic since the sclerosed central portion of the lesion may no longer have ADC values higher than adjacent liver. Several authors have noted that prospective diagnosis of sclerosing hemangiomas is difficult, and this case illustrates some of those challenges, not to mention the potential bias of the incorrect pathologic interpretation of the prior biopsy.

If a sclerosing hemangioma does enter your differential diagnosis, then follow-up imaging or a biopsy could be recommended, which might obviate more invasive intervention. This patient underwent a right hepatectomy for the presumed well-differentiated HCC. Intraoperative US (Figure 1.10.3) was performed and demonstrated a solid, partially calcified mass.

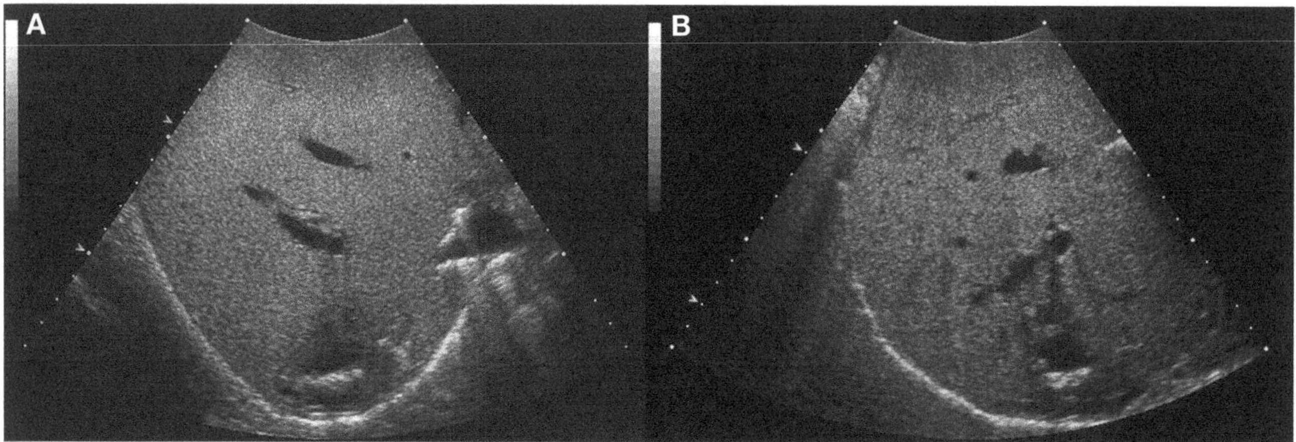

Figure 1.10.3

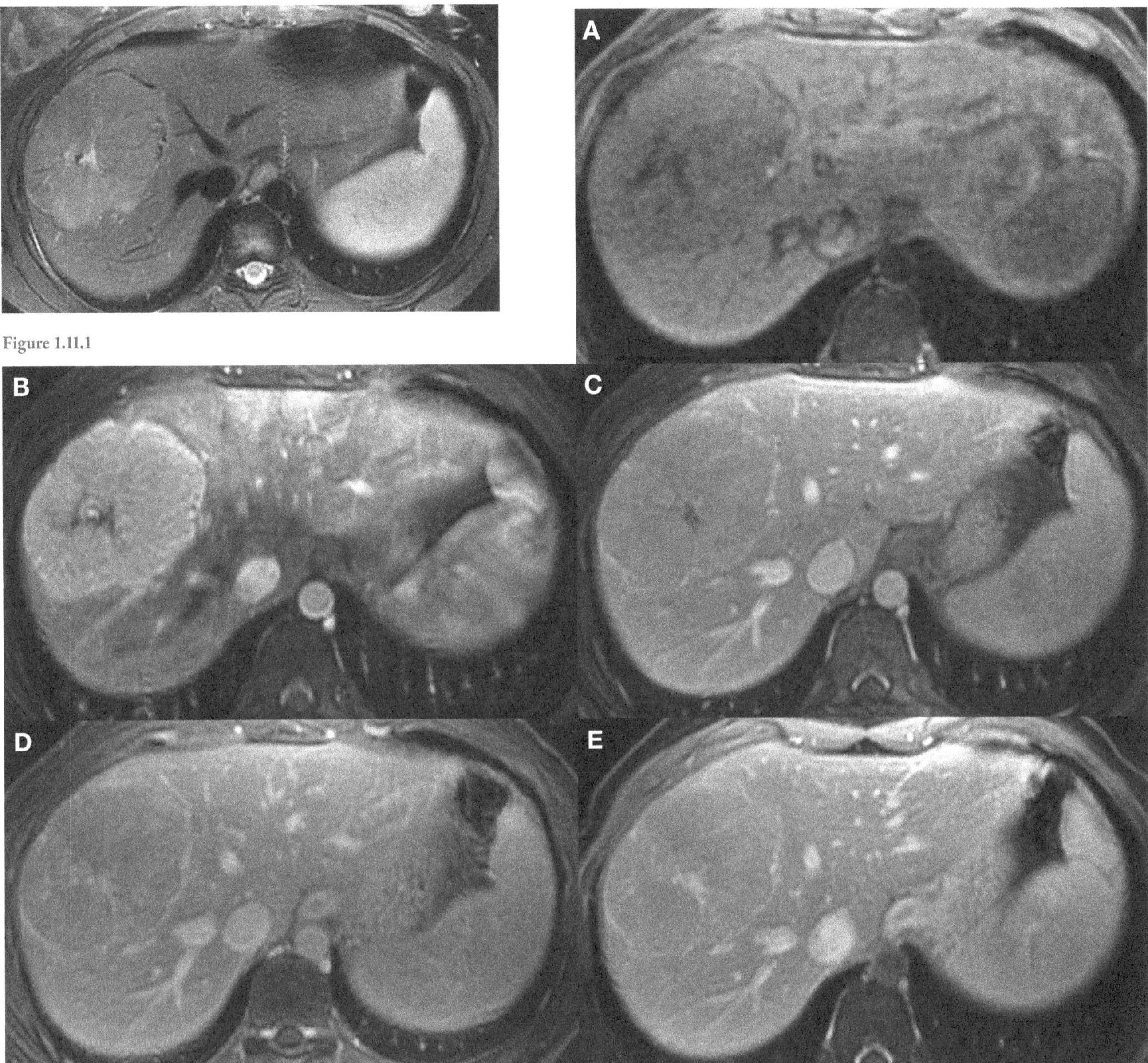

Figure 1.11.1

Figure 1.11.2

HISTORY: 21-year-old woman with a liver mass identified incidentally on CT during work-up for acute appendicitis

IMAGING FINDINGS: Axial fat-suppressed FSE T2-weighted image (Figure 1.11.1) demonstrates a large right hepatic lobe mass with mild hyperintensity relative to liver and a high intensity central scar. IP and OP T1-weighted 2D SPGR images showed no signal dropout to suggest intravoxel fat (images not shown). Pregadolinium and arterial, portal venous, equilibrium, and 5-minute delayed phase postgadolinium 3D SPGR images (Figure 1.11.2) demonstrate marked, uniform arterial phase enhancement within the lesion that rapidly becomes isointense with liver. Note also gradual enhancement of the central scar, as well as peripheral rim enhancement.

DIAGNOSIS: Focal nodular hyperplasia

COMMENT: FNH is the second most common benign tumor of the liver after hemangiomas, accounting for 8% of these lesions and with an estimated prevalence of 0.9%. FNHs consist of hyperplastic hepatocytes and small bile ductules surrounding a fibrovascular central scar that is thought to represent a hyperplastic response to a preexisting vascular malformation rather than a true neoplasm. They are more prevalent in women (usually of reproductive age) than men by an 8:1 ratio and are solitary in 80% to 95% of cases. Since FNHs are benign nonsurgical lesions, the most important job of the imager is to make a confident diagnosis and distinguish them from more potentially unfriendly hypervascular lesions, such as adenoma, HCC, and metastases. Most of the time, this is relatively easy to accomplish.

Classic FNHs (illustrated by this case) are described as invisible or barely perceptible lesions except on postgadolinium arterial phase images; they are typically isointense to liver on T1-weighted images and isointense or mildly hyperintense on T2-weighted images. It is true, however, that FNHs are often at least moderately hyperintense on diffusion-weighted images, which illustrates the general principle that DWI is a technique better used for lesion detection than lesion characterization. Dynamic postgadolinium images show intense uniform enhancement on arterial phase images, which quickly becomes nearly isointense to liver on portal venous and equilibrium phase images. The central scar (seen in this case but not universally identifiable) generally shows high signal intensity on T2-weighted images and gradual enhancement following gadolinium administration. An elaborate set of imaging characteristics of the central scar has been described in the literature as a means of distinguishing FNH from fibrolamellar hepatoma; however, the percentage of lesions that don't follow the rules is high enough that we rarely find these guidelines particularly useful.

This case illustrates the appearance of a very large, but otherwise typical, FNH, obtained with a standard extracellular gadolinium-based contrast agent. The examination was done several years ago and exemplifies one of the problems of advancing technology: We read this case as consistent with FNH and offered no differential diagnosis. If it were to appear today, however, the report likely would contain a differential that included adenoma (the hedge is the radiologist's favorite plant) and suggest that a follow-up examination with a hepatobiliary contrast agent be performed (although the absolutely classic appearance of the central scar might provide enough assurance for bold radiologists to remain firm in their conviction). This is entirely unnecessary; we used to be very certain about what FNH looked like using standard extracellular gadolinium contrast agents and were rarely mistaken. Although it is true that small adenomas can have a nearly identical appearance to FNH, they aren't very common and it's not clear whether missing one of these lesions results in any actual harm.

This case demonstrates another well-established principle: Clinicians (and patients) don't like large masses, regardless of what you say about them. Despite a confident radiologic diagnosis, as well as an absence of symptoms or abnormal laboratory values, much discussion ensued regarding the possibility of fibrolamellar hepatoma and the virtues of resection. Fortunately, surgery was avoided, but an 8-month follow-up examination was performed, which had exactly the same appearance as the first one.

The case was also one of the first abdominal MRI examinations performed at Mayo Clinic with a 3-T magnet. A 3-T system has many real and some theoretical virtues. SNR is proportional to magnetic field strength and therefore in theory is doubled at 3 T (in practice it's usually a little less than this), and the improved signal strength can be used as currency to purchase higher spatial resolution with preserved SNR or faster scans (ie, fewer signal averages or higher acceleration factors with parallel imaging).

There are many limitations, however, including longer T1 and slightly shorter T2 relaxation times, meaning more saturation (and lower signal) for the same TR and more rapid signal decay (and lower signal) for the same TE. More importantly, susceptibility artifacts are greatly increased, as are standing wave and conductivity artifacts, which can lead to severe signal loss in all or part of the image. Although 3-T MRI has become a part of our daily practice and has generated some spectacular images, it is also true that we occasionally need to transfer patients back to a 1.5-T magnet because the 3-T images are uninterpretable.

The next 2 cases—Case 1.12 and Case 1.13—illustrate some normal variations in imaging appearances of FNHs, which are slightly confounded by the clinical histories. These examinations were performed using a hepatobiliary contrast agent, the first one with Multihance and the second one with Eovist. Remember that FNHs can be thought of simplistically as hepatic parenchymal elements arranged slightly differently than the rest of the liver. Bile duct proliferation is a near-universal feature of FNHs and has been divided into 2 categories by some pathologists: well-differentiated proliferative ducts and regions of bile duct metaplasia, with diminished functionality and limited connection to the bile canaliculi. The well-differentiated ductal proliferations may correspond to regions with hyperintense signal intensity and contrast agent accumulation relative to background on hepatobiliary phase images (ie, FNHs become hyperintense on hepatobiliary phase images).

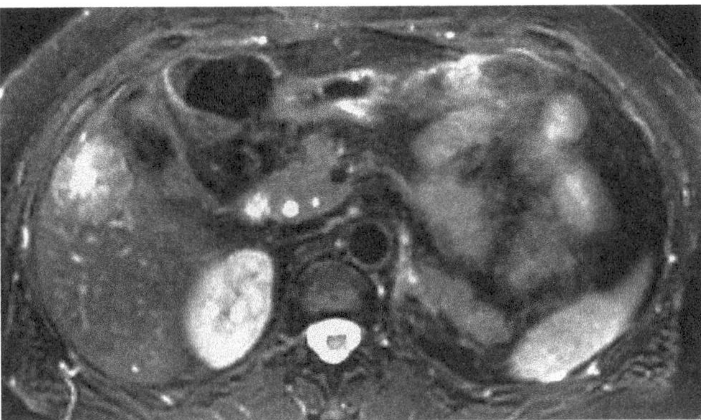

Figure 1.12.1

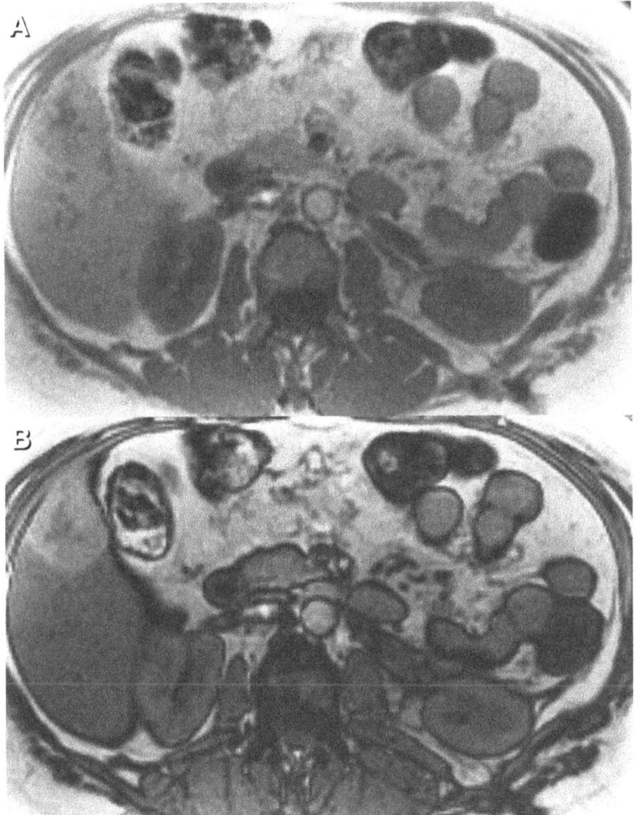

Figure 1.12.2

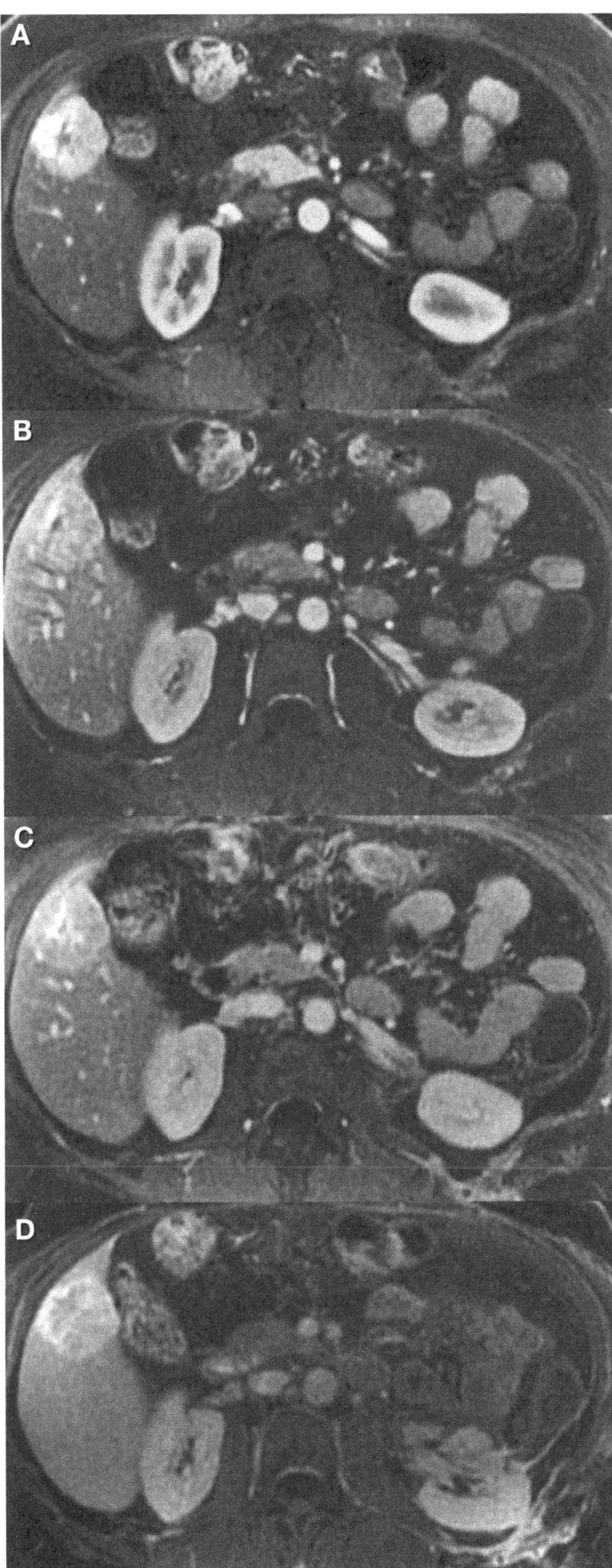

Figure 1.12.3

HISTORY: 58-year-old woman with a mixed epithelial stromal tumor of the left kidney, status post open partial nephrectomy. MRI was requested to assess for metastatic disease. The radiologist chose to use Multihance

IMAGING FINDINGS: Axial fat-suppressed T2-weighted FSE image (Figure 1.12.1) demonstrates a right hepatic lobe mass with mildly increased signal intensity relative to liver and central high signal intensity. There is no signal dropout from IP to OP T1-weighted 2D SPGR images (Figure 1.12.2) to suggest the presence of intravoxel fat within the lesion. The mass is isointense to liver on the IP image, hyperintense on the OP image as a result of hepatic steatosis, with hypointensity of the central component. Axial arterial (Figure 1.12.3A), portal venous (Figure 1.12.3B), and equilibrium (Figure 1.12.3C) phase postgadolinium (Multihance) 3D SPGR images demonstrate initial intense, uniform hyperenhancement except for the center of the lesion, with rapid washout on portal venous and equilibrium phase images, where the lesion becomes slightly hyperintense relative to liver. Notice also the gradual enhancement of the center of the mass. A 60-minute delayed hepatobiliary phase image (Figure 1.12.3D) shows contrast retention within the lesion in a spoke-wheel pattern. There are also postoperative changes from left partial nephrectomy.

DIAGNOSIS: Focal nodular hyperplasia (with Multihance)

COMMENT: This companion case to Case 1.11 illustrates the use of Multihance. Compared with Eovist, Multihance requires a longer delay (60-90 minutes) before hepatobiliary phase images can be acquired, which is logistically challenging in comparison to the relatively short, 15- to 20-minute delay needed for Eovist. The larger percentage of hepatobiliary excretion with Eovist results in greater hepatic parenchymal enhancement (in both cirrhotic and noncirrhotic patients) during the hepatobiliary phase compared with Multihance. Therefore, the hepatobiliary phase images are slightly prettier with Eovist, but there is no convincing evidence that this property leads to a significant advantage in lesion detection or characterization.

CASE 1.13

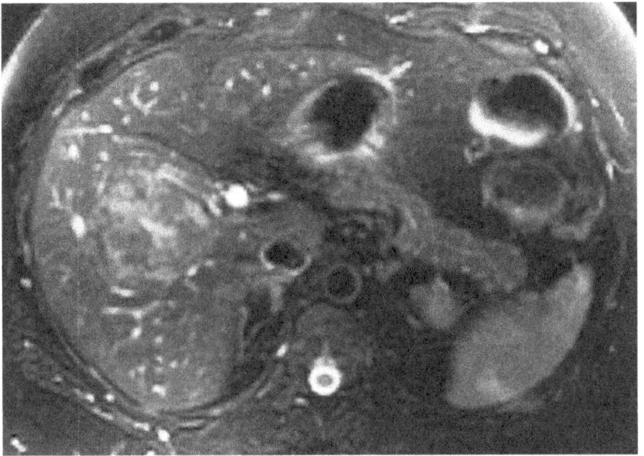

Figure 1.13.1

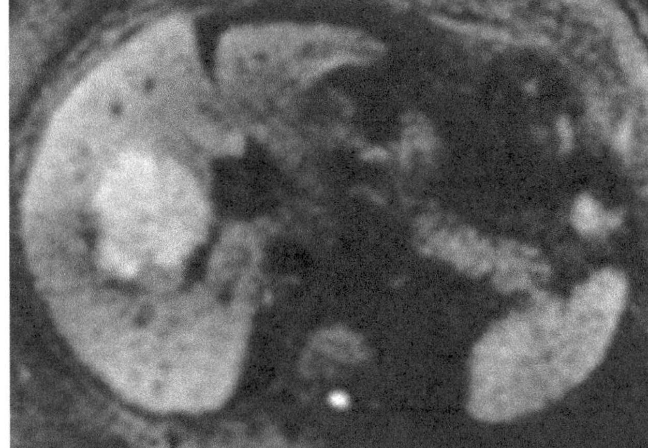

Figure 1.13.2

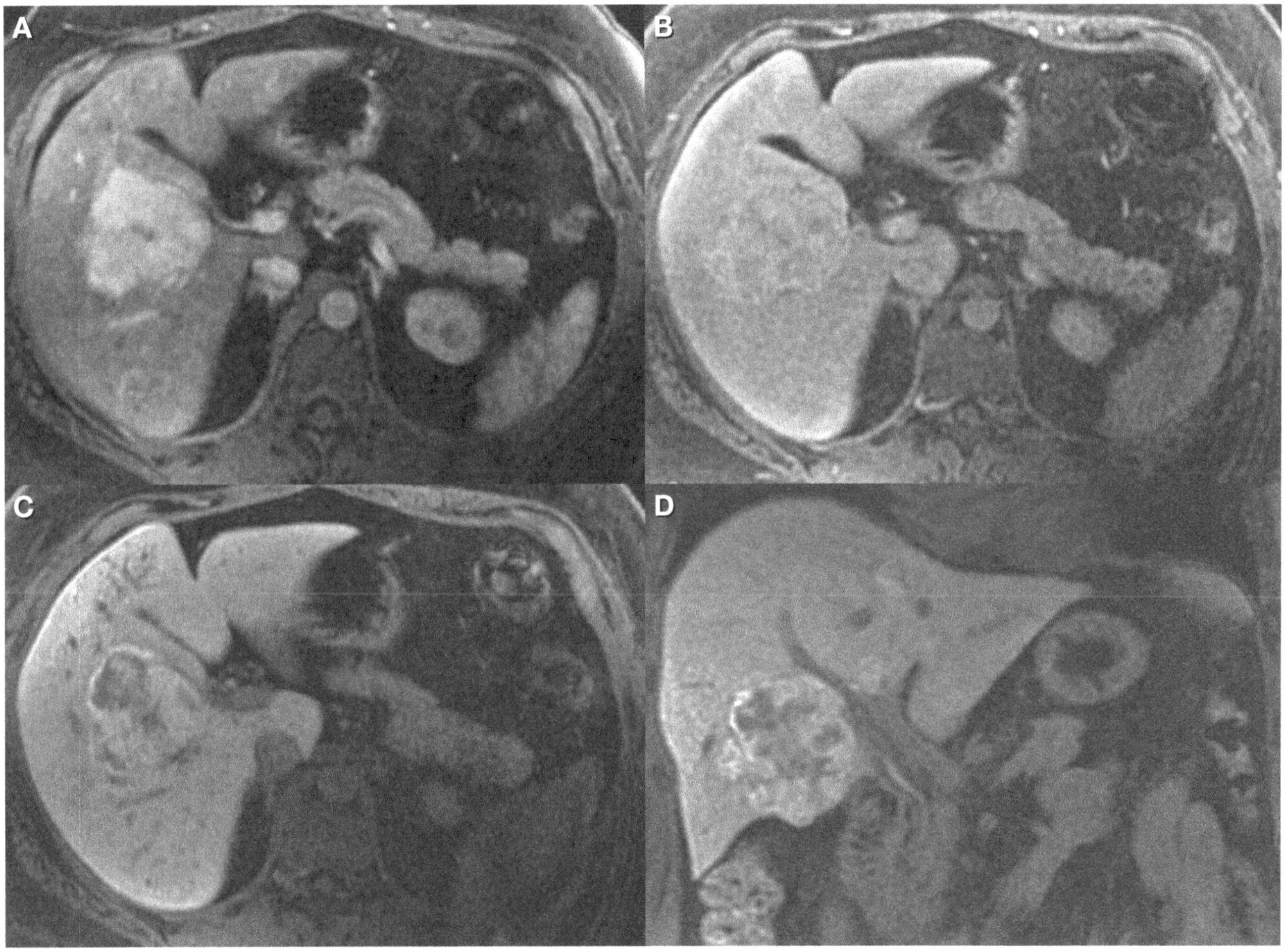

Figure 1.13.3

HISTORY: 51-year-old woman with abdominal pain. The radiologist chose to use Eovist

IMAGING FINDINGS: Axial fat-suppressed FSE T2-weighted image (Figure 1.13.1) and diffusion-weighted ($b=600\ s/mm^2$) image (Figure 1.13.2) demonstrate a right hepatic lobe mass with mild increased signal intensity relative to liver on the FSE image and moderate hyperintensity on the diffusion-weighted image. There was no signal dropout from IP to OP T1-weighted 2D SPGR images (images not shown) to suggest intravoxel fat in the mass. Axial arterial (Figure 1.13.3A) and portal venous (Figure 1.13.3B) phase dynamic postgadolinium (Eovist) 3D SPGR images show intense, uniform arterial phase hyperenhancement with rapid washout and mild persistent hyperintensity on the portal venous phase image. Axial (Figure 1.13.3C) and coronal (Figure 1.13.3D) hepatobiliary phase images obtained 15 minutes after contrast injection reveal patchy hyperenhancement relative to the liver, most prominent in the periphery of the lesion.

DIAGNOSIS: Focal nodular hyperplasia (with Eovist)

COMMENT: The somewhat heterogeneous appearance of the lesion on the hepatobiliary phase images can be disconcerting, but in our experience the appearance is not unusual, particularly when seen in a spoke-wheel configuration (although the central scar should not show hyperenhancement). A few authors have attempted to categorize the patterns of enhancement in FNH on hepatobiliary phase images. In general, uniform hyperintensity in comparison to normal liver is the most common appearance, but inhomogeneous hyperintense, isointense, and predominantly hypointense lesions with rim enhancement have been described.

The patient presented with abdominal pain of 15 years' duration, which coincidentally began at the time of her hysterectomy, during which the hepatic lesions had been noted incidentally. A surgeon attempted to biopsy one of the masses during laparoscopic cholecystectomy but without a pathologic diagnosis.

The consulting surgeon was not convinced that the patient's longstanding abdominal pain could be attributed to the multiple FNHs but nevertheless offered a laparoscopic right hepatectomy to remove the largest lesions. Pathologic evaluation confirmed the diagnosis of FNH.

CASE 1.14

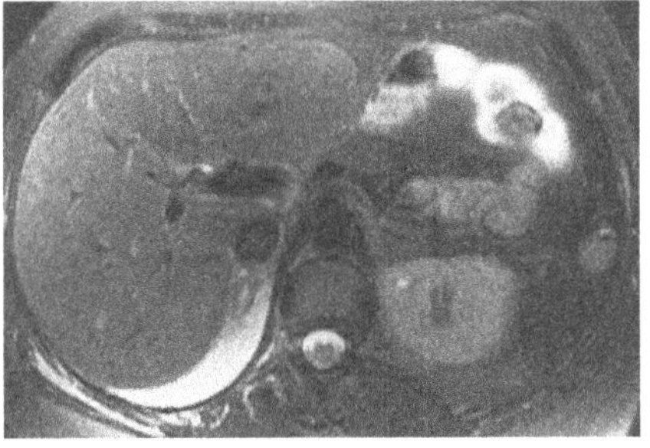

Figure 1.14.1

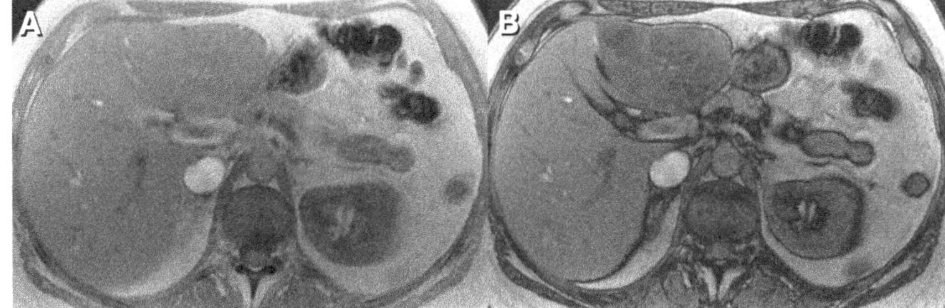

Figure 1.14.2

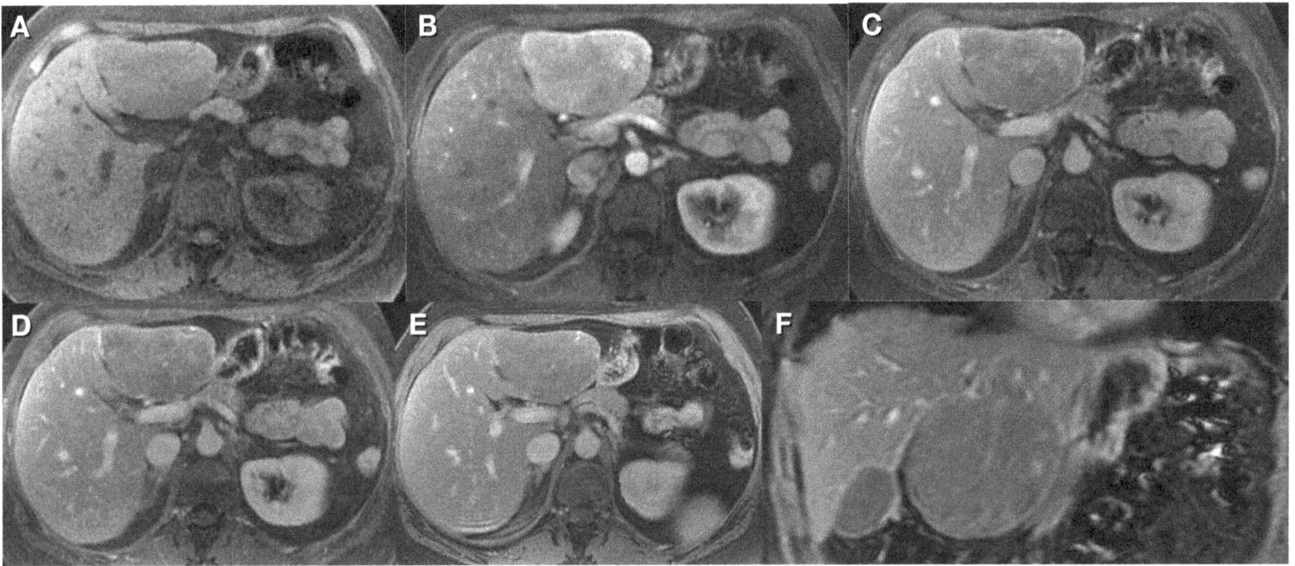

Figure 1.14.3

HISTORY: 50-year-old woman with a hepatic mass discovered incidentally on chest CT

IMAGING FINDINGS: Axial fat-suppressed FSE T2-weighted image (Figure 1.14.1) demonstrates subtle focal enlargement of the lateral left hepatic lobe without an obvious mass. Axial T1-weighted IP (Figure 1.14.2A) and OP (Figure 1.14.2B) 2D SPGR images reveal a large mass with signal dropout on the OP image consistent with the presence of fat. Pregadolinium (Figure 1.14.3A) and arterial (Figure 1.14.3B) and portal venous (Figure 1.14.3C) phase postgadolinium 3D SPGR images demonstrate diffuse, mildly heterogeneous, early enhancement with rapid washout of contrast. Notice also that the mass is hypointense relative to normal liver on the precontrast image, again likely a result of fat suppression. Equilibrium phase postgadolinium (Figure 1.14.3D) and axial (Figure 1.14.3E) and coronal (Figure 1.14.3F) 5-minute delayed 2D SPGR images reveal persistent, mildly heterogeneous hypoenhancement of the mass.

DIAGNOSIS: Hepatic adenoma

COMMENT: Hepatic adenomas, also called *liver cell adenomas*, typically arise in normal or near-normal livers of patients with a history of abnormal hormonal stimulation (usually, oral contraceptives in women and, rarely, anabolic steroids in men) or metabolic conditions, including glycogen storage diseases, Klinefelter syndrome, type 1 diabetes mellitus, and familial polyposis syndromes. Hepatic adenomas most commonly occur in young women taking oral contraceptives, who account for approximately 90% of all lesions. Hepatic adenomas may be single (70%-80%) or multiple and can sometimes be larger than 20 cm. *Adenomatosis* is defined as the presence of more than 10 hepatic adenomas in a patient without a predisposing condition (such as glycogen storage disease) (see Case 1.16).

Pathologically, hepatic adenomas are well-circumscribed encapsulated masses consisting of hepatocytes arranged in plates or cords without an acinar (lobular) architecture and with a paucity or absence of biliary ducts and Kupffer cells. (The absence of bile ducts is the basis of the conventional wisdom regarding the appearance of hepatic adenomas on hepatobiliary phase images following Eovist or Multihance administration, and the fact that this isn't always true helps to explain the occasional adenoma with contrast retention on delayed images.) The hepatocytes within adenomas often contain abundant glycogen, hence the association with type 1 glycogen storage disease, and the fat content within the tumor is often a distinguishing feature on MRI.

Hepatic adenomas have subcapsular feeding arteries that typically flow toward the center of the lesion (ie, centripetal flow). This is in distinction to FNH, which has a central feeding artery that flows away from the center (ie, centrifugal flow). With that being said, however, the direction of the flow of feeding arteries is probably a more useful sign on US, where the vasculature can be directly interrogated, and is less correlative with enhancement patterns seen on CT or MRI. The classic description of adenomas includes modestly increased signal intensity relative to the liver on T2-weighted images; increased or decreased T1-signal intensity, depending on the relative proportions of fat and hemorrhage; and mildly heterogeneous arterial phase enhancement, typically less intense than in FNH, with rapid washout on portal venous phase images. Although many adenomas do exhibit one or more of these characteristics, there are frequent exceptions (giving rise to atypical adenomas). Most of the literature is based on small series of symptomatic patients with relatively large hemorrhagic lesions, and the behavior of small lesions, particularly those without a substantial amount of fat, may be difficult to distinguish from FNH.

Recent histopathologic and genetic analyses of series of adenomas have led to classification of 3 or 4 subtypes. Different classification schemes have been proposed in the literature, but the probable winner comes from a multicenter French experience with 100 to 150 adenomas.

The inflammatory subtype is the most common, accounting for 40% to 50% of all cases, and includes lesions previously classified (and still classified by some Mayo Clinic pathologists) as telangiectatic adenomas. This group is characterized by overexpression of GP 130 and is distinguished histologically by a polymorphous inflammatory infiltrate, prominent sinusoidal dilatation or congestion, and the presence of multiple thick-walled arteries. HNF-1α–mutated adenomas have mutations of the *HNF-1α* gene, represent 30% to 35% of all adenomas, and are characterized by diffuse intratumoral steatosis. Adenomas carrying a mutated β-catenin gene are thought to account for 10% to 15% of adenomas. These occur more frequently in men and are associated with the administration of male hormones, as well as with glycogen storage diseases and familial adenomatous polyposis syndromes. An additional category is termed *unclassified* and includes all adenomas without one of these specific mutations.

The utility of the classification scheme has to do with the relative frequency of complications, as well as the MR imaging appearance. HNF-1α–mutated adenomas have a relatively low risk of bleeding and of malignant transformation and are characterized on MRI primarily by their prominent signal dropout from IP to OP SPGR images, indicating the presence of fat. They generally have a T2 signal that is isointense or mildly hyperintense compared with adjacent liver and show moderate arterial phase hyperenhancement after gadolinium administration, with washout on portal venous and equilibrium phase images.

Inflammatory adenomas have the highest risk of spontaneous bleeding, estimated at 30%, and approximately 10% of these lesions undergo malignant transformation. Inflammatory adenomas are characterized by high T2-signal intensity, particularly in the periphery of the lesion, which is thought to correlate histologically with the presence of dilated sinusoids and is termed the *atoll sign*. These adenomas show no or minimal signal dropout from IP to OP SPGR images (for a striking counterexample, see Case 1.17) and have intense arterial phase hyperenhancement following gadolinium administration, with persistent hyperenhancement on portal venous and equilibrium phase images. β-Catenin–mutated adenomas have no distinctive imaging features but are thought to present the highest risk of malignant transformation. The unclassified category likewise has no distinct imaging characteristics, with an intermediate risk of bleeding and malignant transformation.

This description of the MRI characteristics of adenoma subtypes relies on 2 recent papers that successfully categorized adenomas on the basis of imaging characteristics, with accuracies of 85% to 90%. It is worth noting, however, that neither the histopathologic nor the imaging classification schemes discussed above are universally accepted; a competing group, for example, described their experience with more than 100 adenomas and classified them as *steatotic*, *telangiectatic*, or *unclassified*. They noted that although 100% of telangiectatic lesions had GP 130 overexpression, HNF-1α mutations were present in only 60% of steatotic lesions and as many as 24% of telangiectatic lesions. This finding suggests that identification of HNF-1α–mutated adenomas based solely on visualization of fat may not be entirely straightforward.

This case is a reasonably good example of the HNF-1α subtype, with minimal signal abnormality on T2-weighted images, prominent intratumoral glycogen or fat, and moderate arterial phase hyperenhancement with washout on portal venous and equilibrium phase images. The presence of fat effectively eliminates the possibility of FNH. Although there are a few isolated case reports of lipid-rich FNH, we have not seen any of these in our practice and we continue to ignore the possibility. (One hepatic mass with prominent lipid was biopsied and initially diagnosed as FNH, but when confronted with the imaging appearance, the pathologist reexamined the specimen and revised the report, changing the diagnosis to adenoma.)

The presence of fat within a hepatic mass should not automatically lead to the diagnosis of adenoma. The most important differential diagnosis to keep in mind is HCC. Usually, HCC occurs in patients with cirrhosis, but fibrolamellar HCC has an age distribution similar to that of hepatic adenomas and frequently occurs in normal livers. Distinction between the two is usually possible on the basis of the more heterogeneous and aggressive appearance of fibrolamellar HCC, but not always. Nodular focal fatty infiltration can have a surprisingly masslike appearance, but it should not show enhancement on postgadolinium images.

CASE 1.15

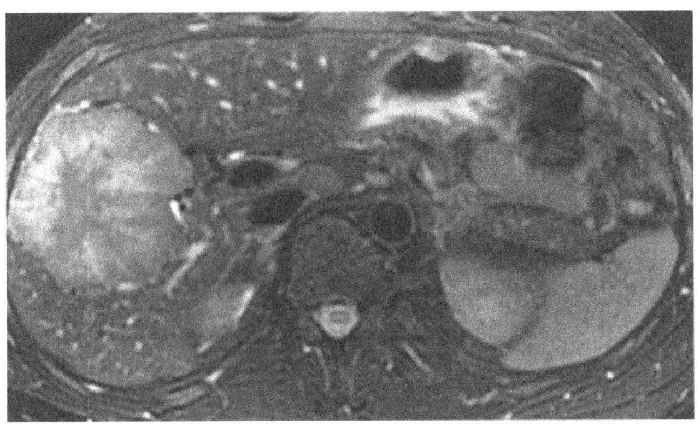

Figure 1.15.1

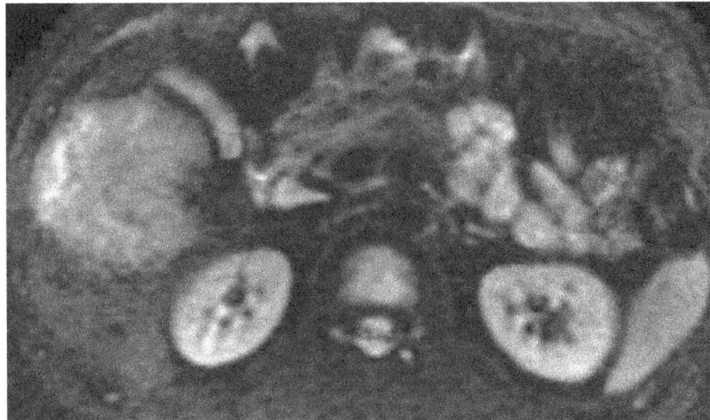

Figure 1.15.2

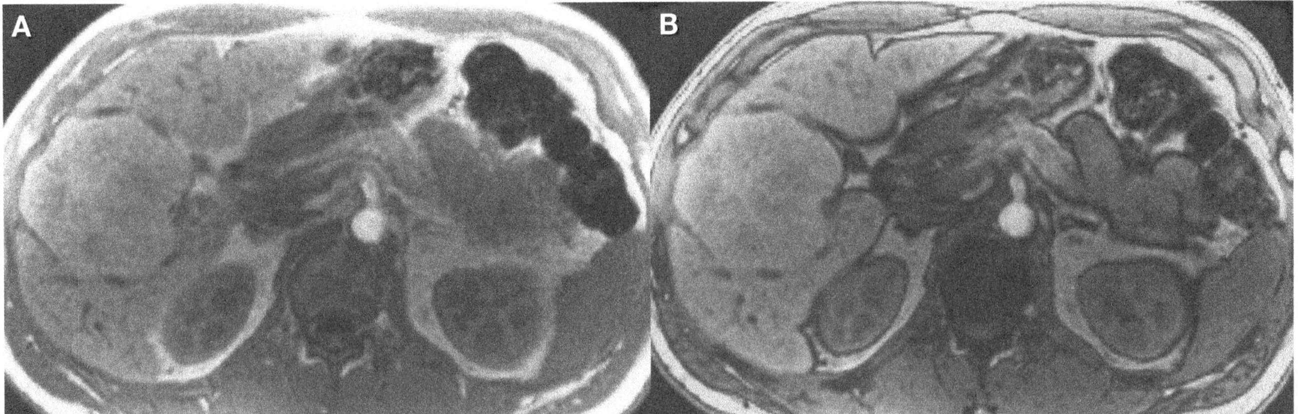

Figure 1.15.3

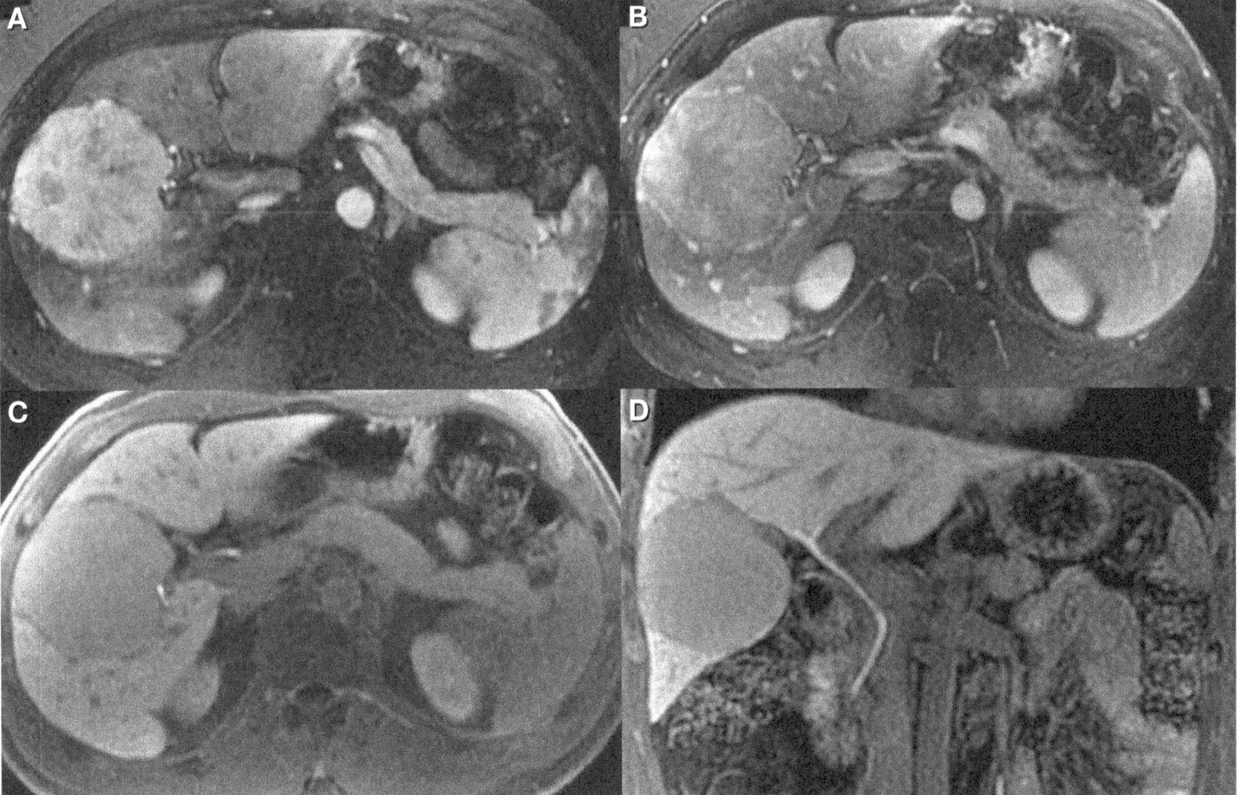

Figure 1.15.4

HISTORY: 39-year-old man with a 6-month history of epigastric and right upper quadrant discomfort with associated intermittent right shoulder pain and nausea. Laboratory tests were unremarkable; specifically, the AFP level was within normal limits. A hepatic mass was seen on CT

IMAGING FINDINGS: Axial fat-suppressed FSE T2-weighted (Figure 1.15.1) and diffusion-weighted (b=100 s/mm^2) (Figure 1.15.2) images demonstrate a well-circumscribed mass with heterogeneous high signal intensity in the right hepatic lobe. Axial T1-weighted IP and OP 2D SPGR images (Figure 1.15.3) show no appreciable signal dropout on the OP image to suggest a fatty component. Axial postgadolinium (Multihance) arterial and portal venous phase 3D SPGR images (Figures 1.15.4A and 1.15.4B) demonstrate heterogeneous enhancement with mixed regions of washout and contrast retention on the portal venous phase image. Axial and coronal hepatobiliary phase 3D SPGR images (Figures 1.15.4C and 1.15.4D) acquired 90 minutes after the initial contrast injection show hypoenhancement of the mass relative to liver. Note also contrast excretion in the biliary tree.

DIAGNOSIS: Hepatic adenoma (with Multihance)

COMMENT: This case does not have classic features of any 1 particular lesion, but adenoma is probably the most reasonable choice. At first glance, the lesion has the kind of spoke-wheel architecture favored by FNH and looks like it might have a central scar, but the T2-signal intensity is higher than one would expect, the arterial phase enhancement is more heterogeneous than is usually seen with FNH, and hypoenhancement on hepatobiliary phase images would be very atypical. Fibrolamellar and well-differentiated HCCs are also a consideration, although these are relatively rare lesions in the otherwise normal liver of an asymptomatic patient without elevated liver enzymes or AFP. Nevertheless, this diagnosis could not be excluded on the basis of the imaging appearance.

Although hepatic adenomas are more typically found in young women taking oral contraceptives, they have also been reported in men using anabolic steroids and, as in this case, in association with antiepileptic medications. This case, performed before genetic phenotyping was routinely obtained, probably represents an inflammatory subtype characterized on MRI by high T2-signal intensity, intense arterial phase hyperenhancement, and persistent hyperenhancement on portal venous and equilibrium phase images. The heterogeneity and partial washout on the portal venous phase image (which increased in the equilibrium phase) lend some ambiguity to this diagnosis, but in our experience this appearance is not uncommon.

The most relevant clinical question in this case was to distinguish between FNH (a leave-alone lesion) and adenoma or fibrolamellar HCC, both of which would require resection. Solitary adenomas of this size are usually removed on the basis of their potential for bleeding, as well as the small risk of malignant transformation, which is increased in male patients.

A hepatobiliary contrast agent (Multihance in this case) is often helpful in making this distinction on the basis of contrast retention within FNH on hepatobiliary phase images, usually with a significant percentage of the lesion showing hyperenhancement relative to adjacent liver. This is in distinction to adenoma and fibrolamellar HCC, which are generally hypointense to liver on hepatobiliary phase images because of absent or reduced functional hepatocytes in the case of HCC and absent or minimal functional biliary ducts in the case of adenomas.

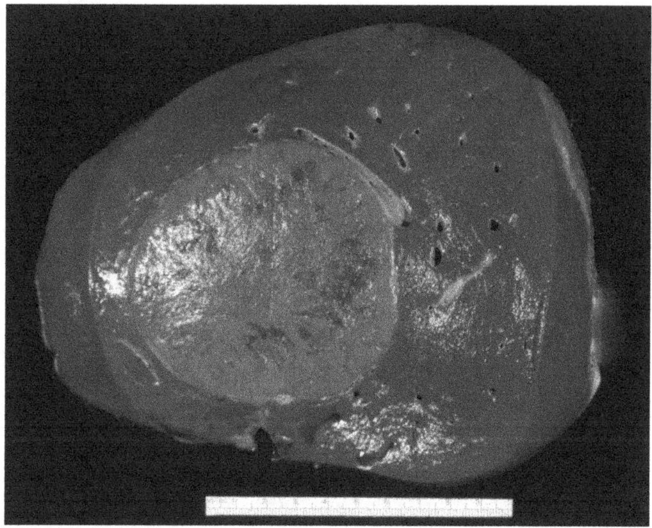

Figure 1.15.5 (Adapted from Lee PU, Roberts LR, Kaiya JK, Lee CU. Hepatic adenomas associated with anti-epileptic drugs: a case series and imaging review. Abdom Imaging. 2010 Apr;35[2]:208–11. Used with permission.)

On the basis of these findings, the patient underwent right hepatectomy and cholecystectomy. Surgical pathology confirmed the diagnosis of hepatic adenoma, with the gross specimen (Figure 1.15.5) showing a circumscribed margin and internal heterogeneity similar to what was seen on MRI.

CASE 1.16

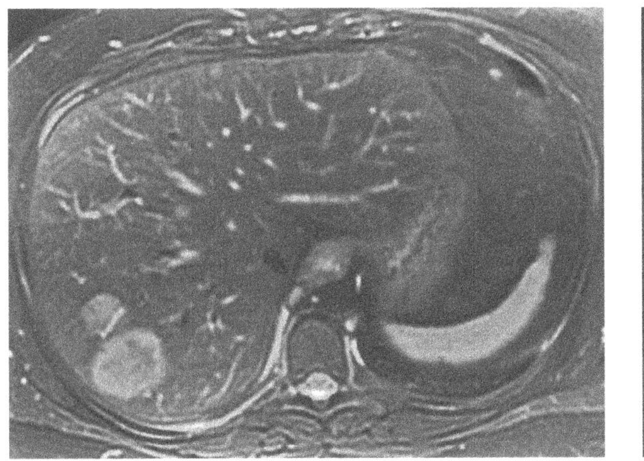

Figure 1.16.1

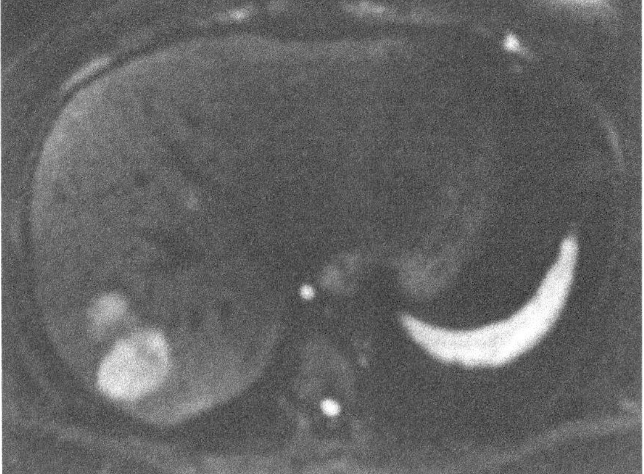

Figure 1.16.2

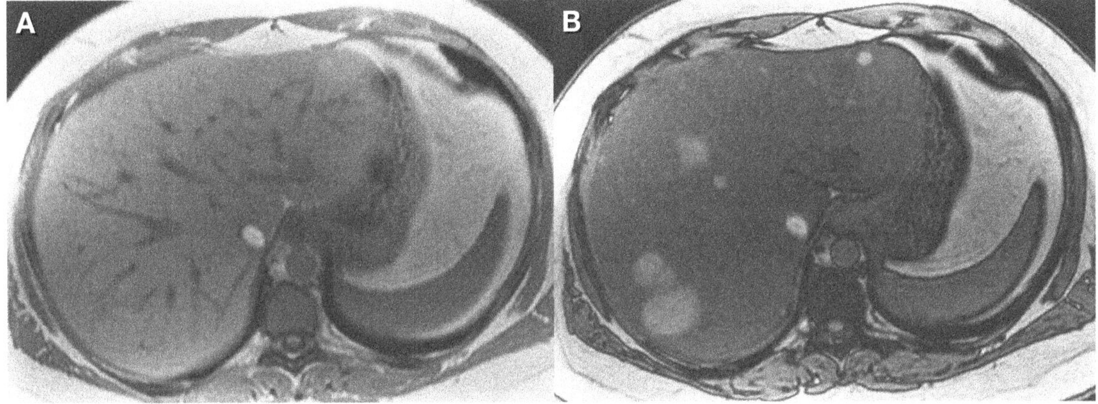

Figure 1.16.3

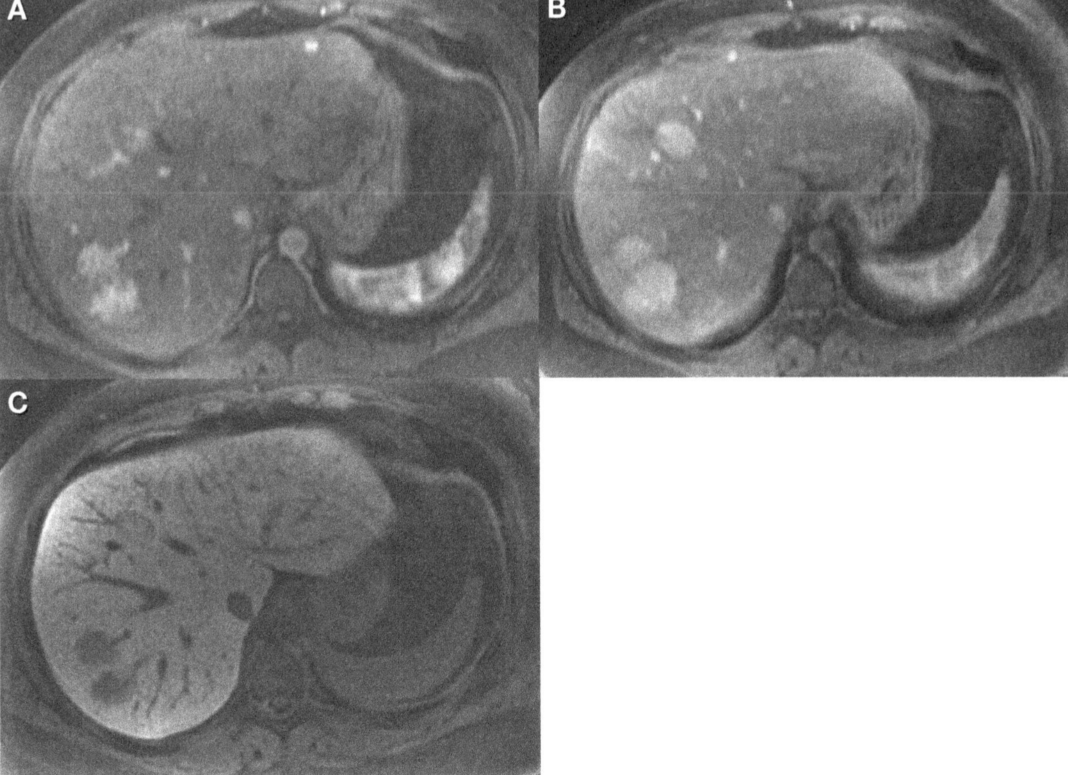

Figure 1.16.4

HISTORY: 22-year-old woman with a history of diabetes mellitus, hyperlipidemia, and polycystic ovarian syndrome; she was involved in a motor vehicle accident, and abdominal CT demonstrated multiple hepatic masses

IMAGING FINDINGS: Axial fat-suppressed FSE T2-weighted image (Figure 1.16.1) demonstrates at least 2 hyperintense masses in the periphery of the right hepatic lobe. Diffusion-weighted image (b=600 s/mm^2) (Figure 1.16.2) also shows increased signal intensity within the lesions. Axial T1-weighted IP and OP 2D SPGR images (Figure 1.16.3) reveal mild-to-moderate diffuse fatty infiltration of the liver with additional lesions visualized on the OP image, none of which show obvious signal loss to suggest a fatty component. Axial arterial (Figure 1.16.4A) and portal venous (Figure 1.16.4B) phase post-gadolinium (Eovist) 3D SPGR images reveal rapid enhancement of the masses with progressive enhancement of the background liver. The masses demonstrate mild hypoenhancement relative to adjacent liver on the hepatobiliary phase image (Figure 1.16.4C).

DIAGNOSIS: Adenomatosis in the setting of diffuse hepatic steatosis

COMMENT: Diagnosis of adenomatosis requires at least 10 lesions in a patient without a predisposing condition (not all of the adenomas can be visualized on the single location included in this case). The risk of complications in patients with adenomatosis is defined primarily by the size and pathology of the lesions and not by the lesion number. In our limited experience with this entity, we have often encountered coexistent FNH, which can be difficult to distinguish from adjacent small adenomas. This is occasionally a problem when a US- or CT-guided biopsy to confirm the diagnosis yields FNH. The lesion in the anterior right hepatic lobe, for example, has early enhancement characteristics identical to the posterior lesions (one of which was biopsied and confirmed as an adenoma); however, it is not clearly seen on the T2- and diffusion-weighted images and shows mild, diffuse contrast retention, albeit slightly below the level of adjacent normal liver, on the hepatobiliary phase image. It's unclear whether this is another adenoma of a different subtype or FNH.

The ability of hepatobiliary contrast agents to distinguish adenomas from FNH, based on the concept that FNH shows contrast retention at or above the level of adjacent liver in the hepatobiliary phase while adenomas have enhancement significantly less than adjacent liver, has been partially addressed by several authors in the past few years. The results have been uniformly excellent, with accuracies of 95% to 100%. It is worth noting, however, that most papers had pathologic proof for only a small percentage of FNH lesions, relying instead on the characteristic imaging appearance and stability of FNH on follow-up examinations, which is somewhat circular reasoning. Two authors have reported an optimal lesion to liver enhancement ratio in the hepatobiliary phase to classify lesions as FNH or adenoma, with values of 0.9 and 0.7. The discrepancy in the numbers may reflect the percentage of patients with fatty infiltration of the liver, as well as the percentage of HNF-1α–mutated adenomas in the 2 studies.

In reality, a spectrum of contrast retention exists within both adenomas and FNH in the hepatobiliary phase. Case reports have described isointense or even hyperintense signal in adenomas (Case 1.17 is our example of this) and corresponding examples of FNH with decreased hepatobiliary phase signal intensity relative to adjacent liver.

Since one of the previously described criteria for distinguishing inflammatory adenomas is persistent hyperenhancement on portal venous and equilibrium phase images, it is worth remembering that both these phases are considerably degraded with Eovist, and therefore categorization of the adenoma, once diagnosed, may be somewhat less accurate.

Several authors have pointed out that use of a 1- to 2-mL test bolus of Eovist can be detrimental to the image quality of the ensuing dynamic acquisition since 1) this bolus can represent as much as 30% of the total dose and 2) rapid hepatocyte uptake occurs in patients with normal liver function, resulting in diffuse, increased signal intensity throughout the liver and thereby reducing the contrast to noise ratio of any hyperenhancing lesions visualized during the arterial phase. Various solutions have been proposed, including fluoroscopically triggered arterial phase acquisition (our favorite), triple arterial phase low-spatial-resolution acquisition acquired with a standard time delay following injection and without fluoroscopic triggering (the favored technique of the majority of our group), and dilution of the Eovist dose with an equal volume of saline, followed by a 1-mL test bolus and standard dynamic acquisition (not a favorite of the technologists who have to dilute the bolus and load the syringes). The triple arterial phase acquisition is occasionally problematic not only because the spatial resolution is poor (the voxel size is more than twice our standard 3D SPGR acquisition), but also because the total acquisition time is long (25-30 seconds). Roughly one-third of the patients don't hold their breath through the third phase, which occasionally is the most useful one (or would be if not degraded by motion artifact).

Fluoroscopic triggering is a better solution. The entire dose of contrast agent is injected at a slightly reduced rate of 1 to 1.5 mL/sec and the arterial phase acquisition can be initiated within 4 to 5 seconds of visualization of the contrast bolus in the abdominal aorta. We acquire dynamic images with spatial resolution considerably higher than the triple arterial phase acquisitions but slightly lower than our standard dynamic 3D SPGR technique, with an acquisition time of approximately 10 seconds, and obtain 3 successive phases within 1 minute. This method is slightly more complex for the technologists, but once learned, fluoroscopic triggering almost always delivers superior image quality.

It should be noted that none of these techniques can do anything about the suboptimal portal phase and absent equilibrium phase caused by rapid hepatic uptake of Eovist. If the primary consideration involves assessment of the portal or hepatic veins or a potential vascular malformation or hemangioma, then a different contrast agent is probably the best solution.

This examination was performed using the triple arterial phase technique and provided clear visualization of the dynamic enhancement of the lesions, although the reduced spatial resolution on arterial and portal venous phase images is easy to appreciate.

At the time of the MRI, the patient was asymptomatic, and short-term follow-up imaging was recommended. The subsequent examination showed minimal enlargement of the masses, after which a biopsy was performed, yielding pathology consistent with an inflammatory (telangiectatic) adenoma in a background of hepatic steatosis.

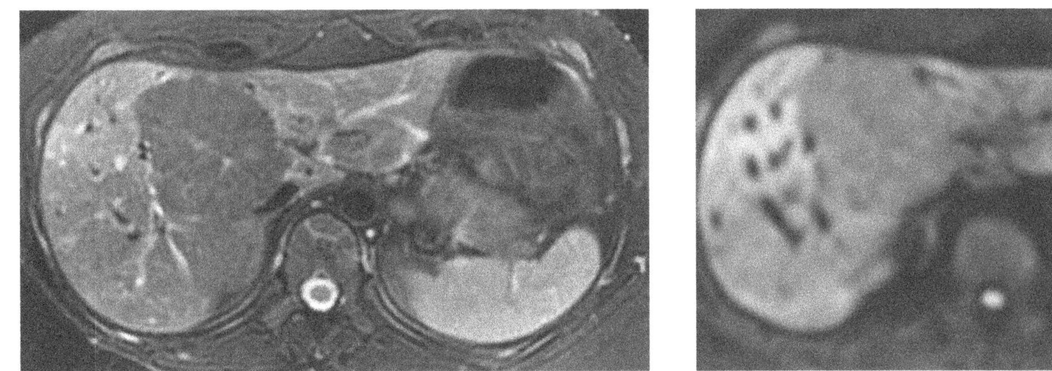

Figure 1.17.1

Figure 1.17.2

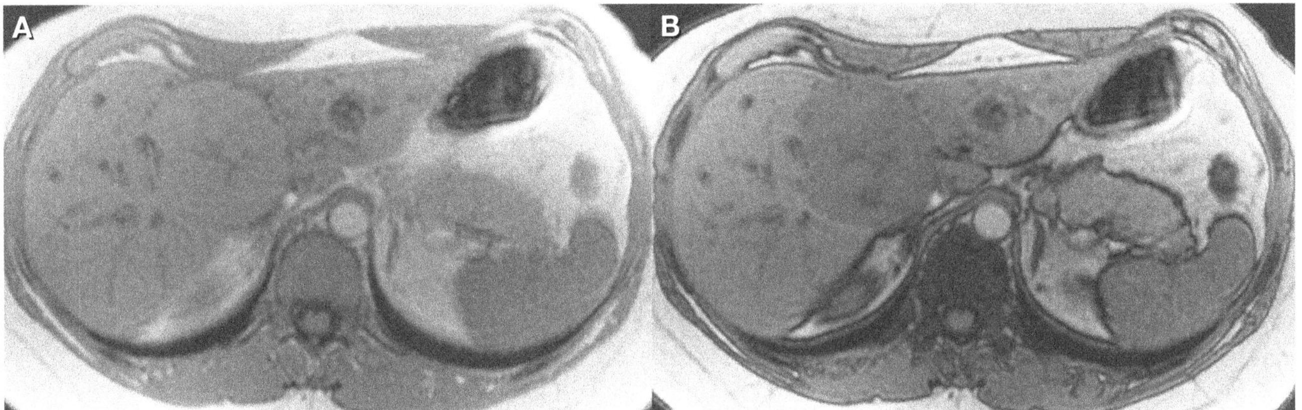

Figure 1.17.3

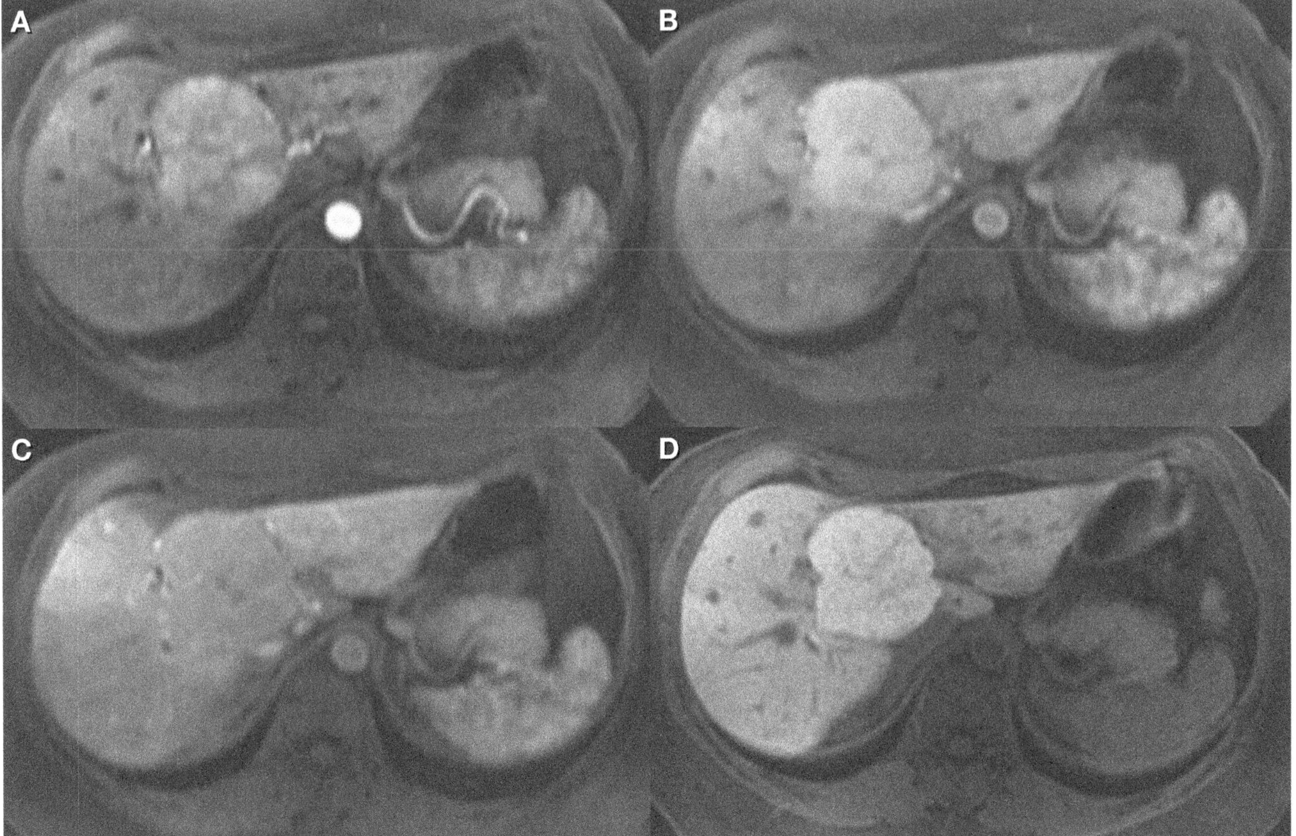

Figure 1.17.4

HISTORY: 33-year-old woman with abnormal liver tests and liver masses seen on CT performed elsewhere

IMAGING FINDINGS: Axial fat-suppressed FSE T2-weighted image (Figure 1.17.1) demonstrates a lobulated hypointense mass in the medial left hepatic lobe. Another similar-appearing mass in the lateral left hepatic lobe is not shown in these images. The lesion is hypointense relative to adjacent liver on a diffusion-weighted image (b=600 s/mm^2) (Figure 1.17.2). Axial IP and OP T1-weighted 2D SPGR images (Figure 1.17.3) reveal signal dropout in the mass on the OP image, suggestive of a fatty component. Three phases of the triple arterial phase postgadolinium (Eovist) acquisition (Figure 1.17.4A-C) reveal rapid uniform hyperenhancement and rapid uniform washout on the last image, where the lesion is isointense relative to adjacent liver. The mass shows diffuse hyperenhancement on the 20-minute delayed hepatobiliary phase image (Figure 1.17.4D).

DIAGNOSIS: Hepatic adenoma (with Eovist)

COMMENT: This case is an example of an atypical adenoma that looks exactly like FNH except for the presence of fat in the lesion. The appearance on postgadolinium 3D SPGR images is classic for FNH, particularly the impressive uniform hyperenhancement on the hepatobiliary phase image. On the other hand, the presence of fat in an FNH is extremely rare. This lesion was reported as likely to be an atypical FNH; however, an adenoma could not be excluded. A US-guided core needle biopsy was performed with histopathology indicating an inflammatory (telangiectatic) adenoma (described in more detail in Case 1.14). Given the size of the masses, the patient underwent left hepatectomy.

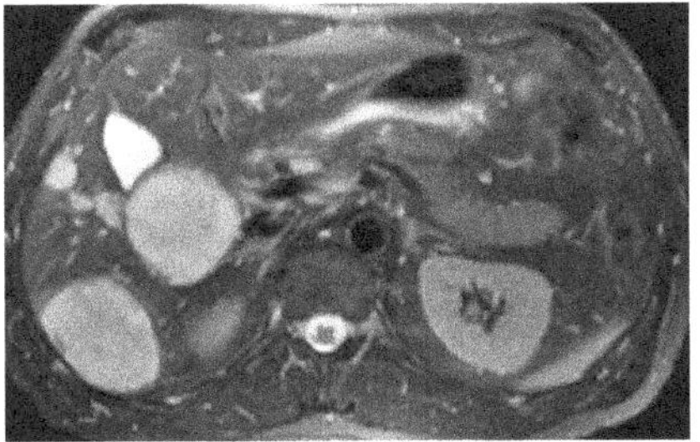

Figure 1.18.1

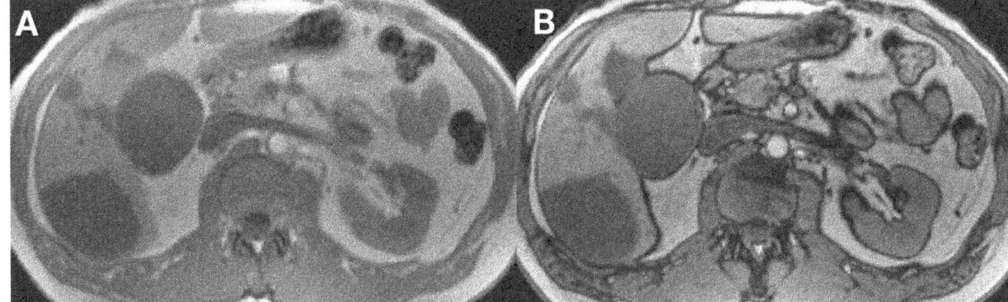

Figure 1.18.2

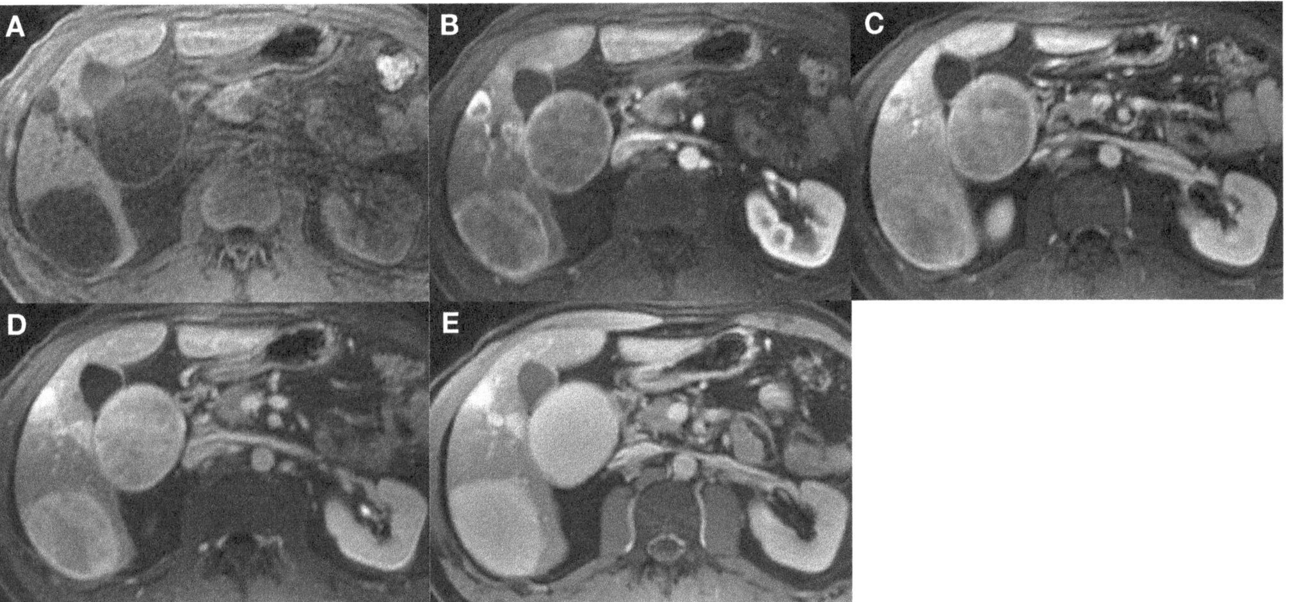

Figure 1.18.3

HISTORY: 45-year-old man with right-sided abdominal pain and multiple indeterminate liver masses initially detected on CT. Various pathologists had read the core biopsies obtained at a separate institution as "positive for malignancy," "low-grade malignancy," "benign liver tissue," and "possible adenoma or atypical FNH"

IMAGING FINDINGS: Axial fat-suppressed FSE T2-weighted image (Figure 1.18.1) demonstrates at least 4 mildly heterogeneous masses in the inferior right hepatic lobe, with markedly increased T2-signal intensity relative to liver and irregular internal septations. No signal dropout from IP to OP T1-weighted 2D SPGR images (Figure 1.18.2) is seen to suggest intravoxel fat, and axial pregadolinium 3D SPGR image (Figure 1.18.3A) demonstrates no increased signal intensity to suggest hemorrhagic or proteinaceous material. Arterial (Figure 1.18.3B), portal venous (Figure 1.18.3C), and equilibrium (Figure 1.18.3D) phase postgadolinium 3D SPGR images and a delayed phase 2D SPGR image (Figure 1.18.3E) reveal well-circumscribed masses with initial rim enhancement followed by gradual internal enhancement.

DIAGNOSIS: Hepatic myxoid adenomatosis

COMMENT: This case is unusual; an extensive literature search revealed only 1 report of a myxoid hepatocellular tumor in the pathology literature, describing a mass characterized by nests and strands of polygonal cells embedded in a myxoid extracellular matrix.

The very high signal intensity of the lesions on T2-weighted images along with initial peripheral enhancement followed by persistent central enhancement near the level of the blood pool are suggestive of hemangiomas, but the peripheral enhancement is not nodular, the progression of enhancement is not particularly centripetal, and the presence of septations is not a feature of hemangiomas. The lesions certainly don't look like FNH, and the only real argument in favor of adenomatosis is that there aren't many other benign hepatic lesions to consider. The possibility of metastases should always be contemplated, even if only on the basis of their relative frequency. The appearance is uncharacteristic of most metastases, although cholangiocarcinoma with intrahepatic metastases might be a remotely plausible diagnosis.

Myxomatous tumors in other organs also tend to have high signal intensity on T2-weighted images, reflecting their high fluid content, and often show gradual enhancement following gadolinium administration as a result of low cellularity, high extracellular and extravascular volumes, and correspondingly slow contrast wash-in and washout rates.

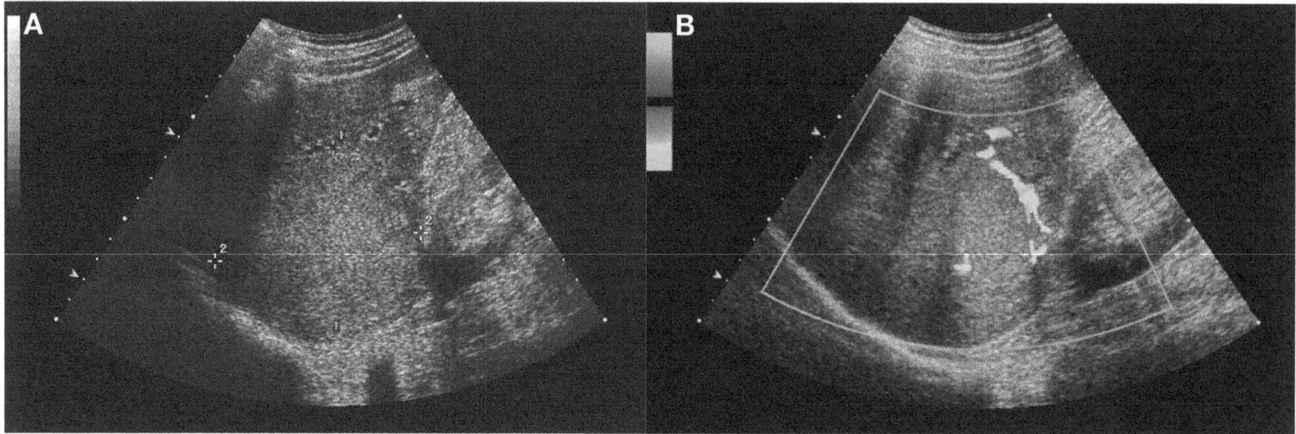

Figure 1.18.4

Preoperative US (Figure 1.18.4) demonstrated multiple homogenous mildly hyperechoic masses with the degree of hyperechogenicity less than typical for cavernous hemangiomas. The patient had no history of anabolic steroid or hormonal use or glycogen storage disease. MRI demonstrated more than 10 similar-appearing masses involving both hepatic lobes; 7 masses were resected and all were myxoid adenomas.

Multiple hepatic adenomas are often seen in patients with glycogen storage disease, which occurs most frequently in young men. The presence of multiple hepatic adenomas does not always imply hepatic adenomatosis, which is characterized by at least 10 masses occurring in equal frequency in men and women and the absence of classic hormonal and metabolic risk factors, such as oral contraceptives and glycogen storage disease.

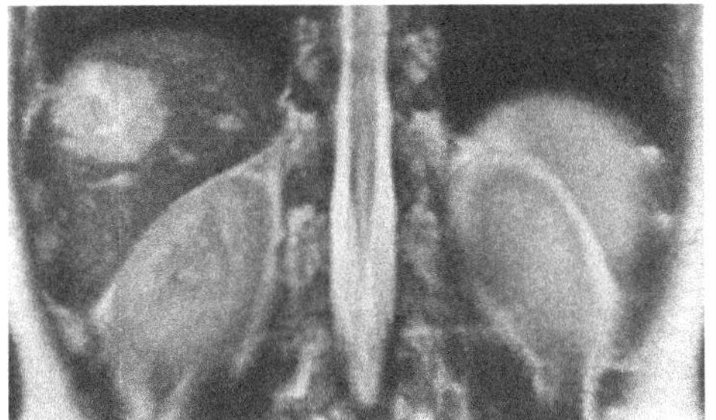

Figure 1.19.1

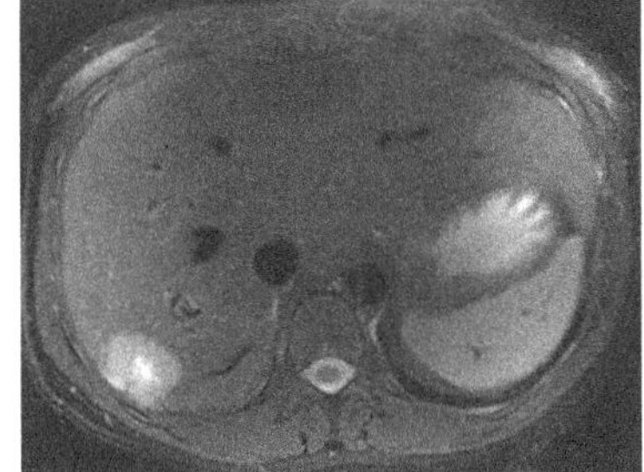

Figure 1.19.2

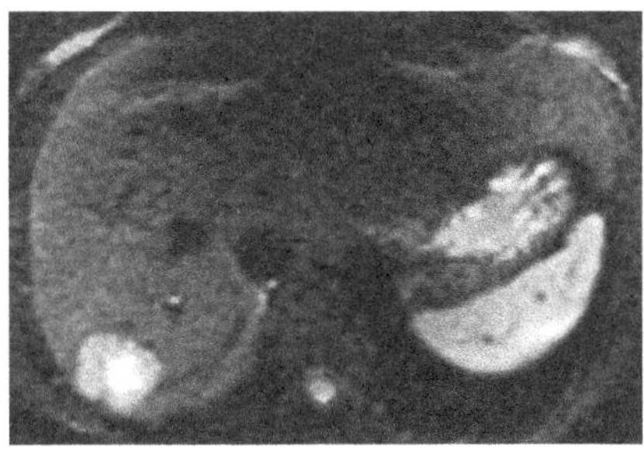

Figure 1.19.3

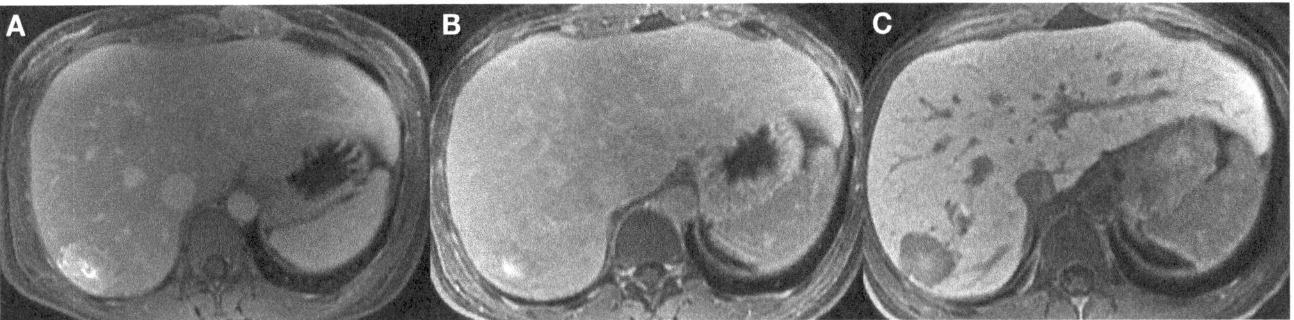

Figure 1.19.4

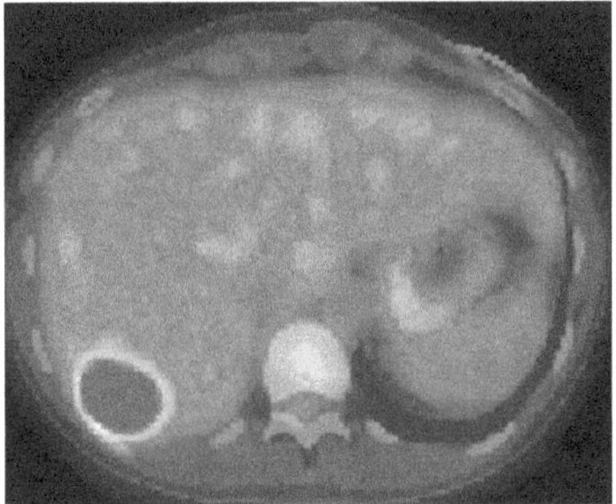

Figure 1.19.5

HISTORY: 30-year-old woman with a long-standing history of palpitations and lightheadedness; she recently was hospitalized for severe hypertension with hypertensive retinopathy

IMAGING FINDINGS: Coronal SSFSE (Figure 1.19.1), axial fat-suppressed FSE T2-weighted (Figure 1.19.2), and diffusion-weighted (b=600 s/mm^2) (Figure 1.19.3) images demonstrate a hyperintense mass in the posterior right hepatic lobe with very high central signal intensity. No associated signal dropout could be seen on IP and OP T1-weighted SPGR images (images not shown). Note the signal loss anteriorly, which is likely secondary to 3-T shading artifact (see Case 17.6). Axial postgadolinium (Multihance) portal venous (Figure 1.19.4A) and delayed (Figure 1.19.4B) phase 3D SPGR images demonstrate gradual hypoenhancement of the mass relative to background liver. A 90-minute delayed hepatobiliary phase image (Figure 1.19.4C) shows only minimal hyperintensity in the center of the lesion. Fused image from PET CT (Figure 1.19.5) demonstrates intense radiotracer activity corresponding to the mass.

DIAGNOSIS: Primary hepatic paraganglioma

COMMENT: There are only a handful of case reports describing primary hepatic paragangliomas; these lesions are, of course, most commonly found in the adrenals, where they are known as *pheochromocytomas*. Approximately 10% of pheochromocytomas are extra-adrenal in location, and 75% of these occur in the organ of Zuckerkandl, the retroperitoneal chromaffin body adjacent to the abdominal sympathetic plexus extending from above the inferior mesenteric artery origin through the aortic bifurcation, with most remaining lesions found in the neck, chest, and bladder.

Patients generally present with signs related to their excessive catecholamine production, including paroxysmal hypertension, flushing, tachycardia, headaches, diaphoresis, and chest pain, although they may also be completely asymptomatic. Paragangliomas are responsible for a very small percentage of hypertension (0.1%-0.5%), and the diagnosis, when clinically suspected, can be made by screening plasma metanephrine (99% sensitivity) or urinary vanillylmandelic acid (95% sensitivity).

The appearance of this lesion is certainly not diagnostic of hepatic paraganglioma. The 2 major differential diagnostic considerations in a patient of this age are FNH and adenoma. The lesion is more hyperintense on the T2-weighted image than the typical FNH, but it does appear to have a central scar. However, the hepatobiliary phase image removes FNH from the differential diagnosis because there is no contrast retention. Although the lesion had no signal dropout from IP to OP images to suggest the presence of fat, there is no convincing evidence on MRI to exclude adenoma from the differential diagnosis.

PET CT was performed after the MRI and following documentation of elevated serum catecholamine levels, since it was considered very unlikely that the hepatic mass represented the primary tumor. The endocrinologists thought it represented either a metastasis or a benign red herring, but PET CT also failed to detect any additional lesions. The patient underwent subsegmental resection of the mass, with pathology demonstrating a paraganglioma without evidence of malignancy.

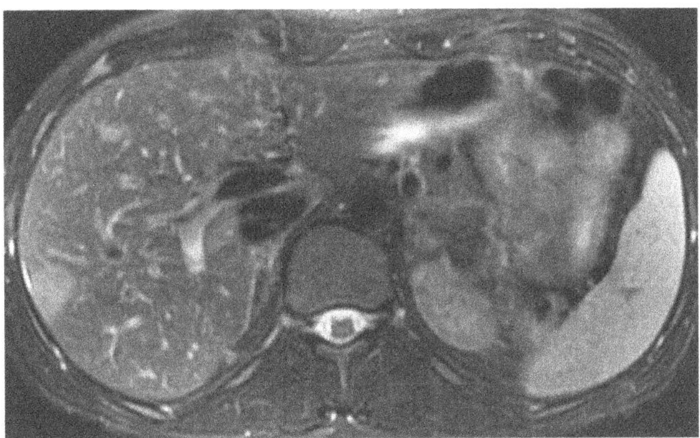

Figure 1.20.1

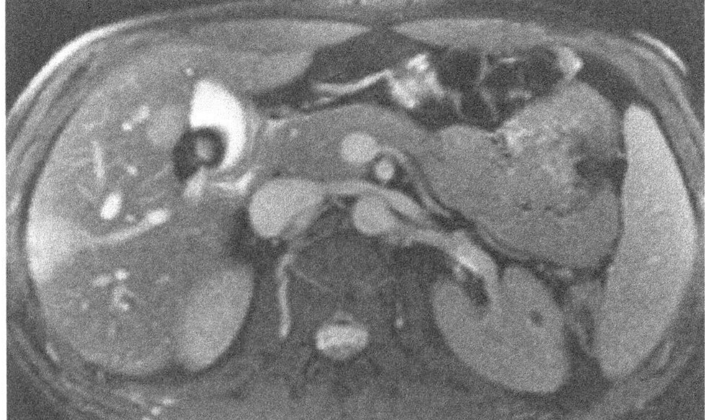

Figure 1.20.2

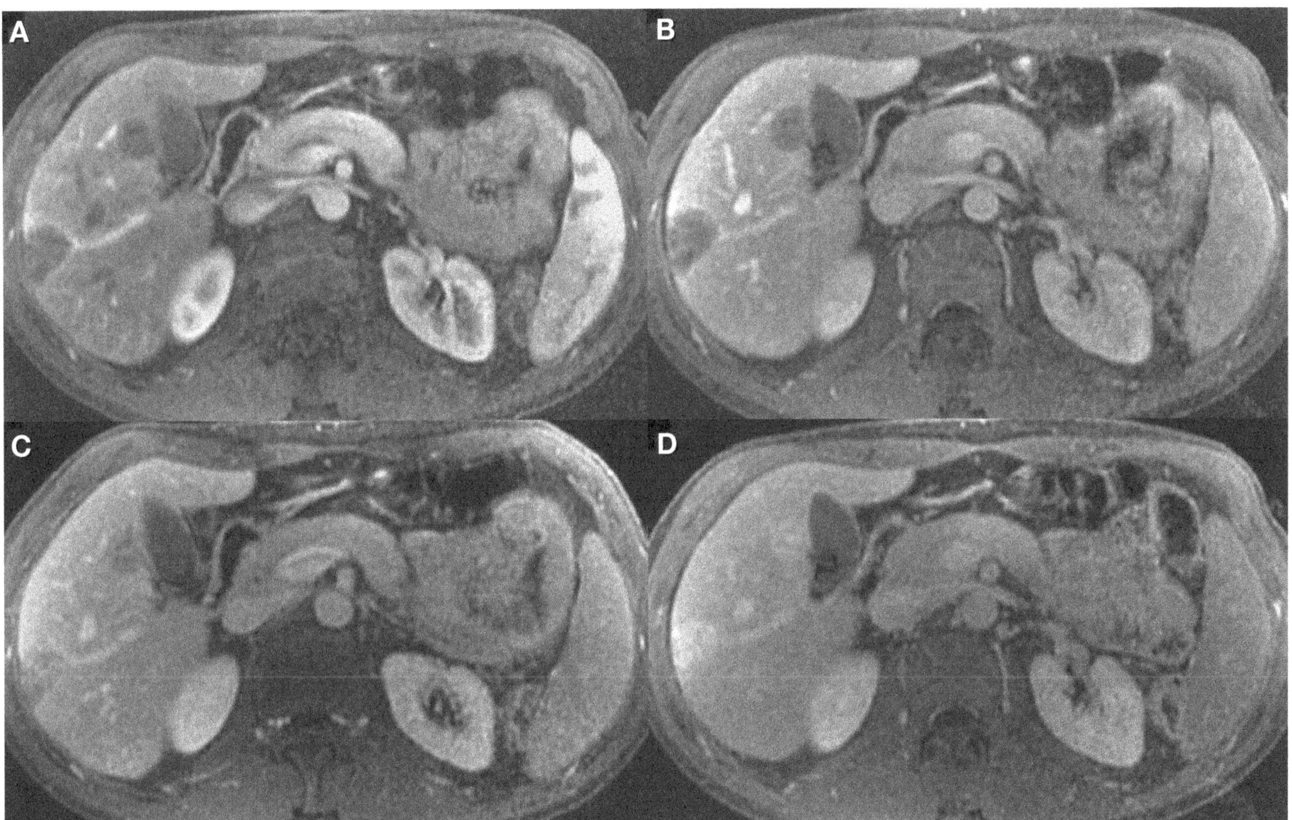

Figure 1.20.3

HISTORY: 27-year-old man with ulcerative colitis and progressive back and abdominal discomfort

IMAGING FINDINGS: Axial fat-suppressed FSE T2-weighted (Figure 1.20.1) and SSFP (Figure 1.20.2) images demonstrate multiple mild-to-moderately hyperintense lesions in the periphery of the liver involving both hepatic lobes. There was no signal dropout from IP to OP T1-weighted 2D SPGR images (images not shown) to suggest intravoxel fat. Axial postgadolinium arterial, portal venous, equilibrium, and 5-minute delayed phase 3D SPGR images (Figure 1.20.3) demonstrate mild rim enhancement of the lesions on the arterial phase image with gradual progressive enhancement. The lesions are hyperintense to adjacent liver on the delayed phase image.

DIAGNOSIS: Epithelioid hemangioendothelioma

COMMENT: EHE is a rare, low-grade, malignant vascular tumor first described in 1982 by Weiss and Enzinger, with the initial report of primary hepatic EHE in 1984. Since then, approximately 200 cases have been described in the literature. There are no known risk factors, although there is a slight female preponderance (60%). Most patients are between the ages of 30 and 50 years at diagnosis. Clinical symptoms are nonspecific and include right upper quadrant pain, weight loss, hepatomegaly, and jaundice, and elevated hepatic enzyme levels (although tumor markers, including AFP, CEA, and CA 19-9, are usually normal), but a significant percentage of patients are asymptomatic and their lesions are detected serendipitously. Budd-Chiari syndrome has been reported in a few cases when the tumors had invaded hepatic veins.

EHE is classified into solitary nodular and diffuse nodular subtypes. The majority of reported cases represent the diffuse nodular subtype (unifocal disease is present at diagnosis in approximately 15% of patients), which likely evolves from an initial solitary lesion. Tumors are composed of a fibrous myxoid stroma with a relatively hypocellular center. The periphery of the tumor contains actively proliferating epithelioid round cells and dendritic spindle-shaped cells in variable proportions. EHE has a propensity for invasion of hepatic sinusoids, terminal hepatic veins, and portal veins. Immunostaining for endothelial markers is essential for diagnosis.

Findings of EHE on MRI include multiple nodules, usually in a peripheral location. Capsular retraction has been reported in a high percentage of cases and has been described as a specific finding for EHE. However, our experience suggests that capsular retraction is often a retrospective diagnosis and that this finding is probably somewhat more common than generally appreciated, occurring in intrahepatic cholangiocarcinoma, confluent hepatic fibrosis, treated metastases, sclerosing hemangiomas, and other fibrotic hepatic lesions.

Most lesions demonstrate peripheral enhancement on arterial phase postgadolinium images, often with increasing enhancement of the rim and gradual central enhancement on later-phase acquisitions. A halo or target sign has been described on postgadolinium images that, depending on whose paper you read, consists of either a hyperenhancing rim surrounding a hypoenhancing center or a hyperenhancing rim sandwiched between a hypointense center and a thin outer hypoenhancing layer, which is thought to represent an avascular zone between tumor and normal liver.

EHE is generally hyperintense to normal liver on T2-weighted images, although usually not to the same degree as typical hemangiomas, and some lesions may display marked central hyperintensity that corresponds to a necrotic core. Halo and target signs have also been applied to T2-weighted images, and a thin hypointense outer layer has been noted in some lesions on T2- and diffusion-weighted images. In advanced disease, the peripheral tumors may coalesce to form large, confluent lesions.

Many cases of EHE are initially misdiagnosed, likely the result of its rarity and its somewhat poorly characterized imaging appearance. The differential diagnosis includes atypical cavernous hemangiomas, metastases, multifocal HCC, cholangiocarcinoma, and angiosarcoma. (Compare this case with Cases 1.7 and 1.10.) The diagnosis can be suggested with the typical appearance of multiple peripheral lesions, moderately increased T2-signal intensity, and initial rim enhancement with gradual accumulation of contrast material on later phase images.

The clinical course of EHE is variable, but in general, the prognosis is favorable in comparison to other malignant primary hepatic tumors. Surgical resection is the treatment of choice and has resulted in 5-year survival rates of 75%; however, most cases are unresectable at diagnosis. Hepatic transplantation is the most common treatment, and extrahepatic disease is not a contraindication. A recent series of 59 patients reported a 10-year survival rate of 72%.

CASE 1.21

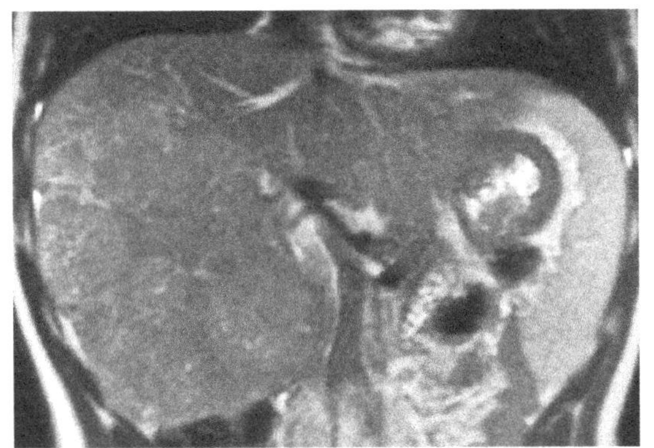

Figure 1.21.1

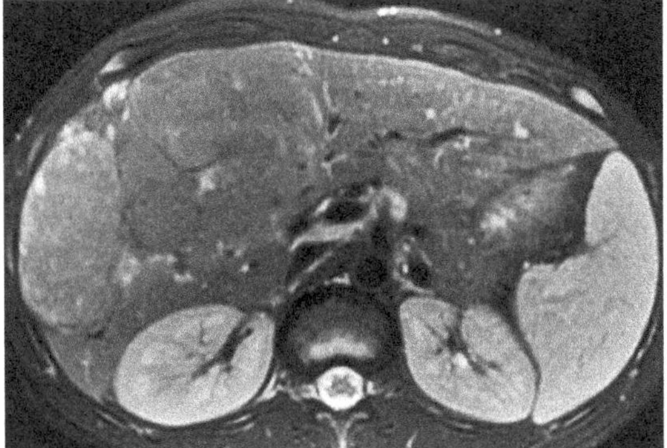

Figure 1.21.2

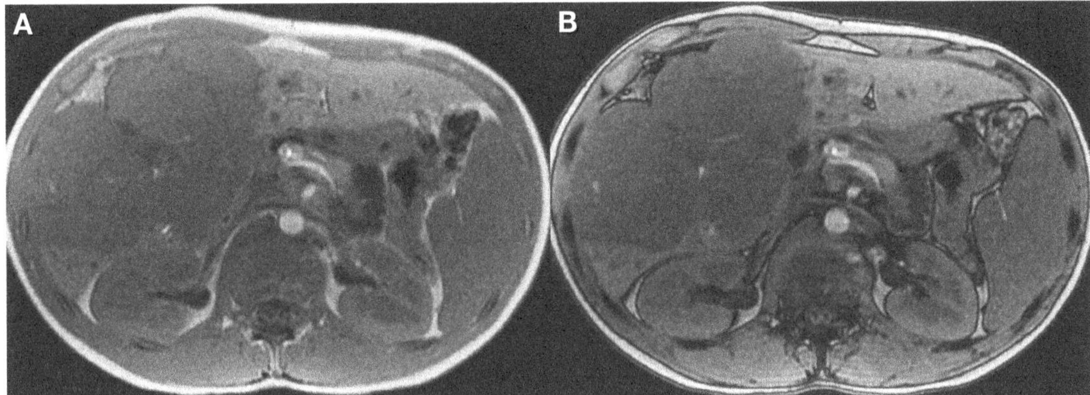

Figure 1.21.3

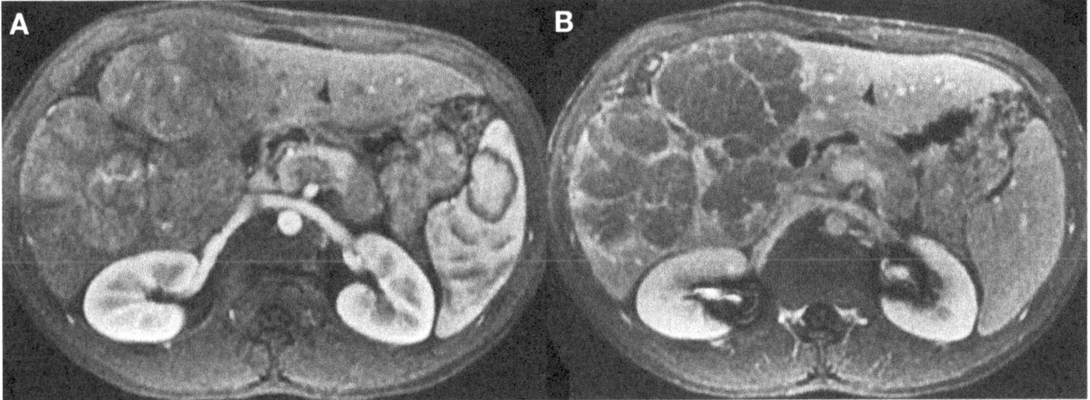

Figure 1.21.4

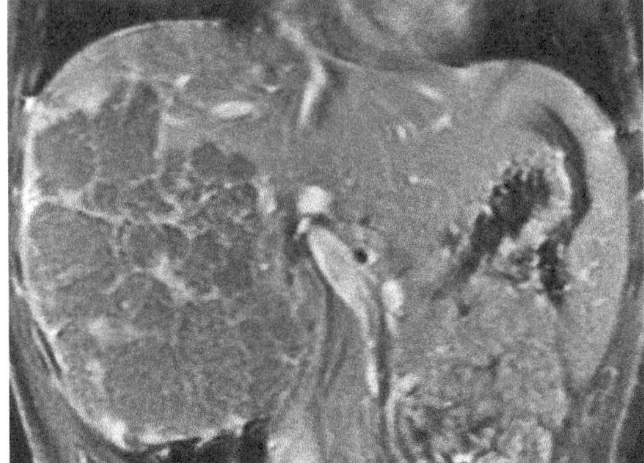

Figure 1.21.5

HISTORY: 14-year-old boy with a 1-year history of episodic fever of unknown origin; he presents with new right-sided abdominal pain

IMAGING FINDINGS: Coronal SSFSE (Figure 1.21.1) and axial fat-suppressed FSE T2-weighted (Figure 1.21.2) images demonstrate a lobulated heterogeneous mass involving both the right and left hepatic lobes with regions of mildly increased signal intensity relative to adjacent liver. The mass is hypointense on axial IP and OP T1-weighted 2D SPGR images (Figure 1.21.3) without signal dropout on the OP image to suggest the presence of intravoxel fat. Arterial and portal venous phase postgadolinium 3D SPGR images (Figure 1.21.4) reveal hypoenhancement of the majority of the mass on both phases, with prominent septations best visualized on the portal venous phase image. Coronal 5-minute delayed 2D SPGR image (Figure 1.21.5) demonstrates similar findings of a septated, hypoenhancing mass with smaller central regions of irregular hyperenhancement.

DIAGNOSIS: Hepatoblastoma, epithelial type

COMMENT: Hepatoblastoma, a mass lying somewhere in the spectrum between hemangioma and angiosarcoma, is the most common primary hepatic malignancy in children and accounts for almost 80% of liver cancer in children younger than 15 years. The incidence is highest in infants (11.2 per 1 million) and 90% of cases appear before 5 years of age. Most patients present with an enlarging abdomen or an abdominal mass and nonspecific symptoms, including anorexia and weight loss. Serum AFP levels are elevated in 90% of patients with hepatoblastoma; the levels may be extremely high (>1,000,000 ng/mL) in patients with metastatic disease or very large tumors but may be in the normal range in patients with undifferentiated lesions. Metastatic disease, when present, most frequently involves the lungs (10%-20% of cases) and, more rarely, the brain and bones. The etiology of hepatoblastoma is unknown, but it has been associated with familial adenomatosis polyposis, Gardner syndrome, Beckwith-Wiedemann syndrome, trisomy 18, and low birth weight.

Hepatoblastoma usually presents as a large solitary mass (80% are at least 12 cm in diameter at diagnosis), often with prominent septations and lobules, and has been classified into 2 broad categories that reflect its histologic composition: epithelial and mixed epithelial-mesenchymal types. The epithelial type is slightly more common, accounting for 56% of cases, and is further subcategorized on the basis of tumor cell differentiation. Mesenchymal elements most commonly found in hepatoblastoma include osteoid, fibrous, and cartilaginous tissue.

The appearance on MRI depends to some extent on the tumor's histologic composition. Tumors are usually large and well circumscribed and often have a lobulated appearance with multiple septations. Epithelial hepatoblastomas in general have a more homogeneous appearance, whereas the various mesenchymal elements present in mixed tumors introduce a greater heterogeneity. Hepatoblastomas generally appear hypointense on T1-weighted images relative to normal liver and hyperintense on T2-weighted images, as is true of most tumors. Septations and fibrous components show gradual enhancement after gadolinium administration, while the bulk of the tumor usually enhances less than adjacent liver. Speckled or amorphous calcification is seen in approximately 50% of tumors on CT but is much more difficult to identify on MRI.

Differential diagnosis depends on the patient's age. In infants, considerations include infantile hemangioendothelioma (ie, much more vascular lesions with persistent enhancement on delayed images) and mesenchymal hamartoma (often predominantly cystic lesions [see Case 1.6 for an example]). In older children and adolescents, the major differential diagnosis is HCC, which may be difficult or impossible to distinguish from hepatoblastoma on the basis of imaging characteristics alone.

Surgical resection is the most effective therapy and is often performed following neoadjuvant chemotherapy to improve the surgical outcome. Currently, 85% of tumors are resectable with or without adjuvant chemotherapy. The overall long-term survival rate for children with hepatoblastoma is in the range of 65% to 70%, with the prognosis primarily determined by the tumor stage.

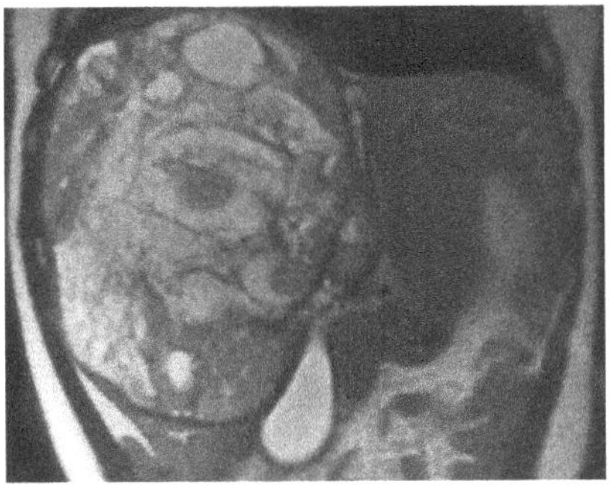

Figure 1.22.1

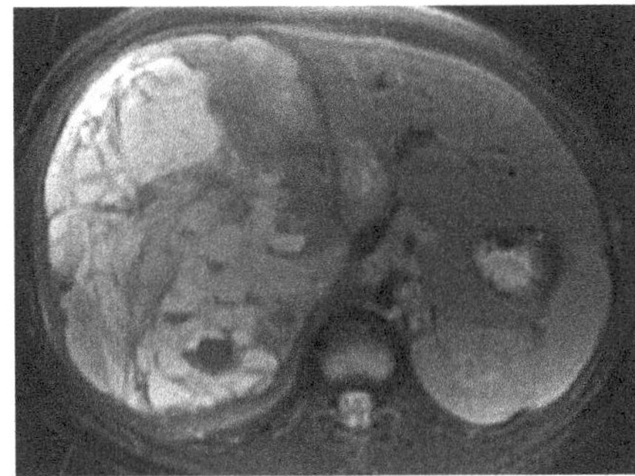

Figure 1.22.2

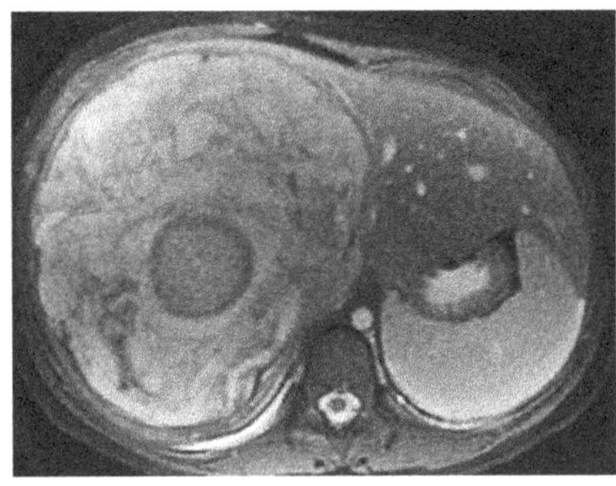

Figure 1.22.3

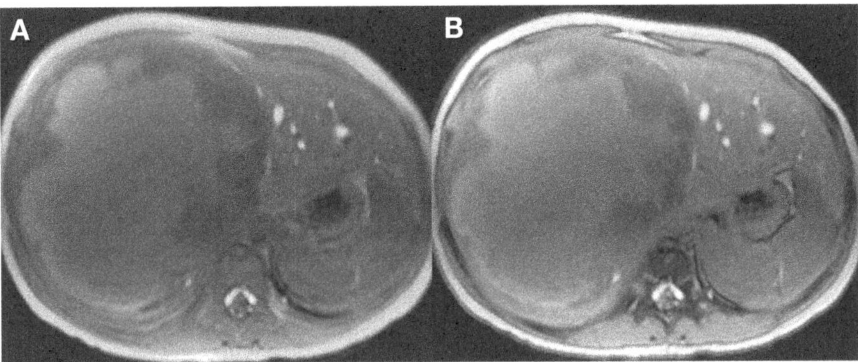

Figure 1.22.4

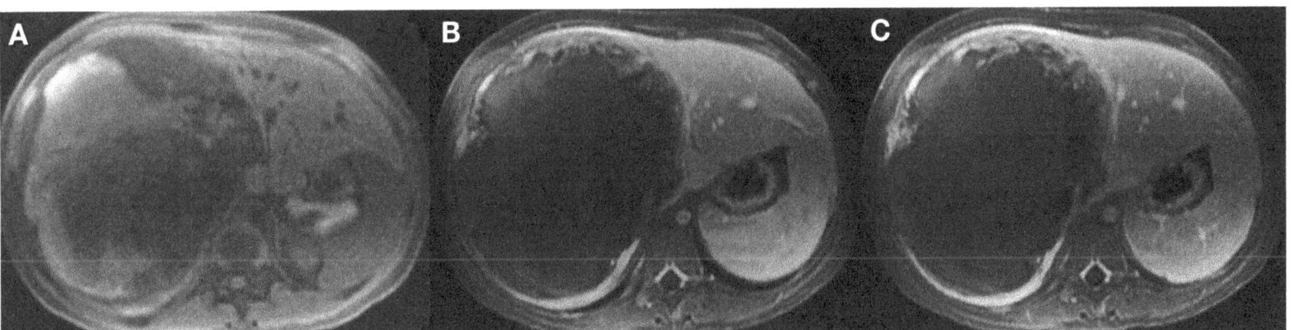

Figure 1.22.5

HISTORY: 8-year-old boy whose sister noticed that the right side of his abdomen was larger than the left

IMAGING FINDINGS: Coronal SSFSE (Figure 1.22.1), axial fat-suppressed FSE T2-weighted (Figure 1.22.2), and axial fat-suppressed 2D SSFP (Figure 1.22.3) images reveal a large, markedly hyperintense, heterogeneous, well-circumscribed mass expanding the right hepatic lobe. The mass has extensive septations and more solid-appearing components in the periphery of the lesion. Axial IP and OP T1-weighted 2D SPGR images (Figure 1.22.4) do not show significant signal dropout to suggest the presence of intralesional fat or lipid. Axial pregadolinium T1-weighted 3D SPGR image (Figure 1.22.5A) shows predominantly low signal intensity within the lesion. Peripheral regions of increased signal intensity could be due to hemorrhagic or proteinaceous components. Portal venous (Figure 1.22.5B) and equilibrium (Figure 1.22.5C) phase postgadolinium 3D SPGR images show irregular enhancement of the periphery of the lesion with minimal central enhancement.

DIAGNOSIS: Undifferentiated embryonal sarcoma

COMMENT: UES is a rare, malignant mesenchymal tumor, with fewer than 200 cases reported in the literature. Nevertheless, it is the third most common malignant neoplasm of the liver in children, after hepatoblastoma and HCC. Most patients with UES present between the ages of 6 and 10 years with an abdominal mass, which may be accompanied by abdominal pain or discomfort.

UES is predominantly composed of sarcomatous stellate or spindle-shaped cells embedded within a prominent myxoid stroma. Lesions are typically large at diagnosis, with an average diameter of 14 cm, and have a predilection for the right hepatic lobe. A highly malignant neoplasm, UES shares many histopathologic and immunohistochemical features with the benign mesenchymal hamartoma (see Case 1.6), and this relation has led to speculation that UES may arise from preexisting mesenchymal hamartomas.

The imaging features of UES are distinctive: a large, markedly T2-hyperintense mass with extensive internal heterogeneity, often containing multiple septations, enhancing soft tissue nodules, and foci of necrosis, cystic degeneration, and hemorrhage. The abundant myxoid tissue is thought to account for the high signal intensity on T2-weighted images and limited enhancement on postgadolinium images, and nearly every UES paper in the literature emphasizes the importance of correlating these findings with sonography, where the lesion typically manifests as a solid mass, in contrast to a more cystic appearance on CT and MRI. Whether this is actually clinically relevant is debatable, since the appearance on MRI is distinctive and usually diagnostic, but this discrepancy was discussed at great length in an early paper and has been faithfully reproduced in subsequent case reports and reviews.

Differential diagnosis includes mesenchymal hamartoma, which usually occurs in a younger age-group (children <2 years of age) and is characterized by a multicystic appearance without hemorrhage and with less overall heterogeneity. Hydatid disease is a consideration in endemic areas, although these lesions are usually characterized by a much less prominent solid component. Hepatoblastoma and HCC rarely have the cystic appearance of UES and may be accompanied by an elevated AFP level, which is not seen in UES.

Until fairly recently, the prognosis of UES was poor, with a mean survival of 12 months after diagnosis; however, recent advances in neoadjuvant chemotherapy have allowed surgical resection in a higher percentage of patients, leading to substantially increased survival. Our patient was treated with complete resection followed by chemotherapy and 4 years later shows no evidence of recurrent disease.

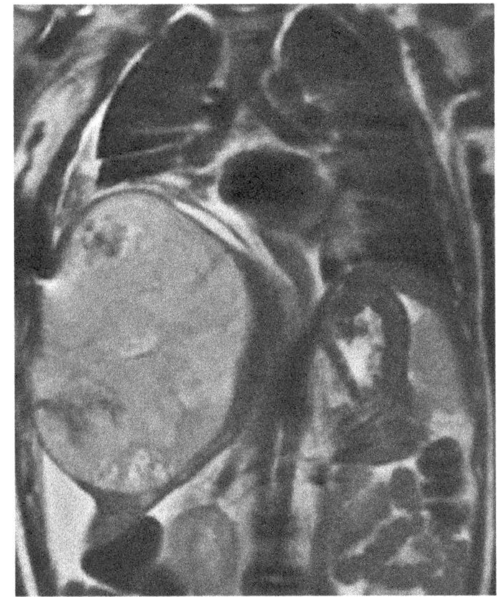

Figure 1.23.1

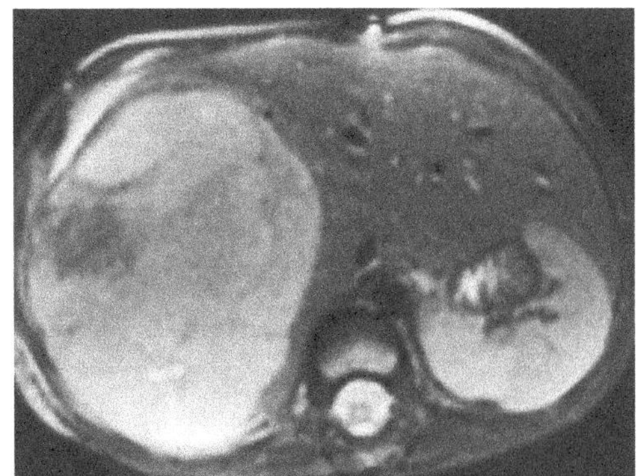

Figure 1.23.2

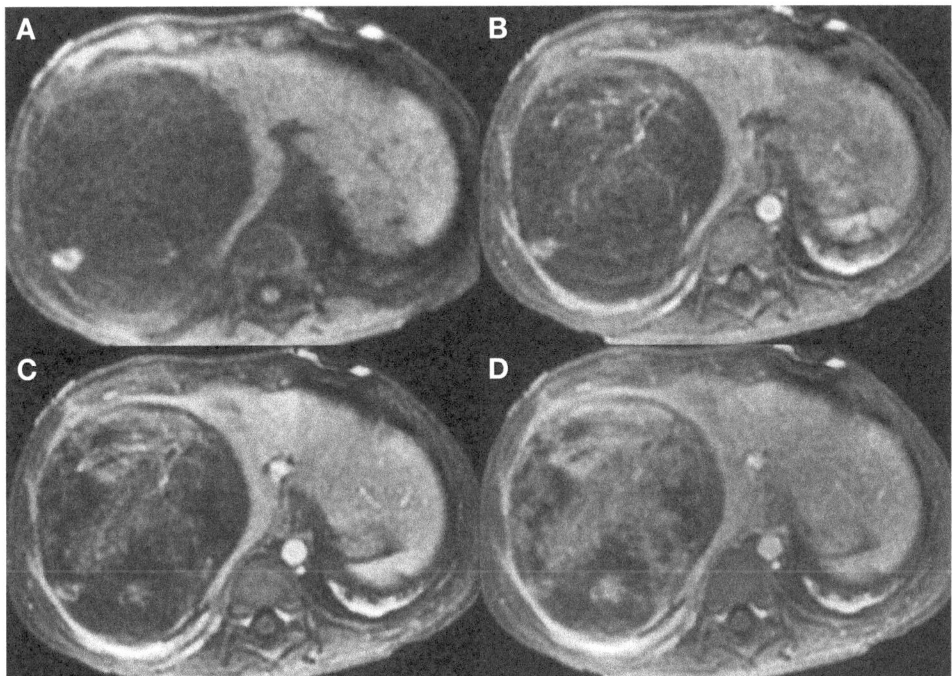

Figure 1.23.3

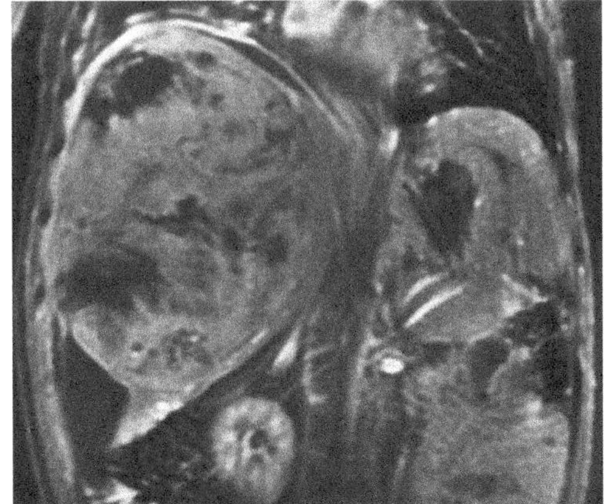

Figure 1.23.4

HISTORY: 4-year-old boy with abdominal pain initially diagnosed as constipation. The pain worsened, and a CT demonstrated a hepatic mass

IMAGING FINDINGS: Coronal SSFSE (Figure 1.23.1) and axial fat-suppressed FSE T2-weighted (Figure 1.23.2) images reveal a large heterogeneous mass in the right hepatic lobe, with markedly increased signal intensity. Axial precontrast and arterial, portal venous, and equilibrium phase postgadolinium 3D SPGR images (Figure 1.23.3) demonstrate gradual heterogeneous enhancement of the lesion. Notice also the focus of high-signal-intensity hemorrhage on the precontrast image. Coronal 2D SPGR image (Figure 1.23.4) acquired 8 minutes after gadolinium injection shows heterogeneous, intense enhancement of the mass.

DIAGNOSIS: Undifferentiated embryonal sarcoma

COMMENT: This is another case of UES, again demonstrating the complex cystic appearance of the lesion on T2-weighted images. Compared with Case 1.22, the postgadolinium images in this case more clearly illustrate the gradual enhancement of the mass, with diffuse intense enhancement on the delayed coronal image. This is the expected enhancement pattern for a lesion with an extensive extracellular matrix—in this case, myxoid stroma. The wash-in and washout rates of gadolinium within a given tissue are determined in part by the volume of distribution available to the contrast agent, which is usually the extravascular extracellular volume. When this volume is large, as in a tumor with extensive stromal elements, the initial distribution of contrast throughout the tissue takes longer and the washout of contrast into the venous system is also delayed relative to tissues that have a smaller volume of distribution.

Similar to the patient in Case 1.22, this patient also had an excellent response to surgery and chemotherapy and has had no recurrence in 5 years following his initial treatment.

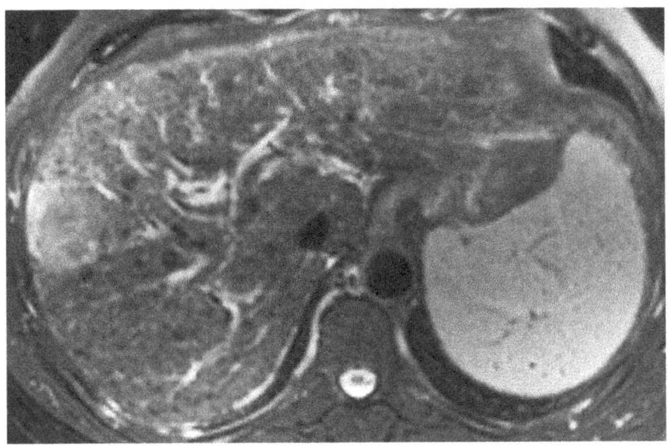

Figure 1.24.1

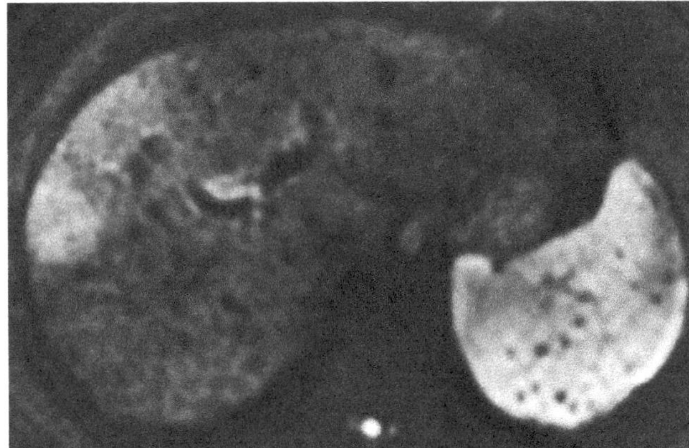

Figure 1.24.2

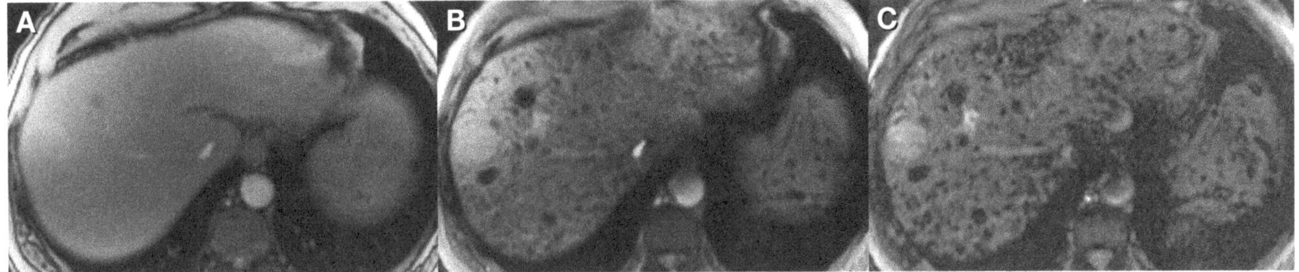

Figure 1.24.3

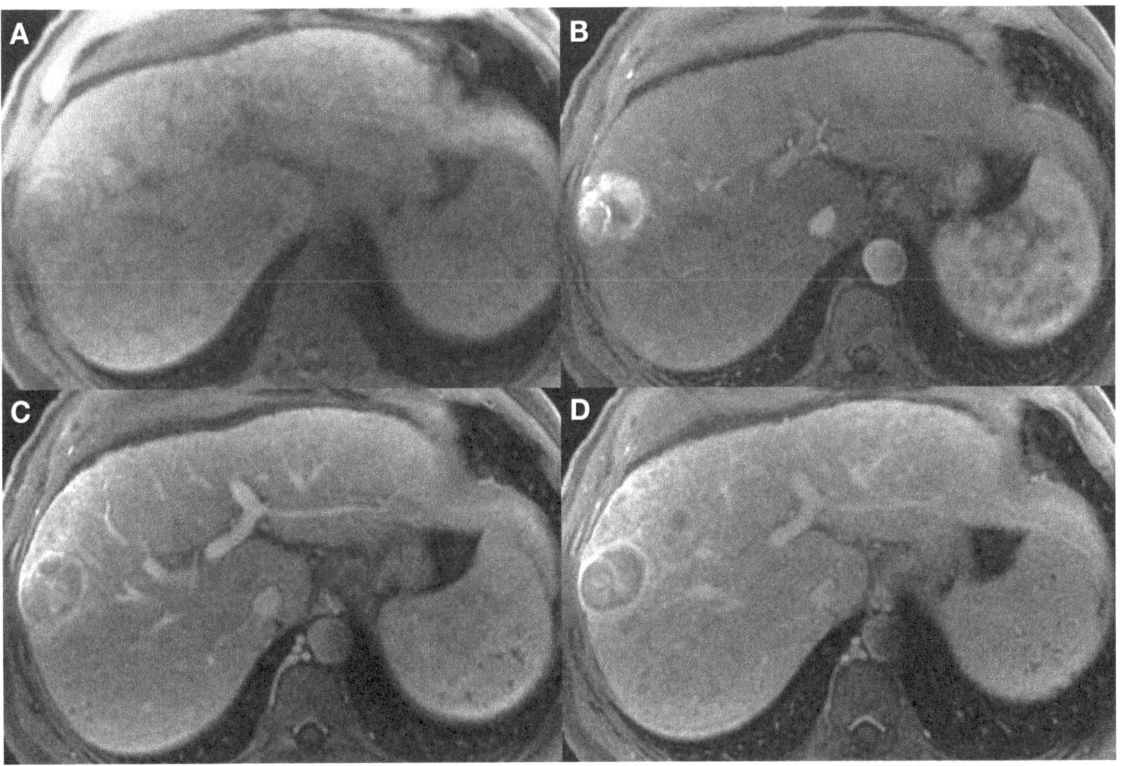

Figure 1.24.4

HISTORY: 57-year-old man with a history of alcoholic cirrhosis

IMAGING FINDINGS: Axial fat-suppressed FSE T2-weighted (Figure 1.24.1) and diffusion-weighted (b=100 s/mm^2) (Figure 1.24.2) images demonstrate a peripheral right hepatic lobe mass that has mildly increased signal intensity relative to adjacent liver. Notice the higher signal intensity and greater contrast on the diffusion-weighted image (b=100 s/mm^2). Axial images from a multiecho 2D GRE acquisition with successively longer TEs (an iron quantification image acquisition) (Figure 1.24.3) demonstrate multiple hypointense foci throughout the liver and spleen that become more prominent as the TE increases. Pregadolinium, arterial, portal venous, and equilibrium phase postgadolinium 3D SPGR images (Figure 1.24.4) reveal intense, fairly uniform enhancement on the arterial phase image and prompt washout on portal venous and equilibrium phase images. Notice also the presence of an enhancing rim. Two small, adjacent hypoenhancing lesions are best seen on the equilibrium phase image and represent siderotic regenerative nodules.

DIAGNOSIS: Hepatocellular carcinoma, hepatic siderosis, and Gamna-Gandy bodies

COMMENT: This case represents the classic appearance of HCC: mildly hypointense on T1-weighted precontrast images, mildly hyperintense on T2-weighted FSE images, hyperintense on diffusion-weighted images, and demonstrating hyperenhancement on arterial phase postgadolinium 3D SPGR acquisitions, which then becomes hypointense (washout) relative to adjacent liver on portal venous or equilibrium phase images. The presence of an enhancing pseudocapsule, usually seen on portal venous or equilibrium phase images, is another classic feature of HCC. All of these findings usually occur against the background heterogeneity of a cirrhotic liver (80% of cases).

HCC is the fifth most common tumor in the world and the third leading cause of cancer-related death (after lung and gastric cancers). The incidence of HCC is increasing precipitously in the United States, largely attributable to the increasing prevalence of hepatitis C virus infection. Cirrhosis is the strongest predisposing factor for HCC development, with an annual incidence of 2% to 7% in the cirrhotic population. Hepatitis B virus infection is the most common etiology of HCC in Asia and Africa; hepatitis C virus infection is thought to account for the majority of disease in the West, as well as in Japan. Additional risk factors include alcoholic cirrhosis, hemochromatosis, biliary cirrhosis, and steatohepatitis.

Extensive literature describes the imaging appearance of HCC, much of it contradictory, but a general consensus regarding some aspects of MRI in HCC has emerged. Although HCC can develop de novo, it most often appears as a result of a progression from regenerative nodule to dysplastic nodule to HCC. The imaging features of dysplastic nodules and HCC overlap to a significant extent, but in general, increased signal intensity on T2-weighted images, arterial phase hyperenhancement, and washout on portal venous and equilibrium phase images are all worrisome features.

Arterial phase enhancement occurs as the dysplastic nodule gradually loses its portal tracts and recruits its own arterial supply (ie, neoangiogenesis). Arterial phase hyperenhancement is the only radiologic criterion on CT and MRI required for noninvasive diagnosis of HCC by the United Network for Organ Sharing before listing the patient for transplantation, but hyperenhancement is present in only 80% to 90% of HCCs. Small well-differentiated lesions may not have developed sufficient neovascularity to appear hyperintense on arterial phase images, and larger lesions that have outgrown their blood supply may become necrotic and likewise fail to enhance during the arterial phase. Another requirement, and an unknown factor in the statistics quoted earlier, is the need for optimal timing of the postgadolinium arterial phase acquisition. Optimal visualization of a small, hyperenhancing HCC might occur within a temporal window lasting only a few seconds, and these lesions can easily be missed if the arterial phase is acquired either too early or too late. Washout (ie, hypoenhancement relative to adjacent liver) on portal venous and equilibrium phase images is highly suggestive of HCC, with a specificity of approximately 95%, but occurs in only about 50% of cases. Visualization of this phenomenon is more difficult in patients with severe cirrhosis and very nodular livers, in whom it can be challenging to find any normal hepatic parenchyma to serve as a basis for comparison.

The appearance of HCC on T2-weighted images is another factor that is critically affected by technique. Increased T2-signal intensity is thought to be quite specific for HCC, but not particularly sensitive. The sensitivity of this sign depends to a great extent on the choice of pulse sequence: Many groups use either an SSFSE or an FRFSE sequence since these both have considerably shorter acquisition times than standard fat-suppressed, respiratory-triggered, or navigator-gated FSE sequences. Unfortunately, however, both of these options are relatively insensitive for detecting solid lesions in the liver. In our practice, they're known as *hepatoma suppression sequences*, and we believe that the few extra minutes spent on a respiratory-triggered (or navigator-gated) FSE acquisition in a cirrhotic patient are well worth the effort.

The importance of T2-weighted imaging is less certain in the era of DWI. In this case, for example, the mass is more conspicuous on diffusion-weighted images, and it seems to be generally true that high signal intensity on diffusion-weighted images is associated with HCC much more frequently than with regenerative and low-grade dysplastic nodules. Notice also in this case that the tumor is very conspicuous on a diffusion-weighted image with low b value (100 s/mm^2). Since T2 shine-through is unlikely to have a strong effect for this lesion (it's only mildly hyperintense on the FSE image), this characteristic may reflect the higher perfusion weighting of the low b-value acquisition. It's often, but by no means universally, true that lesions with strong arterial phase enhancement are better seen on low b-value images.

This case also illustrates the appearance of siderotic nodules in the cirrhotic liver, as well as their splenic equivalent, Gamna-Gandy bodies, which are seen in about 10% of patients with portal hypertension. Accumulation of iron in regenerative or dysplastic nodules leads to the appearance of small, low-signal-intensity lesions on both T1- and T2-weighted images. Their presence is accentuated by heavily T2*-weighted acquisitions—in this case, illustrated by a multiecho GRE sequence. The susceptibility effect increases as TE increases, and T2*-weighted images are sometimes useful in documenting the presence of multiple siderotic nodules in patients with mild cirrhosis and a nearly normal parenchymal appearance on other pulse sequences. Notice also how the conspicuity of HCC increases with increasing TE; this is because hepatomas lack Kupffer cells and therefore don't accumulate much iron in comparison to the rest of the liver. This same principle was used by the SPIO contrast agent (Feridex) before it was taken off the market a few years ago.

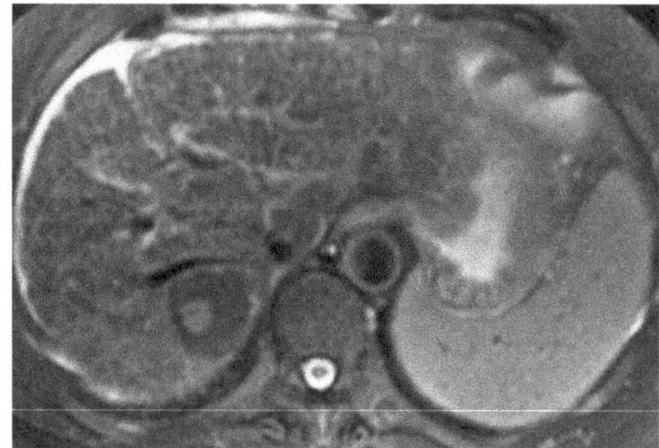

Figure 1.25.1

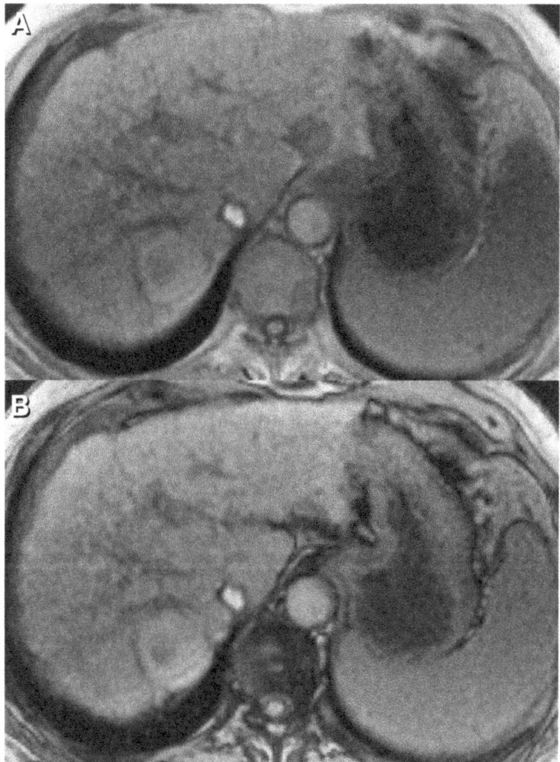

Figure 1.25.2

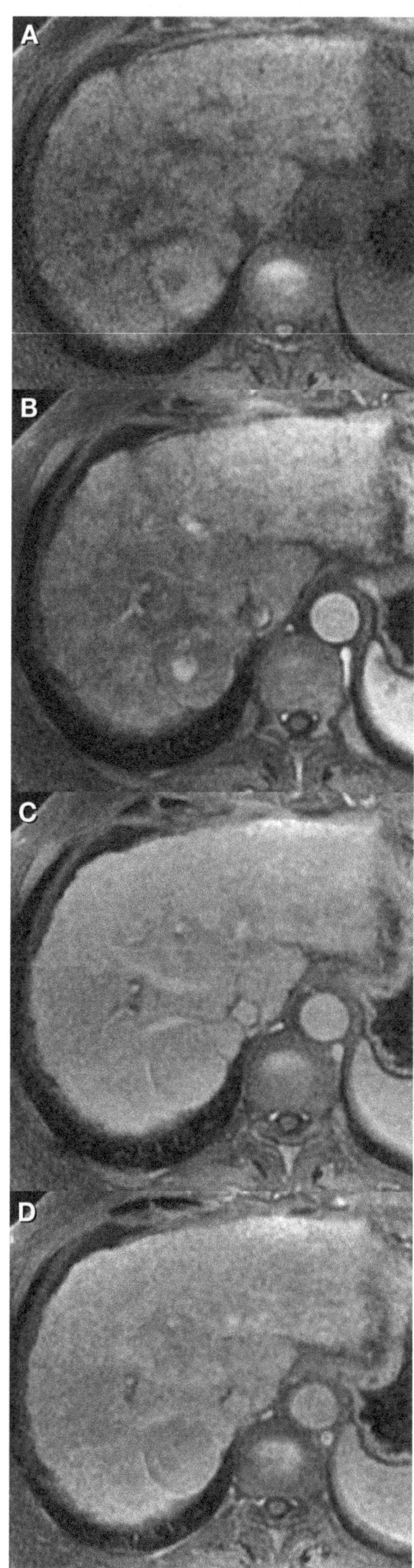

Figure 1.25.3

HISTORY: 68-year-old man with a history of hepatitis diagnosed 40 years ago and gradually worsening hepatic function, now with new lower-extremity swelling and ascites

IMAGING FINDINGS: Axial fat-suppressed T2-weighted image (Figure 1.25.1) demonstrates a cirrhotic liver with perihepatic ascites and a hypointense mass with a hyperintense inner nodule in the posterior medial right hepatic lobe. Axial T1-weighted 2D SPGR IP and OP images (Figure 1.25.2) reveal the larger mass to be hyperintense and the inner nodule hypointense relative to adjacent liver. Pregadolinium and arterial, portal venous, and equilibrium phase postgadolinium 3D SPGR images (Figure 1.25.3) demonstrate uniform arterial phase enhancement of the inner nodule, which then becomes isointense to the larger nodule on portal venous and equilibrium phase images. Note also washout of the larger nodule, most apparent on the equilibrium phase image, as well as mild rim enhancement seen on both portal venous and equilibrium phase images.

DIAGNOSIS: Hepatocellular carcinoma

COMMENT: The "nodule within a nodule" appearance of HCC illustrated in this case is a classic pattern and is thought to represent the development of a focus of frank carcinoma within a larger dysplastic nodule. The small inner nodule exhibits typical imaging characteristics of HCC—namely, increased T2-signal intensity and arterial phase hyperenhancement—while the larger nodule has a more nondescript appearance of increased T1- and reduced T2-signal intensity without significant arterial phase hyperenhancement, reflective of a regenerative or dysplastic nodule.

The appearance of HCC and dysplastic nodules on precontrast T1-weighted images has a long and variable history in the literature. Early papers described hyperintense lesions on T1-weighted imaging as definitely benign and indicative of regenerative or low-grade dysplastic nodules, but it is now recognized that a relatively small percentage (10%-15%) of HCCs are hyperintense on T1-weighted images. The T1-signal intensity has been variously attributed to the presence of fat, glycogen, hemorrhage, protein, copper, zinc, and melanin and is likely multifactorial. A recent paper has suggested that a solitary or dominant T1-hyperintense nodule, even without T2 hyperintensity or arterial phase enhancement, has an increased risk of HCC.

When the background liver tissue demonstrates advanced cirrhosis, as in this case, identification of small HCCs can be challenging—in particular, distinguishing them from the heterogeneous background of regenerative and dysplastic nodules. The presence of a dominant lesion, as well as the fairly classic appearance of the inner nodule, makes the diagnosis relatively straightforward in this case.

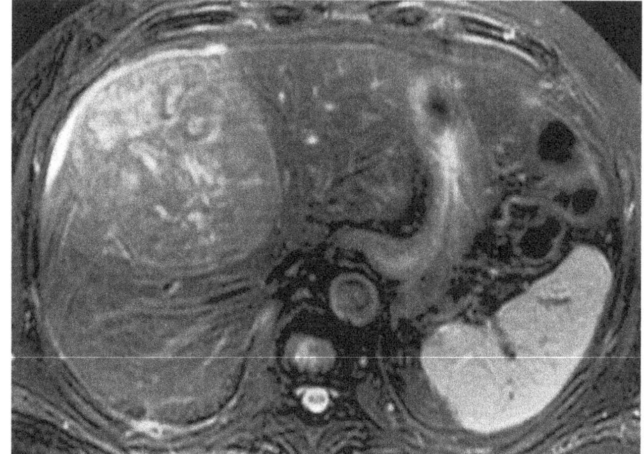

Figure 1.26.1

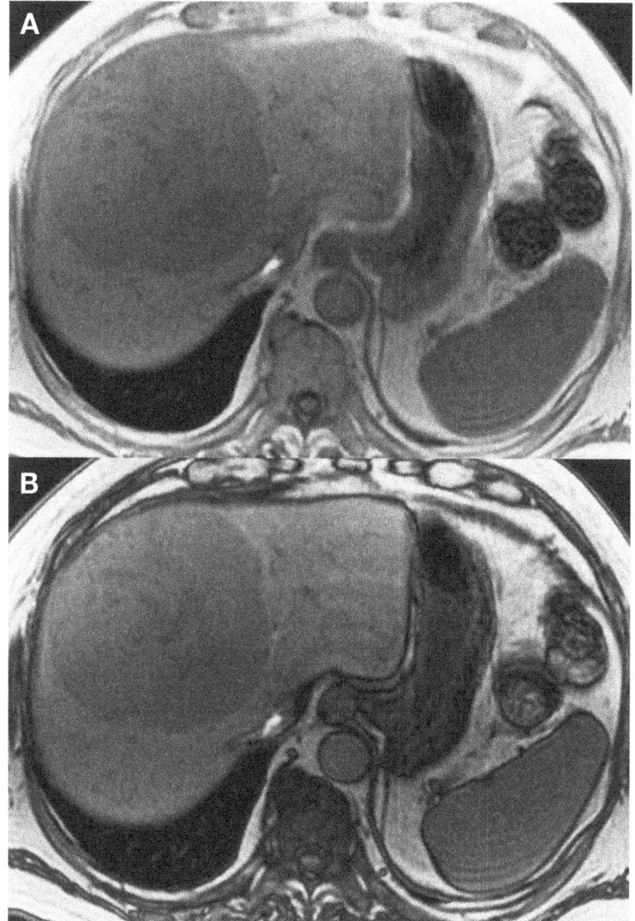

Figure 1.26.2

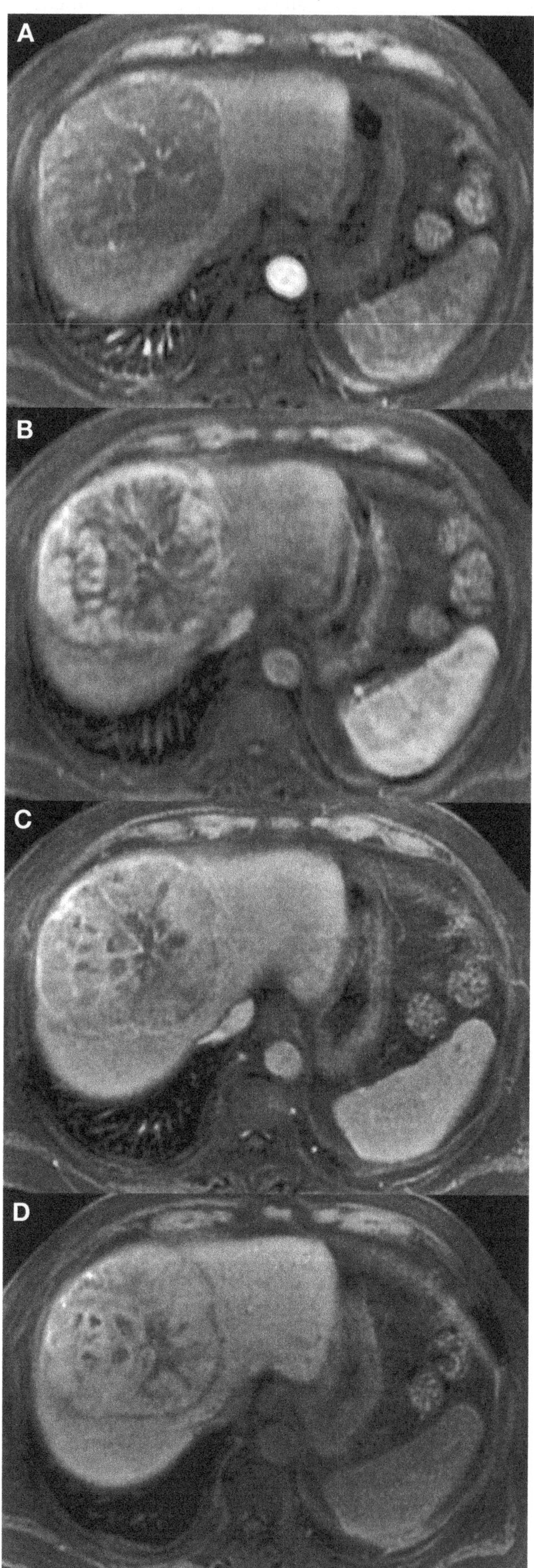

Figure 1.26.3

HISTORY: 83-year-old man with suspected HCC

IMAGING FINDINGS: Axial fat-suppressed FSE T2-weighted image (Figure 1.26.1) demonstrates a large mass in the anterior right hepatic lobe, with heterogeneous increased T2-signal intensity. Axial T1-weighted 2D SPGR IP and OP images (Figure 1.26.2) reveal no signal dropout within the mass on the OP image to suggest intravoxel fat. Axial postgadolinium (Eovist) arterial (Figures 1.26.3A and 1.26.3B), portal venous (Figure 1.26.3C), and hepatobiliary (Figure 1.26.3D) phase 3D SPGR images demonstrate initial peripheral enhancement of the mass, with increasing central enhancement, and diffuse but mildly heterogeneous contrast retention on the hepatobiliary phase image.

DIAGNOSIS: Hepatocellular carcinoma (well differentiated)

COMMENT: Eovist was initially marketed as a contrast agent with a primary function of identifying hepatic metastases: Even small lesions are visible with high contrast on hepatobiliary phase images. It has been applied with increasing frequency for several additional indications, and many experts now advocate its use for nearly all hepatic examinations.

One of the most interesting potential applications of Eovist is in imaging patients with cirrhosis. Although MRI is generally considered the most accurate technique for identifying HCC, the literature does not completely support this view, and the reported sensitivities for HCC detection in hepatic explant studies (which should be the most realistic) are often surprisingly poor, in some cases as low as 50%. In an ideal world, use of Eovist would help to solve this problem by allowing identification of indeterminate lesions on precontrast and dynamic imaging as hypoenhancing masses on hepatobiliary phase images. This is a particularly attractive scenario with regard to the large number of small perfusion abnormalities encountered in cirrhotic livers, which show arterial phase hyperenhancement but cannot be visualized on portal venous or equilibrium phase images or on precontrast images. The vast majority of these lesions are benign, but a small percentage (2%-8%) of them are actually HCCs. The idea that these few malignant lesions could be identified on hepatobiliary phase images is very appealing.

This case illustrates 1 reason why Eovist may not be the perfect solution for imaging the cirrhotic patient. The agent is taken up by functional hepatocytes and excreted into the biliary tree, neither of which is usually found in HCC; however, in a small number of studies, 2.5% to 8.5% of HCCs have shown uptake of Eovist on hepatobiliary phase images. The reasons for this are not entirely clear, with reports of increased uptake in well-differentiated tumors (an animal study without confirmation by other authors) and uptake correlated with expression of the OATP1B3 receptor by tumor cells.

If you were to look only at the hepatobiliary phase image from this case, you might be tempted to diagnose FNH since there is diffuse, albeit slightly inhomogeneous, contrast retention, which in many regions is slightly hyperintense relative to adjacent liver. The 1 worrisome feature is the presence of a hypoenhancing pseudocapsule, which is not characteristic of FNH. It is true, however, that the arterial phase image does not look like FNH, showing heterogeneous nonuniform enhancement, and the T2-weighted image is also slightly more heterogeneous than would be expected of FNH.

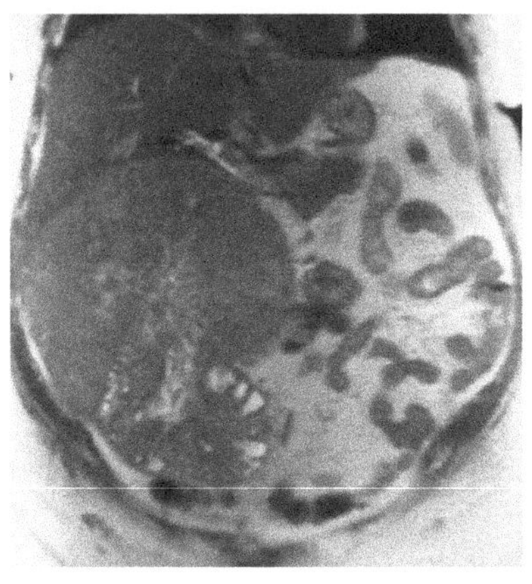

Figure 1.27.1

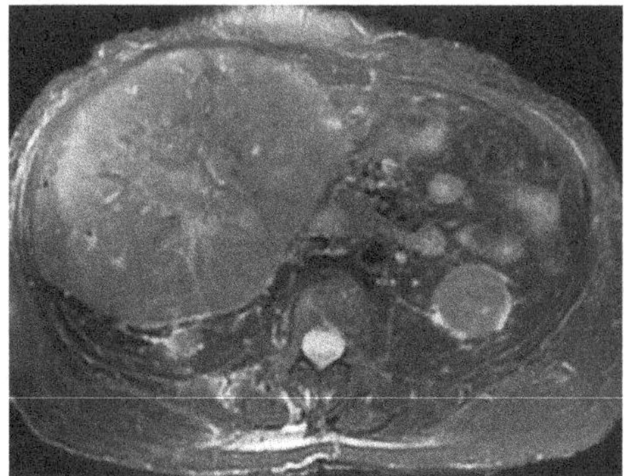

Figure 1.27.2

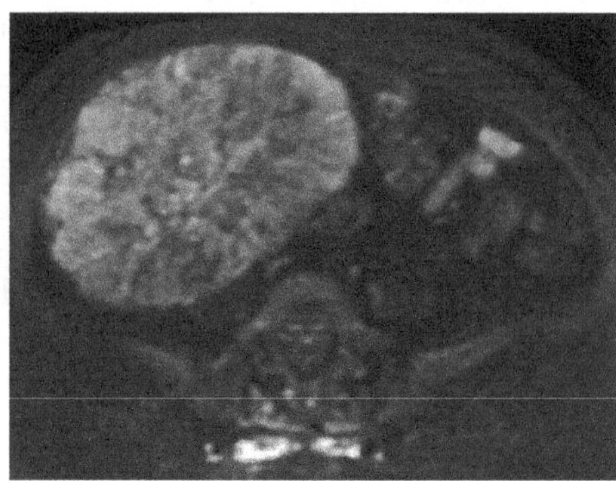

Figure 1.27.3

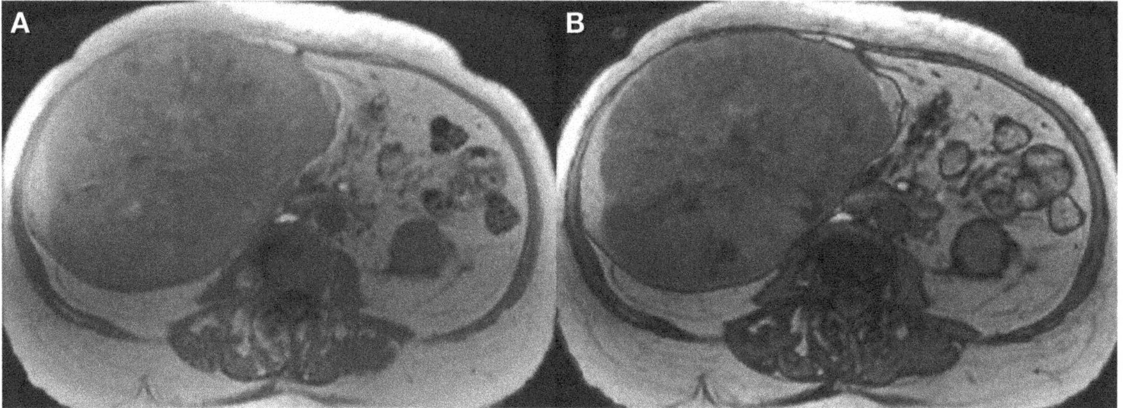

Figure 1.27.4

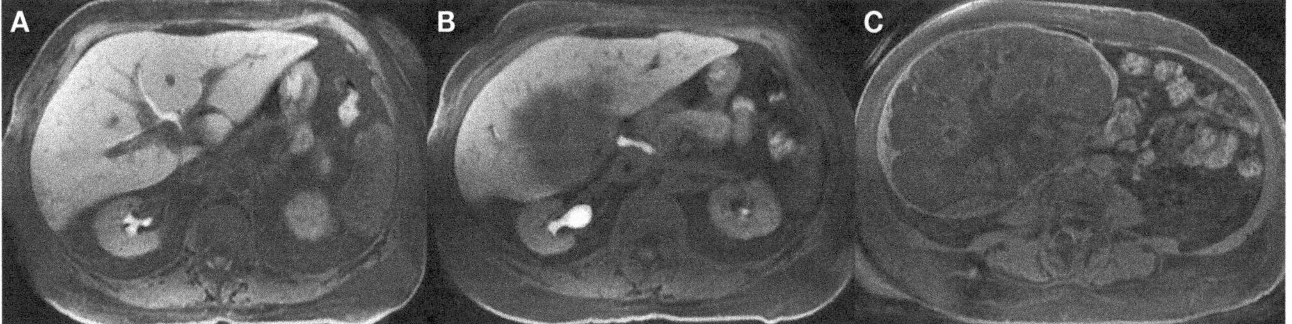

Figure 1.27.5

HISTORY: 75-year-old woman with a history of deep venous thrombosis and pulmonary emboli

IMAGING FINDINGS: Coronal SSFSE (Figure 1.27.1) and axial fat-suppressed FSE T2-weighted (Figure 1.27.2) images reveal a large exophytic mass projecting inferiorly from the right hepatic lobe, with a few scattered foci of mildly increased signal intensity. Axial diffusion-weighted image (b=400 s/mm^2) (Figure 1.27.3) shows heterogeneously increased signal intensity within the mass. Axial IP and OP T1-weighted 2D SPGR images (Figure 1.27.4) demonstrate small regions of signal dropout on the OP image, consistent with intravoxel fat. Axial postgadolinium (Eovist) hepatobiliary phase 3D SPGR images (Figure 1.27.5) obtained 20 minutes after contrast injection demonstrate diffuse hypoenhancement of the mass relative to liver but with a couple of mild hyperenhancing foci in the periphery of the mass. Note also the excretion of contrast into the biliary ducts.

DIAGNOSIS: Hepatocellular carcinoma

COMMENT: This case represents the typical appearance of HCC on hepatobiliary phase images following Eovist or Multihance administration: a hypointense mass without contrast retention, surrounded by uniformly hyperintense liver. Hepatobiliary phase images weren't critical to the diagnosis for this patient; the mass is very large, is too heterogeneous on T2- and diffusion-weighted images to dismiss as benign, and is likely responsible for the patient's venous thrombosis and pulmonary emboli—all indications of an unfortunate conclusion (and a distinction between a solitary metastasis, intrahepatic cholangiocarcinoma, and HCC cannot be made on the basis of its appearance on the hepatobiliary images). On the other hand, this patient was startled by the contrast injection and didn't hold her breath very well for any of the dynamic images (which is why we aren't showing them), but a hepatobiliary contrast agent is forgiving in the sense that multiple second chances are allowed. You can repeat the 3D SPGR acquisition as many times as you want until the patient gets it right, at least in the hepatobiliary phase—an opportunity not provided by the standard extracellular contrast agents.

Another interesting technical feature of this examination was the choice of a b value of 400 s/mm^2 for the diffusion-weighted acquisition. This is somewhat unusual in our practice, where we have settled on b values of 100, 600, and, occasionally, 800 s/mm^2 as our standards for hepatic imaging, but there are surprisingly little data in the literature supporting 1 choice over another. Most DWI experts emphasize the importance of higher b values in overcoming the effects of perfusion and T2 shine-through, in order to achieve true diffusion weighting, but the clinical utility of this approach is uncertain at best. In fact, most of the few studies comparing image quality and lesion detection in the liver over a range of b values have found that low b values (ie, 20-100 s/mm^2) were preferred. Acquisitions with low b values have the virtue of combining the effects of diffusion, perfusion, and T2 weighting, which are often additive and sometimes increase lesion conspicuity. Lower b values (which correspond to smaller diffusion gradients) also have a higher SNR and are less prone to susceptibility artifacts. On the other hand, it is also true that there are many situations in which stronger diffusion weighting (ie, a higher b value) is helpful—for instance, in allowing visualization of discrete lesions within a region of edema or fibrosis or in eliminating signal from adjacent ascites.

Measuring ADC values provides little added benefit in the assessment of hepatic lesions since there is a large overlap between benign and malignant masses. Nearly every solid lesion has restricted diffusion (ie, a lower ADC value) in comparison to normal liver, and so reporting this finding, even though it has become a ubiquitous descriptor in our residents' and fellows' reports, doesn't have any real diagnostic implications. We currently use a respiratory-gated DWI sequence, which allows us to acquire 2 or more b values in the same acquisition and also allows specification of different numbers of signals averaged for different b values—this helps to boost the SNR of higher b-value acquisitions while not wasting time on low b-value acquisitions with adequate SNR.

The original paper describing low b-value hepatic DWI proposed that it could be used in place of standard FSE T2-weighted acquisitions. This is probably true, provided that complete artifact-free coverage of the liver can be obtained. But in our practice, and probably in most others, it has become an addition to the hepatic protocol rather than a replacement, which is a reflection of the general truth that it's much harder to eliminate a pulse sequence from a standard protocol than to add a new one.

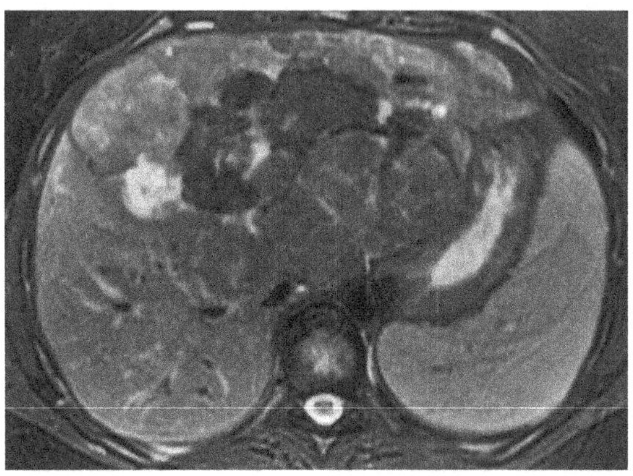

Figure 1.28.1

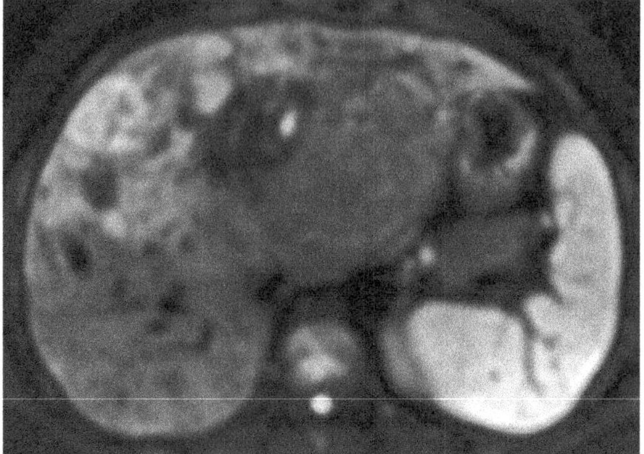

Figure 1.28.2

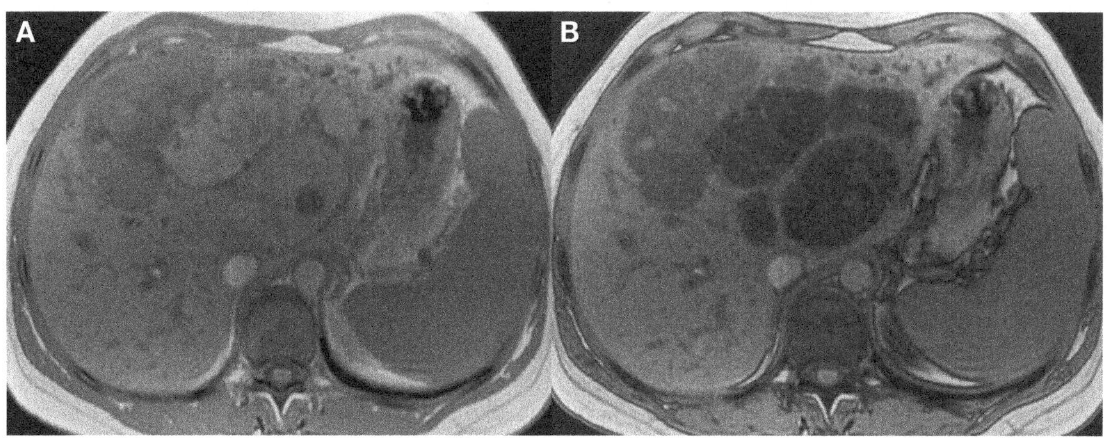

Figure 1.28.3

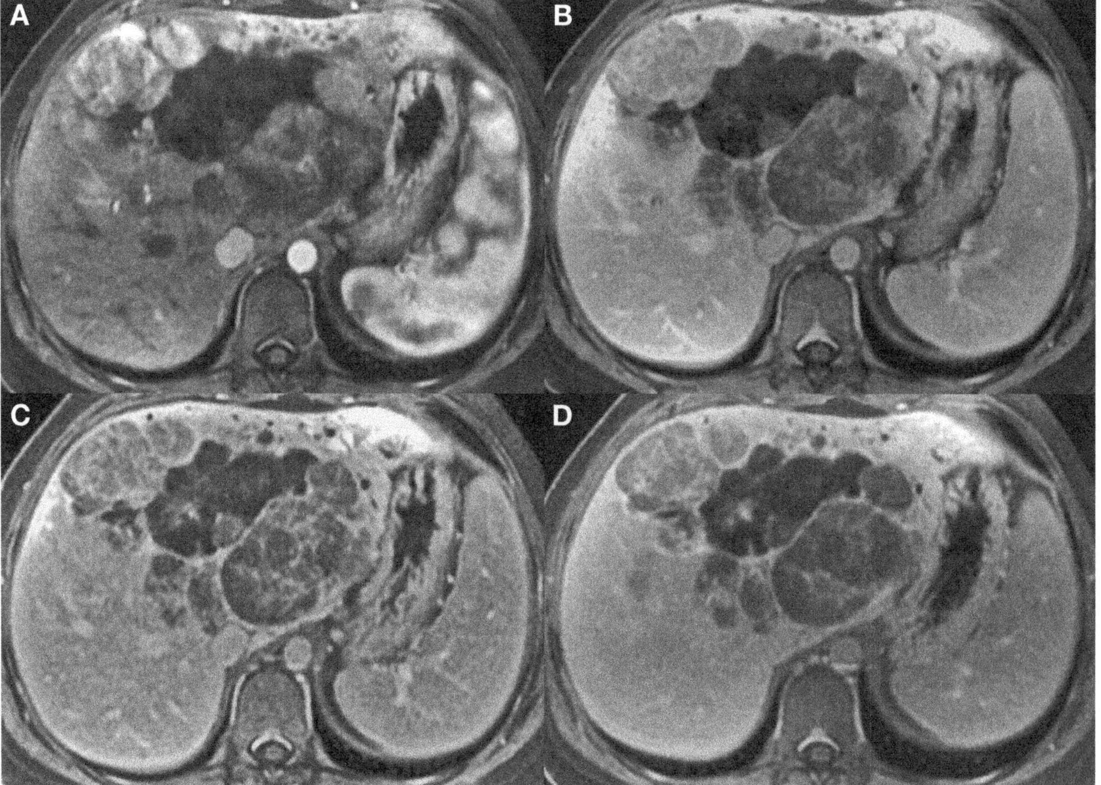

Figure 1.28.4

HISTORY: 20-year-old woman with epigastric pain, episodes of nausea and vomiting, and intermittent diarrhea

IMAGING FINDINGS: Axial fat-suppressed FSE T2-weighted (Figure 1.28.1) and diffusion-weighted (b=600 s/mm^2) (Figure 1.28.2) images reveal a large heterogeneous mass involving the left and anterior right hepatic lobes, with regions of peripheral high signal intensity. Axial IP and OP T1-weighted 2D SPGR images (Figure 1.28.3) show marked signal loss on the OP image, indicating the presence of fat. Axial arterial, portal venous, equilibrium, and 10-minute delayed phase postgadolinium 3D SPGR images (Figure 1.28.4) demonstrate multiple peripheral nodular regions of arterial phase enhancement with washout on portal venous and equilibrium phase images. The central region, corresponding to the fatty component, shows minimal enhancement.

DIAGNOSIS: Moderately differentiated grade 3 (of 4 grades) hepatocellular carcinoma

COMMENT: It is well known that HCCs may contain fat, although we occasionally encounter a resident who is reluctant to make the diagnosis of HCC for this very reason. Several studies have documented fatty change in 15% to 20% of HCCs, with some authors finding a higher incidence in smaller and well-differentiated tumors.

The presence of fat can cause HCCs to appear hyperintense on non–fat-suppressed T1-weighted images; however, high T1-signal intensity may also be attributable to the presence of copper or zinc, protein, or intratumoral hemorrhage. The presence of fat may not be a particularly helpful diagnostic feature since it can be seen in various benign conditions, including focal fatty infiltration, adenomas, angiomyolipomas, and regenerative nodules. However, there are few malignant hepatic lesions that contain fat (excluding rare metastases from liposarcoma and a small number of additional fat-containing primary tumors). In general, it's a good idea to be fairly suspicious of any focal fat-containing lesion in a cirrhotic liver since the baseline probability of HCC is relatively high.

Chemical shift imaging (ie, IP and OP T1-weighted 2D SPGR) is the standard method currently used to assess for the presence of fat (although 2D and 3D Dixon techniques are becoming increasingly popular). Chemical shift imaging relies on the acquisition of images in which the signal from fat and water is either additive (IP images, where the magnetization vectors of fat and water are aligned in the transverse plane) or subtractive (OP images, where the magnetization vectors are oriented in opposing directions). The relative orientation of the fat and water vectors depends on their slightly different precessional (or resonant) frequencies, and the relative contributions of fat and water components within a voxel to the observed signal intensity are dependent on the selected TE.

In this case, the clinical history is not particularly suggestive of HCC, and no evidence of cirrhosis is provided on the images. The main differential diagnosis for a large hepatic mass with prominent fat in a 20-year-old woman would be an adenoma. Features that make this diagnosis less likely include the heterogeneous enhancement pattern; the irregular, lobulated contour of the mass; and the lack of hemorrhage that might be expected in an adenoma of this size.

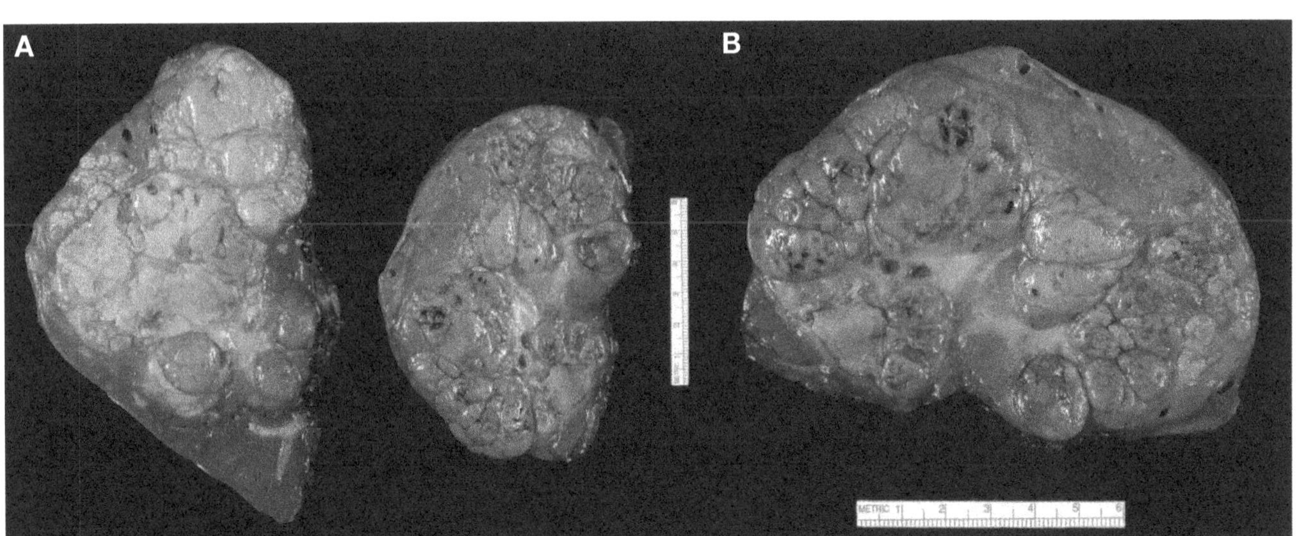

Figure 1.28.5

Gross specimens (Figure 1.28.5) from subsequent extended left hepatectomy (polysegmentectomy I-V and VIII) demonstrate a well-circumscribed heterogeneous, pale tan to red-brown multinodular mass. With a little bit of imagination, one can appreciate the imaging correlation.

CASE 1.29

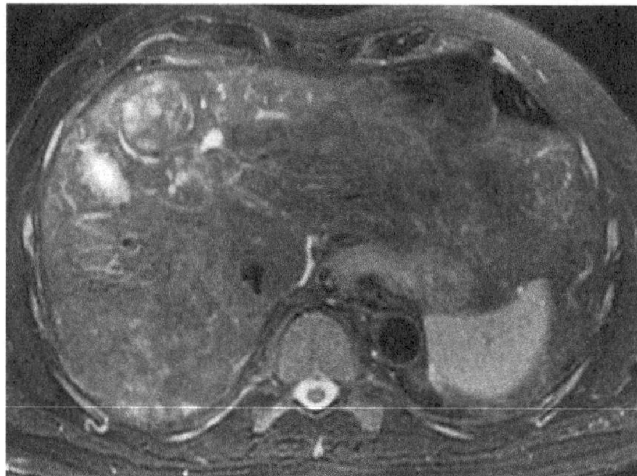

Figure 1.29.1

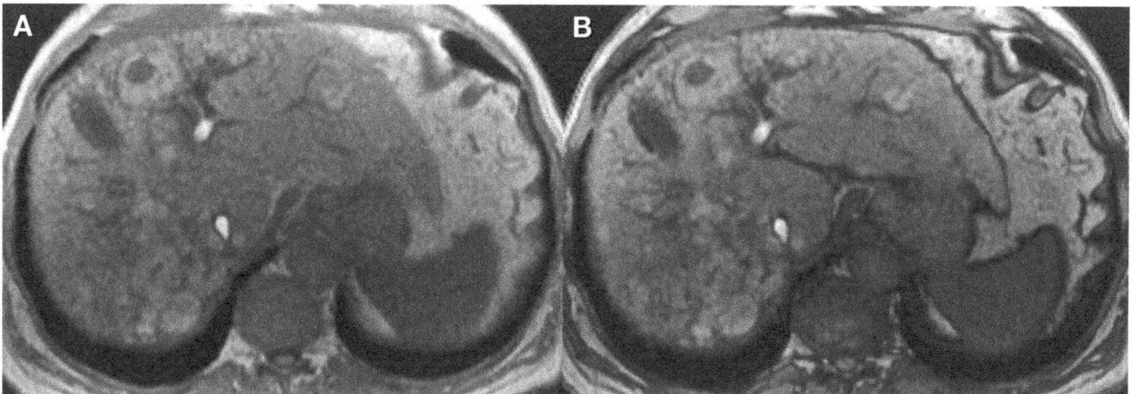

Figure 1.29.2

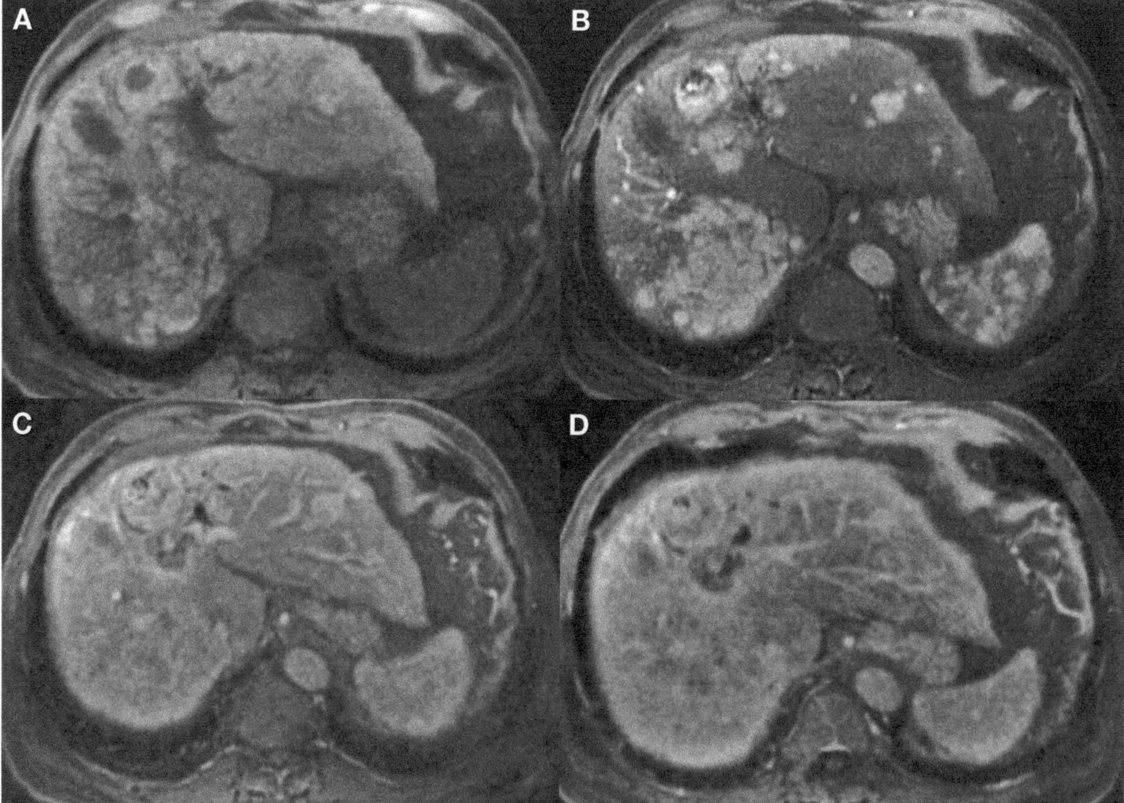

Figure 1.29.3

HISTORY: 72-year-old man with probable alcoholic cirrhosis

IMAGING FINDINGS: Axial fat-suppressed FSE T2-weighted image (Figure 1.29.1) demonstrates a well-circumscribed mass in the medial left hepatic lobe, as well as some subtle, ill-defined, mildly increased signal intensity in the posterior right lobe. Axial IP and OP T1-weighted 2D SPGR images (Figure 1.29.2) reveal that the left lobe nodule is predominantly hyperintense, with a hypointense center. There are additional hyperintense lesions in the left lobe, and the region of subtle, increased T2-signal intensity corresponds to foci of mildly increased T1-signal intensity. The cirrhotic appearance of the liver is probably better appreciated on these images than on the FSE T2-weighted image. Pre- and post-gadolinium arterial, portal venous, and equilibrium phase 3D SPGR images (Figure 1.29.3) show intense enhancement of the left lobe mass, as well as extensive nodular enhancement in both the right and left lobes, with subtle washout visible in several of these regions on portal venous and equilibrium phase images.

DIAGNOSIS: Multifocal hepatocellular carcinoma

COMMENT: This is an advanced case of multifocal HCC, with multiple lesions involving both lobes, and illustrates the general principle that you can often appreciate all of the important findings on the dynamic contrast-enhanced images. In this case, multiple lesions can be seen on the FSE images, but certainly the extent of disease would be grossly underestimated without the arterial phase 3D SPGR acquisition.

There was a brief discussion in the literature several years ago regarding the concept of a limited hepatic examination consisting only of pregadolinium and dynamic post-gadolinium 3D SPGR images. Several authors noted that a clinically significant change in the report was made in only a small percentage of cases by including data from additional precontrast T1- and T2-weighted acquisitions. We suspect that this idea emerged as a consequence of the limited commercial availability of high-quality respiratory-triggered FSE T2-weighted pulse sequences (since then, greatly improved) and the desire to maximize patient throughput. Fortunately, this approach never achieved widespread acceptance; it's not difficult for any abdominal radiologist to recall 1 or more cases within the past day or two in which a patient was unable to hold his breath during 1 or more of the dynamic postgadolinium acquisitions. In addition to the ubiquitous breath-holding problems, there are the occasional mistimed contrast boluses, more frequent in cirrhotic patients, as well as a significant percentage of cases where T1-, T2-, or diffusion-weighted images provide valuable information even when the dynamic contrast-enhanced acquisition is perfect.

Treatment of HCC is based on multiple factors, including the extent of disease, tumor stage, and the patient's performance status. In noncirrhotic patients, resection of a focal mass is the treatment of choice; however, the vast majority of cases occur in patients with cirrhosis. Cirrhosis, particularly in advanced disease, places patients at high risk for perioperative death, and only 5% to 10% of cirrhotic patients are potential surgical candidates. Even with these fairly stringent criteria, the recurrence rate after resection is high, exceeding 70% at 5 years, and thus frequent surveillance imaging is required for these patients. Transplantation is an option for unresectable HCC. Patients with up to 3 lesions, each 3 cm in diameter or smaller, or with a single lesion 5 cm or smaller (the Milan criteria) have a 5-year survival rate of 75%. Patients who are not surgical or transplantation candidates may benefit from localized therapies, including cryoablation, radiofrequency ablation, microwave ablation, and percutaneous ethanol ablation. Treatment options for patients with advanced disease, as in this case, include systemic chemotherapy (Sorafenib), TACE therapy, or radioembolization with Yttrium-90 microspheres.

CASE 1.30

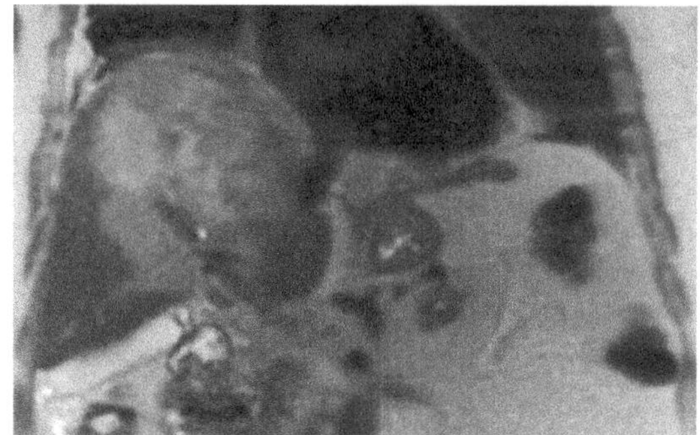

Figure 1.30.1

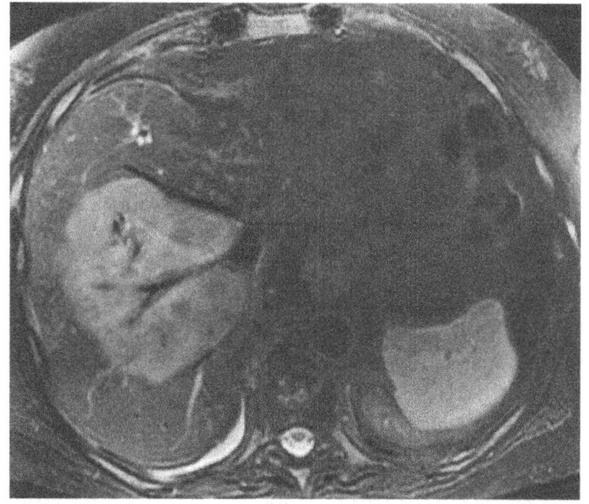

Figure 1.30.2

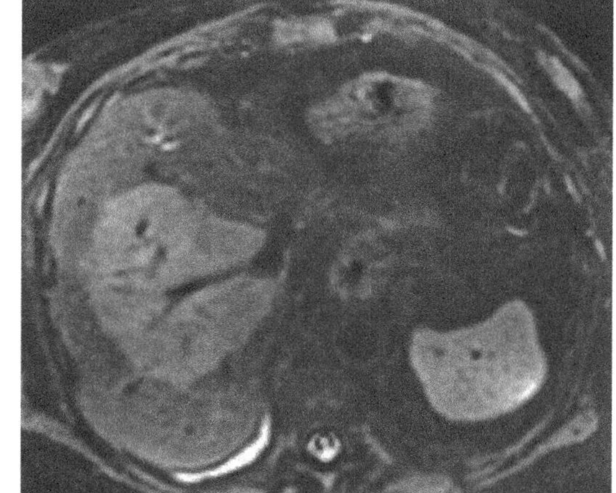

Figure 1.30.3

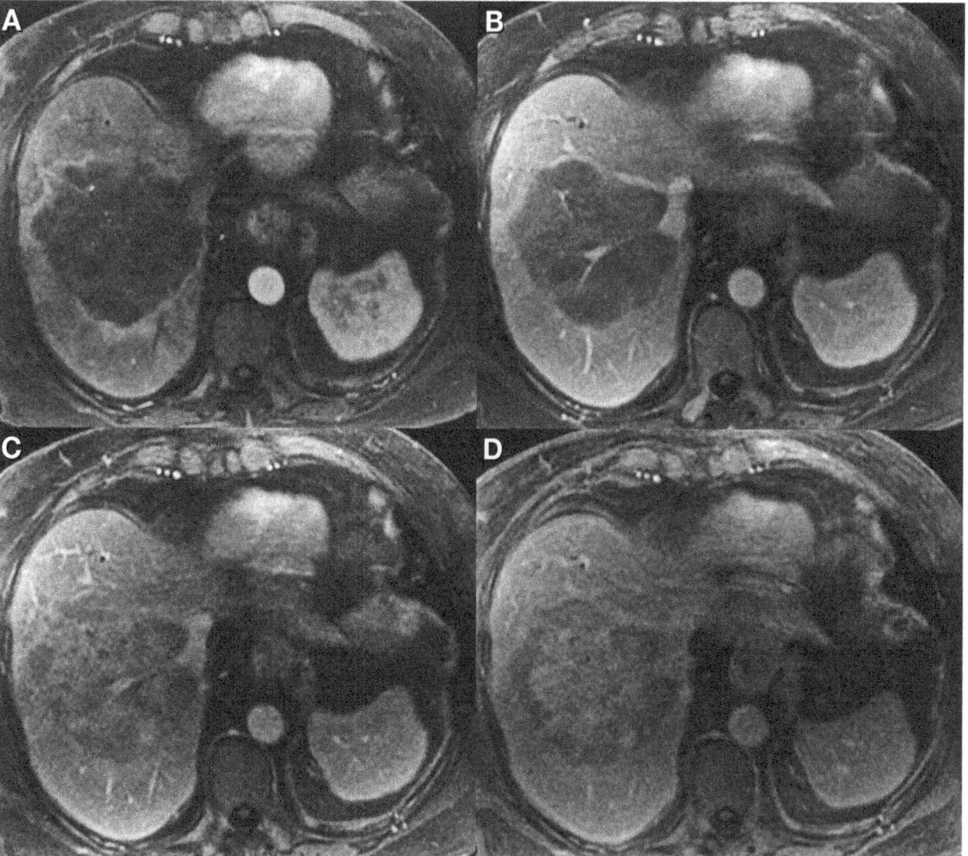

Figure 1.30.4

HISTORY: 82-year-old man with vomiting, jaundice, and abnormal CT

IMAGING FINDINGS: Coronal SSFSE (Figure 1.30.1), axial fat-suppressed T2-weighted FSE (Figure 1.30.2), and axial diffusion-weighted (b=100 s/mm^2) (Figure 1.30.3) images demonstrate a large mass in the central right hepatic lobe surrounding, but not occluding, the right hepatic veins. Axial arterial, portal venous, equilibrium, and delayed phase postgadolinium 3D SPGR images (Figure 1.30.4) demonstrate hypoenhancement of the mass on the arterial phase image with gradual heterogeneous internal enhancement on subsequent phases.

DIAGNOSIS: Diffuse large B-cell lymphoma, primary hepatic involvement

COMMENT: We are all taught that lymphoma can look like anything, and so, fortunately, lymphoma does tend to be in the differential diagnosis for an indeterminate hepatic mass. In this case, the infiltrative nature of the mass with encasement, rather than invasion of the hepatic veins, and the relatively small amount of mass effect for such a large lesion are more suggestive of lymphoma than of other malignant hepatic masses, such as intrahepatic cholangiocarcinoma, HCC, or metastasis. The enhancement characteristics are not typical of HCC or most metastatic lesions but could certainly be seen with intrahepatic cholangiocarcinoma.

Primary hepatic lymphoma (ie, without evidence of extrahepatic disease) is exceedingly rare (0.016% of all non-Hodgkin lymphoma and even less for Hodgkin lymphoma), especially compared with secondary involvement of the liver in both non-Hodgkin (16%-22%) and Hodgkin (6%-20%) lymphoma. In secondary hepatic lymphoma, the lesions are usually diffuse and infiltrative, in which case the only visible sign of hepatic involvement may be hepatomegaly or a diffuse process with nodular (≤1 cm) lesions in about 10% of cases. The few cases of primary hepatic lymphoma reported in the MRI literature generally depict large masses with an appearance similar to the lesion shown in this case.

Biopsy was recommended, and histopathology confirmed diffuse large B-cell lymphoma. Therapeutic guidelines are still under investigation, but chemotherapy is the primary recommendation, with combination surgery and chemotherapy frequently performed. Median survival following diagnosis is 15 to 23 months.

ADC	apparent diffusion coefficient
AFP	α-fetal protein
CA 19-9	carbohydrate antigen 19-9
CEA	carcinoembryonic antigen
CT	computed tomography
DWI	diffusion-weighted imaging
EHE	epithelioid hemangioendothelioma
FNH	focal nodular hyperplasia
FRFSE	fast-recovery fast-spin echo
FSE	fast-spin echo
GP 130	glycoprotein 130
GRE	gradient recalled echo
HCC	hepatocellular carcinoma
HNF-1α	hepatocyte nuclear factor-1α
IP	in-phase
MR	magnetic resonance
MRI	magnetic resonance imaging
OP	out-of-phase
PET	positron emission tomography
SNR	signal to noise ratio
SPGR	spoiled gradient-recalled echo
SPIO	superparamagnetic iron oxide
SSFP	steady-state free precession
SSFSE	single-shot fast-spin echo
TACE	transarterial chemoembolization
TE	echo time
3D	3-dimensional
TR	repetition time
2D	2-dimensional
UES	undifferentiated embryonal sarcoma
US	ultrasonography

2.

LIVER: DIFFUSE DISEASE

CASE 2.1

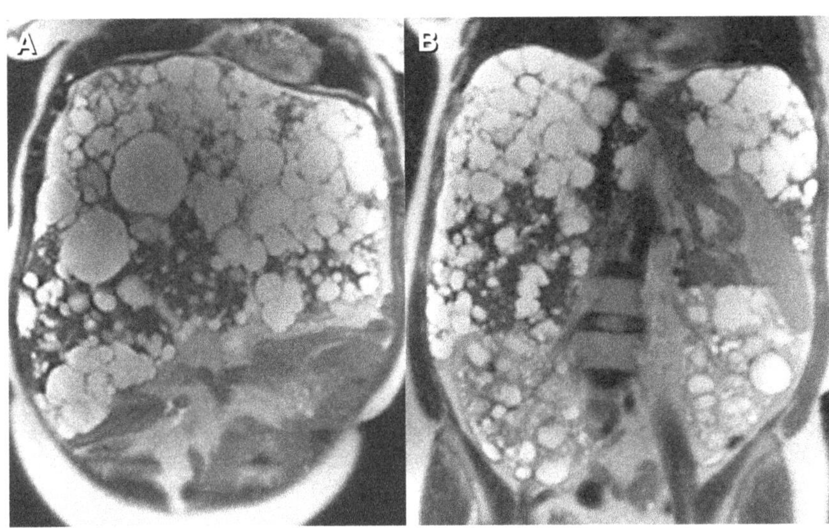

Figure 2.1.1

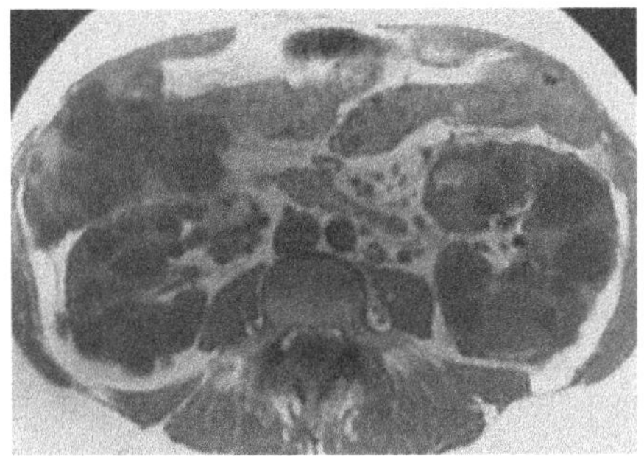

Figure 2.1.2

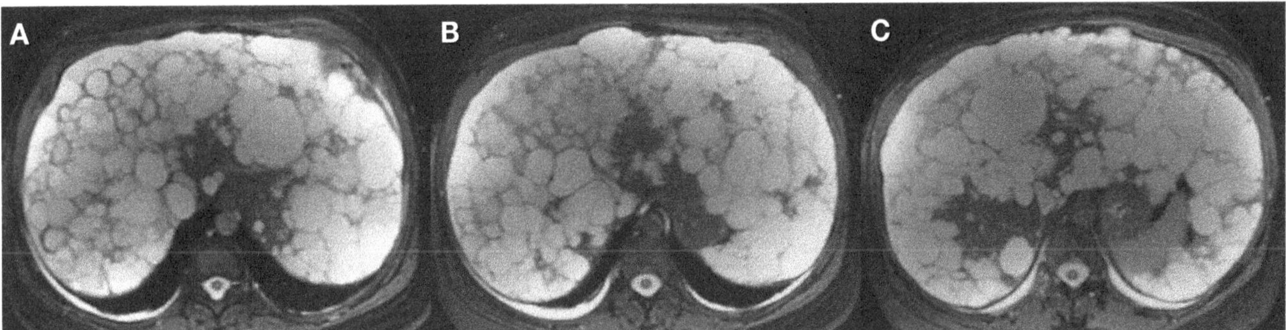

Figure 2.1.3

HISTORY: 47-year-old woman with a genetic disorder

IMAGING FINDINGS: Coronal SSFSE (Figure 2.1.1) and axial T1-weighted FSE (Figure 2.1.2) images demonstrate innumerable variable-sized cysts throughout the liver and kidneys. Some cysts show high T1-signal intensity. Axial fat-saturated 2D SSFP images (Figure 2.1.3) show similar findings and demonstrate patency of the intrahepatic IVC.

DIAGNOSIS: Autosomal dominant polycystic kidney disease

COMMENT: ADPKD is a relatively common hereditary disorder with a prevalence estimated between 1 per 300 to 1 per 1,000 persons. It accounts for approximately 8% to 10% of patients with end-stage renal disease in the United States and Europe. Two separate genetic mutations are responsible for most cases of ADPKD: the *PKD1* gene on chromosome 16 (80%-85%) and the *PKD2* gene on chromosome 4 (15%-20%). Renal function is generally well preserved until the fourth through sixth decades of life, when a rapid decline in renal function occurs; chronic renal failure is present in about 50% of patients by age 60 years. More than 90% of ADPKD patients also have hepatic cysts, although often with less severe hepatic involvement. Unlike in the kidneys, it is uncommon for cystic disease to affect hepatic function. Although renal cysts are virtually always present in ADPKD (hence the name), there are a few reports of patients with isolated hepatic cystic disease.

Although the vast majority of examinations performed on PKD patients at our institution are research studies, occasionally we are asked to scan a patient for an actual clinical indication that generally falls into 1 of 3 categories: screening relatives of patients with known PKD (this is the "Rolls Royce" of screening examinations—US is a lot cheaper but is less aesthetically pleasing); looking for complications of PKD, including hemorrhagic or infected cysts, to explain new onset of pain; and assessing for compression or occlusion of the IVC in patients with abdominal or lower extremity swelling or for compression of biliary ducts in patients with jaundice. The images can also be used as a road map for surgeons interested in resecting dominant or strategically placed cysts in an attempt to relieve symptoms.

Because one of the complications of ADPKD is progressive loss of renal function, MRI scans on ADPKD patients are often performed without intravenous contrast. This presents no real difficulties when looking for a new, large hemorrhagic cyst (high signal intensity on T1-weighted images and low T2-signal intensity in subacute thrombus). Infected cysts are somewhat more problematic, since rim enhancement after gadolinium administration is the classic diagnostic sign, but high signal intensity (ie, restricted diffusion) on diffusion-weighted images with high b values (>600 s/mm^2) can be a useful clue. A high b value is necessary to reduce the amount of T2 shine-through so you can distinguish a simple cyst from an infected one.

Our favorite noncontrast technique for assessing venous patency in the abdomen and pelvis is a 2D fat-suppressed overlapping, thin-section SSFP acquisition, which is fast and highly accurate. This technique is occasionally all that's needed, but in patients with severe disease (unfortunately, most of the patients are in this category), distinguishing cysts with high signal intensity from compressed veins, also with high signal intensity, can be difficult for radiologists and nearly impossible for surgeons. An alternative technique for this situation is a 2D GRE or SPGR sequential acquisition with a superior saturation band. *Sequential acquisition* means that all lines of k-space for a given slice are acquired in succession, which leads to saturation of stationary spins in the slice while blood flowing into the slice remains unsaturated and has higher signal intensity. Addition of a superior saturation band eliminates arterial signal, leaving high signal intensity within the IVC and hepatic veins (Figure 2.1.4). Because this technique works best when the direction of flow is perpendicular to the plane of acquisition, the peripheral hepatic veins are sometimes difficult to image. These acquisitions are generally optimized by using a 20- to 30-degree flip angle, a minimum TE, and a short TR (the TR is, to a certain extent, a method of controlling for the inflow velocity since, as a rule of thumb, you would like the volume of blood within the slice replaced during the TR). We usually start with a TR of 15 msec and increase it if the venous signal is poor—meaning that it is best when the radiologist participates in the optimization.

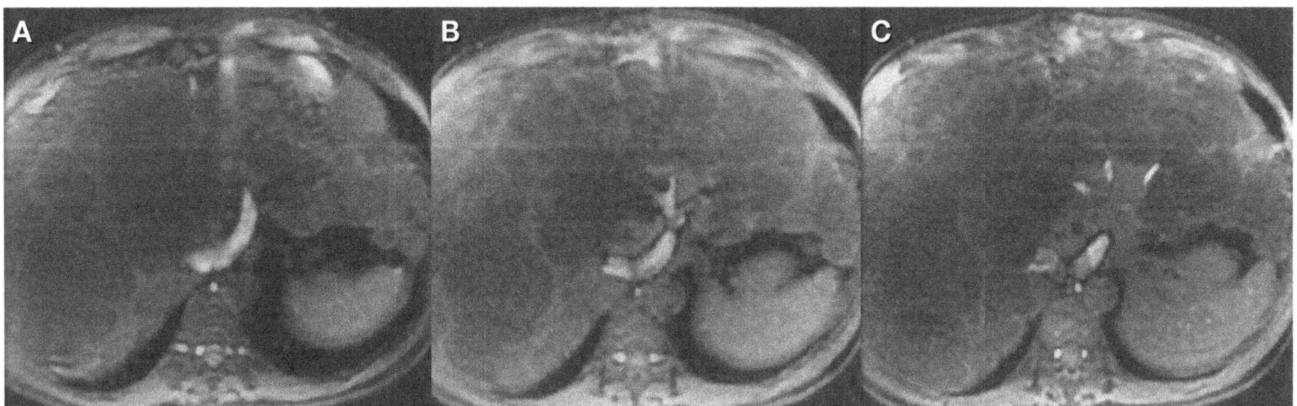

Figure 2.1.4

Axial 2D GRE images (Figure 2.1.4) demonstrate moderate compression of the IVC by adjacent hepatic cysts, but the IVC and the hepatic veins are patent.

SSFSE and SSFP images are generally preferable to respiratory-triggered or navigator-gated FSE images in PKD patients because these are both fast techniques that provide beautiful visualization of cystic lesions. If, however, you are trying to find a solid lesion among the cysts, an FSE acquisition is probably warranted. Remember that livers are often enlarged in patients with severe hepatic cystic disease, and therefore the acquisition times can become quite substantial.

In addition to hepatic cysts, other extrarenal findings associated with ADPKD include asymptomatic pancreatic cysts, cardiac valve disease, colonic diverticula, abdominal wall or inguinal hernias, and cerebral aneurysms.

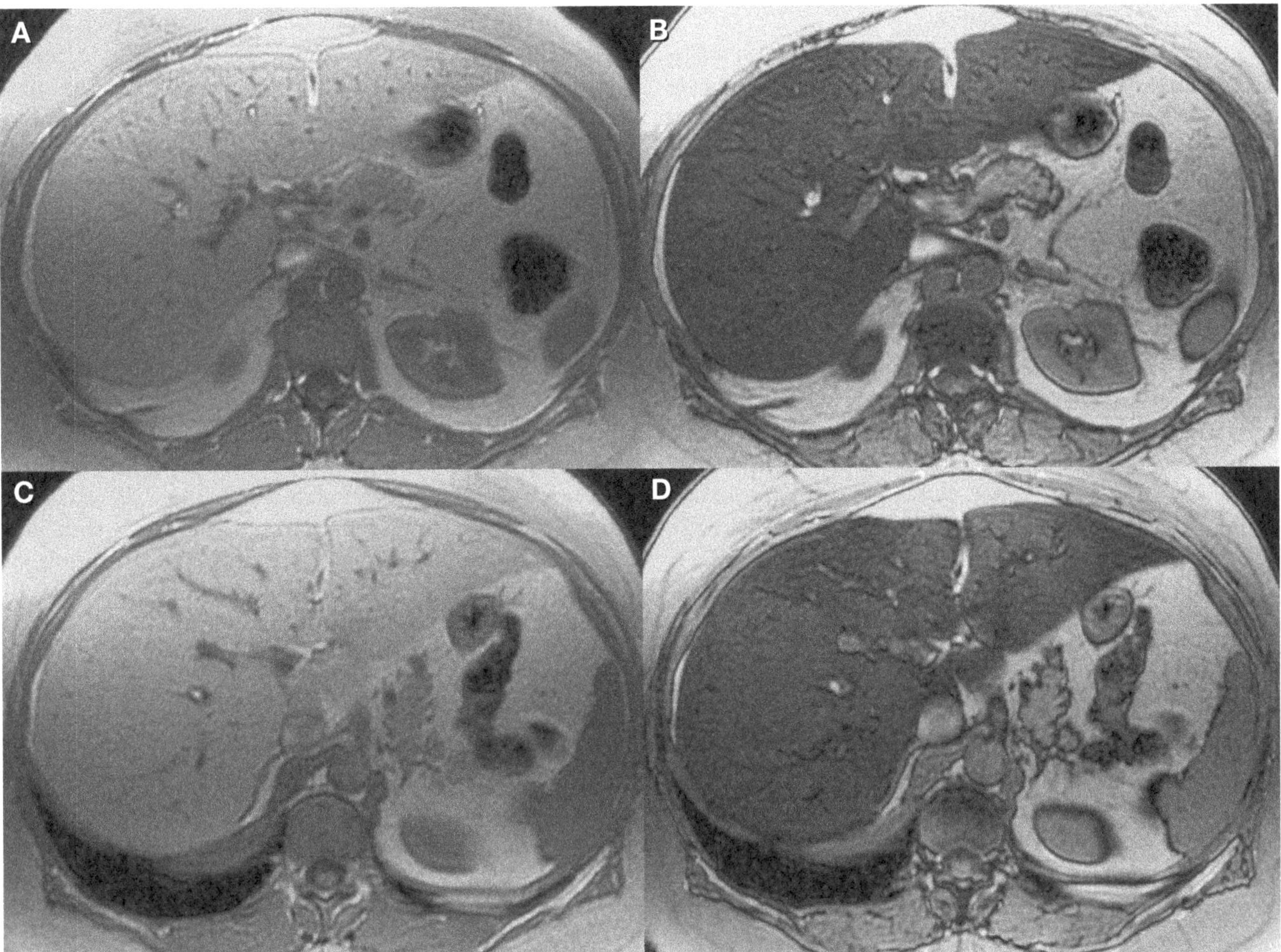

Figure 2.2.1

HISTORY: 52-year-old man with elevated AST and ALT levels

IMAGING FINDINGS: Axial IP and OP T1-weighted 2D SPGR images (Figure 2.2.1) demonstrate diffuse homogeneous signal loss on OP images, consistent with the presence of intravoxel fat.

DIAGNOSIS: Diffuse fatty infiltration of the liver

COMMENT: This case provides a fairly typical example of diffuse fatty infiltration of the liver. *Hepatic steatosis*, *fatty liver*, and *fatty infiltration of the liver* are all terms used interchangeably by most radiologists. Some authors have objected to the term *fatty infiltration* since they believe that the term implies infiltration of fat between hepatocytes rather than accumulation within hepatocytes, but this expression is so widely used that it seems unlikely to disappear.

The most common causes for fatty liver are alcoholic and nonalcoholic liver disease, both of which result in accumulation of triglyceride within hepatocytes. The prevalence of fatty liver in the general population is estimated to be 15%, but it is much more common in patients with obesity (75%), hyperlipidemia (50%), and excess alcohol consumption (45%). In patients with both obesity and excessive alcohol consumption, the prevalence is 95%. Fatty liver associated with nonalcoholic liver disease ranges in increasing severity from steatosis, as described in this discussion, to steatohepatitis, in which the fat causes inflammation and cell injury, and eventually to hepatic fibrosis and cirrhosis, when the inflammation leads to damage and scarring of the liver. With a history of alcohol consumption, there is a similar progression from steatosis, which is reversible, to alcoholic hepatitis, and finally to cirrhosis. Alcohol alone is not sufficient to initiate alcoholic liver disease, and several additional factors, including genetic predisposition as well as multiple environmental stimuli, have a large role. It is probably true, however, that the incidence of alcoholic cirrhosis increases with increasing alcohol intake. Alcoholic hepatitis has considerable variability in its presentation, but the 30-day mortality rate remains 0% to 50%.

The Model for End-Stage Liver Disease (or MELD) score, which originally was the Mayo End-Stage Liver Disease score, is used to estimate the severity of chronic liver disease. A higher score indicates an increasing risk of death and also may cause the patient to move higher up on the transplantation list. The gold standard for determining the severity of hepatic fibrosis in the clinical setting of fatty infiltration is histologic evaluation through liver biopsy, although there is increasing acceptance of the use of MR elastography.

Visualization of hepatic steatosis with MRI relies on inherent differences in the microscopic environment of water protons and fat protons, which in turn leads to small differences in their resonant frequencies. This difference is termed *chemical shift* and reminds us of the spectroscopic origins of MRI, where water and fat peaks are separated by 3.5 ppm on the frequency spectrum. The chemical shift is directly proportional to field strength, so a chemical shift of 3.5 ppm translates to differences of about 220 Hz at 1.5 T and about 440 Hz at 3 T for water and fat protons.

At 1.5 T, fat protons precess about 220 Hz more slowly than water protons (fat is to the right of water on the spectrum), and if we use a double-echo GRE technique, we can set the TEs to coincide with times when fat and water are out of phase (eg, 2.2 msec, 6.7 msec, 11.2 msec) and in phase (eg, 4.5 msec, 9.0 msec, 13.4 msec). A standard IP and OP pulse sequence should be set up by the vendor so that the OP TE is shorter than the IP TE; this ensures that signal dropout from an IP image to an OP image is truly the result of fatty infiltration and not dependent on T2* relaxation. This almost always happens at 1.5 T; however, at 3 T, the first OP TE is fairly short and is technically challenging to obtain, and so some vendors (including ours) switched the order of the IP and OP TEs (apparently hoping that no one would notice). To be fair, it is true that T2* relaxation effects are stronger at 3 T, and therefore using the first IP TE and the second OP TE also has some inherent disadvantages. The solution most vendors have arrived at is to use a Dixon-based technique, where the IP and OP images can be reconstructed from data obtained at different TEs.

There is fairly extensive literature discussing MR methods for quantifying hepatic steatosis. Spectroscopy is probably considered the gold standard, although it is one of the least frequently used, since it's relatively unfamiliar to most abdominal imagers and generally acquires only single voxels (and therefore is prone to sampling error in patients with heterogeneous fatty infiltration). A simple method, and one with excellent reported results, involves an estimation of the fat fraction (FF) from IP and OP images. The FF is defined as follows:

$$FF = (S_{IP} - S_{OP})/2S_{IP}$$

where S_{IP} is the signal from the IP acquisition and S_{OP} is the signal from the OP acquisition. The caveat is that this estimate does not take into consideration T1, T2, or T2* relaxation effects, which are problematic mainly in patients with iron overload (ie, those with hemochromatosis, hemosiderosis, or cirrhosis with siderotic nodules). A multiecho Dixon technique (IDEAL) is less widely available but allows simultaneous estimation of hepatic fat and iron content while accounting for the effects of each substance on measurement of the other.

Diffuse hepatic steatosis is not a diagnostic dilemma, nor is focal fatty infiltration when it occurs in one or more well-known locations, including the porta hepatis and gallbladder fossa and adjacent to the falciform ligament or ligamentum venosum. More challenging are cases with focal nodular or masslike fatty infiltration, and examples of these are illustrated in Cases 2.3, 2.4, and 2.5.

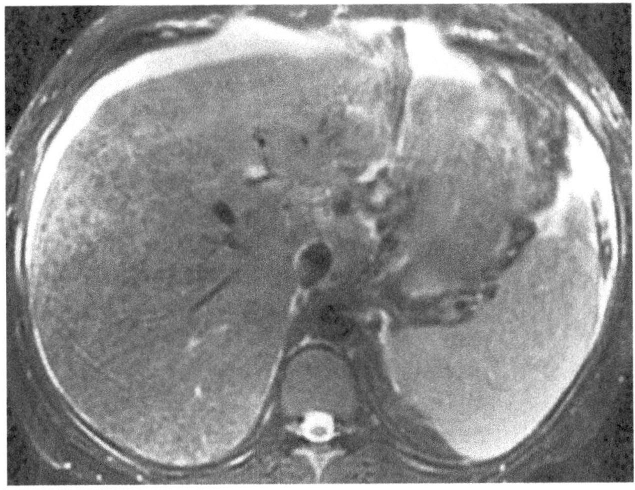

Figure 2.3.1

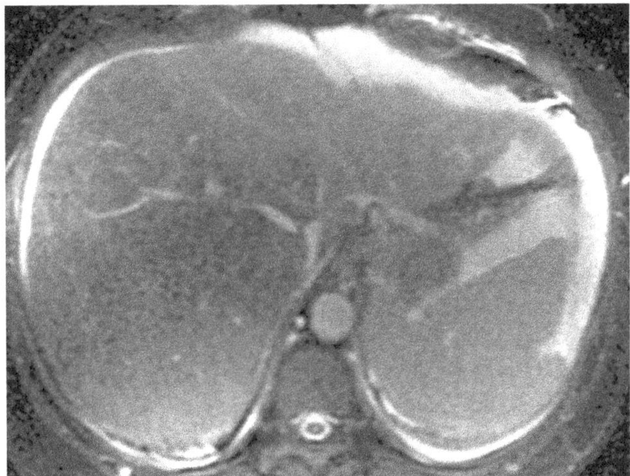

Figure 2.3.2

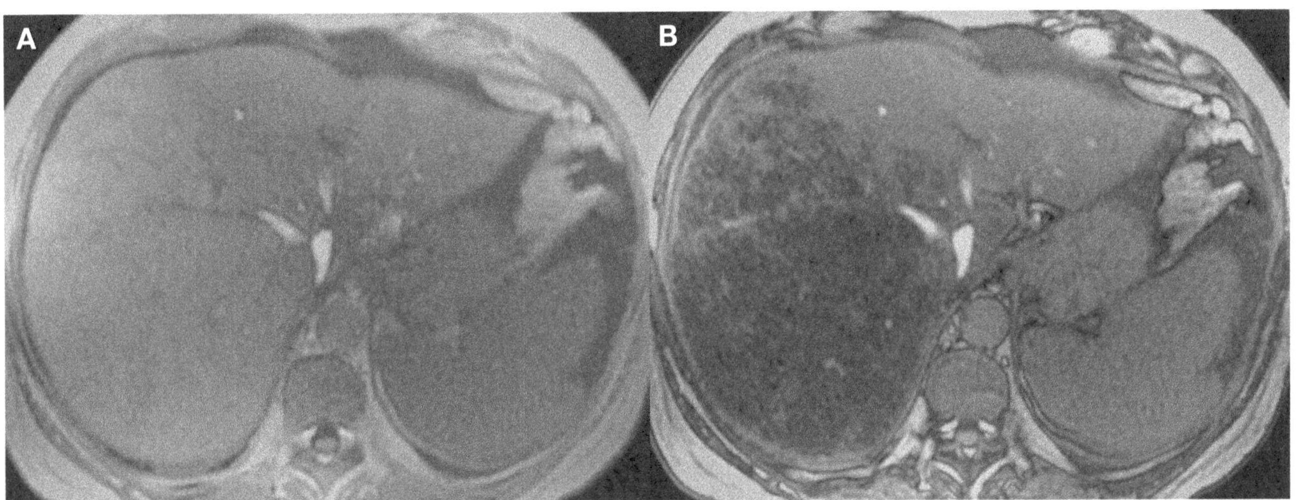

Figure 2.3.3

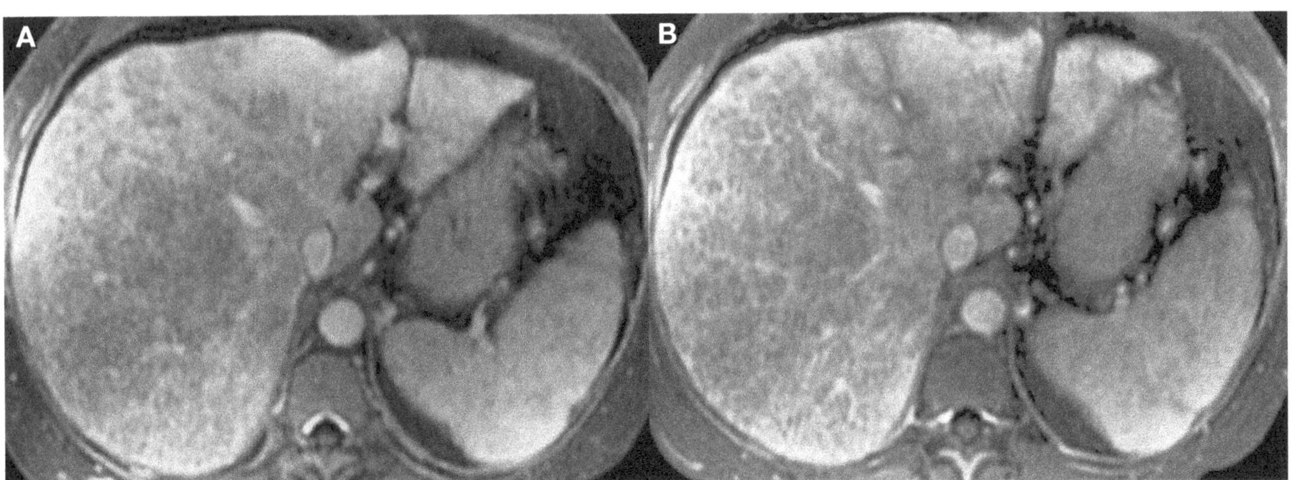

Figure 2.3.4

HISTORY: 42-year-old woman with alcoholic liver disease with new pain, weight loss, and elevated liver function levels; abdominal CT showed a suspicious hepatic mass

IMAGING FINDINGS: Axial fat-suppressed T2-weighted FSE (Figure 2.3.1) and fat-suppressed 2D SSFP (Figure 2.3.2) images demonstrate a nodular hepatic contour and underlying nodularity of the hepatic parenchyma with signal intensity slightly lower in the right hepatic lobe, as well as ascites. Axial T1-weighted IP and OP 2D SPGR images (Figure 2.3.3) show diffuse enlargement of the right hepatic lobe with signal loss on OP images consistent with the presence of fat and relative sparing of the left hepatic lobe. Note also the nodular contour and moderate atrophy of the left lobe. Axial portal venous phase postgadolinium 3D SPGR images (Figure 2.3.4) reveal abnormal enhancement of both right and left hepatic lobes, with persistent heterogeneous enhancement throughout the right lobe. Notice mild distortion of patent hepatic veins in the right lobe.

DIAGNOSIS: Cirrhotic liver with fatty infiltration of the right hepatic lobe

COMMENT: Diagnosis of diffuse steatosis in an otherwise normal liver requires little thought or effort (other than the few seconds needed to assure yourself that you have detected the presence of fat and not iron). Heterogeneous or uncommon distributions of fat can be more problematic, and this is compounded in the cirrhotic liver, where regenerative nodules and HCCs not uncommonly contain fat. This case shows striking asymmetry in the appearance of the right and left hepatic lobes and, given the underlying cirrhosis, should raise some concern for the presence of an infiltrative HCC. Factors mitigating against this include the absence of a discrete mass, as well as the relatively well-preserved course of the hepatic veins through the area in question without obvious mass effect. The absence of tumor thrombus in the hepatic and portal veins is also helpful. Tumor thrombus used to be considered an absolute requirement in patients with infiltrative HCC; however, it is now recognized as a common, but not universal, finding.

This case was read as regional steatosis in a cirrhotic liver, and the patient did undergo biopsy, which revealed moderately active steatohepatitis with advanced septal fibrosis and regenerative nodules. There was no evidence of neoplasm.

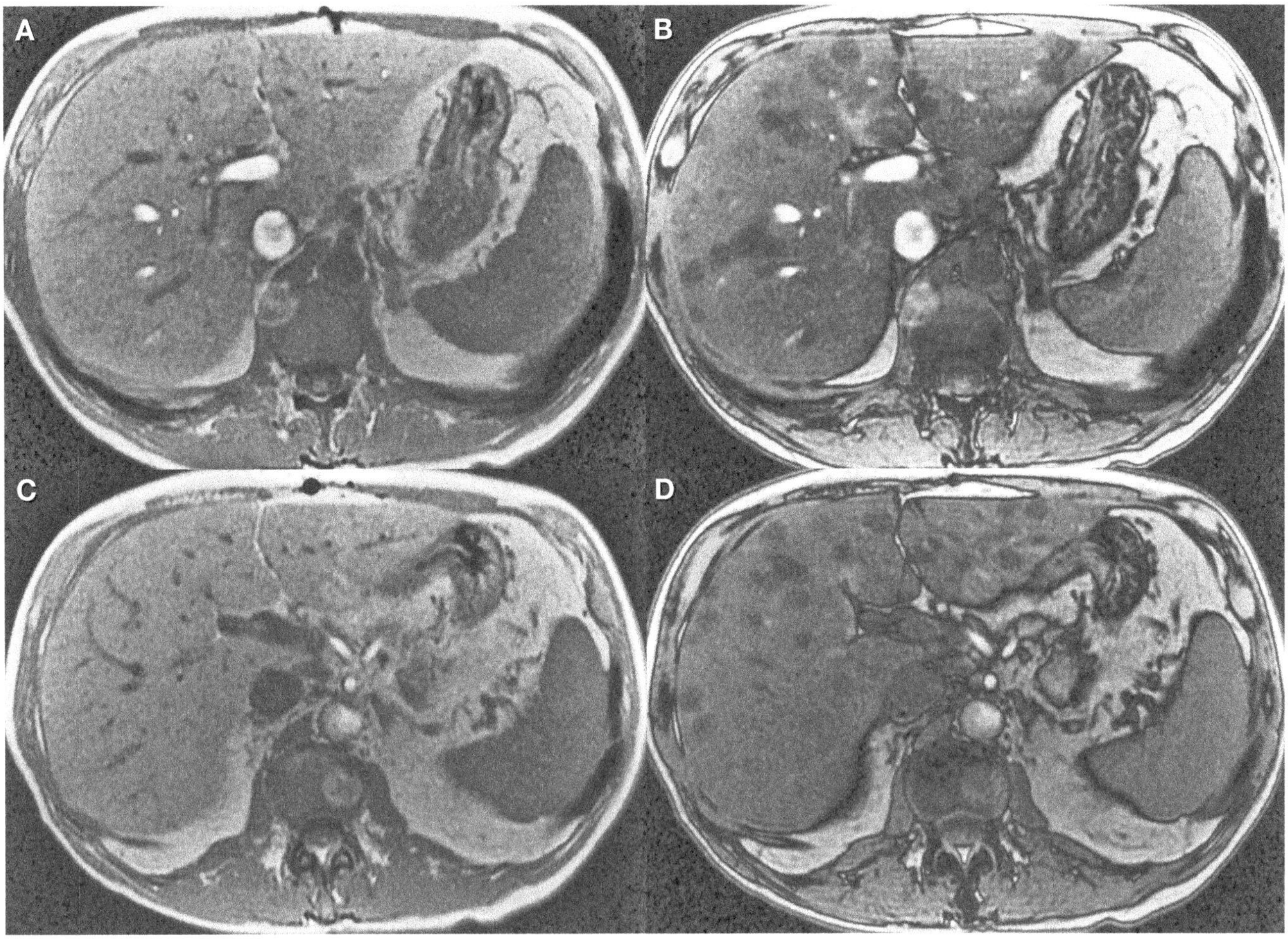

Figure 2.4.1

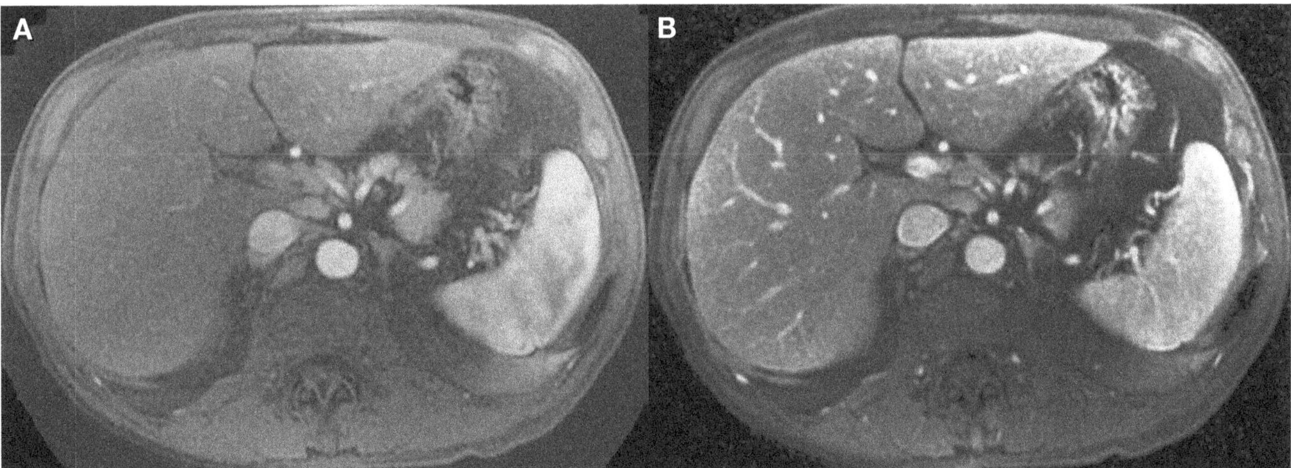

Figure 2.4.2

HISTORY: 58-year-old man with a family history of colon cancer; noncontrast enhanced chest CT showed low-attenuation hepatic masses in the visualized liver

IMAGING FINDINGS: Axial T1-weighted IP and OP 2D SPGR images (Figure 2.4.1) demonstrate multiple low-signal-intensity nodules throughout the liver, visible only on the OP images. These nodules are not apparent on axial arterial and portal venous phase, postgadolinium 3D SPGR images (Figure 2.4.2).

DIAGNOSIS: Nodular focal fatty infiltration

COMMENT: The nodular appearance of the fatty infiltration in this example is striking, and it can be disconcerting for residents, fellows, and young staff radiologists who haven't encountered it before. The key to a confident diagnosis is the absence of any associated abnormalities on T2- or diffusion-weighted images and no abnormal enhancement following gadolinium administration.

This case is an ideal example in that the T2-weighted and dynamic postgadolinium images were uniformly negative, leaving little doubt about the diagnosis. Unfortunately, this doesn't always happen, particularly when the fatty infiltration is associated with steatohepatitis, in which case the arterial phase images can be fairly heterogeneous. It is also worth noting that the question of washout becomes somewhat subjective with fatty lesions—nodular fatty infiltration will be mildly hypointense relative to normal liver on precontrast 3D SPGR images and may or may not be visible. Depending on the lesion size and amount of internal fat, as well as the intensity of the contrast bolus, the nodules may not be perceptible during peak enhancement of the liver (typically, the portal venous phase) but may become faintly visible during the equilibrium phase.

The differential diagnosis for multiple fatty hepatic nodules includes multiple adenomas and multifocal HCC, but both of these lesions should be readily apparent on either T2-weighted or postgadolinium images, or both. Focal fatty deposition may also occasionally occur in regenerative nodules; in this case, the distinction between this entity and nodular focal fatty infiltration may not be possible when the liver is not overtly cirrhotic.

Although the MRI report left no room for doubt, the patient had a strong family history of colon and gastric cancer and neither he nor his primary physician were entirely convinced that the lesions were benign. He eventually had one of them biopsied, with pathology revealing steatosis.

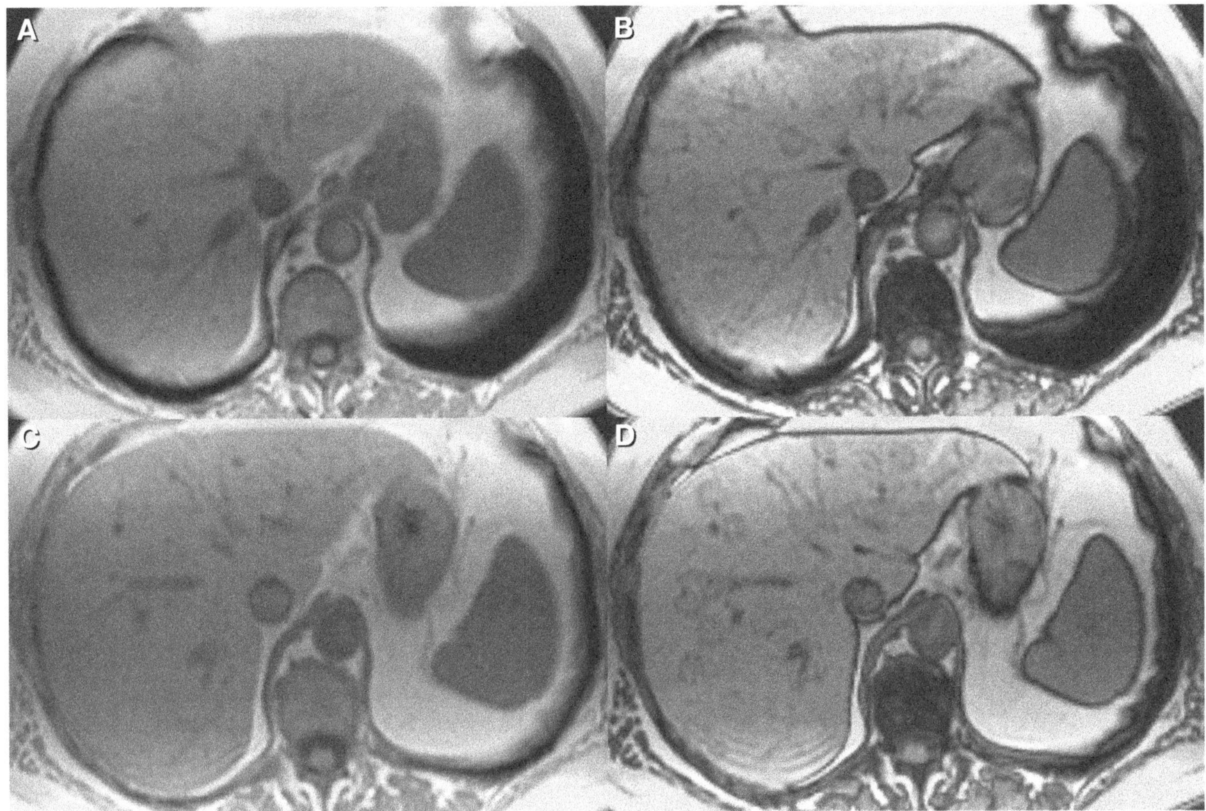

Figure 2.5.1

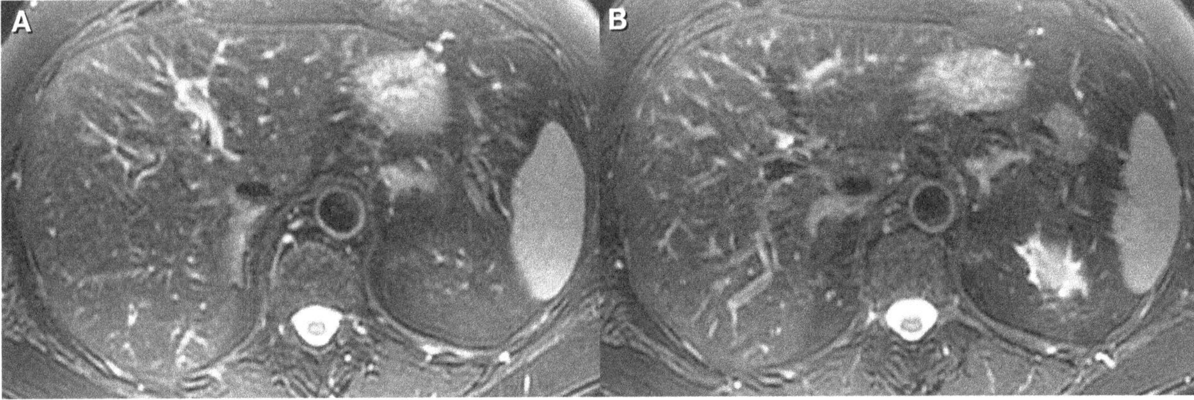

Figure 2.5.2

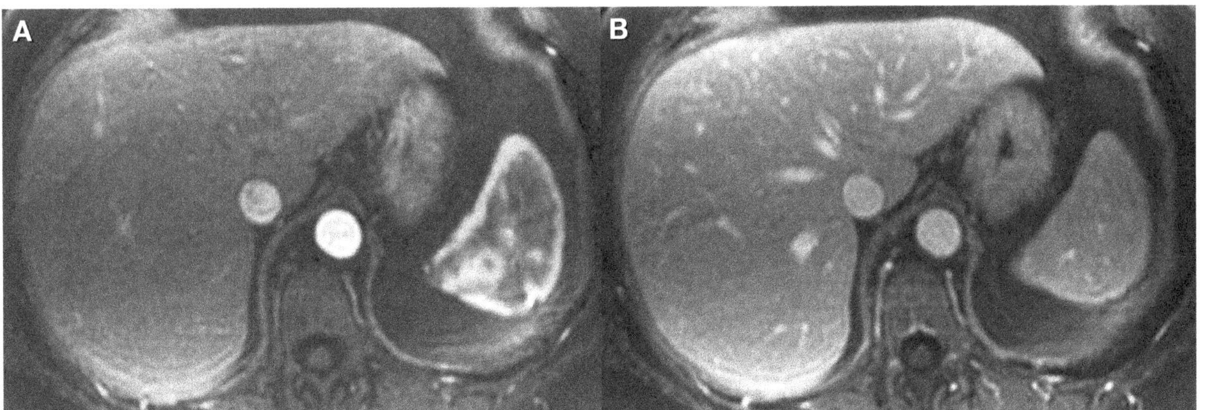

Figure 2.5.3

HISTORY: 69-year-old woman with irritable bowel syndrome and new low back pain; CT showed multiple hepatic lesions suspicious for metastases

IMAGING FINDINGS: Axial T1-weighted IP and OP 2D SPGR images (Figure 2.5.1) demonstrate multiple rounded masses, with peripheral halos of signal dropout seen on only the OP images. Axial fat-suppressed, T2-weighted images (Figure 2.5.2) demonstrate no corresponding abnormalities, and arterial and portal venous phase postgadolinium 3D SPGR images (Figure 2.5.3) are also unremarkable.

DIAGNOSIS: Nodular focal fatty infiltration

COMMENT: This case is another example of an unusual form of fatty infiltration that is also nodular, but with fatty sparing at the center of the lesion and a peripheral halo of fat.

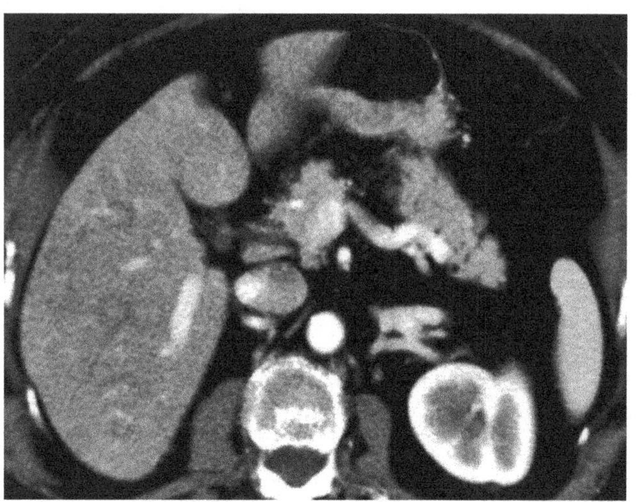

Figure 2.5.4

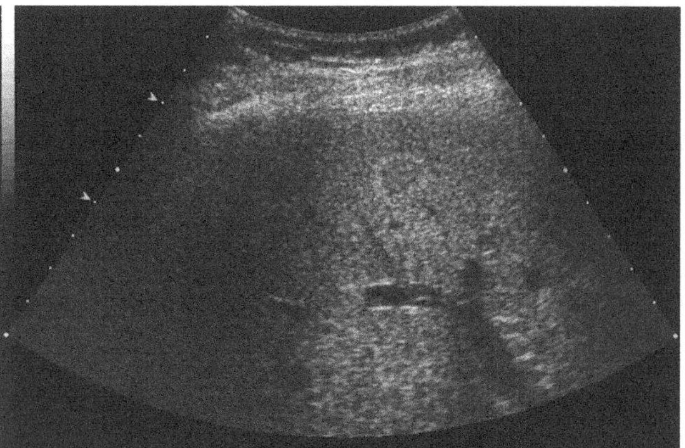

Figure 2.5.5

One of the more challenging aspects of the radiologist's job is making an unexpected diagnosis (particularly one that contradicts a colleague). The CT scan was read as consistent with hepatic metastases (Figure 2.5.4) and a US-guided biopsy (Figure 2.5.5) was negative for malignancy. At the time, this radiologic-pathologic discordance was attributed to sampling error; however, instead of repeating the biopsy, an MRI was performed to better characterize the lesions.

Fatty infiltration is occasionally perivascular in nature, and may appear as halos or tracks (depending on the imaging plane) of fat surrounding the hepatic veins or portal veins, or both. As noted in Case 2.4, a confident diagnosis of nodular focal fatty infiltration rests on the absence of corresponding abnormalities on T2- and diffusion-weighted images in conjunction with unremarkable dynamic postgadolinium images. There are, of course, fat-containing tumors, such as hepatic adenomas and HCCs, that demonstrate imaging features suggestive of a mass. Perilesional fatty infiltration (ie, a halo of fat) has been described in a few case reports as occurring in patients with metastatic insulinoma. This pattern is presumably related to local effects of insulin, but neuroendocrine metastases typically show high signal intensity on T2- and diffusion-weighted images.

In this case, the MRI report listed nodular focal fatty infiltration as the top differential diagnosis but said that neoplasm could not be excluded. This led to a second biopsy, which again demonstrated benign hepatic parenchyma with fatty change. Two years after this examination, a follow-up CT demonstrated radiographic resolution of the multiple liver masses after mild weight loss.

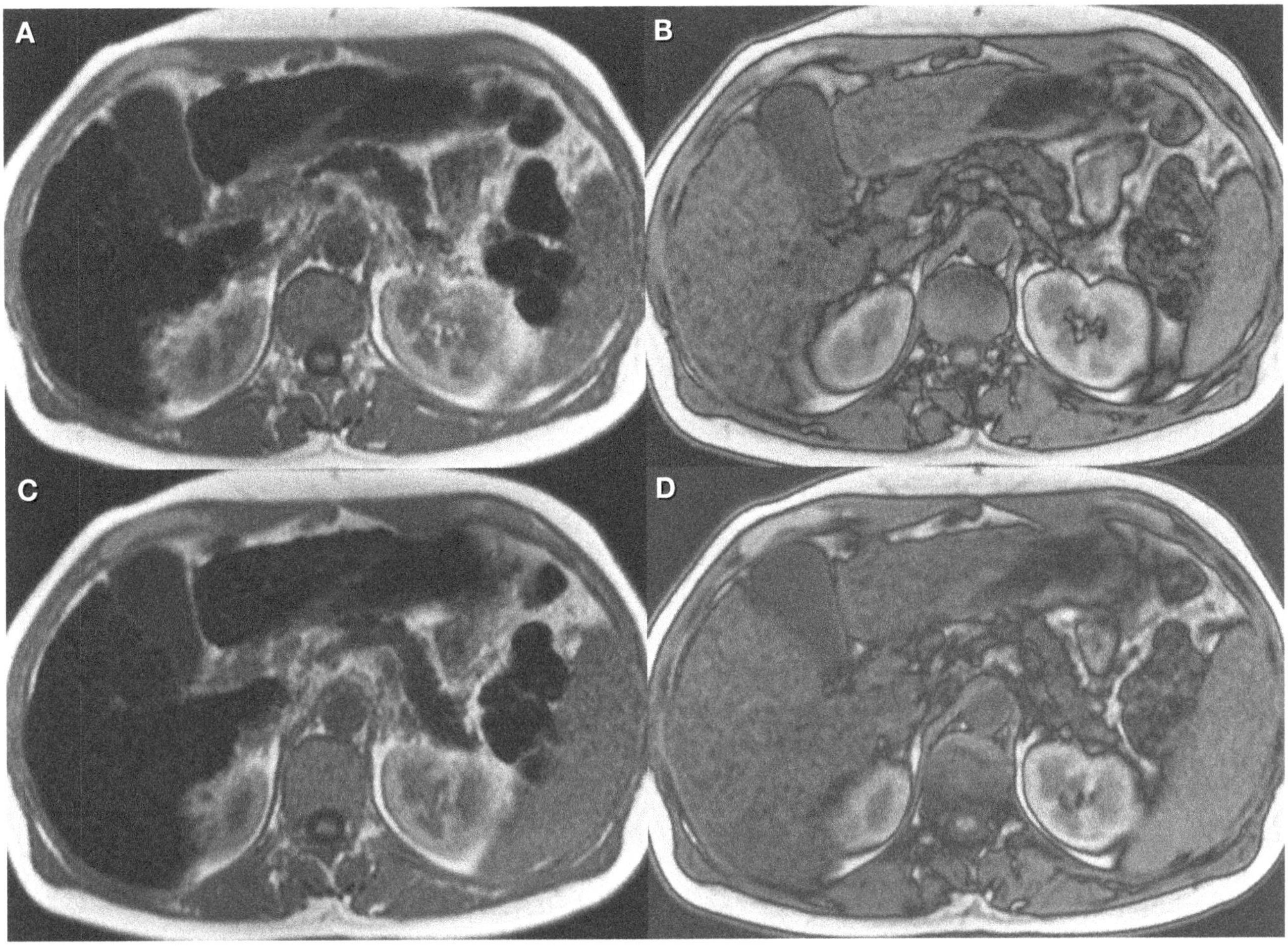

Figure 2.6.1

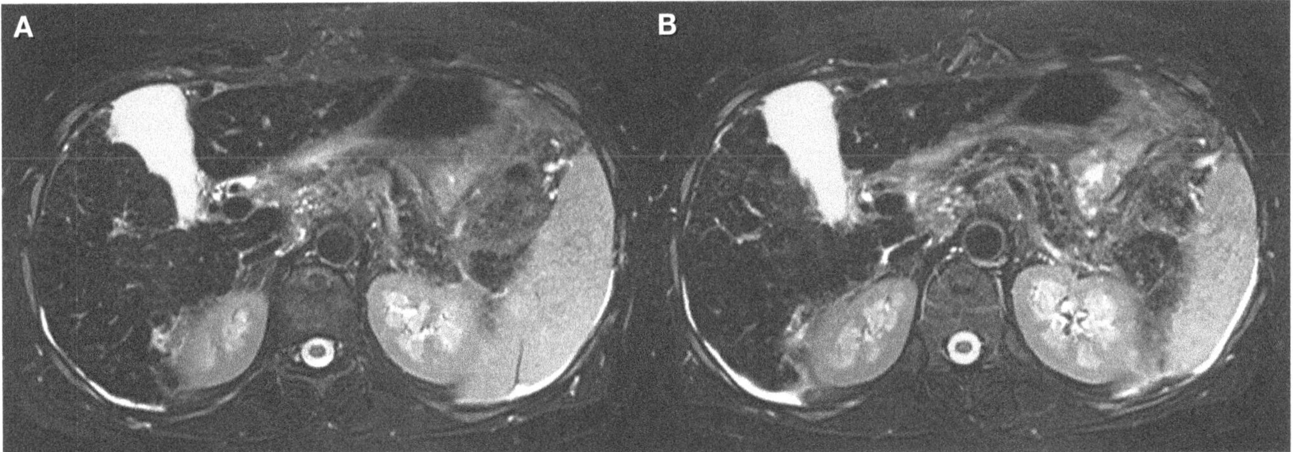

Figure 2.6.2

HISTORY: 52-year-old man with cirrhosis associated with chronic hepatitis C

IMAGING FINDINGS: Axial T1-weighted IP and OP 2D SPGR images (Figure 2.6.1) demonstrate markedly decreased signal throughout the liver and pancreas compared with paraspinal muscle on the IP images. Note also the diffuse parenchymal nodularity of the liver and prominent recanalized paraumbical veins. Axial fat-suppressed T2-weighted FSE images (Figure 2.6.2) also show diffuse low signal intensity throughout the liver and pancreas.

DIAGNOSIS: Hemochromatosis (primary)

COMMENT: Although the term *hemochromatosis* was previously reserved for the primary genetic form of excessive iron deposition in organs, the definition has been broadened to include secondary mechanisms, including multiple blood transfusions or chronic disease. The distinction between *hemosiderosis* and *hemochromatosis* is therefore more confusing than ever. *Hemosiderosis* refers specifically to deposition of hemosiderin in tissues associated with damaged red blood cells and occurring in patients with hemolytic anemias or recipients of multiple blood transfusions and represents a subcategory of secondary hemochromatosis. Primary hemochromatosis is a relatively common genetic disease in the white population (up to 10% for heterozygous disease), and because of its latent clinical manifestations, the incidental finding of iron overload on abdominal MRI is not infrequently the first indicator of disease.

In general, primary or genetic hemochromatosis manifests as decreased signal intensity in the liver and pancreas with sparing of the spleen and bone marrow. Secondary or acquired hemochromatosis (hemosiderosis) results in decreased signal intensity in the liver, spleen, and bone marrow (ie, organs containing cells of the reticuloendothelial system); the pancreas is usually spared unless the blood volume surpasses the iron storage capacity of the reticuloendothelial system. Renal cortical iron deposition with decreased signal in the renal cortices can occur in intravascular hemolysis (eg, from mechanical heart valves), paroxysmal nocturnal hemoglobinuria, or hemolytic sickle cell crises. Different combinations of these patterns can also be seen—for example, in a patient with chronic anemia and findings of primary hemochromatosis (decreased signal intensity in the liver and pancreas) who has received multiple blood transfusions and now has hemosiderosis with additional decreased signal intensity in the spleen and bone marrow.

The criteria for what constitutes reduced signal intensity within an organ are somewhat nebulous. Paraspinous muscle is the favorite internal reference in the literature, although in reality, most radiologists probably don't make this explicit comparison. Instead, they notice that 1 or more organs appear darker than normal or that the usual pattern of relative signal intensity (spleen > kidney > liver and pancreas on fat-suppressed T2-weighted FSE images, for example) is disrupted.

MRI signal loss in iron deposition diseases is explained by the high magnetic susceptibility of iron, which causes local magnetic field inhomogeneities that shorten T1, T2, and T2* relaxation times. T2* effects are generally predominant, meaning that GRE pulse sequences using a relatively longer TE will accentuate the signal drop caused by the susceptibility effects of iron. This is the basis for the common observation of signal dropout from OP to IP images on a T1-weighted dual echo SPGR acquisition; the small difference in TEs (2.2 ms at 1.5 T) is normally insignificant and, absent a substantial amount of fat, the IP and OP signal intensities are essentially equivalent.

In the presence of iron, however, T2* is markedly reduced, and therefore significant relaxation (and signal loss) occurs between the first (out-of-phase) and second (in-phase) echoes. T2-weighted FSE sequences, with their associated long TEs, are also fairly sensitive to the presence of iron. The signal loss of the affected parenchyma is generally proportional to the concentration of iron, and this serves as the basis for quantitative techniques used to estimate hepatic iron levels. The most common method involves a multiecho GRE pulse sequence with 8 to 12 echoes. A region of interest is drawn in the liver (ie, avoiding blood vessels) and then propagated to all of the images with successively longer TEs. This in turn generates a plot of signal intensity vs TE, which should demonstrate exponential decay and can be solved (using a curve-fitting routine) for T2* or R2* (relaxivity or the inverse of T2*) using the following formula:

$$S = S_0 e^{-TE/T2^*} + S_1$$

where *S* represents signal intensity. Several authors have published data relating measurements of hepatic R2* to the iron content obtained from biopsy specimens, with fairly accurate results, and therefore an R2* measurement can be converted to an estimated hepatic iron concentration using one of these tables (this step has been incorporated into the R2* analysis software of some vendors).

Fatty infiltration and iron overload can occur in the same liver. They have opposite effects on signal intensity of IP and OP images, and therefore it may be difficult or impossible to detect the presence of one or both of these conditions on a standard IP and OP SPGR acquisition. A multiecho Dixon technique (IDEAL) can quantify both iron and fat in the same acquisition, and the presence of fat can be inferred on a multiecho GRE iron quantification acquisition by noticing a sinusoidal modulation of the signal intensity vs TE curve.

Primary hemochromatosis is associated with an increased risk (up to 200-fold) for HCC, with most occurring in patients with cirrhosis at the time of diagnosis. If primary hemochromatosis is untreated, the long-term effects of excess iron in various organs can lead to cardiomyopathy, diabetes mellitus, and other endocrinopathies.

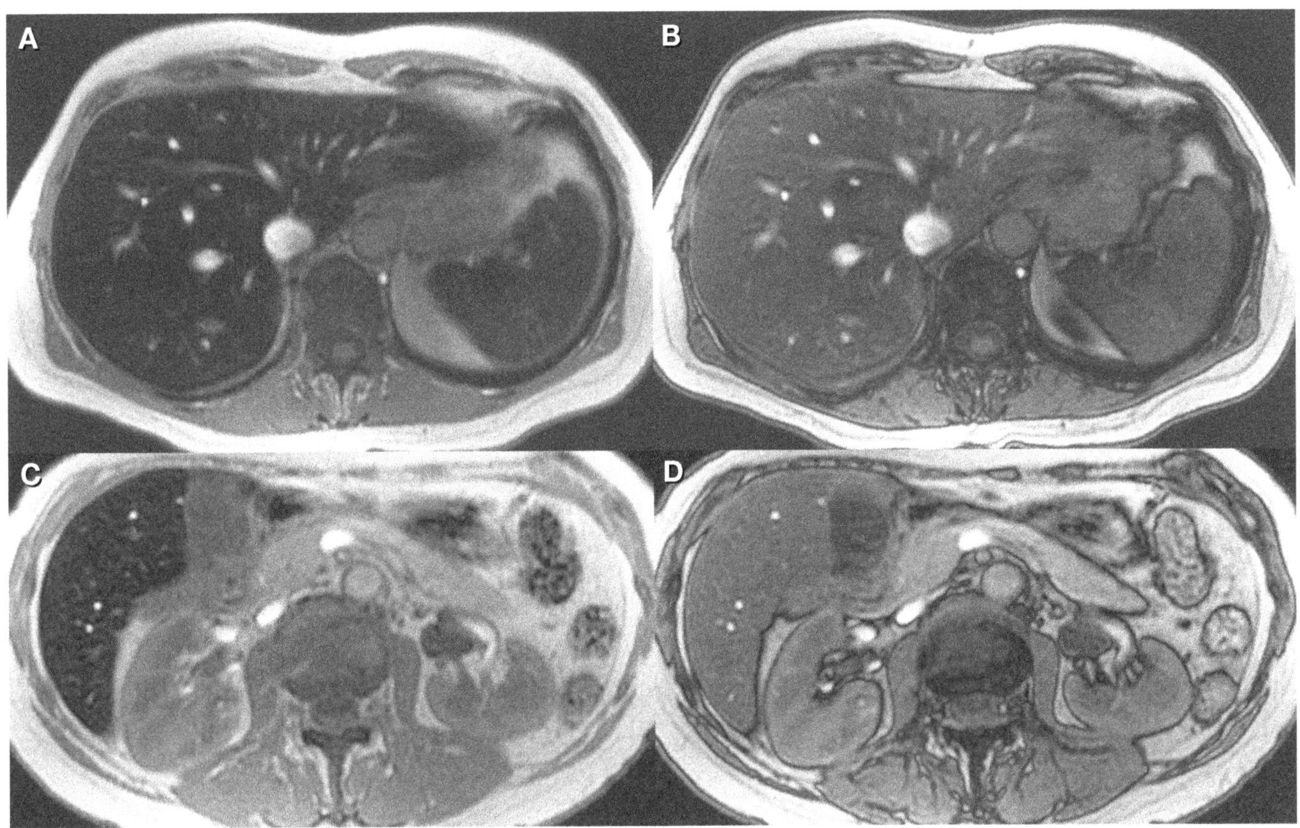

Figure 2.7.1

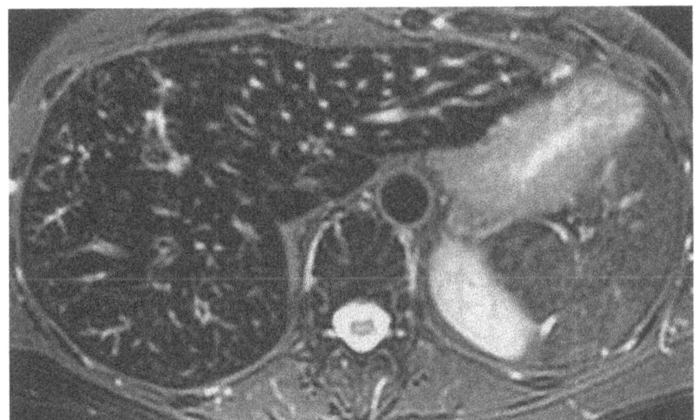

Figure 2.7.2

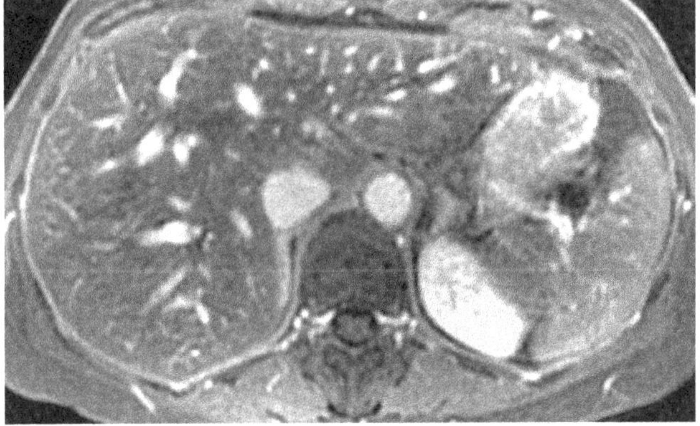

Figure 2.7.3

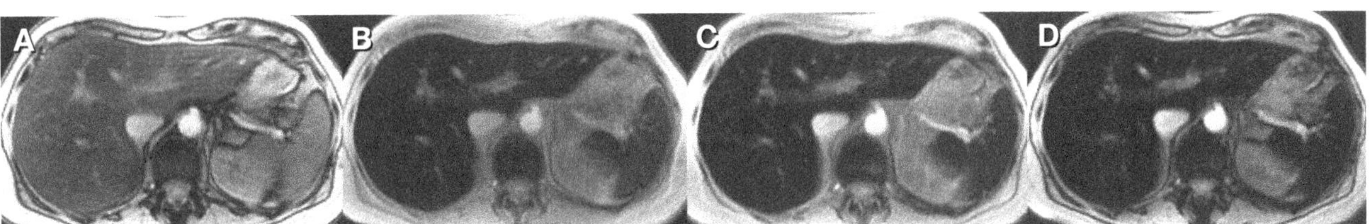

Figure 2.7.4

HISTORY: 52-year-old woman with elevated AST and ALT levels

IMAGING FINDINGS: Axial T1-weighted IP and OP 2D SPGR images (Figure 2.7.1) demonstrate diffuse, decreased signal intensity in the liver and spleen on IP images (which have the longer TE). The pancreas has normal signal intensity. Axial fat-suppressed T2-weighted image (Figure 2.7.2) also shows diffuse, decreased signal intensity in the liver and spleen compared to paraspinal muscles. Axial portal venous phase postgadolinium 3D SPGR image (Figure 2.7.3) demonstrates no suspicious focal hepatic masses and reveals more subtle diffuse signal loss in the liver and spleen. Multiecho GRE images (Figure 2.7.4) demonstrate progressive signal loss with increasing TE throughout the liver, spleen, and bone marrow.

DIAGNOSIS: Hemosiderosis (secondary hemochromatosis)

COMMENT: This case shows marked signal loss throughout the liver, spleen, and bone marrow, with relative sparing of the pancreas. This pattern is consistent with secondary or acquired hemochromatosis. Notice the profound signal dropout on the later echoes of the multiecho GRE acquisition. The abnormal signal intensity of liver, spleen, and bone marrow is difficult to ignore, and this technique represents the most sensitive method for appreciating even relatively mild iron overload.

A liver biopsy demonstrated hemosiderosis without fibrosis. The patient was anemic during her pregnancy 20 years ago and was placed on iron supplementation, which she continued long term. After the liver biopsy and MRI, her iron supplements were replaced with monthly phlebotomies. She is heterozygous for the hemochromatosis gene.

Although the precise details of the time course for development of fibrosis in patients with hemochromatosis are still unknown, some studies have concluded that duration of iron exposure, age, male sex, and alcoholism increase the risk of significant fibrosis. It has also been proposed that certain non–iron-related fibrogenic factors could have a role in the development of hepatic fibrosis in these patients. Similarly, although the association of HCC with hemochromatosis is well known, the pathologic mechanisms are not entirely clear. For patients with primary hemochromatosis, it is estimated that HCC will develop in approximately 5% of men and 1% of women. Periodic phlebotomies to normalize body iron stores and minimize organ dysfunction continue to be the primary therapy for hemochromatosis. The extent to which phlebotomy mitigates the risk of developing cirrhosis or HCC in primary hemochromatosis remains uncertain.

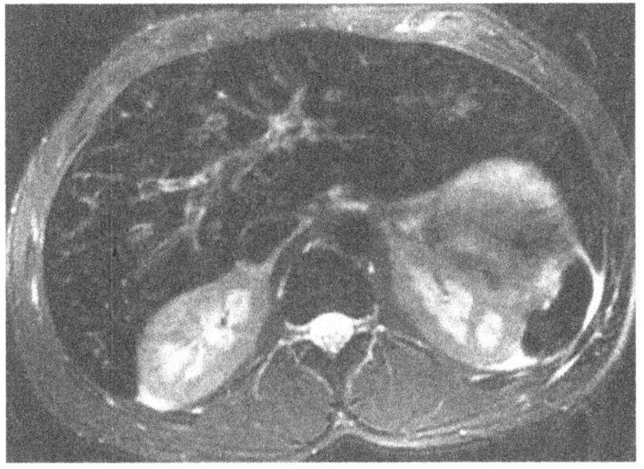

Figure 2.8.1

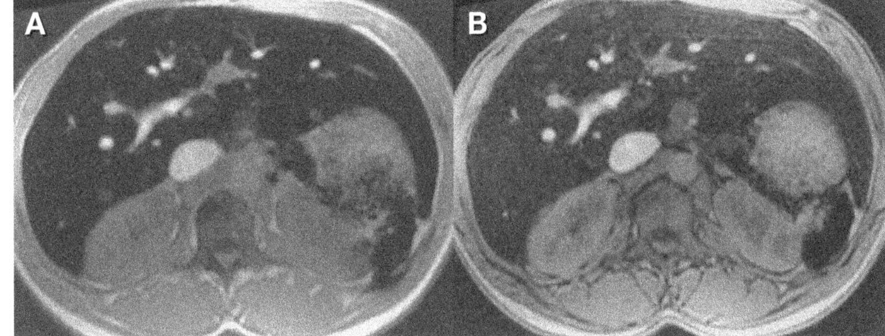

Figure 2.8.2

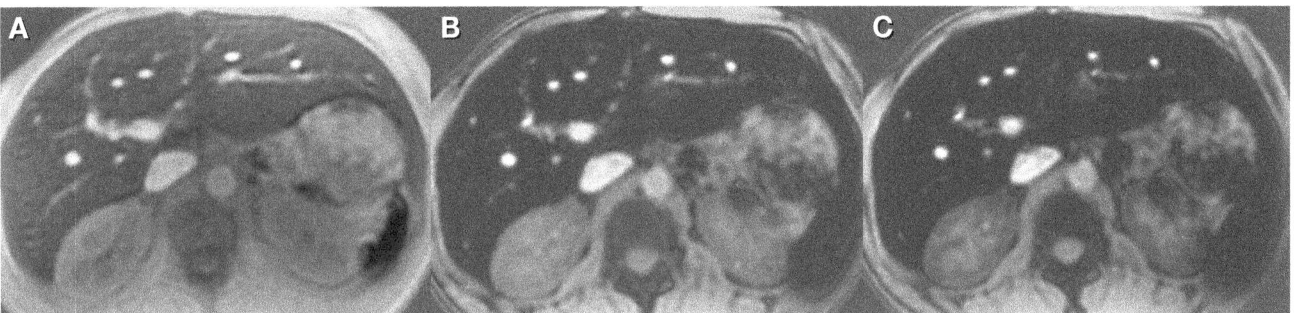

Figure 2.8.3

HISTORY: 24-year-old man with a chronic disease

IMAGING FINDINGS: Axial fat-suppressed FSE T2-weighted image (Figure 2.8.1) demonstrates diffuse, markedly decreased signal intensity in the liver, spleen, and bone marrow compared to paraspinal muscles. Signal intensity in the renal cortex is moderately reduced, suggesting iron deposition. Axial T1-weighted IP and OP 2D SPGR images (Figure 2.8.2) show diffuse, markedly decreased signal intensity in the liver and spleen. Multiecho GRE images (Figure 2.8.3) demonstrate progressively decreased signal intensity throughout the liver with progressively longer TEs. Note that the renal cortex and vertebral bone marrow also show signal loss, which is not apparent on the other images. The spleen is atrophic and has very low signal intensity on all images.

DIAGNOSIS: Hepatic iron deposition in sickle cell disease; autoinfarction of the spleen with secondary calcification

COMMENT: Sickle cell disease results from a mutation in β-globin gene, which leads to production of sickle cell hemoglobin and the generation of fragile, sickle-shaped red blood cells, eventually resulting in hemolytic anemia and episodic small-vessel occlusions.

The consequences of hemolytic anemia are well illustrated in this case, with extensive iron deposition in the reticuloendothelial cells of the liver, spleen, and bone marrow. Although intravascular hemolysis is not a major component of sickle cell disease, it can occur in acute hemolytic crises and lead to iron deposition in the renal cortex. The extent of iron overload in the kidneys, however, is relatively minor in comparison to liver, spleen, and bone marrow.

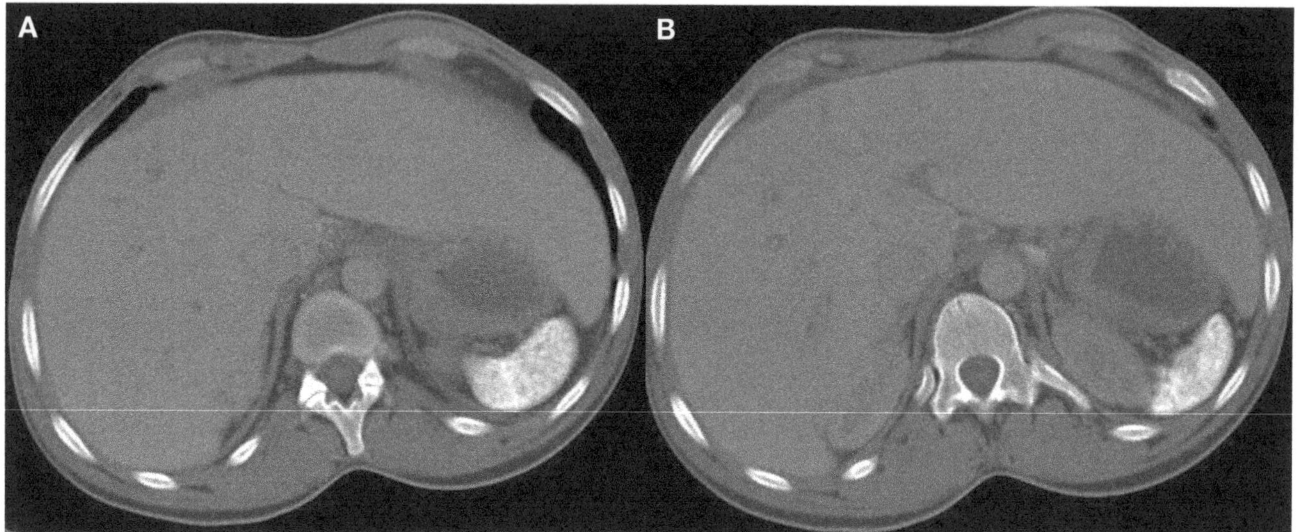

Figure 2.8.4

The distinction between an iron-overloaded spleen and a calcified autoinfarcted spleen is difficult if not impossible to make on MRI but is obvious on the noncontrast CT images (Figure 2.8.4). The fact that the spleen is extremely dark on all images, including the shortest echo of the multiecho GRE sequence, might suggest the presence of calcium; however, severe iron overload could result in an identical appearance (and it's very likely that both effects are involved in this case).

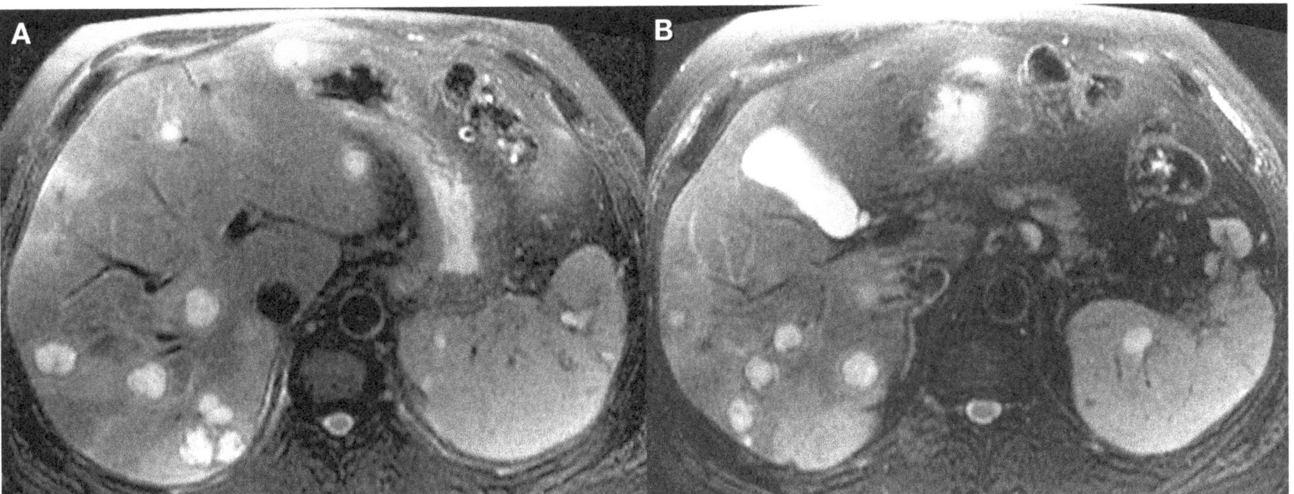

Figure 2.9.1

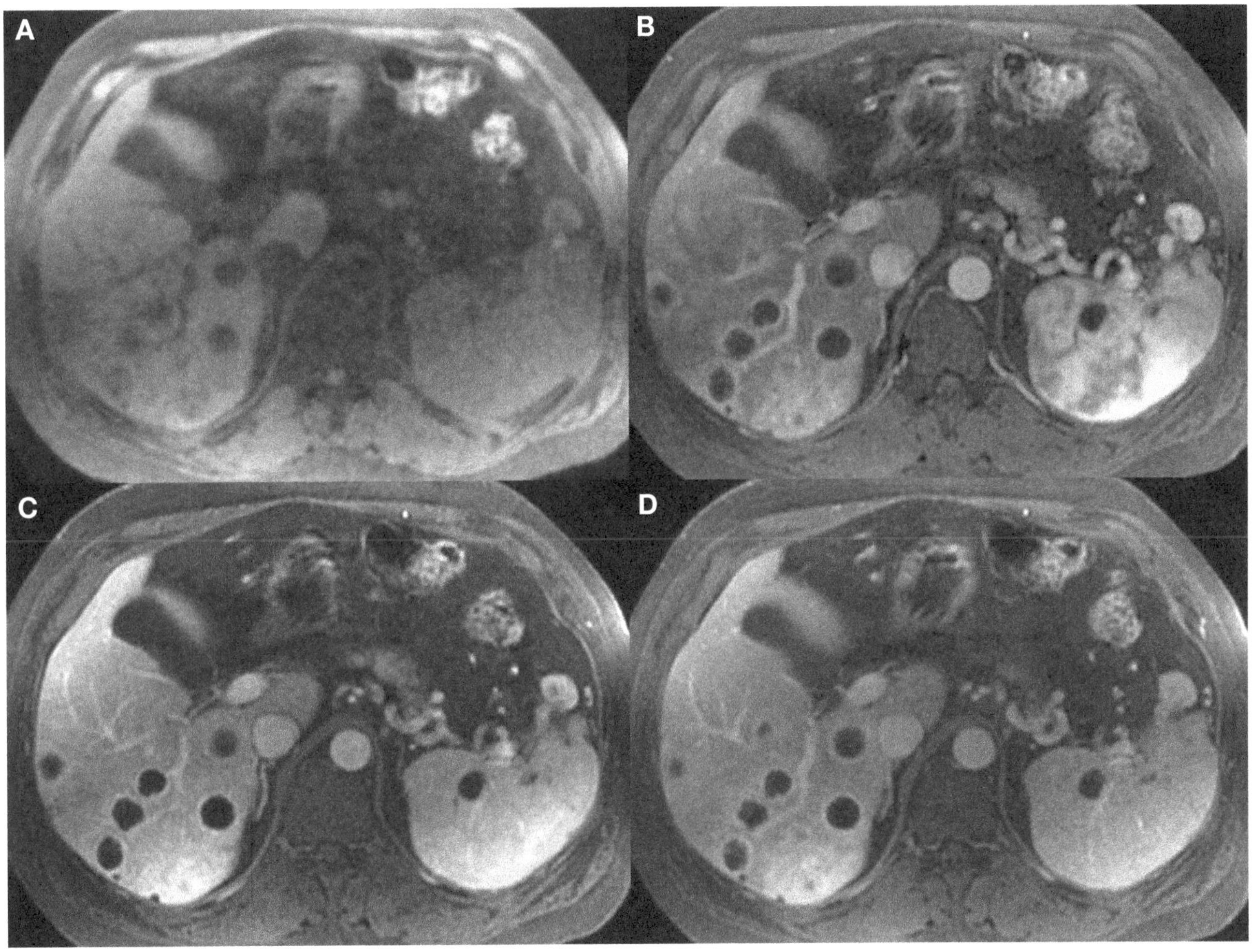

Figure 2.9.2

HISTORY: 45-year-old man with history of vasculitis treated with prednisone and azathioprine, now with fever, chills, and daily sweats

IMAGING FINDINGS: Axial fat-suppressed T2-weighted FRFSE images (Figure 2.9.1) demonstrate multiple complex, hyperintense lesions in the liver and spleen. Axial pregadolinium and arterial, portal venous, and equilibrium phase postgadolinium 3D SPGR images (Figure 2.9.2) demonstrate no internal enhancement, and persistent rim enhancement of the lesions.

DIAGNOSIS: Multiple hepatic and splenic abscesses

COMMENT: Multiple rim-enhancing lesions in the liver and spleen of an immunosuppressed patient with fevers and chills should not present a diagnostic dilemma, and should be considered abscesses until proven otherwise.

Metastatic disease would also be in the differential diagnosis, although given the clinical scenario and the absence of a known primary tumor, this diagnosis is considerably less likely. A few recent papers have investigated the use of DWI for distinguishing between the 2 entities and suggest that abscesses with thick central pus should have restricted diffusion with low ADC values (or high signal intensity on higher-b-value diffusion-weighted images), whereas the centers of necrotic metastases behave more like simple fluid, with high ADC values and low signal intensity on high-b-value diffusion-weighted images. Of course, it's also true that most metastases have more prominent soft tissue components, with thick irregular rims.

Pyogenic hepatic abscesses most often occur through hematogenous spread (the likely mechanism in this case, given the splenic involvement) or biliary obstruction with ascending cholangitis.

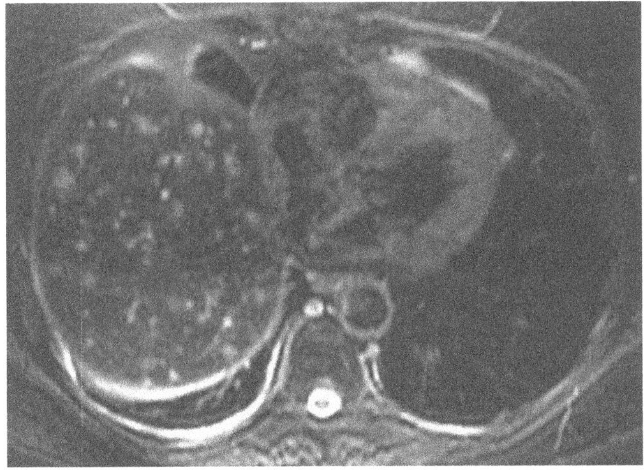

Figure 2.10.1

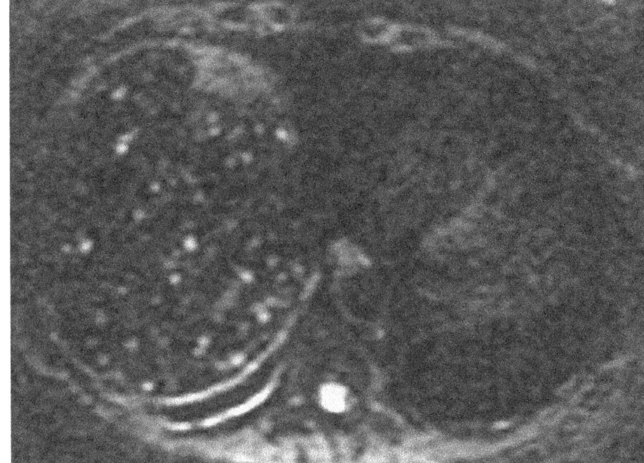

Figure 2.10.2

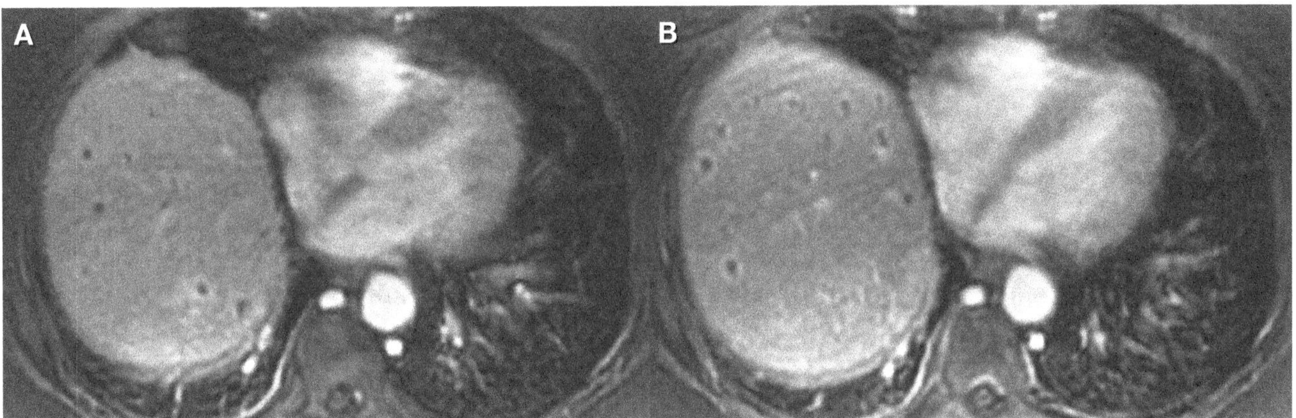

Figure 2.10.3

HISTORY: 57-year-old woman with a history of PBC status post cadaveric liver transplantation 5 years ago

IMAGING FINDINGS: Axial fat-suppressed T2-weighted FSE (Figure 2.10.1) and axial diffusion-weighted (b=100 s/mm^2) (Figure 2.10.2) images demonstrate diffuse, small hyperintense nodules throughout the liver. Axial portal venous phase postgadolinium 3D SPGR images (Figure 2.10.3) reveal rim enhancement of the nodules.

DIAGNOSIS: Hepatic fungal abscesses

COMMENT: Hepatic fungal abscesses typically occur in immunocompromised patients who have had episodes of neutropenia.

The classic appearance of fungal hepatic infection on MRI is microabscesses—multiple small foci with high T2-signal intensity. Several variations of this theme have been described in the literature, likely corresponding to different phases of the disease. In the acute setting, T2-weighted images (or diffusion-weighted images) demonstrate small foci of high signal intensity. Many patients also have transfusional hemosiderosis, and therefore the contrast between the small hyperintense abscesses and the dark background liver is accentuated. In the acute phase, postgadolinium images may be somewhat less sensitive than T2-weighted images when the immune response has not yet been sufficient to generate noticeable rim enhancement. In the subacute phase, rim enhancement becomes more prominent on postgadolinium SPGR images, with persistent hyperintensity on T2-weighted images. Many authors have described a rim of dark signal surrounding the central abscess on all imaging sequences, and this is thought to represent iron-containing macrophages accumulating around the periphery of the abscess (iron storage is in their job description as members of the reticuloendothelial system). This finding is not universally present (it's not seen in this patient, for example) but can be quite impressive, as illustrated by Case 2.11.

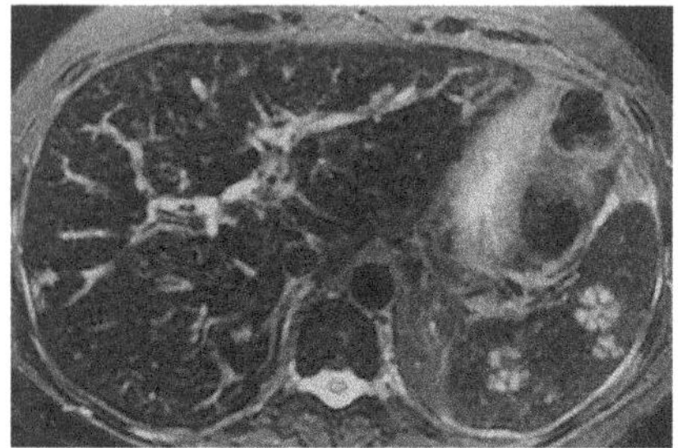

Figure 2.11.1

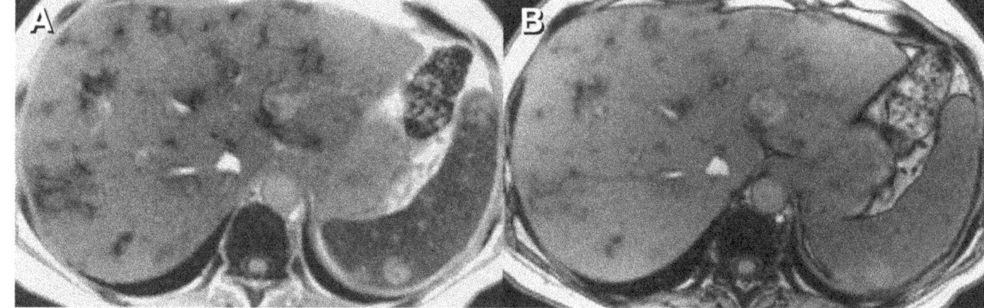

Figure 2.11.2

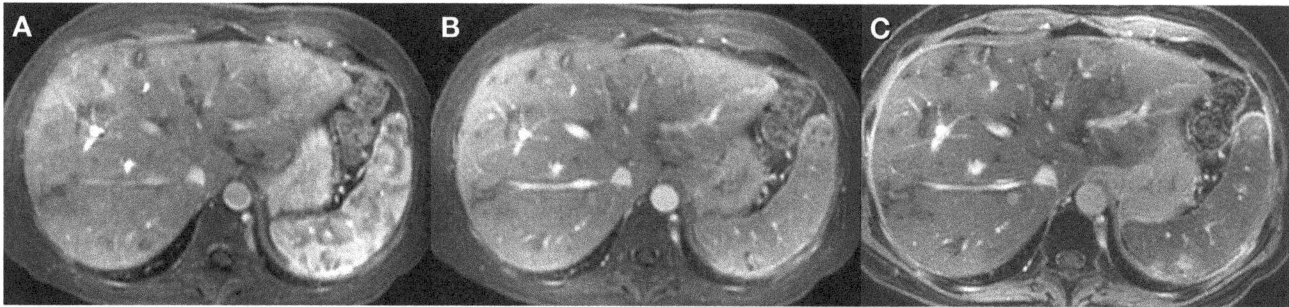

Figure 2.11.3

HISTORY: 45-year-old woman with acute myelogenous leukemia having undergone several chemotherapeutic regimens

IMAGING FINDINGS: Axial fat-suppressed FSE T2-weighted image (Figure 2.11.1) demonstrates several lobulated splenic masses and a more subtle lesion in the periphery of the right hepatic lobe. Axial IP and OP T1-weighted 2D SPGR (Figure 2.11.2), arterial (Figure 2.11.3A) and portal venous (Figure 2.11.3B) phase 3D SPGR, and delayed 2D SPGR (Figure 2.11.3C) postgadolinium images show multiple small hepatic lesions with prominent low-signal-intensity rims, as well as 2 lesions in the spleen with gradual enhancement after gadolinium administration. Notice the signal dropout in the spleen and, to a lesser extent, in the liver from the OP image to the IP image. Note also that the hepatic lesions are much more difficult to detect on the FSE T2-weighted image.

DIAGNOSIS: Hepatosplenic candidiasis

COMMENT: This is an example of subacute-chronic fungal disease in which an immune response has been mounted, and the most striking feature is the peripheral low-signal-intensity rim of hemosiderin, representing iron-containing lymphocytes surrounding the lesions. It's difficult to visualize any rim enhancement; this is also, at least in part, a reflection of the signal dropout caused by hemosiderin, and the amount of central fluid or necrosis is relatively small, evidenced by the relative difficulty in detecting the lesions on the T2-weighted FSE image.

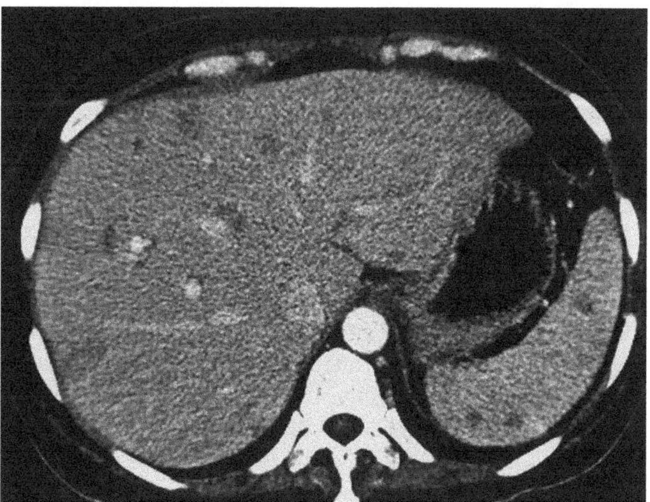

Figure 2.11.4

CT (Figure 2.11.4) is probably somewhat less sensitive for detection of subtle disease, but multiple small hypoenhancing lesions in the liver and spleen of an immunocompromised patient should certainly also suggest fungal infection.

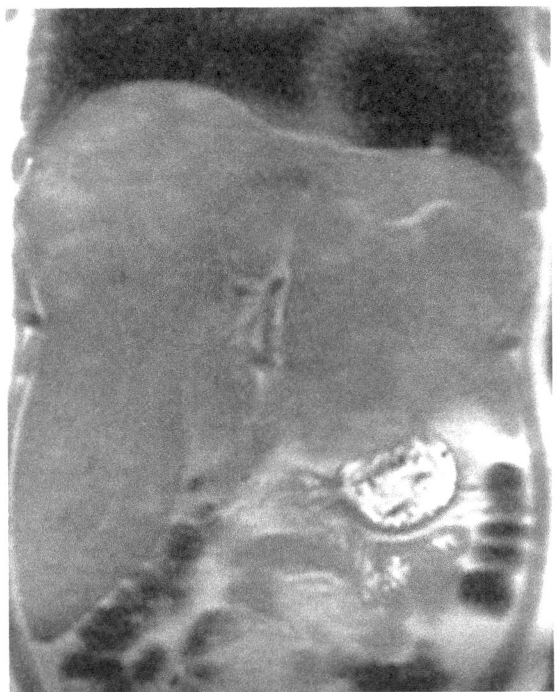

Figure 2.12.1

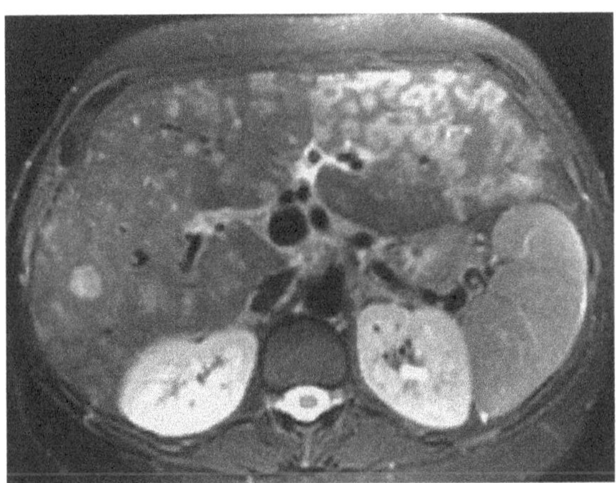

Figure 2.12.2

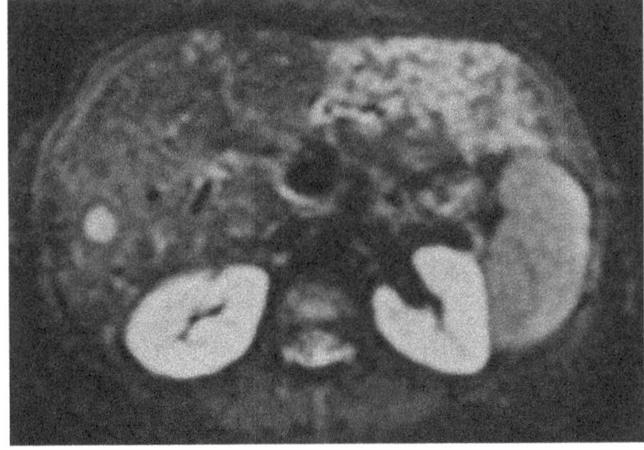

Figure 2.12.3

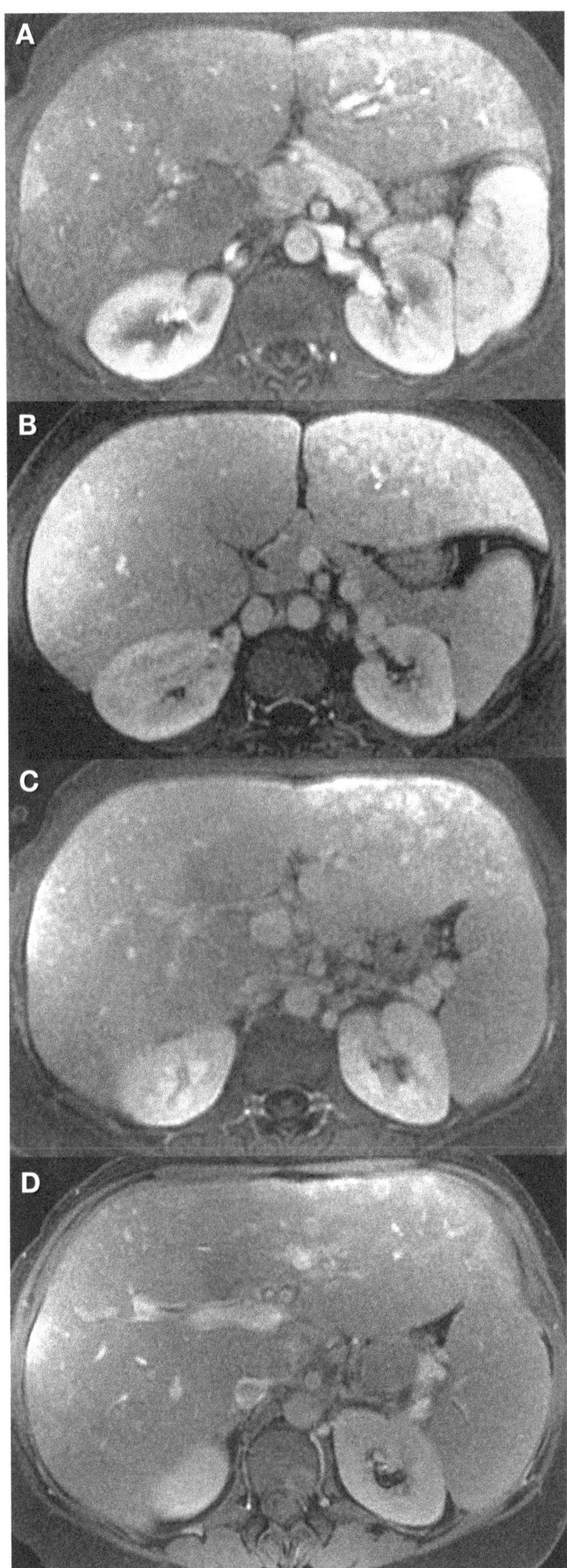

Figure 2.12.4

HISTORY: 34-year-old woman with a systemic disorder

IMAGING FINDINGS: Coronal SSFSE (Figure 2.12.1), axial fat-suppressed T2-weighted FSE (Figure 2.12.2), and axial diffusion-weighted (b=100 s/mm^2) (Figure 2.12.3) images demonstrate hepatomegaly with multiple small hyperintense nodules predominantly involving the left hepatic lobe. Axial arterial (Figure 2.12.4A), portal venous (Figure 2.12.4B), and equilibrium (Figure 2.12.4C) phase postgadolinium 3D SPGR images show gradual enhancement of the nodules, with persistent enhancement on the equilibrium phase image. A delayed postgadolinium 2D SPGR image (Figure 2.12.4D) demonstrates a few persistent ring-enhancing nodules in the left hepatic lobe.

DIAGNOSIS: Hepatic sarcoid

COMMENT: Sarcoidosis is an inflammatory granulomatous disease that primarily affects the lymph nodes, lungs, skin, eyes, liver, and spleen. Histologically, the hallmark of sarcoidosis is noncaseating granulomas. Hepatic involvement has been detected in 50% to 80% of sarcoid patients in autopsy studies; however, demonstration of hepatic disease with cross-sectional imaging is much less frequent and the MRI literature on this topic is limited, with variable descriptions that include hepatomegaly, confluent masses, and multiple subcentimeter nodules, the predominant finding in our case. Long-standing hepatic involvement can lead to fibrosis and eventually cirrhosis. A recent paper described 20 patients with hepatic sarcoidosis and chronic liver disease and noted that large central, regenerative nodules and wedge-shaped regions of peripheral atrophy were common findings.

In this patient, pulmonary sarcoid had already been diagnosed and hepatic involvement was suspected, but there was also concern for an infectious process, since the major treatment for sarcoidosis (corticosteroids) also has immunosuppressive effects. Distinguishing a fungal infection from a sarcoid with MRI is difficult, although the nodules of histoplasmosis are usually (but not always) smaller and more uniform. Bacterial abscesses are more likely to contain a necrotic center. Metastatic disease is another important differential diagnosis and may also be difficult to distinguish from sarcoid, although the persistent hyperenhancement of the nodules on equilibrium phase images would be unusual for metastatic disease.

Transjugular hepatic biopsies in both hepatic lobes demonstrated noncaseating granulomas and confirmed the diagnosis of hepatic sarcoid. All cultures from the biopsies were negative.

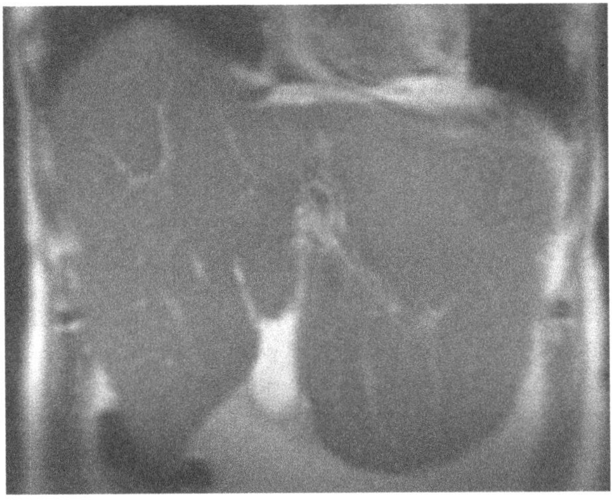

Figure 2.13.1

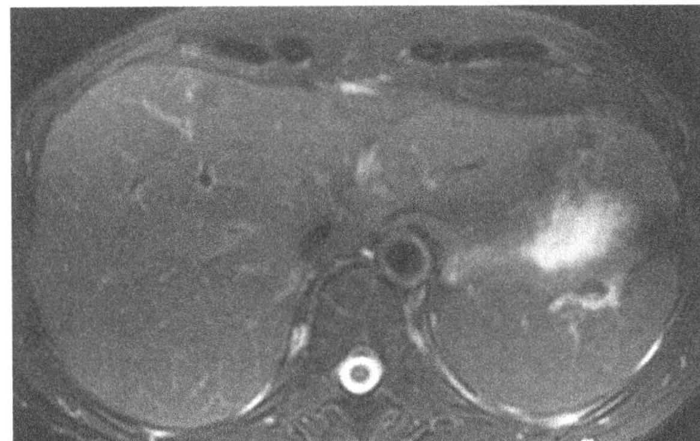

Figure 2.13.2

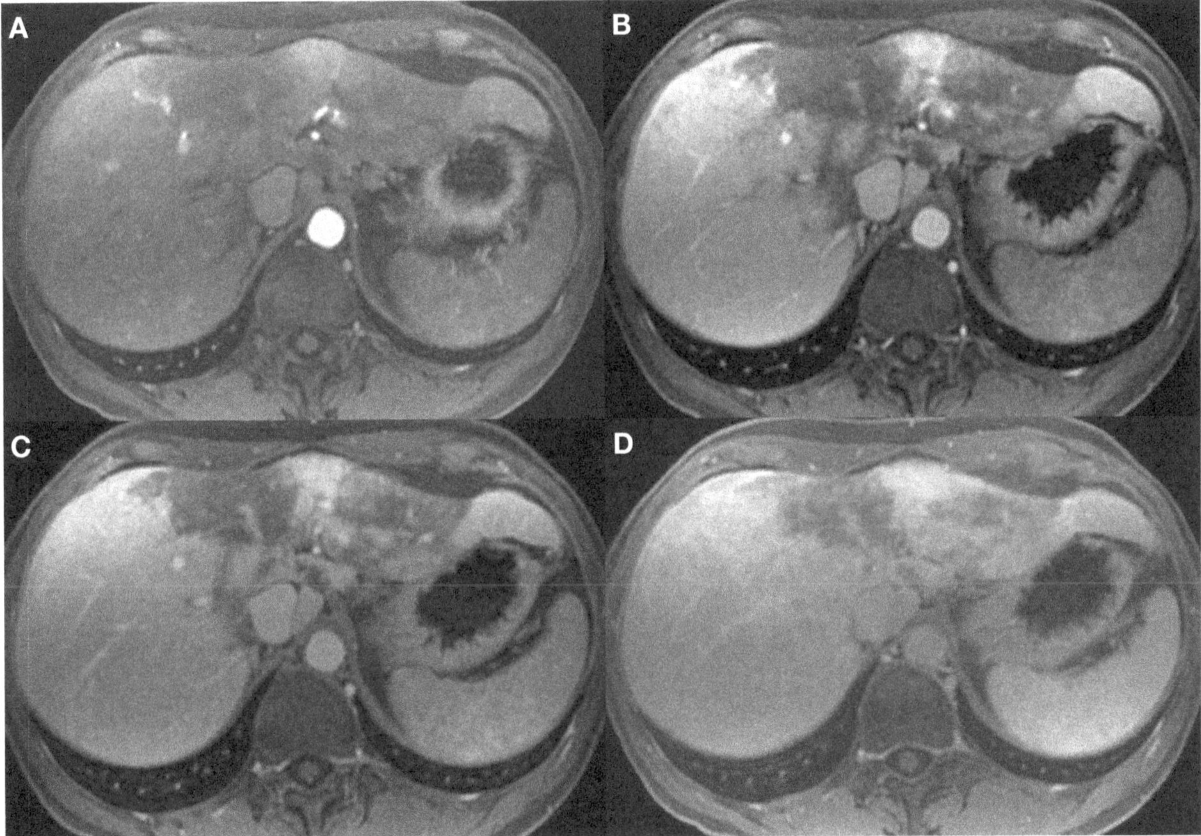

Figure 2.13.3

HISTORY: 54-year-old woman with elevated liver function test levels, abdominal distension, and telangiectasias and purpura on her face, upper chest, and extremities

IMAGING FINDINGS: Coronal SSFSE (Figure 2.13.1) and axial fat-suppressed FSE T2-weighted (Figure 2.13.2) images show hepatomegaly without focal abnormalities. However, axial postgadolinium arterial (Figure 2.13.3A), portal venous (Figure 2.13.3B), and equilibrium (Figure 2.13.3C) phase images demonstrate a geographic region of hypoenhancement in the left hepatic lobe that has begun to fill in on a 5-minute delayed image (Figure 2.13.3D), with mild hyperenhancement along the margins. IP and OP T1-weighted 2D SPGR images demonstrated no signal dropout (images not shown).

DIAGNOSIS: Hepatic amyloidosis

COMMENT: Amyloidosis is a systemic disease whose presentation depends on the organs affected and the severity of involvement. The diagnosis is made when deposits of extracellular amyloid demonstrate an apple-green birefringence with Congo red stain when viewed with polarized light. Primary amyloidosis and secondary amyloidosis are the 2 most common forms, distinguished on the basis of different protein precursors. Primary amyloidosis is associated with plasma cell dyscrasias and multiple myeloma; secondary amyloidosis is associated with chronic inflammatory disease, such as inflammatory bowel disease, rheumatoid arthritis, systemic lupus erythematosus, and Sjögren syndrome.

There is very little guidance in the radiology literature with regard to the appearance of hepatic amyloidosis on MRI. The largest series, of 9 patients, described increased signal intensity on T1-weighted images; however, this finding has not been reliably replicated by subsequent authors. Hepatomegaly is also commonly described, but this is a nonspecific finding. The presence of extensive extracellular protein deposits leads to an increased extravascular, extracellular volume, which in turn should cause changes in the kinetics of contrast agent delivery to the affected organ. In general, the wash-in and washout rates of an extracellular gadolinium contrast agent should be slower in comparison to normal hepatic tissue, and in our limited experience, visualization of heterogeneous regions of initial hypoenhancement that gradually accumulate contrast on delayed images has been a fairly consistent observation in patients with known hepatic amyloidosis. This is also a nonspecific appearance, which can be seen, for example, in patients with cirrhosis and confluent fibrosis. However, this pattern of enhancement in a patient with known or suspected systemic amyloidosis and without a history of cirrhosis might suggest hepatic involvement.

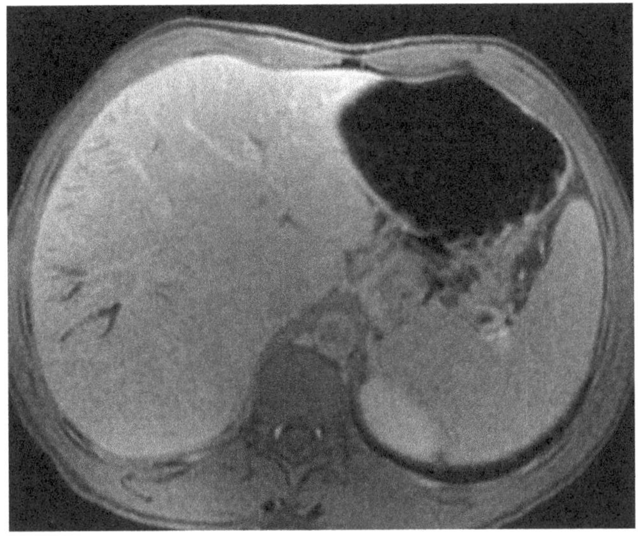

Figure 2.14.1

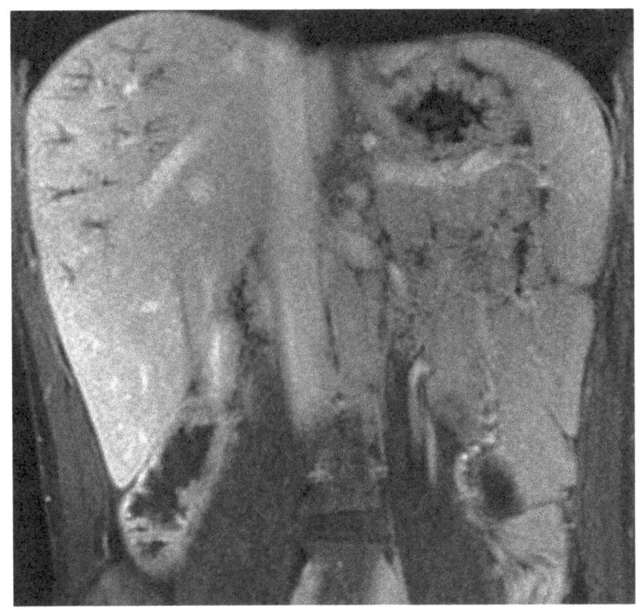

Figure 2.14.2

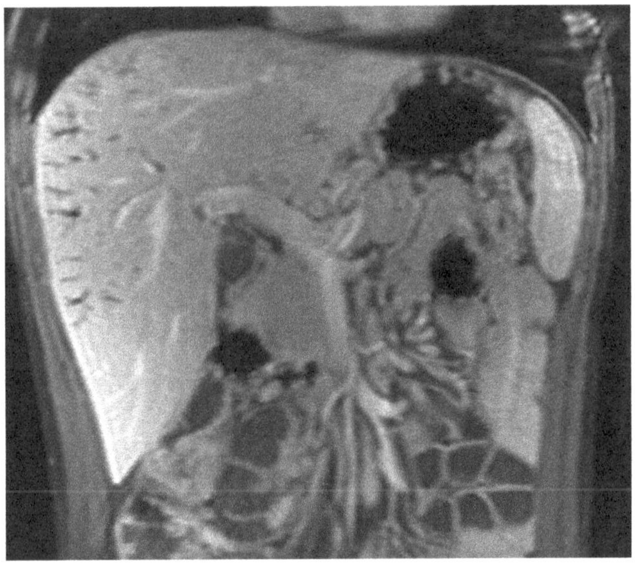

Figure 2.14.3

HISTORY: 22-year-old man with a long history of Crohn disease involving the large and small bowel

IMAGING FINDINGS: Axial (Figure 2.14.1) and coronal (Figure 2.14.2) postgadolinium 3D SPGR images, as well as a coronal postgadolinium 2D SPGR image (Figure 2.14.3) performed during an MR enterography examination, demonstrate signal void in multiple peripheral portal vein branches.

DIAGNOSIS: Portal venous gas

COMMENT: This case illustrates the MRI appearance of a rarely encountered entity and also reflects the change in thinking regarding the prognostic implications of this finding.

Gas within any structure in the body appears as a signal void on essentially all MR pulse sequences since there aren't enough protons available to generate a visible signal. Although appreciation of a signal void sounds like a fairly easy task, detection of small amounts of gas within structures where it normally doesn't reside is not trivial and is much more easily appreciated on CT. (In part, this is a reflection of the fact that MRI is rarely performed in situations where pneumoperitoneum, pneumatosis, or portal venous gas might be an anticipated finding, and so we rarely actively look for it.) Since gas is also a well-known generator of susceptibility artifact, blooming of the signal void can be appreciated on gradient echo–based acquisitions, increasing with longer TEs (greater on IP than OP images) and more prominent on 2D than 3D acquisitions.

In this case, portal venous gas is obvious and the only real differential diagnosis is peripheral biliary dilatation, which could also appear as nonenhancing tubular structures within the liver. The fine peripheral branching pattern without prominent central ducts is much more typical of portal veins, however, and if there is any lingering doubt, inspection of T2-weighted images should solve the problem, since fluid in the biliary tree will be bright and gas will be dark.

The presence of mesenteric or portal venous gas was once considered a sign of impending death because it presumably indicated extensive bowel necrosis. Several papers in the past few years have noted that this is not universally true and that various benign conditions can also cause this finding. This case is an example of an iatrogenic etiology: The patient had a colonoscopy earlier in the day, during which 2 sigmoid strictures were rather aggressively dilated. He had no signs of an acute abdomen and had no complications detected on subsequent clinical visits or follow-up imaging.

CASE 2.15

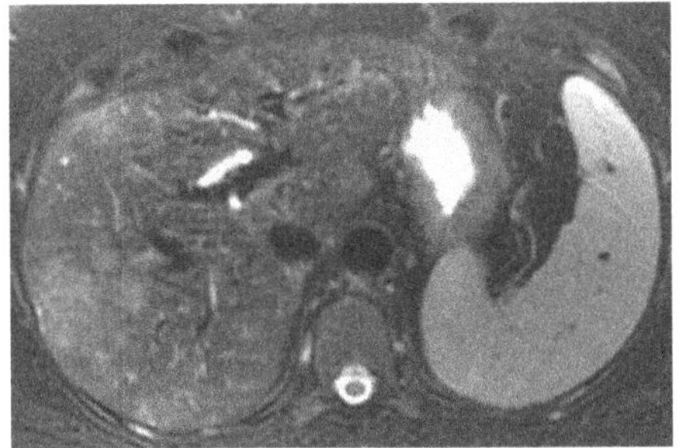

Figure 2.15.1

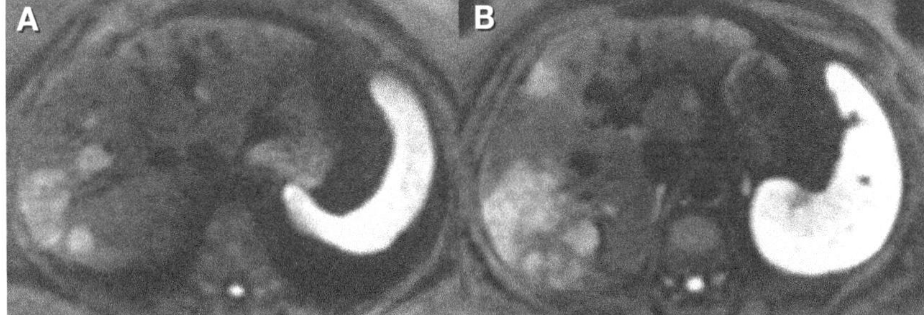

Figure 2.15.2

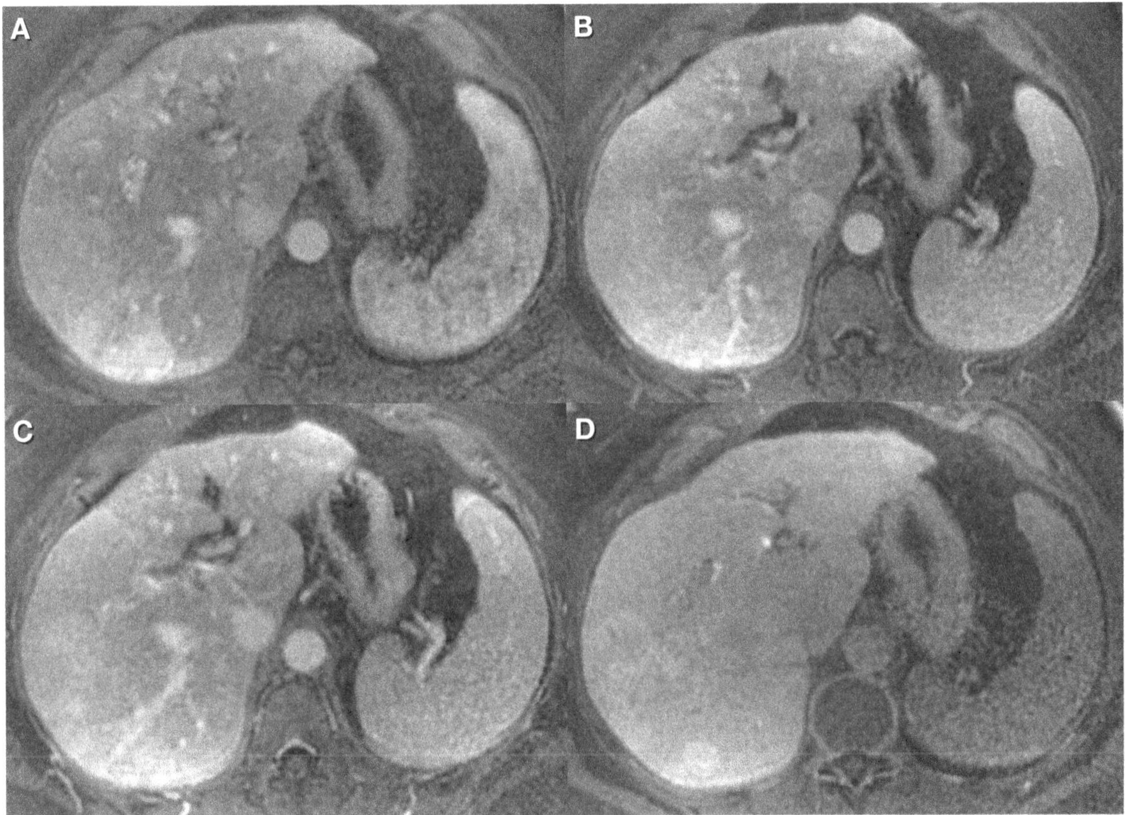

Figure 2.15.3

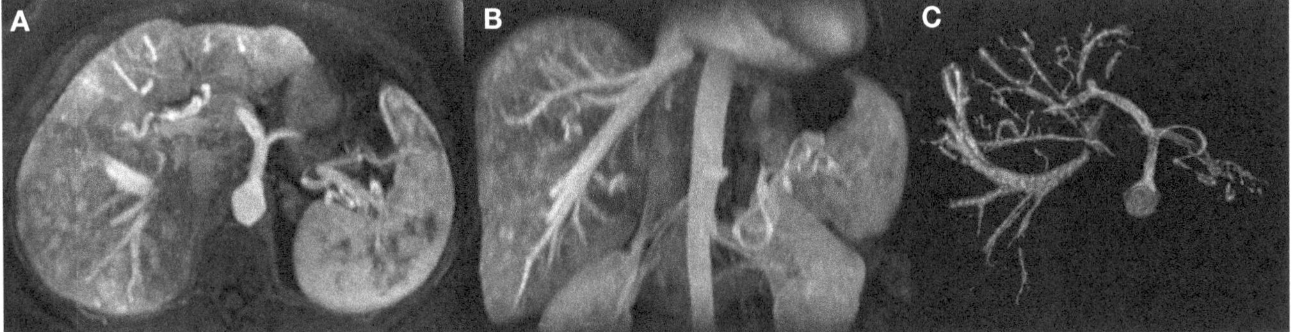

Figure 2.15.4

HISTORY: 55-year-old woman with epistaxis

IMAGING FINDINGS: Axial fat-suppressed T2-weighted FSE image (Figure 2.15.1) demonstrates subtle, ill-defined areas of intermediate increased signal throughout the liver that are more easily visualized on DWI (b=600 s/mm^2) (Figure 2.15.2). Axial arterial, portal venous, equilibrium phase, and delayed hepatobiliary phase 3D SPGR images (Figure 2.15.3) demonstrate heterogeneous nodular hyperenhancement in the arterial phase with prominent early filling hepatic veins. There is persistent hyperenhancement of a few nodular lesions on the hepatobiliary phase image. Subvolume reformatted axial (Figure 2.15.4A) and coronal (Figure 2.15.4B) arterial phase MIP images emphasize the extensive nodular hyperenhancement throughout the liver, as well as the enlarged hepatic artery and hepatic veins, which are also depicted in the VR image (Figure 2.15.4C). A hepatobiliary contrast agent (Multihance) was used; note the contrast in the hepatic duct on the hepatobiliary phase image.

DIAGNOSIS: Hereditary hemorrhagic telangiectasia

COMMENT: HHT is an autosomal dominant hereditary disorder characterized by multiple small telangiectasias of skin, mucous membranes, the gastrointestinal tract, and other organs. Recurrent epistaxis is the dominant clinical symptom in most patients; however, more serious consequences, including cyanosis, hemoptysis, and paradoxical emboli, usually result from pulmonary arteriovenous malformations. Mutations in at least 2 different genes have been associated with HHT and are thought to be involved in regulation of angiogenesis.

Hepatic involvement in HHT has stimulated much interest in recent years. Early investigations concluded that hepatic involvement was relatively infrequent; however, more recent studies using multidetector CT and MRI have demonstrated hepatic manifestations in as many as 85% of patients. Although most patients with hepatic involvement are asymptomatic, 3 clinical syndromes have been described: high-output cardiac failure resulting from intrahepatic shunts; portal hypertension developing in the clinical setting of arterial-portal shunting; and biliary necrosis, also thought to occur as a result of arterial-venous shunting and consequent reduced blood supply to the biliary tree.

Several characteristic findings have been described in HHT patients with hepatic involvement. Enlargement of the hepatic artery (to >6 mm in diameter) has been reported in the US literature as a sensitive and specific finding for HHT and can easily be seen with MRI. Focal arterial aneurysms may also occur, although these are relatively uncommon. Vascular shunts are seen in a majority of patients; hepatic artery–hepatic vein shunting occurs most frequently, in 50% to 65% of patients, and when severe, it may be responsible for high-output cardiac failure. This finding is seen in this patient as rapid filling of mildly dilated hepatic veins on the arterial phase postgadolinium acquisition. Arterioportal and porto-hepatic venous shunts occur somewhat less frequently but are nevertheless fairly common findings.

Telangiectasias are a near-universal finding. They appear as small, hyperenhancing nodules of less than 1 cm on arterial phase images and usually become isointense to hepatic parenchyma on portal venous and equilibrium phase images. These show mild-to-moderate increased signal intensity on T2-weighted images. Less discrete geographic perfusion abnormalities are also commonly seen on arterial and portal venous phase images.

Both nodular regenerative hyperplasia and FNH have been described in HHT patients, and the pathologic and imaging distinctions between the 2 entities are not entirely clear. The classic findings of FNH are isointense to mildly hyperintense signal intensity on T2-weighted images, uniform arterial phase hyperenhancement, and isointensity to adjacent liver on portal venous and equilibrium phase images, with mild-to-moderate hyperenhancement on hepatobiliary phase images if a hepatobiliary contrast agent is used. These findings can also be seen with regenerative nodules, although a prominent central scar should suggest the diagnosis of FNH. Several authors have described an increased incidence (1%-3%) of FNH in HHT patients; however, 1 study with limited pathologic correlation reported an incidence of 47%. Since both entities are thought to be related to regeneration of normal hepatic tissue in response to increased perfusion and both are benign, a clear distinction between the 2 entities at MRI is probably not very important. It is worth remembering, however, that extensive nodular regeneration can occur without parenchymal fibrosis, and therefore a diagnosis of cirrhosis should be made with caution in these patients.

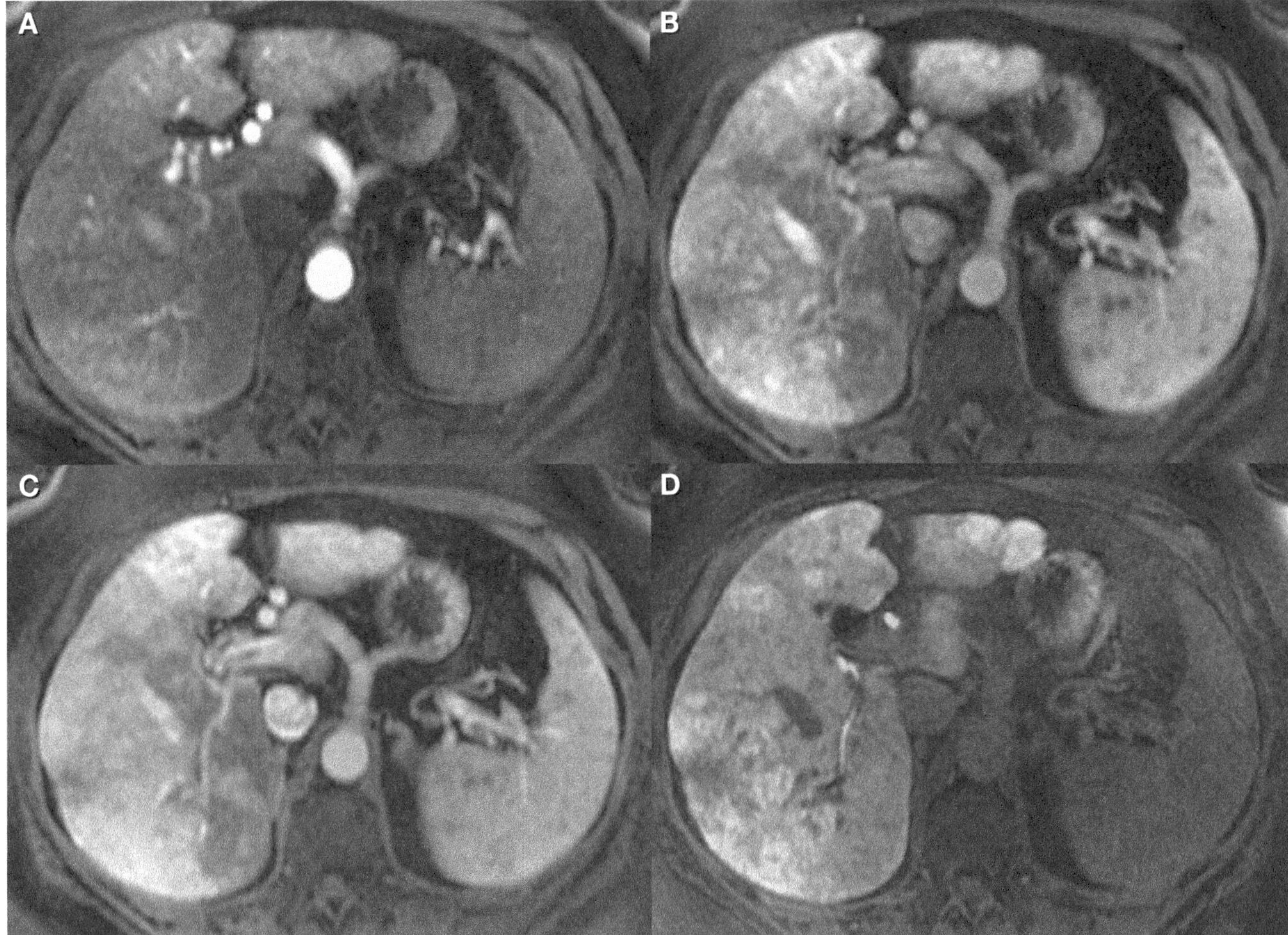

Figure 2.15.5

Two years later, the patient had a follow-up MRI with the hepatobiliary contrast agent Eovist. Axial postgadolinium early (Figure 2.15.5A) and late (Figure 2.15.5B) arterial, portal venous (Figure 2.15.5C), and hepatobiliary phase (Figure 2.15.5D) images demonstrate extensive geographic perfusion abnormalities, as well as more numerous hyperenhancing nodules on the hepatobiliary phase image, consistent with regenerative nodules or FNH.

CASE 2.16

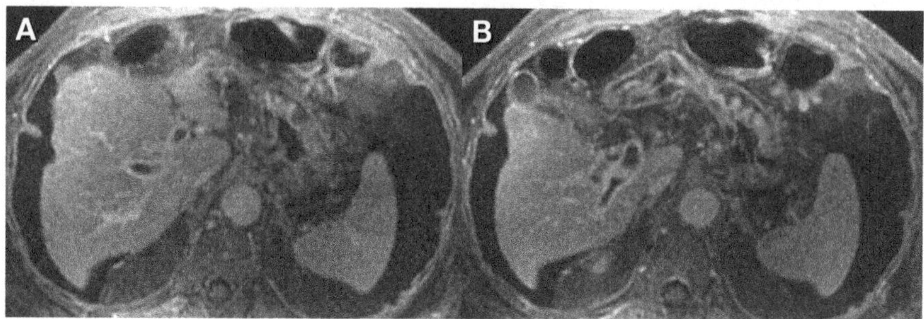

Figure 2.16.1

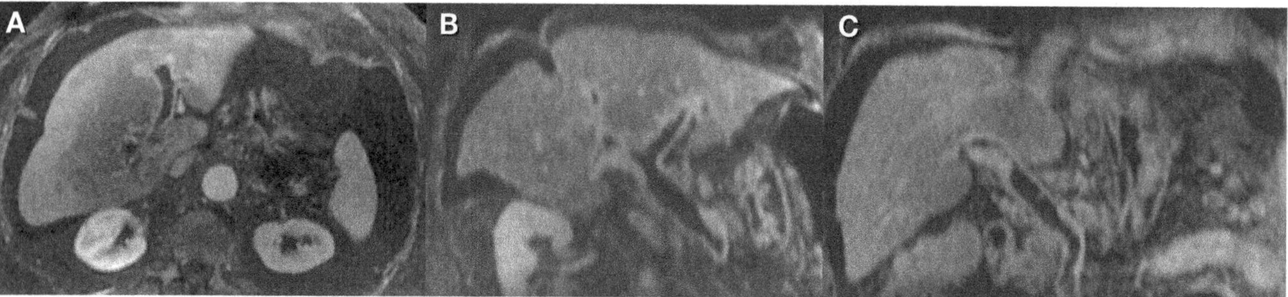

Figure 2.16.2

HISTORY: 83-year-old man being evaluated in the emergency department for abdominal pain

IMAGING FINDINGS: Axial postgadolinium portal venous phase images (Figure 2.16.1) demonstrate nearly occlusive thrombus throughout the main portal vein. Reformatted oblique images (Figure 2.16.2) show thrombus extension into the right and left portal veins and the superior mesenteric vein.

DIAGNOSIS: Acute-subacute portal vein thrombosis

COMMENT: Portal vein thrombosis, when as extensive as in this case, is an easy diagnosis to make with MRI, particularly on postgadolinium images, where the thrombus appears as a dark filling defect within the vein. If gadolinium cannot be administered, 2D or 3D SSFP images are often helpful, demonstrating filling defects with decreased signal intensity relative to adjacent blood. Noncontrast SSFP acquisitions are probably slightly less sensitive for detection of thrombus than postgadolinium 3D SPGR images: A few case reports have described subacute thrombus of exactly the right age to have signal intensity very similar to the adjacent blood pool. In our experience, however, this is a rare occurrence, and SSFP images are in general much more reliable indicators of thrombus than FSE acquisitions, where the absence of a venous flow void can be seen not only in the presence of thrombus, but also with slow flow and in-plane flow. Likewise, diffusion-weighted images are very sensitive for detection of tumor thrombus, which appears as a hyperintense lesion within the portal vein, but may be less successful in the setting of subacute-chronic bland thrombus, which frequently has low signal intensity and may be difficult to distinguish from a normal flow void.

Occlusive portal vein thrombosis that is not quickly recanalized will inevitably lead to portal hypertension and subsequent development of varices. Cavernous transformation of the portal vein occurs when there is incomplete or absent recanalization of the main portal vein accompanied by the development of an extensive network of periportal venous collateral vessels. This is also a straightforward diagnosis with MRI (Figure 2.16.3). In rare instances, we have seen cavernous transformation accompanied by an inflammatory or fibrotic reaction, leading to biliary obstruction (portal biliopathy) and causing an appearance difficult to distinguish from cholangiocarcinoma.

The accessory venous pathways generated by cavernous transformation usually provide much less flow to the liver than a normal patent portal vein, and therefore portosystemic shunts develop in most patients with cavernous transformation.

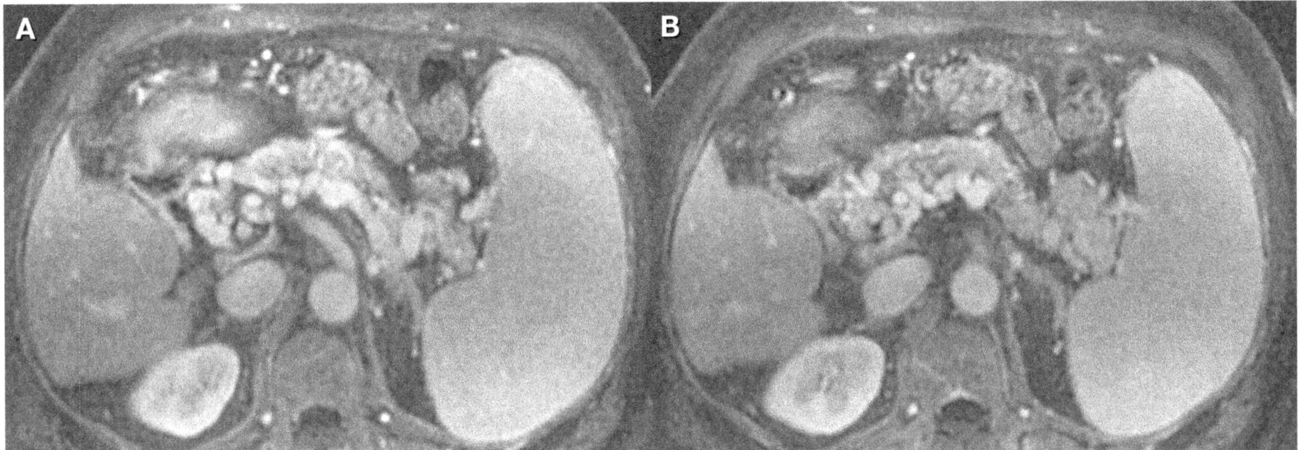

Figure 2.16.3

Axial postgadolinium portal venous phase images (Figure 2.16.3) show a more typical appearance of florid cavernous transformation secondary to portal vein thrombosis.

Risk factors for development of portal vein thrombosis include hypercoagulable states, cirrhosis, pancreatitis, HCC, and prior splenectomy. This patient had no history of chronic liver disease or known malignancy. He was placed on anticoagulation therapy and later had a gastrointestinal bleed from a duodenal ulcer.

CASE 2.17

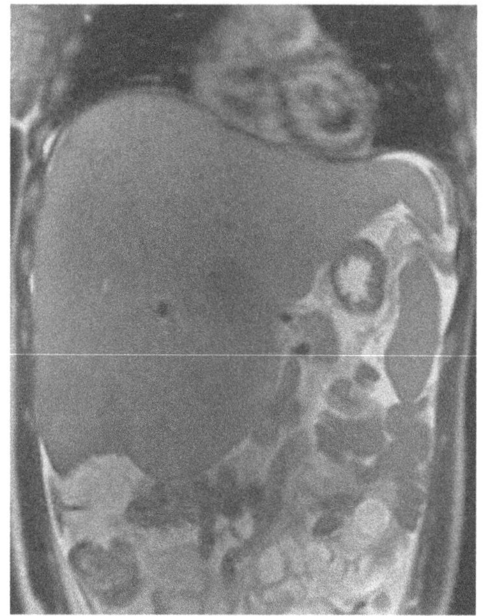

Figure 2.17.1

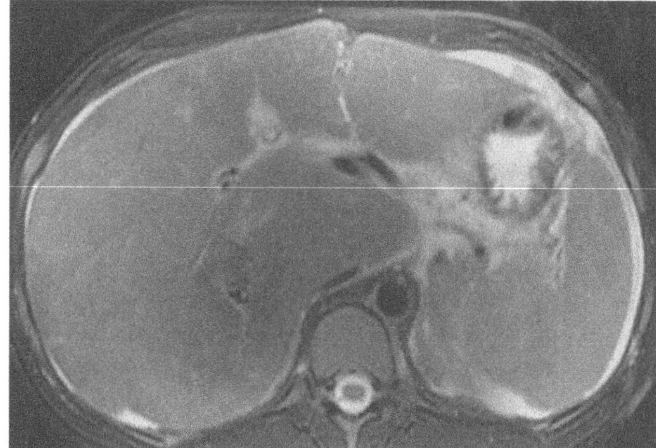

Figure 2.17.2

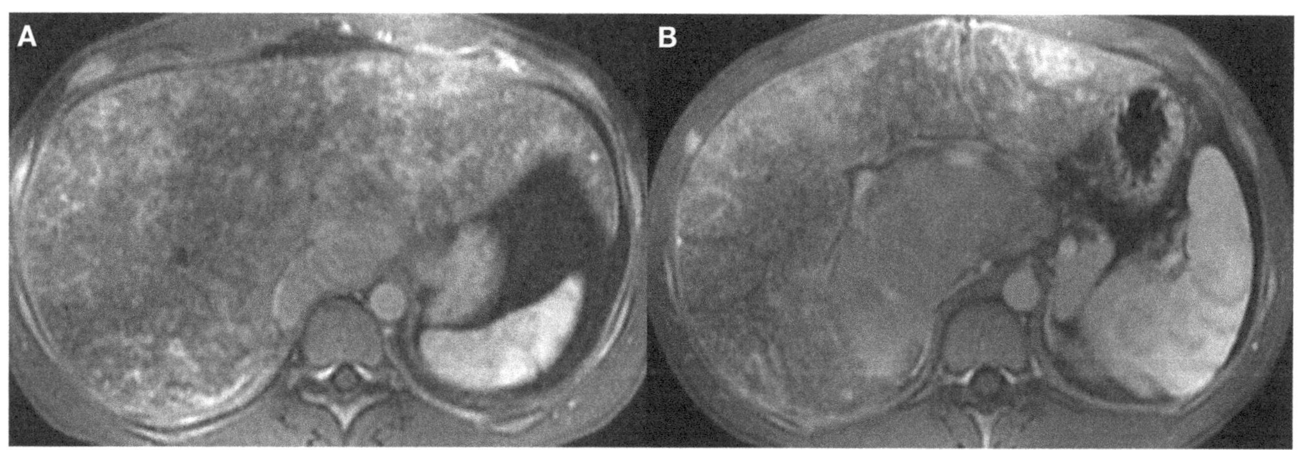

Figure 2.17.3

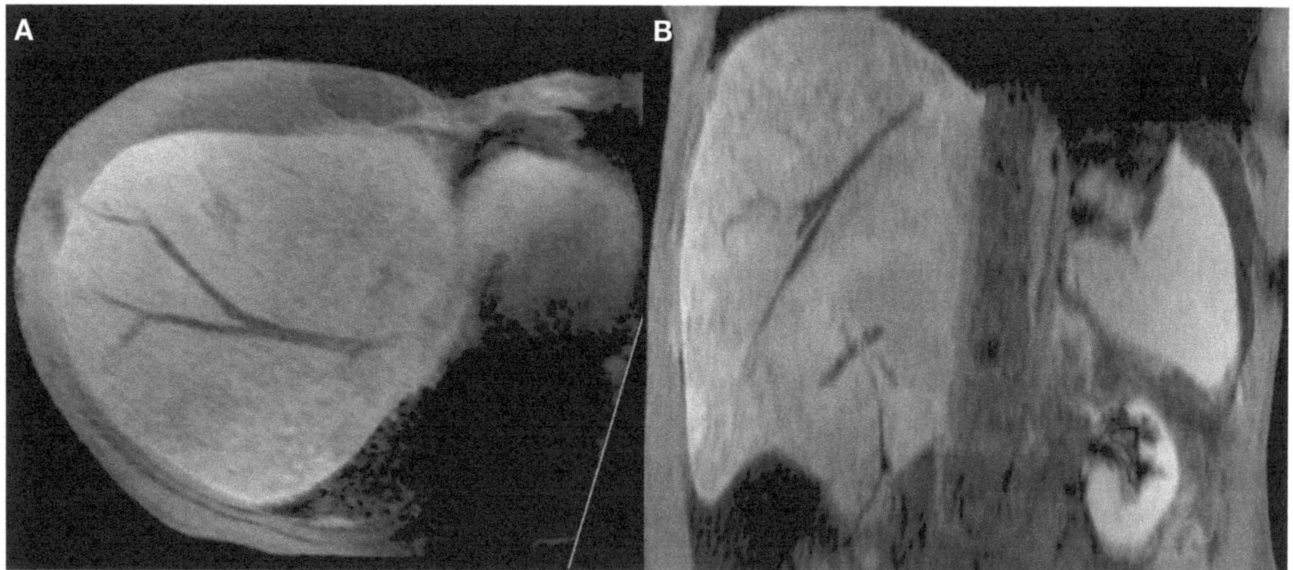

Figure 2.17.4

HISTORY: 19-year-old woman with midabdominal bloating and discomfort

IMAGING FINDINGS: Coronal SSFSE (Figure 2.17.1) and axial fat-suppressed T2-weighted FSE (Figure 2.17.2) images demonstrate marked hepatomegaly with subtle hypointensity of the caudate lobe compared with the remainder of the liver. Axial portal venous phase postgadolinium 3D SPGR images (Figure 2.17.3) show a nutmeg appearance of diffuse heterogeneous enhancement with relative sparing of the caudate lobe. Axial oblique and coronal oblique minimum-intensity projection images (Figure 2.17.4) reconstructed from equilibrium phase data demonstrate hepatic vein thrombosis.

DIAGNOSIS: Budd-Chiari syndrome

COMMENT: BCS is characterized by hepatic venous outflow obstruction, which can occur at the level of the intrahepatic veins, the IVC, or the right atrium. It is named in honor of George Budd, a British internist who described 3 cases of hepatic vein thrombosis in 1845, and Hans Chiari, an Austrian pathologist who published the first pathologic description of BCS in 1899 (and is also responsible for the Arnold-Chiari malformation and the Chiari network).

BCS has been divided into primary and secondary causes. Primary BCS involves intrinsic venous abnormalities, such as thrombosis, stenosis, or webs, and secondary BCS results from extrinsic compression by tumors or other masses. Obstruction of the IVC with or without involvement of the hepatic veins is predominant in Asia; pure hepatic vein obstruction is more commonly seen in Western countries. Risk factors include inherited and acquired hypercoagulable states, and this patient's only risk factor was oral contraceptive use. Clinical presentation depends on the rapidity of onset and can range from fulminant hepatic failure to nearly asymptomatic disease, although most patients have the classic triad of abdominal pain, ascites, and hepatomegaly. Over time, portal hypertension and cirrhosis develop in nearly all untreated patients, and mortality is increased without interventional or surgical treatment.

Dynamic postgadolinium 3D SPGR images typically reveal the most striking findings in patients with BCS, demonstrating thrombosis or stenosis of hepatic veins or the IVC, or both; enlargement of the caudate lobe; and heterogeneous enhancement of the periphery of the liver (*nutmeg liver*), with more uniform enhancement centrally and particularly in the caudate lobe, which generally has separate venous drainage. Prominent collateral veins may be visualized, and Case 2.18 is a good example of this appearance.

BCS is well known for stimulating the development of regenerative nodules or FNH-like lesions that are mildly hyperintense on precontrast T1-weighted images and show intense uniform hyperenhancement in the arterial phase before becoming isointense on portal venous and equilibrium phase images (Figure 2.17.5, from a follow-up examination performed 3 years after initial diagnosis). Development of regenerative nodules is thought to be related to the increased hepatic arterial flow stimulated by elevated portal venous pressures.

Several studies have reported an increased risk of HCC in patients with BCS; however, the range of reported HCC prevalence is extremely wide and the true risk uncertain. Nevertheless, routine surveillance of these patients for development of HCC is probably warranted.

Surgical treatment for BCS patients includes membrane resection, IVC reconstruction, surgical creation of portosystemic or mesoatrial shunts, and hepatic transplantation. Interventional therapy also has proved successful in many patients and includes angioplasty, stent placement, thrombolysis, and TIPS creation.

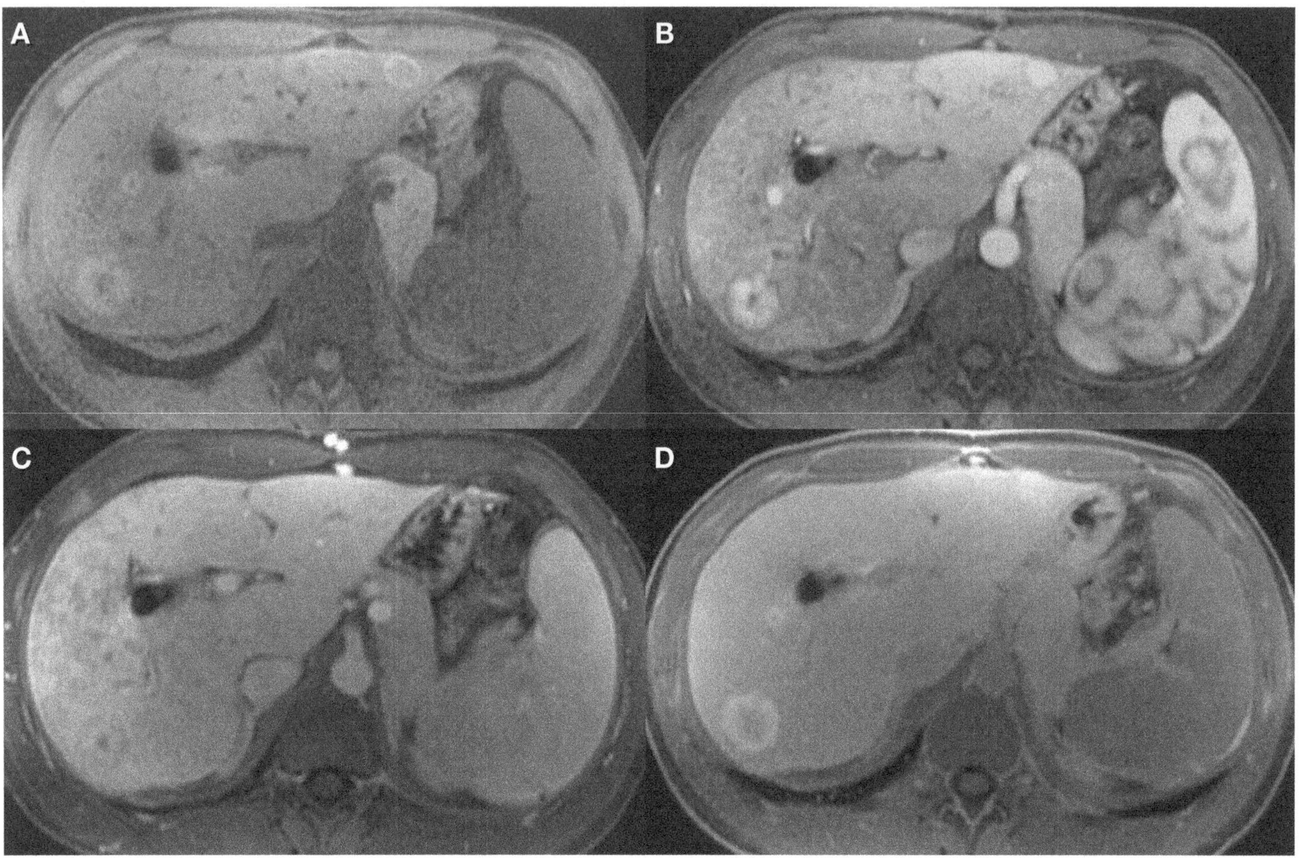

Figure 2.17.5

Precontrast 3D SPGR image (Figure 2.17.5A) demonstrates 3 hyperintense nodules in the liver. Arterial phase postgadolinium 3D SPGR image (Figure 2.17.5B) following Multihance administration shows intense enhancement of the nodules, which become nearly isointense to liver on the portal venous phase image (Figure 2.17.5C). A 90-minute delayed hepatobiliary phase image (Figure 2.17.5D) reveals contrast retention in the nodules, an appearance consistent with regenerative nodules or FNH. Note also metallic artifact in the portal vein consistent with TIPS stent.

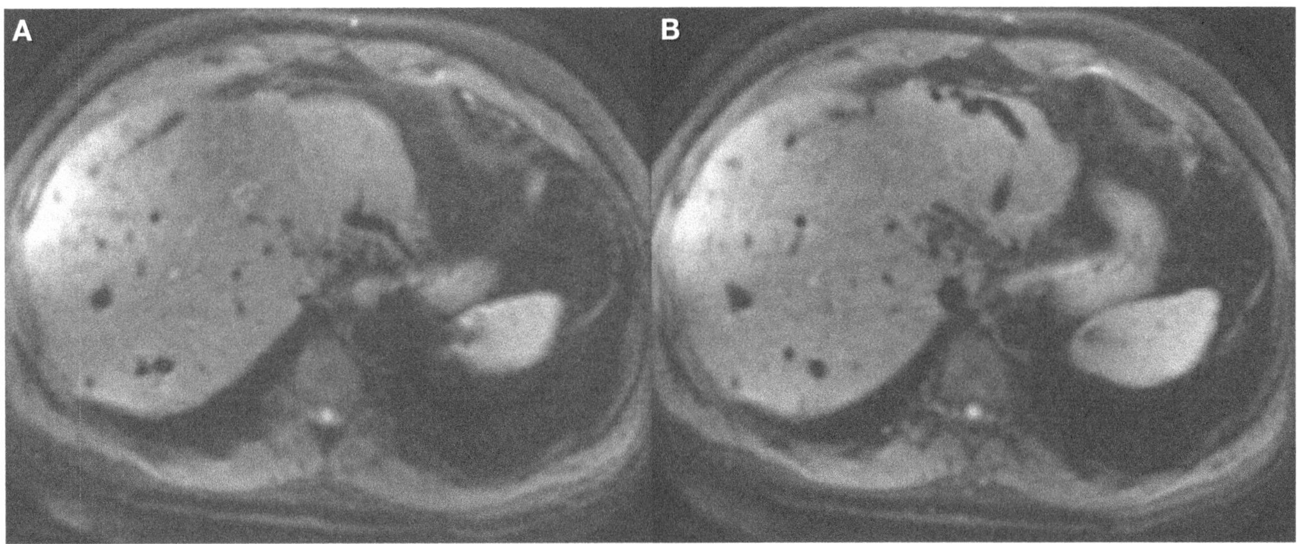

Figure 2.18.1

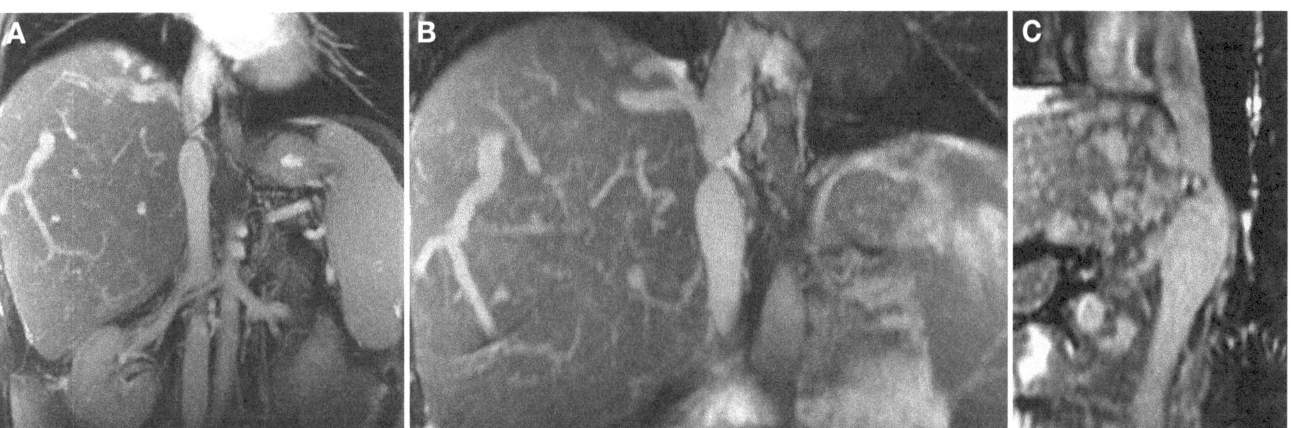

Figure 2.18.2

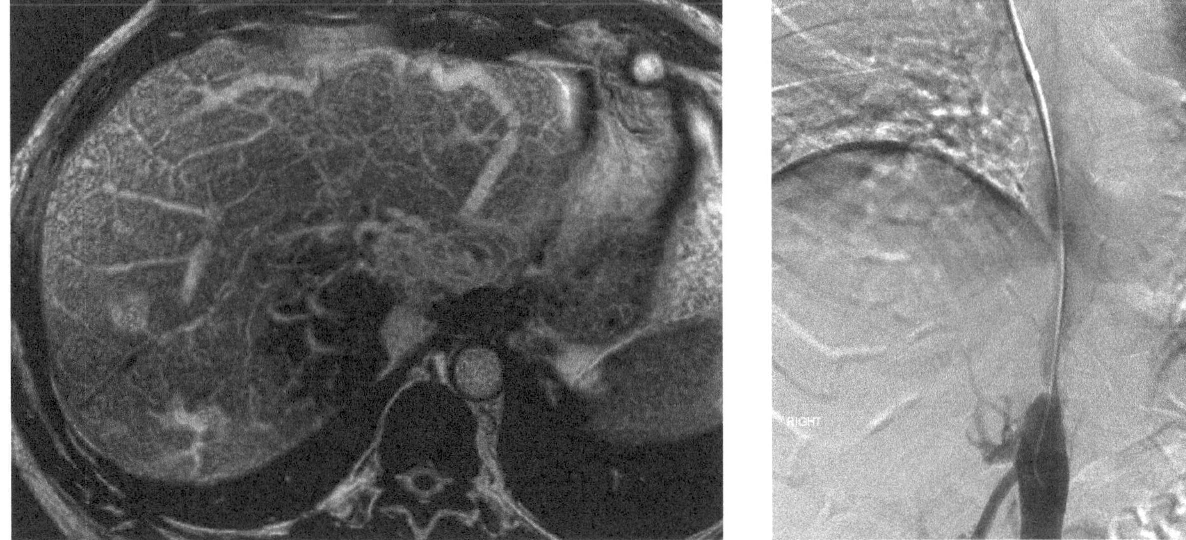

Figure 2.18.3

Figure 2.18.4

HISTORY: 31-year-old man with abdominal pain

IMAGING FINDINGS: Axial diffusion-weighted images ($b=100\ s/mm^2$) (Figure 2.18.1) reveal no normal hepatic veins, prominent collateral veins in the periphery of the liver, and a small tangle of collateral vessels anterior to the IVC. Notice also small, hyperintense filling defects in diminutive hepatic veins (confirmed on postgadolinium images). Coronal fat-suppressed 2D SSFP image (Figure 2.18.2A) demonstrates severe focal narrowing of the intrahepatic IVC. Coronal and sagittal reformatted images from axial 3D SSFP acquisition (Figures 2.18.2B and 2.18.2C) also show severe focal narrowing of the intrahepatic IVC, as well as prominent collateral veins in the periphery of the liver. An additional VR image from a 3D SSFP acquisition (Figure 2.18.3) demonstrates absent hepatic veins, prominent intrahepatic collaterals, and obstruction of the IVC. Image from a conventional IVC venogram (Figure 2.18.4) confirms severe focal stenosis of the intrahepatic IVC, as well as absence of normal hepatic veins. Note the patent small vein draining the caudate lobe, as well as a patent inferior accessory hepatic vein.

DIAGNOSIS: Budd-Chiari syndrome

COMMENT: This case is an example of chronic BCS, with nonvisualization of normal hepatic veins and large intrahepatic collateral veins, and illustrates the IVC subtype of BCS, which is prevalent in Asia and is less common in Western countries. No heterogeneous enhancement or abnormal signal intensity is seen in the periphery of the liver, and there is no enlargement of the caudate lobe—this likely reflects the chronic nature of the process, as well as IVC obstruction occurring above the level of caudate lobe drainage, making it not a particularly useful pathway for hepatic venous return.

This patient was treated with angioplasty of the IVC stenosis, which markedly reduced the pressure gradient across the stricture, and has been asymptomatic since his procedure.

CASE 2.19

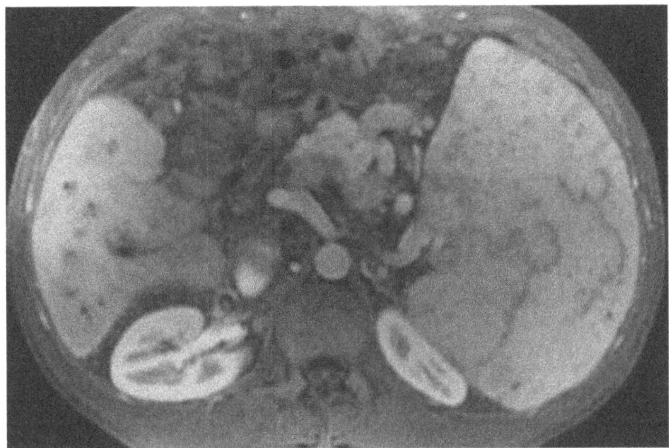

Figure 2.19.1

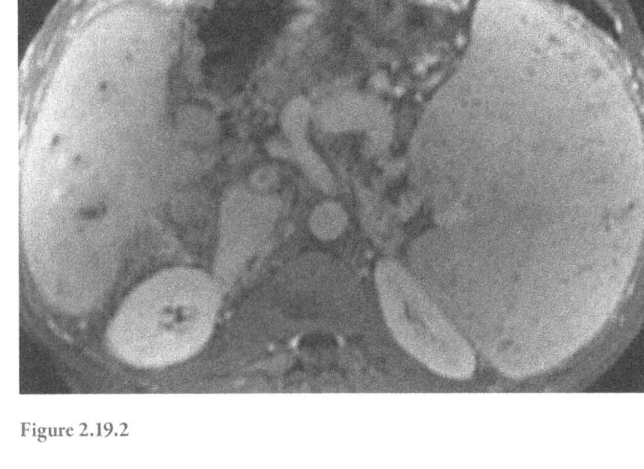

Figure 2.19.2

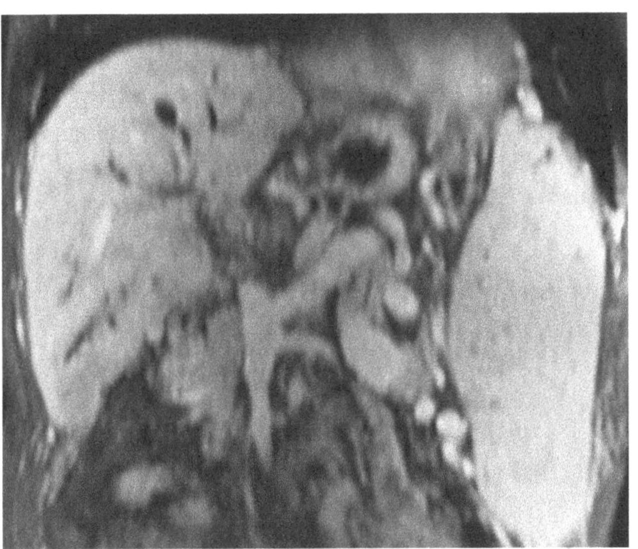

Figure 2.19.3

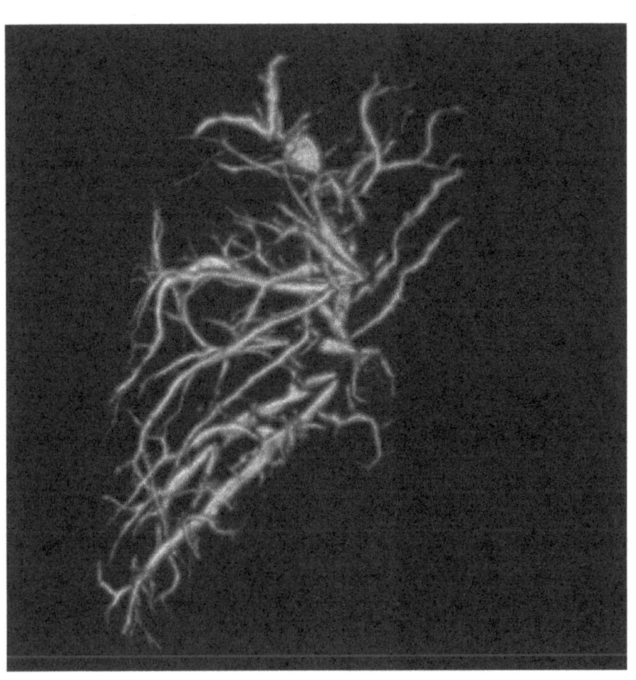

Figure 2.19.4

HISTORY: 32-year-old man status post living donor liver transplantation for PSC

IMAGING FINDINGS: Postgadolinium arterial phase image (Figure 2.19.1) demonstrates a hepatic artery stump (cutoff) at the level of the anastomosis. A subsequent axial portal venous phase image (Figure 2.19.2) at the level of the porta hepatis shows an absent main portal vein, which is confirmed on the coronal reformatted image (Figure 2.19.3). Central biliary strictures with associated moderate biliary dilatation are seen on a VR MRCP image (Figure 2.19.4).

DIAGNOSIS: Liver transplant with hepatic artery thrombosis and biliary strictures, as well as portal vein thrombosis

COMMENT: Transplantation is the treatment of choice for patients with end-stage liver disease with or without HCC. While potentially curative, hepatic transplantation is a complex procedure that requires arterial, venous, and biliary anastomoses and also necessitates long-term immunosuppressive therapy. The incidence of posttransplantation complications remains fairly high, and most centers screen patients frequently, particularly in the first 3 to 4 months following surgery. Sonography is by far the most commonly used imaging modality; it's cheap, portable, and generally sensitive and accurate for detection of most complications.

MRI is most often performed to evaluate a patient with a known or suspected biliary complication, and it is generally agreed that MRCP is the most sensitive and accurate noninvasive technique for this indication, although of course that depends to a large extent on the ability and expertise of the radiologists and technologists and the ability of the patient to cooperate during the examination.

Biliary complications are estimated to occur in 25% to 38% of patients and include anastomotic strictures that are usually related to surgical misadventures or anatomic discrepancies between donor and recipient, nonanastomotic strictures or bilomas that often indicate biliary ischemia and should stimulate a close examination of the arterial supply for hepatic artery stenosis or thrombosis, and more general complications such as stone formation and cholangitis.

In this case, the patient had already undergone repair of a thrombosed donor right hepatic artery, with an interposition graft between the patient's common hepatic artery and the donor right hepatic artery. Unfortunately, the interposition graft also thrombosed, and the thrombosis is seen as an abrupt cutoff of the common hepatic artery on the arterial phase 3D SPGR image. Notice also the severe stenosis of the celiac artery origin. This finding should have been described on preoperative imaging and might have had a role in the subsequent hepatic artery thrombosis.

Hepatic artery thrombosis is the most common vascular complication of orthotopic liver transplantation and occurs in 3% to 9% of cases, usually within the first 4 months following surgery. Duplex sonography has a high sensitivity and a high specificity for detection of hepatic artery thrombosis, and MRI is not typically a first-order test for this indication (small studies have showed that MR angiography is also accurate for detection of hepatic artery thrombosis but tends to overestimate the degree of hepatic artery stenosis). It is worth remembering, however, that the dynamic postgadolinium 3D SPGR images obtained in virtually every patient are generally more than adequate to screen for arterial and venous complications, as illustrated by this case, where both hepatic artery thrombosis and portal vein thrombosis are easily demonstrated.

Portal vein thrombosis occurs in approximately 3% of liver transplantations, most commonly involving the main extrahepatic portal vein. The observation in this case that the thrombosis begins in the region of the anastomosis might suggest a surgical complication.

Given the fact that this patient has seemingly lost his entire blood supply to the transplant, it may seem odd that there is any enhancement of the liver at all. This situation is probably explained by the recruitment of multiple small arterial and venous collaterals from the porta hepatis and diaphragm. Although these vessels can maintain a small blood supply to the liver, they usually are not adequate to prevent biliary necrosis, and this patient was relisted for transplantation.

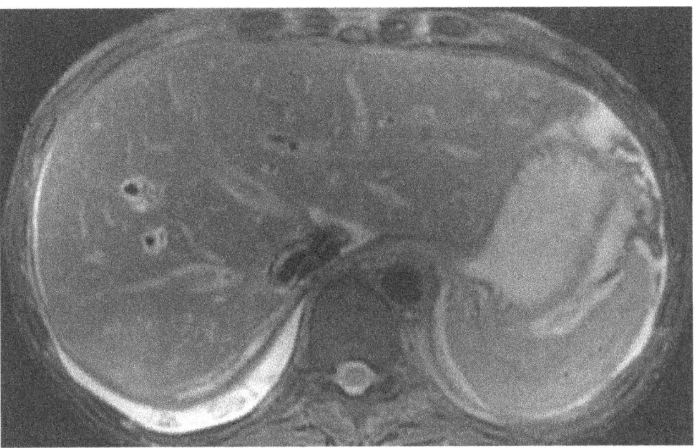

Figure 2.20.1

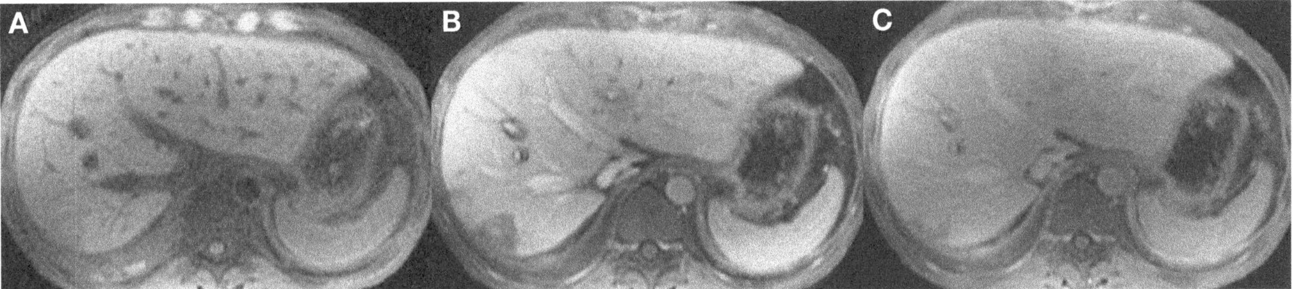

Figure 2.20.2

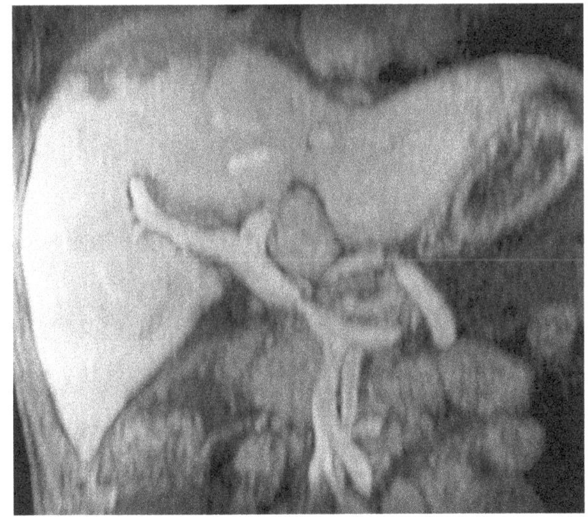

Figure 2.20.3

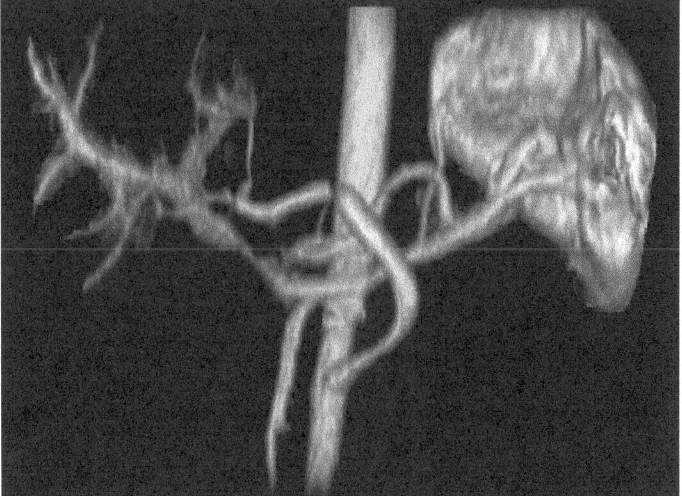

Figure 2.20.4

HISTORY: 29-year-old man with history of liver transplantation for advanced PSC performed 5 weeks ago, now with increasing elevation of hepatic enzymes

IMAGING FINDINGS: Axial fat-suppressed FSE T2-weighted image (Figure 2.20.1) demonstrates a subtle area of mildly increased signal intensity in the periphery of the right hepatic lobe. Biliary ducts were unremarkable on MRCP (images not shown). Pregadolinium, portal venous, and equilibrium phase postgadolinium 3D SPGR images (Figure 2.20.2) show peripheral wedge-shaped perfusion defects that gradually fill in within the posterior right hepatic lobe. Coronal oblique reformatted image (Figure 2.20.3) from portal venous phase postgadolinium 3D SPGR acquisition reveals a more confluent region of minimal enhancement in the hepatic dome, as well as moderate narrowing of the main portal vein at the anastomosis. VR image (Figure 2.20.4) reconstructed from arterial phase 3D SPGR data demonstrates severe focal narrowing at the anastomosis of the graft from the infrarenal aorta to the donor common hepatic artery and again shows narrowing of the portal vein anastomosis.

DIAGNOSIS: Liver transplant with hepatic artery stenosis, portal vein stenosis, and peripheral infarcts

COMMENT: Small peripheral infarcts in a transplant liver are sometimes the result of size differences between the donor and the recipient (ie, the transplant liver is too large and is compressed against the diaphragm of the recipient). The larger confluent infarct seen on the coronal reformatted image is more extensive than expected for this relatively minor complication and suggests a more serious cause, which is confirmed by the severe stenosis at the hepatic artery anastomosis.

It is unlikely that the degree of stenosis can always be accurately determined by reconstructing arterial phase data from a dynamic 3D SPGR acquisition—the spatial resolution is not ideal and the timing of the acquisition is optimized for visualization of the hepatic parenchymal arterial phase rather than for visualization of peak arterial enhancement. Another confounding factor may be the presence of metallic artifact from surgical clips at the anastomosis; this can be verified by inspecting the axial source images for susceptibility artifact extending beyond the arteries. Nevertheless, the severe stenosis seen in this case is quite convincing and was likely responsible for the peripheral infarcts.

The clinical significance of the portal vein stenosis is less certain, but it is clearly visualized and again illustrates the general principle that standard, dynamic 3D SPGR acquisitions can detect most vascular complications of liver transplantation.

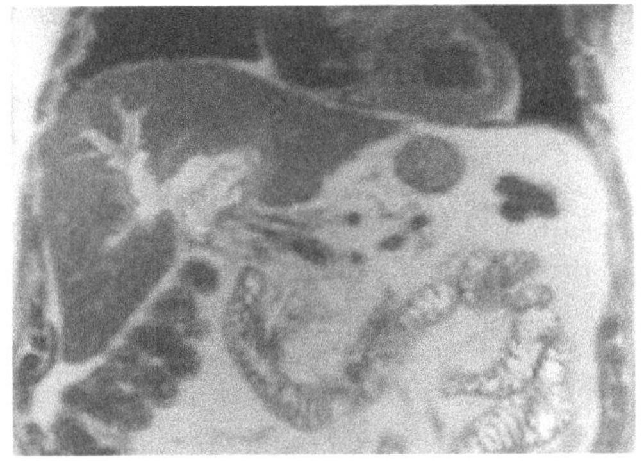

Figure 2.21.1

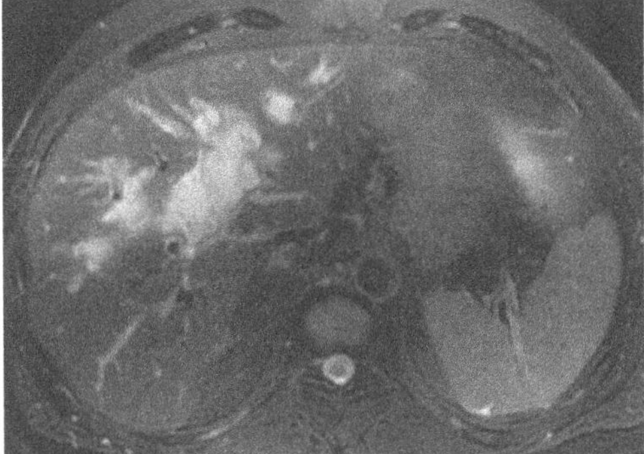

Figure 2.21.2

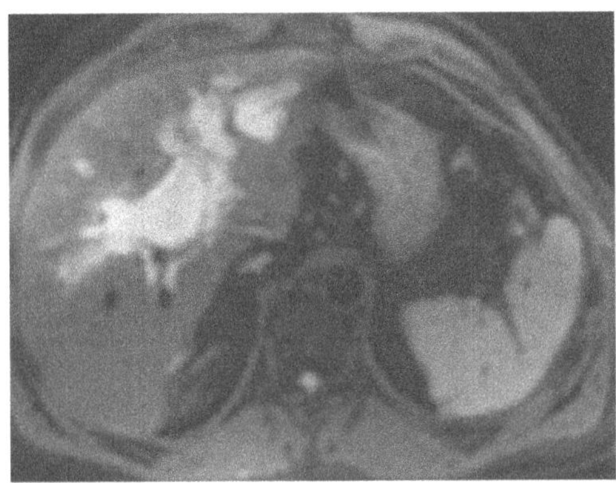

Figure 2.21.3

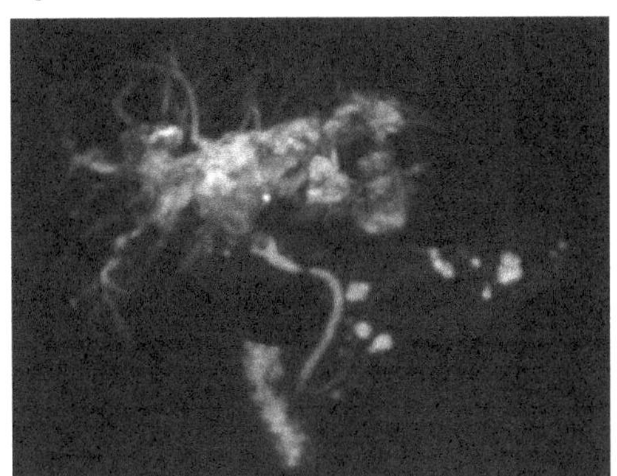

Figure 2.21.4

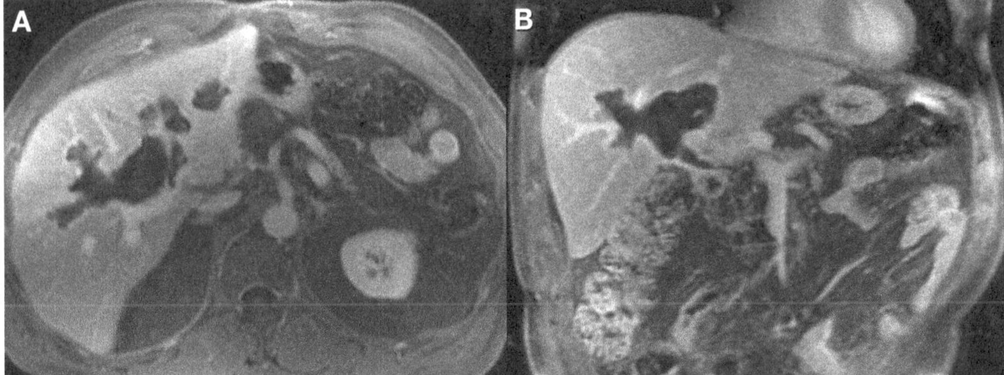

Figure 2.21.5

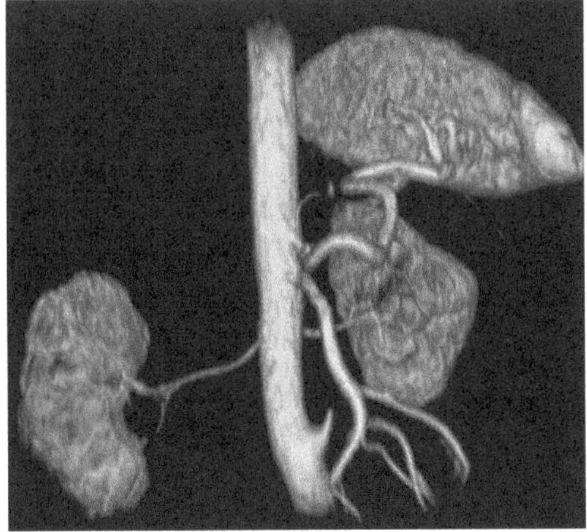

Figure 2.21.6

HISTORY: 57-year-old man status post liver transplantation 13 years ago, now with increasing cholestasis

IMAGING FINDINGS: Coronal SSFSE (Figure 2.21.1), axial fat-suppressed FSE T2-weighted (Figure 2.21.2), and diffusion-weighted (b=600 s/mm^2) (Figure 2.21.3) images demonstrate heterogeneous high signal intensity in the porta hepatis, with mild dilatation of peripheral intrahepatic biliary ducts. MIP image from 3D MRCP (Figure 2.21.4) shows similar findings. Notice also a focal stricture of the common duct at the anastomosis, as well as multiple pancreatic intraductal papillary mucinous neoplasms. Axial oblique and coronal oblique reformatted images from portal venous phase postgadolinium 3D SPGR acquisition (Figure 2.21.5) reveal large rim-enhancing fluid collections in the porta hepatis that follow a ductal distribution. VR image (Figure 2.21.6) from arterial phase 3D SPGR postgadolinium data shows proximal occlusion of a hepatic artery graft originating from the distal abdominal aorta.

DIAGNOSIS: Liver transplant with hepatic artery thrombosis and extensive biliary necrosis

COMMENT: This is another, more impressive illustration of hepatic artery thrombosis causing biliary ischemia. In this case, the central biliary ducts are completely necrotic, resulting in a large biloma in the porta hepatis with associated peripheral biliary dilatation. The focal stricture at the biliary anastomosis is probably not an ischemic complication.

Notice that the arterial phase postgadolinium 3D SPGR data, although not as optimal in spatial resolution and arterial timing as a dedicated MR angiogram would have been, is nevertheless capable of generating reasonable 3D VR images.

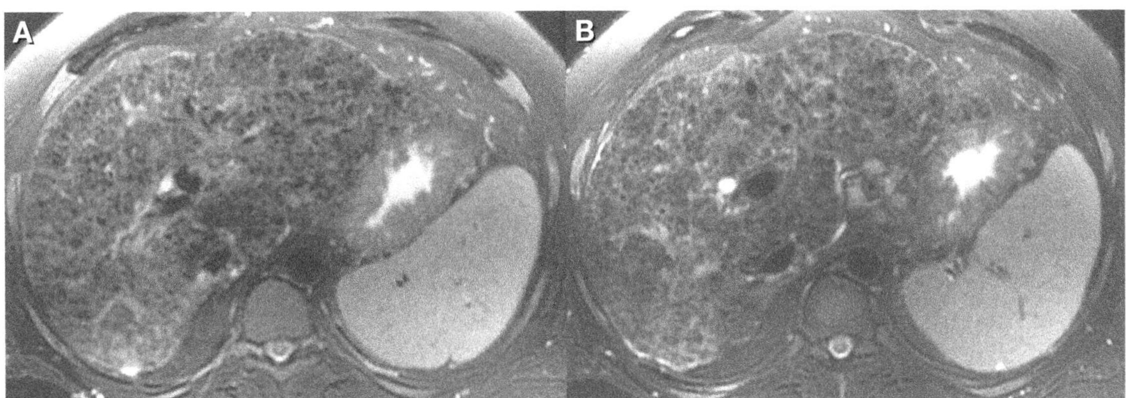

Figure 2.22.1

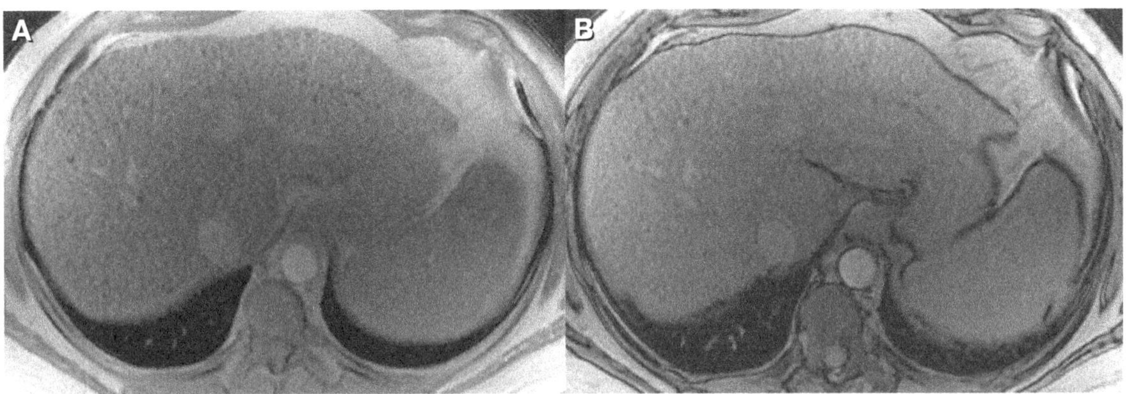

Figure 2.22.2

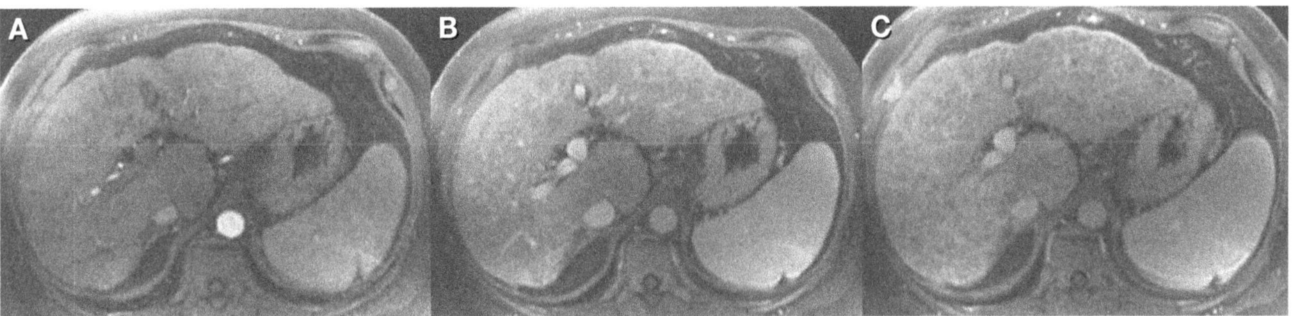

Figure 2.22.3

HISTORY: 52-year-old man with chronic liver disease

IMAGING FINDINGS: Axial fat-suppressed T2-weighted FSE images (Figure 2.22.1) and axial IP and OP T1-weighted 2D SPGR images (Figure 2.22.2) demonstrate a cirrhotic liver with innumerable hypointense nodules. Axial arterial, portal venous, and equilibrium phase postgadolinium 3D SPGR images (Figure 2.22.3) demonstrate underlying parenchymal nodularity but no suspicious focal hepatic mass. Notice the extensive linear and reticular enhancement on the equilibrium phase image, as well as splenic enlargement.

DIAGNOSIS: Cirrhosis

COMMENT: Cirrhosis represents a common pathway for chronic liver injury and is characterized pathologically by bridging fibrosis, nodular transformation, and distortion of the normal hepatic architecture. Repeated injury to the liver causes fibrogenic cytokines to activate collagen-producing hepatic stellate cells. Excess deposition of collagen, proteoglycans, and other macromolecules in the extracellular matrix promote scar formation that bridges adjacent portal triads and central veins. Allowed to progress, these fibrous bands thicken, coalesce, and create the nodularity (regenerative nodules) of a cirrhotic liver.

Cirrhosis can be classified according to the size of the nodules as *micronodular* (diameter <3 mm; most commonly seen in alcoholic liver disease) or *macronodular* (diameter 3 mm-3 cm; characteristic of viral hepatitis). Morphologic changes of advanced cirrhosis are easy to detect and include a shrunken liver with irregular margins and internal nodularity, as well as signs of portal hypertension such as abdominal varices, ascites, and splenomegaly. Several more subtle findings have been described to aid in the detection of early cirrhosis, including enlargement of the hilar periportal space, enlargement of the interlobar fissure, expansion of the gallbladder fossa, and atrophy of the posterior right and medial left lobe with hypertrophy of the caudate lobe and lateral left lobe.

In advanced cirrhosis, bridging fibrosis can be seen on fat-suppressed T2-weighted images as linear or reticulated regions of high signal intensity, illustrated in this case. Similar findings are seen on equilibrium phase or delayed phase postgadolinium images because the fibrotic bands retain gadolinium longer than normal liver parenchyma and appear hyperintense. *Confluent fibrosis* describes broader areas of fibrosis up to several centimeters in size and occasionally confused with focal masses. An example of confluent fibrosis is shown in Case 2.26.

The nodules in this case are larger than 3 mm in diameter and have the additional property of low signal intensity on T2-weighted images, indicating that they probably contain iron and could be classified as siderotic. Iron-sensitive, multiecho GRE pulse sequences are a good way to detect siderotic regenerative nodules, as illustrated in Case 2.28, and may sometimes help to reveal more advanced cirrhosis than can be appreciated on conventional images.

This patient's cirrhosis was the result of nonalcoholic fatty liver disease, which represents a range of disorders characterized by hepatic steatosis in the absence of other causative factors, such as excessive alcohol consumption or viral hepatitis. This disease is extremely common, is related to obesity and type 2 diabetes mellitus, and is estimated to affect as much as 50% of the population of some countries. The histologic spectrum of nonalcoholic fatty liver disease ranges from simple steatosis, characterized by the presence of triglyceride droplets within hepatocytes, to nonalcoholic steatohepatitis (or NASH), typified by liver injury and inflammation, and can progress to cirrhosis.

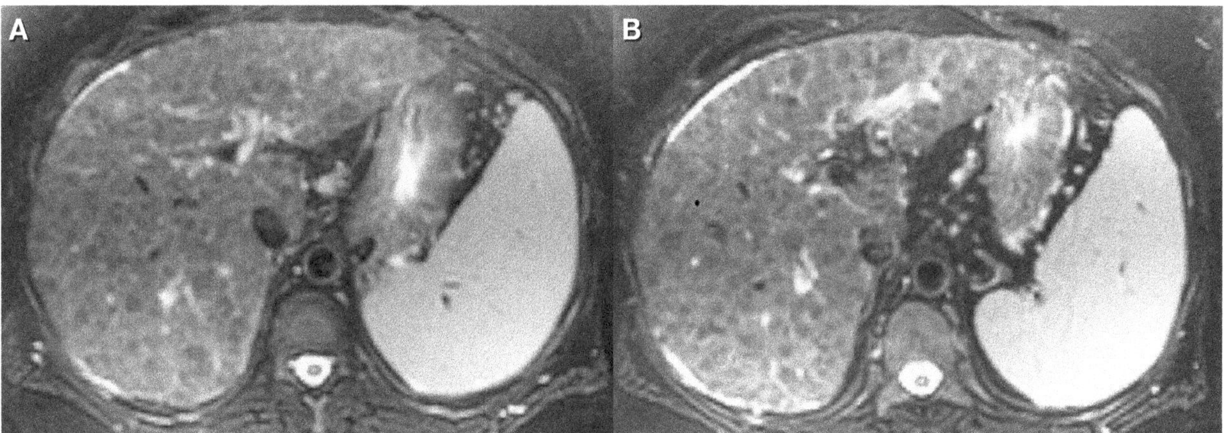

Figure 2.23.1

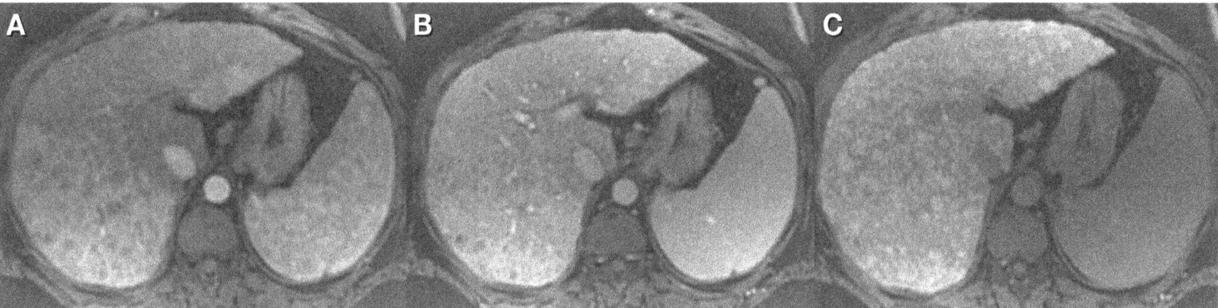

Figure 2.23.2

HISTORY: 55-year-old woman with chronic liver disease

IMAGING FINDINGS: Axial fat-suppressed FSE T2-weighted images (Figure 2.23.1) demonstrate a cirrhotic liver with diffuse, innumerable, small low-signal-intensity nodules. Axial arterial, portal venous, and hepatobiliary phase postgadolinium (Eovist) 3D SPGR images (Figure 2.23.2) demonstrate heterogeneous enhancement of the background parenchyma, particularly in the right hepatic lobe. The multiple nodules are initially hypointense on arterial and portal venous phase images but become hyperintense relative to adjacent liver on the hepatobiliary phase image.

DIAGNOSIS: Cirrhosis with regenerative nodules

COMMENT: This case illustrates the appearance of regenerative nodules in cirrhosis with use of the hepatobiliary contrast agent Eovist. Enhancement of the liver is heterogeneous on the arterial phase image, particularly in the right lobe, with multiple hypoenhancing nodules visible on both the arterial and portal venous phase images. These nodules become hyperintense on the hepatobiliary phase images—in contrast to their appearance with standard extracellular agents, where they are typically isointense or hypointense compared with adjacent liver.

The hepatobiliary phase hyperenhancement of regenerative nodules seen in this case is probably a reflection of the slightly delayed excretion of contrast engendered by the disordered nature of the regenerative nodules and associated biliary radicles, as well as the presence of fibrosis in adjacent hepatic parenchyma, which reduces the total amount of contrast taken up by hepatocytes in a given volume of tissue.

Not all regenerative nodules are hyperintense on hepatobiliary phase images; some are isointense. However, the presence of a hypointense nodule should raise concern for HCC. This appearance is not always indicative of HCC and is illustrated by the small nodule in the right lobe in this patient, which remains hypointense on the hepatobiliary phase images (and has remained stable on follow-up imaging). An arterial phase hyperenhancing lesion that becomes hypointense in the hepatobiliary phase is the most suspicious; however, even a small percentage of these nodules are likely benign. Siderotic regenerative nodules in particular are likely to appear relatively hypointense on hepatobiliary phase images by virtue of their susceptibility effect. Some reassurance can be provided by noting that these nodules are hypointense on precontrast 3D SPGR images.

Hepatobiliary contrast agents may not be the best choice for patients with severe cirrhosis and significantly reduced hepatic function: Hepatic uptake of contrast is diminished and biliary excretion is reduced, generating hepatobiliary phase images of marginal utility. The package insert for Eovist indicates that in patients with severe hepatic impairment, especially patients with abnormally high serum bilirubin levels (>3 mg/dL), the elimination half-life was increased up to 49%, the hepatobiliary excretion decreased to about 5%, and reduced hepatic signal intensity was seen on hepatobiliary phase images. These observations suggest that if your practice routinely uses Eovist in the cirrhotic patient population, some mechanism for screening hepatic function is a good idea.

CASE 2.24

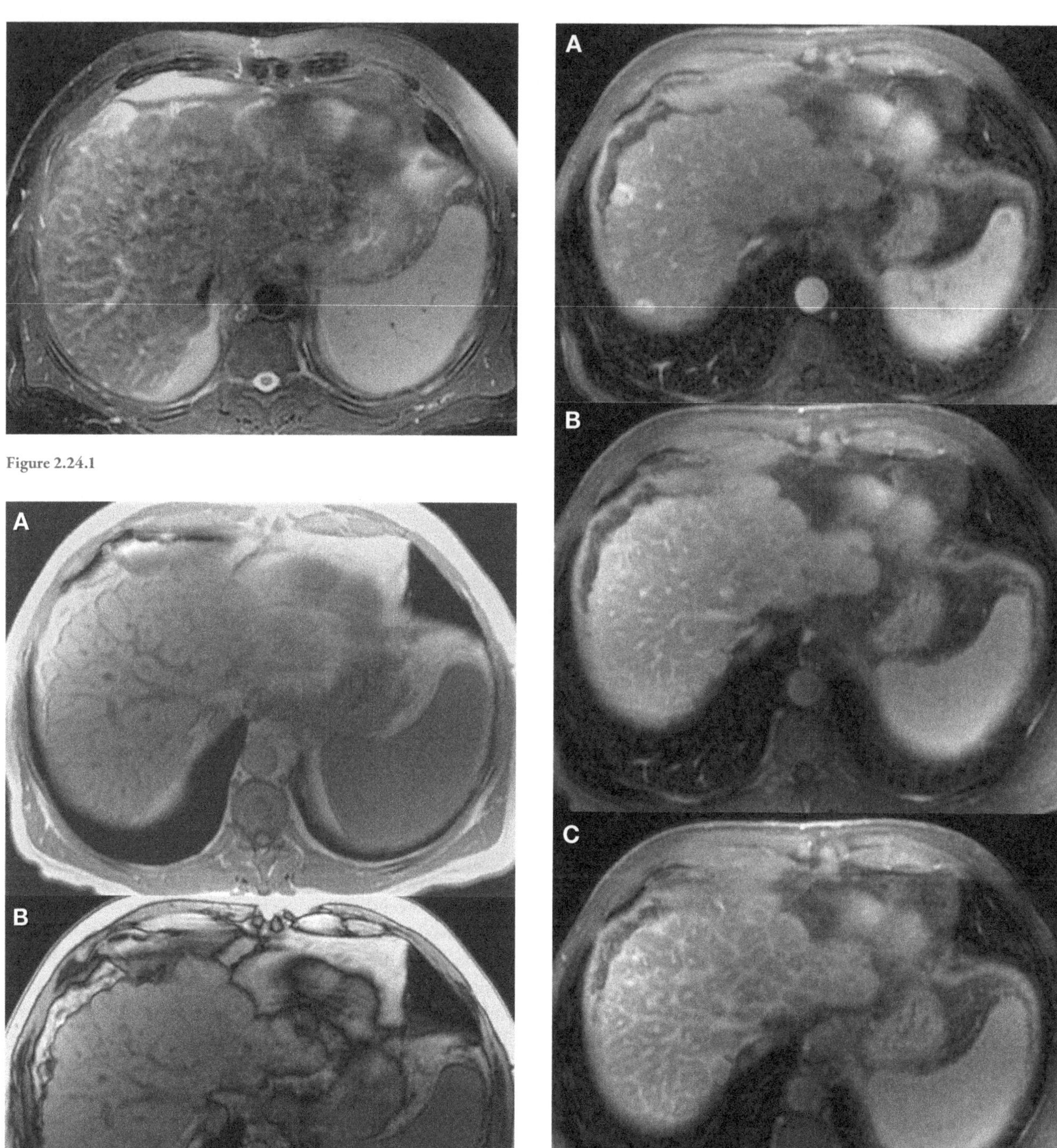

Figure 2.24.1

Figure 2.24.2

Figure 2.24.3

HISTORY: 56-year-old man with chronic liver disease

IMAGING FINDINGS: Axial fat-suppressed FSE T2-weighted (Figure 2.24.1) and axial IP and OP T1-weighted 2D SPGR (Figure 2.24.2) images demonstrate a nodular hepatic contour and parenchymal background. Axial arterial phase postgadolinium 3D SPGR image (Figure 2.24.3A) demonstrates 2 small hyperenhancing lesions in the periphery of the right hepatic lobe that become isointense to background hepatic parenchyma on later portal venous (Figure 2.24.3B) and equilibrium (Figure 2.24.3C) phase acquisitions.

DIAGNOSIS: Transient hepatic intensity defects in the clinical setting of cirrhosis

COMMENT: THIDs are analogous to transient hepatic attenuation defects (or THADs), initially described on CT, and have been ascribed to arterioportal shunts, intrahepatic vascular compression or occlusion, steal phenomenon by adjacent hypervascular tumors, or background inflammatory or infectious processes leading to heterogeneous parenchymal perfusion. The classic THID, illustrated in this case, manifests only on arterial phase postgadolinium images and isn't seen on precontrast T1- or T2-weighted images, and cannot be visualized on portal venous or equilibrium phase postgadolinium images.

THIDs occasionally pose difficulties in interpretation because they are much more common in cirrhotic livers and a small percentage of them are in fact not THIDs at all, but instead are small HCCs. Several initial papers described an incidence of HCC on follow-up imaging that ranged from 2% to 8%. Although the inclusion criteria for some of these papers were probably overly generous, it remains accepted wisdom that a small percentage of these lesions (probably 1%-2%) are actually HCCs or high-grade dysplastic nodules.

A great deal of time and effort has been devoted in recent years to this problem, in particular focusing on the added value of DWI and the use of hepatobiliary contrast agents. Several authors have demonstrated that THIDs not showing high signal intensity on diffusion-weighted images (ie, restricted diffusion) are very unlikely to be malignant. Likewise, THIDs that are not hypointense relative to adjacent liver on hepatobiliary phase images are almost certainly benign. Advocates of both these techniques can point to papers describing essentially perfect accuracy in discriminating benign THIDs from HCCs. Unfortunately, however, a small percentage of HCCs are not hyperintense on DWI and a small percentage are isointense or hyperintense compared to adjacent liver on hepatobiliary phase images acquired after administration of a hepatobiliary contrast agent.

The level of uncertainty probably increases in patients with severely cirrhotic livers. Diffusion-weighted images may be degraded by phase ghosting artifact from ascites or by susceptibility artifact in patients with multiple siderotic nodules, and the heterogeneous signal in patients with extensive fibrosis may make discrimination of small focal lesions more difficult. Similarly, hepatic uptake of hepatobiliary contrast agents is reduced in severe cirrhosis, and discrimination of small regions of low signal intensity becomes more difficult in very nodular and heterogeneous livers.

Patients with THIDs usually have follow-up imaging, typically at an interval of 6 months. This isn't a major imposition since most of them are initially imaged in the setting of cirrhosis surveillance and already require periodic follow-up screening with MRI or CT. Assessing for interval growth of these lesions, however, can be very challenging because the size of the arterial blush is highly dependent on the exact timing of the arterial phase acquisition. Differences of a few seconds can make lesions disappear or grow. Our solution is that although we notice and remark on these changes in size detected on arterial phase images, we pay much more attention to development of increased signal intensity on T2- or diffusion-weighted images, washout on portal venous phase images, or hypointensity on hepatobiliary phase images—all of which are very worrisome signs for HCC.

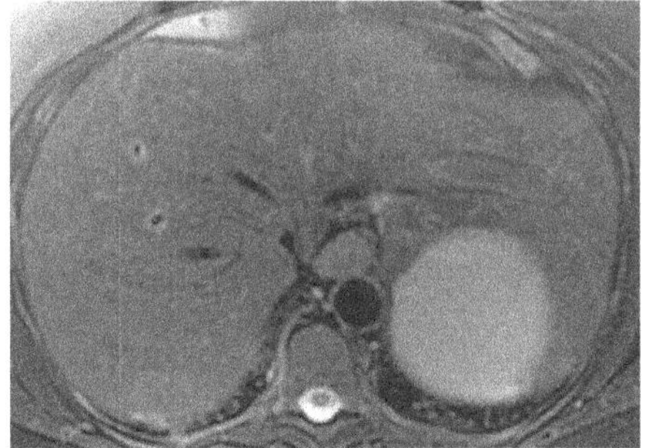

Figure 2.24.4

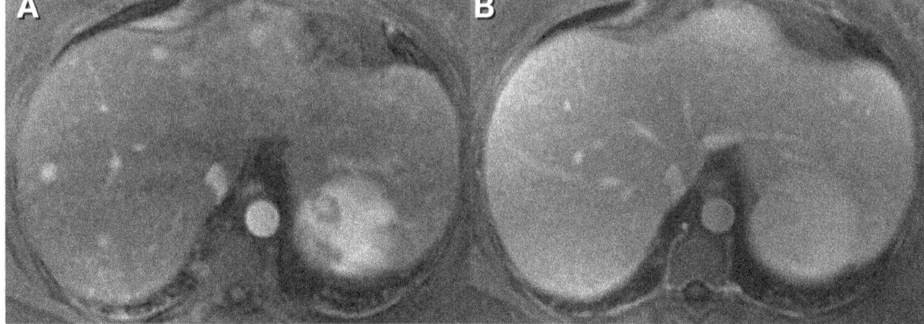

Figure 2.24.5

In this similar case of more obvious THIDs, an axial fat-suppressed T2-weighted image (Figure 2.24.4) demonstrates no findings, and the hyperenhancing foci on the postgadolinium arterial phase image (Figure 2.24.5A) are not present on the portal venous phase image (Figure 2.24.5B).

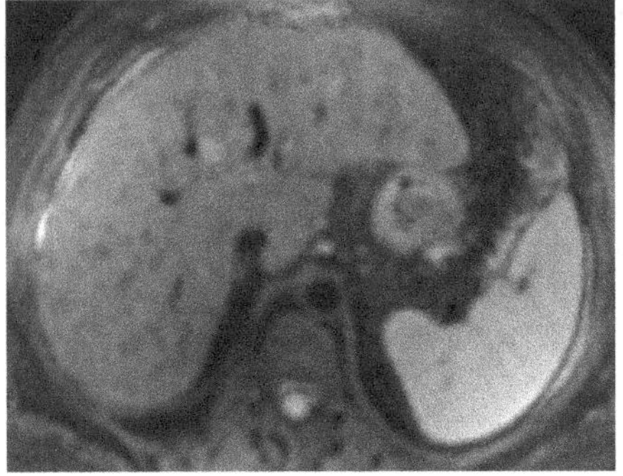

Figure 2.25.1

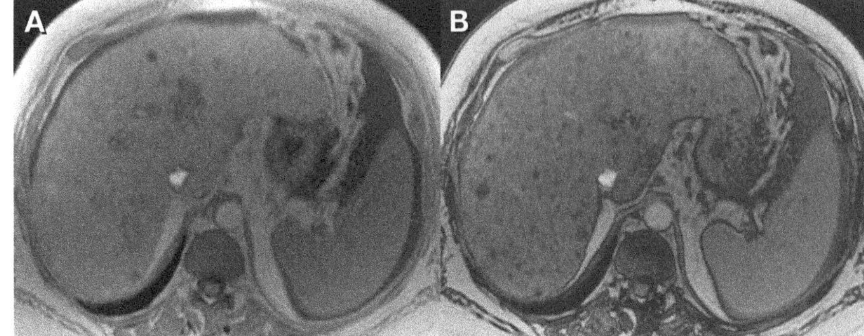

Figure 2.25.2

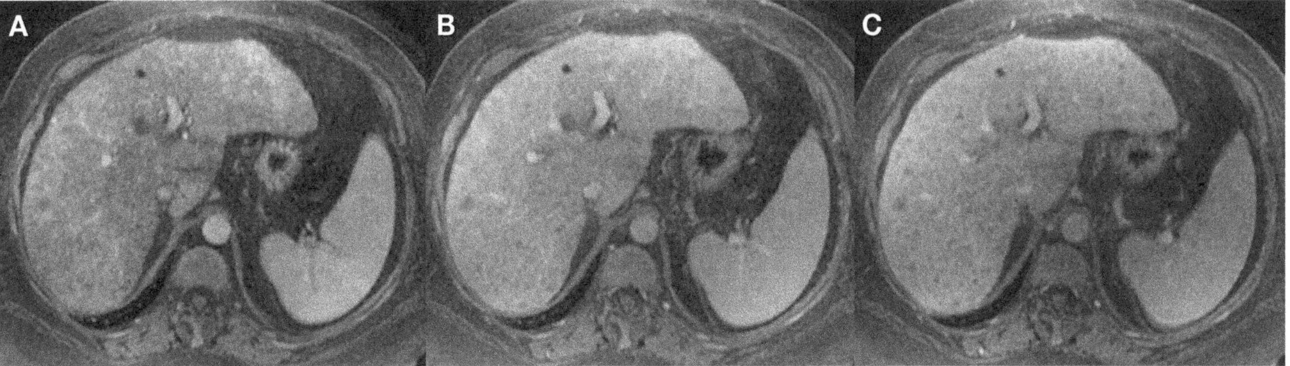

Figure 2.25.3

HISTORY: 60-year-old woman with chronic liver disease

IMAGING FINDINGS: Axial diffusion-weighted image (b=100 s/mm^2) (Figure 2.25.1) demonstrates a mildly irregular hepatic contour with parenchymal nodularity and a hyperintense lesion in the medial left lobe. The IP and OP T1-weighted 2D SPGR images (Figure 2.25.2) show multiple mildly hyperintense nodules on the IP image that become hypointense on the OP image. The left lobe lesion remains mildly hyperintense on the OP image. Note also mild diffuse parenchymal signal loss from the IP image to the OP image. Arterial, portal venous, and equilibrium phase postgadolinium 3D SPGR images (Figure 2.25.3) demonstrate heterogeneous enhancement of the background parenchyma with innumerable hypoenhancing nodules best seen on the equilibrium phase image. The left lobe nodule shows little enhancement on arterial and portal venous phase images, with mild heterogeneous enhancement on the equilibrium phase image. A small cyst is seen in the anterior left lobe.

DIAGNOSIS: Cirrhosis with fatty regenerative nodules and a larger regenerative or dysplastic nodule

COMMENT: The extensive nodularity of the liver is best appreciated on the IP and OP images, which also show the fatty content of the regenerative nodules, as well as a background of mild diffuse hepatic steatosis. The presence of fat in a small percentage of HCCs is a well-known phenomenon, but it is less widely recognized that fat can occasionally be seen within regenerative or dysplastic nodules, with this case representing our most impressive example. A fat-containing lesion in a cirrhotic liver, therefore, should raise the possibility of HCC, but HCC should not always be the presumed diagnosis without additional supportive evidence. In this case, for example, the nodules do not show arterial phase hyperenhancement or increased signal intensity on diffusion-weighted images.

The distinction between fatty regenerative nodules and nodular fatty infiltration is not entirely clear; however, given the clinical history of chronic liver disease, the cirrhotic configuration of the liver, and the presence of innumerable small nodules, the diagnosis of fatty regenerative nodules is more likely correct.

The distinction between regenerative and dysplastic nodules and HCC is also not absolute on MRI, but the features most worrisome for malignant progression are development of increased signal intensity on T2- or diffusion-weighted images and recruitment of an arterial blood supply, resulting in arterial phase hyperenhancement following gadolinium administration. Hyperintensity on T2-weighted images is best appreciated with a respiratory-triggered fat-suppressed FSE acquisition, whereas the non–fat-suppressed SSFSE technique favored by many practices limits visualization of all but the most obvious masses. Contrast washout in nodules is also a useful sign—this requires a drop in the relative signal intensity of the nodule compared to adjacent liver from the arterial phase to the portal venous or equilibrium phase, and its presence is worrisome for HCC.

The dominant nodule in the medial left lobe is somewhat suspicious by virtue of its increased signal intensity on diffusion-weighted images and its mild enhancement on the equilibrium phase image. It remained stable after 2 years of follow-up examinations, however, and likely represents a regenerative or dysplastic nodule.

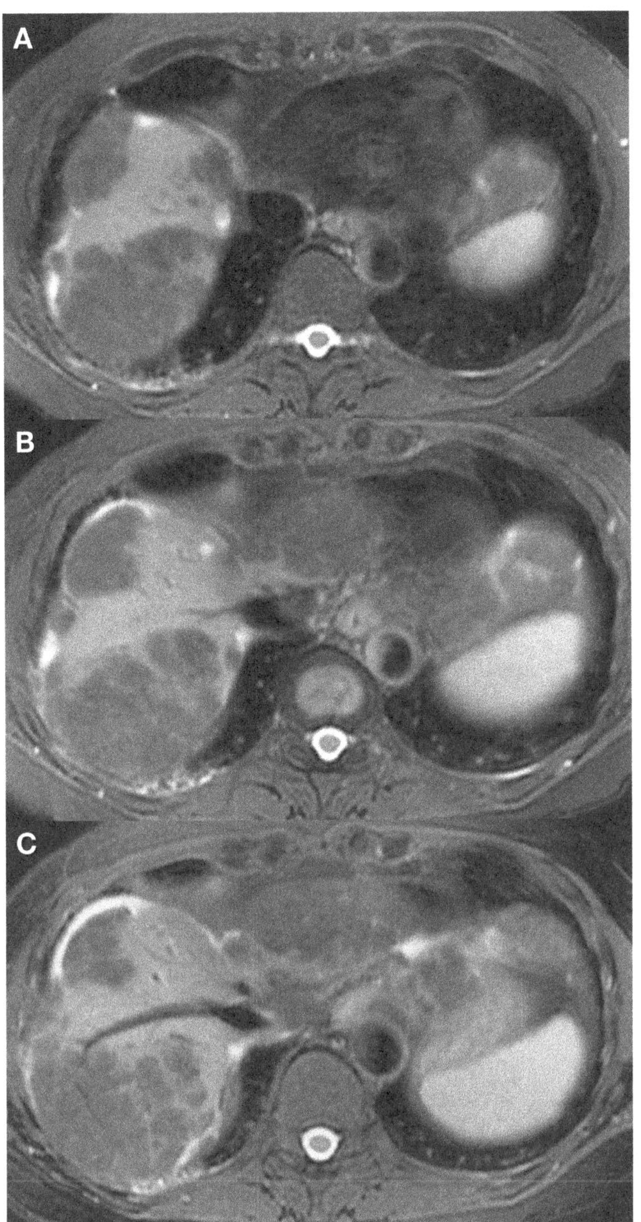

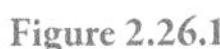
Figure 2.26.1

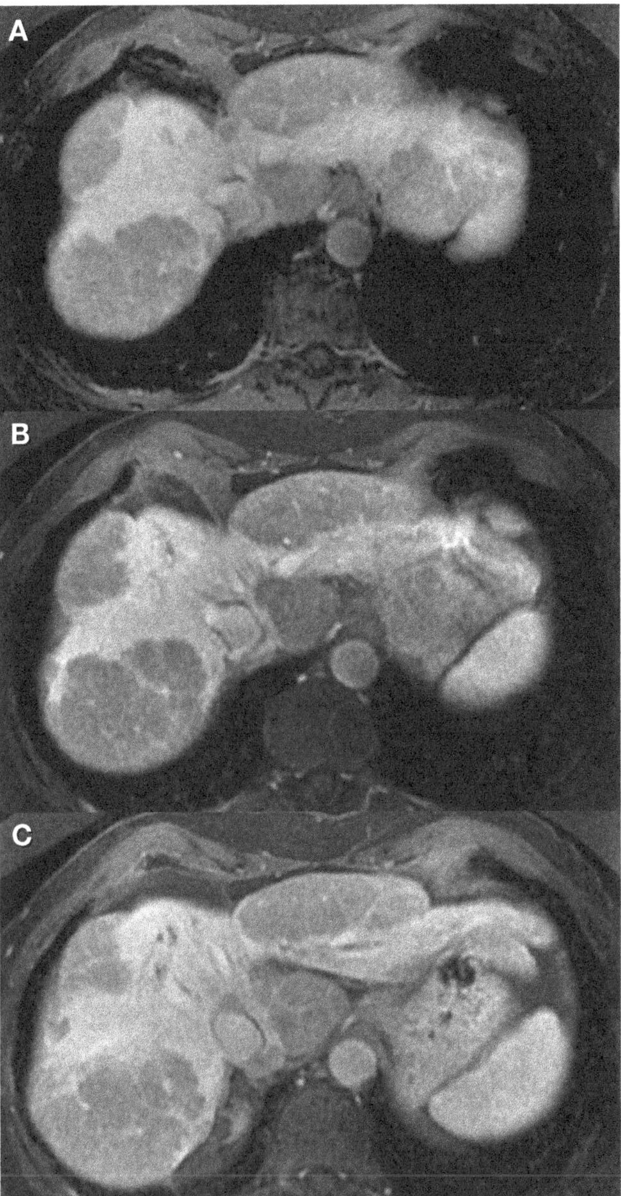

Figure 2.26.2

HISTORY: 60-year-old woman with PSC

IMAGING FINDINGS: Axial fat-suppressed FSE T2-weighted images (Figure 2.26.1) demonstrate a cirrhotic configuration of the liver with bands of increased T2 signal and associated capsular retraction involving the hepatic dome, as well as the anterior right and medial left lobes. Axial equilibrium phase postgadolinium 3D SPGR images (Figure 2.26.2) demonstrate corresponding enhancement of these regions.

DIAGNOSIS: Confluent fibrosis and cirrhosis

COMMENT: Confluent fibrosis is a somewhat subjective description of large regions of fibrosis in a cirrhotic liver. These fibrotic regions generally have a geographic or wedge-shaped distribution and show increased signal intensity on T2-weighted images. Following gadolinium administration, confluent fibrosis appears hypointense compared to adjacent liver on arterial phase images and then gradually accumulates contrast, becoming hyperintense on equilibrium phase images.

Confluent fibrosis is a fairly common finding in PSC patients with advanced disease and may also be seen in other types of cirrhosis. Distinguishing confluent fibrosis from a focal mass is usually possible on the basis of its geographic, rather than masslike, distribution and the relatively minor mass effect. Notice in this case, for example, how the right hepatic vein passes through the region of fibrosis with minimal distortion. There are occasional difficult cases, however, particularly in PSC patients, where cholangiocarcinoma is the major differential diagnosis and may have very similar imaging characteristics.

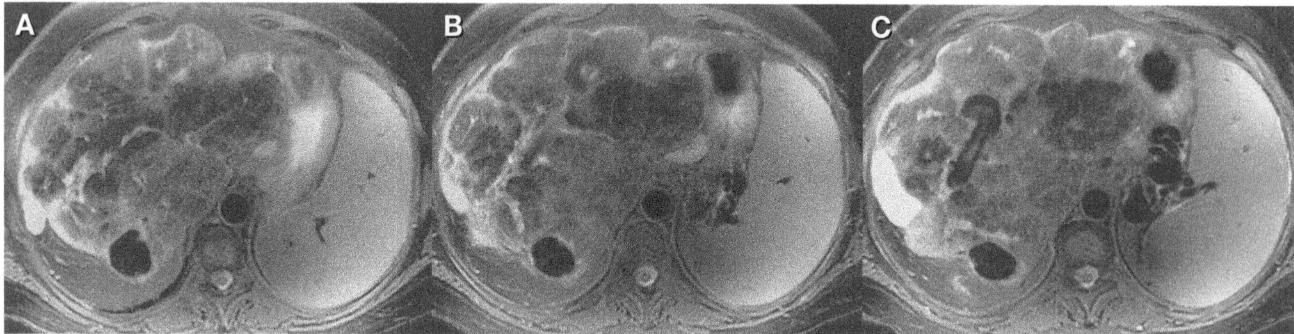

Figure 2.27.1

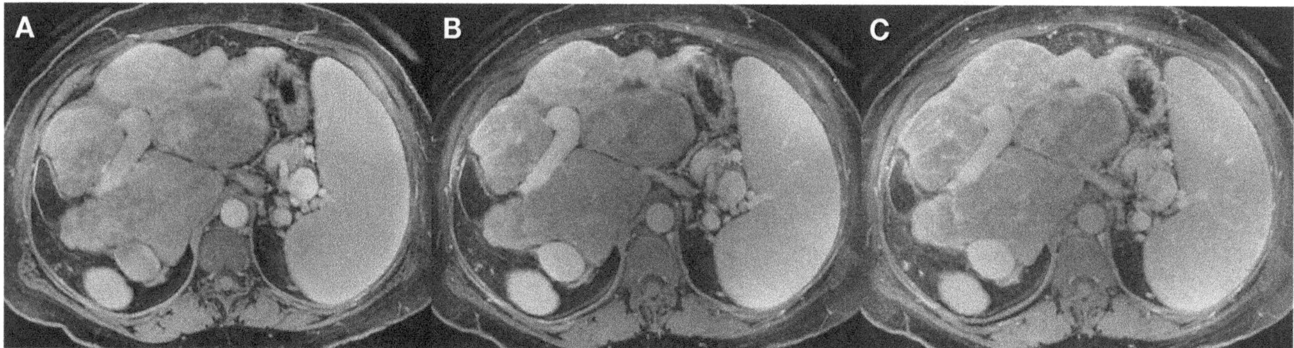

Figure 2.27.2

HISTORY: 51-year-old woman with advanced liver disease

IMAGING FINDINGS: Axial fat-suppressed FSE T2-weighted images (Figure 2.27.1) and axial arterial, portal venous, and equilibrium phase postgadolinium 3D SPGR images (Figure 2.27.2) demonstrate macronodularity of the hepatic parenchyma, marked atrophy of the right hepatic lobe, and hypertrophy of the caudate lobe.

DIAGNOSIS: Macronodular cirrhosis of primary sclerosing cholangitis

COMMENT: The extensive macroscopic nodularity of the liver, as well as the marked hypertrophy of the caudate lobe, is said to be characteristic of cirrhosis resulting from PSC, although the sensitivity and specificity of these findings are uncertain. More characteristic findings of PSC, including multifocal central and peripheral biliary strictures, as well as mural thickening and enhancement of intra- and extrahepatic bile ducts, are generally more helpful in making a confident diagnosis. PSC is also well known for generating impressive confluent fibrosis, and this is illustrated in Case 2.26.

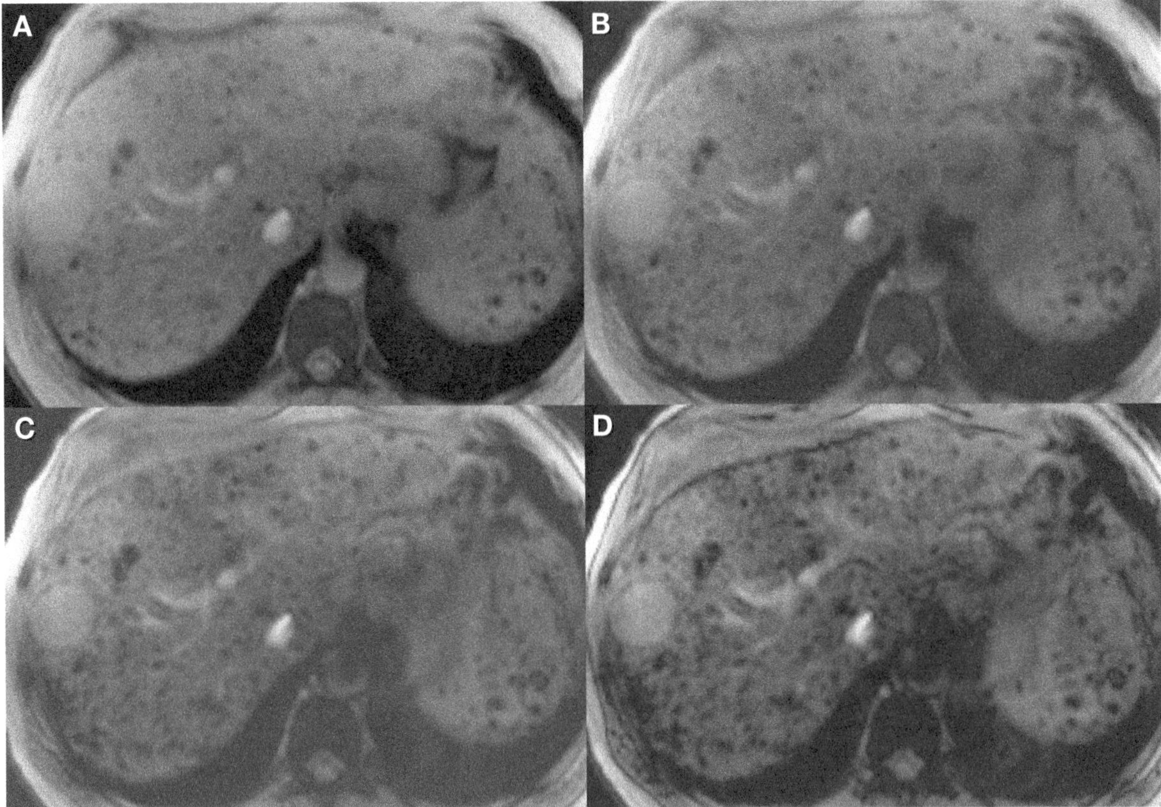

Figure 2.28.1

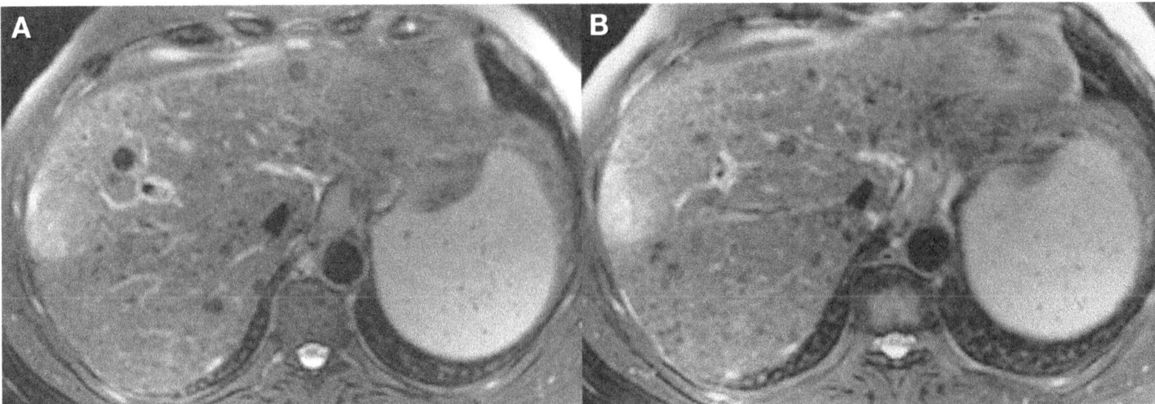

Figure 2.28.2

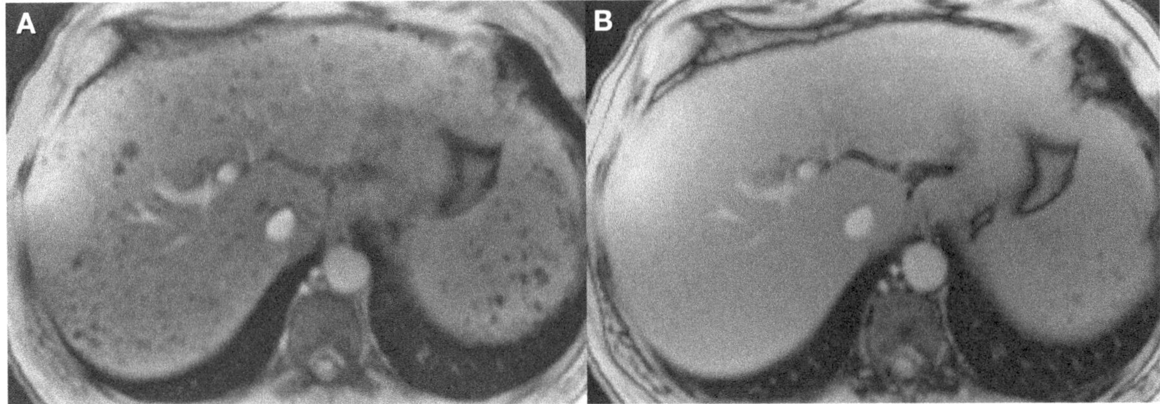

Figure 2.28.3

HISTORY: 57-year-old man with history of chronic hepatitis B virus infection

IMAGING FINDINGS: Axial multiecho (TEs of 2.4, 6.3, 10.0, and 14.2 ms) GRE images (Figure 2.28.1) demonstrate innumerable hypointense nodules throughout the liver and spleen that become more prominent as the TE increases. Notice also the large mass in the lateral right hepatic lobe. Axial fat-suppressed FSE T2-weighted (Figure 2.28.2) and IP and OP (Figure 2.28.3) images reveal similar findings, although the nodules are more difficult to visualize.

DIAGNOSIS: Cirrhosis with siderotic nodules and hepatocellular carcinoma

COMMENT: Siderotic nodules are regenerative nodules containing iron and are best visualized on GRE acquisitions obtained with relatively long TEs to emphasize the T2* susceptibility effect of iron. The multiecho GRE pulse sequence for iron quantification is an excellent technique to demonstrate this effect and shows increasing signal dropout within the nodules with each successively longer TE.

Many years ago, there was a discussion in the literature regarding whether iron within regenerative nodules constituted a risk factor for the development of HCC; although a few authors did find an elevated relative risk, this result has not been widely replicated, and siderotic nodules today are regarded more as an imaging curiosity than a clinically relevant finding. That's not to say that siderotic nodules can be ignored, since the incidence of HCC in patients with cirrhosis is much higher than in persons with normal livers, as illustrated by the large mass in this patient.

Occasionally, the presence of iron is helpful as a diagnostic aid. Notice, for example, how the conspicuity of the HCC increases on the multiecho GRE sequence with longer TEs as the signal intensity from background liver gradually diminishes. A similar, although less prominent, T2 shortening effect also occurs in the FSE images. On the other hand, iron is not particularly helpful for diffusion-weighted acquisitions, where the susceptibility effects can lead to very low signal intensity and can occasionally mask small lesions. Use of the shortest possible TE for DWI of patients with prominent iron deposition in the liver can help to minimize this artifact.

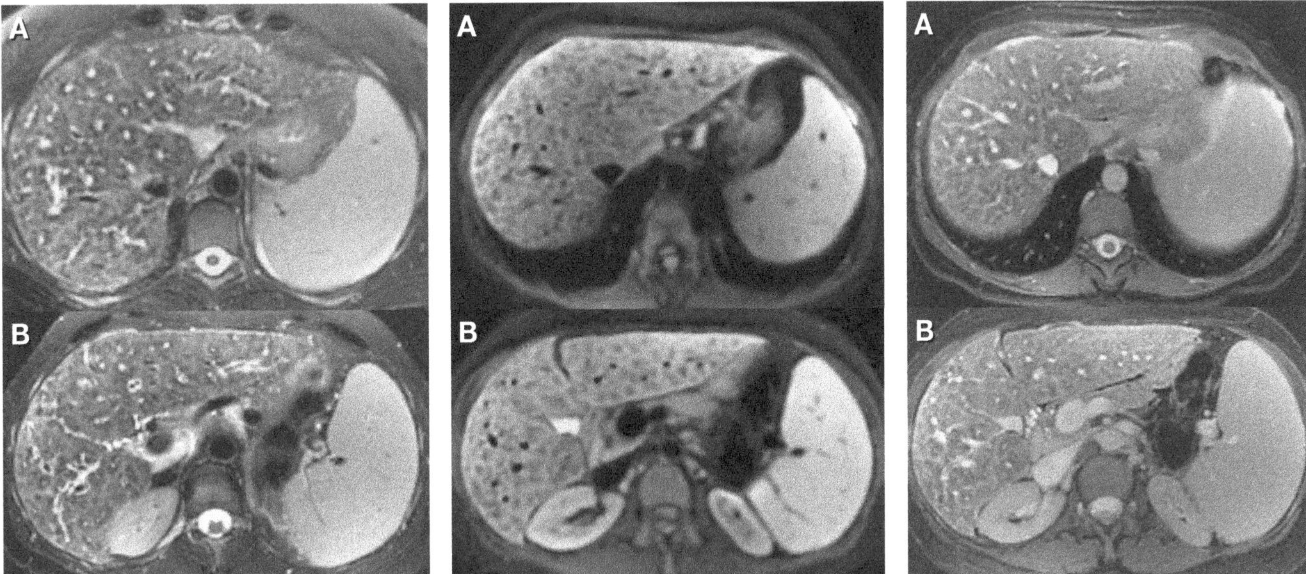

Figure 2.29.1 Figure 2.29.2 Figure 2.29.3

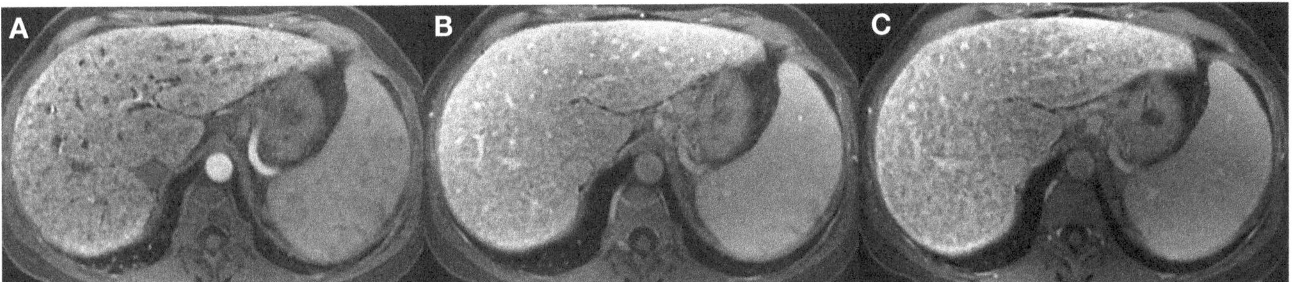

Figure 2.29.4

HISTORY: 47-year-old woman with chronic liver disease

IMAGING FINDINGS: Axial fat-suppressed FSE T2-weighted images (Figure 2.29.1) and diffusion-weighted images (b=100 s/mm^2) (Figure 2.29.2) demonstrate focal, decreased signal intensity surrounding peripheral portal vein branches, or "periportal halos." Axial fat-suppressed 2D SSFP images (Figure 2.29.3) show similar findings. Axial arterial, portal venous, and equilibrium phase postgadolinium 3D SPGR images (Figure 2.29.4) suggest surrounding parenchymal, lacelike fibrosis, particularly on the equilibrium-phase image. There was no associated signal dropout on IP and OP image acquisitions (images not shown).

DIAGNOSIS: Primary biliary cirrhosis

COMMENT: PBC is a rare autoimmune disorder of the biliary ducts occurring predominantly in women (90%), who are usually middle-aged at diagnosis. Four stages of the disease have been characterized at histopathology: Stage 1 constitutes periportal inflammation; in stage 2, the inflammation extends into the hepatic parenchyma; stage 3 includes formation of fibrous septations connecting adjacent portal triads (ie, bridging fibrosis); and stage 4 represents frank cirrhosis. Clinical diagnosis of PBC is based on the presence of chronic biochemical cholestasis, demonstration of antimitochondrial antibodies (found in 90%-95%), and histologic confirmation of destructive nonsuppurative granulomatous (lymphocytic) cholangitis.

The MRI literature regarding PBC is based on a few papers describing a relatively small number of total patients. Two findings have dominated the discussion, both found on T2-weighted images: periportal edema, seen as periportal increased signal intensity, and the periportal halo sign, exemplified by this case and characterized as a region of low signal intensity surrounding the bright central dot of a peripheral portal vein branch. Periportal edema is more commonly seen in early disease (80%-100% prevalence in stage 1 and 30%-65% in stage 4). This is thought to correlate with active periportal inflammation. The periportal halo, however, is more prevalent in late-stage disease (14% in stage 1 and 85% in stage 4, according to the largest study) and is believed to represent periportal fibrotic changes. The periportal halo is considered a specific sign of PBC, although in our experience, the validity of this assumption is questionable in patients with advanced cirrhosis, where distinction between regenerative nodules and periportal halos may be very difficult.

Interestingly, in this case (and in many others we have seen), the periportal halo sign can be appreciated not only on the FSE T2-weighted images but also on DWI and fat-suppressed SSFP sequences (not surprising, given their partial T2 weighting) and even postgadolinium 3D SPGR acquisitions, where the periportal low signal intensity is accentuated by mild enhancement of the adjacent septal fibrosis (this can also be appreciated on the SSFP images, which were obtained at the end of the examination after gadolinium administration).

Another curiosity regarding the MRI literature is the absence of abnormalities reported on MRCP performed in PBC patients. This is in marked contrast to PSC, where multiple biliary strictures, ductal wall thickening and enhancement, and mild peripheral biliary dilatation are diagnostic features. A few authors have noted a paucity of peripheral ducts in PBC patients, but this is a subtle finding that is often very difficult to distinguish from a normal examination unless the gradual disappearance of peripheral ducts can be documented on serial examinations.

After cirrhosis develops, PBC patients are at increased risk for HCC, and autopsy and transplant studies have showed a prevalence of coexistent HCC ranging from 2% to 5%. Liver transplantation is the treatment of choice for advanced PBC, although recurrent disease after transplantation occurs in approximately 15% of patients.

CASE 2.30

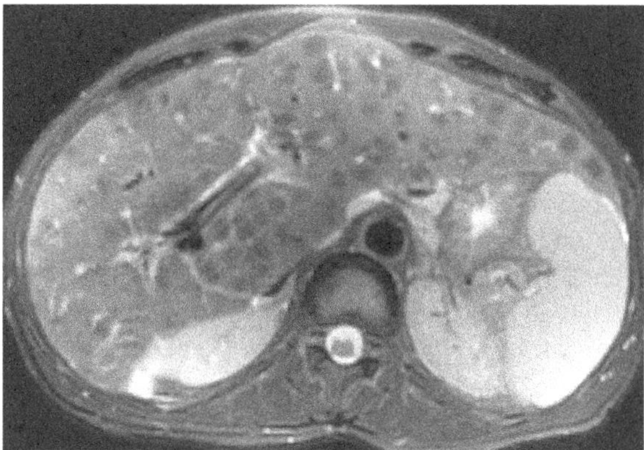

Figure 2.30.1

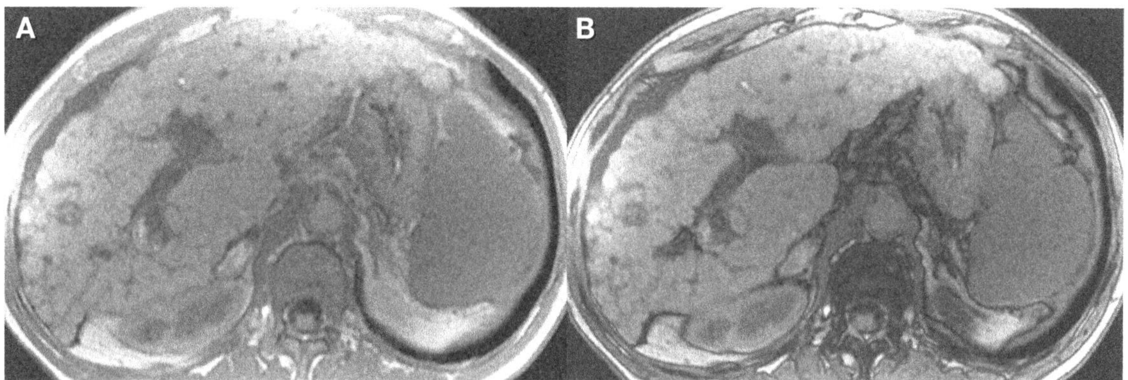

Figure 2.30.2

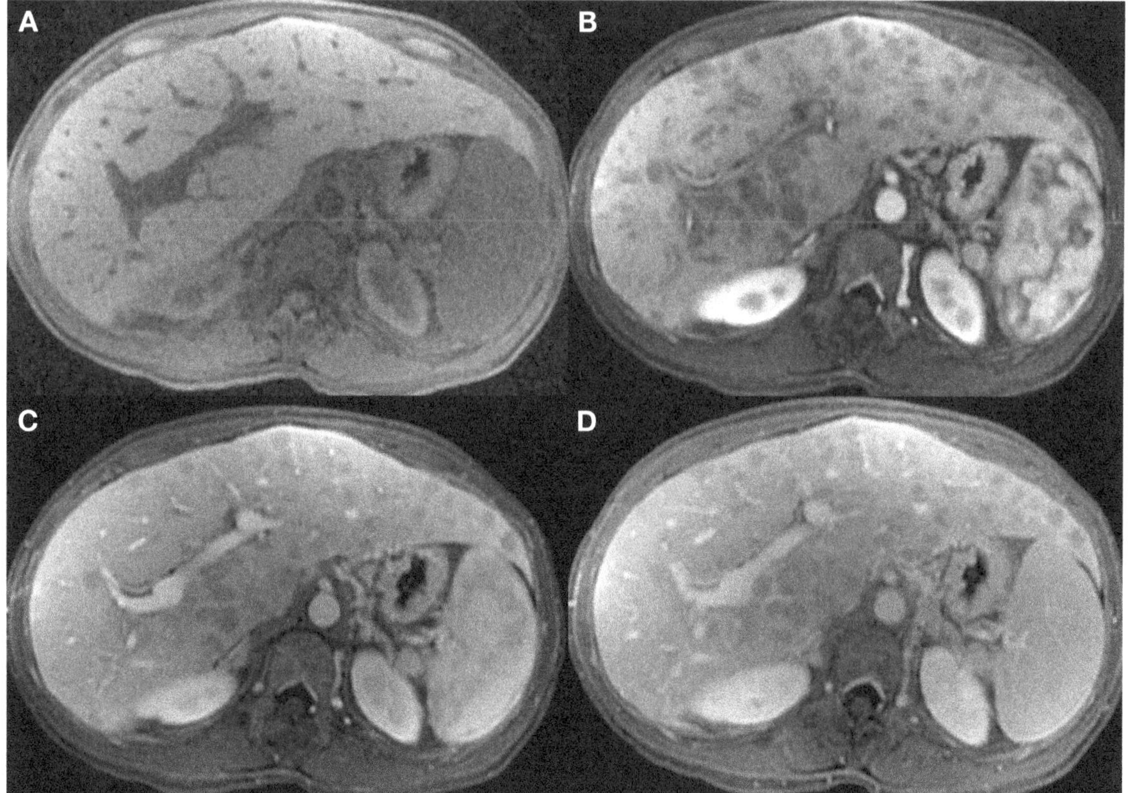

Figure 2.30.3

HISTORY: 60-year-old woman with incidentally noted abnormal liver function tests

IMAGING FINDINGS: Axial fat-suppressed FSE T2-weighted (Figure 2.30.1) and axial IP and OP T1-weighted 2D SPGR (Figure 2.30.2) images demonstrate a cirrhotic configuration of the liver with enlargement of the left hepatic lobe and the caudate lobe (not entirely included here), as well as diffuse, innumerable small hypointense nodules that do not demonstrate appreciable dropout on IP and OP images. The nodules are not seen on the axial T1-weighted pregadolinium 3D SPGR image (Figure 2.30.3A) and are hypoenhancing compared to adjacent liver on arterial (Figure 2.30.3B), portal venous (Figure 2.30.3C), and equilibrium (Figure 2.30.3D) phase postgadolinium images.

DIAGNOSIS: Primary biliary cirrhosis with periportal halos

COMMENT: This is a somewhat unusual example of PBC, with discrete, well-defined periportal halos and little evidence of the bridging fibrosis often seen in association with these lesions. The major differential diagnosis in this case is multiple regenerative nodules. This is a reasonable hypothesis given the mildly cirrhotic appearance of the liver; however, the fact that most of the nodules have a small hyperintense center representing a peripheral portal vein branch makes PBC the most likely diagnosis (supported by subsequent blood tests documenting the presence of antimitochondrial antibodies).

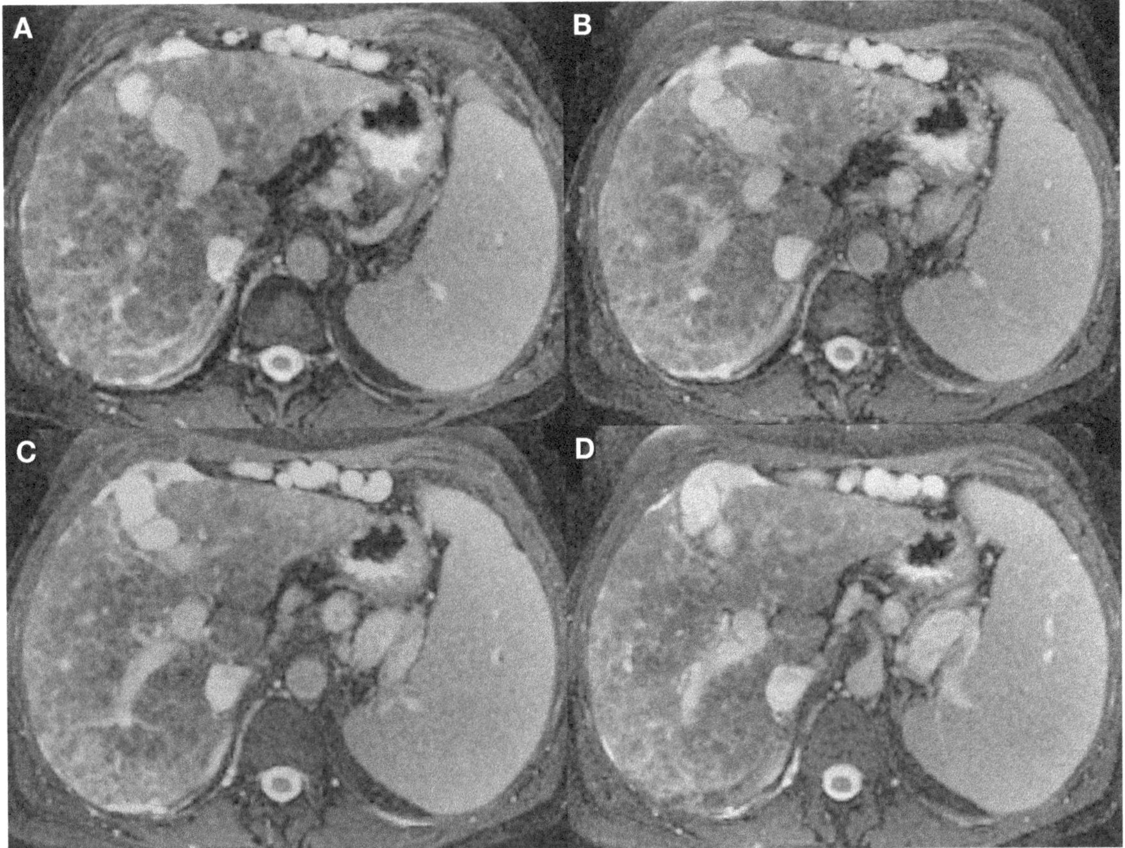

Figure 2.31.1

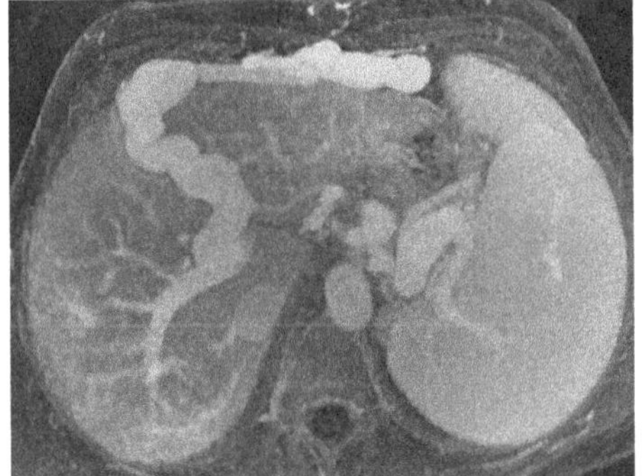

Figure 2.31.2

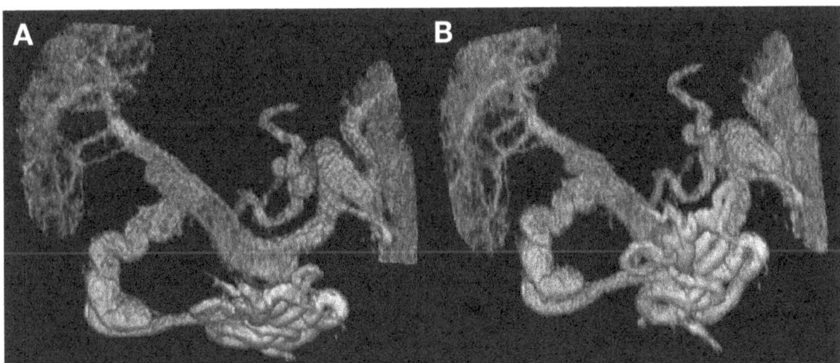

Figure 2.31.3

HISTORY: 53-year-old woman with chronic liver disease

IMAGING FINDINGS: Axial fat-suppressed 2D SSFP images (Figure 2.31.1) demonstrate a nodular cirrhotic liver with splenomegaly and enlarged patent umbilical veins. Subvolume MIP (Figure 2.31.2) and VR (Figure 2.31.3) images reconstructed from a portal venous phase postgadolinium 3D SPGR acquisition again demonstrate large paraumbilical varices.

DIAGNOSIS: Cirrhotic liver secondary to PBC, with varices from portal hypertension

COMMENT: Identification of portosystemic collateral veins in a patient with known or suspected cirrhosis is useful because it provides evidence of portal hypertension and indicates an increased risk of variceal bleeding. Common collateral pathways include gastroesophageal varices, paraesophageal varices, recanalization of the paraumbilical veins, and splenorenal shunts.

Although large collateral veins are easy to detect on virtually any pulse sequence, visualization of smaller varices is usually best on dynamic postgadolinium 3D SPGR images. In patients who are not candidates for gadolinium administration or who have difficulty with breath-holding, a 2D fat-suppressed SSFP acquisition, illustrated here, is an excellent alternative technique. Fluid-filled or vascular structures have high signal intensity on T2/T1-weighted SSFP images, and the short TRs typically used enable rapid sequential image acquisition, which in turn means that image quality in poor breath-holding (or non–breath-holding) patients remains reasonably good. This is not the ideal pulse sequence to use for identifying solid masses in a cirrhotic liver, but it's no worse in this regard than an SSFSE acquisition, which in many practices is the primary T2-weighted sequence in the liver protocol.

The VR images were created by subtracting the portal phase from arterial phase 3D SPGR images to generate a more-or-less pure venous phase data set. These images are not essential for diagnosis, but clinicians and patients appreciate them, and it's worth remembering that reasonable 3D reconstructions of vascular structures can almost always be generated from axial dynamic 3D SPGR acquisitions.

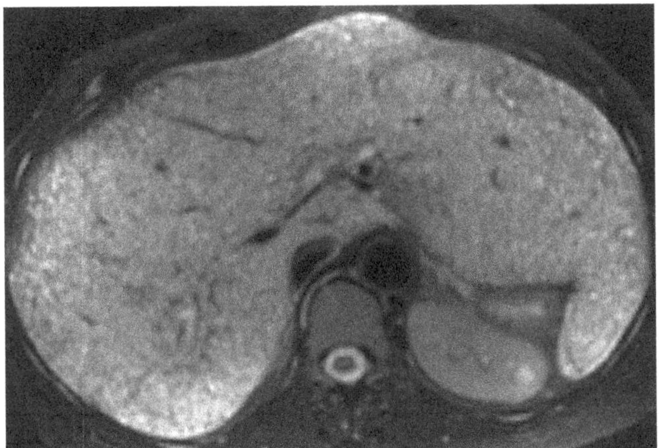

Figure 2.32.1

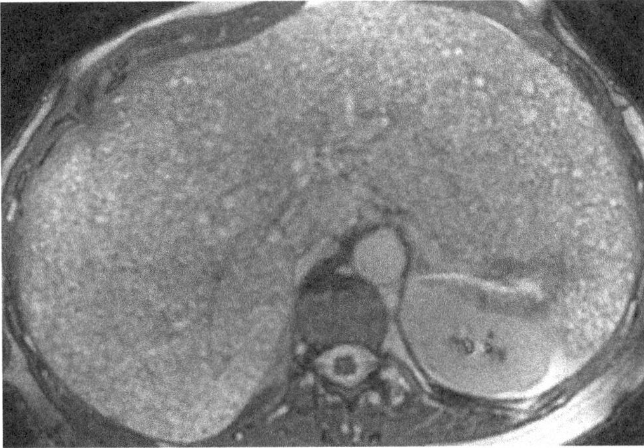

Figure 2.32.2

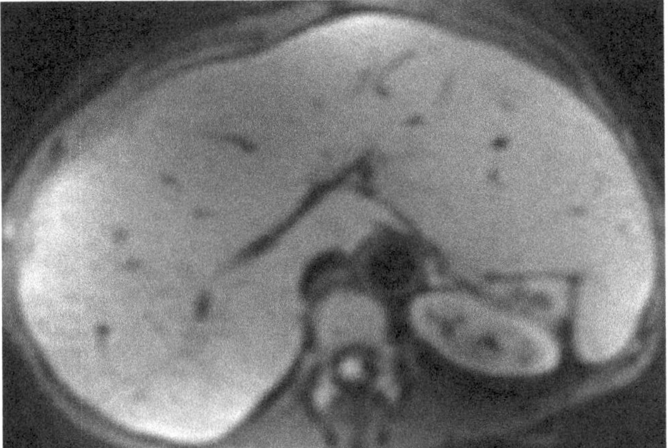

Figure 2.32.3

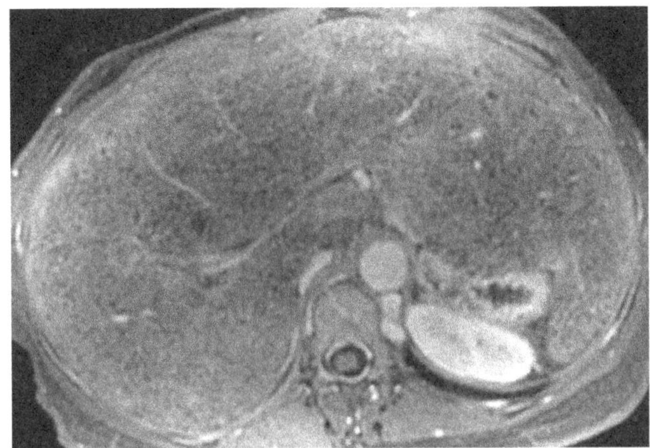

Figure 2.32.4

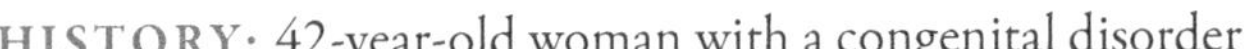

HISTORY: 42-year-old woman with a congenital disorder

IMAGING FINDINGS: Axial fat-suppressed T2-weighted FSE (Figure 2.32.1) and 3D SSFP (Figure 2.32.2) images demonstrate hepatomegaly with innumerable diffuse microcysts throughout the liver. Axial diffusion-weighted image (b=100 s/mm^2) (Figure 2.32.3) also shows hepatomegaly and a lobulated hepatic contour, and an axial postgadolinium portal venous phase 3D SPGR image (Figure 2.32.4) demonstrates diffuse heterogeneity of the hepatic parenchyma.

DIAGNOSIS: Congenital hepatic fibrosis

COMMENT: CHF belongs to the family of fibropolycystic diseases that includes both autosomal dominant and autosomal recessive PKD, as well as Caroli disease. CHF is nearly always associated with autosomal recessive polycystic kidney disease, and in most cases, renal manifestations dominate the initial clinical presentation. One recent series reported that presenting symptoms were related to liver disease in 26% of patients. The genetic defect is a mutation in the *PKHD1* gene located on chromosome 6p12. This gene encodes the protein fibrocystin, which is present on the primary cilia of renal and biliary epithelial cells. The primary defect in the liver is a ductal plate (precursor to intrahepatic bile ducts) malformation occurring at the level of the small interlobular bile ducts and resulting in biliary strictures and periportal fibrosis that then lead to portal hypertension. Clinical manifestations of hepatic disease are usually related to portal hypertension and have a variable onset, ranging from early childhood to the fifth or sixth decade of life, although most patients present as adolescents or young adults.

The imaging features of CHF are also variable. In many patients, cirrhosis is the primary hepatic abnormality, and the specific diagnosis of CHF is only made by noting cystic disease in the kidneys. Some patients have more prominent biliary involvement, and this case is a good (although unusual) example of this, with innumerable, very small peribiliary cysts completely replacing the hepatic parenchyma. The T2-weighted images are much more impressive than the diffusion-weighted images, which have spatial resolution too low to adequately resolve the small cysts. The classic biliary manifestation of CHF is Caroli syndrome, comprising cystic dilatation of the intrahepatic biliary ducts in association with congenital hepatic fibrosis.

This patient had a diagnosis of CHF at age 8 years, presenting with bleeding esophageal varices. She underwent a splenorenal shunt with splenectomy and has had no further symptoms. Her renal disease is also asymptomatic, manifested only by a few cysts and mild proteinuria.

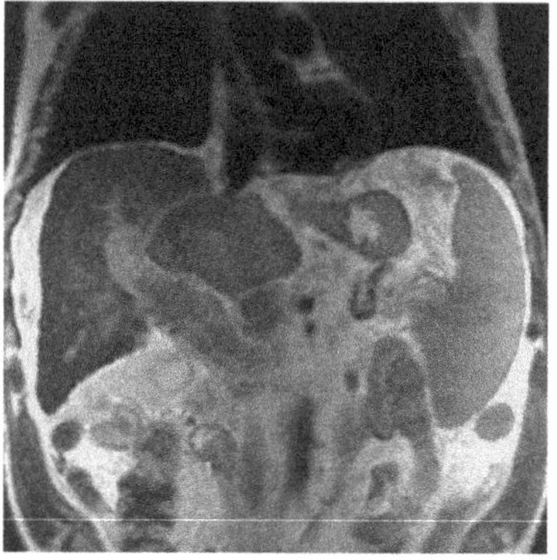

Figure 2.33.1

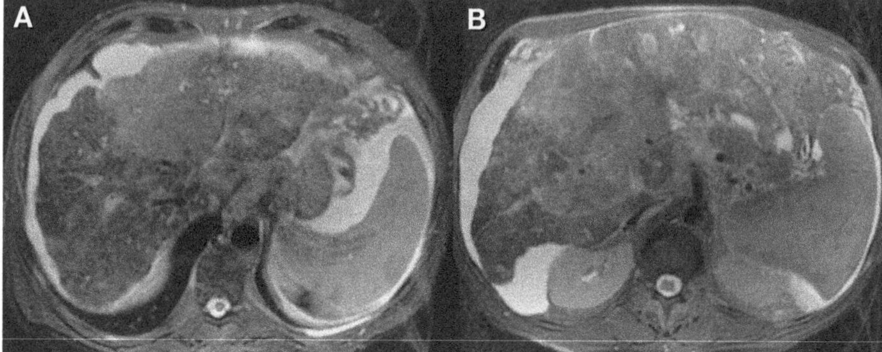

Figure 2.33.2

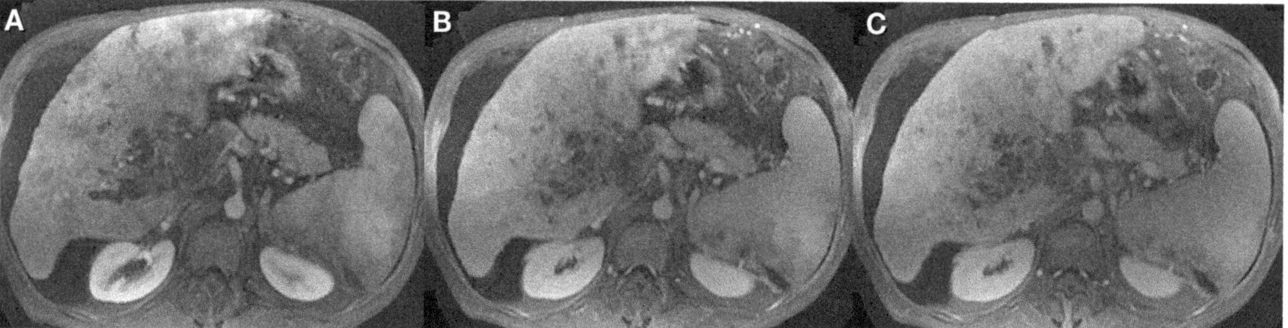

Figure 2.33.3

HISTORY: 62-year-old man with cirrhosis

IMAGING FINDINGS: Coronal SSFSE (Figure 2.33.1) and axial fat-suppressed FSE T2-weighted (Figure 2.33.2) images demonstrate a cirrhotic liver with heterogeneous signal intensity, splenomegaly, and ascites. Ill-defined increased signal intensity in the left hepatic lobe involves nearly all of the liver inferiorly. Note also soft tissue expansion of the main portal vein, depicted in the coronal SSFSE image. Arterial, portal venous, and equilibrium phase postgadolinium 3D SPGR images (Figure 2.33.3) demonstrate diffuse heterogeneous enhancement of the liver, as well as mild enhancement of the portal vein thrombus.

DIAGNOSIS: Infiltrative hepatocellular carcinoma

COMMENT: Infiltrative HCC is a favorite at case conferences, partly because the images shown can be selected to make the diagnosis either very easy (for the good residents) or almost impossible (for the annoying ones). One of the surprising results of the early MRI literature on HCC was that readers missed a high percentage of infiltrative lesions (nearly 80% in some studies). This result was partly a consequence of relatively crude technology but also was undoubtedly related to observational errors. Infiltrative lesions, although often large, frequently have no distinct margins, are less likely to show prominent arterial phase hyperenhancement, and may blend into the heterogeneous background of a cirrhotic liver. Retrospective reviews noted that most of these patients had tumor thrombus in the portal vein, and subsequently it became a standard teaching point that the diagnosis of infiltrative HCC must be accompanied by portal vein tumor thrombus. This isn't always the case, of course, but it's true often enough that a careful inspection of the portal (and hepatic) veins is mandatory anytime a cirrhotic liver is assessed. (A recent review found portal vein tumor thrombus in 70% of patients with infiltrative HCC.)

Infiltrative HCC is generally recognized as a distinct morphologic subtype of HCC, along with focal nodular and massive variants, but it has not been well characterized in part because it's difficult to detect and also likely because the distinction between massive, multinodular, and infiltrative lesions is somewhat in the eye of the beholder. In general, infiltrative HCC is thought to account for 7% to 13% of cases and is associated with hepatitis B virus infection, portal vein thrombosis, and elevated AFP levels. Arterialization of portal vein tumor thrombus (ie, thrombus enhancement during the arterial phase) has been described as a near-universal and classic finding; however, it was reported in only 10% of patients in a recent series from Johns Hopkins Hospital (but it's usually possible to distinguish tumor thrombus from bland thrombus even when this sign is absent). A large percentage of patients with infiltrative HCC have very high AFP levels (>1,000 ng/mL). AFP levels are thought to correlate with overall tumor burden; however, AFP is a specific, but not sensitive, marker and as many as one-third of patients with infiltrative HCC have AFP values within the normal range.

This case is not a particularly subtle example. You can appreciate the expanded portal vein on the SSFSE images, and the axial FSE images clearly show diffuse increased signal intensity throughout the left hepatic lobe, even though it's difficult to point to a discrete lesion. Distinguishing tumor thrombus from bland thrombus is important (since bland thrombus is not uncommon in patients with severe cirrhosis) and usually is fairly straightforward on postgadolinium images. Tumor thrombus enhances, often in a linear pattern, whereas bland thrombus doesn't. In the chronic setting (typically, when MRI is performed), portal vein thrombus shouldn't have high signal intensity at baseline (unlike the high T1-signal intensity from intracellular methemoglobin that can be seen in the subacute setting) and after gadolinium administration appears as a signal void. If gadolinium is contraindicated, thrombus can often be visualized on SSFP images, although the distinction between bland and tumor thrombus is not always easy to make.

The patent main portal vein generally appears as a signal void on respiratory-triggered FSE images, but the absence of a flow void, particularly in cirrhotic patients with slow flow, is not a reliable indicator of thrombus. Tumor thrombus, especially in the main portal vein and proximal branches, appears as a soft tissue lesion with mild-to-moderate increased signal intensity; these findings are occasionally missed when radiologists do not realize that they're looking at the portal vein and not at hepatic parenchyma. Diffusion-weighted images are also very useful in this regard. Diffusion gradients provide a black-blood effect (signal voids in arteries and veins). Whereas bland thrombus can be difficult to appreciate (because of low signal intensity), tumor thrombus should have high signal intensity and its location within a vein may be better appreciated in comparison to FSE images since it is often surrounded by flow voids.

The prognosis of infiltrative HCC is poor, with a median survival following diagnosis of approximately 14 months. There are few therapeutic options; these patients are not candidates for embolization, surgical resection, or transplantation, although both sorafenib and transarterial chemoembolization therapy have shown modest survival benefits in small studies.

CASE 2.34

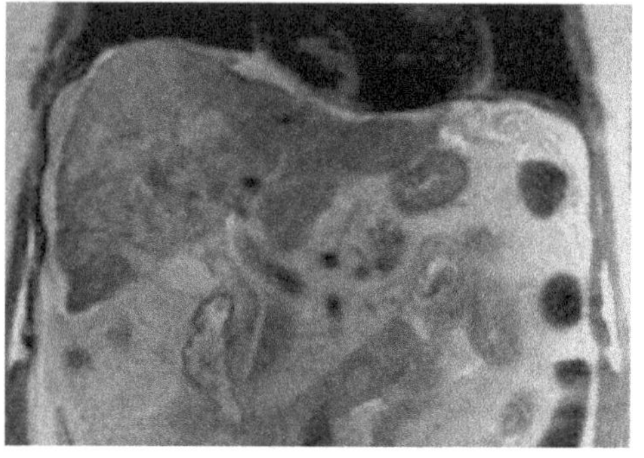

Figure 2.34.1

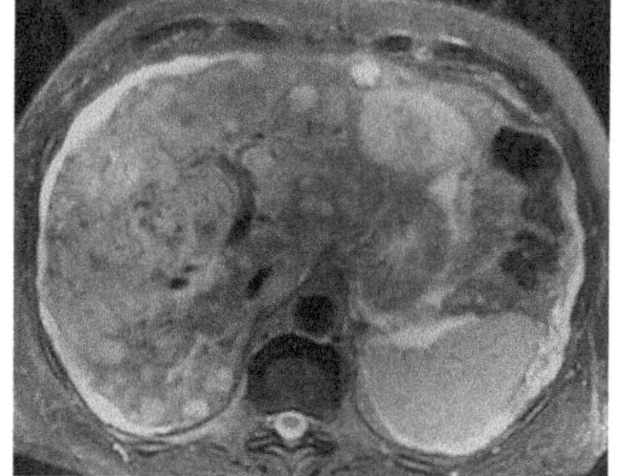

Figure 2.34.2

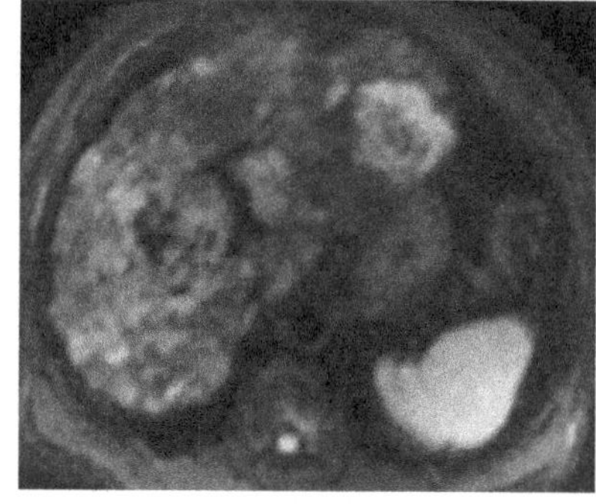

Figure 2.34.3

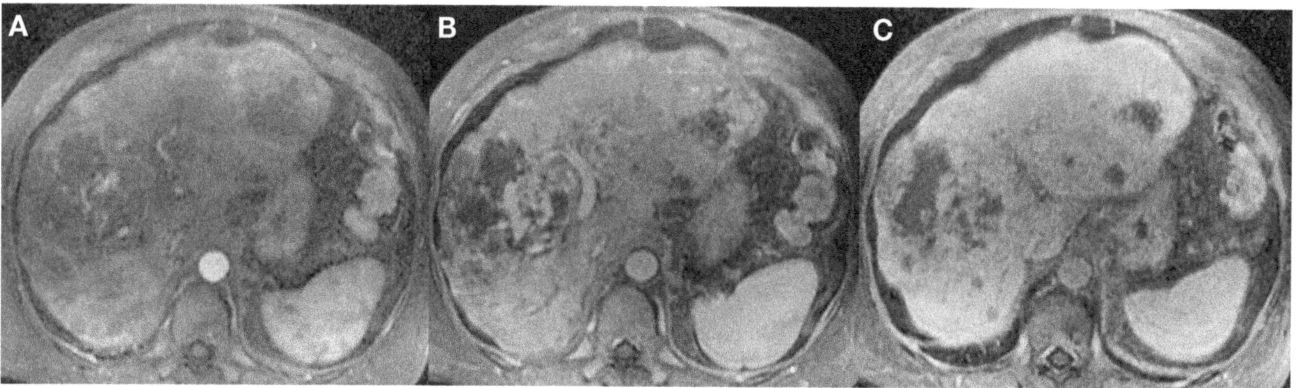

Figure 2.34.4

HISTORY: 80-year-old man with loss of energy and easy fatigability

IMAGING FINDINGS: Coronal SSFSE (Figure 2.34.1), axial fat-suppressed FSE T2-weighted (Figure 2.34.2), and diffusion-weighted (b=100 s/mm^2) (Figure 2.34.3) images demonstrate multiple heterogeneous hyperintense masses in the liver, with a large, poorly defined mass in the right hepatic lobe. Axial arterial, portal venous, and equilibrium phase post-gadolinium 3D SPGR images (Figure 2.34.4) demonstrate mild, predominantly peripheral enhancement of some of the lesions. Notice the progressive enhancement of the hepatic lesions, some of which are isointense to the rest of the hepatic parenchyma in the equilibrium phase.

DIAGNOSIS: Angiosarcoma

COMMENT: Hepatic angiosarcoma is a rare and aggressive neoplasm accounting for approximately 2% of primary hepatic tumors. Nevertheless, it is the most common malignant mesenchymal tumor of the liver. Middle-aged and older men are most frequently affected, with a reported male to female ratio of 4:1.

Angiosarcoma gained a certain notoriety among radiology trainees as the answer to the trivia question regarding which tumors were associated with exposure to thorium dioxide (Thorotrast), a radioactive contrast agent used during the first half of the 20th century primarily for cerebral angiography. Unfortunately, the agent was retained by the reticuloendothelial system with a biological half-life of more than 20 years, thereby exposing adjacent organs to continuous radiation from alpha particles. Angiosarcoma is also associated with exposure to other environmental toxins, including arsenic and vinyl chloride; however, most patients with newly diagnosed angiosarcoma can provide no history of toxic exposure.

Angiosarcomas are composed of malignant endothelial cells that can form rudimentary vessels, line cavitary spaces, grow along vascular channels, or form solid nodules. Immunostaining for endothelial markers is a key element of the pathologic diagnosis. Four typical growth patterns have been described: multiple nodules, a dominant mass, a dominant mass and multiple satellite nodules, and, less commonly, a diffusely infiltrating micronodular tumor.

Approximately 15 to 20 hepatic angiosarcomas have been reported in the MRI literature, with a slight predominance of the multinodular type over the dominant nodule or dominant nodule with satellite lesions. Most lesions show heterogeneous, increased signal intensity on T2- or diffusion-weighted images. Potentially more useful findings include increased signal intensity on precontrast fat-suppressed T1-weighted images, correlating with the presence of hemorrhage, a somewhat unusual finding in cholangiocarcinoma, which is often a differential diagnostic consideration. The enhancement pattern following gadolinium administration is also unusual, consisting of initial heterogeneous hypoenhancement on arterial phase images, with small foci of peripheral enhancement followed by gradual progressive enhancement on portal venous, equilibrium, and delayed phase images—not typical of HCC but certainly possible with cholangiocarcinoma.

A few authors have noted that since HCC and cholangiocarcinoma are often major considerations in the differential diagnosis, the absence of cirrhosis should prompt consideration of angiosarcoma. In our limited experience, however, this has not been particularly helpful since in nearly all of the cases we have seen, the liver was described as cirrhotic in the report either because there was coexisting cirrhosis or because the extensive tumor distorted the hepatic contour into a nodular, pseudocirrhotic appearance.

Patients usually present with nonspecific symptoms, such as abdominal pain, weakness, fatigue, and weight loss. Hematologic abnormalities are frequent and include microangiopathic hemolytic anemia and thrombocytopenia. Red blood cells are thought to be traumatized within the poorly organized neoplastic vessels, and platelets may be trapped, leading to localized coagulopathy and, occasionally, disseminated intravascular coagulation. Case reports have described spontaneous rupture of hepatic angiosarcomas, with massive intra-abdominal bleeding, and caution has been advised when contemplating percutaneous biopsy. However, no significant complications were described in a series from Mayo Clinic that included 9 CT-guided biopsies.

The prognosis of hepatic angiosarcoma is poor, with a median survival of less than 1 year following diagnosis. Metastases are found in 60% of patients at diagnosis, with lung, spleen, and bone marrow frequent targets. Surgical resection may be curative, but this is feasible only in a small percentage of patients, and no effective chemotherapeutic regimen has been established.

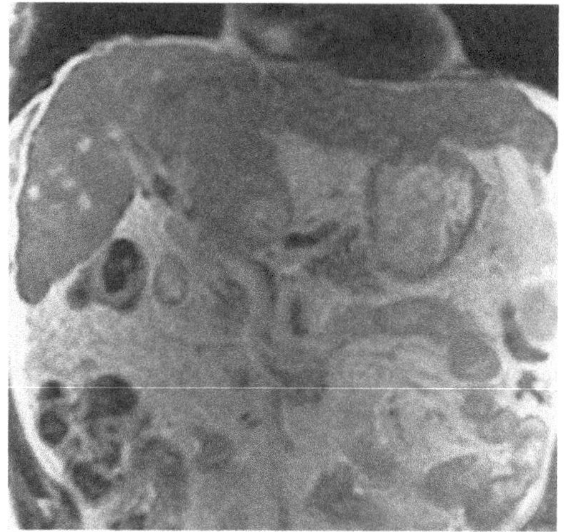

Figure 2.35.1

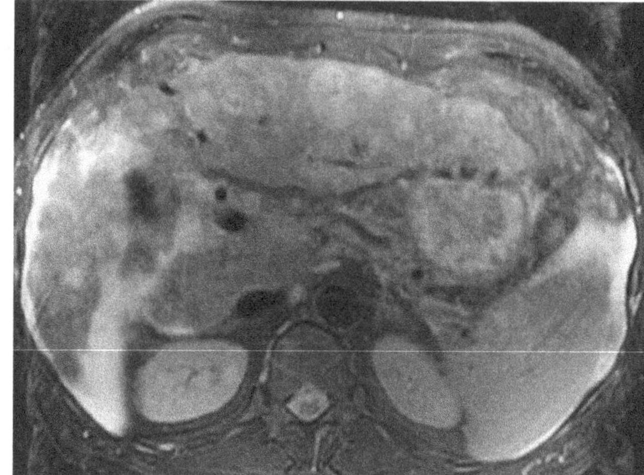

Figure 2.35.2

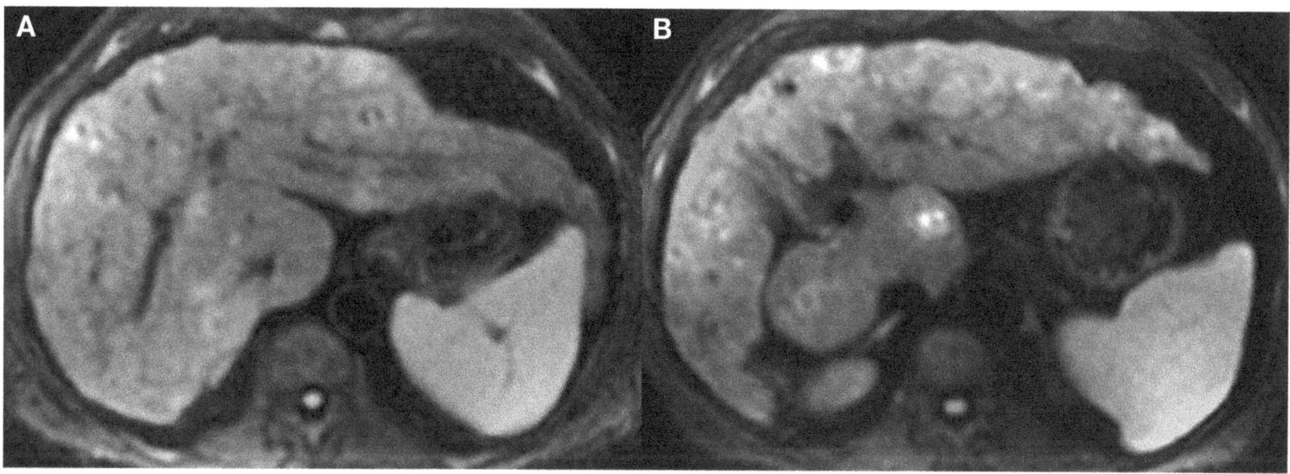

Figure 2.35.3

HISTORY: 57-year-old man with chronic fatigue

IMAGING FINDINGS: Coronal SSFSE (Figure 2.35.1), axial fat-suppressed FSE T2-weighted (Figure 2.35.2), and axial diffusion-weighted (b=600 s/mm^2) (Figure 2.35.3) images demonstrate a nodular hepatic contour and multiple heterogeneous, hyperintense, ill-defined nodules throughout the liver. These findings had appeared since a prior MRI less than a year ago.

DIAGNOSIS: Angiosarcoma in the clinical setting of cirrhosis

COMMENT: The patient in this case presented with a working diagnosis of decompensated cryptogenic cirrhosis. Clinically, the patient had taken a turn for the worse, and this case illustrates the difficulties of making a diagnosis in a cirrhotic liver. Regenerative nodules were not entirely consistent with the clinical picture, so CT was performed, with findings that were similar to the MRI.

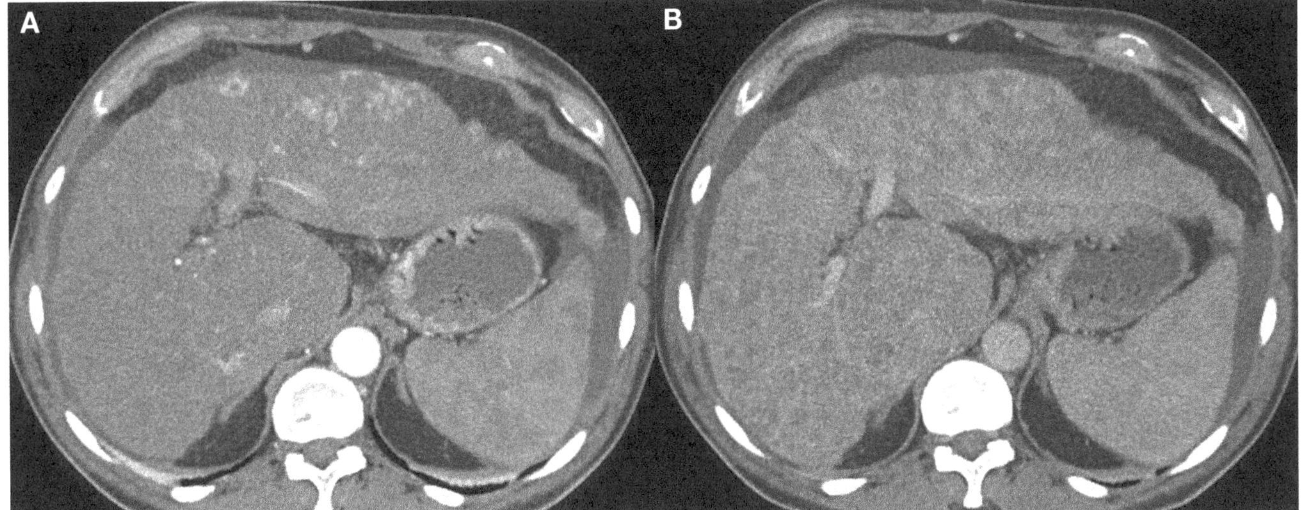

Figure 2.35.4

CT showed multiple hyperenhancing foci (Figure 2.35.4A) throughout the liver on an arterial phase postcontrast image, with diffuse hypoenhancing nodules (Figure 2.35.4B) evident on a 5-minute delayed image. A differential diagnosis of multifocal malignant disease was offered.

A multidisciplinary discussion led to repeat MRI using the hepatobiliary contrast agent Eovist.

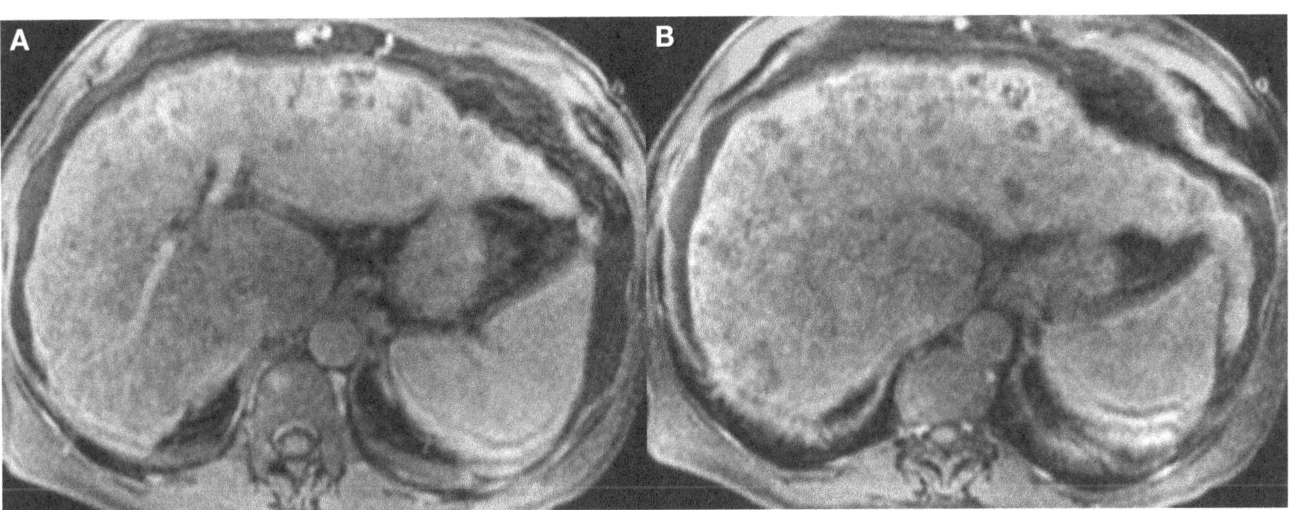

Figure 2.35.5

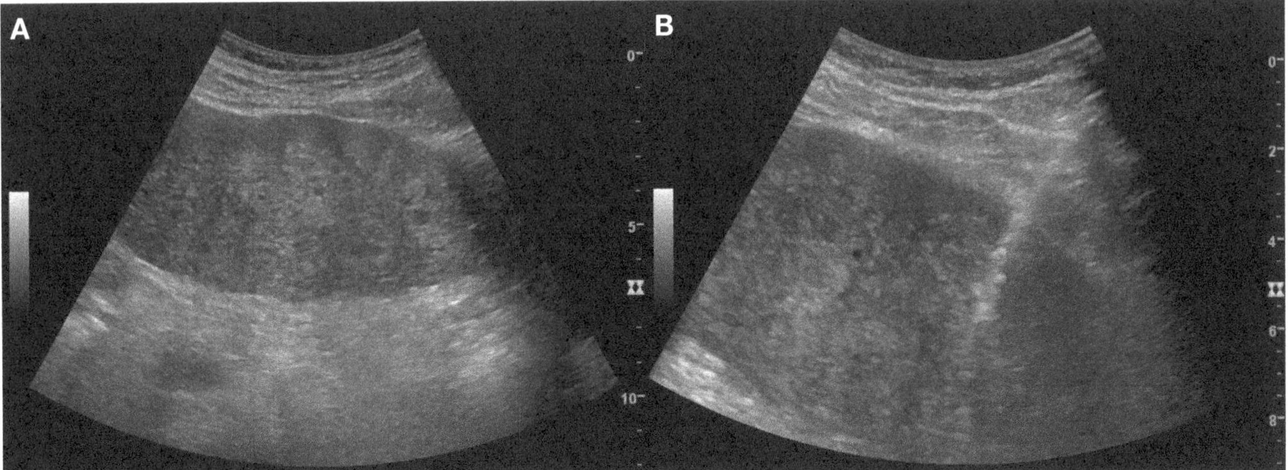

Figure 2.35.6

Image acquisitions are degraded by patient motion, but on the portal venous and equilibrium phase postgadolinium (Eovist) 3D SPGR images (Figure 2.35.5), there is contrast washout of a few of the hepatic lesions. Unfortunately, because of the patient's reduced hepatic function, the hepatobiliary phase images (not shown) were of limited utility; however, many of the lesions in the left hepatic lobe showed persistent hypoenhancement (and this was suggested as a possible target for biopsy if that was being considered). Overall, the MRI appearance was suspicious for infiltrative HCC.

This patient underwent US-guided biopsy (Figure 2.35.6) directed at one of the hyperechoic masses in the left hepatic lobe that corresponded to the MRI findings, with a final diagnosis of angiosarcoma.

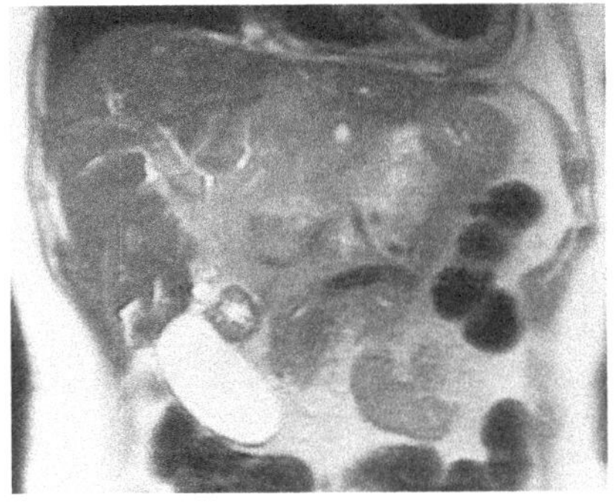

Figure 2.36.1

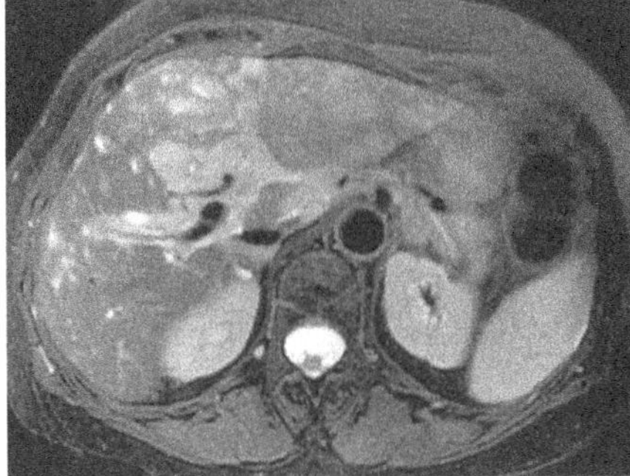

Figure 2.36.2

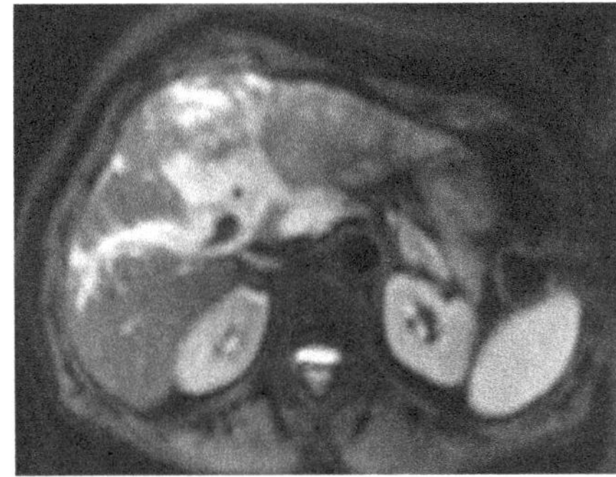

Figure 2.36.3

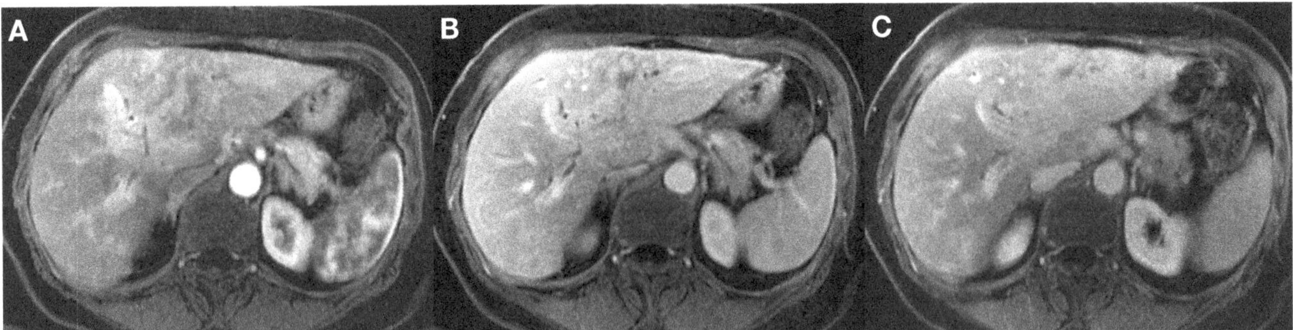

Figure 2.36.4

HISTORY: 74-year-old woman with painless jaundice

IMAGING FINDINGS: Coronal SSFSE (Figure 2.36.1), axial fat-suppressed T2-weighted FSE (Figure 2.36.2), and axial diffusion-weighted (b=600 s/mm^2) (Figure 2.36.3) images demonstrate infiltrative soft tissue predominantly in the central periportal regions and extending along both right and left portal tracts into the liver. Arterial, portal venous, and equilibrium phase images (Figure 2.36.4) demonstrate early and mild persistent enhancement of this infiltrative process. Mild intrahepatic biliary dilatation is present. The spleen is normal in size.

DIAGNOSIS: Low-grade B-cell lymphoma

COMMENT: This is an unusual presentation of lymphoma, particularly because there is no splenic involvement and no adenopathy distinct from the confluent porta hepatis soft tissue mass. The differential diagnosis for an infiltrative mass in the porta hepatis is fairly limited, however, and should include lymphoma. Cholangiocarcinoma is well known for infiltrative growth along biliary ducts, but it would be unusual for a hilar cholangiocarcinoma this large to cause only minimal biliary dilatation; the classic Klatskin tumor causes high-grade biliary obstruction while still small enough to make identification challenging. Lymphatic spread of HCC could present with a similar appearance, although most often in these cases, the primary lesion is obvious and may be coupled with tumor thrombus in portal or hepatic veins. Nerves also travel in the periportal space, and there have been rare cases of plexiform neurofibromas infiltrating along the porta hepatis in patients with neurofibromatosis.

All of these options are fairly obscure, but lymphoma is probably the best diagnostic choice given the large soft tissue mass and relatively mild biliary obstruction.

CASE 2.37

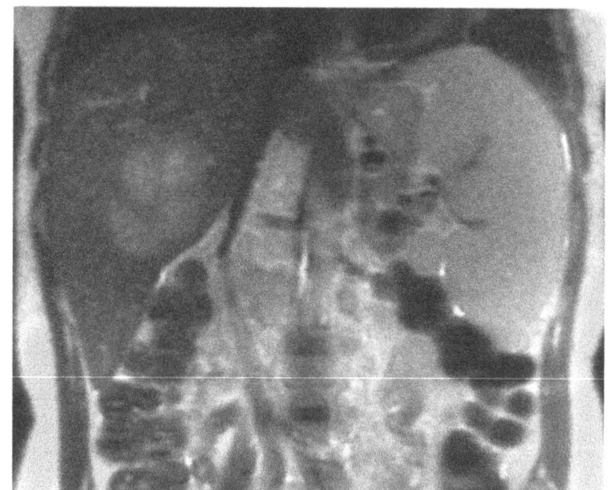

Figure 2.37.1

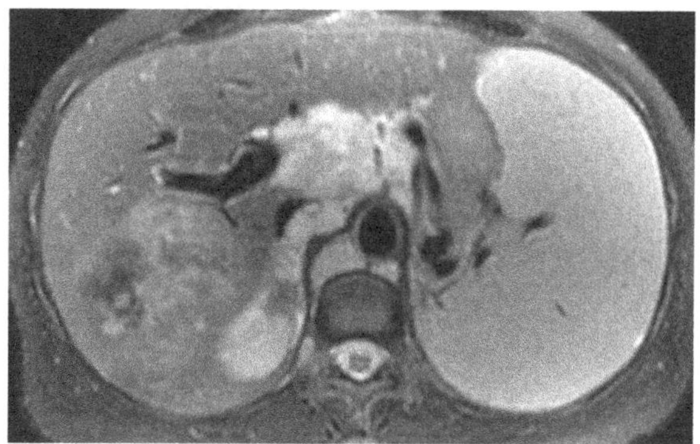

Figure 2.37.2

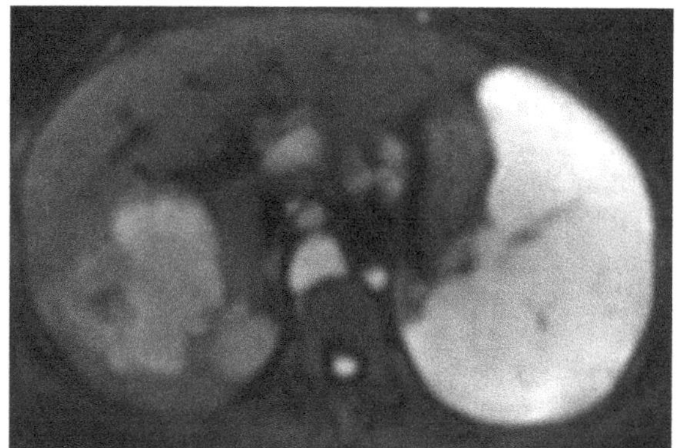

Figure 2.37.3

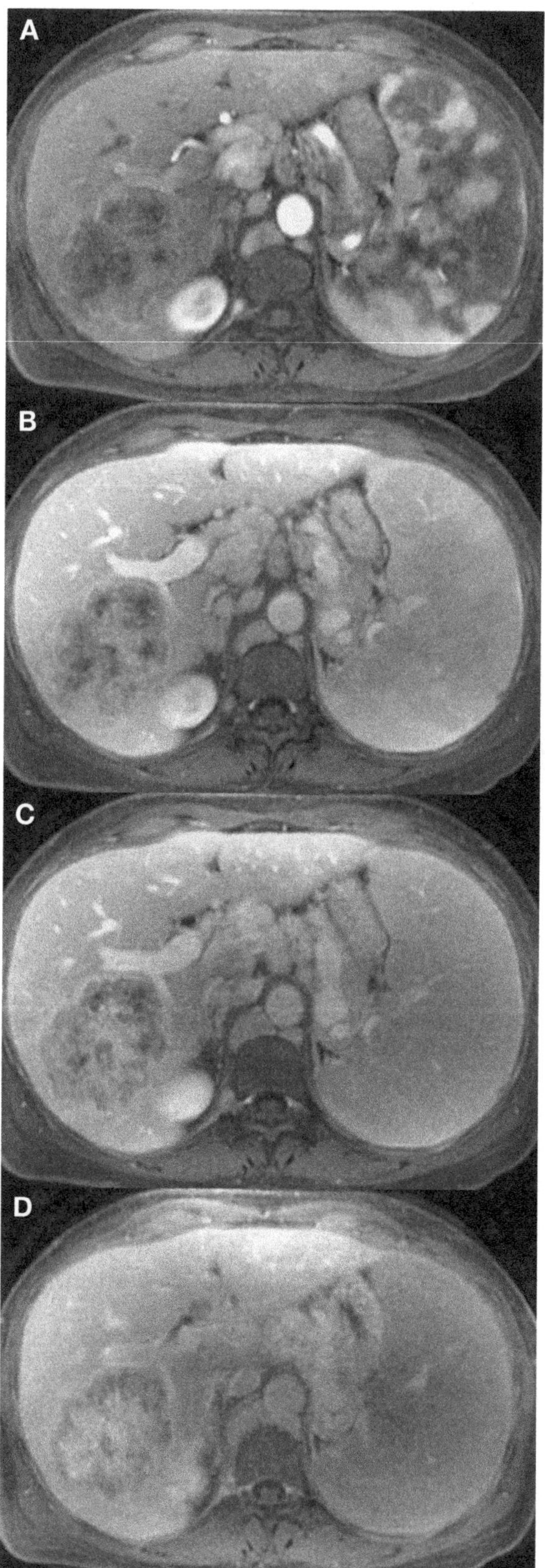

Figure 2.37.4

HISTORY: 50-year-old woman being evaluated for common variable immunodeficiency

IMAGING FINDINGS: Coronal SSFSE (Figure 2.37.1), axial fat-suppressed T2-weighted FSE (Figure 2.37.2), and axial diffusion-weighted (b=100 s/mm^2) (Figure 2.37.3) images demonstrate a heterogeneous mass with lobulated margins in the right hepatic lobe, as well as extensive adenopathy in the celiac axis, porta hepatis, and portocaval space. Note also moderate splenomegaly. Arterial, portal venous, equilibrium, and delayed phase postgadolinium 3D SPGR images (Figure 2.37.4) demonstrate initial hypoenhancement of the mass on the arterial phase image with gradual heterogeneous internal enhancement, which persists on the delayed image. The posterior branch of the right portal vein is slightly attenuated. Adenopathy and splenomegaly are also well seen on the postgadolinium images.

DIAGNOSIS: Lymphoma

COMMENT: Lymphomatous involvement of the liver is relatively common and usually occurs as a secondary process; primary hepatic lymphoma, however, is rare, with fewer than 100 cases reported in the literature. Autopsy studies have shown hepatic involvement in 55% to 65% of patients with Hodgkin disease and non-Hodgkin lymphoma and in 80% of patients with leukemia. Not surprisingly, hepatic involvement is less frequently detected on initial staging examinations in patients with newly diagnosed lymphoma. A recent paper with CT as the primary imaging modality found surprisingly small percentages of patients with detectable hepatic disease: 3% in non-Hodgkin lymphoma and 12% in Hodgkin disease. This is probably a reflection of the limited sensitivity of CT (and also MRI, to some extent) for detection of diffuse infiltrative disease, which may manifest only as hepatomegaly or even as a normal liver.

The most common manifestation of hepatic lymphoma seen on CT or MRI is single or multiple masses. The imaging appearance is often not distinctive unless, as in this case, there is accompanying splenomegaly and adenopathy to suggest the diagnosis. Several occasionally helpful features of lymphomatous lesions have been described, including a lack of prominent arterial phase hyperenhancement, mild but not markedly increased T2-signal intensity, and relatively little mass effect on adjacent vessels. Central necrosis or hemorrhage are relatively infrequent but can occur in larger lesions. Similarly, invasion of the portal or hepatic veins is much more frequently seen in HCC and cholangiocarcinoma, but it has been reported in lymphoma. The gradual central enhancement of the mass seen in this case is not unusual for lymphoma but is not necessarily a distinctive feature. This pattern can also be seen in cholangiocarcinoma, some metastases, granulomatous infections, amyloidosis, and angiosarcoma.

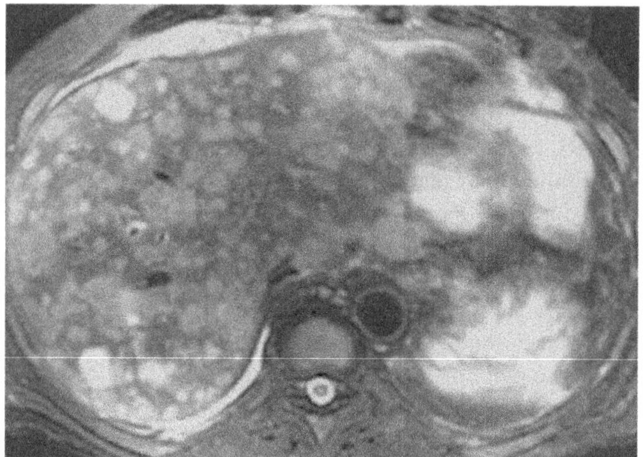

Figure 2.38.1

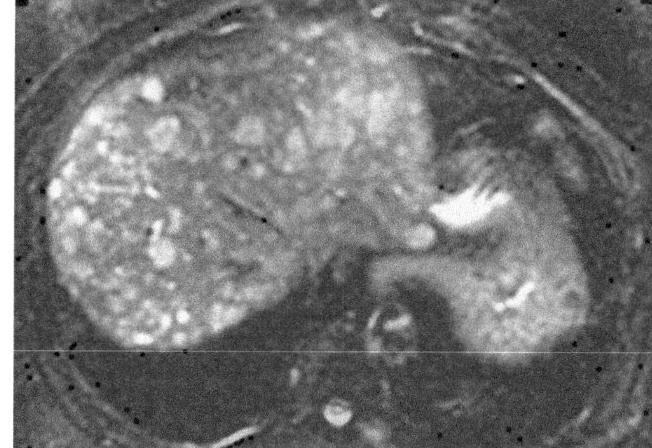

Figure 2.38.2

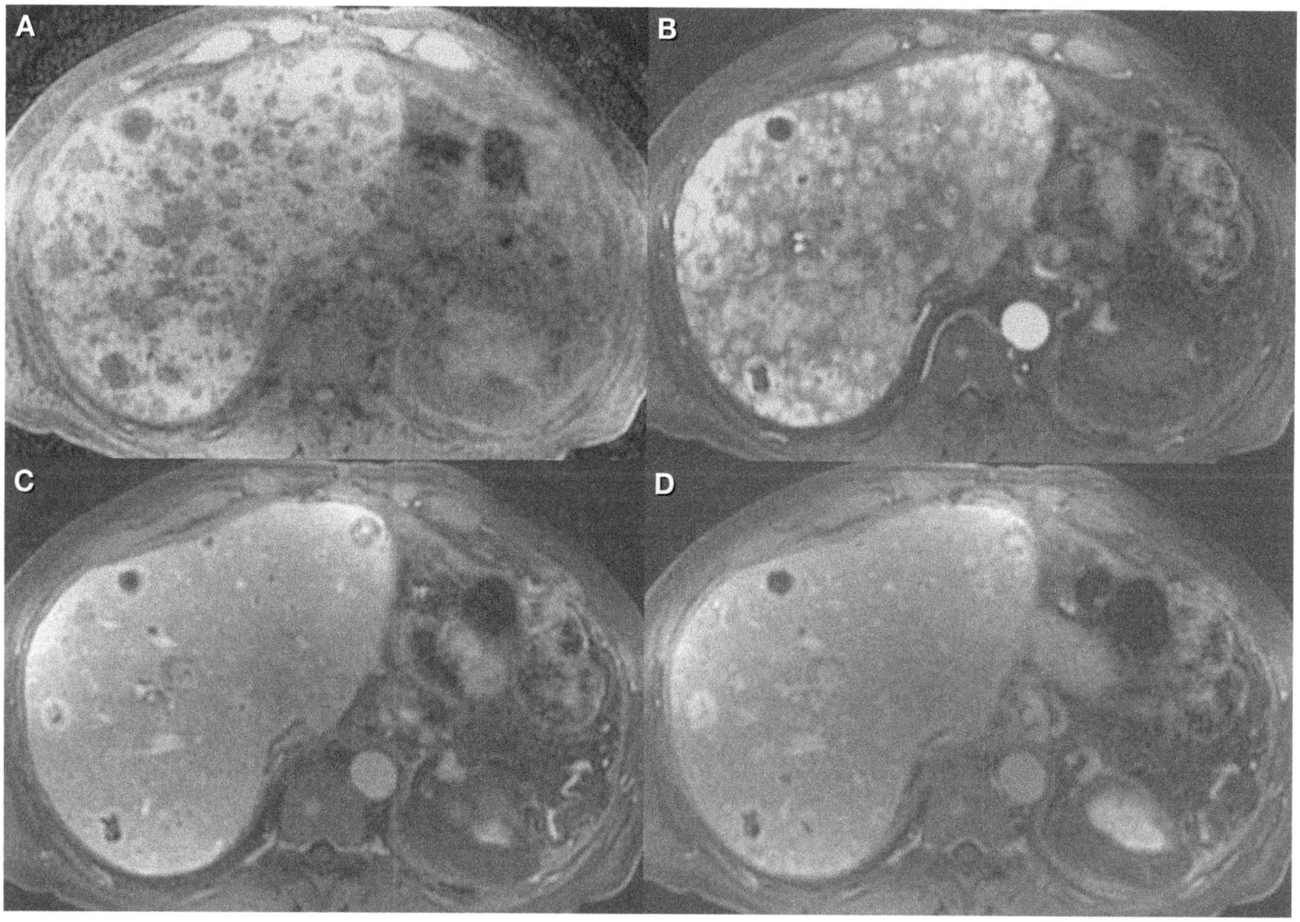

Figure 2.38.3

HISTORY: 57-year-old man with known disease

IMAGING FINDINGS: Axial fat-suppressed FSE T2-weighted (Figure 2.38.1), and diffusion-weighted (b=100 s/mm^2) (Figure 2.38.2) images demonstrate innumerable hyperintense lesions throughout the liver. Axial precontrast, arterial, portal venous, and equilibrium phase images (Figure 2.38.3) show that most of these lesions have intense arterial phase hyperenhancement and become isointense relative to liver on portal venous and equilibrium phase images. A few lesions have central necrosis; others show more gradual contrast enhancement.

DIAGNOSIS: Neuroendocrine metastases (pancreatic neuroendocrine tumor primary)

COMMENT: Assessment for metastatic disease is one of the most common indications for hepatic MRI, and many studies have shown that MRI is generally more sensitive than CT or US for detection of hepatic metastases. This largely has to do with the greater lesion-to-liver contrast on MRI and with the variety of available pulse sequences with different contrast weightings, thereby offering multiple opportunities within the same examination to find lesions.

Neuroendocrine tumor metastases, for example, often exhibit a propensity for intense arterial phase hyperenhancement followed by near invisibility on portal venous and equilibrium phase images. This can be problematic for CT where, if the arterial phase acquisition is mistimed by a few seconds, many lesions cannot be identified. With MRI, on the other hand, not only do the lesions have greater conspicuity against background liver on arterial phase images, but they also are well seen on respiratory-triggered FSE images, an important advantage for patients with limited breath-holding ability. Diffusion-weighted images are also useful, particularly for detection of neuroendocrine tumor metastases; these appear as markedly hyperintense lesions, almost always with greater contrast relative to background liver than obtained with FSE images. In a recent paper, investigators evaluated 162 metastases (152 with surgical histopathology) in 41 patients, using DWI with b values up to 600 s/mm^2. They determined a sensitivity of about 71% compared with roughly 52% for both T2-weighted and dynamic gadolinium-enhanced MRI. The specificity of DWI, T2-weighted FSE, and dynamic gadolinium-enhanced MRI in the patient population who have primary neuroendocrine tumors was comparable and ranged from 89% to 100%.

Hepatobiliary contrast agents represent an additional advantage of MRI compared with CT. Hepatobiliary phase images show metastases as hypoenhancing lesions with high contrast against the hyperenhancing background liver, and even very small lesions can be detected with high sensitivity. The hepatobiliary phase also has a long half-life, which means there are effectively no time constraints on the timing of the acquisition, so that higher spatial resolution images can be obtained and multiple acquisitions can be performed in patients with limited breath-hold capacity.

ABBREVIATIONS

ADC	apparent diffusion coefficient
ADPKD	autosomal dominant polycystic kidney disease
AFP	alpha fetoprotein
ALT	alanine aminotransferase
AST	aspartate aminotransferase
BCS	Budd-Chiari syndrome
CHF	congenital hepatic fibrosis
CT	computed tomography
DWI	diffusion-weighted imaging
FNH	focal nodular hyperplasia
FRFSE	fast-recovery fast-spin echo
FSE	fast-spin echo
GRE	gradient-recalled echo
HCC	hepatocellular carcinoma
HHT	hereditary hemorrhagic telangiectasia
IDEAL	iterative decomposition of water and fat with echo asymmetry and least-squares estimation
IP	in-phase
IVC	inferior vena cava
MIP	maximum intensity projection
MR	magnetic resonance
MRCP	magnetic resonance cholangiopancreatography
MRI	magnetic resonance imaging
OP	out-of-phase
PBC	primary biliary cirrhosis
PKD	polycystic kidney disease
PSC	primary sclerosing cholangitis
SPGR	spoiled gradient-recalled echo
SSFP	steady-state free precession
SSFSE	single-shot fast-spin echo
TE	echo time
THID	transient hepatic intensity defect
3D	3-dimensional
TIPS	transjugular intrahepatic portosystemic shunt
TR	repetition time
2D	2-dimensional
US	ultrasonography
VR	volume-rendered

3.

BILIARY

CASE 3.1

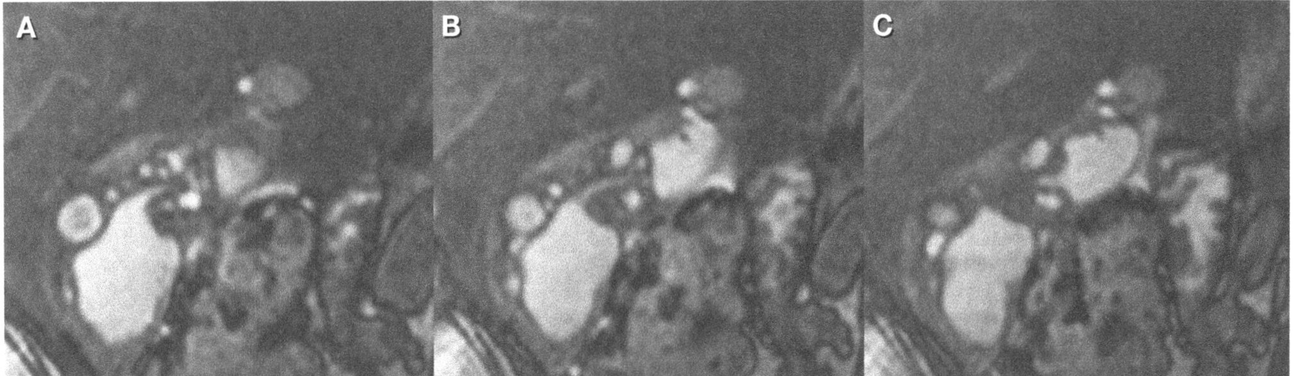

Figure 3.1.1

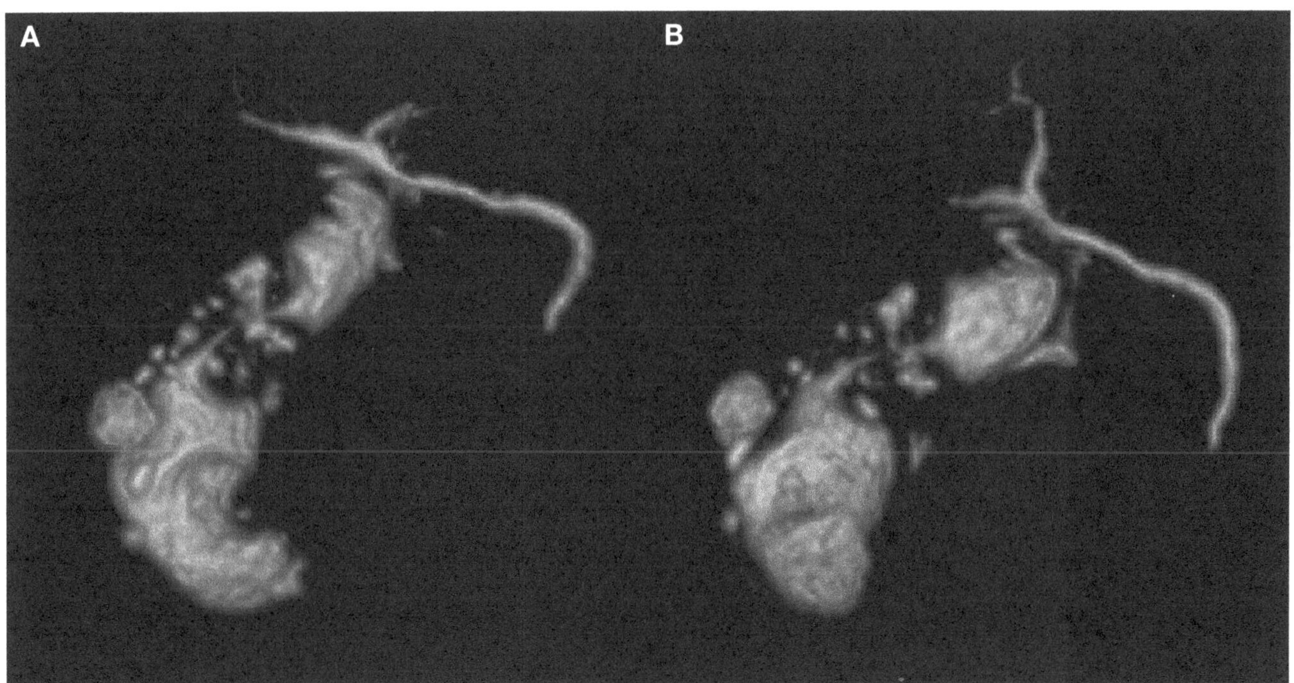

Figure 3.1.2

HISTORY: 51-year-old woman with severe right upper quadrant pain; US revealed focal, masslike mural thickening of the gallbladder with differential considerations including adenomyomatosis, gallbladder neoplasm, and cholecystitis

IMAGING FINDINGS: Coronal images from 3D SSFP acquisition (Figure 3.1.1) demonstrate heterogeneous gallbladder wall thickening interspersed with multiple small mural cysts. Volume-rendered images from the 3D SSFP acquisition (Figure 3.1.2) show distortion of the gallbladder lumen, again with multiple cysts within the wall.

DIAGNOSIS: Adenomyomatosis

COMMENT: Adenomyomatosis is a common disorder reported in 2% to 8% of cholecystectomy specimens. It is characterized by hyperplasia of the gallbladder mucosa, which develops invaginations through the thickened muscular layer to generate the characteristic Rokitansky-Aschoff sinuses. Adenomyomatosis is considered an acquired disease. The most common theory regarding its etiology is that increased intraluminal pressure within the gallbladder, due to abnormalities of contraction, leads to development of Rokitansky-Aschoff sinuses, similar to diverticular disease in the colon.

Adenomyomatosis has been classified into 3 subcategories: focal, segmental, and diffuse. Focal adenomyomatosis may mimic gallbladder carcinoma, particularly when Rokitansky-Aschoff sinuses cannot be identified. In the segmental subtype, an annular stricture may be seen dividing the gallbladder into 2 compartments.

Adenomyomatosis is more common in women than men. Many patients present with right upper quadrant pain, and a high percentage (up to 90%) have coexistent gallstones; however, it also can be an incidental finding. Although adenomyomatosis is not considered a premalignant condition, there have been a few reports of gallbladder carcinoma developing in these patients—this is thought to result from the presence of stones and chronic inflammation, rather than adenomyomatosis per se.

Much of the literature regarding imaging of adenomyomatosis has focused on US, with the classic appearance of cystic spaces in the gallbladder wall and echogenic reverberation "ring-down" artifact. The MRI literature on adenomyomatosis is not extensive, but the consensus is that MRI is probably at least as good as US and significantly better than CT for detection and characterization of these lesions. Standard MRCP sequences (2D SSFSE and 3D FRFSE) are useful for visualizing fluid-filled Rokitansky-Aschoff sinuses and gallbladder wall thickening.

Difficulties typically arise when something strange about the gallbladder is noticed after a standard hepatic MRI has been performed, in which case you may be left with images of the gallbladder that have relatively low spatial resolution, are centered on other structures, and often have relatively poor fat suppression. If, however, you know from the beginning that you're looking at the gallbladder, then the examination can be tailored to answer the question, using thinner slices centered over the gallbladder with better shimming. Don't forget about SSFP sequences: A 3D SSFP acquisition is shown in this case (Figure 3.1.1) and provided the most diagnostic images from the examination. The images were obtained in a 20-second breath-hold and beautifully demonstrate gallbladder wall thickening, luminal distortion, and multiple Rokitansky-Aschoff sinuses. These data were also used to generate the 3D reconstructions.

If you don't see Rokitansky-Aschoff sinuses, it doesn't necessarily mean that the diagnosis cannot be adenomyomatosis, but your specificity may be poor.

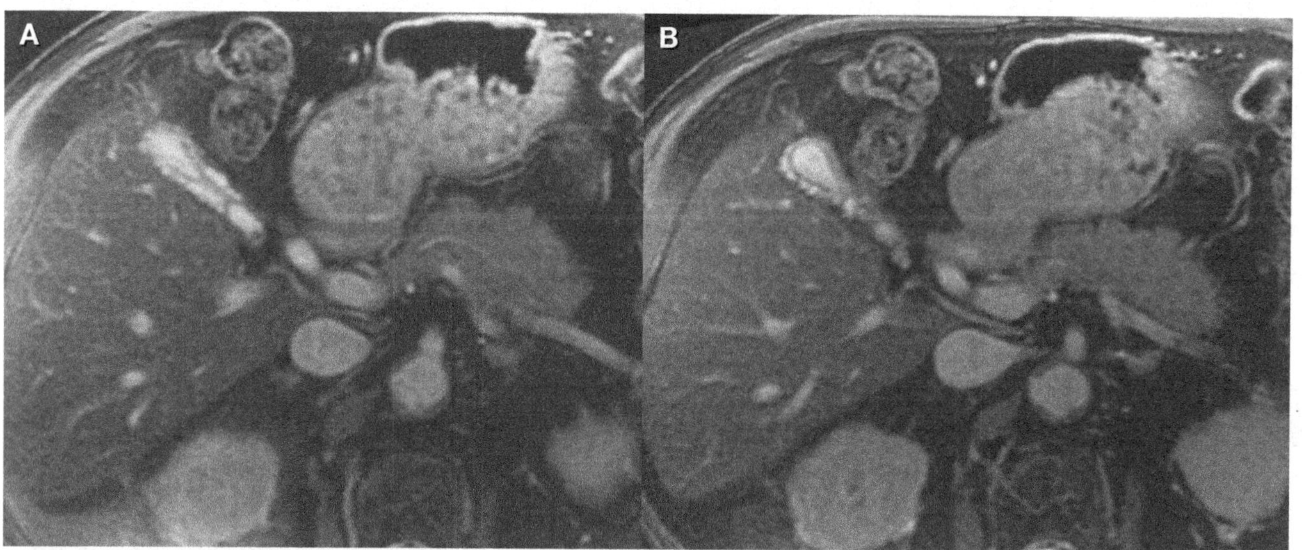

Figure 3.1.3

In a second example of adenomyomatosis, an SSFP technique again provided the best images—this time, a 2D fat-suppressed sequence (Figure 3.1.3) obtained with overlapping thin sections. Relatively little mural thickening or luminal distortion is seen; the appearance is dominated by diffuse small, uniform Rokitansky-Aschoff sinuses.

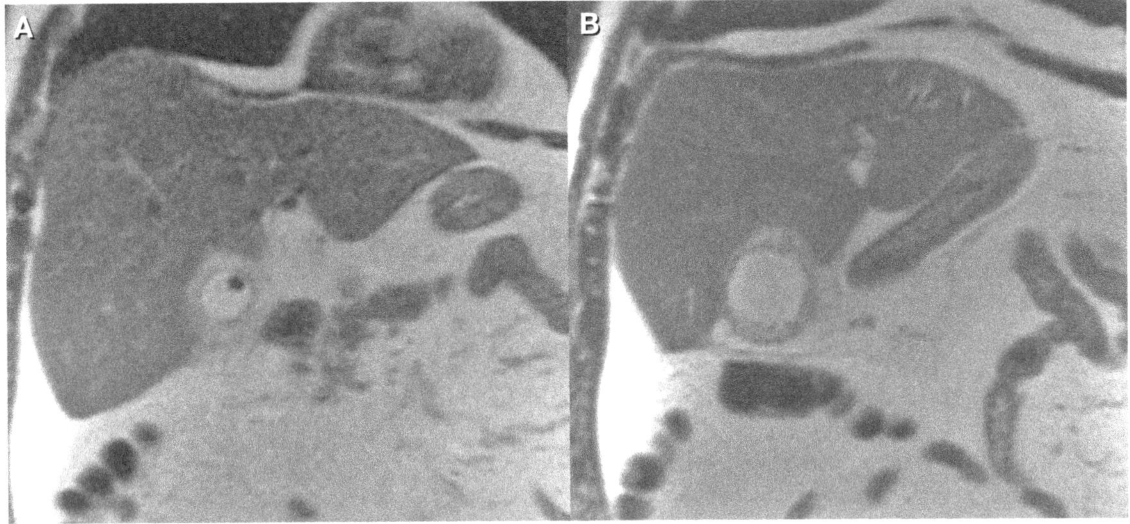

Figure 3.2.1

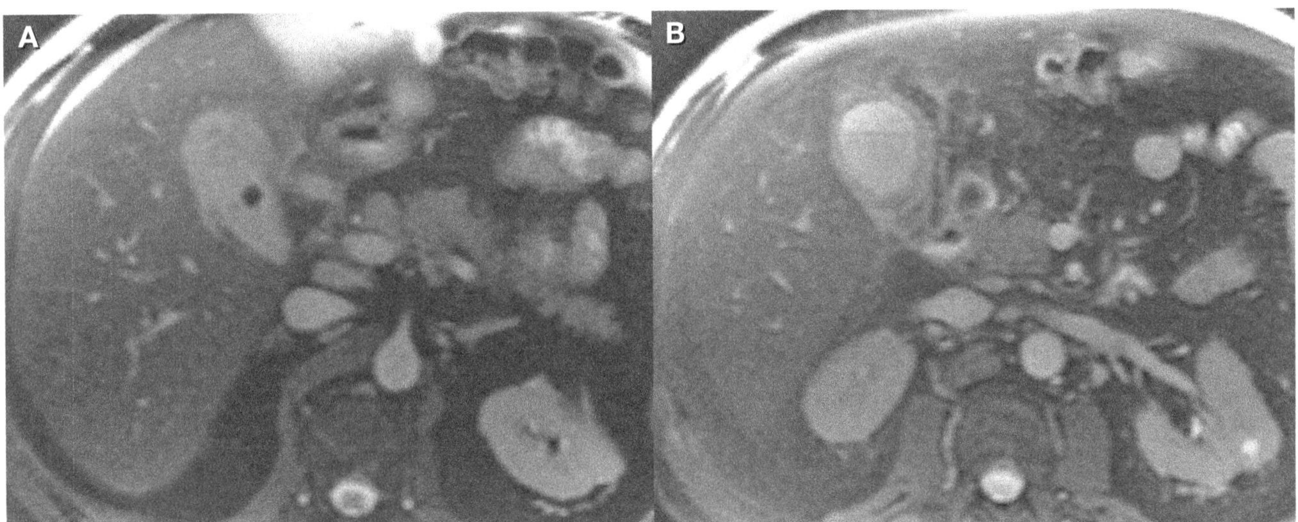

Figure 3.2.2

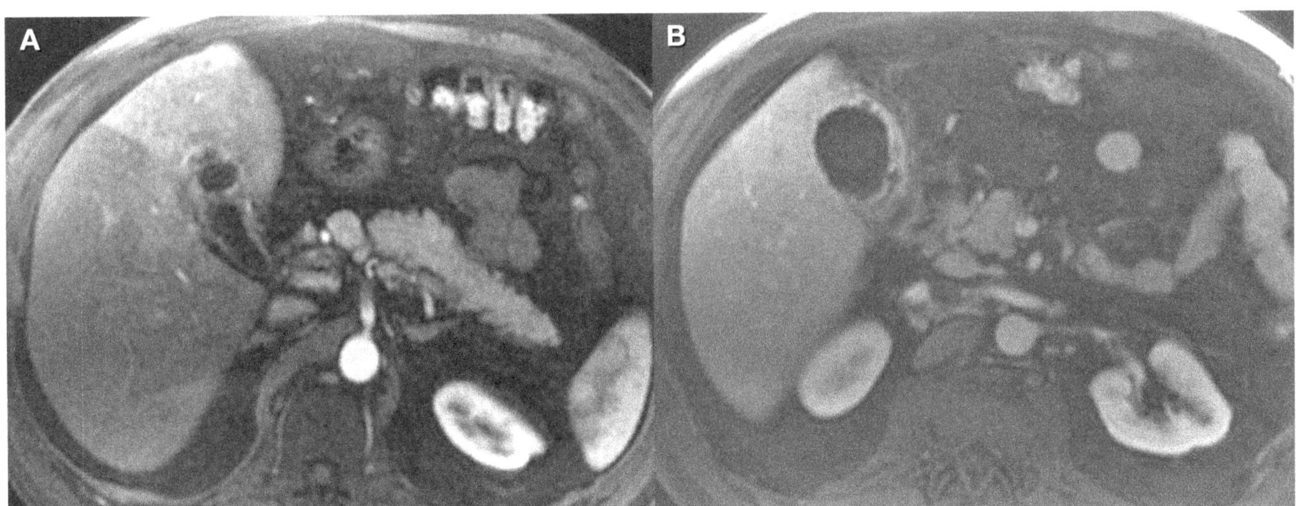

Figure 3.2.3

HISTORY: 49-year-old man with a history of prior intrahepatic biliary stone disease and new onset of right upper quadrant pain

IMAGING FINDINGS: Coronal SSFSE (Figure 3.2.1) and axial fat-suppressed SSFP (Figure 3.2.2) images show moderate gallbladder wall thickening with mural edema and a gallstone in the gallbladder neck. Of note, a smaller stone, probably impacted in the cystic duct, and the bile fluid-fluid level can be seen on axial SSFP images. Axial postgadolinium 3D SPGR images (Figure 3.2.3) show irregular mucosal enhancement of the gallbladder wall, as well as patchy enhancement of the liver adjacent to the gallbladder fossa.

DIAGNOSIS: Acute cholecystitis

COMMENT: MRI is not the primary imaging test for patients with right upper quadrant pain and suspected cholecystitis. US is much more readily available, is cheaper, and is reasonably accurate, and we certainly agree with the American College of Radiology Appropriateness Criteria for this indication, although the criteria lump MRI, CT with or without contrast medium, and scintigraphy as secondary options with equal validity (a questionable conclusion). Nevertheless, in cases where US is indeterminate or there are other potential diagnoses, MRI can be helpful. In this case, since the patient had known intrahepatic biliary stones, it was thought that MRI would be the more useful test.

Acute cholecystitis usually results from obstruction of the cystic duct or gallbladder neck by an impacted gallstone. Acalculous cholecystitis occurs in 5% to 10% of cases and may be incited by a gallbladder polyp, neoplasm, or adenomyomatosis. MRI findings in acute cholecystitis include impacted gallstones in the gallbladder neck or cystic duct, gallbladder wall thickening >3 mm, gallbladder wall edema, gallbladder distention (diameter >40 mm), pericholecystic fluid, and fluid around the liver. The presence of 1 or more of these 6 criteria was predictive of cholecystitis, with a sensitivity of 88% and specificity of 89% in 1 study. These results are dubious, however, because most of the criteria are nonspecific and have long differential diagnostic lists (ie, not all cirrhotic patients have acute cholecystitis), but in the appropriate clinical setting, they may be useful findings. We would also add to the list the presence of mucosal or mural enhancement, a near universal indication of inflammation. Hyperenhancement of the adjacent hepatic parenchyma, seen in this case, is a nonspecific finding but is suggestive of adjacent inflammation.

Another option in assessing patients with suspected cholecystitis is to use gadoxetate disodium (Eovist) and essentially perform the MR equivalent of nuclear scintigraphy. On hepatobiliary phase images, you should be able to see excreted contrast in the cystic duct and gallbladder. If you don't, its absence implies obstruction of the cystic duct and cholecystitis.

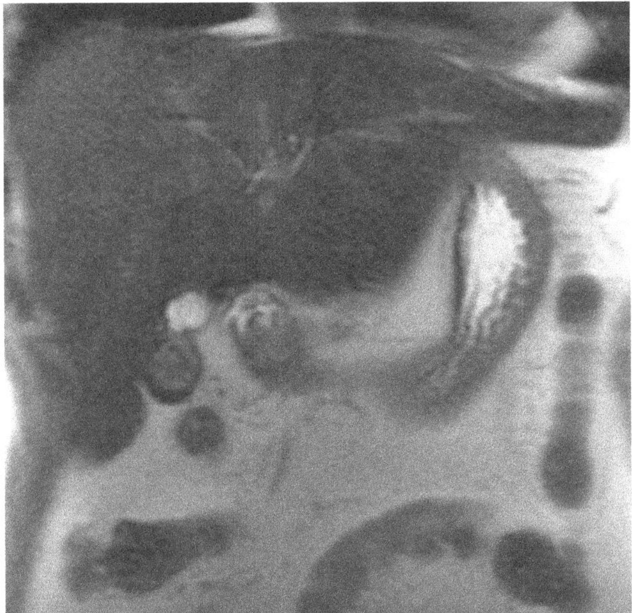

Figure 3.3.1

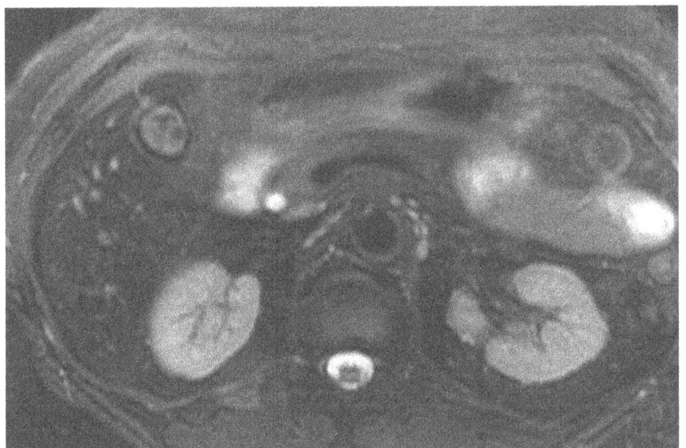

Figure 3.3.2

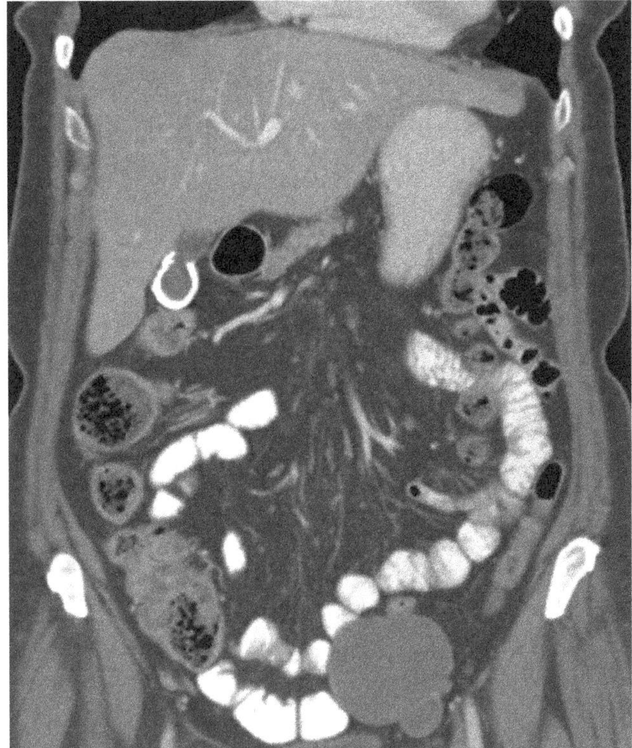

Figure 3.3.3

HISTORY: 65-year-old woman with rectal cancer and indeterminate hepatic lesions on CT

IMAGING FINDINGS: Coronal SSFSE (Figure 3.3.1) and axial FSE T2-weighted (Figure 3.3.2) images demonstrate low signal intensity in the gallbladder fundus, with a markedly hypointense rim. Coronal reformatted image from contrast-enhanced CT (Figure 3.3.3) shows diffuse calcification of the gallbladder fundus corresponding to the hypointense rim on MRI.

DIAGNOSIS: Porcelain gallbladder

COMMENT: *Porcelain gallbladder* is used to describe diffuse calcification of the gallbladder wall and has long been thought to constitute a significant risk factor for gallbladder carcinoma. For that reason, prophylactic cholecystectomy has been advocated for patients with porcelain gallbladder, whether or not they have symptoms. This thinking was based largely on papers published in the 1960s, one of which reported a 61% incidence of gallbladder carcinoma in patients with porcelain gallbladder. This association has been called into question more recently; 2 larger studies published in 2001 showed much lower incidences of 0% and 5%, respectively. The explanation for the large discrepancies is not clear but likely has to do with the rapid proliferation of US and CT and the subsequent detection of gallbladder calcification as an incidental finding leading to cholecystectomy. It also is possible that the epidemiology of gallbladder carcinoma is changing.

Whatever the case, the finding of porcelain gallbladder should still be reported, but without the dire prognostic implications once ascribed to it. MRI is well known as the test of choice if you don't want to see calcification, but calcification can sometimes be appreciated by the careful observer, generally as a nonenhancing, hypointense structure on both T1- and T2-weighted images. This case illustrates this principle: The gallbladder wall is hypointense in the fundus, corresponding to the calcification on CT. It should be noted that this is not universally true but probably is the more common presentation.

Porcelain gallbladder is strongly associated with chronic inflammation and the presence of gallstones (60%-100%), and the ongoing inflammatory process is thought to be responsible for mucosal dysplasia and eventual calcification.

CASE 3.4

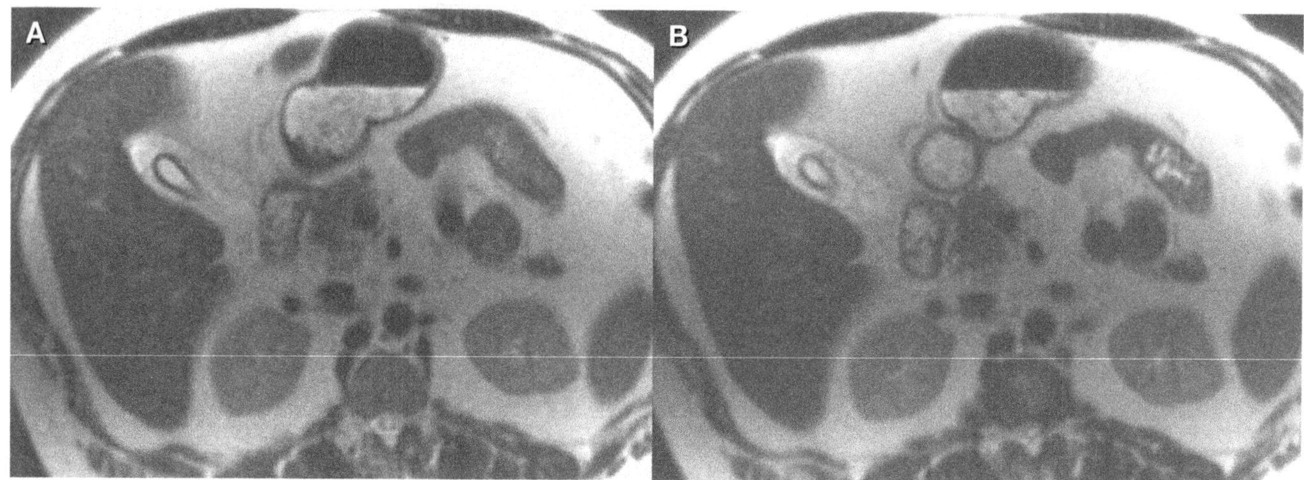

Figure 3.4.1

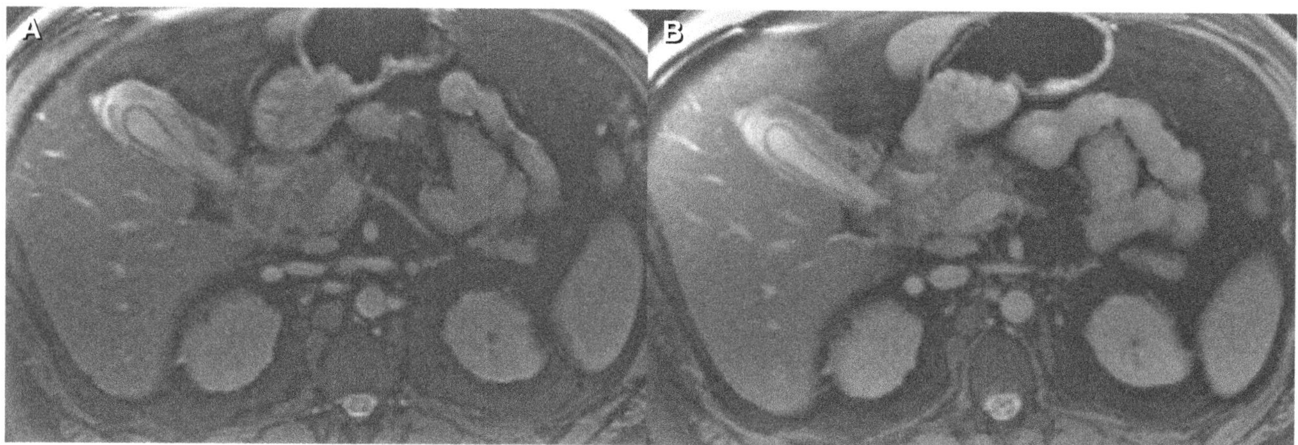

Figure 3.4.2

HISTORY: 32-year-old man with chronic hepatitis C and recent elevation of liver enzyme levels

IMAGING FINDINGS: Axial SSFSE (Figure 3.4.1) and fat-suppressed SSFP (Figure 3.4.2) images demonstrate marked diffuse thickening of the gallbladder wall.

DIAGNOSIS: Hepatitis with marked gallbladder wall thickening

COMMENT: Gallbladder wall thickening is associated with a large number of pathologic conditions, including cirrhosis, acute and chronic cholecystitis, ascites, hypoalbuminemia, viral hepatitis, chronic renal failure, and heart failure. The physiologic mechanism responsible for diffuse gallbladder thickening in the presence of systemic or diffuse hepatic disease is uncertain but probably is related to elevated portal venous pressure or decreased intravascular osmotic pressure, or both.

The main point to remember is that a thickened gallbladder doesn't always mean cholecystitis, even in patients with right upper quadrant pain (a frequent symptom in patients with cirrhosis and hepatitis).

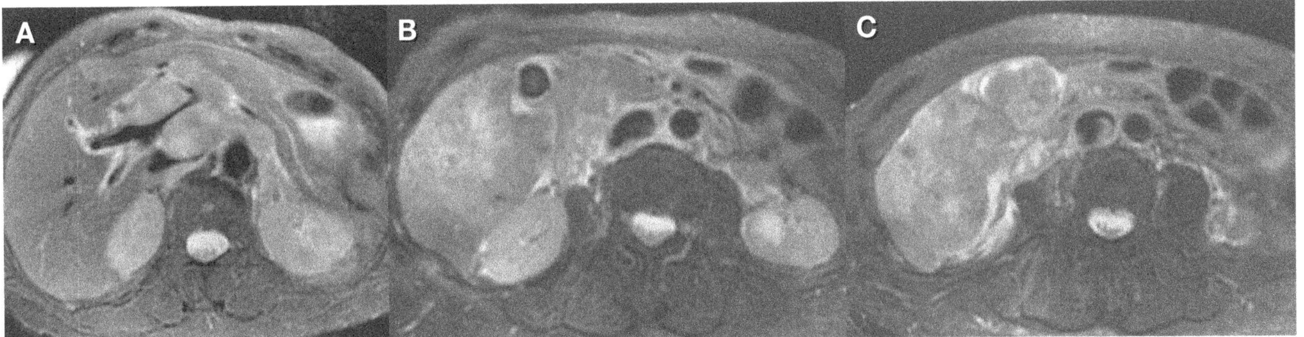

Figure 3.5.1

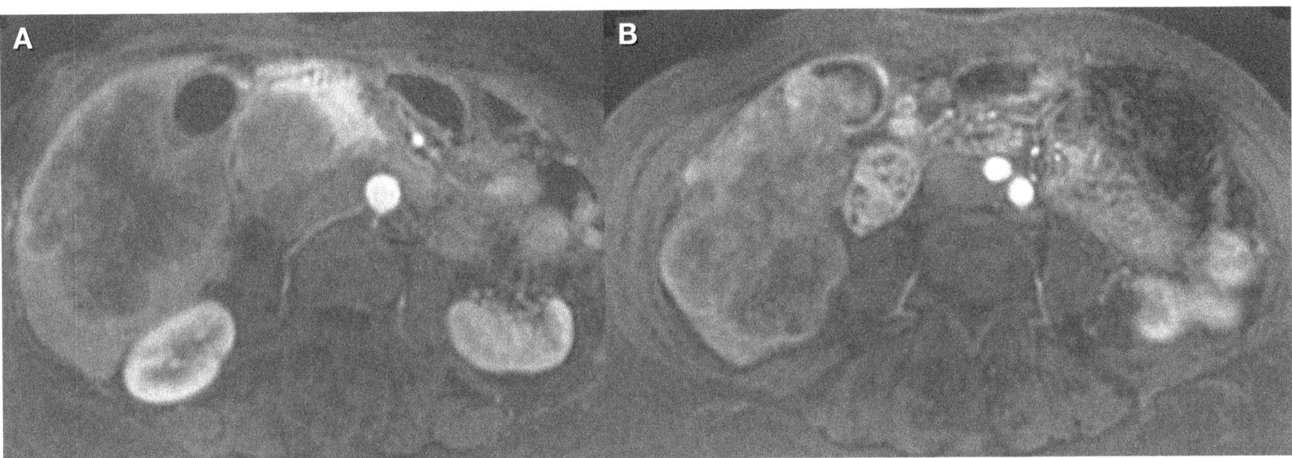

Figure 3.5.2

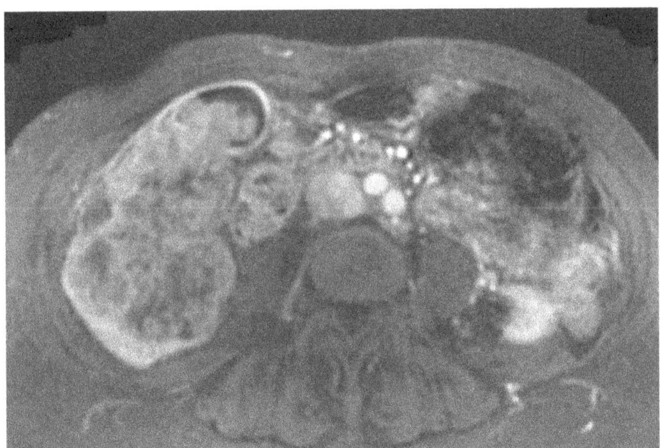

Figure 3.5.3

HISTORY: 69-year-old woman with epigastric and retrosternal pain and jaundice

IMAGING FINDINGS: Axial fat-suppressed FSE T2-weighted images (Figure 3.5.1) demonstrate extensive adenopathy in the porta hepatis, as well as heterogeneous, mildly hyperintense masses in the gallbladder and adjacent right hepatic lobe. Note the large gallstone in Figure 3.5.1B. Axial arterial phase (Figure 3.5.2) and portal venous phase (Figure 3.5.3) postgadolinium 3D SPGR images show a heterogeneously enhancing mass centered in the gallbladder and extending through the gallbladder wall to directly invade the liver.

DIAGNOSIS: Gallbladder carcinoma with invasion of the liver

COMMENT: Adenocarcinoma of the gallbladder is a rare lesion that nevertheless is the most common malignant neoplasm of the biliary tract and the seventh most common gastrointestinal cancer. Gallbladder carcinoma affects women more frequently than men, and although there are multiple risk factors, its incidence is highly correlated with cholelithiasis. The vast majority of patients with gallbladder carcinoma have gallstones, and the presence of gallstones is thought to increase the risk of gallbladder carcinoma 4 to 5 times over the risk in patients without cholelithiasis (although only about 1% of persons with gallstones develop gallbladder carcinoma).

Porcelain gallbladder was once thought to represent a significant risk for development of gallbladder carcinoma, but this view has changed in recent years. The most recent studies indicate no additional risk or a slight additional risk (see Case 3.3 for further discussion of porcelain gallbladder). Gallbladder polyps rarely may transform into frank carcinomas; the risk increases with increasing lesion diameter, increasing patient age, and presence of a solitary polyp or gallstones. Other risk factors for gallbladder carcinoma include xanthogranulomatous cholecystitis, adenomyomatosis, and inflammatory bowel disease.

Most gallbladder cancers are adenocarcinomas, and these have been subdivided into papillary, tubular, and nodular variants, with papillary tumors having the least aggressive behavior. The modified Nevin system is commonly used for staging gallbladder carcinoma. Stage I disease is limited to the mucosa; stage II has tumor invasion into the muscularis layer; stage III, direct extension into the liver; stage IV, lymph node metastases; and stage V, distant metastases. Five-year survival rates are poor: 39% for stage I, 15% for stage II, and 5% or less for stages III through V.

In general, symptoms of gallbladder carcinoma are nonspecific and include abdominal pain, nausea and vomiting, jaundice, anorexia, and weight loss. At least 20% of patients receive the diagnosis at cholecystectomy performed for biliary colic and cholelithiasis.

The appearance of this case is unfortunately a fairly typical one: a heterogeneously enhancing polypoid mass in the gallbladder that is growing through the wall and directly invading the liver. These lesions are usually hypointense relative to the liver on arterial phase dynamic 3D SPGR images and show greater enhancement on portal venous and equilibrium phase images. They generally are mildly to moderately hyperintense on T2-weighted images. The hepatic invasion and lymph node metastases in this case constitute stage IV disease—inoperable and with a poor prognosis.

The differential diagnosis for an appearance like this one is limited. Occasionally, the gallbladder is difficult to visualize among the large hepatic metastases, but the hepatic lesions are often clustered around the gallbladder fossa, which is suggestive of the diagnosis. Less advanced or more subtle lesions (see Case 3.6) have a differential diagnosis that includes benign focal gallbladder masses.

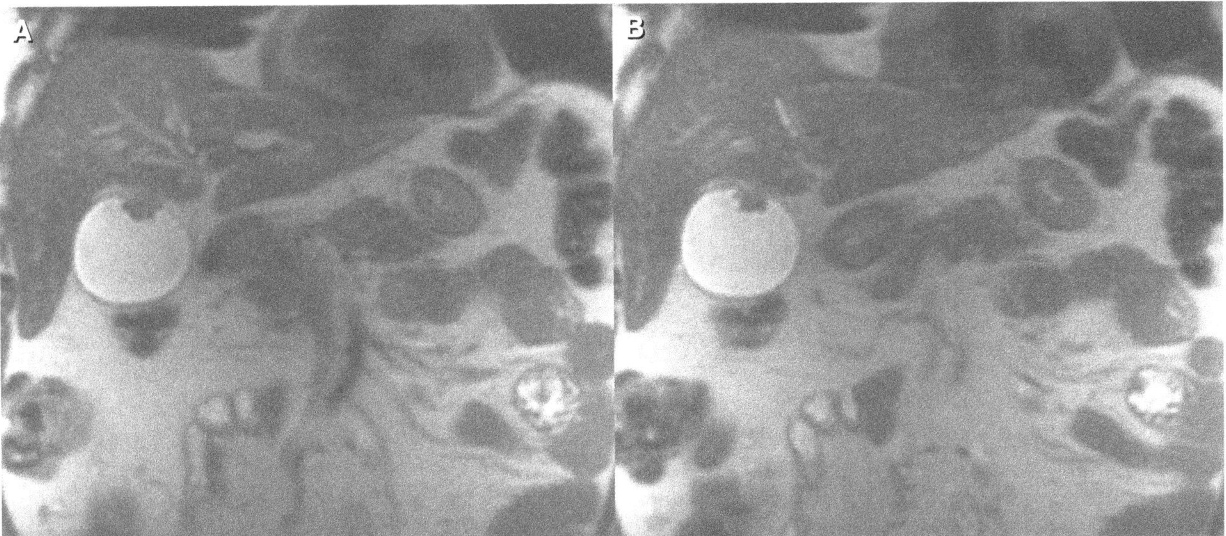

Figure 3.6.1

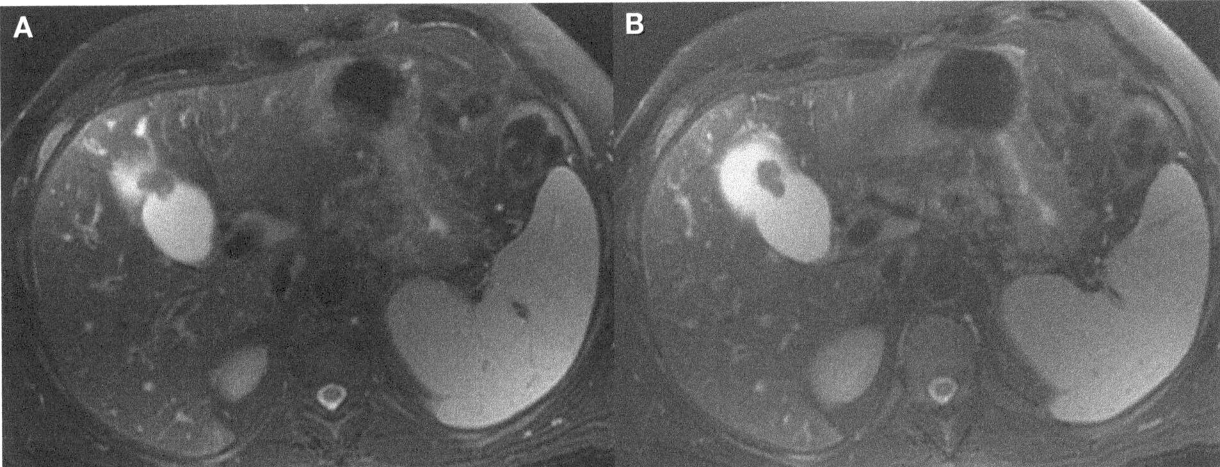

Figure 3.6.2

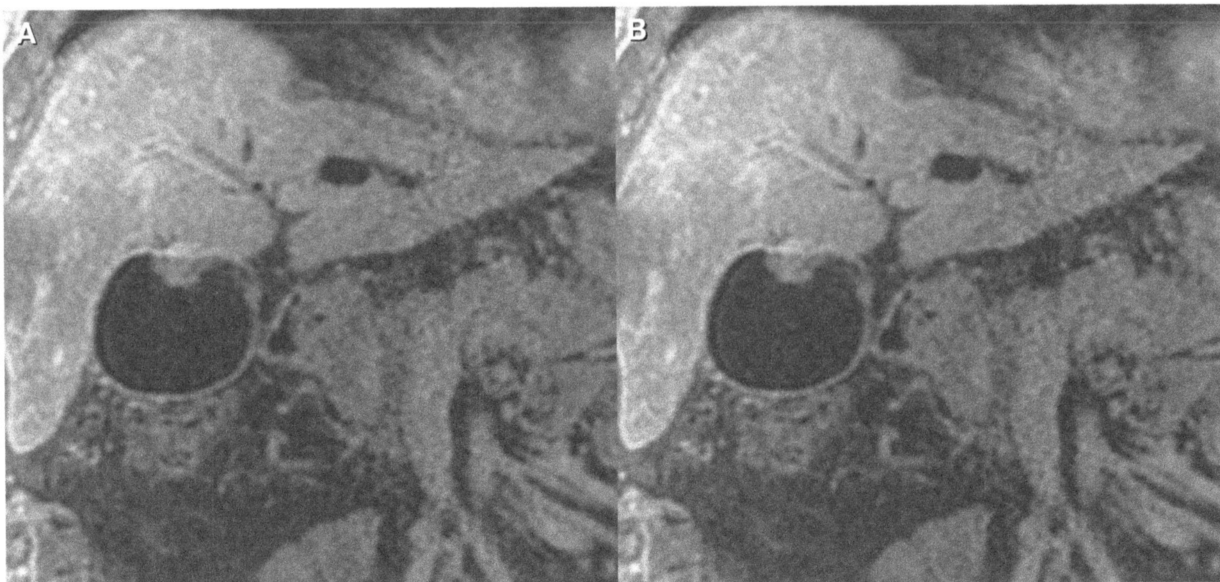

Figure 3.6.3

HISTORY: 54-year-old man with a chronic biliary disorder; MRI was performed for routine surveillance

IMAGING FINDINGS: Coronal SSFSE (Figure 3.6.1) and axial fat-saturated FSE (Figure 3.6.2) images demonstrate an irregular lesion in the gallbladder, abutting the superior wall. Coronal, delayed phase 3D SPGR images (Figure 3.6.3) show transmural extension of the lesion. Note the dilated left hepatic lobe biliary duct and irregular generalized parenchymal enhancement in the liver, suggestive of fibrosis.

DIAGNOSIS: Gallbladder carcinoma

COMMENT: The lesion in this case is much smaller than in Case 3.5 and the diagnosis is a little more difficult. However, the coronal delayed phase images show transmural extension of the mass, which shouldn't be seen for a benign gallbladder polyp. This finding was confirmed at surgery, and no direct invasion of the liver was identified. The patient unfortunately developed metastatic disease within 2 years of surgery and subsequently expired. This outcome emphasizes the poor prognosis of even low-stage lesions (stage II in this case).

The main differential diagnosis in this case (especially if it had no mural invasion) would be a gallbladder polyp or adenoma. Most benign polyps are small and round and have uniform low signal intensity on T2-weighted images and minimal enhancement. They are often difficult to distinguish from gallstones except that you might see them in nondependent locations. A rule of thumb from US that should apply equally well to MRI is that the level of suspicion becomes higher for lesions greater than 1 cm in diameter, with surgical consultation often recommended. An example of a gallbladder adenoma (benign at surgery but definitely a worrisome imaging appearance) and a coexisting polyp are shown in Figures 3.6.4, 3.6.5, and 3.6.6.

Diagnosis of gallbladder carcinoma can be trickier in the setting of focal or diffuse gallbladder wall thickening without hepatic invasion, in which case adenomyomatosis, as well as chronic inflammatory conditions such as xanthogranulomatous cholecystitis, should also be considered. In general, gallbladder carcinoma tends to show greater wall thickening and a more heterogeneous appearance, although this description is relatively nonspecific. Recently, some authors have suggested that diffusion-weighted imaging may help to discriminate these lesions; gallbladder carcinoma tends to have more restricted diffusion and a lower apparent diffusion coefficient than inflammatory conditions. This conclusion is based on very little data, however, and it seems likely that apparent diffusion coefficient criteria for gallbladder carcinoma will be about as useful as those for other biliary and hepatic masses (ie, not at all).

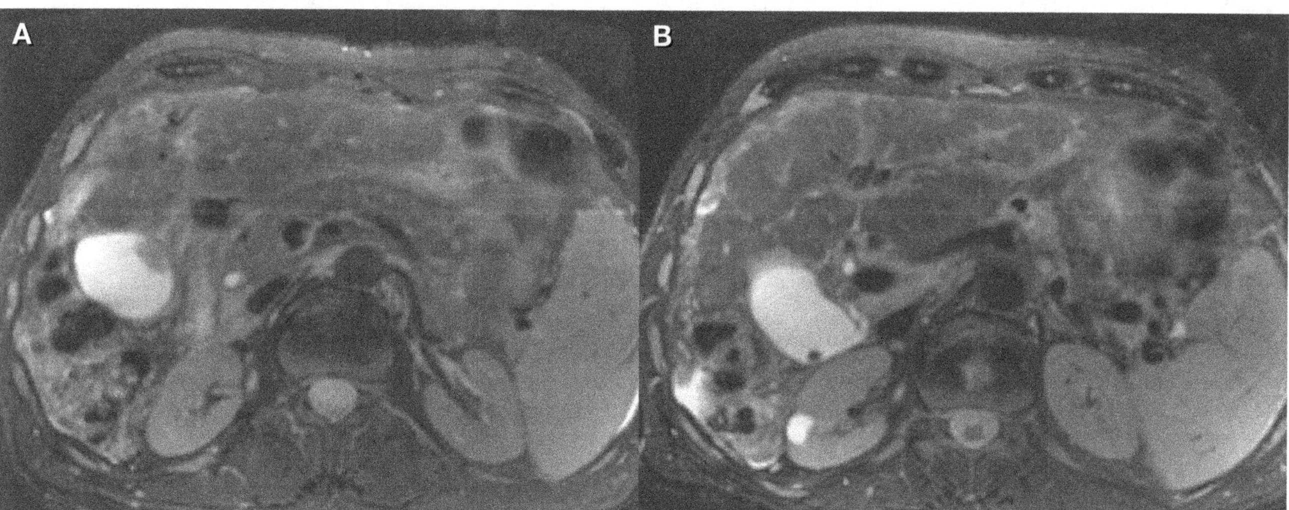

Figure 3.6.4

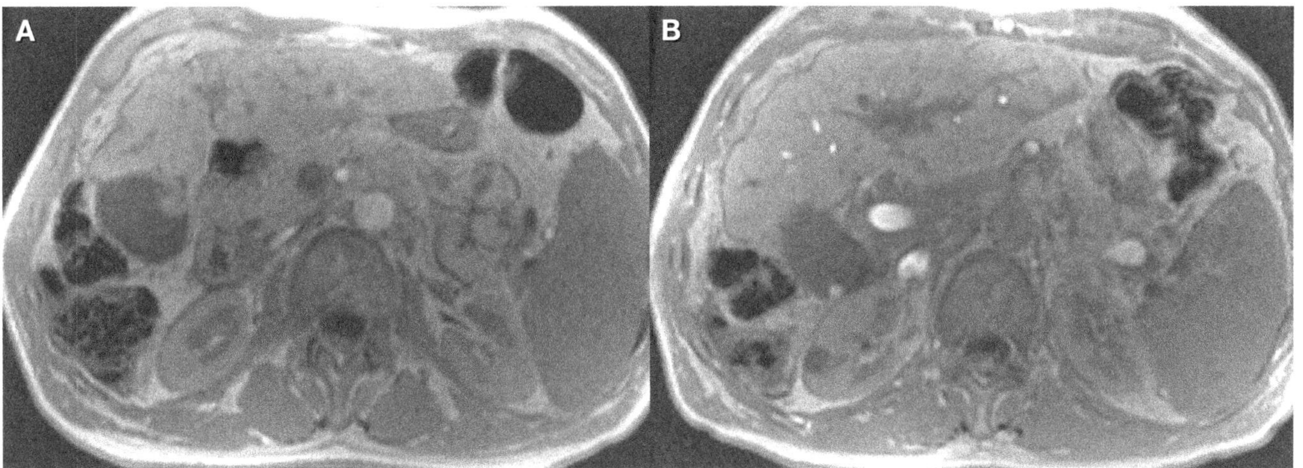

Figure 3.6.5

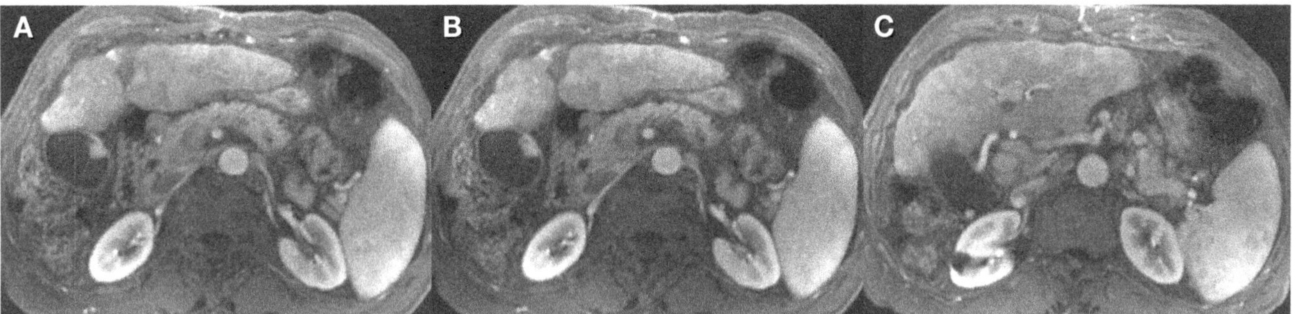

Figure 3.6.6

Axial fat-suppressed FSE T2-weighted images (Figure 3.6.4) from an examination performed after incidental detection of a gallbladder lesion on abdominal CT in a 75-year-old man show an irregular lesion (adenoma) along the anterior surface of the gallbladder, as well as a much smaller, round, hypointense lesion (polyp) posteriorly. Corresponding in-phase 2D SPGR images (Figure 3.6.5) demonstrate that the small polyp has a relatively high T1-signal intensity and the larger adenoma has an intermediate signal. Arterial phase post-gadolinium 3D SPGR images (Figure 3.6.6) show moderate enhancement of the adenoma, with associated mild thickening and enhancement of the adjacent gallbladder wall. The gallbladder polyp has minimal enhancement, which is difficult to appreciate because of its high signal intensity before contrast administration.

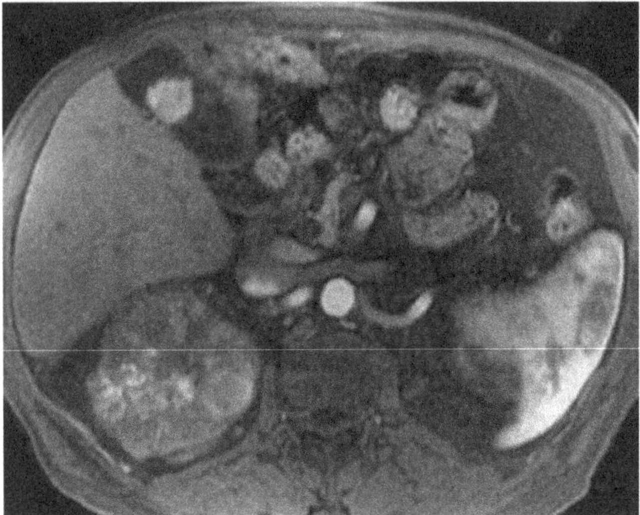

Figure 3.7.1

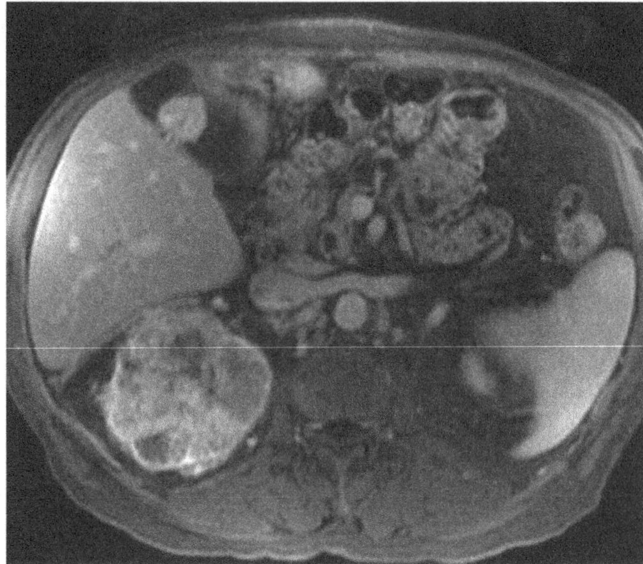

Figure 3.7.2

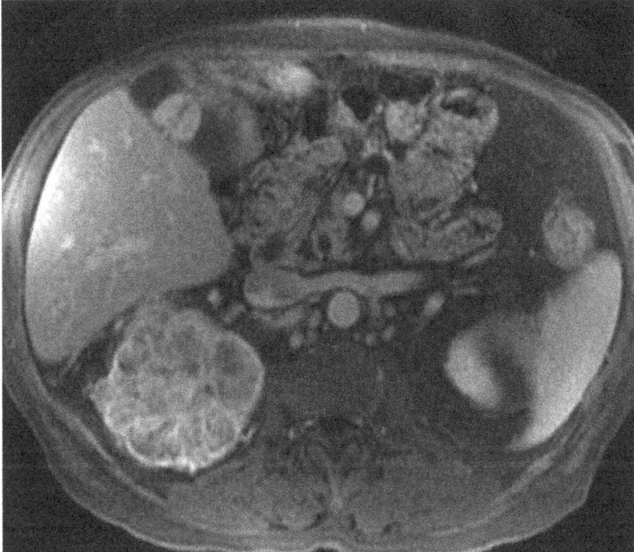

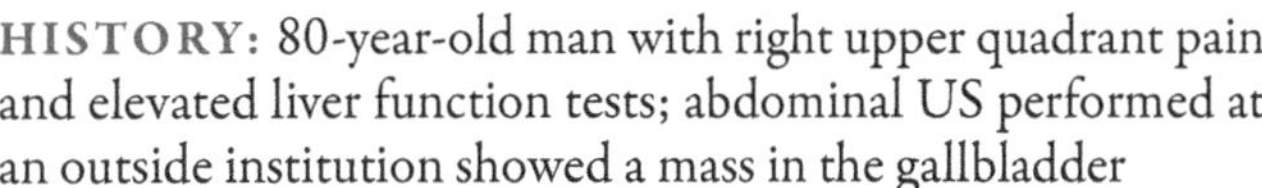

Figure 3.7.3

HISTORY: 80-year-old man with right upper quadrant pain and elevated liver function tests; abdominal US performed at an outside institution showed a mass in the gallbladder

IMAGING FINDINGS: Arterial (Figure 3.7.1), portal venous (Figure 3.7.2), and equilibrium phase (Figure 3.7.3) postgadolinium 3D SPGR images demonstrate a hyperenhancing mass within the gallbladder lumen. Note also the large heterogeneous mass seen in the upper pole of the right kidney.

DIAGNOSIS: Gallbladder metastasis from renal cell carcinoma

COMMENT: Metastatic disease in the clinical setting of RCC is unfortunately fairly common. At the time of diagnosis, approximately one-third of patients have metastases, and the prognosis in this group is poor, with 5-year survival rates of 5% to 10%. Gallbladder metastases, on the other hand, are extremely rare, documented in only 0.6% of cases in a large autopsy review. They seem to be a little more common in our practice. We recently reviewed 60 cases of RCC and found gallbladder metastases in 3 patients, so it's probably worth keeping an eye on the gallbladder when performing MRIs of patients with renal masses. A review of 24 cases of metastatic RCC to the gallbladder noted that in nearly all patients, the appearance was of a hyperenhancing polypoid mass, with the major differential diagnosis being gallbladder carcinoma. The presence of a large renal mass, as seen in this case, and the knowledge that RCC is notorious for spreading to virtually every organ make the diagnosis of gallbladder metastasis straightforward.

Some benefit may be gained in resecting metastases in patients with RCC, particularly solitary lesions, in whom 5-year survival rates of 40% to 50% have been reported. A similar survival trend is noted in the series on gallbladder metastases; no patient who underwent cholecystectomy was reported to have local recurrence in the liver or bile ducts.

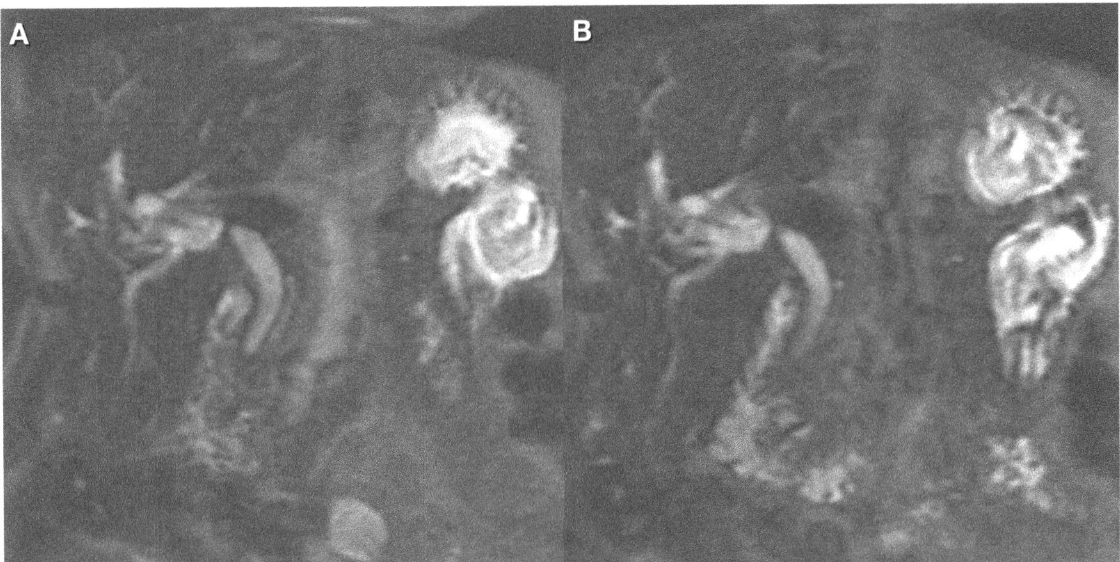

Figure 3.8.1

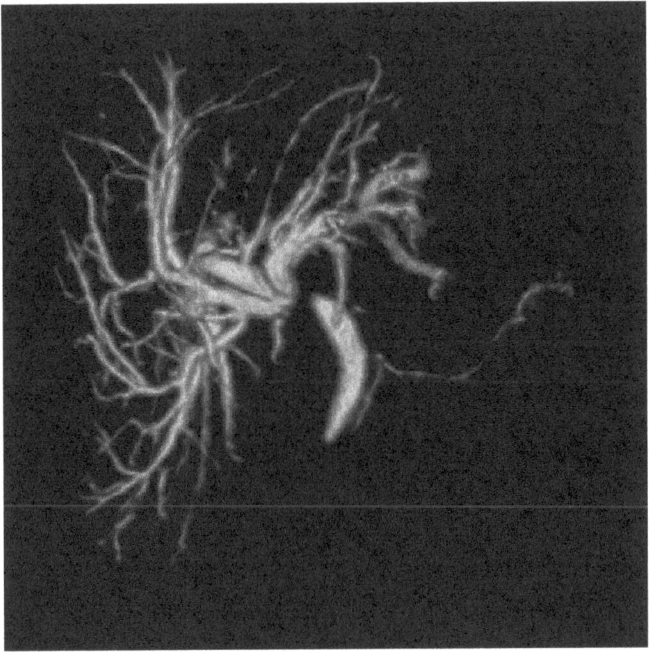

Figure 3.8.2

HISTORY: 68-year-old woman who developed abdominal pain 6 months previous, had an abnormal HIDA scan, and subsequently underwent laparoscopic cholecystectomy at an outside institution; since the surgery, she has had intermittent abdominal pain and cramping, as well as a 20-lb weight loss

IMAGING FINDINGS: Coronal SSFSE images (Figure 3.8.1) and a volume-rendered image from 3D FRFSE MRCP (Figure 3.8.2) show a high-grade focal stricture of the proximal CBD, with moderate intrahepatic biliary dilatation.

DIAGNOSIS: Iatrogenic CBD injury during laparoscopic cholecystectomy

COMMENT: Happy, well-adjusted gastroenterology surgical residents or fellows are something of a rarity in our experience. CBD injury during laparoscopic cholecystectomy is a good example of the kind of thing that can make their lives miserable. The first laparoscopic cholecystectomy was performed in 1985, and after a brief period of initial skepticism, the technique was widely embraced, along with the potential benefits of reduced postoperative pain and shorter hospital stay. Laparoscopic surgery is not a trivial procedure, however, and the challenge of educating and training surgeons beyond their residency in a new technique is a difficult one. Weekend courses in laparoscopic surgery using pigs or plastic models are no doubt better than nothing, but it's also true that you don't want to be your surgeon's first case, or probably even the 99th, just as you would never want to get sick in July.

Despite expectations that the rate of bile duct injury would decrease over time as the learning curve of laparoscopic cholecystectomy flattened, large studies have shown a complication rate of 0.5%—well above the 0.1% rate obtained in the era of open surgery. In the United States, an estimated 34% to 49% of surgeons have caused a major bile duct injury. Most injuries occur during the surgeon's first 100 laparoscopic cholecystectomies; however, one-third result after the surgeon has performed more than 200 operations. Most injuries are thought to result from misidentification of the biliary anatomy.

Bile duct injury is associated with significant morbidity and death, reduced quality of life, and high rates of subsequent litigation. Although these cases are probably best managed by experienced hepatobiliary surgeons at tertiary centers, 55% to 75% of injuries are still repaired by the surgeon responsible for the initial injury.

Many bile duct injuries are not detected during the initial surgery and instead are recognized on development of classic symptoms and signs of biliary leak or transection, including jaundice, biloma, sepsis, biliary fistula, and biliary peritonitis. Optimal timing of definitive repair is somewhat controversial. Some evidence shows that early repair is associated with shorter duration of treatment and improved quality of life; other authors have noted that initial percutaneous or endoscopic biliary drainage followed by a delay to control inflammatory or infectious conditions results in fewer complications during reparative surgery. Even under the best of circumstances, management of these cases remains challenging. The largest series of bile duct injuries from Johns Hopkins Hospital reported a mortality rate of 1.7% and a complication rate of 43%.

The patient in this case had a complex, but not atypical, course. Further investigation showed that CBD injury was noted during the initial surgery, where a T tube was placed. The tube was removed a few weeks later, and a severe stricture subsequently developed. At Mayo Clinic, she initially underwent ERCP, which was unsuccessful in crossing the stricture, followed by percutaneous transhepatic cholangiography with stent placement. Stents were replaced a few times when they became obstructed, but eventually the stricture resolved and the stent was removed, and currently the patient is symptom free.

MRCP is a useful technique in evaluating patients with known or suspected biliary complication after laparoscopic cholecystectomy. The entire anatomy of the biliary tree can be shown and any fluid collections can be identified for subsequent drainage. If you're interested in confirming through a noninvasive manner that a fluid collection is truly a biloma, you can use a hepatobiliary contrast agent to demonstrate a bile leak. It's also important to remember to assess the hilar vessels because some series have reported associated vascular injuries in 25% to 30% of patients. This finding is yet another reason why we almost never perform an MRCP as a stand-alone examination. If something is wrong with the biliary tree, then often there are associated abnormalities in the liver, pancreas, duodenum, or blood vessels—none of which are well assessed by standard MRCP pulse sequences.

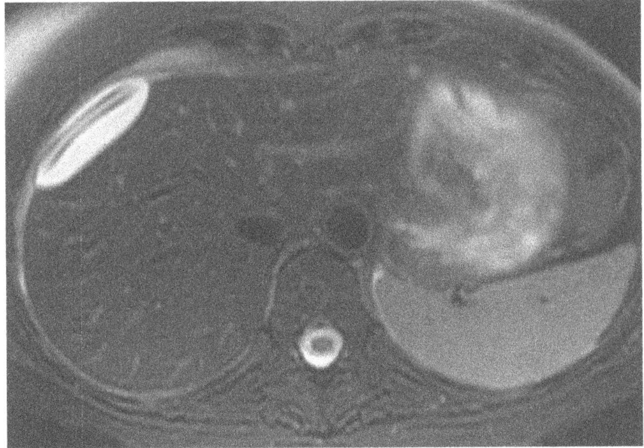

Figure 3.9.1

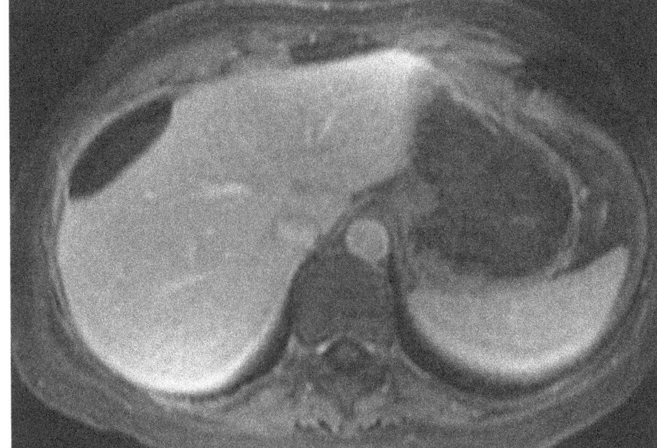

Figure 3.9.2

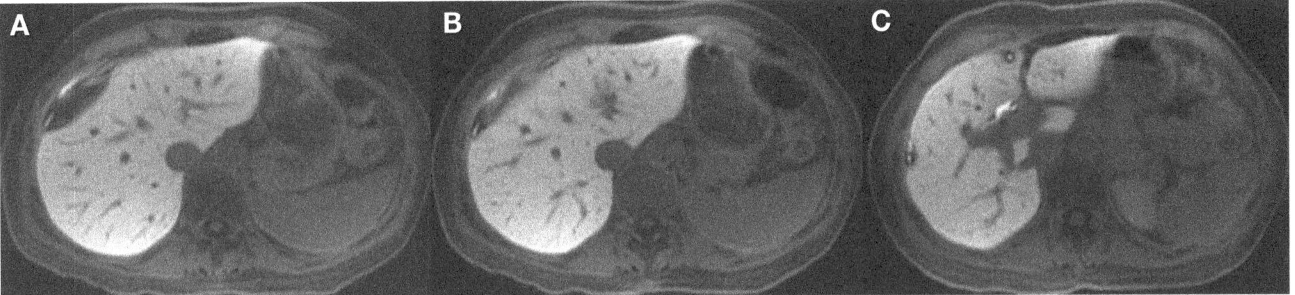

Figure 3.9.3

HISTORY: 52-year-old woman who underwent laparoscopic cholecystectomy at an outside institution 1 month ago; bilious drainage has been noted through a surgically placed drain, and subsequent ERCP showed complete cutoff of the distal CBD

IMAGING FINDINGS: Axial FSE (Figure 3.9.1) and portal venous phase (Figure 3.9.2) post–gadoxetate disodium (Eovist) 3D SPGR images reveal a small subcapsular fluid collection along the anterolateral margin of the liver. A small drain passing through the collection is visible on the FSE image. Axial hepatobiliary phase 3D SPGR images (Figure 3.9.3) demonstrate hyperintense extravasated contrast within the margin of the collection, as well as in the drain. A slightly more inferior image demonstrates extravasated contrast in the hepatic hilum.

DIAGNOSIS: Bile leak following laparoscopic cholecystectomy and bile duct injury

COMMENT: Case 3.8 provides a more thorough discussion of bile duct injuries during laparoscopic cholecystectomy. This case illustrates the use of hepatobiliary contrast agents to document a bile leak. Although it can be argued (and frequently has been by our interventional radiologists) that if you find a fluid collection on CT or US in a symptomatic patient following hepatobiliary surgery, you're going to end up putting a needle or drain in it anyway, so why spend an extra $2,000 to document the presence of bile? This is a valid point, and in general we advocate this technique in patients who are already being scanned for another indication (in this case, for example, to document the site of CBD injury and to assess the intrahepatic ducts).

The available literature regarding imaging bile leaks with MRI is limited, and most of these investigators used mangafodipir trisodium (Teslascan), a manganese-based contrast agent no longer commercially available, with sensitivities ranging from 86% to 95% and specificities near 100%. Today, it makes the most sense to use gadoxetate disodium (Eovist) simply because it has a higher biliary excretion (50%) than the other available agent, gadobenate dimeglumine (Multihance), which has an excretion of 5%. This characteristic results in a shorter wait to obtain hepatobiliary phase images (15-20 minutes vs 60-90 minutes). However, either agent works (see Figures 3.9.4 and 3.9.5 for a second example using Multihance), and after you've waited the appropriate length of time, you will see T1 hyperintense contrast in the biliary tree and extravasation into the peritoneum or biloma if a bile leak is present.

Several papers have attempted to sell the premise that Eovist MRCP has advantages over conventional noncontrast, heavily T2-weighted techniques. For the most part, we're underwhelmed, except for the opportunity to detect bile leaks. Eovist MRCP requires the use of 3D SPGR sequences; the commercially available versions of these (eg, LAVA [GE Healthcare], VIBE [Siemens Medical Solutions], THRIVE [Philips Healthcare]) are all breath-hold acquisitions, which means that the obtainable spatial resolution is limited in comparison to respiratory-gated 3D FRFSE. A few investigative respiratory- or navigator-gated versions of 3D SPGR have been reported, nearly all with marginal image quality at best. Another point to keep in mind is that while the signal to noise ratio of a 3D SPGR sequence is generally higher than 3D FRFSE images obtained with a long TE, the bile-to-liver contrast to noise ratio is much smaller, which means that generating high-quality 3D reconstructions is considerably more difficult. This technique may have applications in functional evaluation of the gallbladder and biliary tree or perhaps in assessment of biliary anatomy in potential living liver donors who have small, nondilated ducts, but these arguments are not compelling.

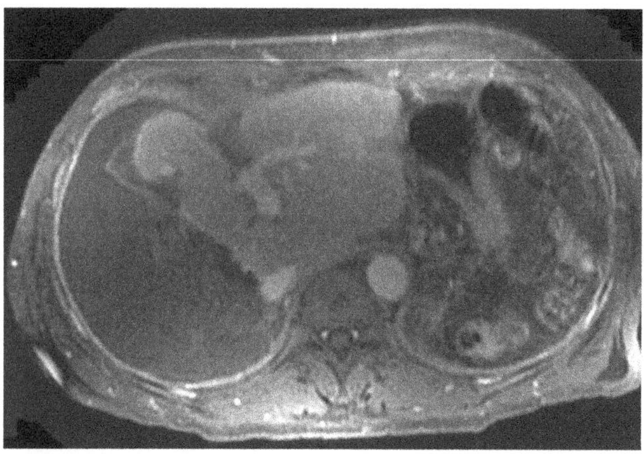

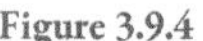

Figure 3.9.4

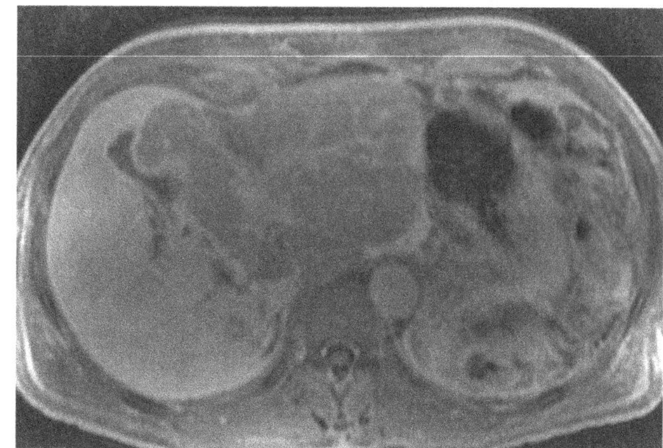

Figure 3.9.5

Axial portal venous phase 3D SPGR image (Figure 3.9.4) following gadobenate dimeglumine (Multihance) injection from a patient who had a recent right hepatectomy for resection of islet cell carcinoma metastases demonstrates a large, rim-enhancing fluid collection adjacent to the resection margin. Two-hour delayed 3D SPGR image (Figure 3.9.5) obtained at approximately the same location shows intense enhancement of the fluid, consistent with bile leak and biloma.

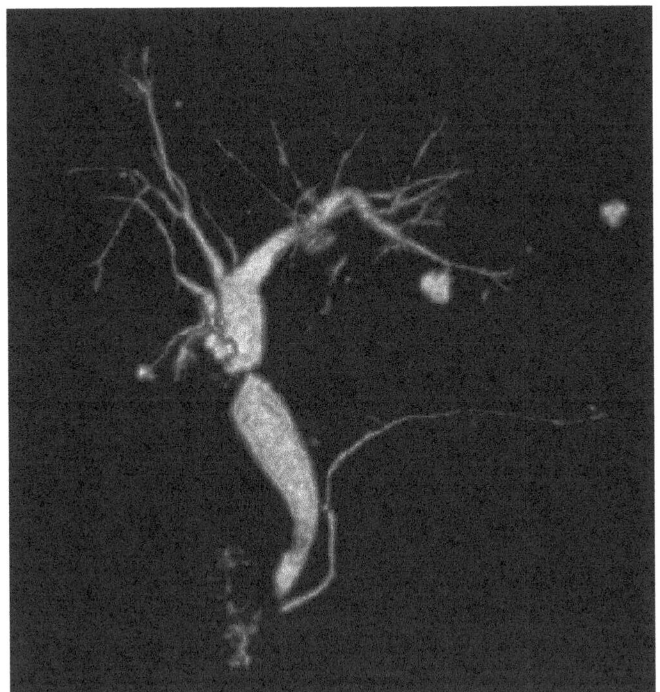

Figure 3.10.1

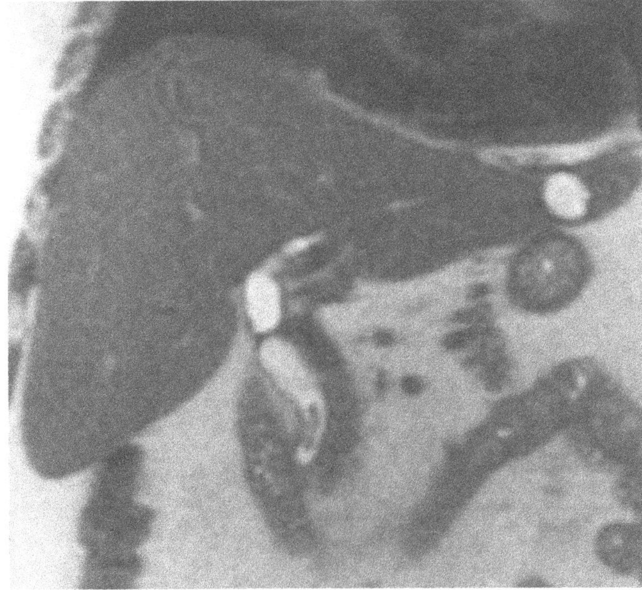

Figure 3.10.2

HISTORY: 76-year-old woman status post liver transplant 5 years ago for cirrhosis secondary to hepatitis B

IMAGING FINDINGS: Volume-rendered image from 3D FRFSE MRCP (Figure 3.10.1) and coronal SSFSE image (Figure 3.10.2) demonstrate an abrupt high-grade stricture in the mid CBD at the site of biliary anastomosis. Note also the filling defect in the distal CBD on the SSFSE image.

DIAGNOSIS: Post–liver transplant biliary anastomotic stricture

COMMENT: This case looks just like the laparoscopic cholecystectomy misadventure described in Case 3.8 but for very different reasons. Complications following liver transplant are unfortunately not rare, and biliary complications occur in 5% to 15% of patients. Most often, they are seen within the first 3 months of surgery and include biliary obstruction, anastomotic stricture, stone formation, bile leak, biloma, biliary necrosis, and cholangitis. As in this case, most strictures are extrahepatic and occur at the anastomosis secondary to scar formation. Nonanastomotic strictures are usually the result of ischemia (typically caused by hepatic artery stenosis or thrombosis) or cholangitis.

Although US is the standard test for routine assessment of posttransplant patients, accurate evaluation of the extrahepatic biliary tree and blood vessels is sometimes difficult. CT generally obtains greater spatial resolution than MRI and is a lot faster, and questions about the hepatic artery can be answered readily with CT angiography. MRI has the advantage of combining reasonably good vascular assessment with excellent visualization of the biliary tree and hepatic parenchyma, without the radiation exposure required for a multiphase CT. The accuracy of MRI in detecting vascular, parenchymal, and biliary problems in posttransplant patients is good to excellent in most studies.

The stones and/or debris in the distal CBD are presumably related to bile stasis induced by the upstream stricture. This case is a good example of the principle that the easiest way to miss small intraductal stones or masses on MRCP is to look only at the 3D reconstructions.

CASE 3.11

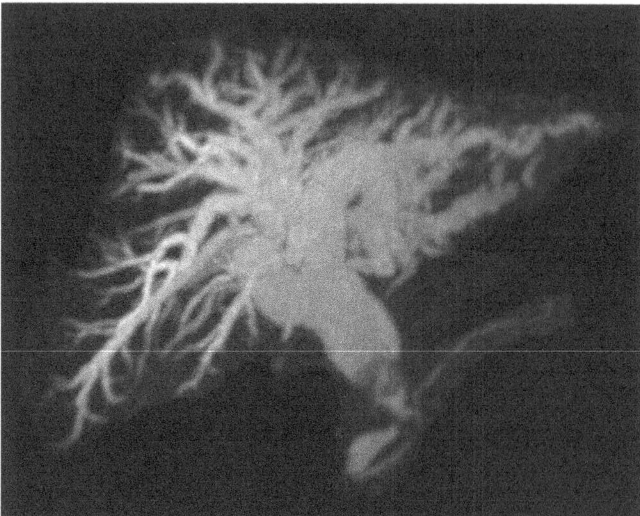

Figure 3.11.1

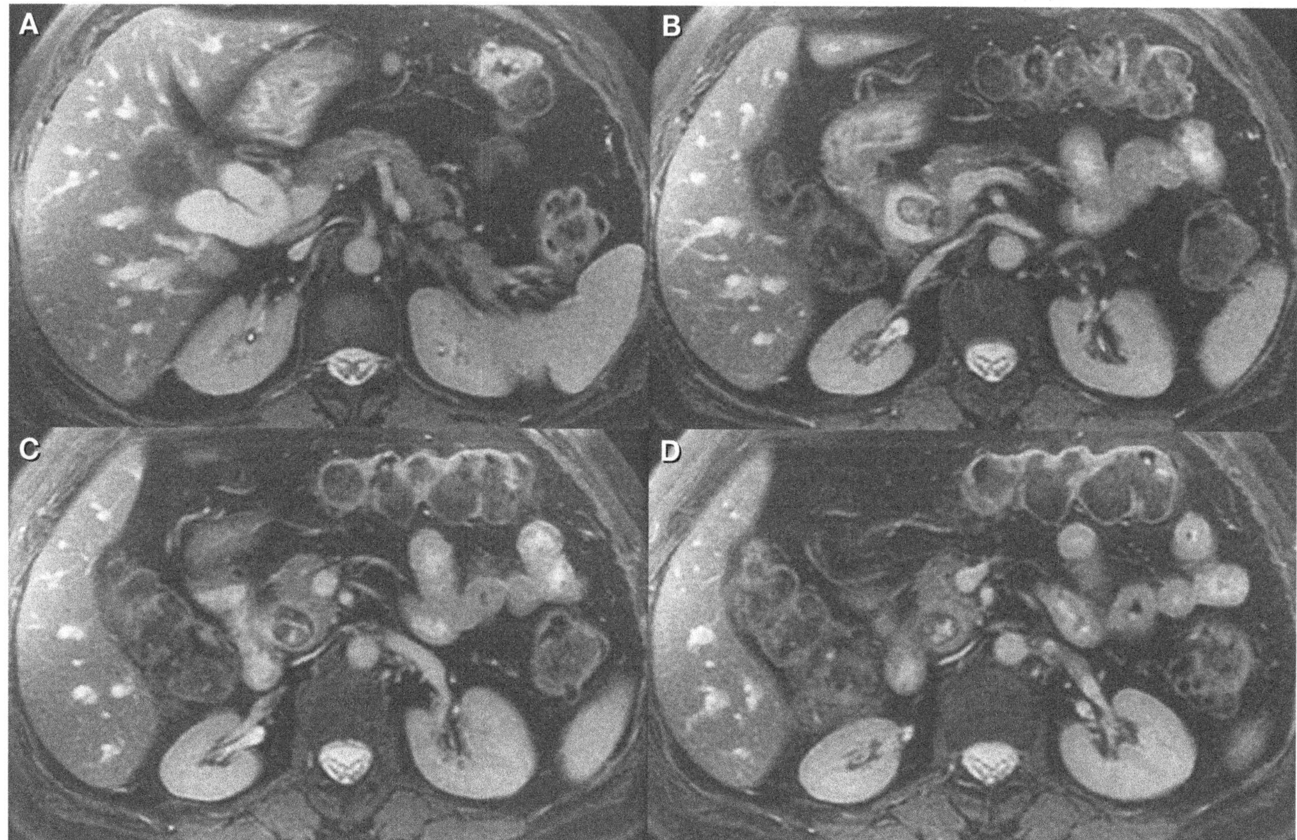

Figure 3.11.2

HISTORY: 66-year-old woman with upper abdominal pain radiating to her back, jaundice, nausea, and chills; CT demonstrated intra- and extrahepatic biliary dilatation

IMAGING FINDINGS: MIP image from 3D FRFSE MRCP (Figure 3.11.1) demonstrates diffuse intra- and extrahepatic biliary dilatation extending to the distal CBD, which shows focal narrowing. An intraductal filling defect is seen immediately above the narrowing. Axial fat-suppressed SSFP images (Figure 3.11.2) show polygonal predominantly hypointense filling defects in the distal CBD.

DIAGNOSIS: Choledocholithiasis and distal CBD stricture

COMMENT: Most radiologists (and even most clinicians) believe that MRCP is an effective technique for identifying stones in the CBD, and much of the radiology literature addressing this topic has reported sensitivities and specificities of 95% or greater for detection of CBD stones. However, a few studies have produced less favorable results. For example, a recent evaluation of patients with gallstone pancreatitis found the sensitivity of MRCP to be only 62%. Even though some of these discouraging results have come from papers written by gastroenterologists, it is worth remembering that the success of any technique depends on the skill of the imagers and the ability of the patient to cooperate. A patient with acute pancreatitis, for example, probably will not have beautiful respiratory-triggered images. With that in mind, we have built a few layers of redundancy in our MRCP protocol.

The respiratory-triggered 3D FRFSE sequence is the mainstay, and when it works, the images are beautiful, 3D reconstructions are easily generated, and the spatial resolution is high enough to identify even small filling defects. Thin-section SSFSE acquisitions are also included because they provide landmarks to prescribe the 3D sequence and are generally effective in identifying biliary abnormalities. (Most of the successful results in the literature were published before the 3D techniques were widely available and relied almost exclusively on 2D SSFSE images.) Thick-slab SSFSE images are useful for identifying the level of biliary obstruction when the 3D sequence doesn't work but aren't that helpful for visualizing small filling defects. (This statement is also true of the MIP or volume-rendered reconstructions from 3D FRFSE images; never look only at 3D reconstructions since this is a good way to miss important findings.) We also include 2D fat-suppressed SSFP acquisitions in our standard MRCP protocol. These have many of the same advantages as thin section SSFSE images, including rapid sequential acquisition, which means that poor breath holding is not a critical issue. The occasional low-signal intensity, pseudo filling defect that may be seen in the middle of the duct on SSFSE images because of biliary flow artifact is never a problem with SSFP images, and the contrast between bright bile and dark stones is just as high. Problems may occur with SSFP images near surgical clips, embolization coils, and prominent bowel gas, all of which generate considerable susceptibility artifact, in which case SSFSE images are the better option.

Notice that in this case, the stones in the distal CBD are completely impacted and no longer surrounded by fluid. Although that's not a problem in this case, you can imagine if the stone was 2 or 3 mm in diameter it might make the diagnosis very challenging. If this situation happens to you, remember that stones are generally darker than masses or normal anatomic structures on conventional MRCP sequences (and SSFP sequences) and to add thin-section SSFSE and SSFP acquisitions as needed. Also remember that noncontrast 3D SPGR images can be helpful. Often (but not always), biliary stones are bright on these fat-suppressed T1-weighted images, and sometimes this sequence is the easiest way to spot a distal CBD stone.

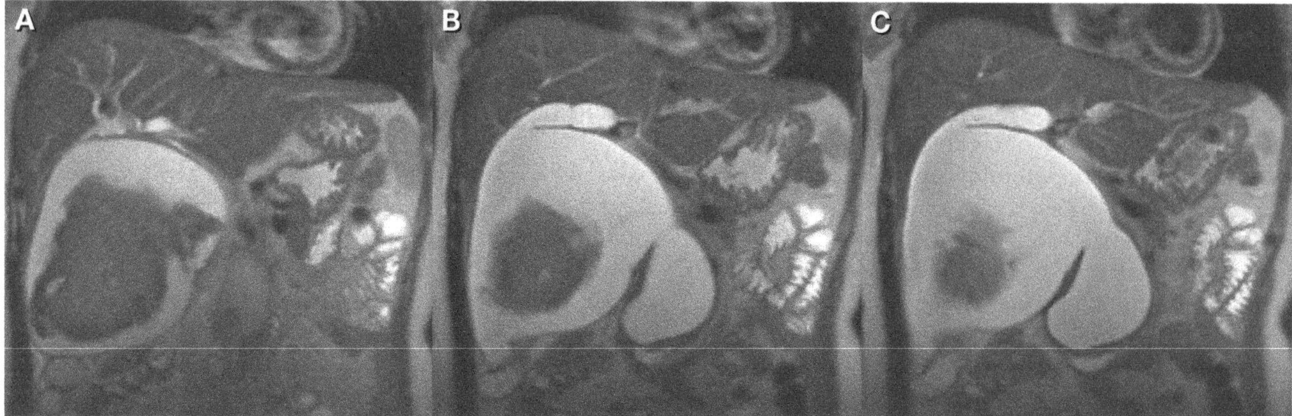

Figure 3.12.1

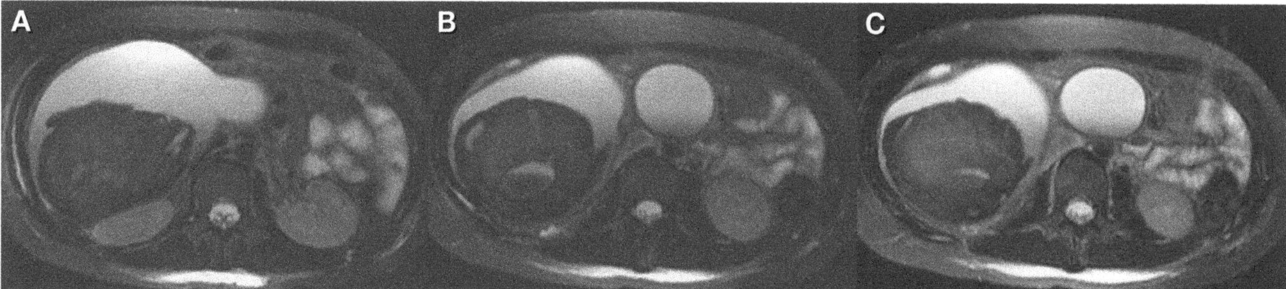

Figure 3.12.2

HISTORY: 19-year-old pregnant woman with a 2-week history of right upper quadrant pain

IMAGING FINDINGS: Coronal SSFSE (Figure 3.12.1) and axial T2-weighted FSE (Figure 3.12.2) images demonstrate massive dilatation of the CBD at the bifurcation, as well as the distal duct. Dilatation of perihilar intrahepatic ducts can be seen. Within the duct, there is a large filling defect or nodule, which is predominantly hypointense on the T2-weighted images and contains a central cystic region with a fluid-fluid level.

DIAGNOSIS: Choledochal cyst with intraductal hematoma and debris

COMMENT: Choledochal cysts are rare entities, with an estimated incidence in the Western population of 1 in 100,000 to 150,000 live births. Rates are much higher in Asia, where the reported incidence is 1 in 1,000 live births. Choledochal cysts are more common in women, with a female to male ratio of 4:1.

The etiology of choledochal cysts remains a controversial topic. The most popular theory is that they are the result of an abnormal pancreaticobiliary duct junction where the 2 ducts join outside the ampulla of Vater and form a long, common channel that then allows mixing of pancreatic and biliary contents. Activated pancreatic enzymes reflux into the biliary ducts and cause inflammation and deterioration of the biliary duct walls, leading to progressive dilatation. In support of this theory are several studies documenting increased levels of amylase in the bile of patients with choledochal cysts. Animal studies also have demonstrated that surgical creation of an abnormal pancreaticobiliary junction leads to cystic dilatation of the biliary ducts. Nevertheless, skeptics have been unable to show an abnormal pancreaticobiliary junction in as many as 20% to 50% of patients with choledochal cysts, which implies that this mechanism is probably not the only one involved.

The classification scheme generally used for choledochal cysts is the Todani modification of the original system proposed by Alonso-Lej in 1959. Type I cysts involve the extrahepatic biliary tree and are the most common, representing 50% to 80% of all choledochal cysts, with type IA describing cystic dilatation of most or all of the extrahepatic biliary tree; type IB, focal segmental dilatation; and type IC, fusiform dilatation of the extrahepatic ducts. Type II cysts are discrete diverticuli of the extrahepatic ducts connected to the common duct by a narrow stalk. Type III cysts represent choledochoceles—focal dilatation at the ampulla of Vater that projects into the duodenum. Type IVA cysts have multiple intra- and extrahepatic dilatations; in type IVB cysts, the multiple dilatations involve only the extrahepatic ducts. Type V represents Caroli disease, defined as multiple saccular or cystic dilatations of intrahepatic ducts.

This classification system, although widely used, is not without controversy. If you have already read the discussion of Caroli disease, for example, you might remember that although Caroli disease is technically defined as intrahepatic biliary dilatation, a notable percentage of patients (in fact, probably a majority) also have involvement of the extrahepatic ducts, which makes the type IVA and type V classifications somewhat redundant. Some authors doubt whether Caroli disease belongs in this classification at all, since its frequent autosomal recessive inheritance and association with renal cystic disease and hepatic fibrosis are not shared by any other group of patients with choledochal cysts. Other authors have questioned whether type II cysts (diverticuli) and type III cysts (choledochoceles) are true choledochal cysts, since type II cysts generally have minimal inflammatory response and carcinogenic potential and there are alternative theories for the origin of choledochoceles.

Choledochal cysts are considered a premalignant state, with cancers occurring more often in these patients and at an earlier age. The overall risk of cancer has been reported to be 10% to 15%, and the incidence rises with age (up to 75% for patients aged 70-80 years). Adenocarcinoma (cholangiocarcinoma) is by far the most common histologic type. Development of carcinoma is thought to result from chronic inflammation that leads to cellular regeneration and dysplasia and, eventually, frank malignancy.

This case might be classified as a type IVB choledochal cyst, with multiple (at least 2) regions of focal dilatation in the CBD. The large filling defect should probably raise some concern for neoplasm, and normally dynamic contrast-enhanced 3D SPGR images would answer that question. However, this patient was pregnant and so there was reluctance to give intravenous contrast. (Gadolinium-based contrast agents do cross the placenta, but there is little evidence to suggest that they are harmful to the fetus. Then again, there isn't much evidence that they are completely safe either, and it is unlikely that anyone will ever perform the definitive experiment.) At surgery, this filling defect turned out to be a large hematoma.

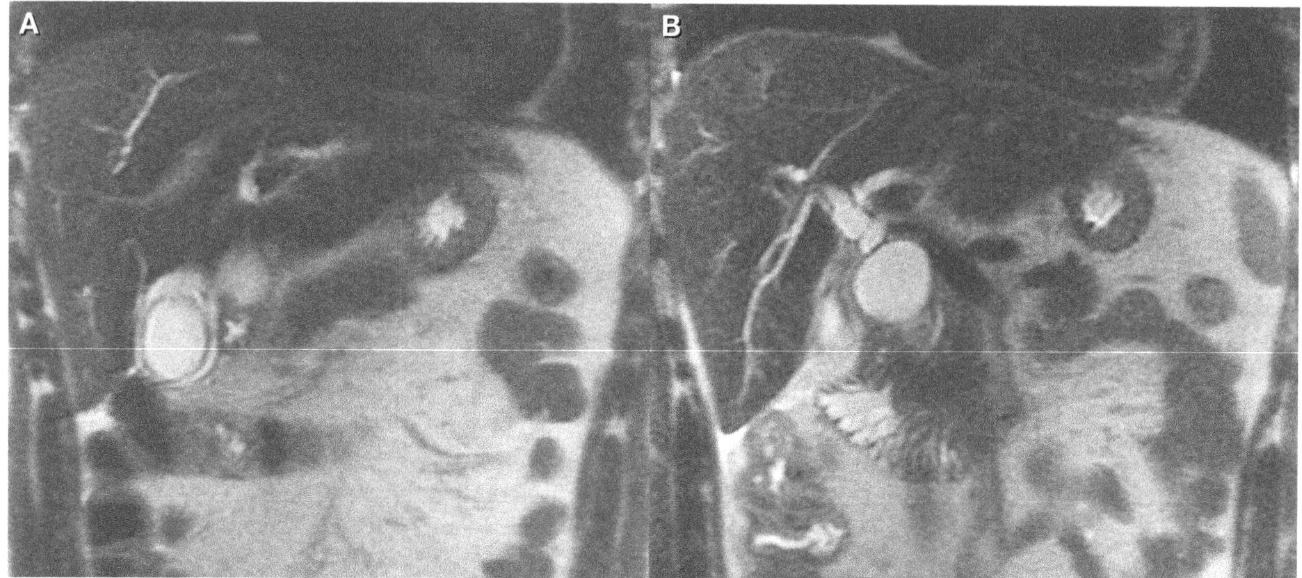

Figure 3.13.1

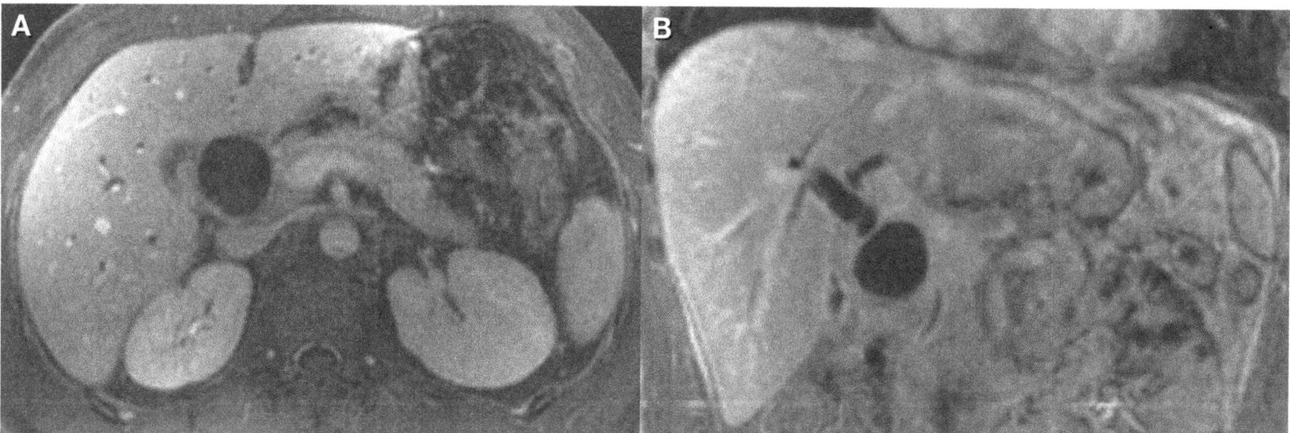

Figure 3.13.2

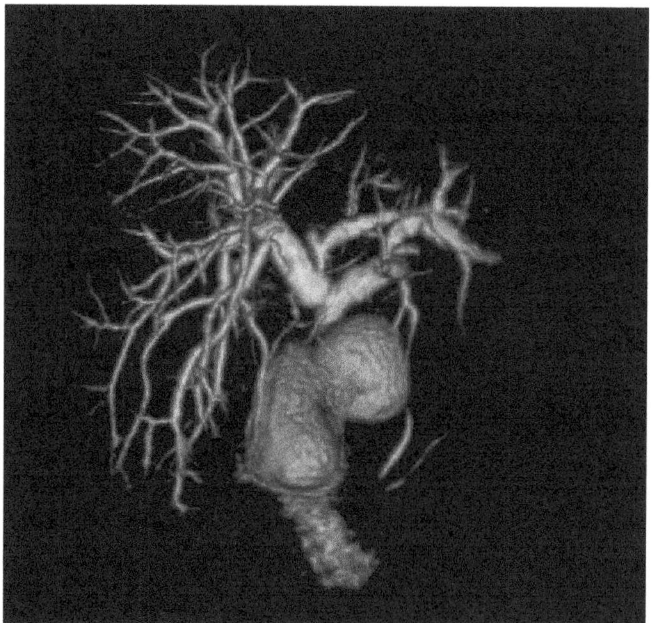
Figure 3.13.3

HISTORY: 25-year-old man who had an episode of severe abdominal pain following a meal; abdominal CT was abnormal

IMAGING FINDINGS: Coronal SSFSE images (Figure 3.13.1) demonstrate focal dilatation of the mid CBD, as well as moderate gallbladder wall thickening. Axial and coronal 3D SPGR images (Figure 3.13.2) again show marked focal dilatation of the mid CBD. Volume-rendered image from 3D FRFSE MRCP (Figure 3.13.3) demonstrates similar findings, along with moderate intrahepatic biliary dilatation.

DIAGNOSIS: Choledochal cyst with associated chronic cholecystitis

COMMENT: This case illustrates a more typical appearance of a choledochal cyst—in this patient, type IB—with additional (but not uncommon) complications of chronic cholecystitis, likely due to obstruction of the cystic duct by the cyst, and cholangitis. Notice the mural thickening and enhancement of some intrahepatic ducts on the 3D SPGR images.

The clinical presentation of choledochal cysts is variable and depends to some extent on the location of the cysts. Most patients (80%) present before age 10 years. The classic triad of abdominal pain, jaundice, and a palpable mass occurs in less than 20% of patients, although most patients have at least 2 of these 3 symptoms. Neonatal patients are more likely to have obstructive jaundice and an abdominal mass; adults more commonly present with pain, fever, nausea, vomiting, and jaundice.

The complications of choledochal cysts result from bile stasis, stone formation, and recurrent infection and inflammation. Chronic obstruction and infection may lead to secondary biliary cirrhosis, which can occur in 40% to 50% of patients. As noted in Case 3.12, patients with choledochal cysts have a significant risk of developing cholangiocarcinoma that increases over time, and therefore, whenever feasible, the cysts are surgically resected. Even after surgery, these patients have an increased incidence of biliary cancers—in the range of 0.7% to 6%—which is thought to be due to remnant choledochal cyst tissue or subclinical malignant disease not detected before surgery. All patients, and especially those who are not surgical candidates, require careful surveillance throughout their lives.

MRI with MRCP is now considered the gold standard for noninvasive imaging of this condition. Given a cooperative patient, 3D MRCP images can be obtained with excellent spatial resolution and complete visualization of the biliary tree, and complications such as intraductal stones and debris, cholangitis, and hepatic abscesses can be detected with a high degree of accuracy. Early detection of cholangiocarcinoma can be difficult regardless of the imaging modality, but MRI is likely a little better than anything else.

Differential diagnosis for choledochal cysts includes recurrent pyogenic cholangitis (oriental cholangitis), which can look exactly like Caroli disease with chronic superinfection. Diagnosis of type I cysts is usually straightforward; however, a diligent search should always be performed to exclude a site of distal obstruction that could account for dilatation of the extrahepatic ducts. Making the diagnosis of choledochal cyst in a patient postcholecystectomy is challenging, since mild to moderate dilatation of the common duct is an expected finding, and no rigorous size criteria are available for distinguishing a fusiform choledochal cyst from a postcholecystectomy dilated CBD at the upper end of the bell curve.

CASE 3.14

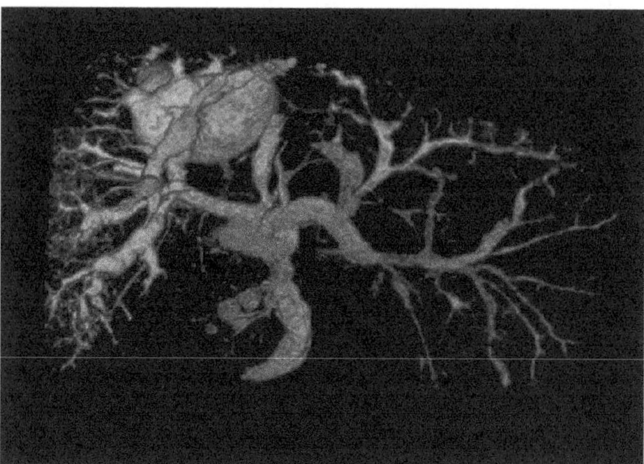

Figure 3.14.1

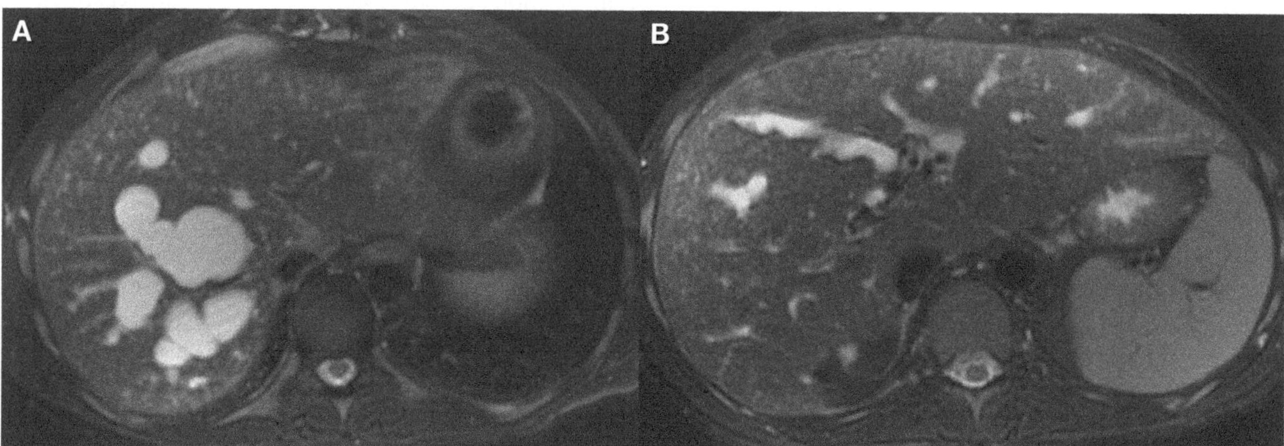

Figure 3.14.2

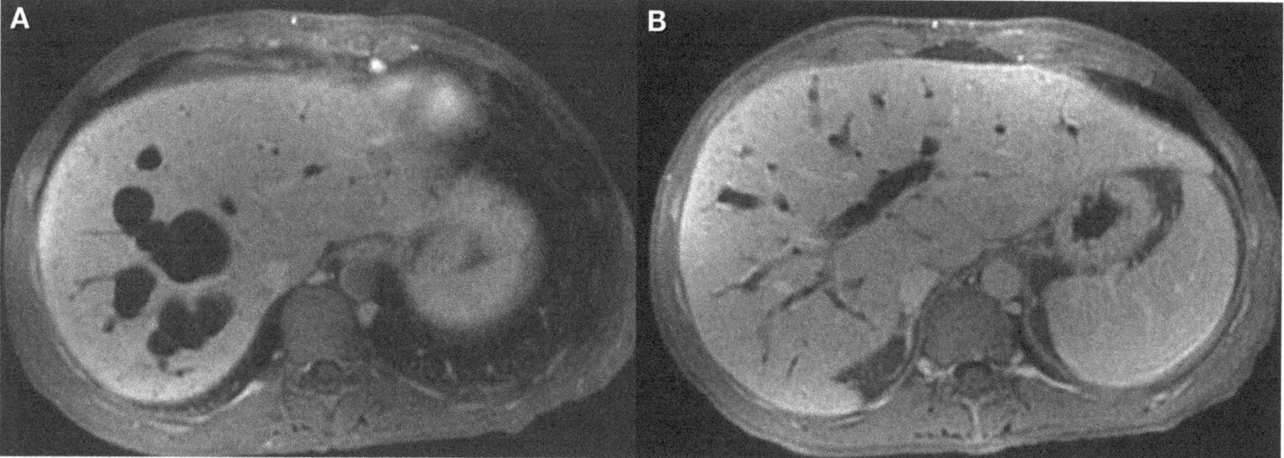

Figure 3.14.3

HISTORY: 28-year-old man with a known syndrome

IMAGING FINDINGS: Volume-rendered image from 3D FRFSE MRCP (Figure 3.14.1) demonstrates diffuse intra- and extrahepatic biliary dilatation, most prominently in the right hepatic lobe. Axial T2-weighted FSE images (Figure 3.14.2) and axial portal venous phase postgadolinium 3D SPGR images (Figure 3.14.3) also show marked dilatation of intrahepatic biliary ducts in the right hepatic lobe, with lesser dilatation in the left lobe. No significant mural enhancement is seen.

DIAGNOSIS: Caroli disease

COMMENT: Caroli disease (and Caroli syndrome) was first described in 1958 by Caroli, who reported a series of patients with communicating cystic dilatation of the intrahepatic biliary ducts, and is included in a number of different classification schemes, including fibropolycystic liver disease, ductal plate malformations, and choledochal cysts. This rare disorder has an estimated incidence of one per million.

This entity has been further divided into 2 subtypes: Caroli disease, which describes only dilated biliary ducts, and Caroli syndrome, which is associated with congenital hepatic fibrosis. Caroli syndrome is better understood as belonging to the continuum of ductal plate malformations ranging from biliary hamartoma to polycystic liver disease. The ductal plate is a cylindrical layer of cells that surrounds a branch of the portal vein. Biliary ducts are normally formed from remodeling and partial involution of the ductal plates; when this process is incomplete or interrupted, a ductal plate malformation occurs. The pathologic abnormality encountered depends on the level of the biliary tree affected. Involvement of large-sized ducts can result in Caroli disease (and some authors include choledochal cysts); involvement of medium-sized ducts, in autosomal dominant polycystic liver disease; and involvement of small ducts, in congenital hepatic fibrosis or biliary hamartomas. The concept of ductal plate malformations helps to explain the association of Caroli disease with congenital hepatic fibrosis.

Caroli disease, although technically defined as intrahepatic biliary ductal ectasia, is often associated with dilatation of the extrahepatic ducts as well. This is certainly true in our experience and has been described in the literature in 20% to 50% of patients. The presence of extrahepatic dilatation is often a stumbling block for our residents, who frequently revert to the next item on their differential diagnosis whenever they see a dilated CBD in association with Caroli disease. Caroli disease is included in the Todani classification as a type V choledochal cyst, although this classification is somewhat controversial. Other types of choledochal cysts are not associated with renal disease or autosomal recessive inheritance.

Persons with Caroli disease are often asymptomatic during the first 20 years of life, and some persons have undiagnosed disease for much longer. Intrahepatic ductal ectasia leads to stagnation of bile that, in turn, can cause stone formation, cholangitis, and hepatic abscesses. Acute cholangitis is thought to be the most common presentation, occurring in 64% of patients.

Imaging in patients with known Caroli disease is useful for detecting these complications. In addition, an increased incidence of cholangiocarcinoma is associated with the diagnosis, for which frequent surveillance is required.

MRCP is the most useful technique for diagnosis of Caroli disease, although this diagnosis is typically not a subtle one and biliary dilatation can often be seen on virtually every pulse sequence. Intraductal stones or debris can be appreciated on 3D FRFSE MRCP images or on SSFSE or SSFP sequences included in standard MRCP protocols. However, don't neglect to look at your precontrast 3D SPGR images; intrahepatic biliary stones often appear as hyperintense foci (see Cases 3.15 and 3.16). The central dot sign (ie, dilated biliary duct surrounding the adjacent portal vein radical) is always included in discussions like this as the diagnostic hallmark of Caroli disease, although frankly we don't see it that often and rarely find it useful.

Differential diagnosis for Caroli disease includes PSC, recurrent pyogenic cholangitis, choledochal cyst (other than types IVA and V), and biliary papillomatosis. PSC usually doesn't have the same level of intrahepatic biliary dilatation seen with Caroli disease (unless a cholangiocarcinoma or dominant stricture is also present), and biliary strictures are a much more prominent feature. Recurrent pyogenic cholangitis can be difficult to distinguish from Caroli disease since it encompasses many of the same imaging features.

CASE 3.15

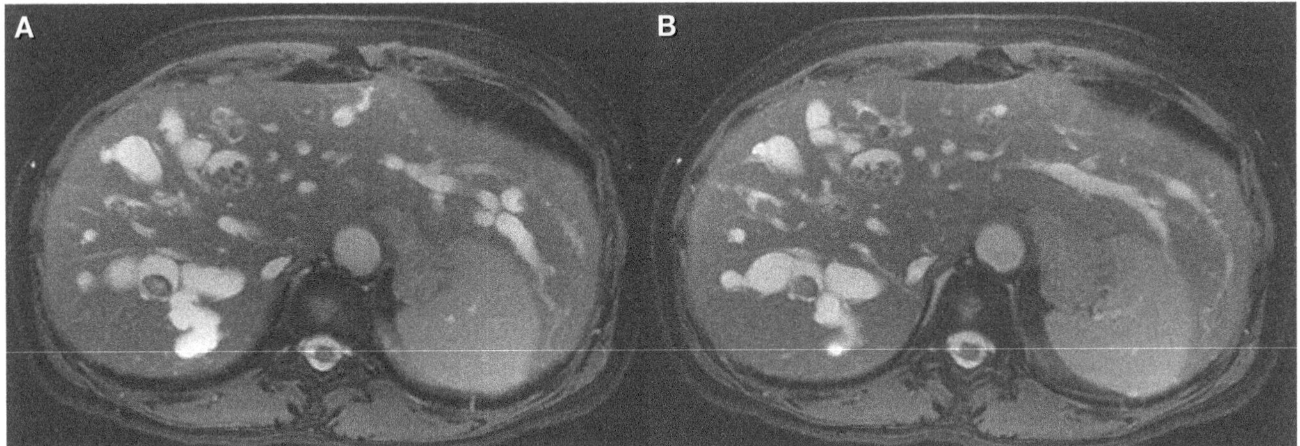

Figure 3.15.1

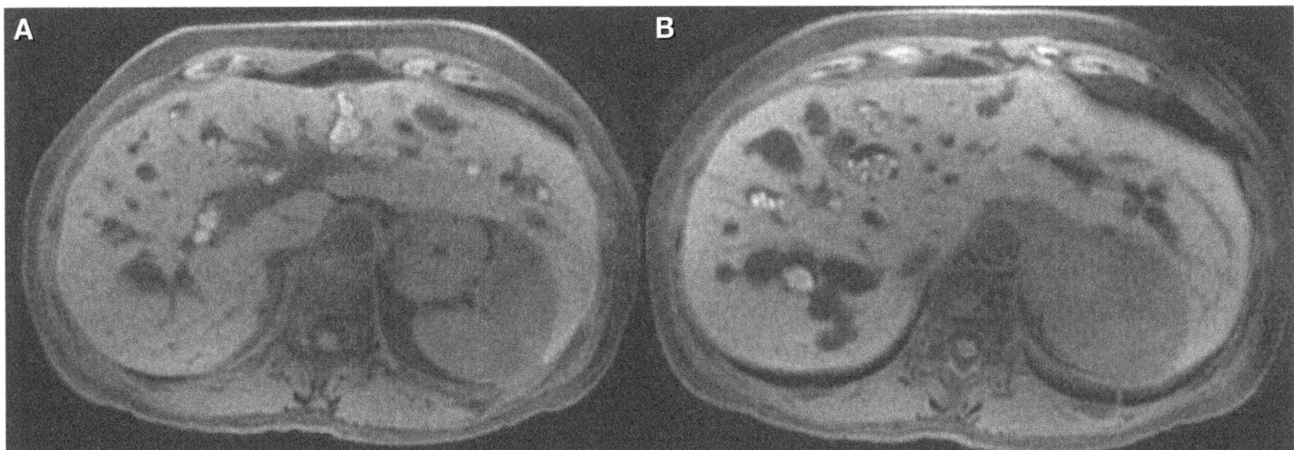

Figure 3.15.2

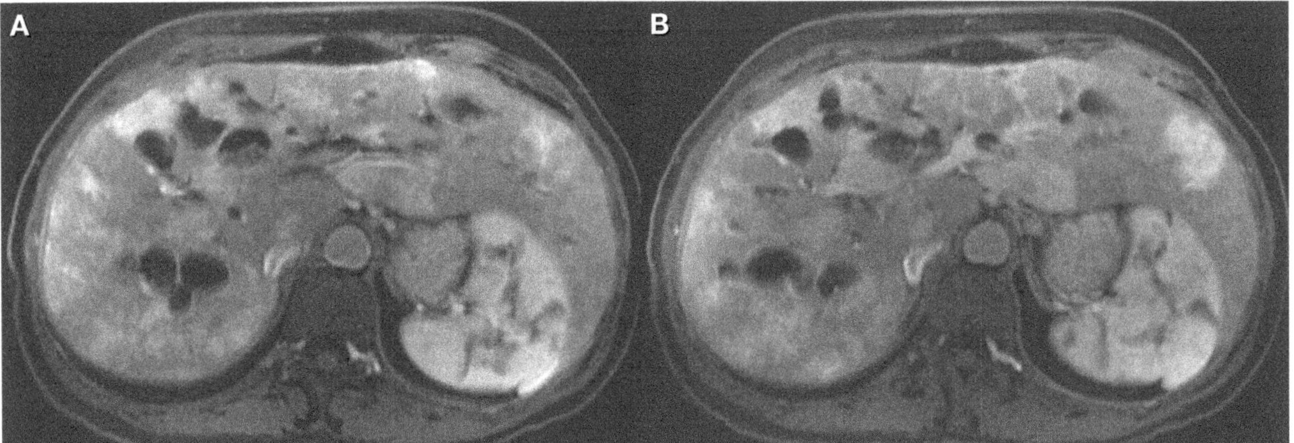

Figure 3.15.3

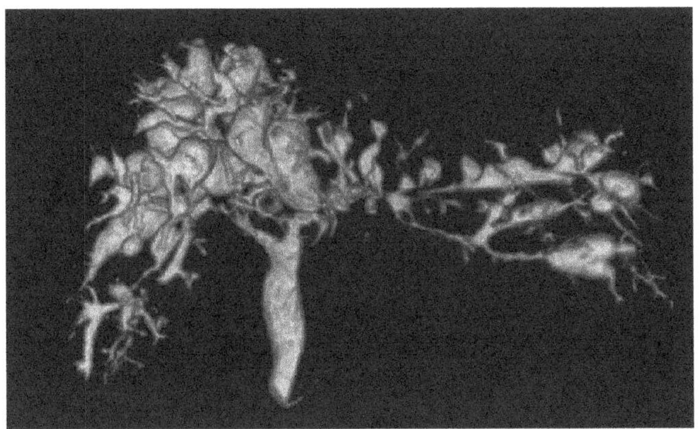

Figure 3.15.4

HISTORY: 52-year-old woman with a recent episode of right upper quadrant pain, fever, and chills

IMAGING FINDINGS: Axial fat-suppressed SSFP images (Figure 3.15.1) and axial pre- (Figure 3.15.2) and arterial phase postgadolinium (Figure 3.15.3) 3D SPGR images demonstrate diffuse dilatation of intra- and extrahepatic biliary ducts. Note the numerous intraductal stones (bright on precontrast T1-weighted 3D SPGR images) in intrahepatic ducts. Arterial phase postcontrast images demonstrate patchy parenchymal enhancement and mild periductal enhancement, indicative of acute inflammation. A volume-rendered image from 3D FRFSE MRCP (Figure 3.15.4) shows diffuse dilatation of intra- and extrahepatic biliary ducts, with regions of stricturing most prominent in the left lobe.

DIAGNOSIS: Caroli disease with extensive intrahepatic biliary stones and cholangitis

COMMENT: This is a companion case to Case 3.14 and illustrates the common complications of intraductal stone formation and associated cholangitis. Intrahepatic biliary dilatation makes it fairly easy to identify the stones on SSFP images because they stand out as dark, well-defined structures surrounded by bright fluid. Notice also how well you can see the stones on the precontrast 3D SPGR images as hyperintense intraductal nodules. T1 hyperintensity is not a universal finding, however, and when stones don't appear bright on T1-weighted images, you're much better off reverting to the standard heavily T2-weighted MRCP sequences. Occasionally, stones or debris may completely fill a duct with no surrounding fluid; they can then be very difficult to see on standard MRCP sequences, and your best bet may be the precontrast 3D SPGR images.

The heterogeneous parenchymal enhancement on arterial phase postgadolinium images is an indication of inflammation—in this case, likely the result of resolving cholangitis. The biliary strictures in the left hepatic lobe, by comparison, are indications of chronic recurrent cholangitis. Cholangitis may be associated with hepatic abscesses, so it's important to look for these, which probably are seen best on postgadolinium 3D SPGR images. Thickening and enhancement of biliary ductal walls are often prominent features of cholangitis, although not to the same extent that you might see in PSC.

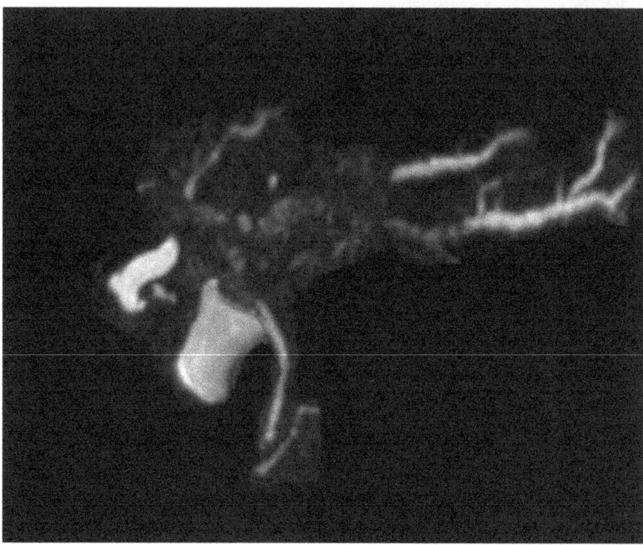

Figure 3.16.1

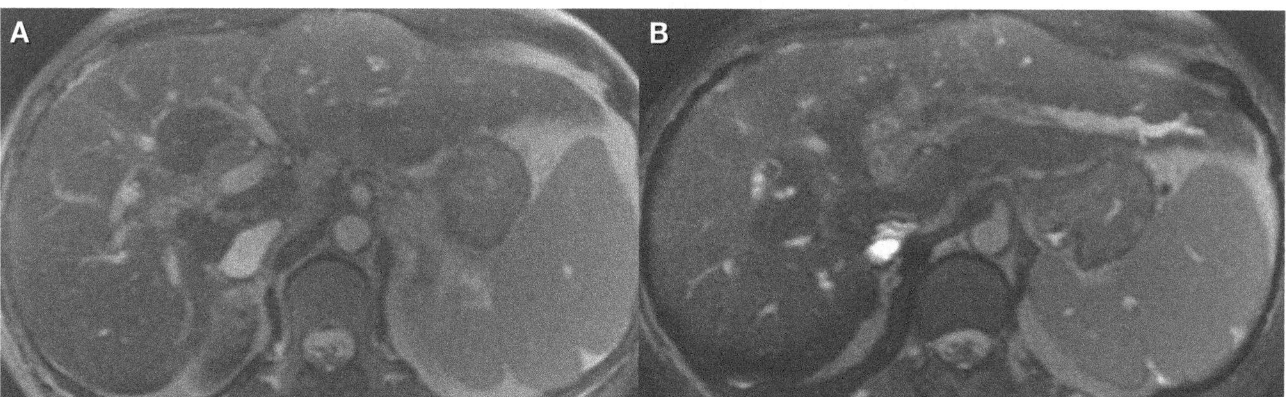

Figure 3.16.2

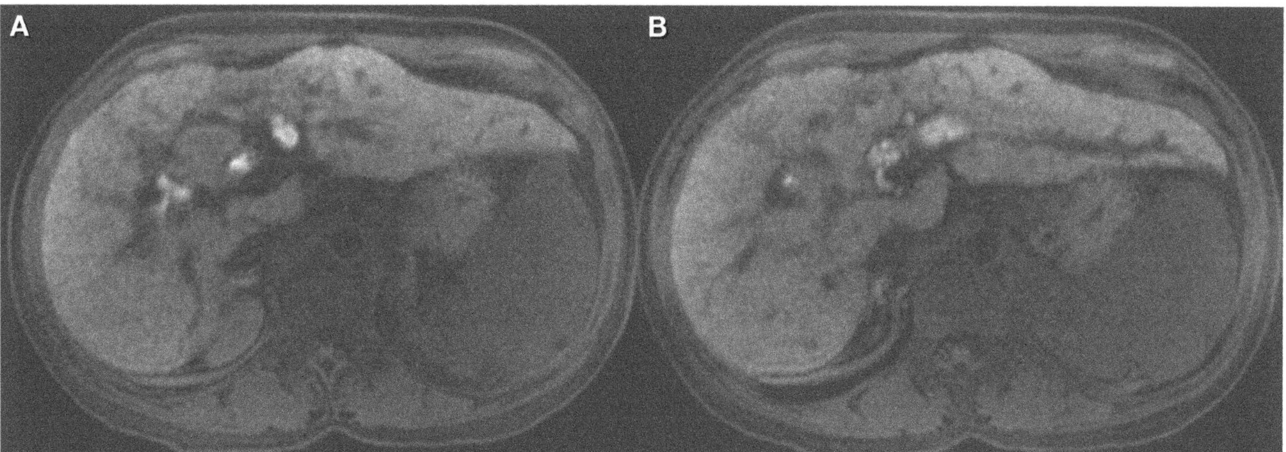

Figure 3.16.3

HISTORY: 57-year-old woman who had an ERCP at an outside institution with diagnosis of PSC potentially complicated by cholangiocarcinoma

IMAGING FINDINGS: MIP image from 3D FRFSE MRCP (Figure 3.16.1) demonstrates dilatation of peripheral biliary ducts in the right and left lobes, with central obstruction. Note also the deformed gallbladder. Axial 2D fat-suppressed SSFP images (Figure 3.16.2) reveal that the central ducts are packed with low-signal-intensity stones and debris. Precontrast axial 3D SPGR images (Figure 3.16.3) demonstrate corresponding intrahepatic biliary stones with high signal intensity.

DIAGNOSIS: Recurrent pyogenic cholangitis

COMMENT: Also known as *oriental cholangitis*, recurrent pyogenic cholangitis is characterized by intrahepatic, pigmented biliary stones and recurrent attacks of cholangitis. It is equally common in men and women, and most patients present between ages 30 and 50 years. Although the exact cause is unknown, there is a strong association with parasitic infections, most commonly *Ascaris lumbricoides* and *Clonorchis sinensis*. These organisms are not identified in all cases, however, and other risk factors include *Escherichia coli* cholangitis and nutritional deficiency. Chronic inflammation from multiple episodes of cholangitis induces a fibrotic response in biliary ductal walls that in turn causes strictures, bile stasis, and intraductal stones. Intraductal stones worsen the obstruction and lead to recurrent infection and intrahepatic abscesses. In severe cases, progressive parenchymal destruction, cirrhosis, and hepatic failure may result.

MRI with MRCP is probably the optimal imaging technique for initial diagnosis and follow-up of these patients. Characteristic findings of recurrent pyogenic cholangitis include dilatation of intra- and/or extrahepatic ducts, multiple intrahepatic biliary strictures, and mural thickening of bile ducts. Pigmented biliary stones are found in nearly all patients; the size and distribution are variable, but the most common appearance is multiple small stones.

The diagnosis is usually suggested by biliary dilatation with multiple intrahepatic stones in a patient without another diagnosis that might account for these findings (such as Caroli disease, choledochal cyst, or PSC). Hepatic parenchymal abnormalities are frequently encountered, including intrahepatic abscesses (in approximately 20% of patients), hepatic atrophy, and cirrhosis. Patients with recurrent pyogenic cholangitis are at increased risk for cholangiocarcinoma, which occurs in 2% to 5%.

This case illustrates some of the typical features of recurrent pyogenic cholangitis. The multiple stones are packed tightly in the central right and left biliary ducts, with little surrounding fluid. This makes the diagnosis of central obstruction fairly easy on 3D FRFSE MRCP, but the cause of the obstruction is difficult to figure out on the basis of these images alone. Conventional T2-weighted 2D FSE or, in this case, 2D SSFP images may be more helpful, showing the round or polygonal appearance of the stones without any obvious extension beyond the ducts to suggest malignancy. Once again, the precontrast 3D SPGR images are helpful in showing the high signal intensity of the intraductal stones. Although blood products or other debris might have similar signal intensity, this appearance effectively excludes tumor or other infiltrative soft tissue process. That's not to say there couldn't be a central tumor, and you do have to worry about this since these patients are at increased risk for cholangiocarcinoma.

The differential diagnosis includes Caroli disease or choledochal cyst (type IVA or V), as well as PSC. Intraductal stones are common in these disorders (Case 3.15, for example) but tend to be more numerous in recurrent pyogenic cholangitis. The degree of biliary dilatation is generally greater in Caroli disease than recurrent pyogenic cholangitis and PSC, but this finding may not always be a useful discriminatory factor.

Treatment options of patients with recurrent pyogenic cholangitis include antibiotic therapy for acute attacks, stricture dilatation, biliary drainage, stone removal, biliary bypass, hepatic resection, and transplantation. A multidisciplinary approach is usually required, and there is often more than enough work to satisfy both endoscopists and interventional radiologists.

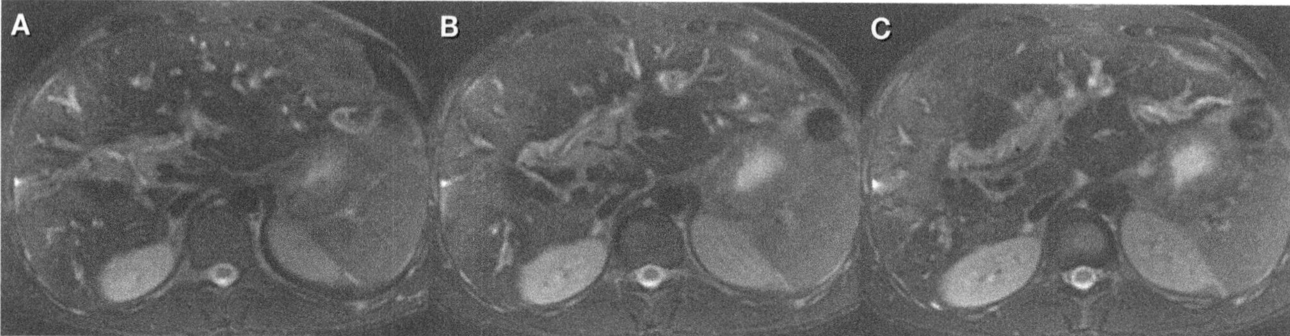

Figure 3.17.1

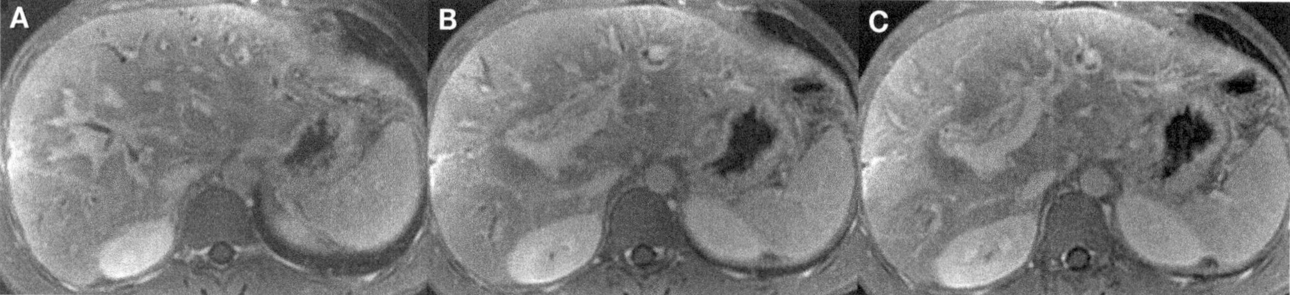

Figure 3.17.2

HISTORY: 27-year-old man with ulcerative colitis and recent history of intermittent fever, chills, and dilated biliary ducts on CT

IMAGING FINDINGS: Axial T2-weighted FSE images (Figure 3.17.1) show diffuse soft tissue thickening in the hepatic hilum encasing the central biliary ducts. Note the mild peripheral intrahepatic biliary dilatation. Axial equilibrium phase 3D SPGR images (Figure 3.17.2) demonstrate diffuse enhancement of this soft tissue process, again with mild peripheral intrahepatic biliary dilatation.

DIAGNOSIS: Primary sclerosing cholangitis

COMMENT: PSC is a chronic disease of the bile ducts and liver that primarily affects young and middle-aged men (approximately two-thirds of patients with PSC are male), particularly those with underlying inflammatory bowel disease. The association with inflammatory bowel disease is highly variable depending on geography and varies from 20% in Asia to 80% in Northern Europe. The cause of PSC is not known, but current theory suggests that it is an autoimmune process.

Many patients with PSC are asymptomatic at presentation, and the diagnosis is suggested by elevated liver function tests or abnormalities on imaging performed for another indication. Fatigue, jaundice, pruritis, and right upper quadrant pain are common and nonspecific initial symptoms. PSC results in damage, atrophy, and loss of medium-sized and large intra- and extrahepatic bile ducts. The characteristic pathologic feature is concentric periductal fibrosis progressing to narrowing and then obliteration of small bile ducts, leaving a bile duct scar. Liver biopsy often yields nonspecific results, and therefore the diagnosis must be reached with consideration of pathologic, clinical, and radiologic findings.

PSC is generally a progressive disease and eventually leads to biliary cirrhosis and its associated complications. Liver transplantation is the treatment of choice for patients with end-stage disease due to PSC. Excellent 5-year survival rates of 80% to 90% have been achieved, although recurrent PSC develops in up to 40% of patients. The median transplantation-free survival after diagnosis is approximately 18 years, and mortality rates have not changed markedly over the past 25 years, indicating that the various attempted medical management strategies have been largely unsuccessful. Patients with PSC have a high risk of cholangiocarcinoma: The lifetime risk of cholangiocarcinoma is 7% to 15%, with an annual incidence of approximately 1%. Interestingly, a high percentage of cholangiocarcinoma cases (40%-50%) occur within 1 year of the initial PSC diagnosis.

Diagnosis of cholangiocarcinoma is tricky enough on its own, but it can be very challenging in the clinical setting of PSC since many radiologic features overlap and small tumors can be hidden within regions of periductal fibrosis. Lesions are generally detected either when they are too large to miss (not good) or, in the slightly better alternative scenario, when changes are noticed on serial imaging that suggest presence of a mass—for example, development of focal biliary dilatation. It is true, however, that a dominant biliary stricture is a frequent occurrence in PSC, appearing in up to 45% of patients at some point in the course of their disease, and therefore, a dominant stricture, while always suspicious, is more often benign than malignant. PSC patients also have a 10-fold increased risk of developing gallbladder carcinoma.

This case emphasizes the appearance of periductal fibrosis in PSC, and Case 3.18 illustrates the classic appearance on MRCP. The extensive periductal soft tissue in the hilum seen in this case is a somewhat extreme example. It's relatively easy to spot on the T2-weighted images because this study was performed when Feridex (a superparamagnetic iron oxide [SPIO] contrast agent) was still available; normal hepatic parenchyma with Kupffer cells takes up the agent and loses signal intensity by virtue of T2/T2* shortening. Under ordinary circumstances (ie, without Feridex), the periductal soft tissue thickening of PSC appears minimally hyperintense (or often essentially identical) relative to adjacent hepatic parenchyma and therefore is difficult to delineate.

The appearance of periductal fibrosis on dynamic gadolinium-enhanced 3D SPGR images is similar to that of fibrosis anywhere else and unfortunately is similar to cholangiocarcinoma: hypoenhancing on arterial and portal venous phase images, with gradual accumulation of contrast on equilibrium phase and delayed images. This isn't always true: In the setting of active cholangitis (and *cholangitis* is, after all, in the name of the disease), you will often see fairly intense arterial phase enhancement of ductal walls and periductal soft tissue, a good indication of active inflammation, but unfortunately not useful for excluding cholangiocarcinoma, which can also elicit an inflammatory response. When hepatobiliary contrast agents (Eovist and Multihance) are used, the appearance of periductal fibrosis is hypointense relative to the liver on hepatobiliary phase images. This feature makes it easy to distinguish from adjacent liver tissue but difficult to distinguish from the portal vein and other vascular structures, which generally have about the same signal intensity.

As a general (and only occasionally helpful) rule of thumb, fibrosis in PSC tends to be diffuse and fairly symmetrical. If you see fibrotic soft tissue concentrated around one lobe or one segment, then you should probably ask yourself whether this could be cholangiocarcinoma, particularly if it's a new finding.

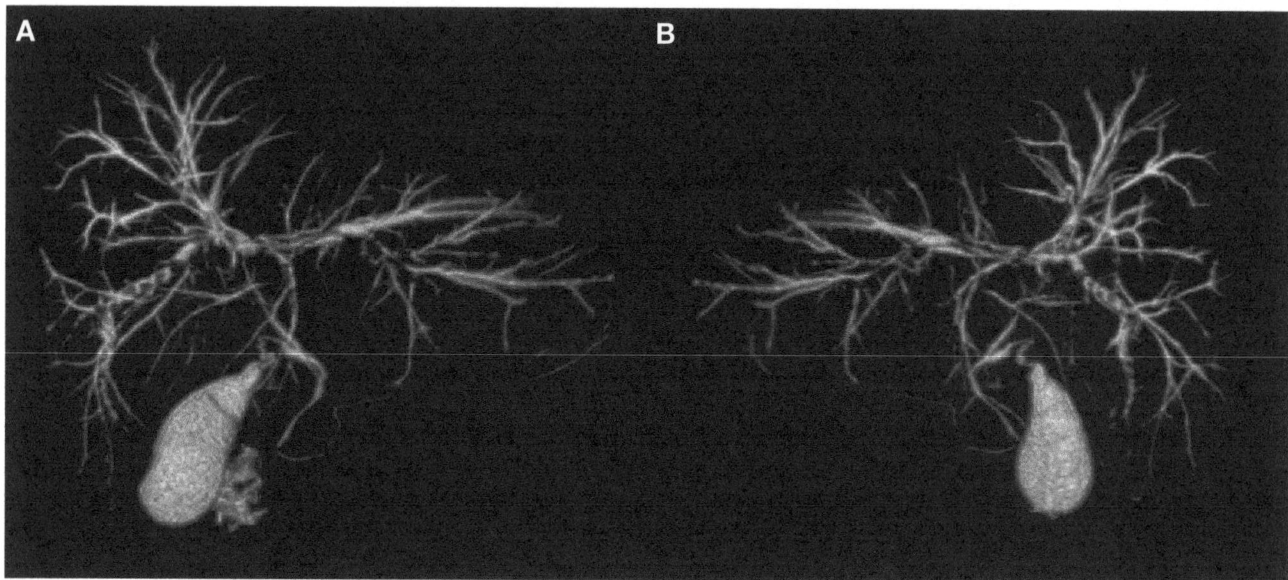

Figure 3.18.1

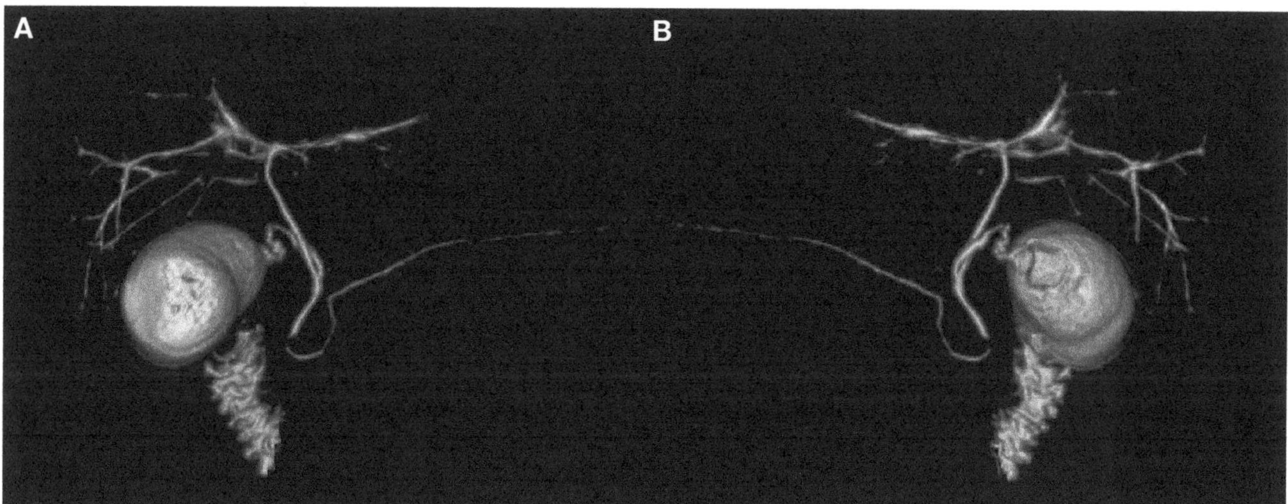

Figure 3.18.2

HISTORY: 52-year-old man with ulcerative colitis and renal failure secondary to chronic glomerulonephritis; new onset of right upper quadrant pain, fever, jaundice, and elevated liver function tests

IMAGING FINDINGS: Volume-rendered images from 3D FRFSE MRCP in anterior and posterior projections (Figure 3.18.1) demonstrate mild to moderate dilatation of intrahepatic biliary ducts with multiple strictures. Multiple calculi are visible in a posterior right duct. Follow-up volume-rendered MRCP images from an examination performed 4 years later (Figure 3.18.2) show progression of disease with only central ducts visible, again with multiple strictures.

DIAGNOSIS: Primary sclerosing cholangitis

COMMENT: This case illustrates the typical appearance of PSC on MRCP, as well as the progression of this disease. Initial examination shows mild dilatation of peripheral intrahepatic ducts and, as you look more carefully, you can see multiple central strictures, as well as a mildly obstructed right-sided duct containing multiple stones. The alternating appearance of strictures and normal or dilated segments within the same duct has led to the nearly universally applied descriptor, *beading*. We're not really fond of this description—*beading* to us is fibromuscular dysplasia and not the kind of picture seen here—but if it helps you reach the correct diagnosis, so be it.

Remember that PSC is a progressive disease resulting in the destruction of biliary ducts. This is nicely illustrated on the follow-up examination, where only a few central intrahepatic ducts are visible (Figure 3.18.2). One could argue that this appearance is simply a result of fewer dilated ducts, and we're just not seeing nondilated peripheral ducts that are below the spatial resolution of the acquisition. This consideration will always be true to some extent; very small ducts containing minimal fluid are not seen on a heavily T2-weighted acquisition. However, in this case, it should be obvious that something pathologic is happening. And if you were to look at the parenchymal images (2D FSE and 3D SPGR), you would see that the liver has become atrophic and cirrhotic, with increasing peripheral and central fibrosis.

The classic appearance of PSC at MRCP is that of mild to moderate intrahepatic biliary dilatation (although remember that extrahepatic ducts are also affected). Severe dilatation, especially when focal, should raise concern of cholangiocarcinoma, particularly if you notice the dilatation appearing on serial imaging. However, as noted in Case 3.17, most dominant strictures in PSC are benign.

Autoimmune pancreatitis is often associated with autoimmune sclerosing cholangitis, which can have an identical appearance to PSC. It's a useful differential diagnosis to keep in mind: Autoimmune pancreatitis generally occurs in older men (vs the younger population of PSC) and typically shows an excellent response to corticosteroid therapy, which is rarely successful in PSC. So take a look at the pancreas, kidneys, and retroperitoneum in any patient with known or suspected PSC. A diagnosis of autoimmune pancreatitis gives a much happier prognosis and is not always suspected by the ordering physician (Case 4.10 features an example and a more detailed discussion).

In the early days of MRCP, there was a lot of discussion about whether MRCP was really adequate for identifying PSC compared to the gold standard of ERCP. For the most part, that question has been answered affirmatively. Most studies show MRCP to have sensitivities of 80% to 90%, and the majority of these studies were performed before the 3D FRFSE respiratory-triggered sequences—with much higher spatial resolution and better image quality—became available. Nevertheless, it is probably true that MRCP will miss a few early cases with nondilated ducts and minimal strictures, but that may be a reasonable tradeoff to make in comparison to the 5% incidence of post-ERCP pancreatitis.

It's also possible to overcall PSC when motion artifact on the long respiratory-triggered acquisitions leads to the appearance of pseudo-strictures. For this reason, it's always worth acquiring breath-hold 2D SSFSE or SSFP sequences or thick-slab breath-hold SSFSE sequences, or both, to verify subtle findings on respiratory-triggered images. Another common pseudo-stricture occurs in the hilum where the hepatic artery crosses the CBD. This artifact is usually more prominent on SSFSE images than SSFP images, and if you see it, you can correlate with axial anatomic 2D or 3D images (which should always be obtained) to verify the proximity of the hepatic artery.

CASE 3.19

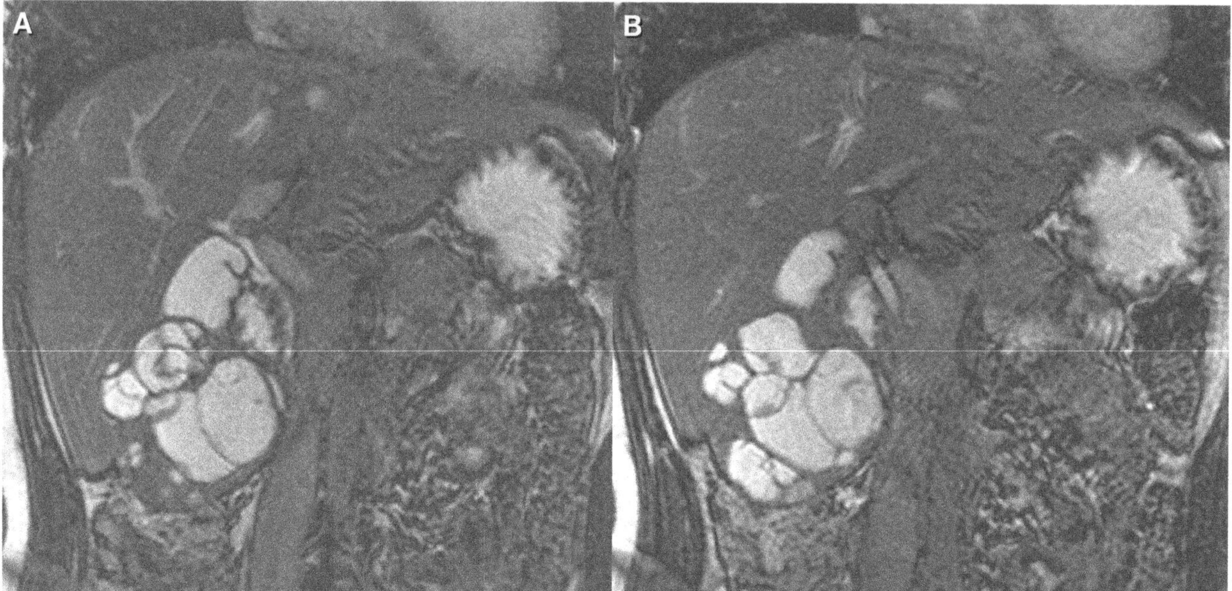

Figure 3.19.1

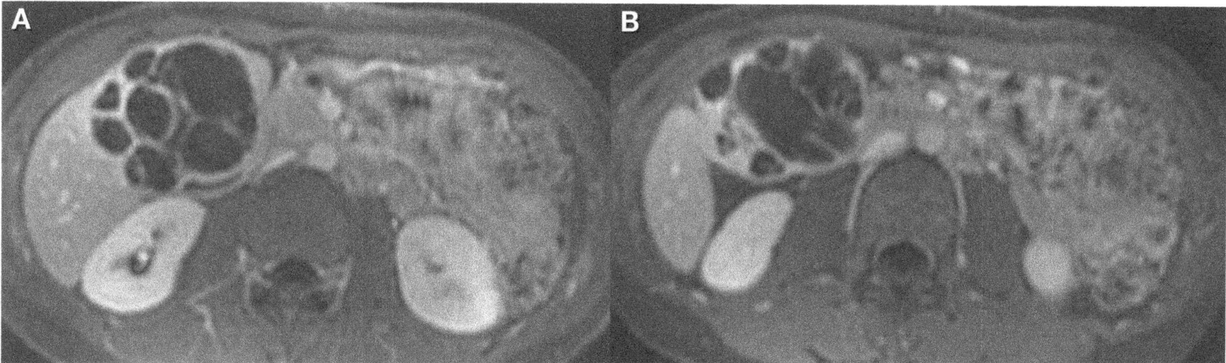

Figure 3.19.2

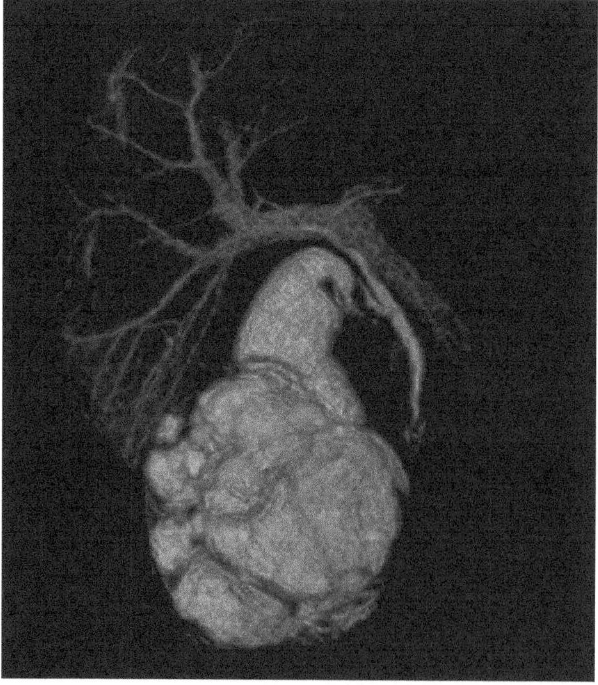

Figure 3.19.3

HISTORY: 21-year-old woman who noticed a right upper quadrant bulge, which her physician thought was a hernia; eventually, CT was performed, revealing a complex hepatic mass

IMAGING FINDINGS: Coronal 3D SSFP images (Figure 3.19.1) and axial postgadolinium 3D SPGR images (Figure 3.19.2) demonstrate a multicystic lesion with multiple mildly enhancing septations. The inferior axial image shows a more prominent enhancing soft tissue component along the lateral margin of the mass. A volume-rendered image reconstructed from 3D SSFP source data (Figure 3.19.3) again reveals the cystic septated lesion without significant intra- or extrahepatic biliary dilatation.

DIAGNOSIS: Biliary cystadenoma

COMMENT: Biliary cystadenomas are rare neoplasms accounting for less than 5% of hepatic cystic lesions of biliary origin, with 150 to 200 cases reported in the literature. Most biliary cystadenomas arise from intrahepatic biliary ducts, although cases have been reported in which the lesion developed from extrahepatic ducts or from the gallbladder. Communication with the biliary tree is rare but has been reported. The typical biliary cystadenoma patient (and our example doesn't quite fit into this categorization) is a middle-aged woman. There is a striking female preponderance, accounting for 90% to 95% of lesions. Clinical manifestations of biliary cystadenomas are nonspecific. Many lesions are detected as incidental findings at abdominal sonography, CT, or MRI performed for vague indications; however, some patients present with abdominal pain or mass.

Histologic evaluation of biliary cystadenomas reveals lesions similar to mucinous cystic tumors arising in the pancreas and ovary. The largest series of biliary cystadenomas and cystadenocarcinomas (from the Armed Forces Institute of Pathology) divided tumors according to presence or absence of a band of spindle cells beneath the epithelium, resembling ovarian stroma. Most cases had ovarian stroma, ovarian stroma was found only in female patients, and cystadenocarcinoma with ovarian stroma was associated with a better prognosis. (The reliability of descriptive papers from the Armed Forces Institute of Pathology is always difficult to gauge, since by definition they have a strong referral bias.) Our rule of thumb is that the more uncommon the lesion, the more believable the results.

The classic appearance of biliary cystadenoma is a large (average diameter, 10-12 cm) solitary, multilocular cystic lesion. A relatively thick fibrous capsule and multiple internal septations can usually be visualized. Since biliary cystadenomas are generally considered premalignant lesions, it would be helpful to distinguish them from cystadenocarcinomas. Although making this distinction with great accuracy is not possible, the presence of enhancing mural nodules favors cystadenocarcinoma. Notice that in this case, some prominent enhancing soft tissue can be seen along the inferior lateral margin of the lesion. Whether this appearance would technically qualify as a mural nodule is not clear, but it is somewhat worrisome for malignant degeneration and illustrates the overlap in the imaging appearance of biliary cystadenoma and cystadenocarcinoma. Coarse mural calcification has also been described as a feature of malignant degeneration, although it is difficult to detect on MRI.

Most standard hepatic MRI protocols should be adequate for making the diagnosis since the lesions are not small or subtle. MRCP sequences (heavily T2-weighted 3D FRFSE, and 2D or 3D SSFP and SSFSE) generate the most photogenic images. 3D SPGR dynamic contrast-enhanced images are useful in the search for enhancing mural nodules.

Differential diagnosis includes hepatic abscess, hydatid disease, and complex cysts. Since hydatid disease is not endemic in Rochester, Minnesota, this is not usually a problem for us, although hydatid cysts often have thicker walls and smaller, more regular daughter cysts. Abscesses usually are clinically apparent and may have thicker rims with intense enhancement. That's not to say that this is always an easy diagnosis.

In the 2 cases presented below, biliary cystadenoma was the working diagnosis, but they turned out to be something else entirely: a complex cyst and a mesothelial cyst, respectively.

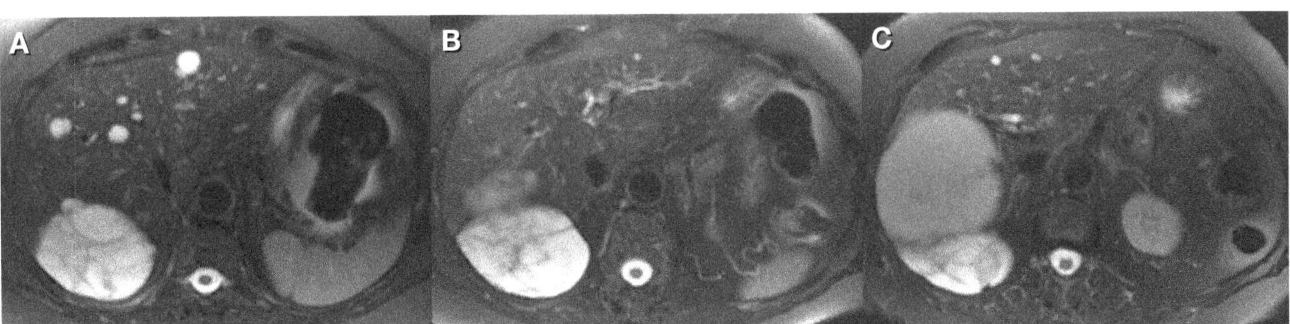

Figure 3.19.4

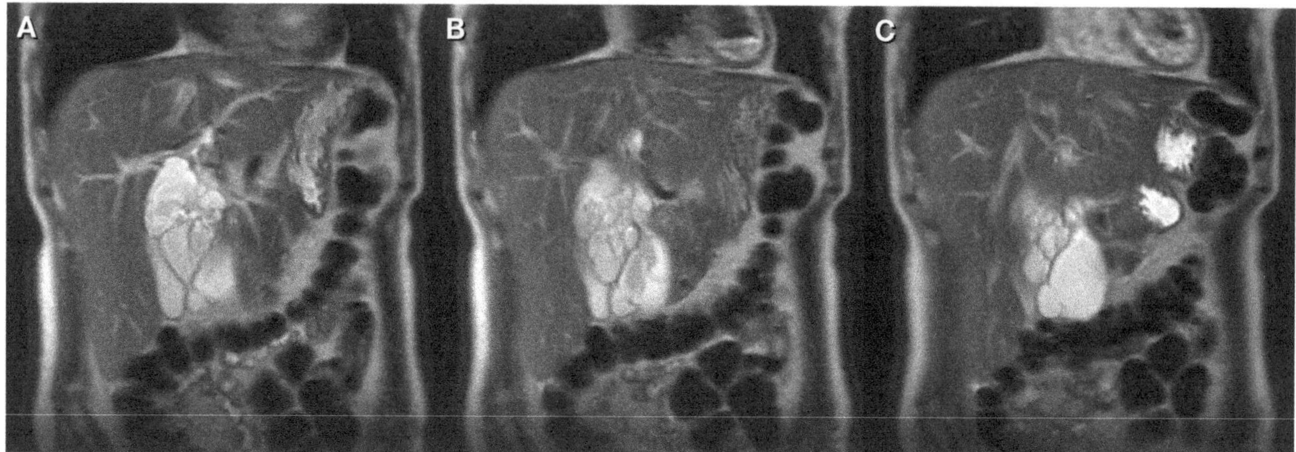

Figure 3.19.5

Axial FSE T2-weighted images (Figure 3.19.4) demonstrate a multiseptated cystic lesion in the posterior right hepatic lobe, with a larger complex cyst immediately adjacent that contains a nodular septation. This was a complex hemorrhagic cyst at pathology. Note the presence of several additional simple cysts in the liver. In the second case, coronal SSFSE images (Figure 3.19.5) show a large multilocular cystic lesion in the hepatic hilum that does not cause biliary obstruction. This was a mesothelial cyst at pathology.

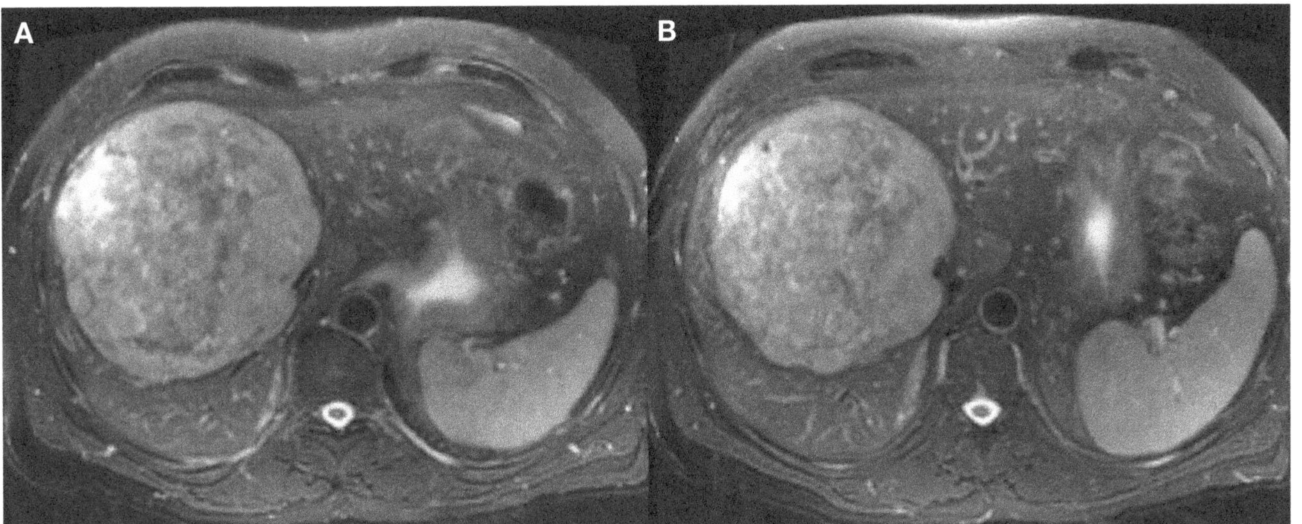

Figure 3.20.1

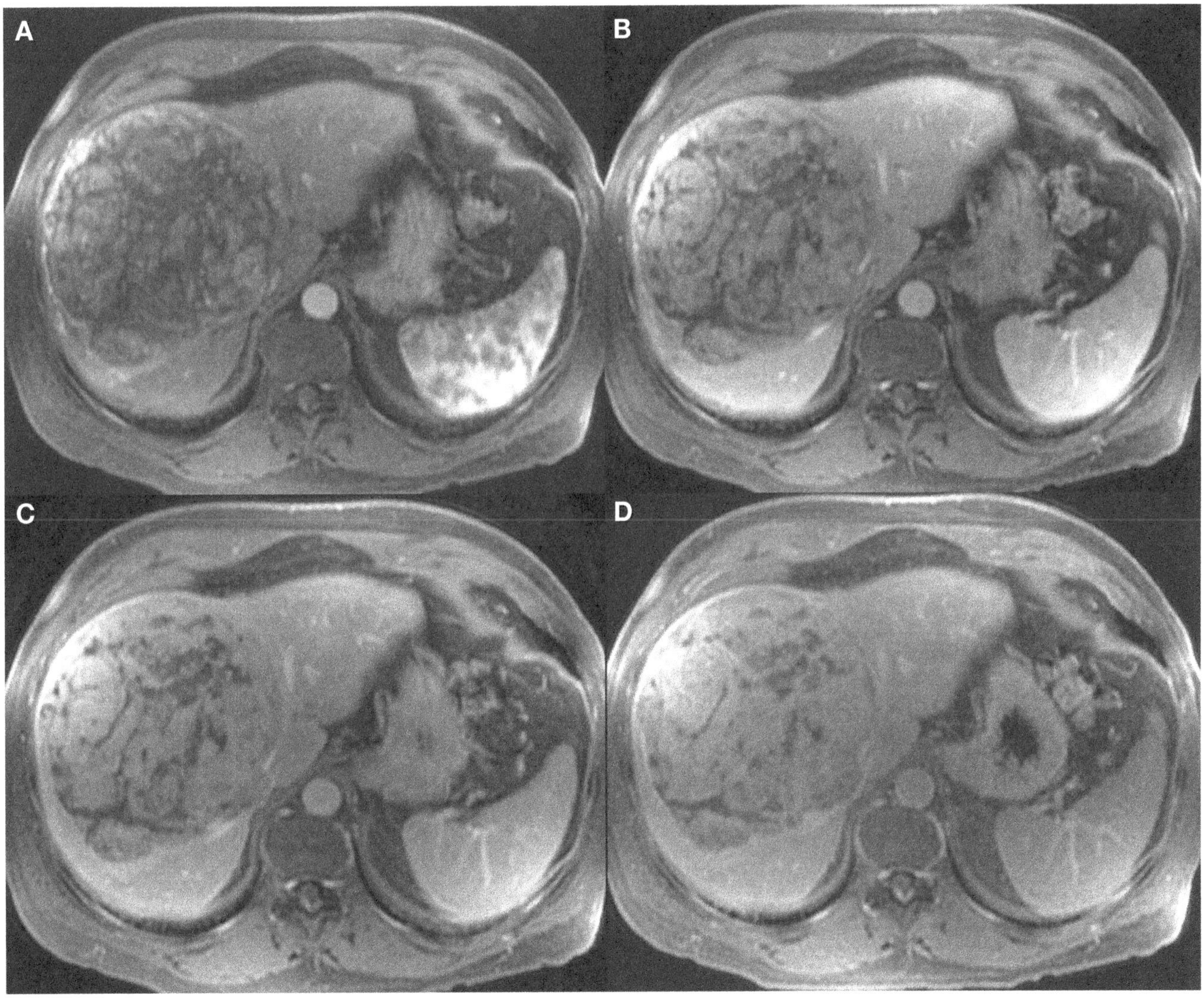

Figure 3.20.2

HISTORY: 56-year-old man with abnormal liver function tests; abdominal US revealed a large hepatic mass

IMAGING FINDINGS: Axial fat-suppressed FSE T2-weighted images (Figure 3.20.1) demonstrate a large heterogeneous, hyperintense mass in the right hepatic lobe. Arterial, portal venous, equilibrium, and delayed-phase postgadolinium 3D SPGR images (Figure 3.20.2) show heterogeneous enhancement of the lesion with gradual accumulation of contrast on later images.

DIAGNOSIS: Combined hepatocellular carcinoma and cholangiocarcinoma

COMMENT: Primary liver carcinomas can be classified broadly as either HCC derived from hepatocytes or cholangiocarcinoma arising from intrahepatic biliary epithelium. cHCC-CC was first described in 1903 by Wells, with a more rigorous description provided by Allen and Lisa in 1949. The World Health Organization tumor classification system defines cHCC-CC as a tumor in which both HCC and cholangiocarcinoma components coexist in either the same tumor or the same liver. Allen and Lisa classified cHCC-CC into 3 categories: 1) separate tumors each composed of only 1 cell type, 2) contiguous tumors each with a different cell type that may commingle as they grow together, and 3) individual lesions having both types of cells. This case is an example of the third type. A second classification scheme, introduced by Goodman et al, includes type I (collision tumors), type II (transition tumors), and type III (fibrolamellar tumors).

The incidence, demographic characteristics, and natural history of cHCC-CC are not well understood. These tumors are thought to be rare, accounting for 1% to 14% of primary hepatic tumors. The 2 largest series of cHCC-CC have reported somewhat discrepant results; one suggested the tumors more closely resemble HCC and the other noted that tumor markers (low AFP and elevated CEA or CA 19-9 levels) more closely followed cholangiocarcinoma, although both series found that the prognosis of patients with cHCC-CC was significantly worse than patients with HCC.

This case shows a large heterogeneous mass in a liver that is not grossly cirrhotic. Differential diagnosis includes metastasis (not a typical appearance but not unheard of), HCC, cholangiocarcinoma, and other, less common primary hepatic tumors. One element that might suggest cholangiocarcinoma or cHCC-CC is the pattern of gradual enhancement on successive phases of dynamic 3D SPGR images.

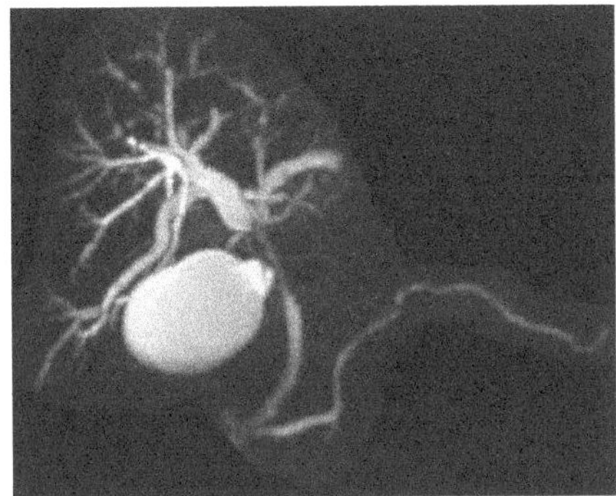

Figure 3.21.1

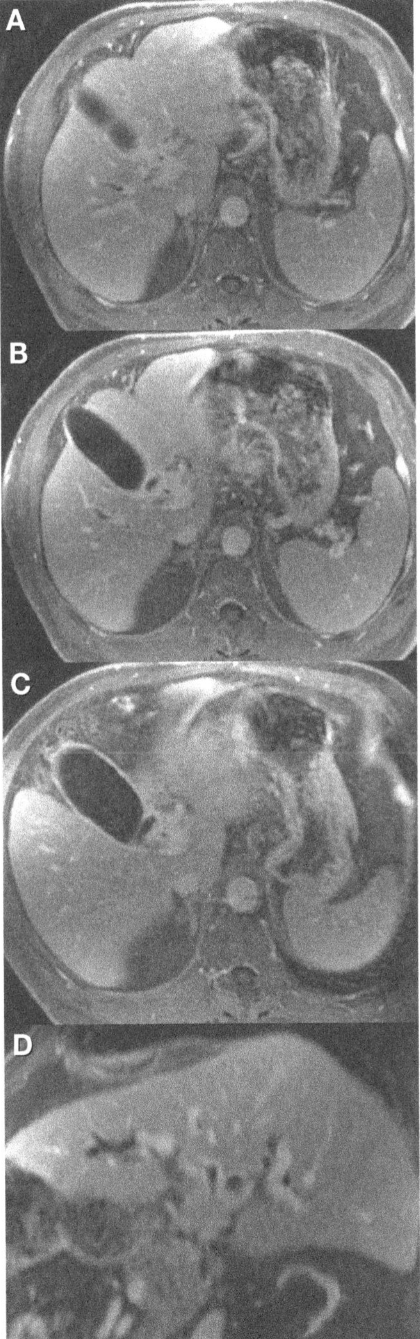

Figure 3.21.2

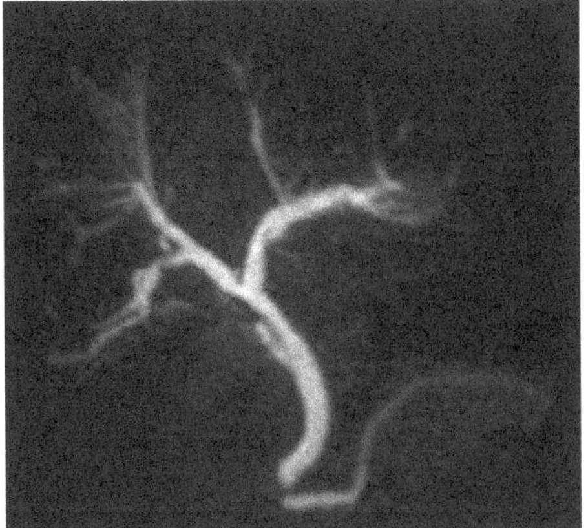

Figure 3.21.3

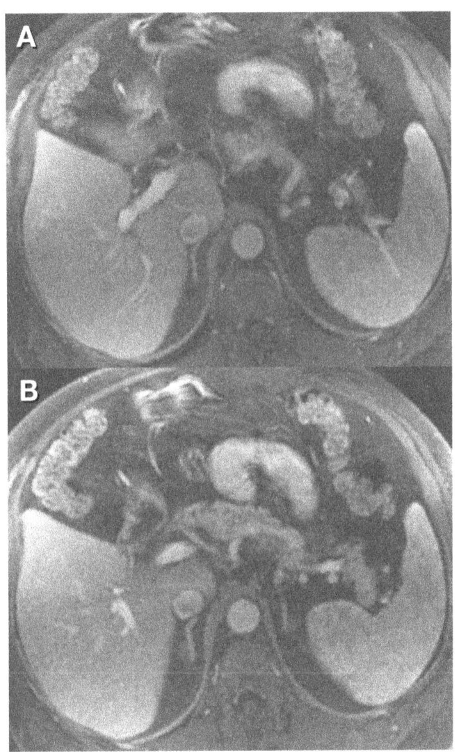

Figure 3.21.4

HISTORY: 63-year-old man with recent fever, chills, and jaundice. ERCP performed at an outside institution revealed a hilar stricture concerning for cholangiocarcinoma; a biliary stent was placed

IMAGING FINDINGS: MIP image from 3D FRFSE MRCP (Figure 3.21.1) demonstrates marked focal narrowing of the proximal CBD in the hepatic hilum with intrahepatic biliary dilatation. Axial equilibrium phase postgadolinium 3D SPGR images (Figures 3.21.2A-C) and a coronal oblique, reformatted delayed-phase image (Figure 3.21.2D) demonstrate focal soft tissue thickening that surrounds the CBD at the hilum and accounts for the focal narrowing. MIP image from MRCP (Figure 3.21.3) and axial portal venous phase postgadolinium 3D SGPR images (Figure 3.21.4) from 3-month follow-up examination show that all these abnormalities have resolved. (The patient also has undergone a cholecystectomy, performed during staging laparotomy.)

DIAGNOSIS: Biliary sarcoid

COMMENT: This case is very unusual; only 4 previous reports in the literature describe hepatobiliary sarcoid mimicking cholangiocarcinoma. This patient had no prior diagnosis of sarcoid and had no other manifestations visible on imaging other than some mildly prominent porta hepatis nodes. (He had a normal chest radiograph and no splenic lesions.) The presence of a hilar stricture with an associated soft tissue mass demonstrating late enhancement is highly suggestive of cholangiocarcinoma, even though the patient had no risk factors for this disease. We don't intend this case to suggest that you start including sarcoid in your differential diagnosis for cholangiocarcinoma. But it is a useful exercise in humility and reminds us of many unfortunate episodes in resident conferences where we said a variation of "This could only be 1 thing" and turned out to be wrong more often than not. More common mimics of cholangiocarcinoma include PSC, autoimmune pancreatitis, benign inflammatory biliary stricture, and metastatic disease to the porta hepatis.

Sarcoidosis is a systemic granulomatous disease of unknown cause. The liver is frequently involved (the third most common site after lymph nodes and lung, with 50% to 80% of livers involved by biopsy and around 70% by autopsy), but most patients are asymptomatic. Of patients with hepatic sarcoid, 35% have abnormal liver function tests and about 20% have hepatomegaly. Histologic abnormalities include noncaseating granulomas, chronic intrahepatic cholestasis, periportal fibrosis, and, eventually, micronodular biliary cirrhosis. The appearance of hepatic sarcoid on MRI is often nonspecific; you may see only changes of cirrhosis or hepatomegaly, with visible T2 hypointense or hypoenhancing granulomas present in only 5% to 15% of patients.

This patient had an excellent response to corticosteroid therapy and has had no recurrent symptoms.

CASE 3.22

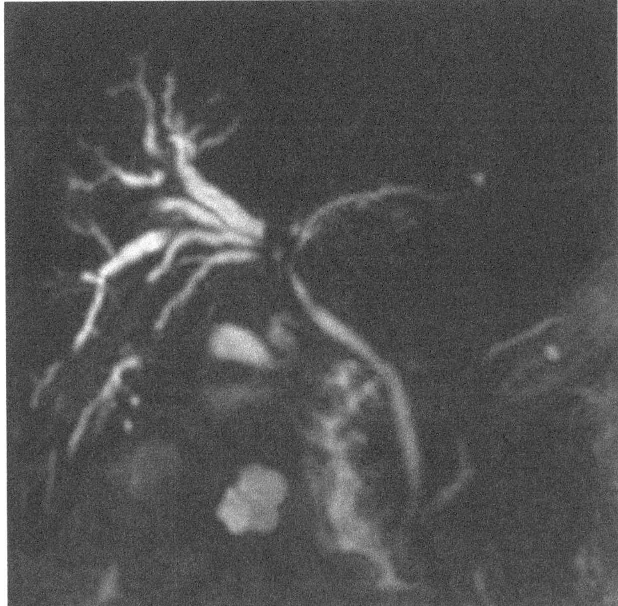

Figure 3.22.1

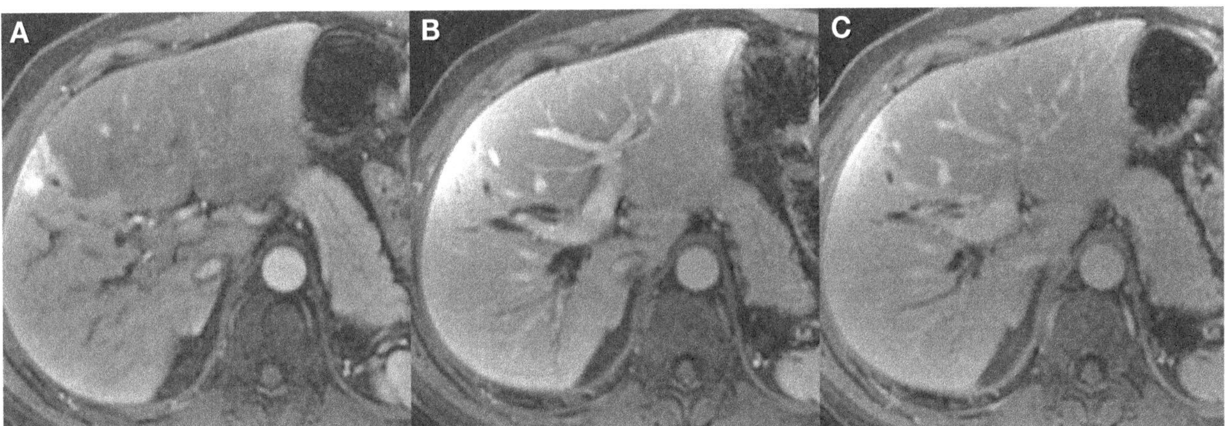

Figure 3.22.2

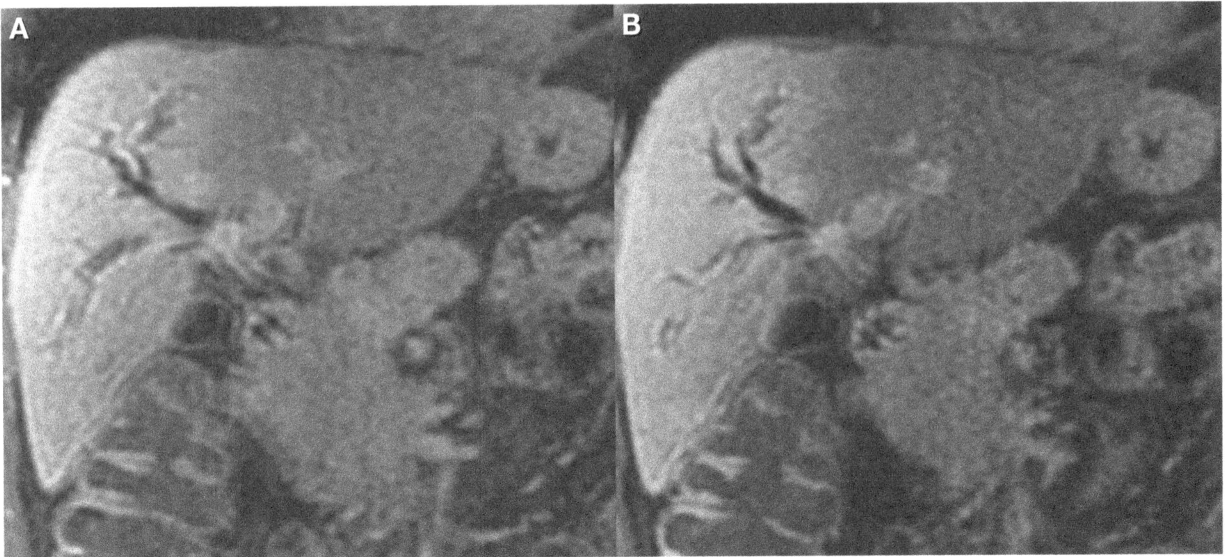

Figure 3.22.3

HISTORY: 53-year-old man with an elevated level of alkaline phosphatase; US revealed intrahepatic biliary dilatation

IMAGING FINDINGS: A partial volume MIP image from 3D FRFSE MRCP (Figure 3.22.1) shows dilatation of right-sided intrahepatic ducts with obstruction in the hilum at the level of the right duct division. Left-sided ducts are normal in caliber. Axial arterial (Figure 3.22.2A), portal venous (Figure 3.22.2B), and equilibrium phase (Figure 3.22.2C) postgadolinium 3D SPGR images demonstrate a small spiculated mass centered at the right main duct bifurcation that shows gradual enhancement. Notice on the arterial phase image that the hepatic artery traverses the mass and there is a discrepancy in enhancement between the right and left hepatic lobes. Coronal 8-minute delayed 3D SPGR images (Figure 3.22.3) again show a spiculated hyperenhancing lesion centered in the hilum at the bifurcation of the right main duct.

DIAGNOSIS: Hilar cholangiocarcinoma (Klatskin tumor)

COMMENT: Cholangiocarcinoma is an uncommon neoplasm arising from the epithelial cells of bile ducts anywhere along the biliary tree except the gallbladder and the ampulla of Vater (carcinomas in these latter locations are classified separately). Accounting for less than 3% of all cancers, cholangiocarcinoma is nevertheless the most common primary malignancy of the biliary tract and the second most common primary malignant hepatobiliary neoplasm, responsible for approximately 15% of liver cancers.

Cholangiocarcinomas are classified as intrahepatic or extrahepatic (ductal), and extrahepatic tumors usually are divided into those occurring near the hilum (perihilar or Klatskin tumors) and those arising in the distal extrahepatic duct. Klatskin tumors account for a majority (50%-60%) of cholangiocarcinomas, with 20% to 30% located within the distal extrahepatic duct and 10% arising within the liver. To complicate matters further, the Liver Cancer Study Group of Japan has distinguished 3 macroscopic growth types for cholangiocarcinoma: mass forming, periductal infiltrating, and intraductal growth. Intrahepatic and extrahepatic cholangiocarcinomas usually have different presentations: Patients with extrahepatic tumors have early development of biliary tract obstruction and jaundice, while those with intrahepatic tumors have more nonspecific signs and symptoms of a hepatic mass. Etiology, risk factors, natural history, and response to therapy also differ somewhat between the 2 phenotypes.

Prognosis for patients with cholangiocarcinoma is poor. Most patients become symptomatic after the disease is advanced. Approximately half of untreated patients die within 3 to 4 months of presentation, and the 5-year survival for all patients is less than 5%. Surgical resection of early-stage tumors is potentially curative; however, few patients are surgical candidates, and even after surgery the 5-year survival rates are 30% to 40% for intrahepatic tumors and 50% for extrahepatic lesions. A second approach in carefully selected patients combines systemic chemotherapy and radiation therapy with liver transplantation and has resulted in 5-year survival rates approaching 70%.

Most cases of cholangiocarcinoma occur sporadically. However, there is evidence that chronic inflammation and injury of the biliary epithelium induced by chronic obstruction results in the release of cytokines, which may lead to malignant transformation. Approximately 10% of cholangiocarcinomas arise in the setting of well-known risk factors, which include PSC, choledochal cysts, Caroli disease, recurrent pyogenic cholangitis, cirrhosis of any cause, and exposure to toxic substances, including nitrosamines, dioxin, asbestos, Thorotrast, and radon. In a large Swedish trial, 8% of PSC patients developed cholangiocarcinoma within 5 years of the initial diagnosis, and 70% to 89% of these patients also had ulcerative colitis. In patients with PSC, cholangiocarcinoma develops at an earlier age, is more often multifocal, and is less amenable to resection.

Diagnosis of cholangiocarcinoma can be difficult, and although MRI is by no means ideal, it is probably the best option currently available. Levels of such tumor markers as CA 19-9 and CEA are sometimes elevated in patients with cholangiocarcinoma, but these markers are not very sensitive (CA 19-9 level >100 U/mL has a sensitivity of 76% and a specificity of 92%). For patients with biliary obstruction, ERCP is often performed and brush cytology obtained, but the sensitivity is extremely poor—by some reports, as low as 20%. The addition of chromosomal analysis using FISH improves the sensitivity to 47% and the specificity to 97% for cholangiocarcinoma detection in patients with PSC.

Most cholangiocarcinomas are perihilar tumors. Most of these tumors are small at presentation (although paradoxically, many of the small lesions are inoperable) and most are of the periductal infiltrating type, all of which means that they are difficult to visualize.

MRI is probably the best technique for finding these lesions because of its combination of biliary imaging and superior soft tissue contrast. You can use MRCP to localize the level of biliary obstruction and then use your best parenchymal imaging techniques in this general area. Most cholangiocarcinomas (roughly 80%) show arterial phase hypoenhancement with gradual accumulation of contrast over time. This feature has led to the ubiquitous delayed acquisition acquired 8 to 10 minutes after gadolinium injection, which is a good idea, and has inspired some experts to downplay the role of traditional dynamic imaging (ie, skipping the test bolus to optimize the arterial phase), which is not.

Cholangiocarcinomas generally are slightly hyperintense on T2-weighted images relative to hepatic parenchyma. Known or suspected cholangiocarcinoma is definitely an indication for which you should spend the extra time on a respiratory-triggered fat-suppressed FSE sequence rather than a breath-hold SSFSE or FRFSE technique with marginal soft tissue discrimination (2D FRFSE is also known to us as the *hepatoma suppression sequence*). Diffusion-weighted imaging also may be helpful on occasion. It generally works best with a relatively high b value (ie, ≥600 s/mm^2); at low b values, fluid in the obstructed biliary tree is also bright by virtue of T2 shine-through and therefore difficult to distinguish from a small tumor.

We also include overlapping fat-suppressed 2D SSFP images in our protocol. These images may not be critical for identifying the lesion (although soft tissue discrimination is improved when the images are obtained after gadolinium administration between the dynamic and delayed acquisitions). However, they allow for visualization of the bile ducts, portal and hepatic veins, and, sometimes, the mass all on a single acquisition, which can be helpful in tumor staging.

Your main job when performing MRI of a patient with suspected cholangiocarcinoma is to find the lesion, but remember that staging is also important. Staging is discussed more comprehensively in Case 3.23. As a general rule, however, when there is prominent extension into both hepatic lobes, the tumor is inoperable. Involvement of biliary ducts is generally assessed with MRCP. Amputated, invisible ducts are involved with the tumor; dilated fluid-filled ducts are not. Vascular involvement is usually best appreciated on dynamic contrast-enhanced 3D SPGR images or overlapping 2D SSFP images. Venous involvement (ie, narrowing or thrombosis of portal or hepatic veins) is fairly easy to spot in most cases. Detecting arterial encasement is trickier with MRI because spatial resolution is somewhat limited in comparison to CT. In this case, the striking perfusion discrepancy on arterial phase images suggests vascular involvement. If you carefully inspect the tumor margins on all 3 phases, you can see that the small right hepatic artery is encased by the posterior margin of the tumor.

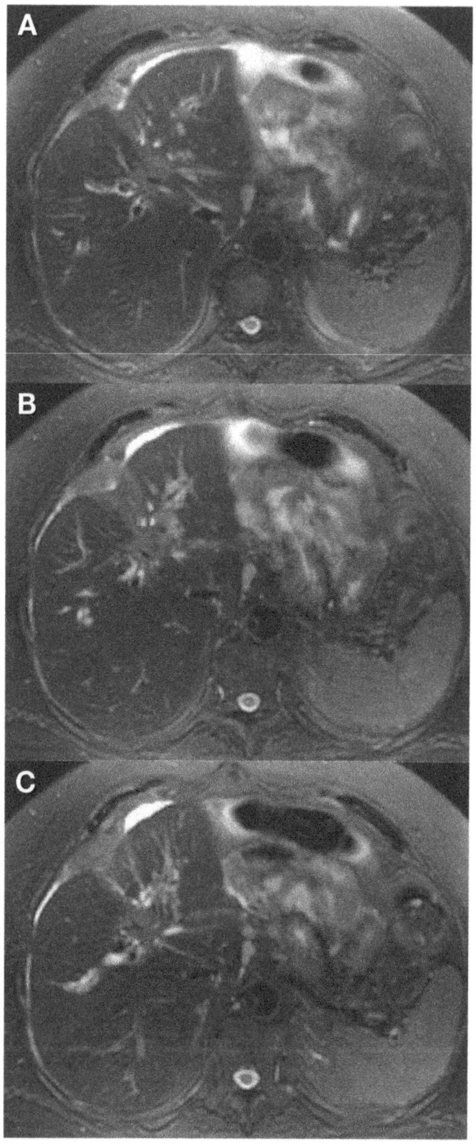

CASE 3.23

Figure 3.23.1

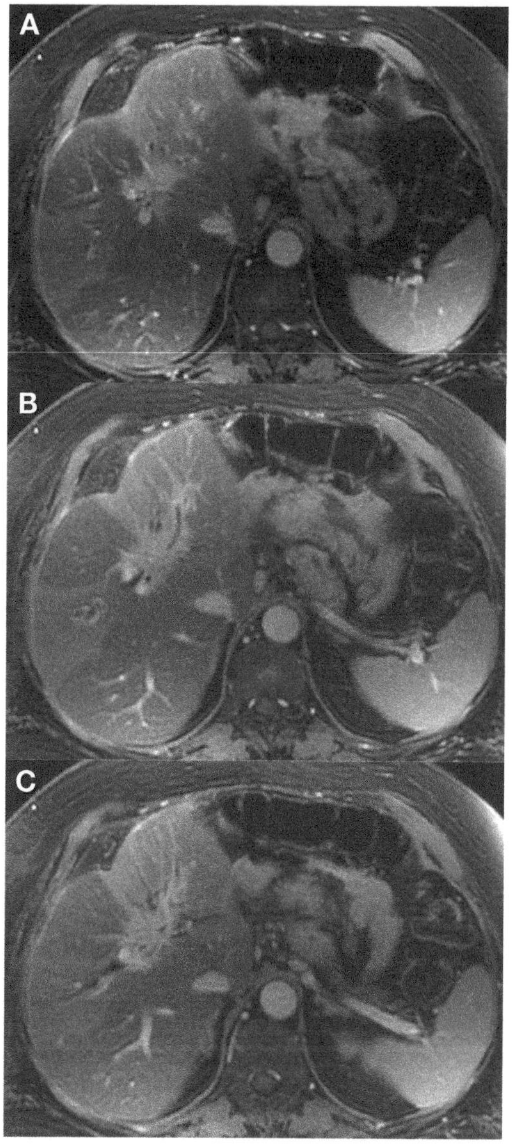

Figure 3.23.2

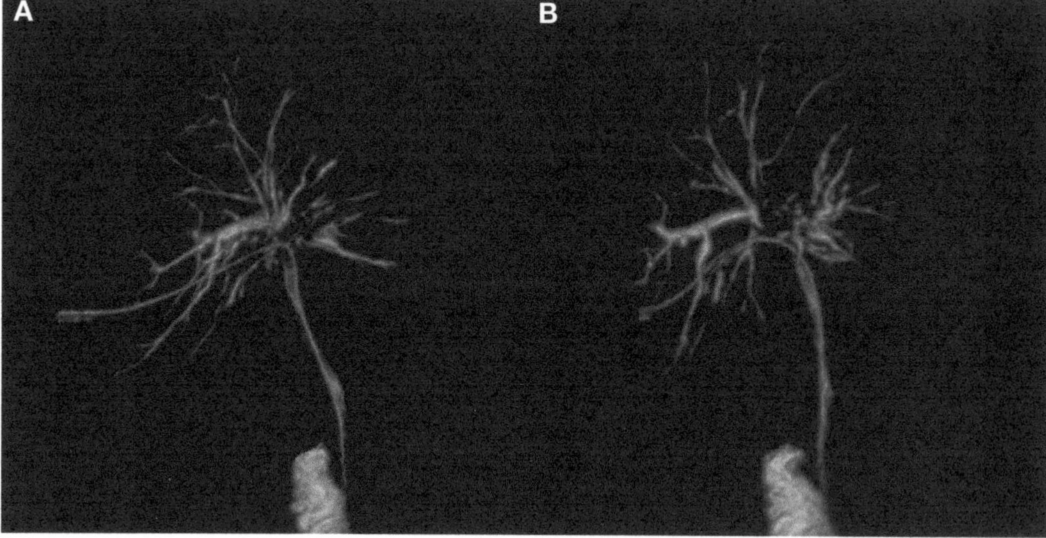

Figure 3.23.3

HISTORY: 62-year-old man with jaundice, an elevated CA 19-9 level, and a porta hepatis mass on CT performed at an outside institution

IMAGING FINDINGS: Axial fat-suppressed FSE T2-weighted images (Figure 3.23.1) reveal an ill-defined, spiculated mass in the hepatic hilum encasing the central biliary ducts, with peripheral intrahepatic biliary dilatation. Axial 2D SPGR images obtained 8 minutes after gadolinium injection (Figure 3.23.2) demonstrate diffuse enhancement of the central mass. Note encasement and narrowing of the left portal vein in the inferior image, as well as prominent anterior capsular retraction. Volume-rendered images from 3D FRFSE MRCP (Figure 3.23.3) demonstrate occluded central biliary ducts extending beyond the bifurcation of the right and left main ducts.

DIAGNOSIS: Unresectable hilar cholangiocarcinoma (Klatskin tumor)

COMMENT: Staging cholangiocarcinoma can be challenging not only because the imaging is difficult, but also because a number of different staging systems are currently in use—and none are entirely successful. Our strategy, therefore, is to describe the relevant findings in detail and then leave it up to the surgeon to decide whether the lesion is resectable.

The Bismuth-Corlette system is probably the most popular staging scheme for extrahepatic cholangiocarcinoma. Type I tumors are confined below the confluence of right and left hepatic ducts, type II tumors extend to the confluence, type III tumors extend to the bifurcation of either the right (type IIIa) or the left (type IIIb) hepatic duct, and type IV tumors involve the bifurcation of both right and left ducts. In the absence of other problems (eg, vascular involvement, intrahepatic metastatic disease), lesions of types I to III are potentially resectable. Type IV lesions are generally considered inoperable, although recently some surgeons have attempted resections in cases where the tumor remained within 2 cm of the hilum.

The Memorial Sloan-Kettering system also includes vascular involvement: T1 lesions are tumors involving the biliary confluence with or without unilateral extension to second-order biliary radicals; T2 lesions include ipsilateral portal vein involvement or ipsilateral lobar atrophy, or both; and T3 lesions include those with bilateral extension to second-order biliary radicals, with unilateral extension to second-order biliary radicals with contralateral portal vein involvement or lobar atrophy or with main or bilateral portal venous involvement. In this classification, T1 and T2 lesions are potentially resectable; T3 lesions are not.

Most studies have shown MRI to be accurate in staging hilar cholangiocarcinomas. The level of biliary involvement is predicted by amputation, stenosis, or irregularity of bile ducts on MRCP. This approach potentially can understage lesions since cholangiocarcinomas have a tendency to spread between the hepatocyte plates, along the biliary duct walls, and adjacent to the nerves. Perineural invasion is very common, found in as many as 80% of tumors. This infiltrative extension can sometimes be appreciated on MRI as mural thickening and/or enhancement of biliary ducts. However, an identical appearance can be seen in PSC, in cholangitis resulting from biliary obstruction by the central tumor, and in periductal fibroblastic and inflammatory reaction, all of which can result in overstaging of tumor extension. Venous involvement is usually identified fairly easily on MRI as 1) a narrowing of the lumen or a frank invasion of the vessel with tumor thrombus or 2) tumor contact of greater than 90° around an adjacent vessel. Arterial invasion has a similar appearance, although the involved vessels are considerably smaller and thus optimization of technique (ie, maximizing spatial resolution and ensuring that you are acquiring good arterial phase images) is very important for accurate assessment.

This case illustrates common features of unresectable hilar cholangiocarcinoma. On MRCP, neither the right nor left biliary confluence is identified, indicating tumor involvement of both sides. Postgadolinium images show a narrowed left portal vein surrounded by tumor, with associated atrophy of the left hepatic lobe. Capsular retraction, also evident in this case, was once considered a specific sign of cholangiocarcinoma because of its fibrotic tendencies. It continues to be an observation worth noting but can also be seen in other neoplastic and inflammatory lesions.

In general, understaging cholangiocarcinoma is better than overstaging, since after it is classified as inoperable, there is little to offer a patient. This is not trivial surgery, however, and the morbidity and mortality rates are high. Approximately 40% of patients with hilar cholangiocarcinoma undergo surgery, and 1 long-term study in the United Kingdom showed that roughly half of patients undergoing potentially curative laparotomy had unresectable disease. This result is somewhat at odds with the much higher sensitivities and specificities quoted in the MRI literature, but it might be a more accurate reflection of current reality.

CASE 3.24

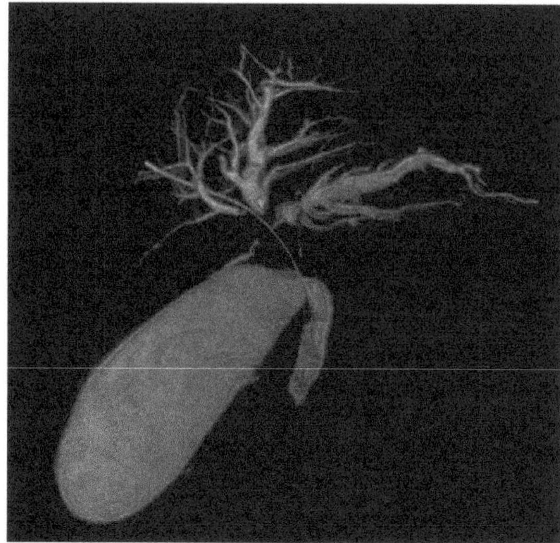

Figure 3.24.1

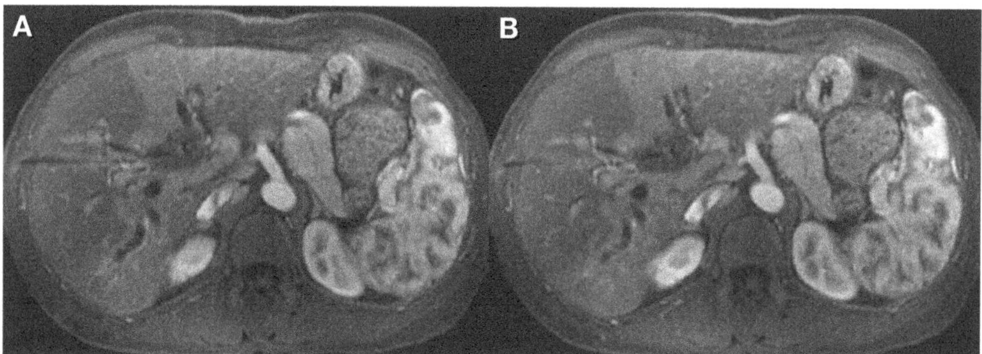

Figure 3.24.2

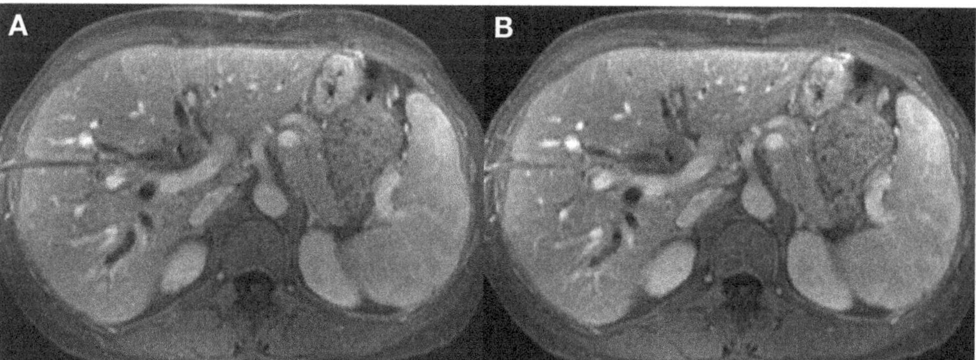

Figure 3.24.3

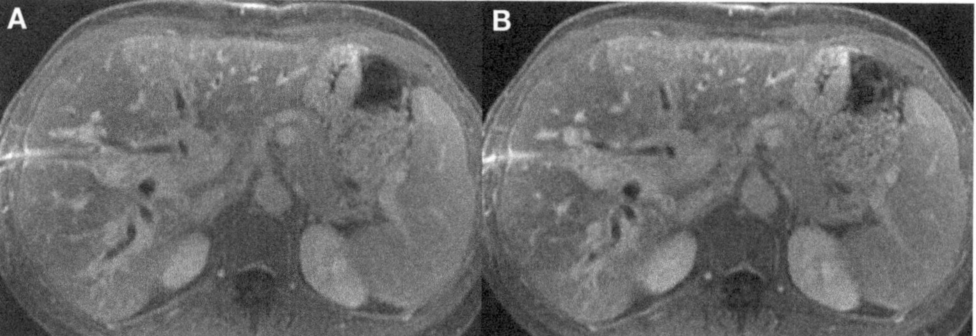

Figure 3.24.4

HISTORY: 58-year-old woman who has fatigue and jaundice; ERCP at an outside institution revealed an obstructive hilar lesion

IMAGING FINDINGS: Volume-rendered image from 3D SSFP MRCP (Figure 3.24.1) demonstrates central biliary obstruction extending to the bifurcation of the right and left ducts. Axial arterial (Figure 3.24.2), portal venous (Figure 3.24.3), and 8-minute delayed phase (Figure 3.24.4) postgadolinium 3D SPGR images reveal a soft tissue mass encasing the central biliary ducts that is initially hypoenhancing and gradually accumulates contrast. Note also the percutaneous biliary tube entering the right hepatic lobe laterally.

DIAGNOSIS: Hilar cholangiocarcinoma (Klatskin tumor)

COMMENT: This case is an example of a hilar cholangiocarcinoma better seen on arterial and portal venous phases than on delayed phase images. This appearance is more common than you might think and is another reason (in addition to vascular staging) why good dynamic 3D SPGR images are important. The central hypoenhancing mass can be visualized against a background of enhancing parenchyma. This appearance is accentuated by vascular encasement of the left portal vein and hepatic artery, which led to hyperenhancement of the left hepatic lobe on arterial and portal phase images. A consistent limitation of delayed phase images also is illustrated in this case: The tumor becomes nearly isointense to the adjacent portal vein, and distinguishing the tumor from the vein is difficult.

Notice the presence of the transhepatic biliary drain in this case. Relief of biliary obstruction before a staging examination may limit its accuracy but unfortunately is a frequent occurrence. In our practice, well over 90% of MRIs performed for cholangiocarcinoma staging occur in patients with internal or external biliary drains. These are problematic for a couple of reasons. First, identifying the site and extent of biliary involvement is often more difficult on MRCP after the obstruction has been relieved, and second, drain placement can result in an inflammatory response that may mimic tumor infiltration or in perfusion abnormalities also seen in vascular encasement. There is no evidence that relief of biliary obstruction before definitive surgery has any benefit and, in fact, it sometimes leads to complications that can delay surgery, but biliary drainage is a tempting procedure for gastroenterologists or interventional radiologists to perform and seems reasonable to patients and their families.

The patient in this case was not considered a surgical candidate but did undergo successful chemoradiation therapy followed by hepatic transplantation.

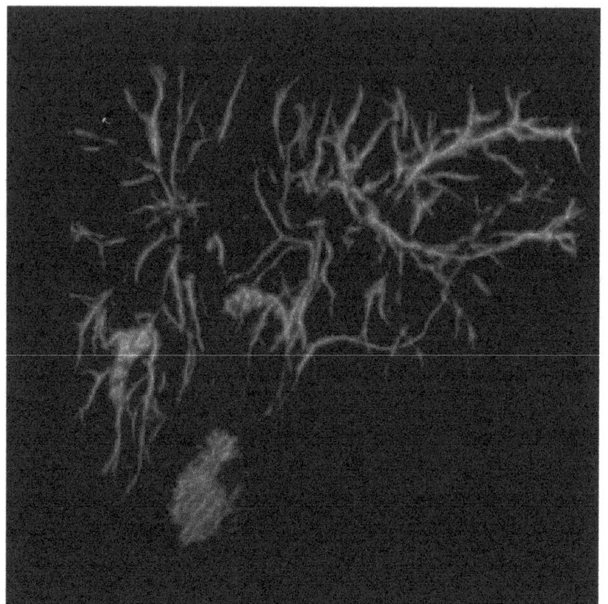

Figure 3.25.1

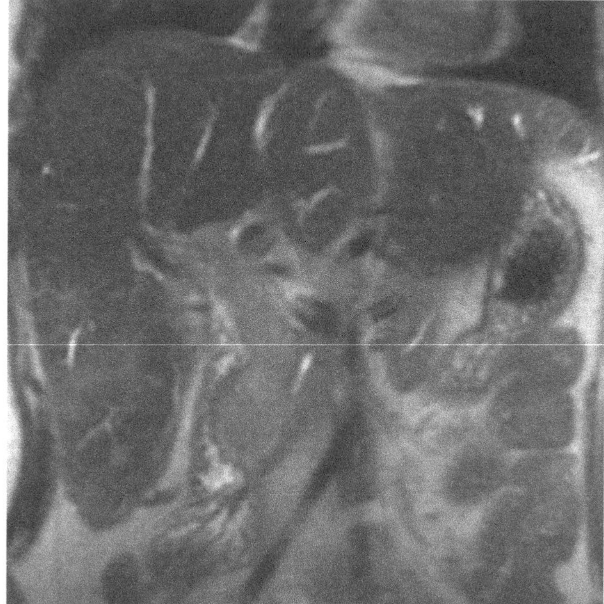

Figure 3.25.2

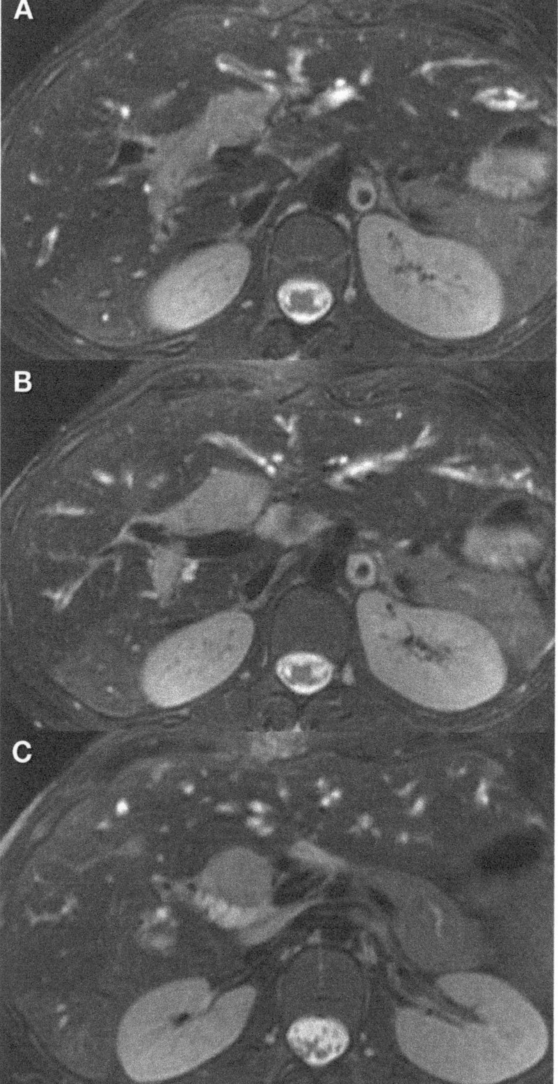

Figure 3.25.3

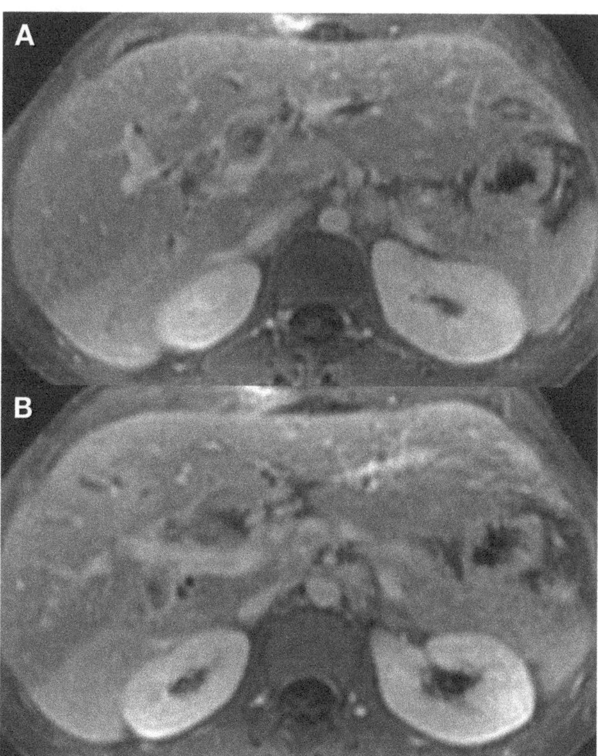

Figure 3.25.4

HISTORY: 29-year-old woman with a history of Crohn disease and neurofibromatosis with jaundice and abdominal pain

IMAGING FINDINGS: A volume-rendered image from 3D FRFSE MRCP (Figure 3.25.1) reveals diffuse intrahepatic biliary dilatation with central obstruction. Coronal SSFSE image (Figure 3.25.2) demonstrates an expansile soft tissue mass involving the entire extrahepatic CBD. Axial fat-suppressed FSE images (Figure 3.25.3) show the soft tissue mass extending from the CBD primarily into right-sided intrahepatic ducts. Axial portal venous phase 3D SPGR images (Figure 3.25.4) show mild heterogeneous enhancement of the intraductal mass.

DIAGNOSIS: Intraductal cholangiocarcinoma

COMMENT: Intraductal cholangiocarcinoma represents the least common variant of cholangiocarcinoma and, when detected early, is thought to have a more favorable prognosis. Unfortunately, this case represents advanced disease with tumor extension throughout the extrahepatic ducts and involving both right and left ducts beyond the first bifurcation. Staging can proceed as for any other extrahepatic tumor, although in this case the determining factor is the extent of ductal involvement. Vascular involvement and hepatic parenchymal invasion are less common for intraductal tumors than for the more typical periductal infiltrating lesions. Intraductal masses should be fairly specific for cholangiocarcinoma; however, rare cases of HCC with biliary ductal growth or invasion have occurred, and there are even reports of metastatic disease to biliary ducts.

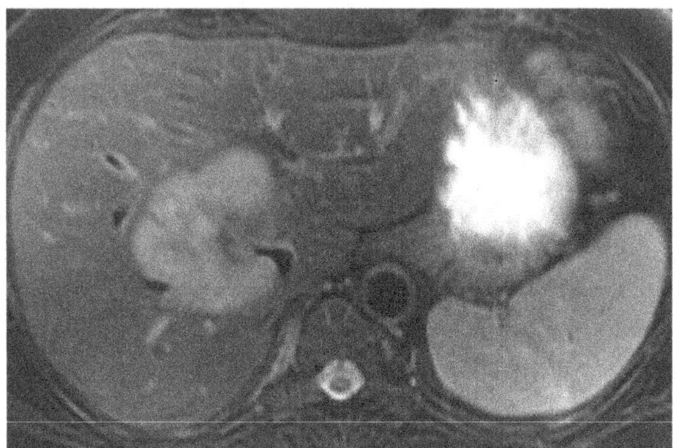

Figure 3.26.1

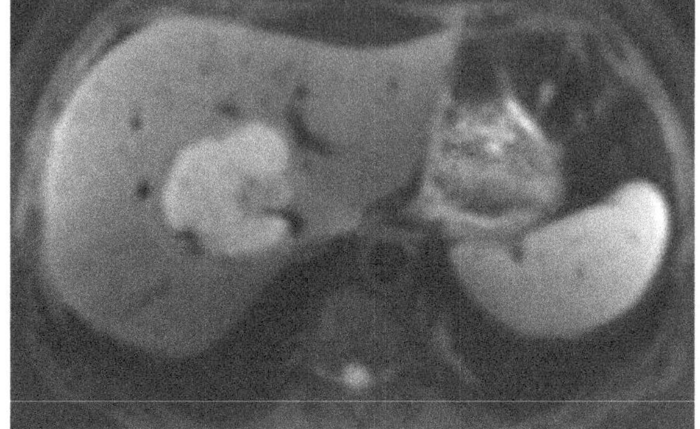

Figure 3.26.2

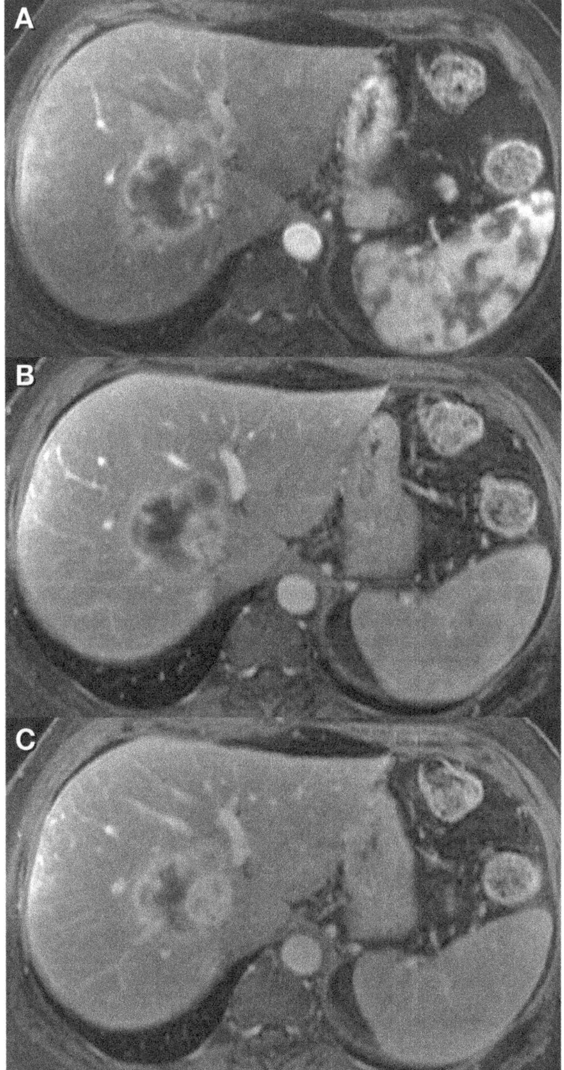

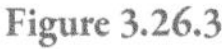

Figure 3.26.3

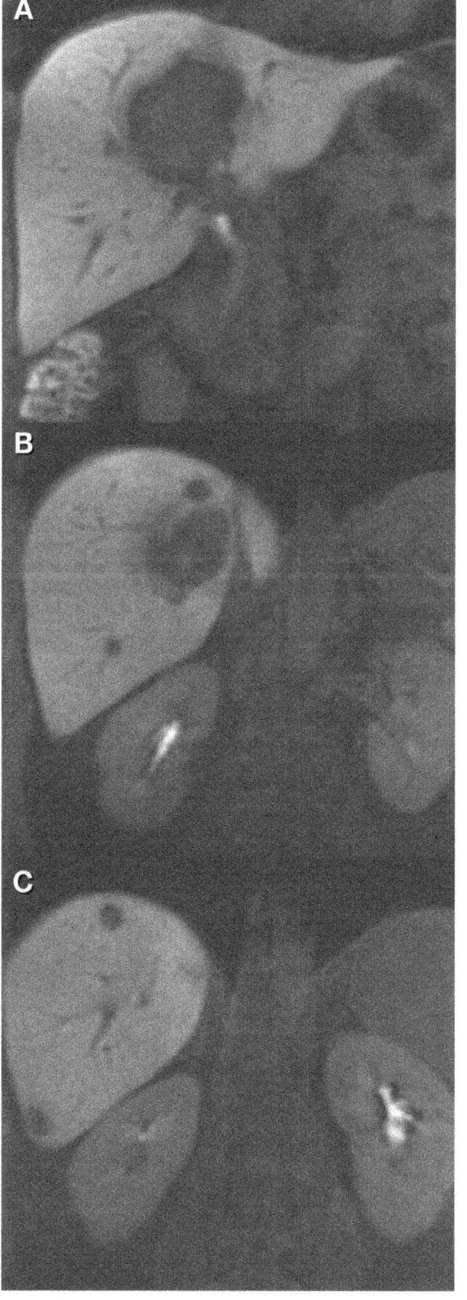

Figure 3.26.4

HISTORY: 52-year-old woman with abdominal discomfort and abnormal results on liver function tests

IMAGING FINDINGS: Axial fat-suppressed FSE T2-weighted image (Figure 3.26.1) and diffusion-weighted image (b=600 s/mm^2) (Figure 3.26.2) reveal a large mass with increased signal intensity partially surrounding the right hepatic vein and inferior vena cava. Axial arterial, portal venous, and equilibrium phase postgadolinium 3D SPGR images (Figure 3.26.3) demonstrate heterogeneous enhancement of the mass, with some accumulation of contrast on the equilibrium phase image. Coronal hepatobiliary phase images (Figure 3.26.4) show diffuse hypoenhancement of the mass with additional smaller lesions in the right hepatic lobe, consistent with metastases.

DIAGNOSIS: Intrahepatic cholangiocarcinoma with hepatic metastases

COMMENT: Intrahepatic cholangiocarcinomas represent 10% of all cholangiocarcinomas. In contrast to patients with perihilar lesions who have early obstruction and jaundice, those with intrahepatic tumors present with nonspecific symptoms, such as abdominal pain, malaise, night sweats, and cachexia. Intrahepatic cholangiocarcinomas usually have similar imaging characteristics to extracellular lesions on dynamic contrast-enhanced 3D SPGR images: early hypoenhancement followed by progressive contrast agent uptake through equilibrium and delayed images. In our experience, intrahepatic lesions tend to have higher signal intensity on T2- and diffusion-weighted images and generally are much larger at diagnosis than extrahepatic tumors. Differential diagnosis includes HCC, which more often arises in cirrhotic livers and classically shows arterial phase hyperenhancement with washout on portal venous and equilibrium phase images (examples are included in Chapter 1). Metastatic disease is also a consideration, although few metastases show the gradual enhancement typically seen with cholangiocarcinoma. Atypical hemangiomas, particularly the sclerosing variety, can have an appearance similar to cholangiocarcinoma if you don't see the diagnostic lobulated, peripheral arterial phase enhancement.

Hepatic resection with negative margins is the best curative option, although unfortunately, many patients are not surgical candidates at presentation. Following resection, the 5-year survival rate is 25%, with prognosis affected by the margin status, lymph node involvement, and vascular invasion.

In this case, we used gadoxetate disodium (Eovist)—the hepatocyte-specific gadolinium agent. Several experts (including some in our department) advocate its use for almost any indication involving the liver. We have had some unfortunate experiences imaging extrahepatic cholangiocarcinoma with Eovist, however. The most important consideration is hepatic function. In patients with obstructed ducts and poor hepatic function (bilirubin >5 mg/dL), very little contrast will be taken up by hepatocytes and excreted into the biliary tree, so that no true hepatobiliary phase is ever obtained. In addition, the quality of the dynamic images is generally reduced compared to standard extracellular contrast agents because of the small doses used, and the resulting examination may be almost as bad as, or even worse than, a CT scan.

In the ideal case, there is strong contrast uptake by hepatocytes and prompt biliary excretion so that, on hepatobiliary phase images, the hypointense tumor surrounds the narrowed or obstructed ducts, which contain gadolinium. Even under ideal conditions, however, these tumors often have a signal intensity similar to the hilar vessels on hepatobiliary phase images, a similar problem (but with the opposite signal) encountered on delayed images obtained with standard extracellular gadolinium agents. On the other hand, Eovist is an excellent agent for identifying small intrahepatic metastases, as demonstrated in this case.

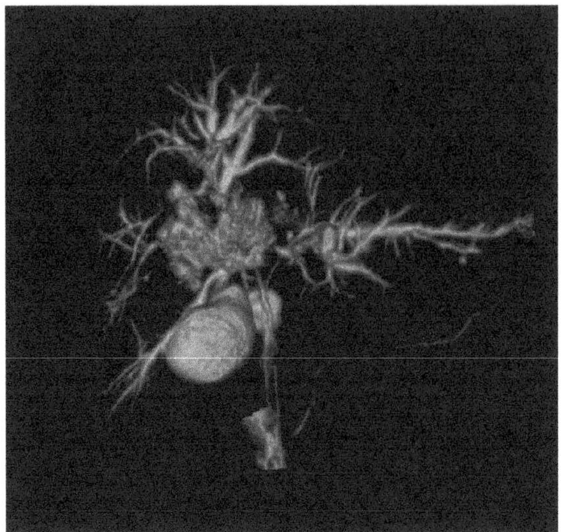

Figure 3.27.1

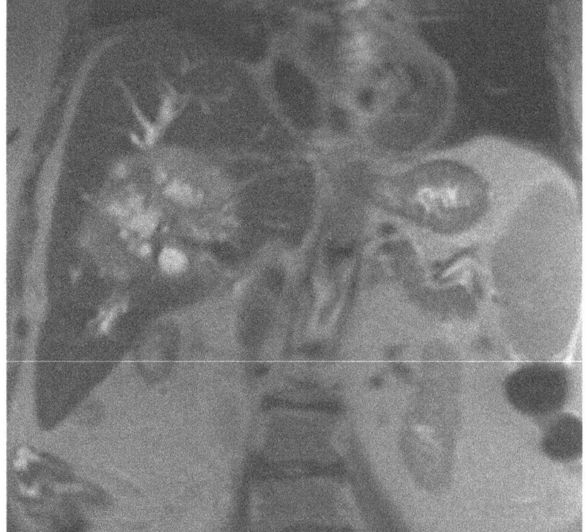

Figure 3.27.2

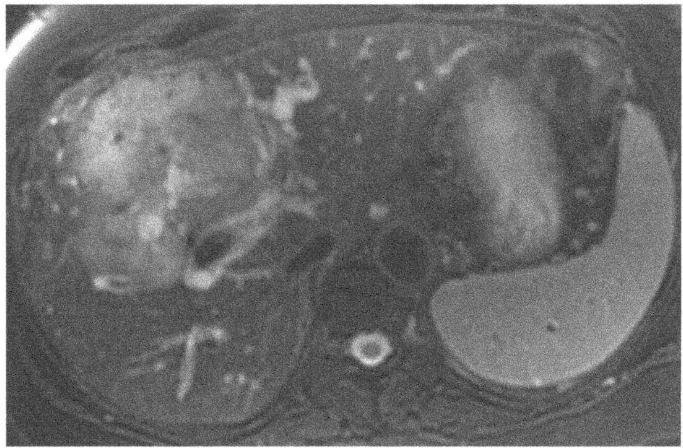

Figure 3.27.3

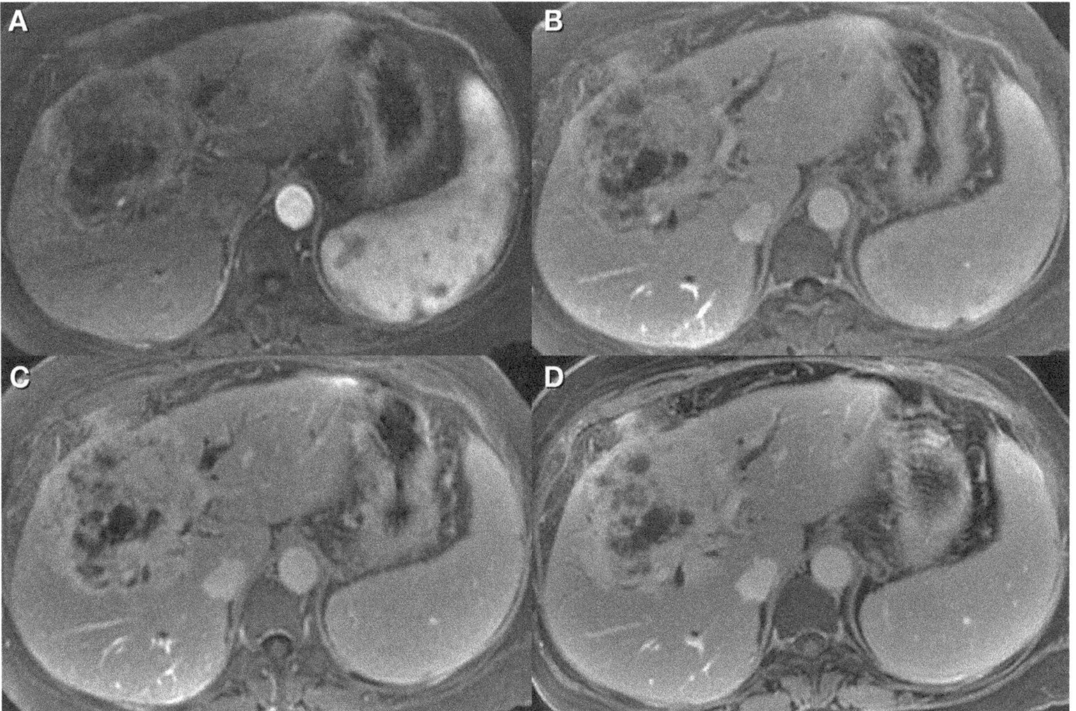

Figure 3.27.4

HISTORY: 75-year-old woman with jaundice

IMAGING FINDINGS: Volume-rendered image from 3D FRFSE MRCP (Figure 3.27.1) demonstrates central biliary obstruction. Coronal SSFSE (Figure 3.27.2), axial fat-suppressed FSE (Figure 3.27.3), and axial arterial (Figure 3.27.4A), portal venous (Figure 3.27.4B), equilibrium (Figure 3.27.4C), and delayed phase (Figure 3.27.4D) postgadolinium 3D SPGR images show a large hilar mass with regions of central necrosis causing biliary obstruction. Note the regions of high signal intensity within the central mass on T2-weighted images. Postgadolinium images show gradual contrast accumulation in the lesion. Note also irregular enhancement in the peritoneum along the anterior margin of the lesion.

DIAGNOSIS: Necrotic cholangiocarcinoma with peritoneal metastases

COMMENT: This case illustrates a large lesion with regions of central necrosis and a classic enhancement pattern following gadolinium administration. Deciding whether this is an extrahepatic or intrahepatic lesion is difficult; it does seem to be centered at the hilum, with obstruction of peripheral intrahepatic ducts, but it is very large for a typical Klatskin tumor. The distinction in this case is a moot point since metastatic disease is present in the peritoneum, the result of direct extension of the tumor. Peritoneal extension is best seen as hazy enhancement on portal venous, equilibrium, and late phase images extending from the anterior tumor margin.

ABBREVIATIONS

AFP	alpha fetoprotein
CA	carbohydrate antigen
CBD	common bile duct
CEA	carcinoembryonic antigen
cHCC-CC	combined hepatocellular carcinoma and cholangiocarcinoma
CT	computed tomography
ERCP	endoscopic retrograde cholangiopancreatography
FISH	fluorescence in situ hybridization
FRFSE	fast-recovery fast-spin echo
FSE	fast-spin echo
HCC	hepatocellular carcinoma
HIDA	hepatobiliary iminodiacetic acid
MIP	maximum intensity projection
MR	magnetic resonance
MRCP	magnetic resonance cholangiopancreatography
MRI	magnetic resonance imaging
PSC	primary sclerosing cholangitis
RCC	renal cell carcinoma
SPGR	spoiled gradient-recalled echo
SSFP	steady-state free precession
SSFSE	single-shot fast-spin echo
TE	echo time
3D	3-dimensional
2D	2-dimensional
US	ultrasonography

4.

PANCREAS

CASE 4.1

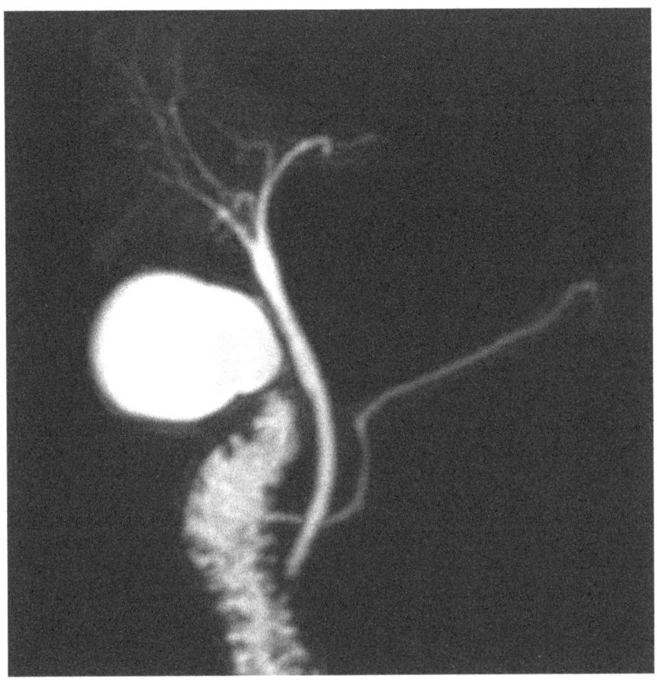

Figure 4.1.1

HISTORY: 51-year-old man with possible cholangiocarcinoma

IMAGING FINDINGS: MIP image from 3D FRFSE MRCP (Figure 4.1.1) demonstrates that the main pancreatic duct drains into the duodenum at the minor papilla, separate from the common bile duct.

DIAGNOSIS: Pancreas divisum

COMMENT: Pancreas divisum is the most common pancreatic developmental anomaly, with an estimated prevalence of 4% to 15%. It occurs when the ducts of the dorsal and ventral pancreatic buds fail to fuse. This results in the main pancreatic duct draining into the duodenum at the minor papilla via the duct of Santorini, separate from the common bile duct, which drains into the major papilla. (With normal development, the ventral duct of Wirsung fuses with the main pancreatic duct of the body and tail and drains into the major papilla with the common bile duct.)

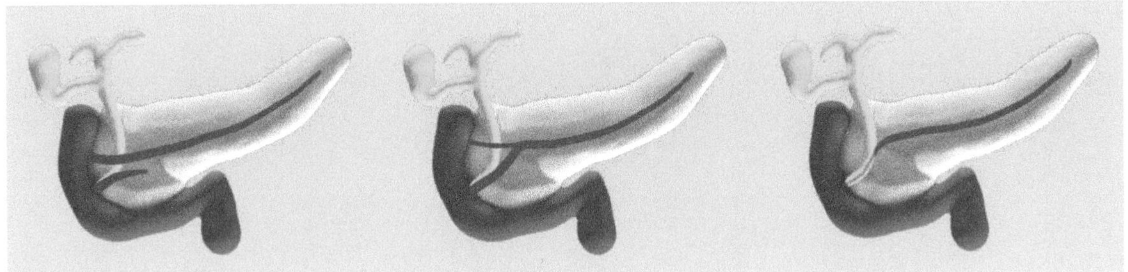

Figure 4.1.2 (Used with permission of Benjamin H. Lee.)

Variants of pancreas divisum can be seen, including a type with a small communicating branch between the dorsal and ventral pancreatic ducts. Figure 4.1.2 illustrates the most common variants in pancreatic ductal anatomy.

The relatively small size of the minor papilla and the potential for obstruction have long been cited as an explanation for the development of recurrent pancreatitis in a small percentage of patients with pancreas divisum. The association of pancreas divisum with recurrent pancreatitis is controversial, although the trend in the most recent literature seems to support the opinion that there is not an increased incidence of pancreatitis in patients with pancreas divisum. This is by no means a universal consensus, however, and many gastroenterologists continue to treat symptomatic patients, most often with minor papilla sphincterotomy and occasionally with stent placement. Reported rates of successful therapy have a broad range, but in general, patients with acute pancreatitis are more likely to have a good response than patients with CP.

Pancreas divisum is usually an easy diagnosis to make with MRI and MRCP. The pancreatic duct is seen to drain into the duodenum at a separate location from the common duct. There are a few instances, however, in which the diagnosis is missed or can be difficult:

1) Pancreas divisum may be a serendipitous finding on an abdominal MRI performed for some purpose other than MRCP and assessment of the pancreatic duct. (It's certainly arguable that missing this diagnosis is not a great tragedy, since it would be an incidental finding in an asymptomatic patient. But it's nice to impress referring clinicians, and we have found that the combination of coronal SSFSE images obtained at the beginning of every abdominal examination and overlapping 2D fat-suppressed SSFP images at the end nearly always give us a good look at the ductal anatomy of the pancreatic head).
2) Some patients for one reason or another (bad luck, pancreatic atrophy, CP and ductal stricture, etc) have a poorly visualized pancreatic duct. Sometimes this result is your fault (poor technique), and sometimes it's the patient's fault (motion artifact from bowel gas, peristalsis, poor breath holding, etc), but it's very difficult to visualize a duct that doesn't contain any fluid. Secretin can help in these situations by stimulating exocrine secretion. Within a couple of minutes, the amount of fluid in the duct increases, allowing better visualization of the main duct and, sometimes, the side branches. Secretin can also be used for functional assessment of the pancreas and pancreatic duct. If the duct doesn't distend and a reasonable amount of fluid is not secreted into the duodenum, these findings are suggestive of pancreatic dysfunction. Some institutions use secretin routinely for all cases calling for imaging of the pancreatic duct. This is probably more elaborate than absolutely necessary, but it can be helpful in many cases. Secretin should be used with caution or not at all in patients with acute pancreatitis.

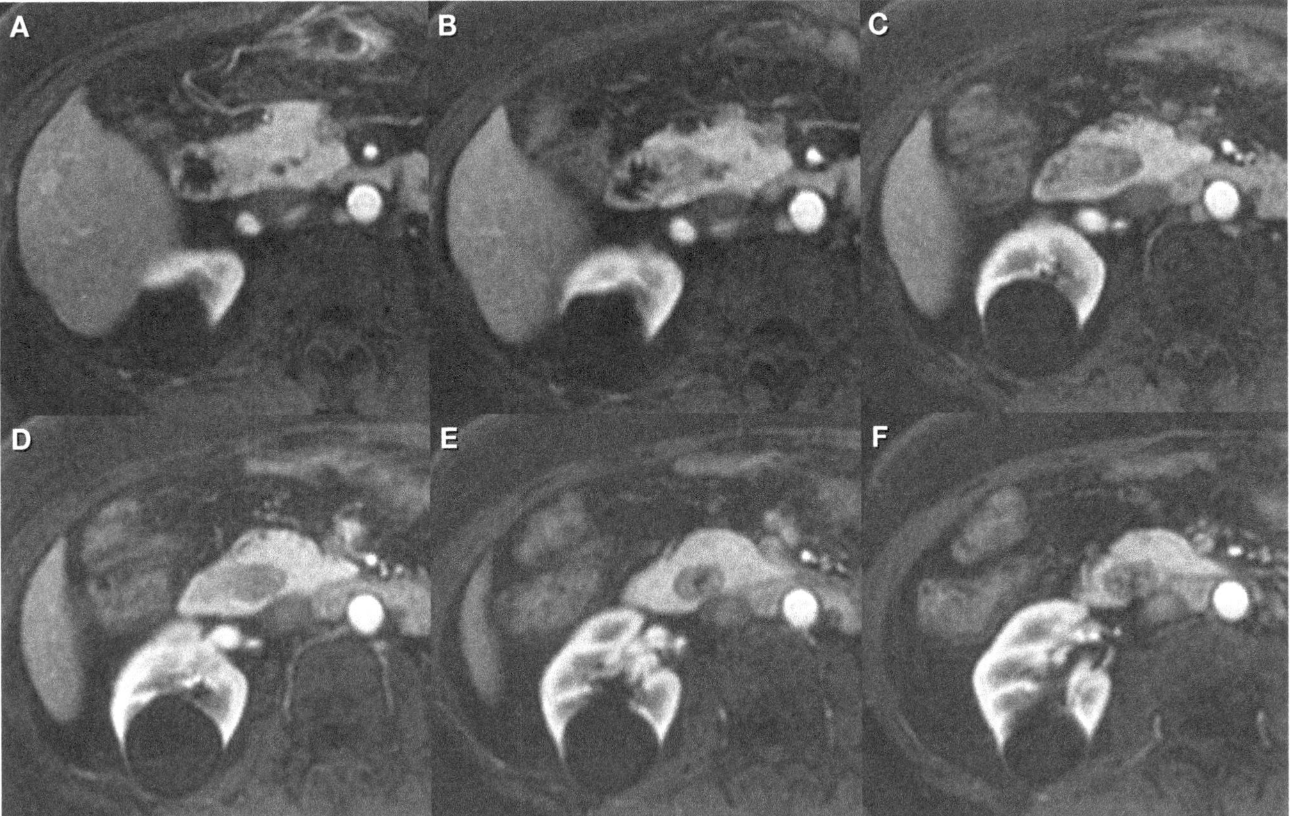

Figure 4.2.1

HISTORY: 56-year-old woman with previously resected ileal neuroendocrine tumor; MRI was performed to assess for hepatic metastases

IMAGING FINDINGS: Axial arterial phase postgadolinium 3D SPGR images (Figure 4.2.1) demonstrate enhancing soft tissue extending from the pancreatic head and uncinate process and encircling the second portion of the duodenum. Note also a hyperenhancing metastasis in the inferior right hepatic lobe (Figure 4.2.1A).

DIAGNOSIS: Annular pancreas

COMMENT: While annular pancreas is a favorite differential diagnosis for gastric outlet obstruction in resident conferences, we have never actually seen a case of symptomatic obstruction from an annular pancreas in an adult (at least not one discovered with MRI). What we have seen are a few instances in which an annular pancreas was misdiagnosed as an invasive pancreatic mass or a circumferential duodenal mass. Needless to say, this is much more likely when image quality is marginal or when coverage of the pancreatic head is incomplete.

Annular pancreas is a congenital abnormality in which pancreatic tissue encircles the duodenum (the second portion in 85% of cases and the first and third portions in the remainder). The ringlike extension of pancreatic tissue around the duodenum was first described by Tiedemann in 1818 and later named by Ecker in 1862. There is no broad consensus on the exact developmental mechanism responsible for annular pancreas, but most anatomists agree that the annular tissue originates from the ventral pancreatic bud. The most widely accepted explanation is probably Lecco's theory, proposed in 1910, which suggests that the free end of the ventral bud becomes fixed to the duodenal wall and results in duodenal encirclement during subsequent duodenal rotation.

Annular pancreas has long been considered a rare anomaly, although it is the second most common developmental pancreatic abnormality after pancreas divisum. One autopsy study found only 3 cases in 20,000 autopsies. As is true of many other previously rare entities, however, the incidence seems to be increasing in our age of frequent cross-sectional imaging, and more recent studies have estimated a frequency of 1 in 1,000.

Clinical manifestations are distinct among different age groups. Most patients (50%-65%) present during infancy with symptoms of gastric outlet obstruction, including bilious vomiting, abdominal distention, and feeding intolerance. Annular pancreas in these patients is associated with Down syndrome, cardiac anomalies, esophageal and duodenal atresia, tracheoesophageal fistula, malrotation, Meckel diverticulum, Hirschsprung disease, and imperforate anus.

Symptomatic adults with annular pancreas usually present between the ages of 20 and 50 years with symptoms related to duodenal obstruction, including epigastric pain, nausea, vomiting, and early satiety, or they may present with an initial diagnosis of peptic ulcer disease or pancreatitis. Treatment of severely symptomatic patients typically involves gastrojejunostomy or duodenojejunostomy to bypass the affected segment, since surgeons are not generally fond of partial pancreatic resections. Many adult patients, including the patient in this case, are asymptomatic, and the annular pancreas is detected incidentally in the course of cross-sectional imaging performed for another indication, which, in this case, was screening the liver for metastatic disease.

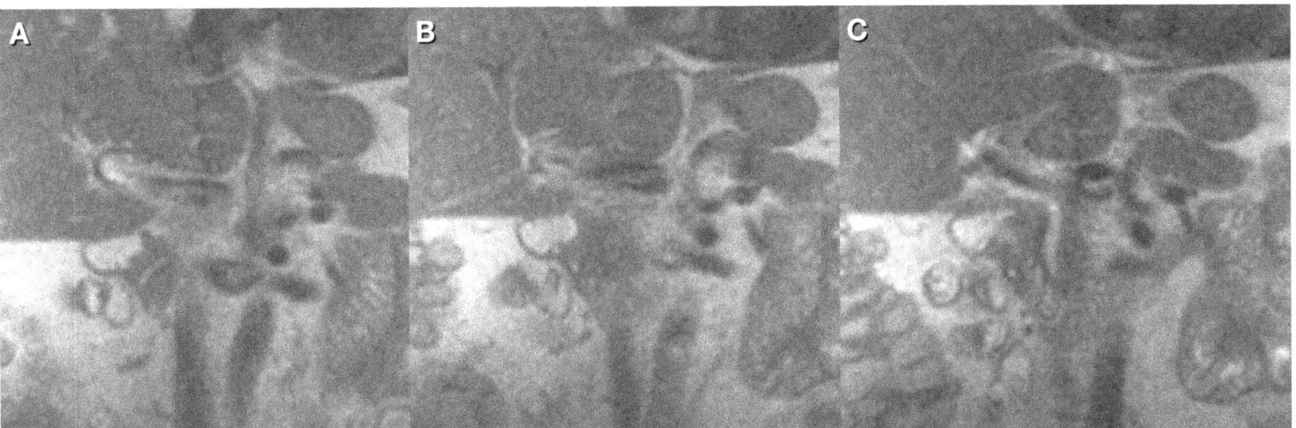

Figure 4.3.1

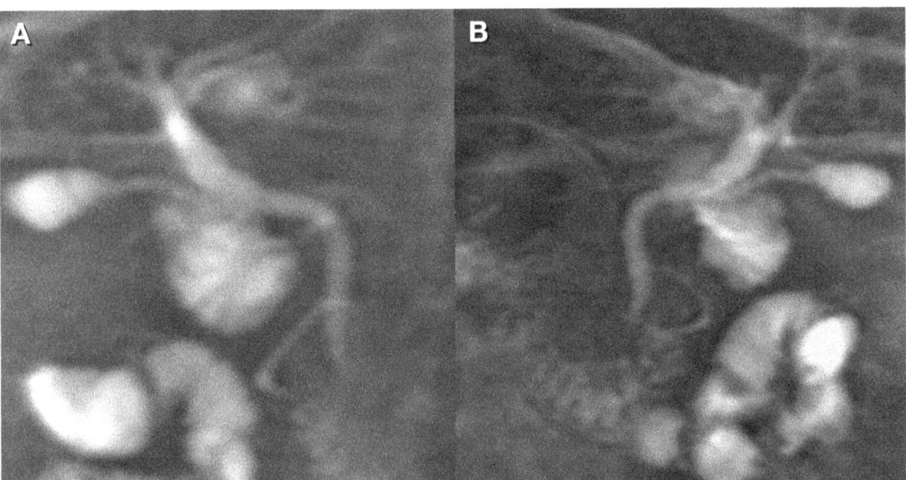

Figure 4.3.2

HISTORY: 50-year-old man with abdominal pain

IMAGING FINDINGS: Coronal SSFSE images (Figure 4.3.1) demonstrate pancreatic tissue and the pancreatic duct wrapping around the duodenum on successive images. Thick slab anterior (Figure 4.3.2A) and posterior (Figure 4.3.2B) SSFSE images reveal similar findings, again showing the pancreatic duct in the pancreatic head wrapping around the duodenum.

DIAGNOSIS: Annular pancreas

COMMENT: This companion case to Case 4.2 illustrates the appearance on MRCP when the pancreatic duct continues into the annular tissue and sweeps posteriorly around the second portion of the duodenum to enter the ampulla. A duct may not always traverse the annular tissue, or it may be too small to visualize with MRCP, but when it is present, the appearance (although somewhat bizarre) should be diagnostic.

This is another illustration of a serendipitous diagnosis. The patient had vague abdominal pain, and a diagnosis of mesenteric panniculitis was made on CT enterography, along with a questionable diagnosis of annular pancreas, which led to the MRI and MRCP request. The patient had no duodenal obstruction or other abnormalities at endoscopy of the upper gastrointestinal tract. His pain eventually resolved; presumably, it was unrelated to the annular pancreas.

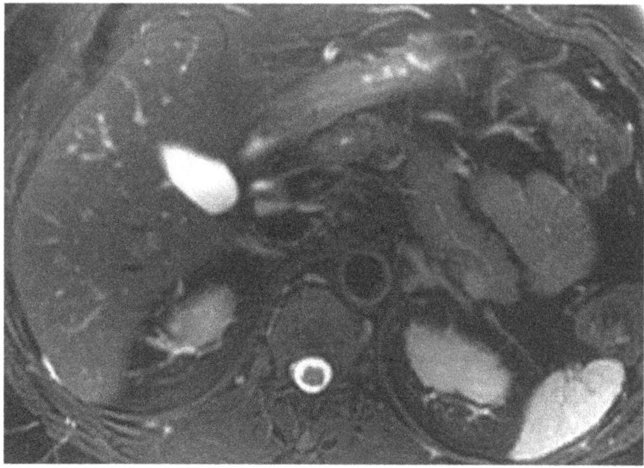

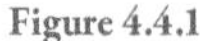

Figure 4.4.1

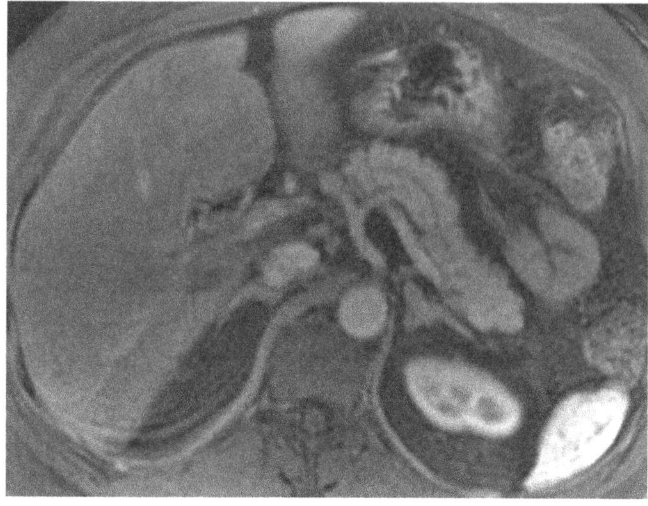

Figure 4.4.2

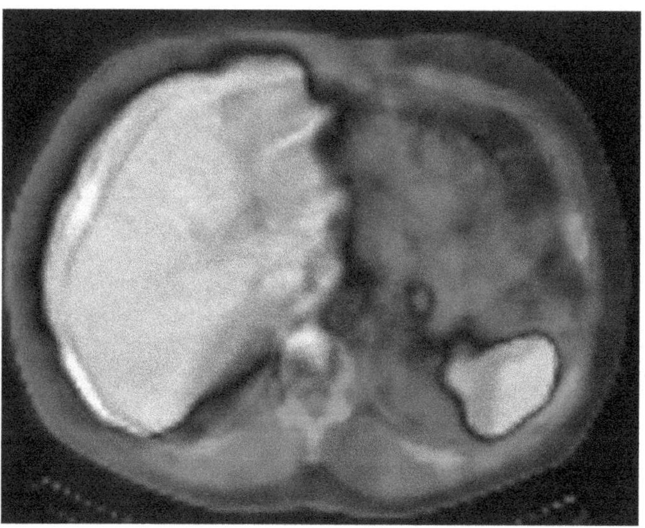

Figure 4.4.3

HISTORY: 56-year-old man with abdominal pain; sonography was unrevealing except for a possible mass in the pancreatic tail, and MRI was suggested for further assessment

IMAGING FINDINGS: Respiratory-triggered fat-suppressed FSE T2-weighted image (Figure 4.4.1) reveals a small hyperintense lesion in the pancreatic tail, which demonstrates mild hyperenhancement on arterial phase postgadolinium 3D SPGR image (Figure 4.4.2). Image from a liver-spleen sulfur colloid scan (Figure 4.4.3) shows radiotracer uptake in the lesion.

DIAGNOSIS: Pancreatic splenule (IPAS)

COMMENT: Splenules are extremely common and almost always irrelevant (which is probably why they're the second most frequently reported finding, after hiatal hernias, on abdominal CT). They show up occasionally in unexpected places, such as the pancreatic tail, where they may present diagnostic dilemmas.

In 2 autopsy studies, at least 1 accessory spleen was found in 10% and 20% of patients. The splenic hilum is, as might be expected, the most common location of the accessory splenic tissue, but the pancreatic tail is a surprisingly frequent runner-up, accounting for 11% and 17% of lesions in the 2 studies. This is somewhat at odds with the radiology literature, which provides relatively little information on the subject, and with our general experience, in which pancreatic accessory spleens are rarely detected (perhaps because we frequently miss them).

Most authors have noted that the IPAS signal should closely mirror the signal of adjacent splenic tissue on all imaging sequences. Some authors have also stated that the moiré, or zebra-stripe pattern, of the spleen seen on arterial phase postgadolinium images is faithfully reproduced in the IPAS. In our experience, these are helpful guidelines, but they are somewhat optimistic and easier to apply retrospectively. Limited pathologic data have shown that the relative percentages of red and white pulp are frequently different in an IPAS compared to a normal spleen. Therefore, relative signal intensities on T1- and T2-weighted images may be slightly different. In this case, for example, the IPAS has relatively high T2-signal intensity compared to the adjacent pancreas, but it is hypointense compared to the spleen. It's also true that most lesions are small (1-3 cm in diameter), and visualization of a distinct moiré pattern within such a small lesion may be difficult or impossible. Dynamic contrast-enhanced images may be helpful since neuroendocrine tumors and hypervascular metastases (the 2 main differential diagnoses) usually show the most intense hyperenhancement on arterial phase images and may show washout or significant fading during the portal venous phase. In contrast, an IPAS is more likely to remain hyperintense in the portal venous phase. This is occasionally true, especially among patients who have moderate fatty atrophy of the pancreas and a low background pancreatic parenchymal signal intensity on fat-suppressed T1-weighted images.

The MRI in this case was read as indeterminate, but *splenule* was listed as a leading possibility. A liver-spleen scan confirmed the diagnosis. As noted above, the appearance of the lesion is nonspecific and could just as easily represent a neuroendocrine tumor or a hypervascular metastasis. In the absence of a neoplastic history, however, splenule should be a leading consideration for a small, solid, hyperenhancing pancreatic tail lesion.

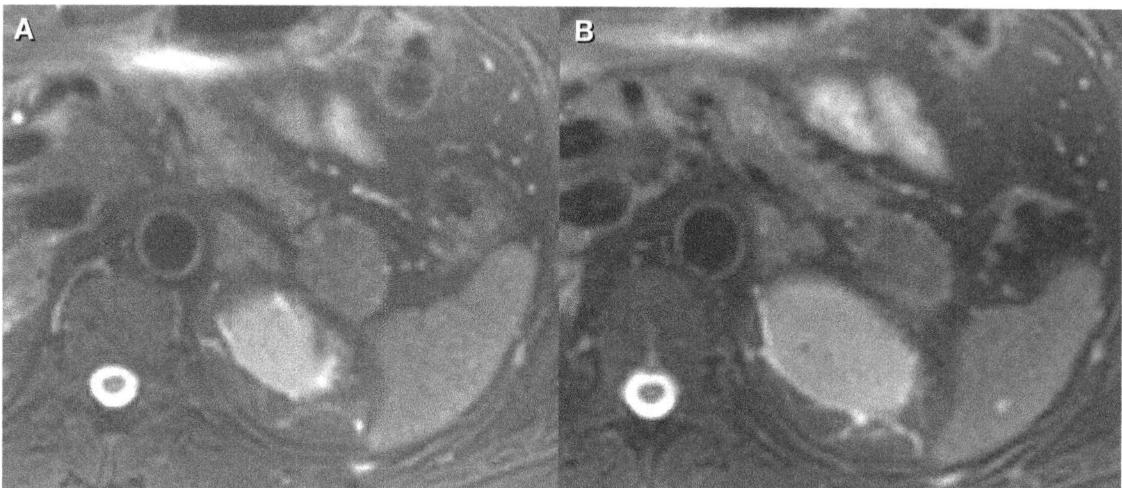

Figure 4.5.1

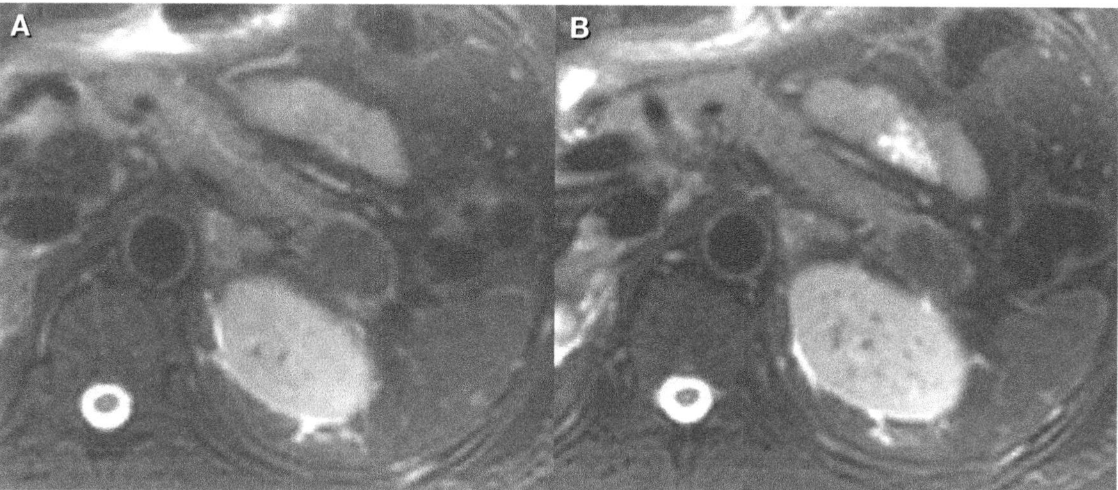

Figure 4.5.2

HISTORY: 58-year-old man with a history of prostate cancer and a possible pancreatic mass on CT

IMAGING FINDINGS: Axial fat-suppressed FSE T2-weighted images obtained before (Figure 4.5.1) and after (Figure 4.5.2) administration of an SPIO contrast agent demonstrate an ovoid mass in the pancreatic tail with intermediate signal intensity that becomes significantly hypointense after SPIO administration and matches the signal intensity of the spleen.

DIAGNOSIS: IPAS

COMMENT: The MRI equivalent of the liver-spleen scan is unfortunately no longer available in the United States since there are currently no US Food and Drug Administration–approved SPIO contrast agents on the market. These agents were intended primarily for hepatic imaging. Uptake of SPIO particles by phagocytic cells of the reticuloendothelial system leads to a dramatic decrease in T2* in the liver, spleen, and bone marrow and consequent signal dropout of normal liver tissue on T2- or T2*-weighted images. This in turn results in increased conspicuity of solid hepatic lesions, with no SPIO uptake, compared to the background normal liver tissue. SPIO agents performed similarly to gadolinium agents in lesion detection in most studies but were probably less effective in lesion characterization and had the additional limitation of requiring slow infusion over 30 minutes, occasionally accompanied by severe back pain. SPIO agents may be making a comeback as lymph node agents for cancer staging (uptake and signal dropout in negative nodes, and no uptake and no signal dropout in malignant nodes); preliminary studies have been promising. More esoteric but potentially useful applications include identification of inflammatory atherosclerotic lesions in the aorta and other arteries as well as stem cell labeling. If these agents again become available, keep in mind their utility for identifying ectopic splenic tissue.

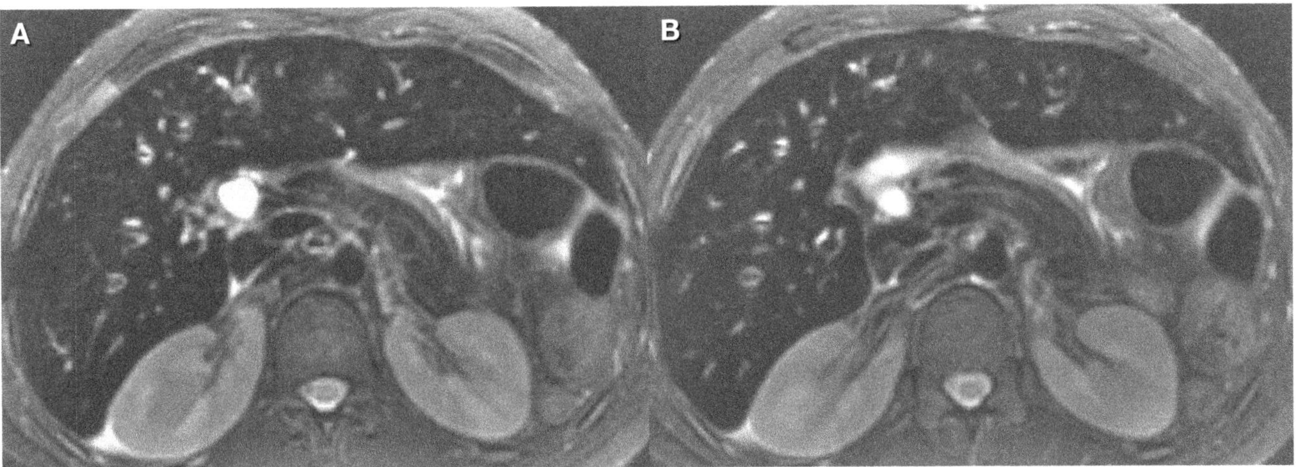

Figure 4.6.1

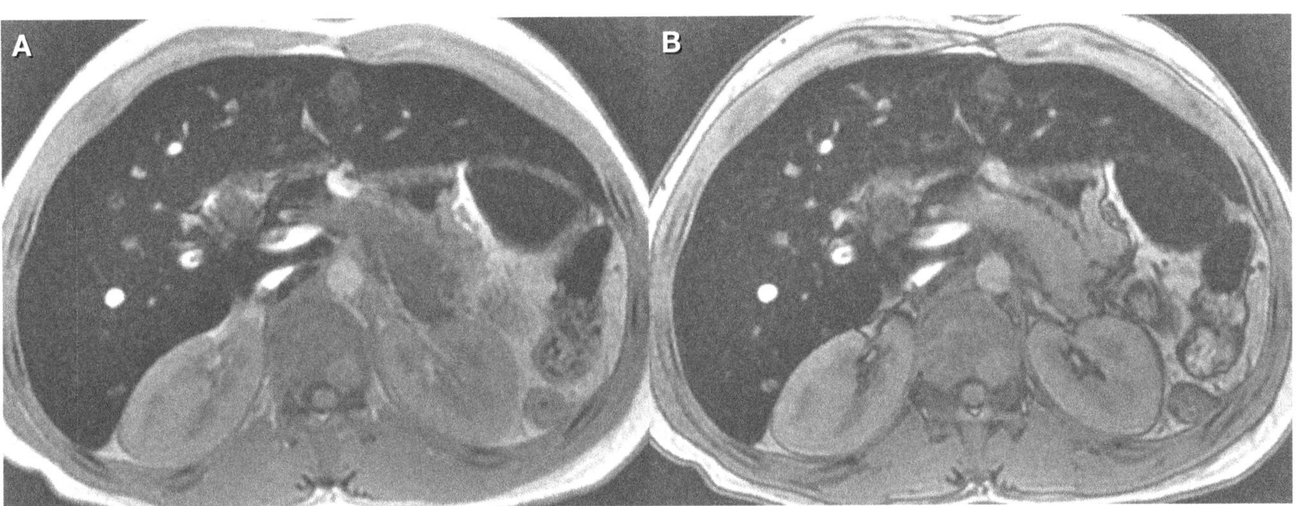

Figure 4.6.2

HISTORY: 21-year-old woman with thalassemia major

IMAGING FINDINGS: Axial fat-suppressed FSE T2-weighted images (Figure 4.6.1) demonstrate low signal intensity throughout the liver and pancreas. The spleen is absent (as a result of splenectomy). In-phase (Figure 4.6.2A) and out-of-phase (Figure 4.6.2B) 2D SPGR images reveal markedly low signal intensity in the liver, which changes little from in-phase to out-of-phase images. Signal intensity is lower within the pancreas on the in-phase image than on the out-of-phase image.

DIAGNOSIS: Thalassemia with iron deposition in the liver and pancreas

COMMENT: The thalassemias are a group of autosomal recessive disorders characterized by absent or decreased synthesis of 1 of the 2 polypeptide chains (α or β) that form the normal hemoglobin molecule, resulting in decreased red cell hemoglobin levels and anemia. Thalassemia is classified both by genotype and phenotype (clinical severity). While stem cell transplant offers a potential cure, this therapy is not widely available and has variable outcomes. The mainstay of clinical treatment is transfusion and chelation therapy.

Long-term transfusion therapy has significantly increased the life expectancy of patients with thalassemia; however, it also delivers a large amount of excess iron to the body. Initially, the excess iron is handled by the cells of the reticuloendothelial system in the liver, spleen, and bone marrow. These are the first organs to show the classic signs of iron overload on MRI, including decreased signal intensity on T2- and T2*-weighted images, and signal dropout from out-of-phase to in-phase SPGR images (a T2* effect resulting from the slightly longer TE of the standard in-phase acquisition).

When the reticuloendothelial cells are overwhelmed, iron also accumulates in the parenchymal cells of the liver, heart, pancreas, and other endocrine organs. The entry of iron into myocardial and endocrine tissue is thought to be mediated by nontransferrin-bound iron. At normal iron levels, plasma iron is bound to transferrin, which prevents catalytic activity and free radical production. When transferrin is fully saturated, surplus iron appears as nontransferrin-bound iron and more easily enters parenchymal cells.

Without appropriate chelation therapy, the accumulation of iron in the myocardium can lead to heart failure, which is the most common cause of death among patients with thalassemia. Likewise, iron deposition in the pancreas can cause endocrine and exocrine dysfunction. Diabetes mellitus is present in 10% to 24% of thalassemic patients and is only partially reversible with chelation therapy.

Relatively little work has been done in quantifying iron deposition within the pancreas; however, quantification can be accomplished with the same techniques more frequently applied to hepatic iron measurement. A multi-echo gradient echo pulse sequence acquires multiple images with successively longer TEs, and then plots of signal intensity versus TE can be fitted to the expected single exponential decay to solve for T2* and its inverse, R2*, both of which have been related via tissue calibration curves to the concentration of iron in liver and myocardium.

Interestingly, pancreatic R2* has been proposed as a surrogate marker of myocardial iron (the liver is less useful since it initially accumulates iron through its reticuloendothelial cells). A few small studies have demonstrated fairly good correlation in iron content between the heart and the pancreas.

Hemochromatosis, another autosomal recessive disorder, is the classic differential diagnosis for a dark signal within the pancreas on T2*-weighted images (Case 2.6). In this disorder, iron accumulates primarily within the parenchymal cells of the liver and to a lesser extent in the pancreas, other endocrine glands, and myocardium, sparing the cells of the reticuloendothelial system. Therefore, low T2* signal intensity in the liver and pancreas, but not the spleen, suggests hemochromatosis rather than transfusional hemosiderosis. (The distinction is difficult in this case since the spleen is absent, but a review of the clinical history also solves the problem.)

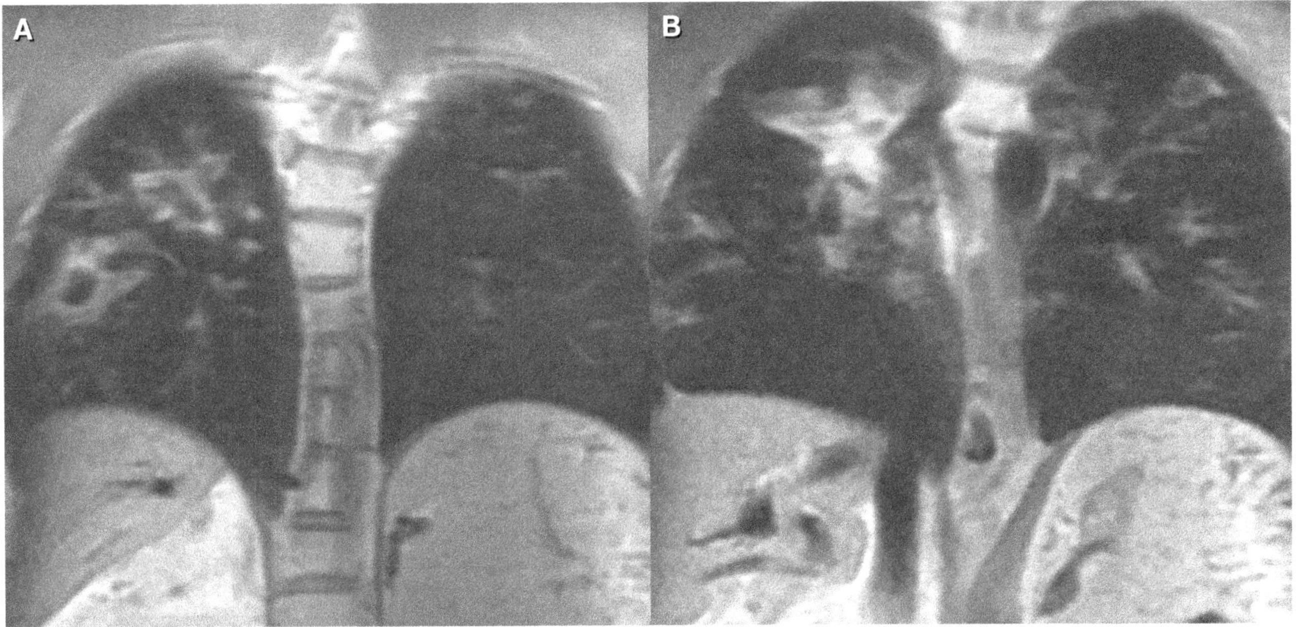

Figure 4.7.1

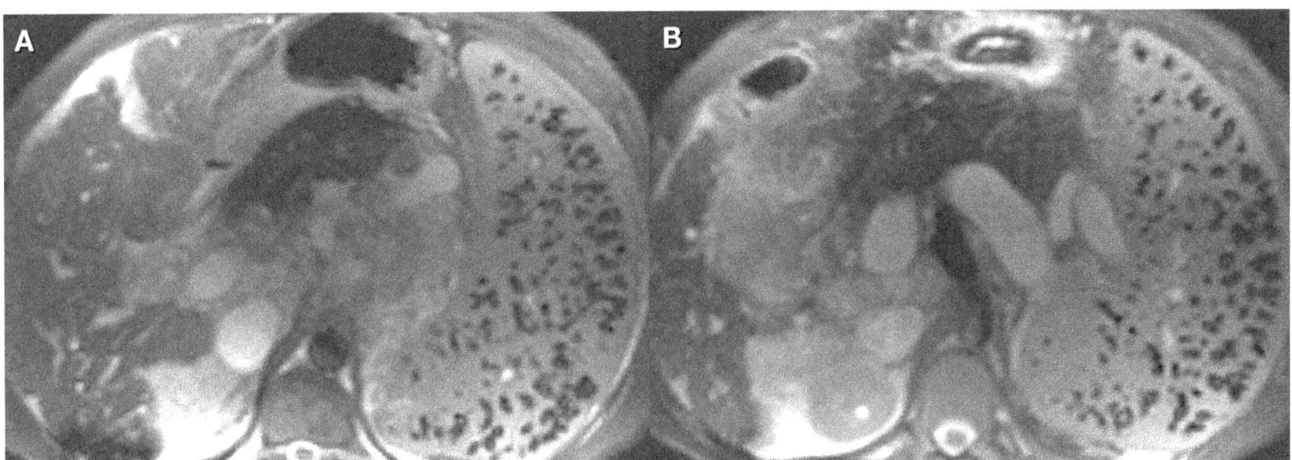

Figure 4.7.2

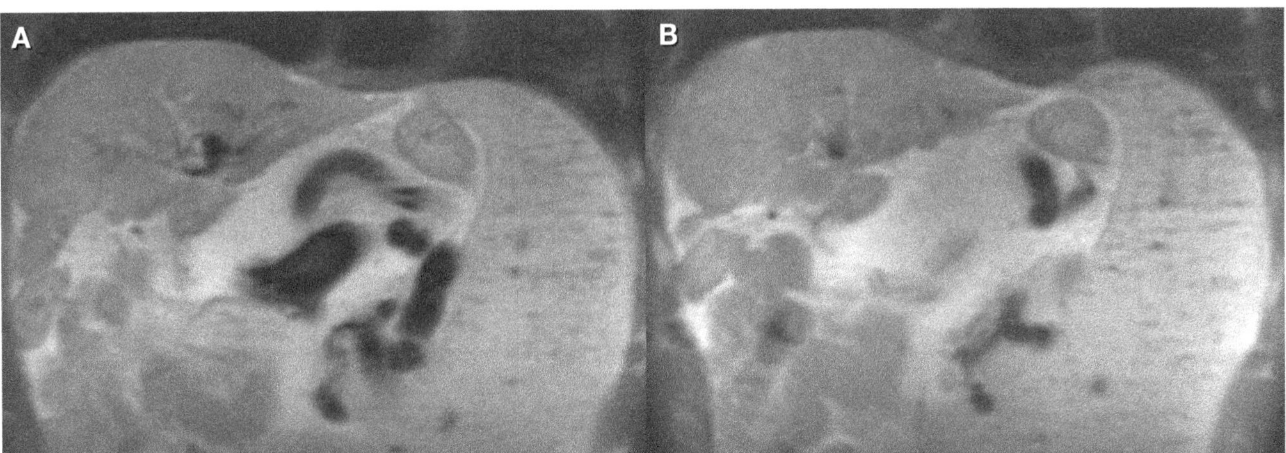

Figure 4.7.3

HISTORY: 33-year-old man with a chronic illness

IMAGING FINDINGS: Coronal SSFSE images through the posterior lungs (Figure 4.7.1) reveal chronic peribronchial infiltrates and bronchiectasis. Axial fat-suppressed SSFP images (Figure 4.7.2) and coronal SSFSE images (Figure 4.7.3) through the upper abdomen demonstrate a cirrhotic liver, splenomegaly, splenic siderotic nodules (Gamna-Gandy bodies), and complete fatty replacement of the pancreas.

DIAGNOSIS: CF with cirrhosis and fatty replacement of the pancreas

COMMENT: It's commonly said (and somewhat true) that it's easier to notice an abnormal structure than to detect its absence. This case in particular has many findings in both the chest and the abdomen, and the complete fatty replacement of the pancreas might easily be overlooked. Nevertheless, it is a useful observation and one that should clinch the diagnosis.

While most of the emphasis on imaging in CF is correctly placed on pulmonary abnormalities, CF is truly a systemic disease, with manifestations affecting the bowel (meconium ileus, intussusception, obstruction, and pneumatosis), the liver (steatosis, cirrhosis, and portal hypertension), the biliary tree (cholelithiasis, strictures, and microgallbladder), and the pancreas. Pathologic features generally result from the accumulation of viscous glandular secretions within hollow organs or ducts.

Pancreatic abnormalities are common in CF, which is the most common cause of exocrine pancreatic insufficiency in pediatric patients and young adults. Viscous pancreatic secretions (resulting from a genetic defect in epithelial chloride ion permeability) produce duct obstruction, acinar atrophy, fibrosis, and progressive fatty replacement. Clinically apparent exocrine insufficiency is present in 85% to 90% of patients with CF and endocrine deficiency in 30% to 50%. Complete fatty replacement is one of the more common pancreatic manifestations of CF, occurring in 50% to 75% of patients. The differential diagnosis for this finding is relatively short, particularly for younger patients, and includes Shwachman-Diamond syndrome and metaphyseal dysostosis, with diabetes mellitus, obesity, Cushing syndrome, and CP generally resulting in less complete fatty replacement.

Quantification of pancreatic fatty replacement is just beginning to receive attention and is an offshoot of the techniques developed to quantify hepatic steatosis. Such quantification may have clinical value in assessing patients with CP and has the added benefit of allowing academic radiologists to apply the same technique to a different organ and write another set of papers. (See Chapter 2, "Liver: Diffuse Disease," for a discussion of these methods.)

CASE 4.8

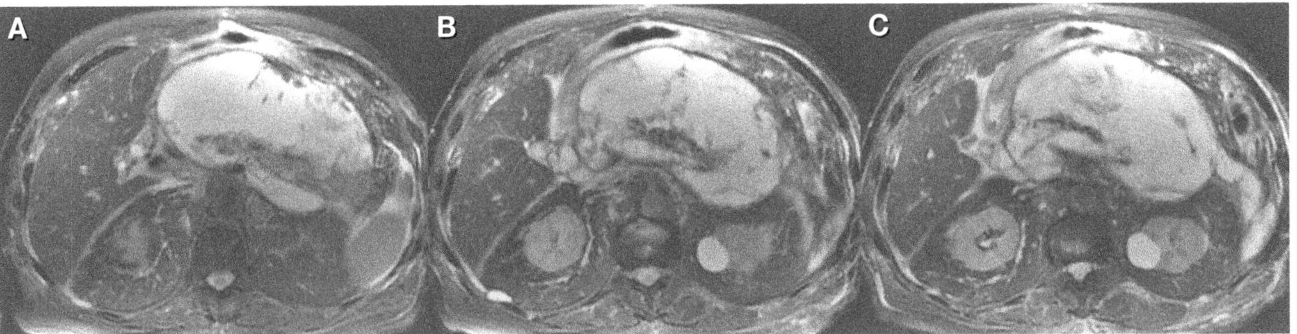

Figure 4.8.1

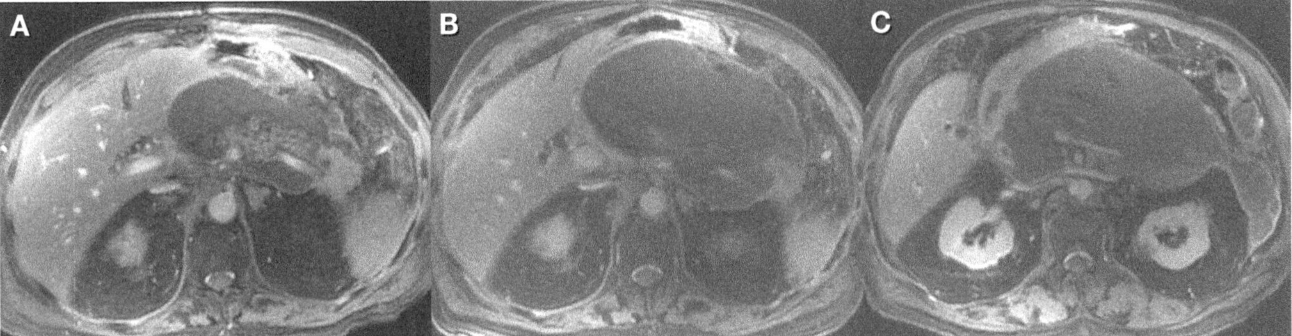

Figure 4.8.2

HISTORY: 74-year-old man with abdominal pain

IMAGING FINDINGS: Axial fat-suppressed FSE T2-weighted images (Figure 4.8.1) reveal a small residual pancreas surrounded by a large, complex fluid collection that extends into the right paracolic gutter and contains extensive internal debris. Axial portal venous phase postgadolinium 3D SPGR images (Figure 4.8.2) demonstrate peripheral enhancement of the fluid collection with minimal enhancement of the residual pancreatic tissue.

DIAGNOSIS: Necrotizing pancreatitis with walled-off pancreatic necrosis

COMMENT: Both acute pancreatitis and CP are relatively common diseases, at least in comparison to the pancreatic tumors constituting the bulk of this chapter. Approximately 300,000 patients are hospitalized annually for acute pancreatitis in the United States, with mortality ranging from 1% to 3%. Severe acute pancreatitis is strongly associated with pancreatic necrosis, and mortality is as high as 50% in some series. Gallstones and alcohol abuse account for approximately 90% of all cases of acute pancreatitis, with alcohol abuse also responsible for 70% to 90% of CP cases.

Acute pancreatitis is diagnosed in patients who have at least 2 of the following: sudden onset of upper abdominal pain, serum amylase or lipase level greater than 3 times the upper limit of normal, and findings on cross-sectional imaging consistent with the diagnosis. Most cases of acute pancreatitis are relatively mild; however, 15% to 20% of patients have severe disease, often associated with multiple organ failure.

Acute pancreatitis has been divided into 2 morphologic types: interstitial edematous pancreatitis and necrotizing pancreatitis. Necrotizing pancreatitis occurs in 6% to 20% of patients, with an associated mortality of 12% to 30%, depending on the presence or absence of infection within the necrotic tissue.

Imaging findings of acute pancreatitis are similar with CT and MRI. Both demonstrate enlargement of the pancreas, often with an irregular contour, effacement of the peripancreatic fat planes, and peripancreatic fluid collections. Necrotizing pancreatitis is demonstrated with MRI (as it is with CT) by minimal or no enhancement of the pancreas after contrast administration.

Evolving terminology has become somewhat more specific in describing peripancreatic fluid collections. In *necrotizing pancreatitis*, fluid collections associated with necrosis occurring in the first 4 weeks are known as *postnecrotic pancreatic fluid collections* and contain both fluid and necrotic debris. In the late phase (ie, >4 weeks after the initial presentation), when postnecrotic pancreatic fluid collections become walled off and organized, they are then termed *walled-off pancreatic necrosis*.

In this case, the walled-off pancreatic necrosis involves nearly the entire gland. When these collections involve the central gland they are almost always associated with disruption of the main pancreatic duct, and any secretions from residual viable pancreatic tissue drain into the fluid collection. These collections often do not resolve and require prolonged cystogastrostomy or partial or complete pancreatic resection.

CT is probably the test of choice for initial diagnosis of acute pancreatitis and assessment of complications. Patients are often very ill, sometimes clinically unstable, and almost never interested in spending 30 to 40 minutes in the magnet. MRI, with no radiation exposure, does have an important role in serial follow-up of patients who have complex disease. MRI may also be important when drainage of peripancreatic fluid collections is contemplated. The presence of necrotic debris within a peripancreatic fluid collection often means that standard percutaneous drainage will be unsuccessful and may in fact increase the risk of superinfection. This is much more easily appreciated with MRI and can be seen in this case as multiple dark filling defects within the high-signal-intensity encapsulated central fluid on T2-weighted images. Precontrast T1-weighted images are also frequently useful for demonstrating high-signal-intensity subacute blood products within these fluid collections.

MRCP images are almost always worth acquiring in patients with necrotizing pancreatitis and may demonstrate a disconnected pancreatic duct, communication of the duct with a central or peripancreatic fluid collection, strictures of the pancreatic or common bile duct, and choledocholithiasis or pancreatic ductal calculi.

Dynamic contrast-enhanced images are important not only for demonstrating a necrotic pancreas, but also for assessing for relatively common associated vascular complications, such as splenic or portal vein thrombosis and splenic artery or gastroduodenal artery pseudoaneurysms.

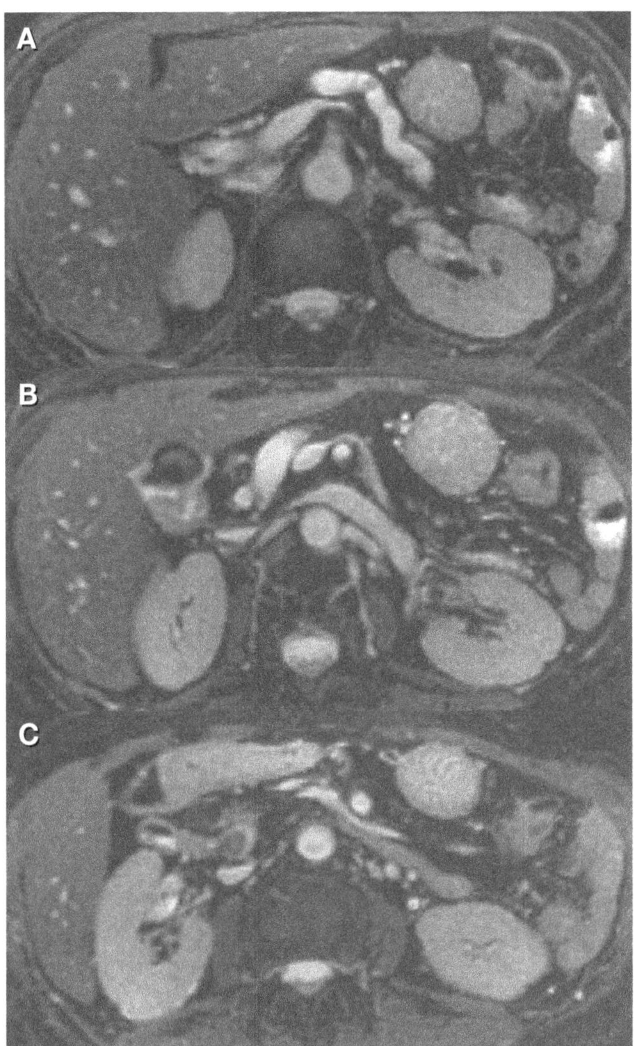

Figure 4.9.1

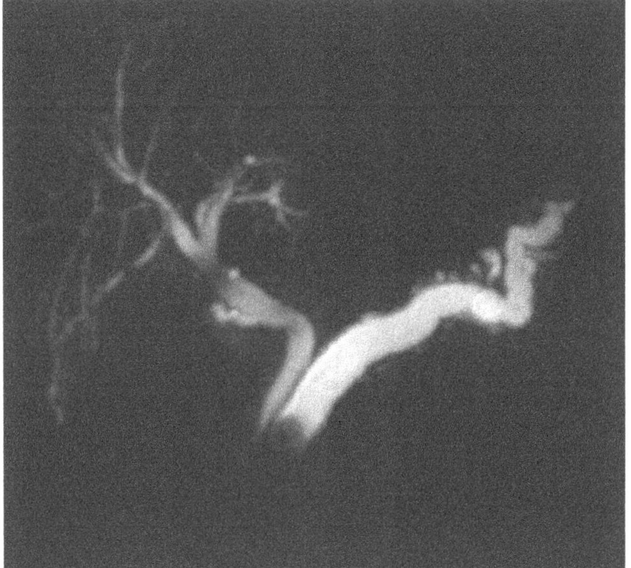

Figure 4.9.2

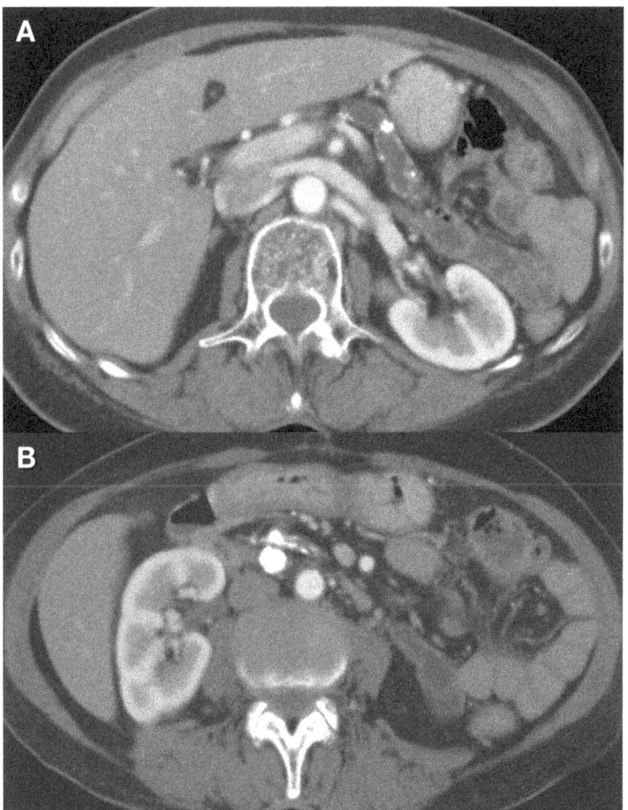

Figure 4.9.3

HISTORY: 72-year-old woman with chronic abdominal pain and a previous episode of pancreatitis 5 years ago

IMAGING FINDINGS: Axial fat-suppressed 2D SSFP images (Figure 4.9.1) reveal marked diffuse dilatation of the pancreatic duct without any visible pancreatic parenchyma. Note also a large filling defect in the duct at the pancreatic head and a smaller filling defect in the body of the pancreas. MIP image from 3D FRFSE MRCP (Figure 4.9.2) reveals similar findings, demonstrating a large filling defect within the pancreatic duct near the ampulla. Axial images from a contrast-enhanced CT (Figure 4.9.3) show similar findings, with a dilated duct, calcified ductal stones, parenchymal calcifications, and marked parenchymal atrophy.

DIAGNOSIS: CP with large intraductal stone

COMMENT: Chronic inflammation of the pancreas can lead to progressive and permanent endocrine and exocrine dysfunction, as illustrated in this case, in which essentially nothing is left of the pancreas except for a dilated duct. The incidence of CP is estimated at 3.5 to 10 cases per 100,000. While alcohol abuse and gallstones are the leading causes, many additional etiologies have also been implicated, including genetic disease, neoplasms, cigarette smoking and other toxic exposures, infection, and vascular disease.

Alcohol abuse is thought to account for 70% to 90% of CP cases, and although the mechanism of injury is not entirely understood, calcifications within the pancreatic parenchyma and pancreatic duct are prominent features seen in 30% to 70% of patients. Parenchymal atrophy and ductal dilatation are also common (present in >50% of cases). Only a few papers discuss the relative sensitivities of CT and MRI for detection of intraductal stones in CP, but CT is obviously much more sensitive for detecting calcium, and pancreatic ductal stones are more frequently calcified than gallstones, particularly in CP. However, MRI is a more effective tool for visualizing gallstones and choledocholithiasis as a cause of CP.

The differential diagnosis for a diffusely dilated pancreatic duct includes main-duct IPMN as well as a pancreatic head or ampullary tumor, but the extensive calcifications on CT and near-complete parenchymal atrophy make the diagnosis of CP far more likely. It is important to remember, however, that the incidence of pancreatic carcinoma is much higher among patients with CP than in the general population, with a cumulative incidence of 1% at 5 years after initial diagnosis; therefore, a relatively high level of suspicion is warranted.

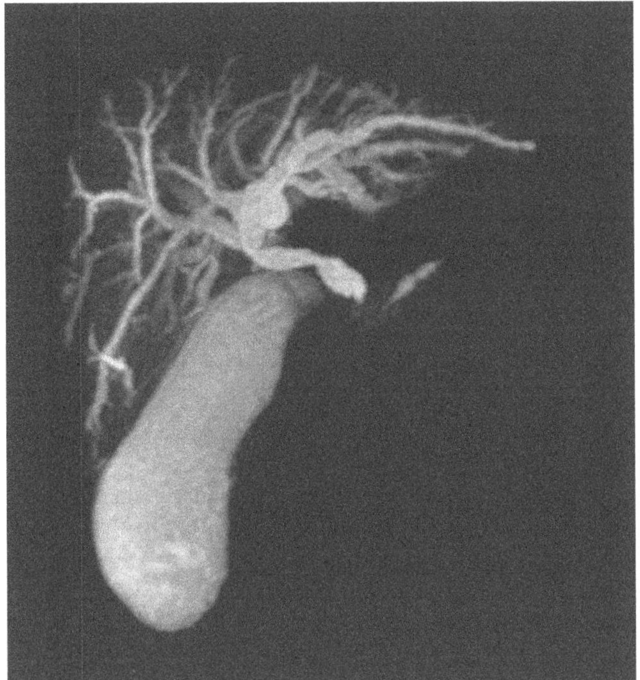

Figure 4.10.1

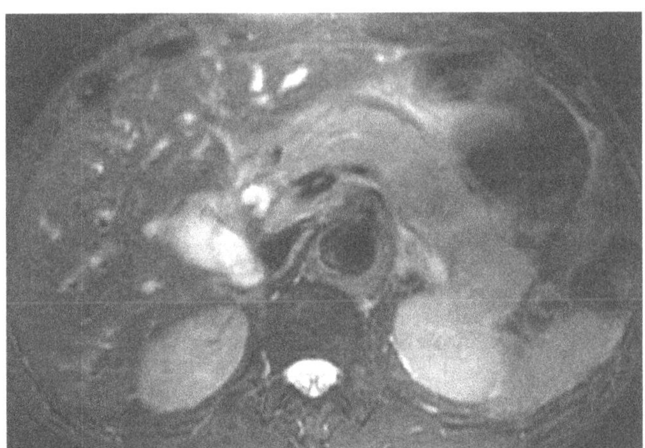

Figure 4.10.2

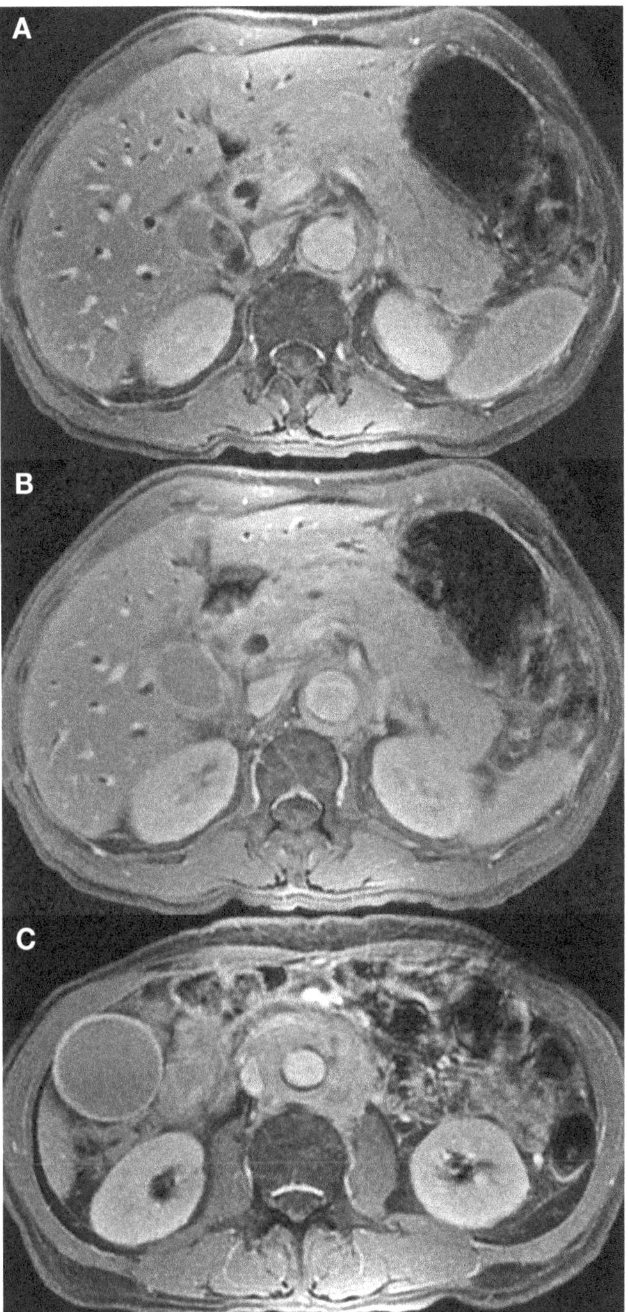

Figure 4.10.3

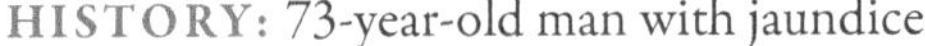

HISTORY: 73-year-old man with jaundice

IMAGING FINDINGS: MIP image from 3D FRFSE MRCP (Figure 4.10.1) demonstrates dilated intrahepatic and extrahepatic biliary ducts, a distended gallbladder, and irregular narrowing of the pancreatic duct. Axial fat-suppressed FSE T2-weighted image (Figure 4.10.2) and axial venous phase postgadolinium 3D SPGR images (Figure 4.10.3) demonstrate diffuse enlargement of the pancreas and loss of normal pancreatic lobulations. Additionally, massive circumferential soft tissue thickening surrounds the distal abdominal aorta. Note also a hypointense rim along the anterior margin of the pancreas on the T2-weighted image.

DIAGNOSIS: AIP with retroperitoneal fibrosis

COMMENT: AIP, previously known as lymphoplasmacytic sclerosing pancreatitis, is a form of CP that often resolves completely with corticosteroid therapy, and therefore a correct diagnosis can be curative. Imaging findings are often subtle, however, and may be confused with ordinary pancreatitis, pancreatic neoplasms, and primary sclerosing cholangitis. MRI is often helpful in accentuating important diagnostic clues that might be more difficult to detect on CT or sonography.

AIP is a distinct form of CP characterized by periductal infiltration of a mixed inflammatory cell infiltrate consisting predominantly of CD4-positive T lymphocytes and IgG4 plasma cells. AIP is thought to account for 2% to 11% of all CP and is a disease that primarily affects older patients, with a mean age of 60 years at presentation. Men are affected 2 to 7 times more frequently than women. Presenting symptoms, which are characteristically more typical of pancreatic carcinoma than pancreatitis, include jaundice, abdominal pain, weight loss, steatorrhea, and diabetes mellitus. The serum IgG4 level is frequently elevated in AIP, and while some authors have reported high sensitivity and specificity for the diagnosis based on cutoff values of serum IgG4, these results have not been universally replicated, and others have noted that IgG4 values are also occasionally elevated in patients with pancreatic cancer. Several sets of clinical criteria for diagnosis of AIP have been published. The Mayo Clinic criteria require 1 or more of the following: histologic findings diagnostic of AIP, characteristic imaging findings along with elevated serum IgG4 levels, and response to corticosteroid therapy.

Three patterns of AIP have been described: diffuse, focal, and multifocal. The diffuse form, shown in this case, is probably the easiest to recognize. The pancreas is typically enlarged, with loss of its normally lobulated contour, and may show mildly decreased signal intensity on T1-weighted images and increased signal intensity on T2-weighted images. These signal changes have been variably attributed to fibrosis, decreased protein-rich secretions within the pancreatic acinar cells, and edema, but the distinctions can be difficult to make in the real world. In most papers, the pancreatic signal intensity is compared to that of the liver, which on T2-weighted images often has lower signal intensity than the normal pancreas in older patients who have had 1 or 2 blood transfusions. Similarly, while the pancreas is generally described as having higher signal intensity than the liver on T1-weighted images, older patients with age-related fatty atrophy often show lower signal intensity on fat-suppressed T1-weighted acquisitions. The pancreas may appear hypointense on postgadolinium arterial phase images, with gradually increasing enhancement on portal venous and equilibrium phase acquisitions. The presence of a hypointense halo on T2-weighted images with late enhancement after gadolinium administration is a specific but probably not highly sensitive finding.

In early disease, the pancreatic duct is typically stenotic or strictured and may be difficult to visualize on MRCP, although in long-standing cases pancreatic atrophy and ductal dilatation may predominate. Again, the fact that you cannot clearly visualize the entire pancreatic duct with MRCP should not be taken as strong evidence in and of itself for the presence of AIP, since the normal duct is small and may be incompletely filled with fluid; however, a combination of the above findings in the appropriate clinical setting is very suggestive of the diagnosis.

Focal or mass-forming AIP is considered less common than the diffuse variety, although there is considerable variation in the relative frequencies among reported series. Focal AIP can be a diagnostic dilemma since it can have an appearance similar to if not identical to pancreatic carcinoma and it occurs in a similar patient population with similar presenting symptoms. A few MRI findings are more characteristic of focal AIP: hyperenhancement relative to adjacent pancreas on portal venous and equilibrium phase images, the presence of a hypoenhancing capsule, the penetrating duct sign (the pancreatic duct extends into the focal lesion rather than being amputated at the margin), absence of distal pancreatic atrophy, and relatively mild upstream ductal dilatation. DWI with quantification of ADC values has also been described as a useful technique, with AIP exhibiting significantly lower ADC values than pancreatic carcinoma. The problems of measurement standardization are evident in this limited literature: The cutoff ADC value that 1 author used to achieve 100% sensitivity and specificity would have stratified 60% to 70% of the AIP cases from a second paper as carcinoma. It would therefore be a bad idea to apply these threshold values to your practice without first performing a careful internal validation.

AIP is well-recognized as a systemic disease, and manifestations in other organ systems have been described. The biliary system is the most common site of extrapancreatic involvement, occurring in as many as 88% of patients. The appearance is similar to or identical to primary sclerosing cholangitis, with multifocal intrahepatic and extrahepatic biliary strictures. Renal involvement affects up to one-third of patients, most frequently as multiple bilateral cortical hypoenhancing lesions. Retroperitoneal fibrosis or periaortitis, of which this case is an impressive example, is less common and occurs in 10% to 20% of patients. The presence of 1 or more sites of extrapancreatic involvement is an important clue to the diagnosis, particularly in subtle cases.

Most patients show a dramatic response to corticosteroid therapy. Clinical and imaging signs often resolve within a few weeks; however, recurrent disease is relatively common and occurs in 20% to 40% of patients when the use of corticosteroids is tapered or discontinued.

CASE 4.11

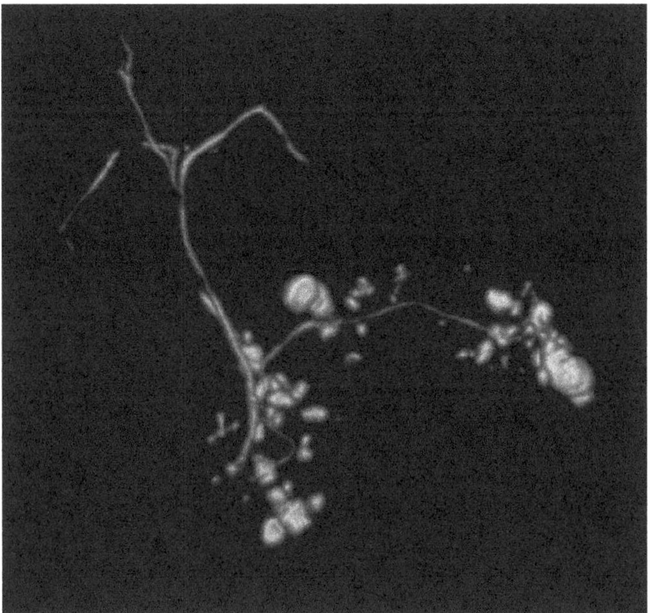

Figure 4.11.1

HISTORY: 58-year-old woman with suspected mesenteric ischemia

IMAGING FINDINGS: VR image from 3D FRFSE MRCP (Figure 4.11.1) reveals multiple small cystic lesions throughout the pancreas, many connecting to the pancreatic duct.

DIAGNOSIS: Multiple side-branch IPMNs

COMMENT: Diagnostic imaging of IPMN provides an interesting case study of the effect of imaging technology on disease prevalence. In the 1990s, IPMN was a rare and exotic diagnosis, leading to case reports and excited presentations at imaging conferences. As magnetic resonance technology improved and the use of abdominal MRI and MRCP increased, IPMN became a more pedestrian diagnosis. (In our practice, if we're not reporting a potential IPMN at least 2 or 3 times a day, it probably means that we're forgetting to look at the pancreas again.)

IPMNs are neoplasms of the mucinous cells lining the pancreatic ducts and are typically classified as side-branch or main-duct lesions (some include mixed or combined lesions, which are usually treated the same as main-duct tumors). IPMN was first described by Ohashi et al in 1982 and formally recognized in 1996 by the WHO, which then recategorized the lesion in 2000 to include terms that describe tumor aggressiveness (*adenoma, borderline, carcinoma in situ*, and *invasive carcinoma*).

Most IPMNs (70%) occur in men, most commonly in older men between the ages of 60 and 70 years; the average age of all patients at diagnosis is 65 years. Patients with side-branch IPMNs are often asymptomatic, and the IPMNs are common incidental findings at cross-sectional imaging, particularly MRI, which is better than CT for detecting small cystic lesions in the pancreas (or any organ). Patients with main duct lesions are more often symptomatic; presenting symptoms may include nausea, vomiting, abdominal pain, and weight loss. Many patients present with symptoms of chronic recurring pancreatitis because the thick mucin generated by IPMNs can cause ductal obstruction that results in pancreatitis.

Side-branch IPMNs appear as small cystic lesions, often with a visible connection to the main pancreatic duct. This feature is distinctive and diagnostic since other cystic pancreatic neoplasms rarely if ever communicate with the main duct. Several papers have attested that MRI shows the ductal connection in nearly every IPMN, but clinically this is not always true, particularly since many of the lesions are detected incidentally during examinations in which the pancreas is not the center of attention, and for which high-resolution heavily T2-weighted imaging of the pancreas may not be performed. If you are looking specifically for an IPMN, a respiratory-triggered 3D FSE or FRFSE heavily T2-weighted MRCP (centered on the pancreatic duct, not the liver) usually provides the highest sensitivity and also helps to demonstrate the connection to the main pancreatic duct. Respiratory-gated techniques are not ideal for every patient, however, and in this group, breath-held overlapping thin-section fat-suppressed 2D SSFP or SSFSE images can be helpful, as can breath-held 3D SSFP acquisitions. Postgadolinium 3D SPGR images are probably somewhat less sensitive for detecting very small cystic lesions but are useful for visualizing mural nodules and mural enhancement within larger lesions, which are signs that are worrisome for malignant degeneration.

Side-branch IPMNs are multifocal in approximately one-third of cases; more importantly, most are low-grade neoplasms with indolent growth. The malignant potential of side-branch IPMNs is somewhat controversial. Most large series have reported malignant transformation in 5% to 30% of cases, with much lower rates for smaller lesions without worrisome imaging or clinical features (1 recent study that carefully excluded main-duct lesions found no instances of malignant degeneration in 50 cases followed for 10 years). The Sendai criteria, reported in 2006, provide guidelines for management of IPMNs and recommend that all main-duct IPMNs be resected in patients who are reasonable surgical candidates. Side-branch lesions less than 3 cm in diameter can be followed, unless the patient is symptomatic or 1 of the following is present: mural nodules, dilated main duct, or positive cytologic findings on aspiration.

The surge of interest in IPMNs has stimulated a closer examination of the pancreas and led to the recognition that small pancreatic cystic lesions are much more common than was previously thought. There has been a 20-fold increase in detection of these lesions since the late 1990s. One paper reported an incidental detection rate of 2.6% by CT in patients without known pancreatic disease, and a similar investigation described an incidence of 13.5% by MRI. Autopsy studies have found cystic pancreatic lesions in up to 25% of cases, of which roughly 5% are neoplastic. More worrisome are reports that the incidence increases with age and that as many as 60% of cysts in patients older than 70 years are malignant or potentially malignant.

The question of what to do with the incidental small cystic pancreatic lesion is similar in many ways to the question of what to do with the incidental pulmonary nodule. The absence of widely accepted guidelines for follow-up has led to a proliferation of institutional recommendations. The guidelines from Mayo Clinic are not unreasonable, although diameters of lesions have been split into rather fine categories (<5 mm, 5-10 mm, 11-15 mm, and >15 mm), which lean toward the obsessive end of the spectrum and probably overestimate the measurement skills of most radiologists. In general, larger lesions should be followed more frequently. Most recommendations include annual or biannual examinations for 2 years, followed by less frequent follow-up for stable lesions.

The differential diagnosis for IPMN includes CP with main-duct or focal side-branch dilatation or CP with small pseudocysts. A definitive diagnosis may not always be possible, especially if there is 1 small cystic lesion and a questionable history of prior pancreatitis (fortunately, in those cases it doesn't really matter). Occasionally, a serous or mucinous cystadenoma might have an appearance similar to an IPMN, although neither of these lesions should have a connection to the pancreatic duct.

Main-duct IPMNs are more serious lesions. They have a higher incidence of malignant degeneration, and they may be more difficult to distinguish from CP. These lesions are discussed in Cases 4.12 and 4.13.

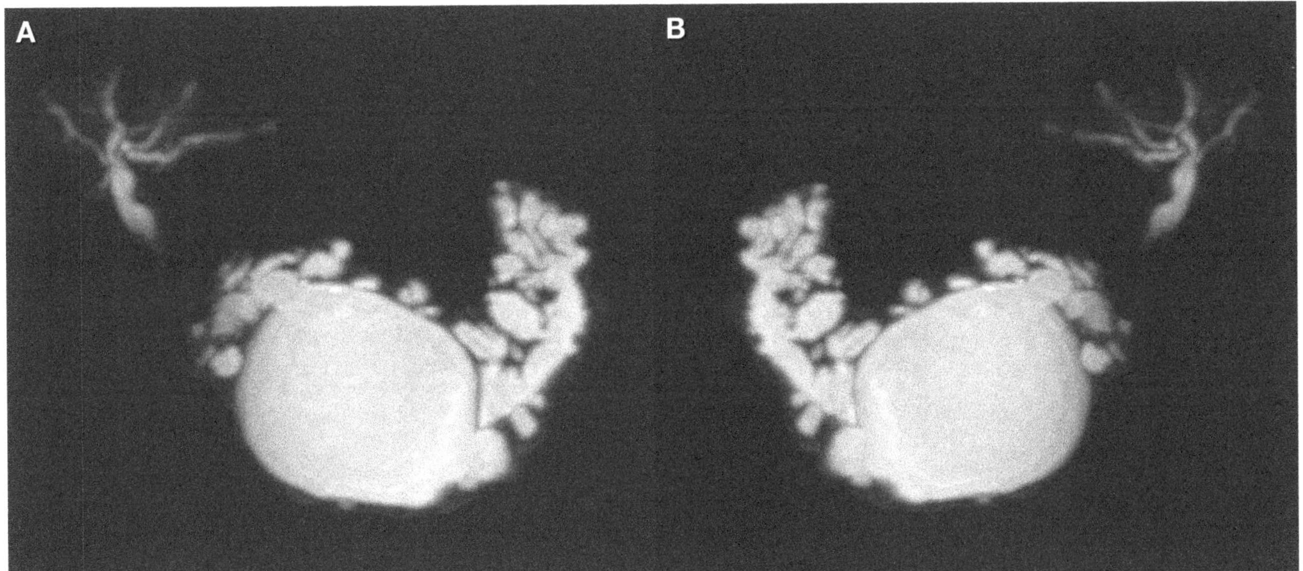

Figure 4.12.1

HISTORY: 71-year-old woman with a possible pseudocyst

IMAGING FINDINGS: Anterior (Figure 4.12.1A) and posterior (Figure 4.12.1B) MIP images from 3D FRFSE MRCP reveal marked irregular cystic dilatation of the main pancreatic duct and dilatation of multiple side-branch ducts.

DIAGNOSIS: IPMN involving the main pancreatic duct

COMMENT: IPMN of the main pancreatic duct is characterized by moderate to severe diffuse or segmental dilatation of the duct, often with papillary projections or mural nodules. The classic appearance of these lesions on endoscopic retrograde cholangiopancreatography is a distended papilla projecting into the duodenal lumen and secreting mucin. Contrast-enhanced imaging is useful for showing enhancement of mural nodules, thereby distinguishing them from stones or debris within the duct and helping to differentiate this entity from ductal dilatation resulting from CP.

Histologically, IPMNs are characterized by intraductal proliferation of neoplastic ductal epithelium accompanied by abundant mucin production. Lesions are classified according to whether the main duct or the branch ducts are involved and according to the degree of dysplasia.

Approximately 60% to 70% of patients with main-duct IPMN have high-grade dysplasia, and 45% have an associated invasive carcinoma. While any patient with a main-duct IPMN is a surgical candidate, the presence of mural nodules or mural enhancement (or both) is worrisome for malignant degeneration. When enhancing mural nodules are not present, main-duct IPMN may occasionally be difficult to distinguish from CP, which also frequently results in ductal dilatation. Two imaging features more often associated with IPMN than with CP are ductal dilatation without stricture (seen in this case) and a bulging ampulla. Multiple strictures, a mildly dilated duct, and intraductal stones are all more suggestive of CP.

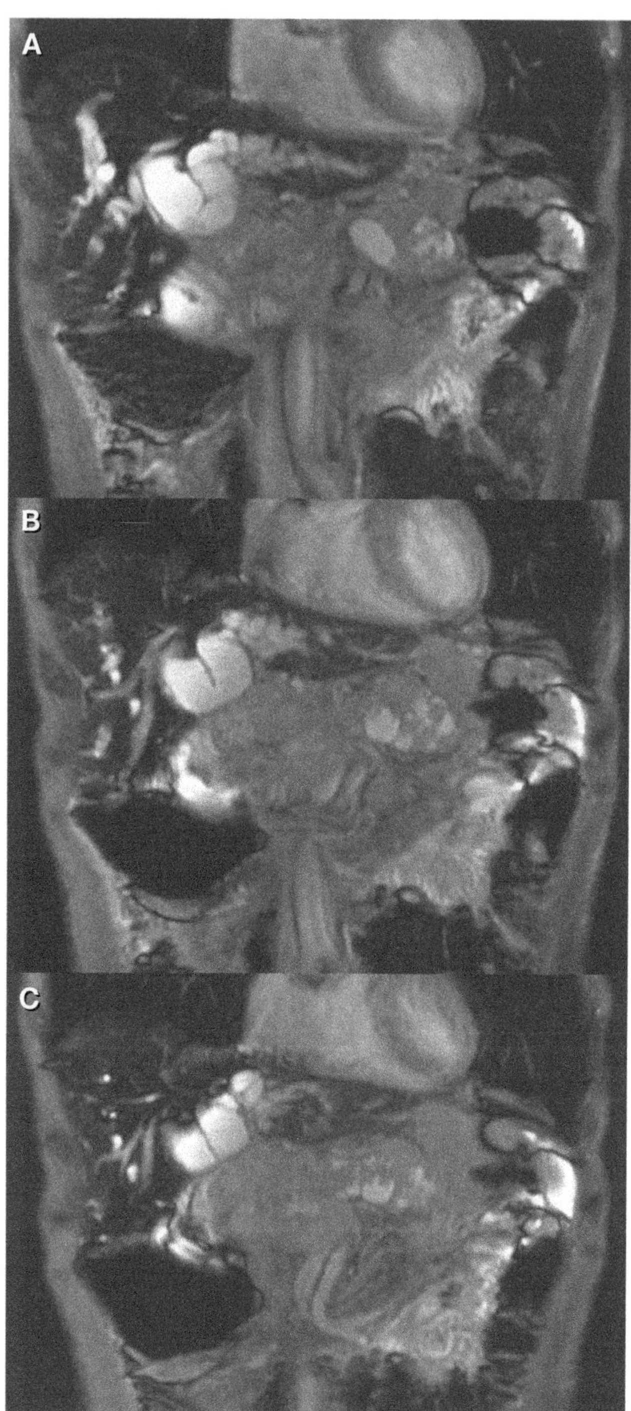

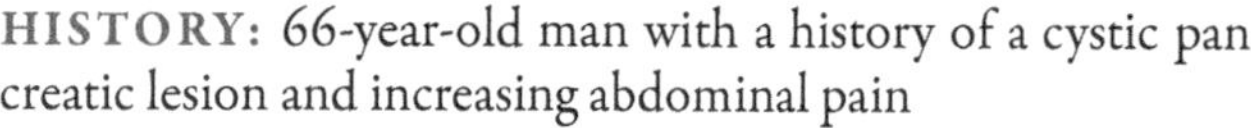

Figure 4.13.1

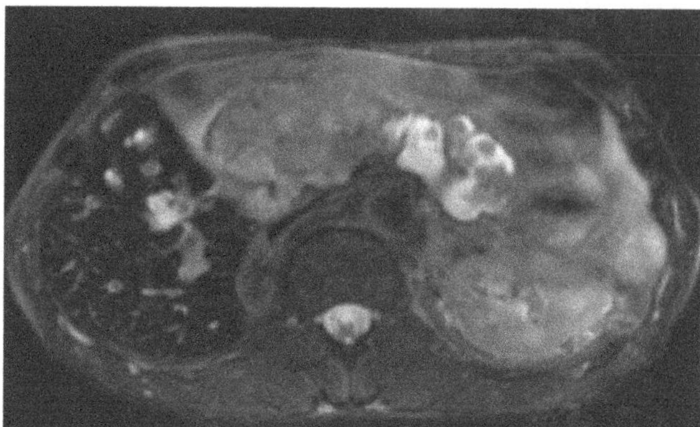

Figure 4.13.2

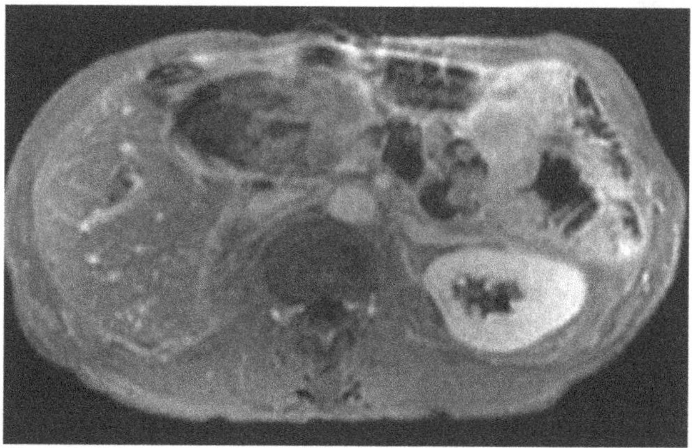

Figure 4.13.3

HISTORY: 66-year-old man with a history of a cystic pancreatic lesion and increasing abdominal pain

IMAGING FINDINGS: Coronal fat-suppressed 2D SSFP images (Figure 4.13.1) reveal marked biliary and pancreatic ductal dilatation. Note also the large soft tissue nodules in the proximal and distal pancreatic duct and the small nodules at the bifurcation of the common duct. Axial fat-suppressed T2-weighted FSE image (Figure 4.13.2) demonstrates mural nodules throughout the distended pancreatic duct, and postgadolinium venous phase 3D SPGR image (Figure 4.13.3) shows that these nodules enhance. The hepatic parenchyma has diffuse decreased signal intensity on T2-weighted images, likely reflecting hemosiderosis resulting from prior blood transfusions.

DIAGNOSIS: Invasive main-duct IPMN

COMMENT: Main-duct IPMNs have the highest malignant potential, with 60% to 70% showing high-grade dysplasia and 45% invasive carcinoma. This case has many features that are worrisome for carcinoma, including multiple enhancing mural nodules, a prominent soft tissue mass, a large-diameter main pancreatic duct, and biliary obstruction.

The prognosis for patients with IPMNs is strongly dependent on the presence of invasive carcinoma. The 5-year survival for patients with surgically resected noninvasive IPMN is greater than 90% (perioperative surgical mortality is generally about 3%). The 5-year survival decreases to 30% to 60% for patients with an associated invasive carcinoma.

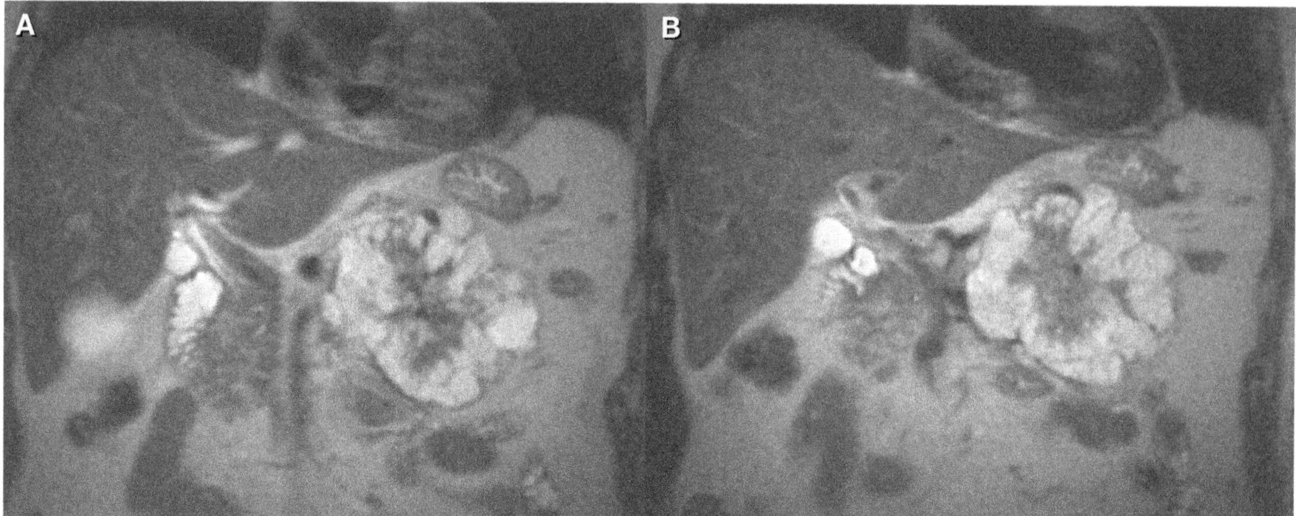

Figure 4.14.1

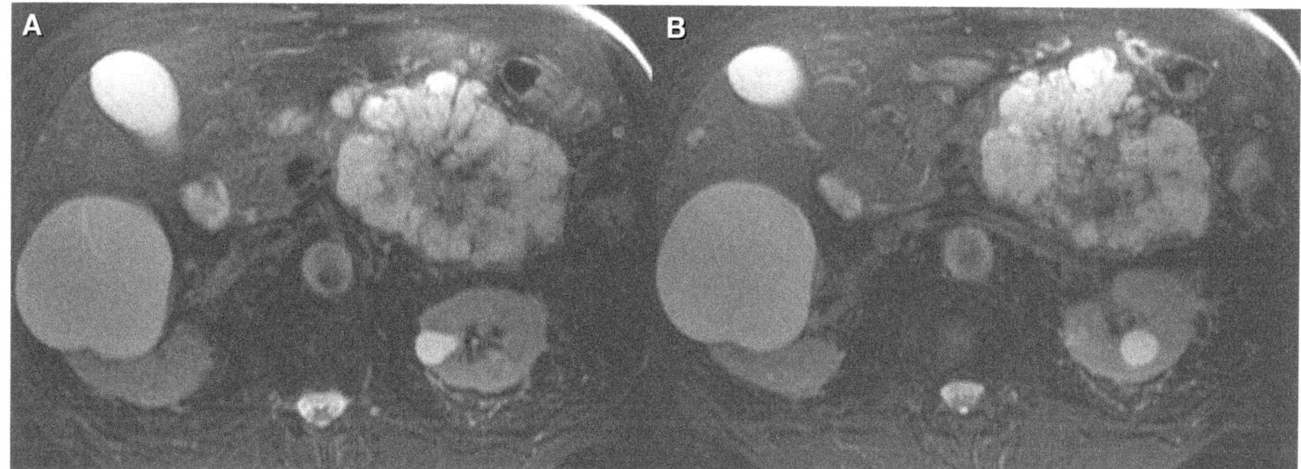

Figure 4.14.2

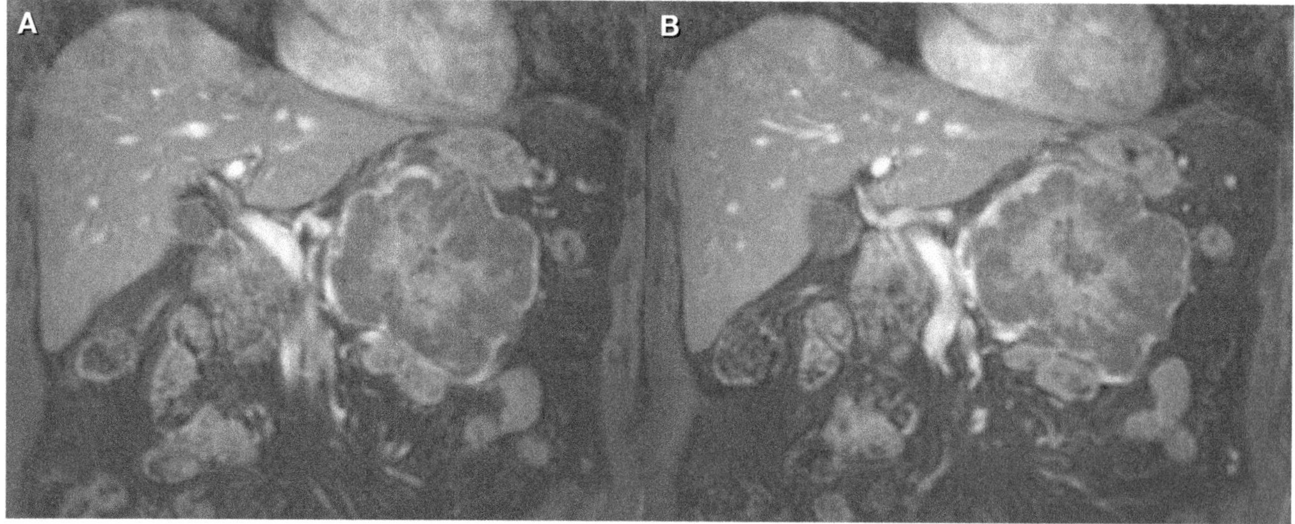

Figure 4.14.3

HISTORY: 87-year-old man with an abdominal mass

IMAGING FINDINGS: Coronal SSFSE (Figure 4.14.1) and axial fat-suppressed FRFSE T2-weighted (Figure 4.14.2) images reveal a large multilocular cystic mass centered in the pancreatic tail with a central scar. Postcontrast coronal 2D SPGR images (Figure 4.14.3) demonstrate mild enhancement of the central scar and capsule.

DIAGNOSIS: Serous cystic neoplasm

COMMENT: SCNs, formerly known as serous cystadenomas, comprise approximately 1% of all pancreatic neoplasms and occur predominantly in older women. The peak age of incidence is 65 years, and 60% to 85% of patients are female (but remember that SCNs are also common in younger patients with VHL syndrome). SCNs are composed of multiple small cysts ranging from 0.1 to 2.0 cm in diameter and separated by fibrous septations. The septations typically radiate from a central scar that may calcify. The cysts are filled with serous fluid and lined by glycogen-rich epithelium.

The appearance on MRI is usually diagnostic, and often the best images are obtained with SSFSE or SSFP acquisitions. These have T2-weighting; therefore, the cysts are bright, and the thin septations separating the cysts are often seen better on these rapidly acquired images than in respiratory-triggered or contrast-enhanced series. The fibrous central scar may enhance on delayed images, or it may not (approximately 30% of lesions have calcification in the central scar, which won't enhance no matter how long you wait). The appearance of SCNs tends to be symmetrical and well ordered as opposed to MCNs, which have larger cysts and appear more irregular. Other lesions in the differential diagnosis include clustered IPMNs and complex pancreatic pseudocysts.

The well-ordered honeycomb appearance is the classic and most common appearance of SCNs; however, other patterns have been described, including a macrocystic or oligocystic variant with fewer than 6 cysts, typically between 1 and 2 cm in diameter and lacking a central scar. Oligocystic SCNs probably account for 10% to 20% of all lesions and may be difficult to distinguish from MCNs, although MCNs are much more likely to contain internal septations and mural nodules. A less common solid variant has also been reported in large series and probably comprises 1% to 3% of all tumors.

Most SCNs are benign and the patients asymptomatic. If pain, biliary or pancreatic obstruction, or recurrent pancreatitis develops, patients become surgical candidates. Malignant degeneration is extremely rare, but descriptions of approximately 25 cases have been published.

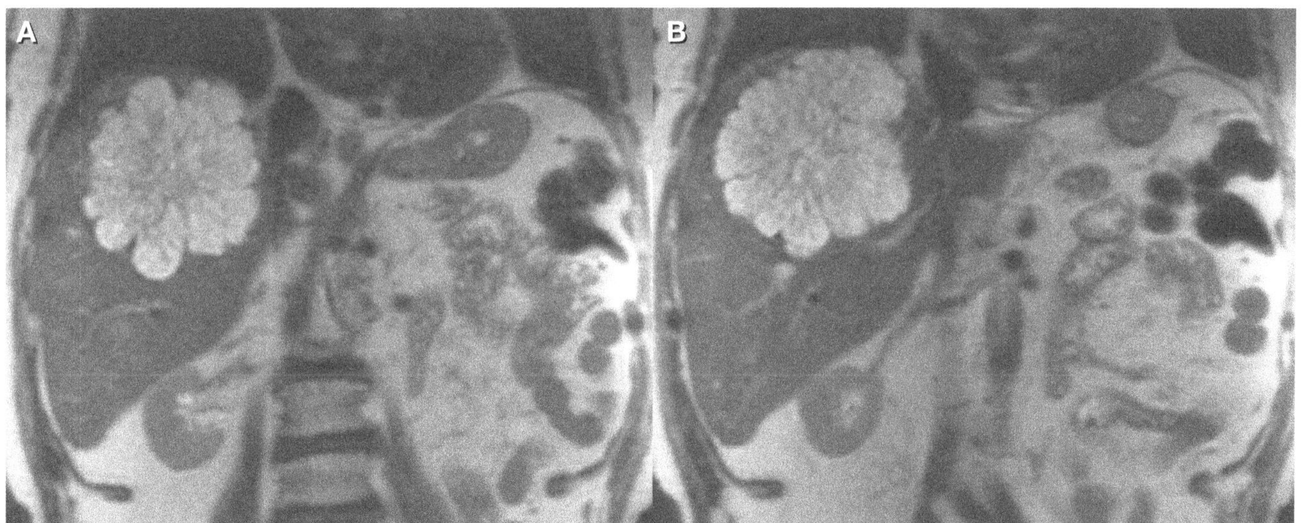

Figure 4.14.4

The 1 case of serous cystadenocarcinoma that we have seen was in a 90-year-old man who had a pancreatic lesion resected 15 years earlier and then had hepatic metastases that looked exactly like a serous cystadenoma, but in the wrong organ (Figure 4.14.4—coronal SSFSE images show a large markedly hyperintense multilocular hepatic mass consistent with metastatic pancreatic cystadenocarcinoma).

In the ongoing struggle between advocates of MRI and advocates of CT, the pancreas remains unsettled territory. While the most devoted MRI partisans would almost never willingly recommend that a patient undergo CT (and experience the "rays of death"), we believe that for most patients CT is probably a better choice for detecting and staging pancreatic adenocarcinoma. Lesion contrast often is not any better with MRI, spatial resolution is worse, and since the patient population is older, concerns about radiation exposure are minimal. However, even 1 of our colleagues, who once said that he could not recall a single instance when abdominal MRI had detected a clinically relevant finding that couldn't be seen just as well or better with properly performed CT, might have to admit that MRI is much better at distinguishing cystic from solid pancreatic lesions, an important distinction that is not always trivial with CT.

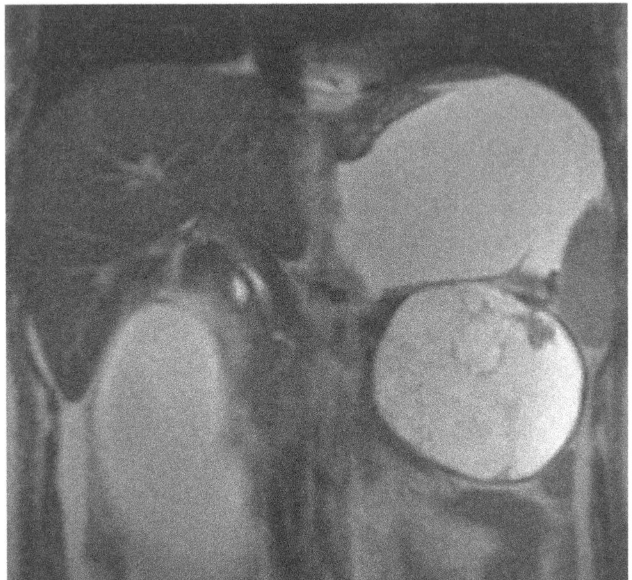

Figure 4.15.1

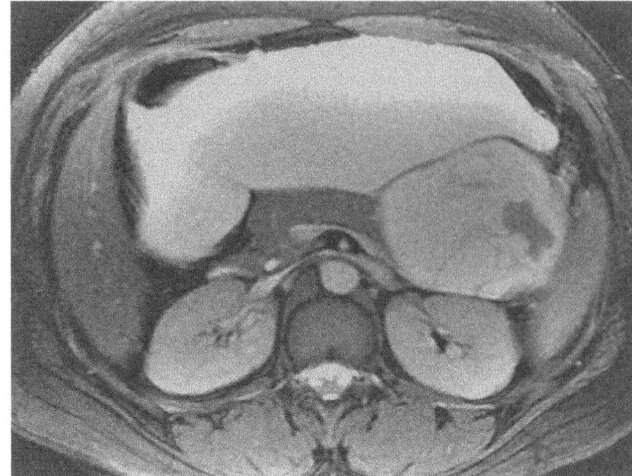

Figure 4.15.2

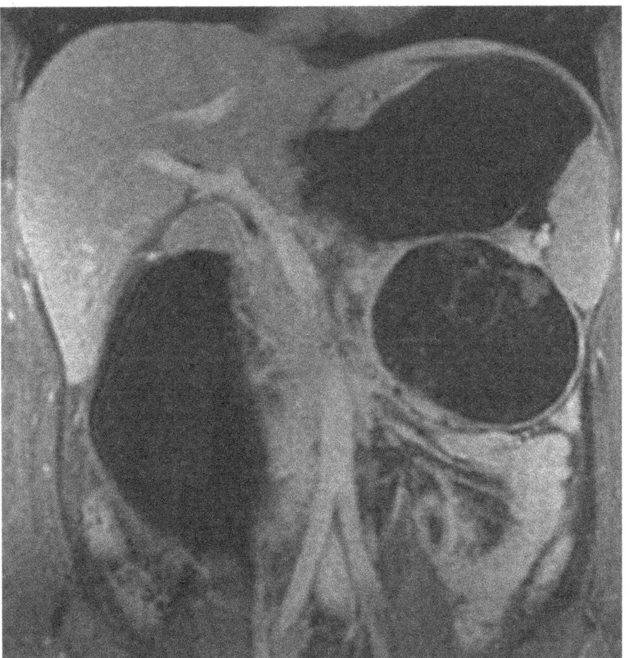

Figure 4.15.3

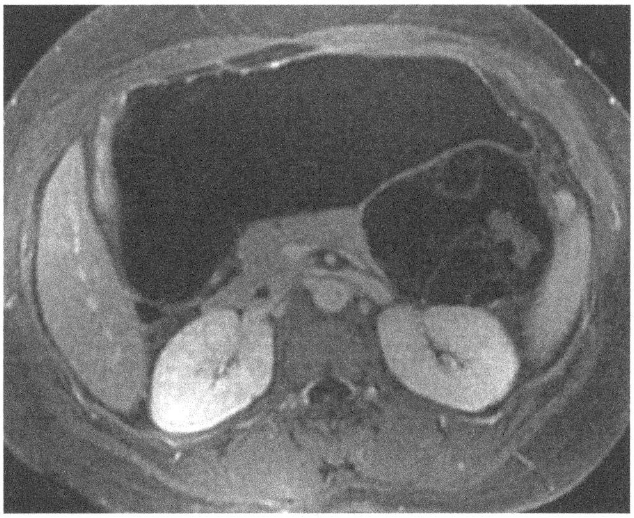

Figure 4.15.4

HISTORY: 44-year-old woman with pancreatitis

IMAGING FINDINGS: Coronal SSFSE (Figure 4.15.1) and axial fat-suppressed 2D SSFP (Figure 4.15.2) images reveal a complex cystic mass in the tail of the pancreas containing multiple septations and a focal nodule. A large encapsulated fluid collection surrounds the anterior aspect of the pancreas. Coronal (Figure 4.15.3) and axial (Figure 4.15.4) venous phase postgadolinium 3D SPGR images demonstrate enhancement of the rim of the lesion and mild enhancement of the septations and internal nodule.

DIAGNOSIS: MCN and pancreatic pseudocyst

COMMENT: MCNs account for approximately 2% of all pancreatic neoplasms and occur almost exclusively in women aged 40 to 60 years. Approximately 95% of the lesions are located in the pancreatic body and tail. In contrast to SCNs, MCNs do possess significant malignant potential.

While patients who have MCNs are more frequently symptomatic at presentation than patients with SCNs, asymptomatic incidental detection is not unusual. Symptoms are typically vague, including abdominal pain, fullness, and nausea, although approximately 10% of patients (including the one in this case) have episodes of pancreatitis.

MCNs consist of 1 or more (but usually <6) large (>2 cm in diameter) cysts lined by mucinous columnar epithelium. The cysts are often complex, containing thick septations, papillary excrescences, or frank nodules. The pathologic hallmark of MCN is the presence of an ovarian-type stroma forming the mesenchymal component of the tumor (which probably explains its extreme rarity in men), and this feature reliably distinguishes MCNs from side-branch IPMNs, which occasionally have a similar appearance. There is no universally accepted explanation for the presence of ovarian stroma in a pancreatic tumor; however, the close proximity of the ovary and pancreas during embryogenesis has been postulated as a mechanism whereby ovarian cells could infiltrate into the pancreas. The cysts of MCNs contain abundant mucin, carcinoembryonic antigen, and carbohydrate antigen 19-9, all of which can help in distinguishing MCNs from SCNs.

MCNs are classified into 1) mucinous cystadenomas, comprising approximately 65% of lesions and containing only benign cells; 2) noninvasive proliferative MCNs (approximately 30%), with various degrees of atypia, dysplasia, and carcinoma in situ; and 3) mucinous cystadenocarcinomas, with 1 or more foci of frank invasive carcinoma, likely accounting for 6% to 20% of cases.

The imaging appearance of MCNs reflects the pathology, with 1 or more large cysts often containing thick enhancing septations and mural nodules. The lesions are usually hypointense compared to adjacent pancreas on T1-weighted images; however, T1 hyperintensity has been reported, probably reflecting the proteinaceous content of the cysts (and invalidating the rule that only solid pseudopapillary neoplasms have high signal intensity on T1-weighted images). Oligocystic SCNs can have a similar if not identical appearance, although as the internal complexity of the lesion increases, so too does the probability of an MCN. Features worrisome for malignancy include large size (>8 cm), focal mass or large mural nodules, focal thickening or enhancement of a wall or septations, and evidence of local invasion or metastatic disease. Eccentric calcifications, best seen on CT, are present in approximately 20% of cases and are also thought to suggest malignant degeneration.

The distinction between SCNs and MCNs sounds easy but is not always straightforward in practice. In general, however, MCNs are more disorganized and asymmetrical and have a more worrisome appearance, with thick irregular septations and internal nodules. In addition, although these lesions do not arise from the pancreatic duct, MCNs may occasionally be difficult to distinguish from IPMNs.

This case also illustrates the relatively common occurrence of more than 1 diagnosis in a single patient. The large peripancreatic fluid collection was the result of a previous episode of pancreatitis that was probably related to the presence of the MCN. It is tempting to try to find a single explanation for everything, which might lead to the conclusion that these findings represent evolving pancreatic pseudocysts, 1 simple and 1 complex. However, closer examination would reveal that the internal nodules in the MCN enhance, which should never occur in a pseudocyst.

Surgical resection is the treatment of choice for all MCNs. When MCNs lacking an invasive component are completely resected, the patient is cured and routine follow-up examinations are probably not indicated. The prognosis for patients with invasive carcinoma is relatively poor, with 5-year survival rates of 15% to 35%. Most authors believe that mucinous cystadenocarcinomas develop from previously existing mucinous cystadenomas over the course of several years, emphasizing the opportunity for detection and definitive treatment of these lesions before they become invasive.

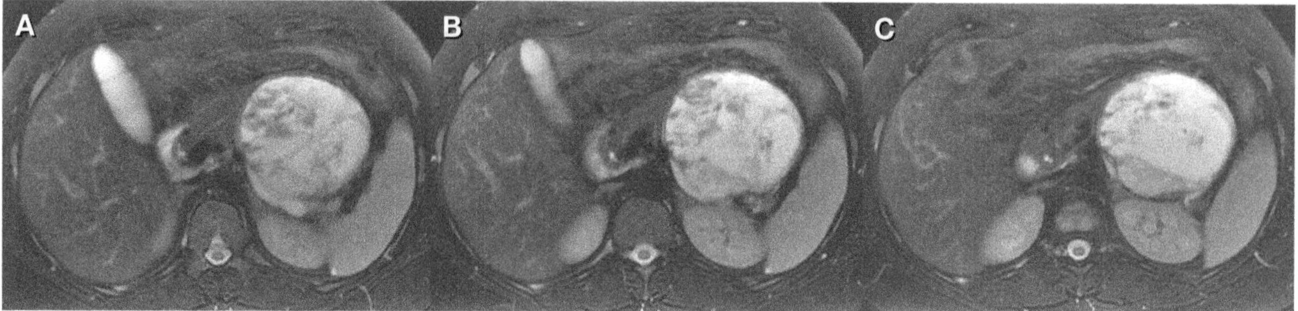

Figure 4.16.1

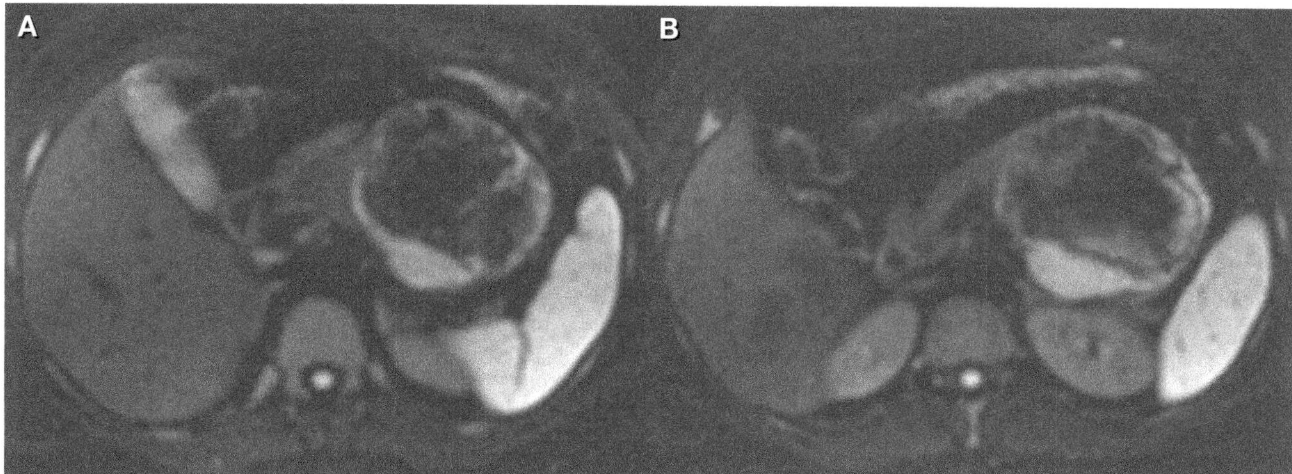

Figure 4.16.2

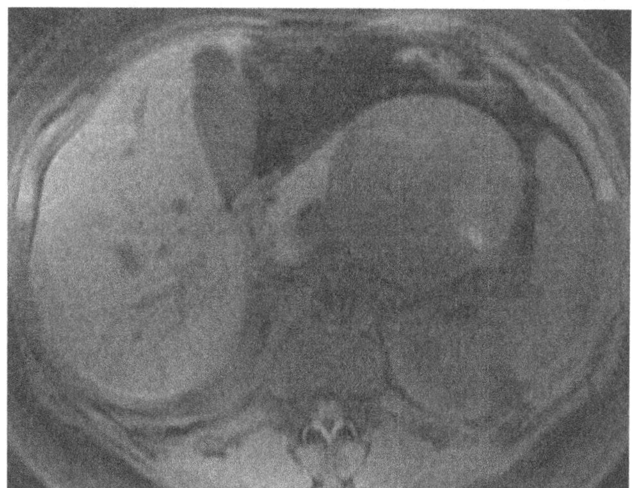

Figure 4.16.3

HISTORY: 32-year-old pregnant woman with an abdominal mass; MRI was performed without intravenous contrast

IMAGING FINDINGS: Axial fat-suppressed FSE T2-weighted images (Figure 4.16.1) reveal a complex predominantly cystic mass in the pancreatic body and tail with a prominent solid component along the posterior margin. Note the multiple small fluid-fluid levels within the lesion. Axial diffusion-weighted images (b=600 s/mm^2) (Figure 4.16.2) emphasize the nodular solid component posteriorly, with minimal signal within the cystic portion of the lesion. Axial fat-suppressed T1-weighted 3D SPGR image (Figure 4.16.3) shows a small focus of increased signal intensity within the mass, with most of the lesion demonstrating decreased signal intensity relative to the pancreas.

DIAGNOSIS: Solid pseudopapillary neoplasm

COMMENT: SPNs of the pancreas are rare lesions thought to comprise 1% to 2% of exocrine pancreatic neoplasms. They were initially described by Franz in 1959 as *papillary tumor of the pancreas, benign or malignant*. Subsequent case reports and larger series used various synonyms, including *solid and papillary epithelial neoplasm*, before the WHO settled on the name *solid pseudopapillary tumor of the pancreas* in 1996 (in 2010, the WHO reclassified the lesion as SPN).

These lesions occur most often in young women, with the highest incidence in the second and third decades of life and a female to male ratio of 10:1. Approximately one-third of patients are asymptomatic at diagnosis, and the tumor is found on routine physical examination or during cross-sectional imaging performed for another indication. When symptoms are present, they are typically vague (abdominal pain, nausea, or a palpable mass). SPNs are usually large at diagnosis (average diameter, 6-8 cm) and occur with nearly equal frequency in the head and the tail of the pancreas.

The histopathologic features of SPN are fairly distinctive, consisting of degenerating pseudopapillae and noncohesive tumor cells with round nuclei and eosinophilic cytoplasm. Hemorrhagic degeneration is frequent and is often reflected in the imaging appearance.

MRI typically shows a large, well-defined encapsulated mass with a complex internal architecture containing both solid and cystic elements. Several authors have emphasized 2 features of SPNs that are helpful in diagnosis: 1) the presence of a capsule that is hypointense on T1- and T2-weighted images and shows early enhancement after gadolinium administration, and 2) the presence of hemorrhagic debris (ie, high precontrast T1-signal intensity, occasionally with fluid-fluid levels), which is thought to be extremely rare in most other pancreatic tumors. In our experience, these signs are helpful but by no means exclusive to SPNs. Hemorrhage is occasionally seen in various neoplasms, including NETs, and in non-neoplastic lesions (eg, pseudocysts) in the differential diagnosis. High precontrast T1-signal intensity is also seen with tumors that have a high protein content, such as the occasional MCN. In general, SPNs have solid components that are much more prominent than those of MCNs and show enhancement after gadolinium administration (unlike the internal components of pseudocysts). SPNs also occur in a distinctly younger population than most other pancreatic tumors. Approximately 30% of lesions contain peripheral calcification, which is difficult to appreciate on MRI but more apparent on CT. Some authors have linked this finding with a higher risk of malignancy, but this association has not been widely confirmed.

One recent paper described a series of smaller, predominantly solid SPNs occurring in middle-aged women. These SPNs were difficult to reliably distinguish from NETs, but the diagnosis could be suggested on the basis of their strikingly high T2-signal intensity and their heterogeneous and slowly progressive enhancement.

The prognosis for patients with SPN is excellent, particularly compared to that for patients with pancreatic adenocarcinoma, and the overall 5-year survival is approximately 95%. Surgical resection is the treatment of choice and is generally curative, although recurrence has been reported in less than 10% of cases. Approximately 10% of SPNs have malignant features, including local invasion or hepatic metastases.

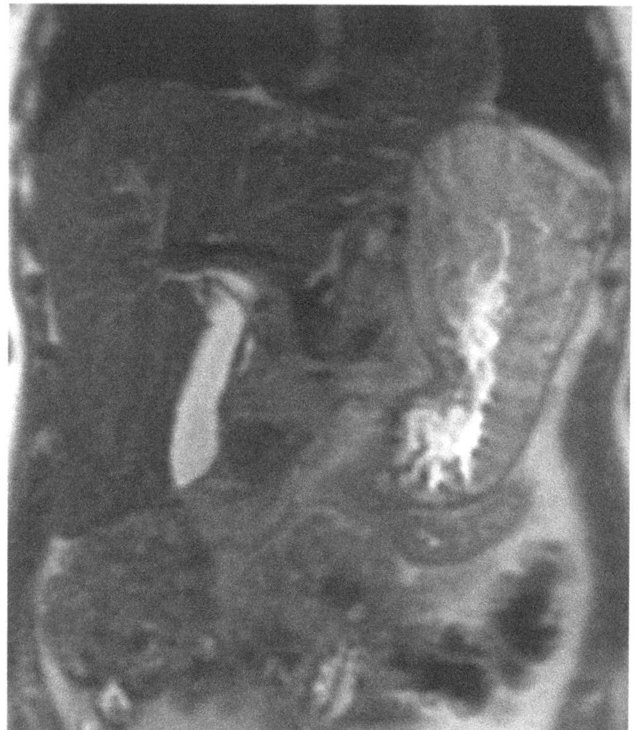

Figure 4.17.1

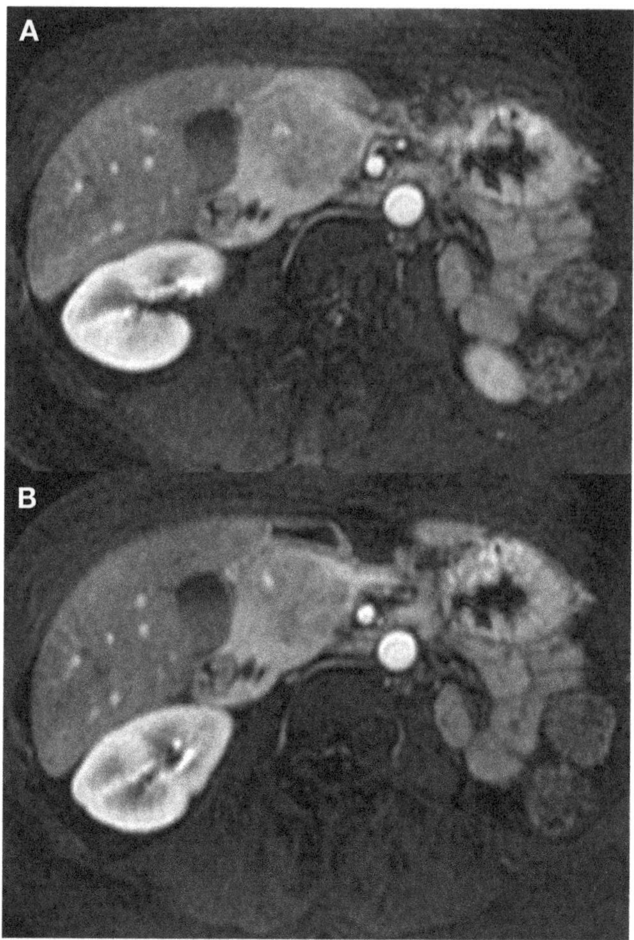

Figure 4.17.3

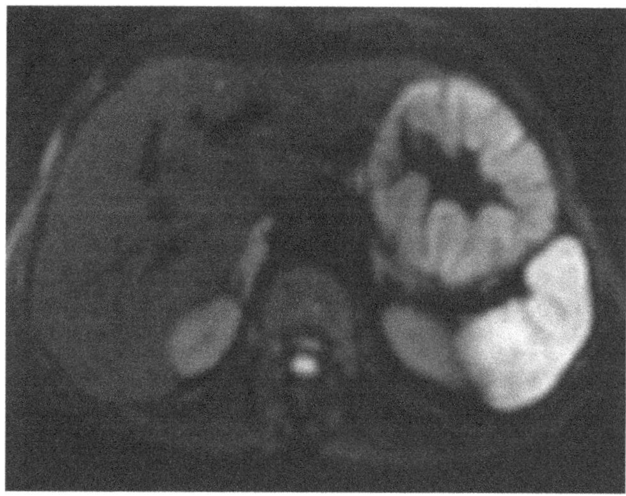

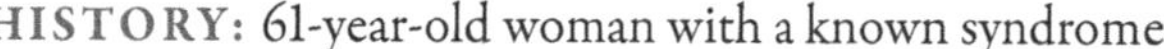

Figure 4.17.2

HISTORY: 61-year-old woman with a known syndrome

IMAGING FINDINGS: Coronal SSFSE (Figure 4.17.1) and axial diffusion-weighted images (b=600 s/mm^2) (Figure 4.17.2) demonstrate marked rugal fold thickening in the fundus and body of the stomach. A heterogeneous hypoenhancing mass at the neck of the pancreas is seen on arterial phase postgadolinium 3D SPGR images (Figure 4.17.3). A thin rim of pancreatic tissue extends around the anterior and posterior margins of the duodenum.

DIAGNOSIS: Pancreatic gastrinoma with Zollinger-Ellison syndrome (and incidental annular pancreas)

COMMENT: Pseudo–gastric fold thickening is a common diagnosis made by our residents (the folds look thick in a collapsed stomach, but the finding disappears when the patient drinks a glass of water). Experienced radiologists are less likely to fall into this trap, not so much because they are actually better at distinguishing real from imaginary fold thickening on CT or MRI but because they remember all the normal endoscopy reports emailed to them by their helpful gastroenterology colleagues. The folds in this case are too thick to ignore, though, and the persistence of the finding over the course of a 30- to 45-minute MRI examination is another indication of the pathologic nature of the stomach. The differential diagnosis for isolated gastric mural thickening includes gastric carcinoma, metastases, lymphoma, and inflammation; however, with a pancreatic mass or any mass within the gastrinoma triangle (defined by vertices at the cystic duct, at the junction of the neck and body of the pancreas, and at the junction of the second and third portions of the duodenum), Zollinger-Ellison syndrome is the most likely diagnosis.

Pancreatic NETs were previously referred to as islet cell tumors because they were thought to have originated from the islets of Langerhans. More recent evidence, however, suggests an origin from pluripotential stem cells in the ductal epithelium; in 2000, the WHO replaced the term *islet cell tumor* with the more generic classification *NET*. NETs account for 1% to 2% of all pancreatic neoplasms and are generally divided into functional and nonfunctional categories, based on whether the tumor does or does not produce pancreatic hormones in sufficient quantity to cause clinical symptoms. Published estimates of the relative percentages of functional and nonfunctional NETs vary widely, with most authors concluding that functional tumors are less common, accounting for 15% to 50% of lesions.

Patients with pancreatic NET are generally middle-aged or older, with peak incidence between 50 and 70 years. Most pancreatic NETs occur sporadically; however, they also can occur in association with several syndromes, including multiple endocrine neoplasia type 1, VHL, neurofibromatosis 1, and tuberous sclerosis. Gastrinomas are gastrin-secreting NETs, and gastrin is responsible for the ulceration and thickening of the stomach and duodenal walls. In general, a higher percentage of nonfunctional NETs are malignant compared to functional tumors, but gastrinomas are an exception since approximately 70% are malignant.

The classic imaging appearance of a NET is that of a fairly homogeneous lesion with moderately to markedly increased T2-signal intensity compared to normal pancreas and with intense arterial phase enhancement on dynamic postgadolinium 3D SPGR images. These guidelines are useful, except for when they do not apply, as in this case, where the mass is hypointense relative to adjacent pancreas on arterial phase postgadolinium images. In general, larger lesions are less likely to follow the rules: they may outgrow their blood supply and fail to show early enhancement, or they may develop central necrosis and occasionally be mistaken for cystic pancreatic neoplasms. Diffusion-weighted images can be useful for detecting NETs, with an appearance even more hyperintense against the dark background of normal pancreas in comparison to standard FSE T2-weighted images. In spite of numerous attempts, though, measurement of ADC values has not proved particularly reproducible in characterizing the various pancreatic tumors, or in distinguishing benign from malignant lesions. The main differential diagnosis is ductal adenocarcinoma. Adenocarcinoma generally is more infiltrative with a less well-defined border, is less likely to enhance on arterial phase images, and is much more likely to cause significant obstruction of the pancreatic duct or biliary ducts (or both).

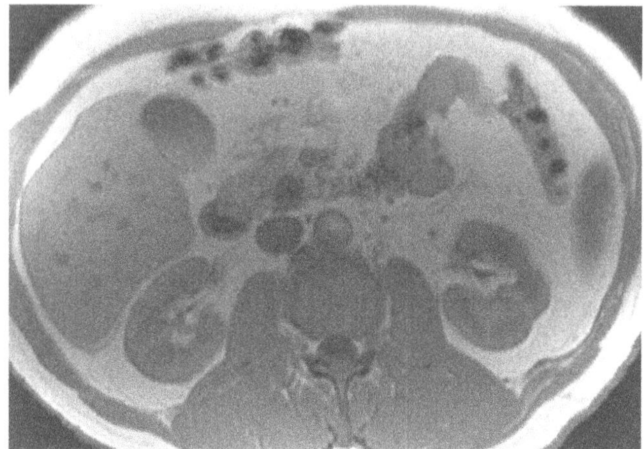

Figure 4.18.1

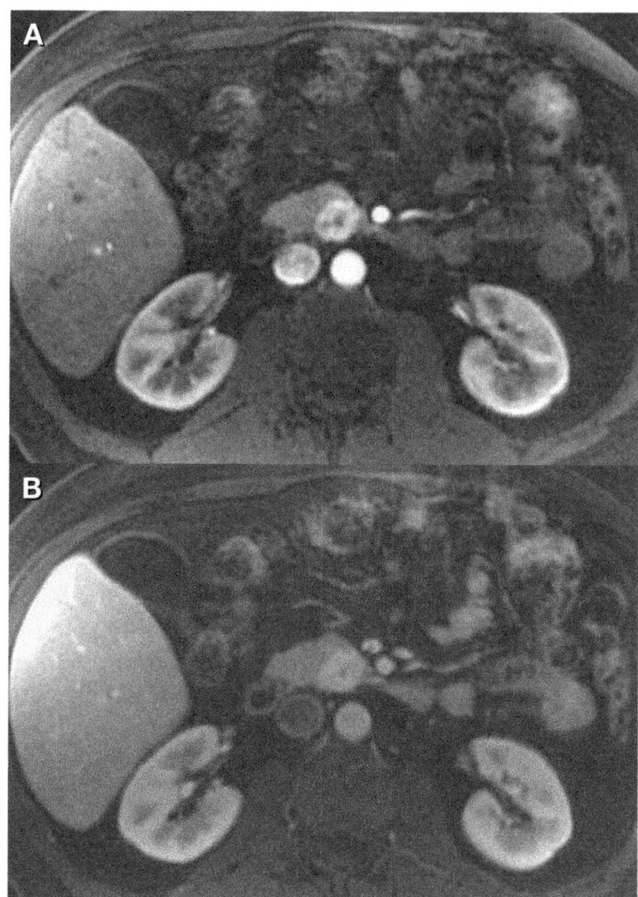

Figure 4.18.4

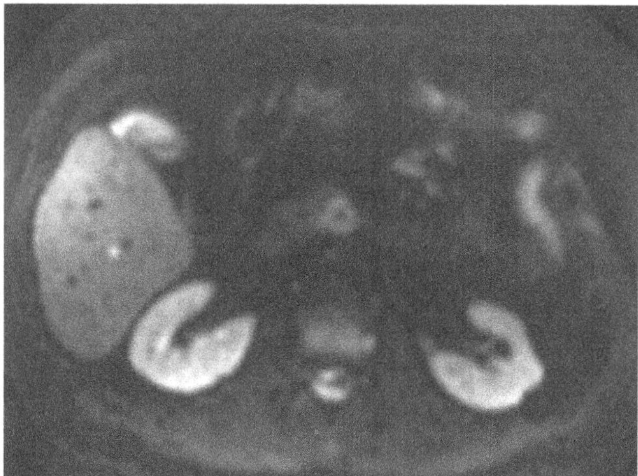

Figure 4.18.2

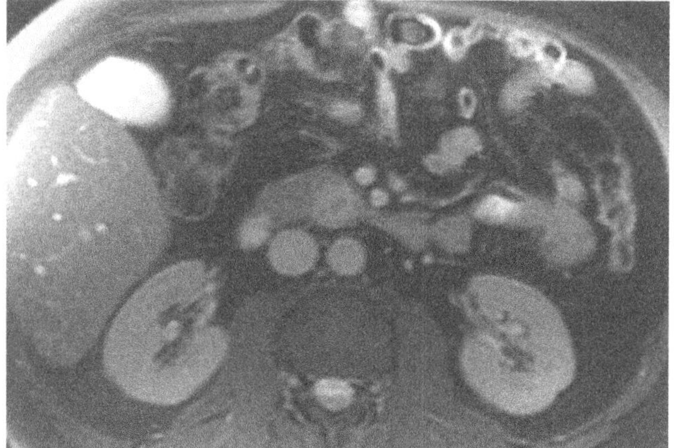

Figure 4.18.3

HISTORY: 52-year-old man with severe mitral insufficiency; an incidental pancreatic mass was detected on preoperative CT angiography

IMAGING FINDINGS: Axial T1-weighted in-phase 2D SPGR image (Figure 4.18.1) demonstrates a round low-signal-intensity mass in the pancreatic uncinate process. Axial diffusion-weighted image (b=600 s/mm^2) (Figure 4.18.2) and axial fat-suppressed SSFP image (Figure 4.18.3) reveal high-signal-intensity within the lesion. Arterial phase (Figure 4.18.4A) and portal venous phase (Figure 4.18.4B) postgadolinium 3D SPGR images show intense enhancement of the mass relative to adjacent normal pancreatic parenchyma. Note also the small hyperintense lesion in the inferior right hepatic lobe on the diffusion-weighted image, which shows enhancement on the arterial phase postcontrast image.

DIAGNOSIS: NET, nonfunctional, with hepatic metastases

COMMENT: This case is an example of the classic appearance of pancreatic NET: a well-circumscribed mass with low signal intensity on precontrast T1-weighted images, high signal intensity on diffusion-weighted images (and the somewhat T2-weighted SSFP image), and intense uniform arterial phase hyperenhancement.

This lesion is fairly easy to distinguish from the typical adenocarcinoma, which has a more infiltrative appearance and is generally hypointense relative to adjacent pancreas on arterial phase and portal venous phase postgadolinium images. It is also likely that an adenocarcinoma of this size and in this location would have caused significant obstruction of the pancreatic duct or common bile duct (or both).

Patients with nonfunctional NETs are often asymptomatic until the NET becomes large enough to generate symptoms on the basis of mass effect or metastatic disease. This probably also explains the overall higher risk of malignancy with nonfunctional tumors compared to functional tumors, since the risk increases with the size of the lesion.

The propensity of NETs for vascular invasion and thrombosis is probably underappreciated. While adenocarcinomas are notorious for arterial and venous encasement, NETs frequently invade the splenic and superior mesenteric veins. A recent CT study found tumor thrombus in 33% of patients with NET and also noted that this finding was frequently missed in the initial report.

Notice that the small hepatic metastasis is a subtle finding on all but the diffusion-weighted image, where it appears as a high-signal-intensity lesion adjacent to a vascular flow void. The lesion is hyperintense on the arterial phase postgadolinium image and fades slightly on the portal venous phase image, but it would be easy to dismiss as a vessel on end without careful inspection of the adjacent images. DWI is a great technique for identifying these small hypervascular metastases either as a stand-alone method or preferably as a supplement to standard dynamic contrast-enhanced 3D SPGR acquisitions.

CASE 4.19

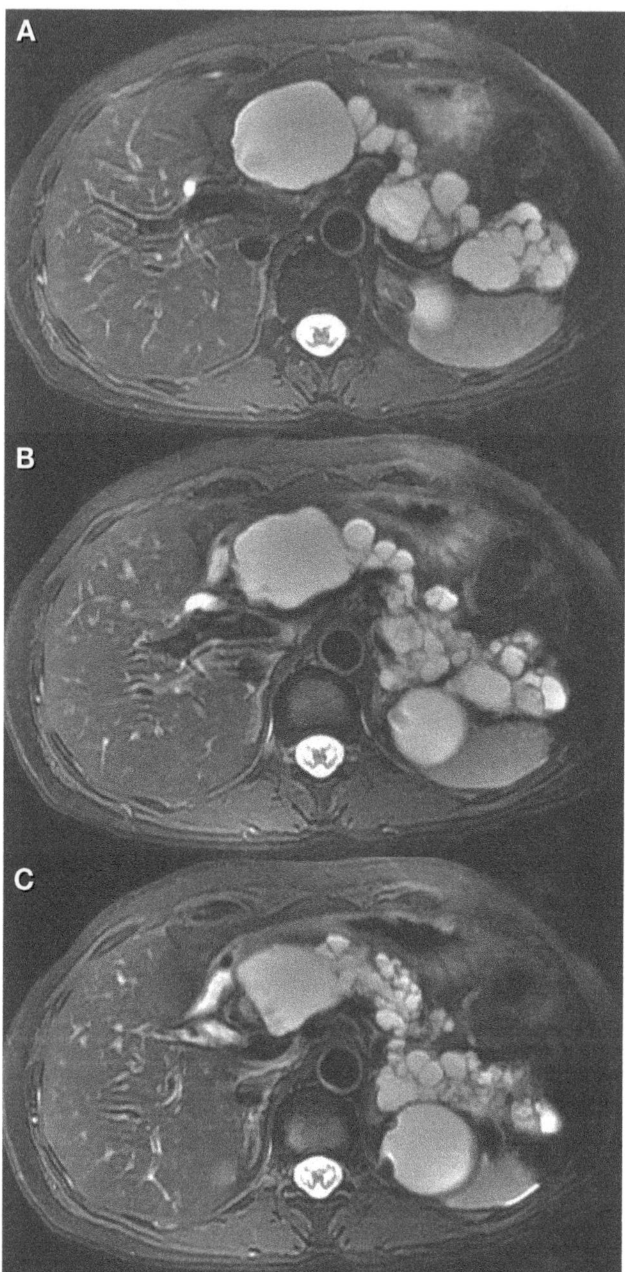

Figure 4.19.1

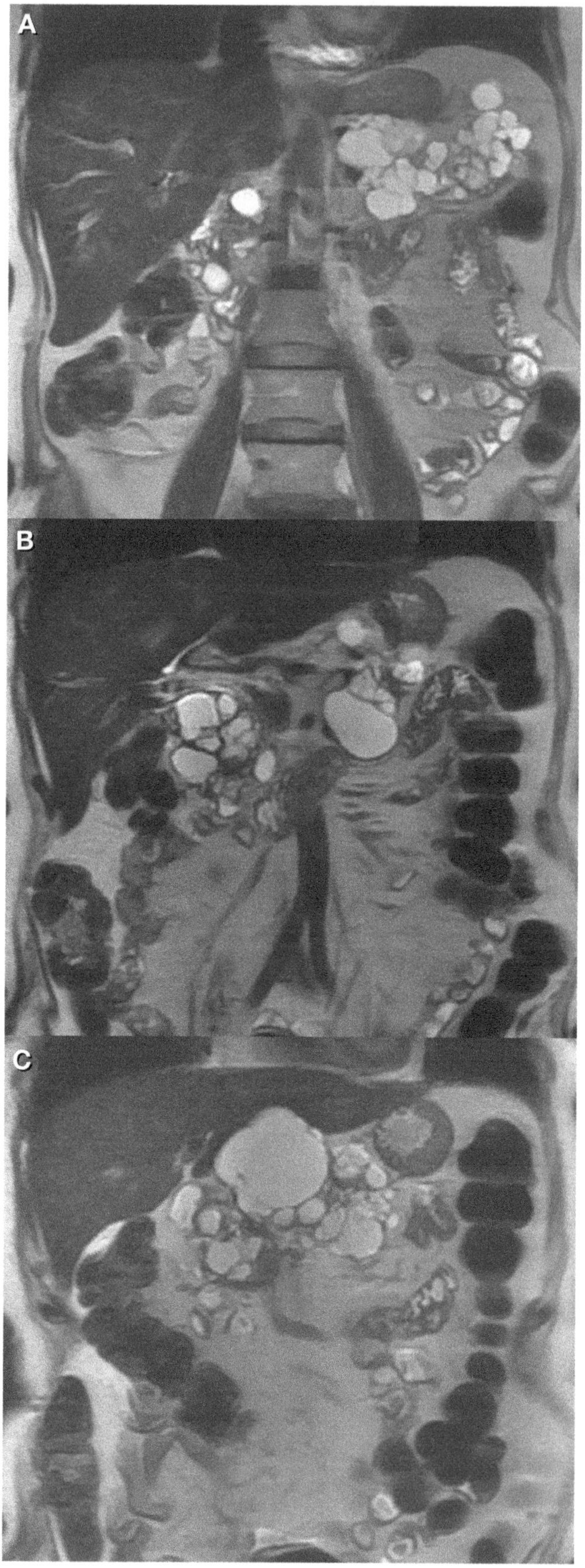

Figure 4.19.2

HISTORY: 62-year-old woman with a systemic disorder

IMAGING FINDINGS: Axial fat-suppressed FSE T2-weighted (Figure 4.19.1) and coronal SSFSE images (Figure 4.19.2) demonstrate innumerable pancreatic cysts.

DIAGNOSIS: VHL syndrome with cystic pancreas

COMMENT: Pancreatic involvement in VHL syndrome is not exactly an afterthought in many texts, but it does tend to be the last abdominal manifestation mentioned. This case is somewhat unusual in that the kidneys were almost completely spared in spite of extensive pancreatic involvement, but this can occur and should not dissuade anyone from making the correct diagnosis.

Pancreatic manifestations of VHL syndrome include cysts (in 72% of patients in 1 autopsy series), serous cystadenomas (11%), and nonfunctional NETs. Nonfunctional NETs occur in approximately 15% of patients with VHL syndrome; however, the behavior of NETs is generally less aggressive than that of sporadic tumors in the general population. Metastatic disease is seen in 10% to 15% of VHL syndrome patients with NETs and in 60% to 90% of patients with sporadic NETs. Even in this subgroup of patients with VHL syndrome, survival times are often relatively long. Since renal cell carcinoma (typically clear cell) occurs in 25% to 40% of patients with VHL syndrome, metastatic renal cell carcinoma is an important differential diagnostic consideration for an enhancing pancreatic mass.

VHL syndrome is an autosomal dominant neurocutaneous disorder with high penetrance (80%-100%) and an incidence of approximately 1 in 36,000 in the United States. The genetic defect in VHL syndrome is a mutation in a tumor suppression gene located on chromosome 3. Patients with VHL syndrome are predisposed to retinal angiomas, central nervous system hemangioblastomas, pheochromocytomas, renal cell carcinoma, NETs, endolymphatic sac tumors, and renal, pancreatic, pulmonary, and epididymal cysts.

Cysts are the most common pancreatic lesions in patients with VHL syndrome. When the cyst burden is relatively high, as in this case, confidently distinguishing adjacent cysts from serous cystadenomas can be difficult, although generally the distinction is not a clinically important problem.

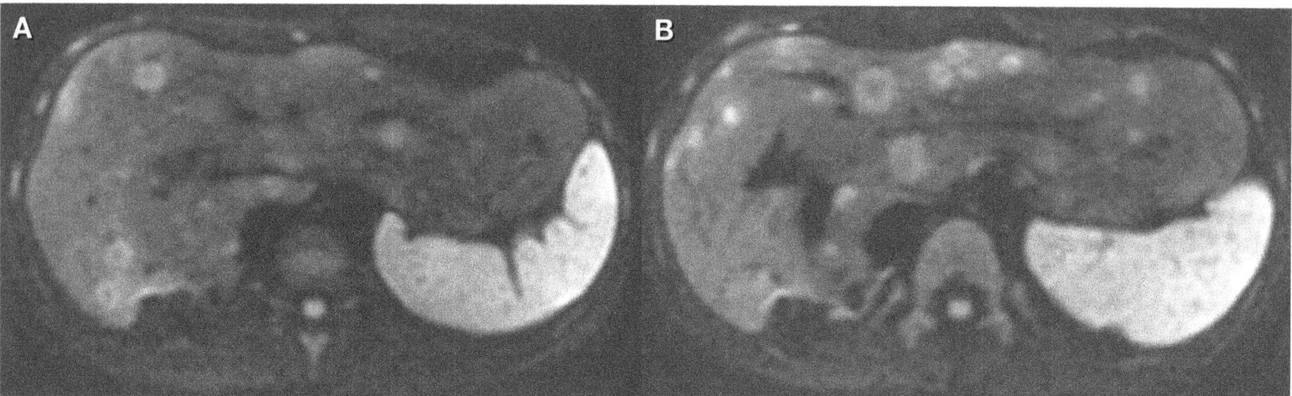

Figure 4.20.1

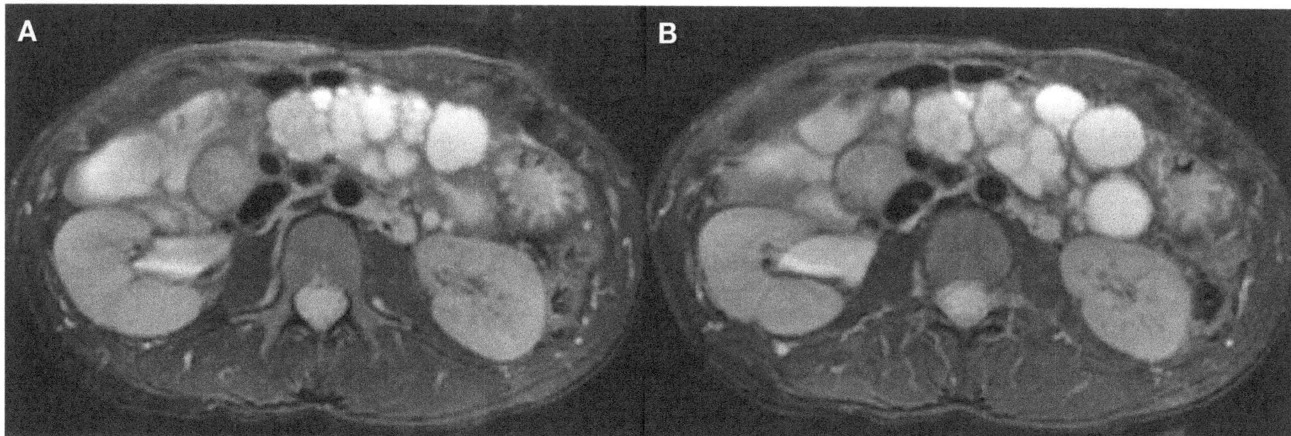

Figure 4.20.2

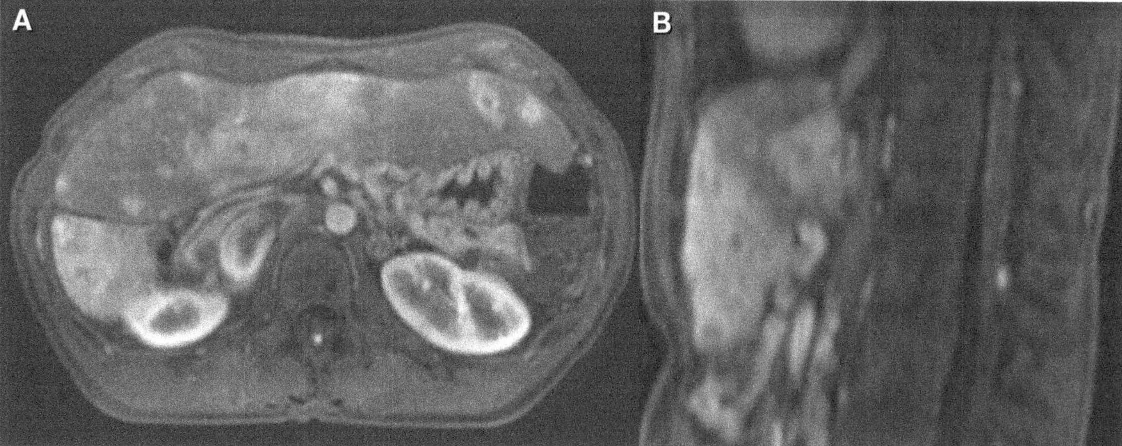

Figure 4.20.3

HISTORY: 30-year-old woman with VHL syndrome and prior pancreatic surgery

IMAGING FINDINGS: Axial diffusion-weighted images (b=100 s/mm^2) (Figure 4.20.1) reveal multiple hyperintense hepatic lesions. Axial fat-suppressed FSE T2-weighted images (Figure 4.20.2) demonstrate extensive cystic disease involving the pancreas. Note also that several lesions consist of clustered cysts. Axial (Figure 4.20.3A) and sagittal (Figure 4.20.3B) reformatted arterial phase postgadolinium 3D SPGR images show hyperenhancing hepatic masses, hepatic perfusion abnormalities, and small hyperenhancing lesions along the margins of the spinal canal.

DIAGNOSIS: VHL syndrome with pancreatic cysts and serous cystadenomas, hepatic metastases from previously resected pancreatic NET, and spinal hemangioblastomas

COMMENT: This companion case to Case 4.19 illustrates the presence of multiple pancreatic serous cystadenomas (clusters of cysts, some with a small central scar) and simple cysts in a patient with VHL syndrome. This case also demonstrates the importance of including the liver in surveillance imaging in this patient population.

NETs are relatively common in patients with VHL syndrome, and while it is true that their behavior is generally less aggressive than that of de novo pancreatic NETs, they are nevertheless metastatic in 10% to 15% of patients. The presence of hepatic metastases could in theory result from renal cell carcinoma, pancreatic NET, or, less likely, another primary tumor; however, the patient in this case had no significant renal involvement. Therefore, the diagnosis of metastatic NET could be made fairly confidently even before a lesion was biopsied.

The large portocaval lymph node seen on the FSE T2-weighted images had been called the primary pancreatic tumor on several of the patient's annual or semiannual examinations until someone read a clinical note and discovered that the patient had had a Whipple procedure 10 years earlier to resect a NET in the uncinate process. (This case illustrates the principle that inspection of previous reports, while generally a good idea, can also on occasion lead to serial error propagation.) Frequent imaging surveillance (typically performed at 6-month or yearly intervals) is obviously important for patients with VHL syndrome. Abdominal examinations should focus on the kidneys, pancreas, and adrenals, but the liver should always be included to assess for metastatic disease. This case also illustrates the typical appearance of spinal hemangioblastomas, which are best appreciated as small enhancing lesions within the canal or neuroforamen on arterial phase postgadolinium images.

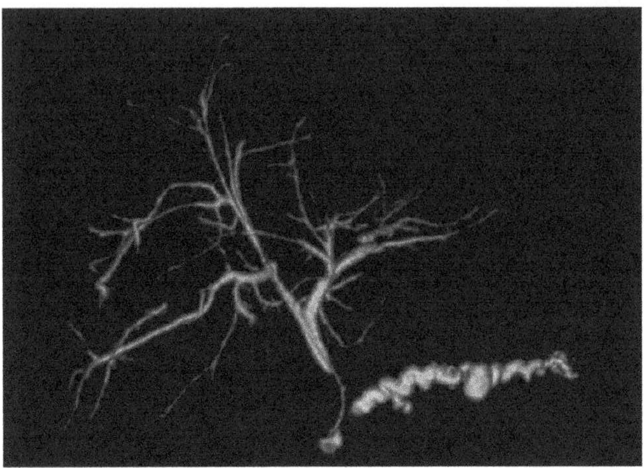

Figure 4.21.1

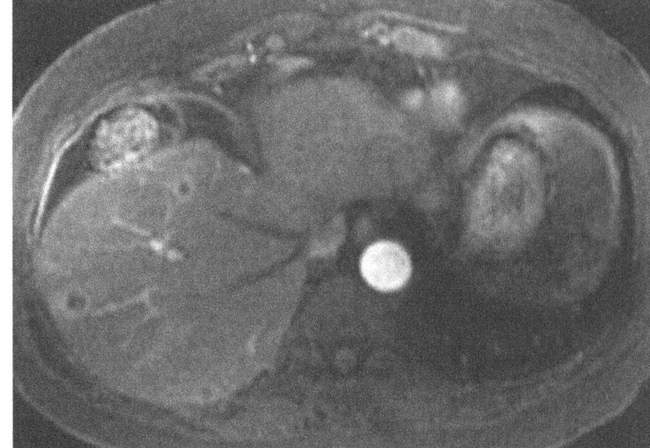

Figure 4.21.2

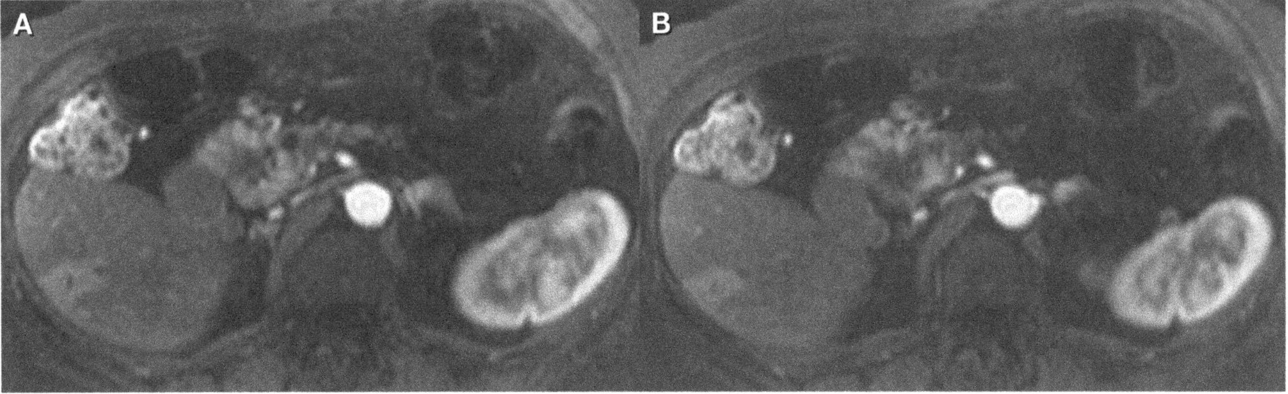

Figure 4.21.3

HISTORY: 68-year-old woman with pruritus, jaundice, and generalized weakness

IMAGING FINDINGS: VR image from 3D FRFSE MRCP (Figure 4.21.1) demonstrates biliary and pancreatic ductal dilatation, with obstruction at the level of the pancreatic head, and a small biliary stent extending into the duodenum. Axial arterial phase postgadolinium 3D SPGR image through the hepatic dome (Figure 4.21.2) reveals 3 small ring-enhancing lesions. Additional arterial phase 3D SPGR images at the level of the pancreatic head (Figure 4.21.3) show an ill-defined spiculated hypoenhancing mass. Note also a wedge-shaped perfusion abnormality in the peripheral right hepatic lobe.

DIAGNOSIS: Pancreatic adenocarcinoma with hepatic metastases

COMMENT: Adenocarcinoma accounts for 85% to 95% of all pancreatic malignancies and is the fourth leading cause of cancer-related death. Most patients are 60 to 80 years old when pancreatic adenocarcinoma is initially diagnosed; men are affected approximately twice as often as women. Abdominal pain, weight loss, and jaundice are the most frequent presenting symptoms; however, these usually occur late in the disease after local invasion or metastatic spread. In 75% of patients, the tumor is nonresectable at presentation. The overall prognosis is poor, with a 1-year survival rate of less than 20% and a 5-year survival rate of 5%. Even for patients who are surgical candidates, the 5-year survival is only 20%.

Since early diagnosis and surgery offer the only hope of long-term survival, much emphasis in the radiology literature has been placed on early detection of pancreatic adenocarcinoma with high sensitivity. CT is the primary imaging technique for assessment of patients with known or suspected pancreatic carcinoma. CT has the important advantage of high spatial resolution, with concerns about the radiation dose being somewhat muted since the patient population is older. Most carcinomas are hypoattenuating on arterial phase images; hepatic metastases are optimally detected on portal venous phase images. In approximately 10% of cases, no mass is detected with CT, and this has led some authors to suggest that MRI could have a primary role in detection and staging of pancreatic carcinoma. Indeed, 1 paper noted that MRI enabled visualization of 80% of tumors which appeared isodense to pancreas on multiphase contrast-enhanced CT.

There is some truth to this point of view. However, it is important to realize that adenocarcinomas are often subtle lesions on MRI as well and are not infrequently visualized on only 1 series. Therefore, optimal technique and patient cooperation (including adequate breath-holding) are critical for a successful examination.

In this case, for example, the mass is visualized only on the arterial phase postgadolinium 3D SPGR images as an indistinct hypoenhancing spiculated lesion in the pancreatic head. Precontrast T2-weighted images were not helpful, diffusion-weighted images were not obtained (this is a slightly older case), and the lesion could not be identified on additional precontrast or postcontrast T1-weighted acquisitions. What is useful in this case is the MRCP image, which shows the classic double-duct sign (and which would have been even more impressive absent the biliary stent) indicating an obstruction in the pancreatic head and stimulating a careful search of this region.

The appearance of adenocarcinoma on dynamic 3D SPGR images is variable. Most lesions are hypointense to normal pancreas on arterial phase images and often on portal venous phase images as well. Some tumors demonstrate slow enhancement, which is likely a result of the desmoplastic reaction stimulated by the lesion, and may be isointense or even slightly hyperintense to adjacent pancreas on equilibrium phase images. Many lesions have well-defined borders, but the presence of a poorly marginated mass, as in this case, is more indicative of adenocarcinoma than other lesions in the differential diagnosis, such as NET or metastasis. The classic adenocarcinoma has mildly increased T2-signal intensity and moderately increased signal intensity on diffusion-weighted images, and it is hypointense relative to normal pancreas on precontrast T1-weighted images.

Adenocarcinomas, even very small lesions, are notorious for causing obstruction of the pancreatic duct and biliary ducts, and the presence of a high-grade obstruction, even without an obvious mass, should raise suspicion for this diagnosis. Many authors also emphasize the importance of this sign in the differential diagnosis of pancreatic masses (ie, a mass causing only mild obstruction is unlikely to be an adenocarcinoma); however, in our experience, while this is true more often than not, it is probably not reliable enough to make us reconsider our diagnosis.

MRI is likely more sensitive than CT for detection of hepatic metastases from pancreatic carcinoma, and it may increase the level of confidence in your diagnosis. In this case, for example, CT showed fewer lesions and no ring enhancement, making the diagnosis much easier with MRI. Hepatobiliary contrast agents (in particular, gadoxetate disodium [Eovist]) are favored by some of our colleagues to provide optimal sensitivity for detection of hepatic metastases in the hepatobiliary phase. Keep in mind, however, that the relatively small doses of Eovist, in comparison to standard extracellular contrast agents, may decrease the quality of the arterial phase images and may therefore limit visualization of the primary tumor. Eovist is also contraindicated in patients with severe biliary obstruction—hepatic excretion of the contrast agent may be greatly reduced, resulting in poor-quality hepatobiliary phase images.

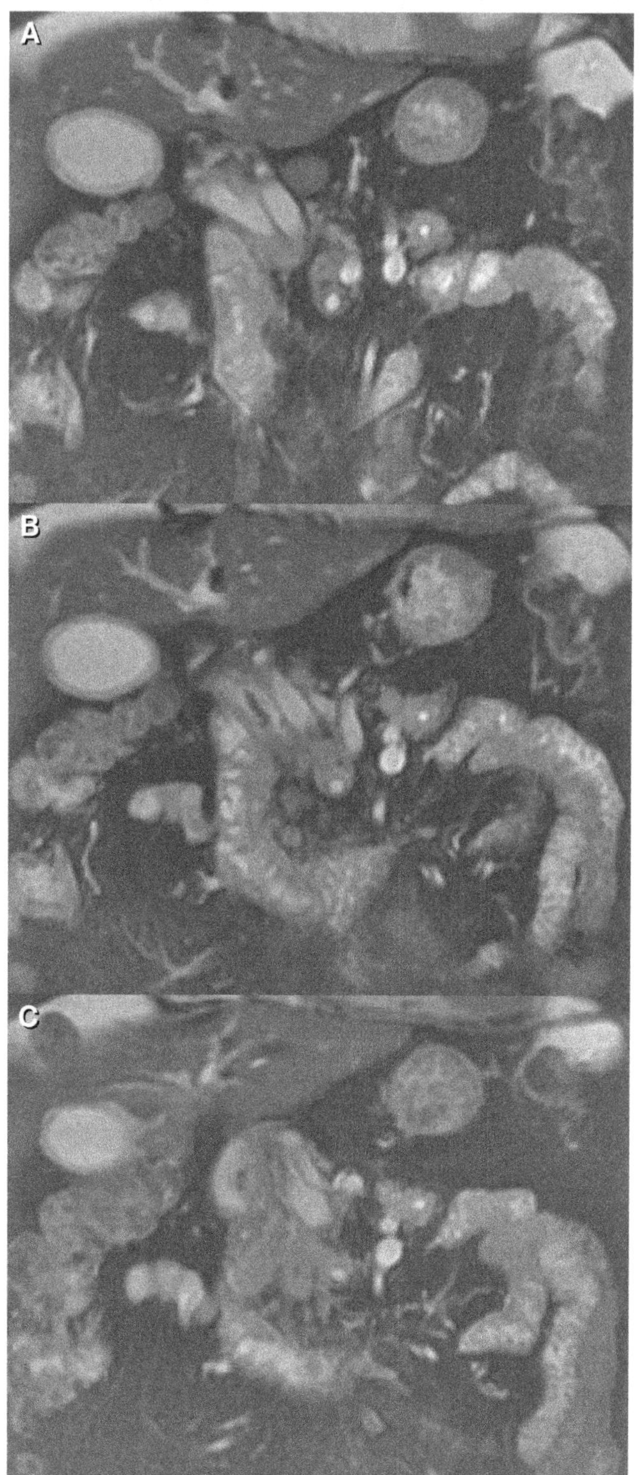

Figure 4.22.1

Figure 4.22.2

HISTORY: 76-year-old man with weight loss and jaundice

IMAGING FINDINGS: Coronal fat-suppressed 2D SSFP images (Figure 4.22.1) reveal an ill-defined mass involving the pancreatic uncinate process and completely encasing the superior mesenteric artery. Note also multiple small lymph nodes and associated soft tissue stranding adjacent to the duodenum. Axial portal venous phase postgadolinium 3D SPGR images (Figure 4.22.2) demonstrate a subtle minimally enhancing mass extending from the uncinate process and encasing the superior mesenteric artery.

DIAGNOSIS: Pancreatic adenocarcinoma with vascular encasement

COMMENT: This case, an example of arterial encasement in pancreatic adenocarcinoma, illustrates the principle that 1 pulse sequence may be particularly valuable in any given examination. In this case, the fat-suppressed SSFP acquisition most clearly shows the extensive circumferential encasement of the superior mesenteric artery.

Both arterial involvement and venous involvement are common features of pancreatic adenocarcinoma. In the past, they were considered absolute contraindications to surgery, but advances in surgical reconstructive techniques now allow fairly extensive venous resections. In fact, staging criteria have been revised to emphasize arterial involvement while eliminating references to venous extension. The definition of disease that is resectable or unresectable is somewhat controversial and differs from center to center. Generally, it is most useful to group patients into disease categories such as 1) clearly resectable disease (ie, small tumors confined to the pancreas without metastatic disease); 2) clearly unresectable disease (ie, tumors with extensive circumferential arterial encasement, distant metastases, or adenopathy outside the surgical field); and 3) borderline disease. Borderline disease may have tumor abutting but not encircling the celiac and superior mesenteric arteries with common hepatic artery involvement limited to short segment encasement (allowing for placement of an arterial bypass graft). Likewise, venous involvement in resectable disease is generally limited to short segment occlusion with patent veins above and below (allowing for resection and reconstruction).

Arterial and portal venous phase postgadolinium 3D SPGR images are generally the most useful for delineating vascular encasement and occlusion, but occasionally venous opacification is poor, or image quality is limited by motion artifact, for which fat-suppressed SSFP acquisitions can be helpful. In this case, the primary tumor is exophytic and shows only minimal enhancement on the postgadolinium images. Its extension around the superior mesenteric artery is visible but quite subtle. The tumor is much more apparent on the coronal SSFP images, and the extensive arterial encasement (intermediate-signal-intensity tumor surrounding the bright vessel) is obvious. These images are also useful for detection of duodenal invasion, since the rapid sequential acquisition frequently reduces or eliminates motion artifact from peristalsis—notice how well seen are the small nodes and soft tissue stranding adjacent to the medial margin of the duodenum.

CASE 4.23

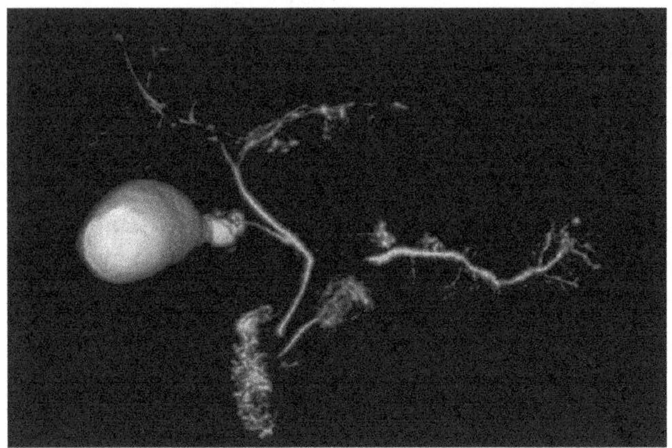

Figure 4.23.1

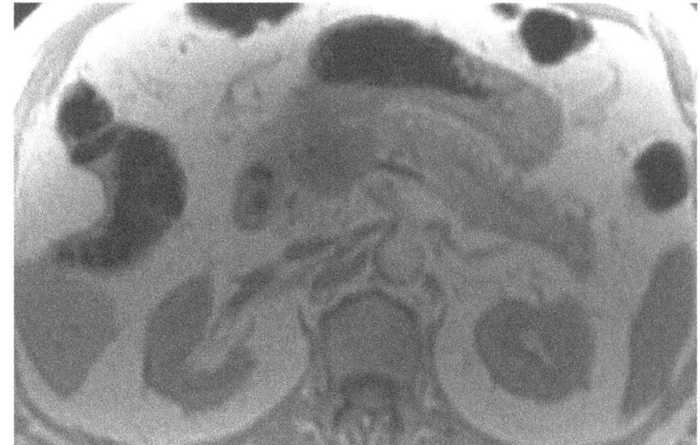

Figure 4.23.2

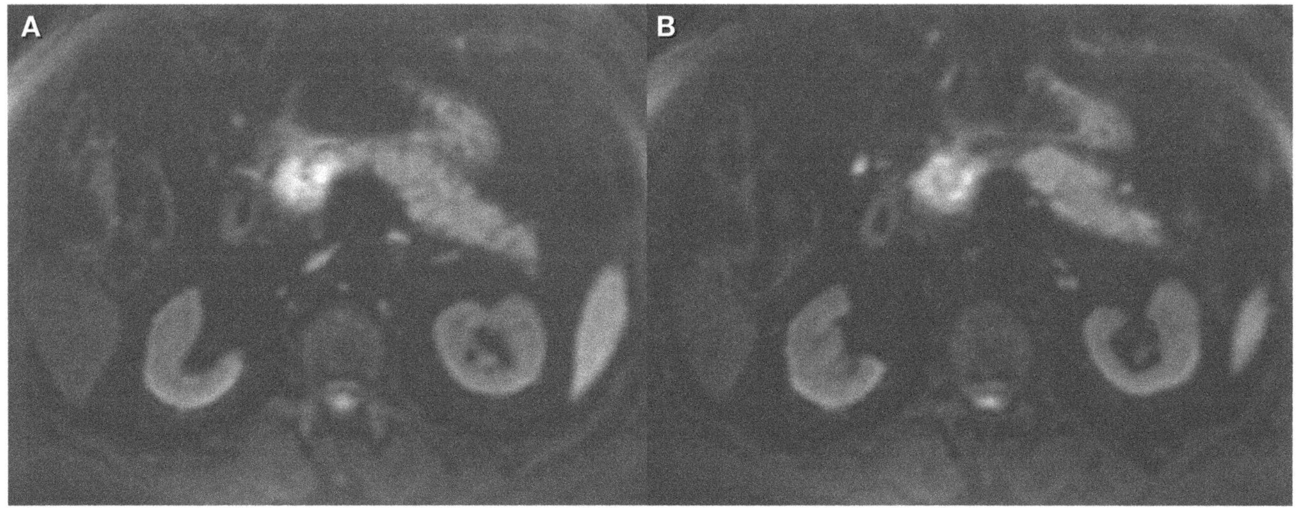

Figure 4.23.3

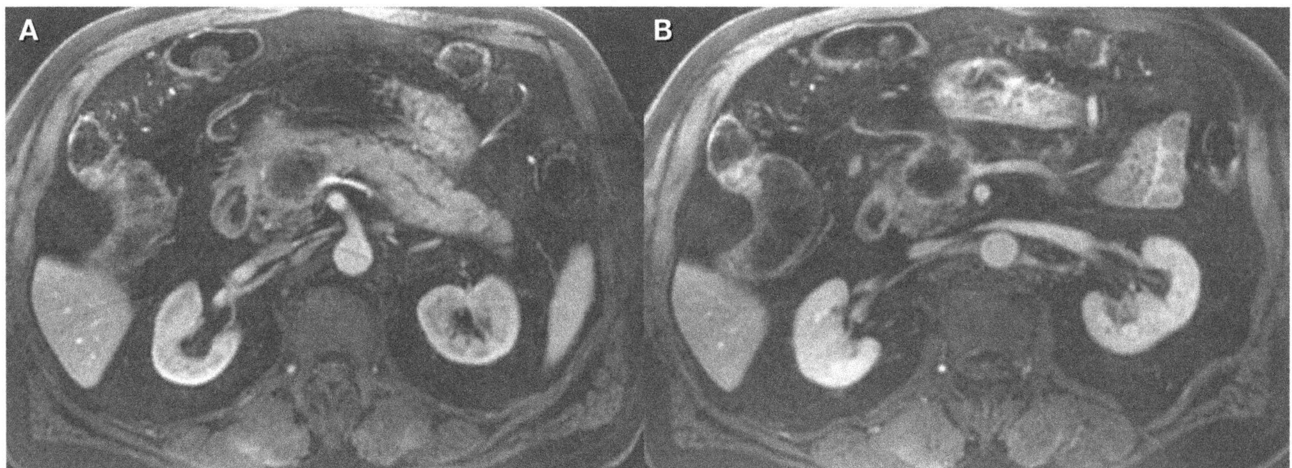

Figure 4.23.4

HISTORY: 69-year-old man with a recent onset of upper abdominal pain

IMAGING FINDINGS: VR image from 3D FRFSE MRCP (Figure 4.23.1) reveals abrupt cutoff of the pancreatic duct in the neck of the pancreas with mild proximal dilatation. Axial T1-weighted in-phase 2D SPGR image (Figure 4.23.2) demonstrates an ill-defined mass in the pancreatic neck that is slightly hypointense to adjacent pancreas. Axial diffusion-weighted images (b=800 s/mm^2) (Figure 4.23.3) show a high-signal-intensity lesion corresponding to the pancreatic neck mass, and axial portal venous phase postgadolinium 3D SPGR images (Figure 4.23.4) reveal a hypoenhancing mass with compression and occlusion of the portal confluence.

DIAGNOSIS: Pancreatic adenocarcinoma

COMMENT: This case shows many of the classic MRI findings of pancreatic adenocarcinoma. The mass is mildly hypointense to adjacent pancreas on the precontrast T1-weighted image; it shows marked hyperintensity on the diffusion-weighted images; and it has only minimal internal enhancement on portal venous phase postgadolinium images, which also demonstrate venous occlusion at the level of the portal confluence.

The excellent visibility of the tumor on diffusion-weighted images is the ideal appearance, but unfortunately many lesions are only faintly visible, and some cannot be identified at all. Several papers have described the appearance of pancreatic adenocarcinoma on DWI, most with more favorable results than we have seen in our clinical practice. However, 1 author has noted the extensive variability in delineation of the tumor and, in particular, reported that in nearly 50% of lesions the signal intensity and ADC values of pancreatic parenchyma upstream from the site of ductal obstruction were essentially identical to those of the mass. Nevertheless, DWI is an important technique that should be included in every examination, not only for identification of the primary lesion but also for detection of hepatic and peritoneal metastases as well as enlarged lymph nodes.

This tumor shows the expected hypointensity relative to pancreas on precontrast T1-weighted images. The conspicuity of the mass may be accentuated or reduced depending on whether fat suppression is applied. With a mildly or moderately atrophic gland, fatty infiltration of the parenchyma results in higher signal intensity (and greater contrast with the tumor) on images obtained without fat suppression; however, the normal nonatrophic pancreas often has relatively high T1-signal intensity on the basis of acinar protein, and the contrast between tumor and normal tissue is accentuated by fat suppression. In-phase and out-of-phase 2D or 3D SPGR acquisitions can also be helpful for focal fatty infiltration with or without focal pancreatitis. This relatively uncommon abnormality can appear as a contour deformity and may show mild enhancement differences from normal parenchyma. Therefore, it can be difficult to distinguish from an infiltrative lesion on other pulse sequences; however, the presence of fat (ie, signal drop-out from in-phase to out-of-phase images) effectively excludes the diagnosis of adenocarcinoma.

The one arguably atypical feature of this case is that the degree of pancreatic ductal obstruction is relatively small considering the size of the tumor. Nevertheless, the mild dilatation of the upstream duct and its abrupt cutoff are suggestive of the diagnosis.

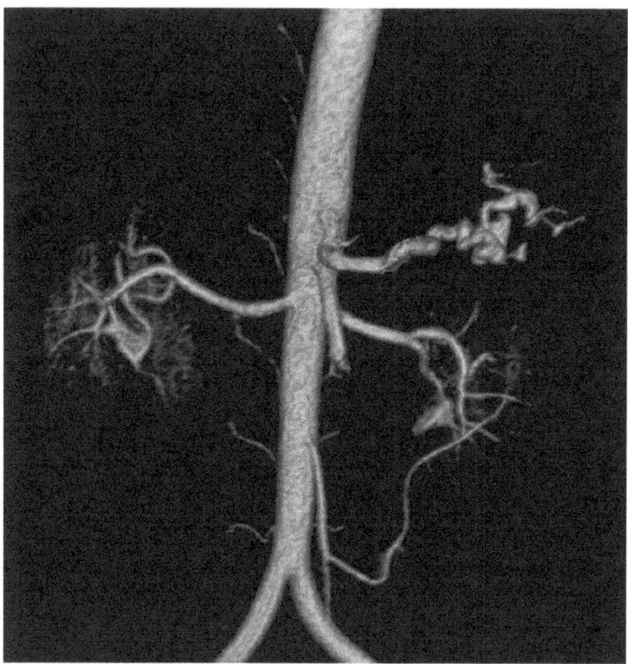

Figure 4.24.1

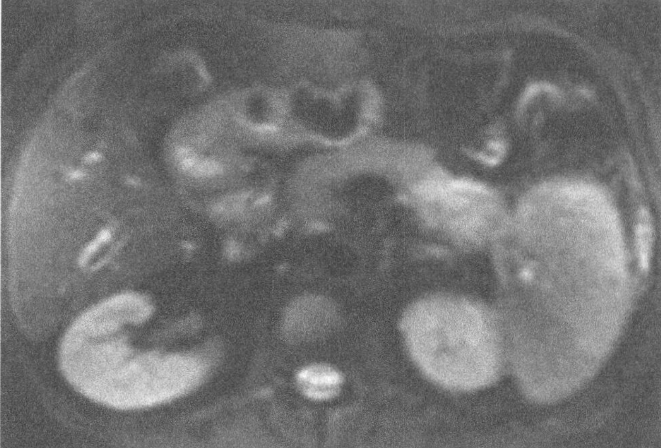

Figure 4.24.2

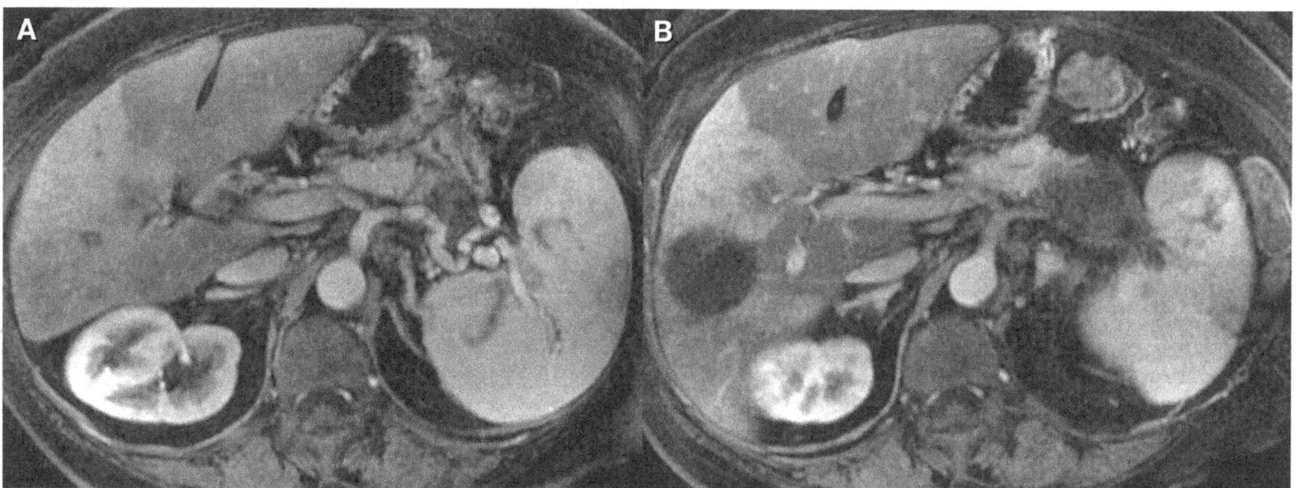

Figure 4.24.3

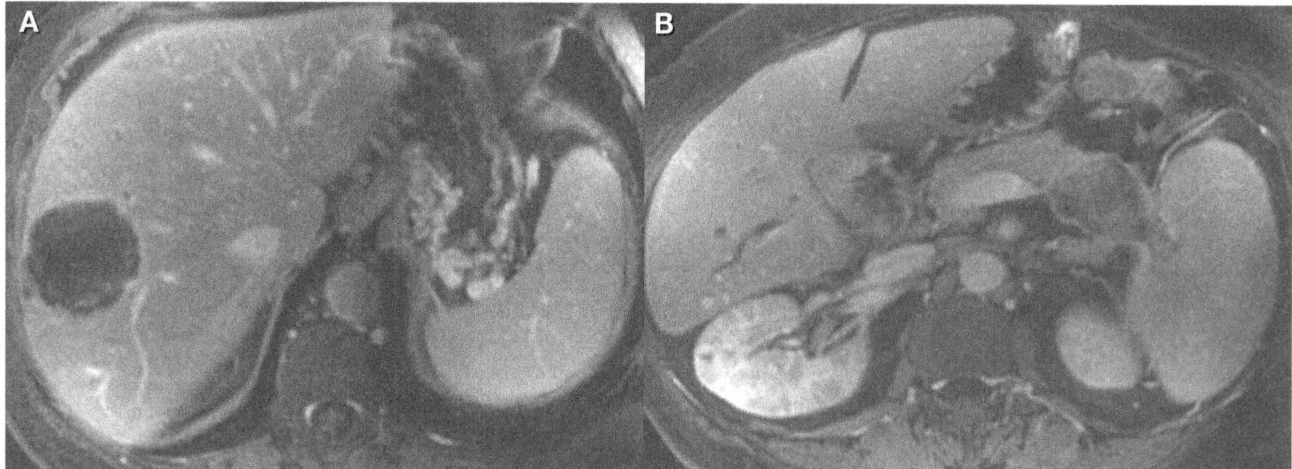

Figure 4.24.4

HISTORY: 66-year-old woman with loss of appetite, weight loss, fatigue, and upper abdominal pain

IMAGING FINDINGS: VR image from 3D contrast-enhanced MRA (Figure 4.24.1) shows marked irregularity of the distal splenic artery. Axial diffusion-weighted image (b=600 s/mm^2) (Figure 4.24.2) reveals a hyperintense mass in the pancreatic tail. Axial arterial phase postgadolinium 3D SPGR images (Figure 4.24.3) demonstrate a hypoenhancing mass in the tail of the pancreas and a large hypoenhancing lesion in the right hepatic lobe with associated perfusion abnormality. Notice also irregularity of the distal splenic artery as it crosses the pancreatic tail. Equilibrium phase postgadolinium 3D SPGR images (Figure 4.24.4) reveal multiple gastric varices, ring enhancement of the hepatic mass, and mild internal and rim enhancement of the distal pancreatic lesion. The splenic vein is absent.

DIAGNOSIS: Pancreatic adenocarcinoma with encasement of the splenic artery, splenic vein thrombosis, and hepatic metastases

COMMENT: This case illustrates a typical appearance of adenocarcinoma in an atypical location—roughly 70% of these lesions occur in the head and neck. Both arterial encasement and venous occlusion are nicely illustrated. The MRA demonstrates extensive irregularity and beading of the distal splenic artery, and the arterial phase 3D SPGR images show the artery passing through the body of the tumor in the pancreatic tail. The tumor also occludes the splenic vein, and the classic sign of isolated gastric varices is well seen on the portal venous phase postgadolinium images.

The primary tumor is straightforward to identify on arterial phase and portal venous phase postgadolinium images, and it shows high signal intensity on diffusion-weighted images. The large hepatic metastasis would be difficult to miss with any imaging technique. It has a large associated segmental perfusion abnormality on arterial phase images and ring enhancement on portal venous phase images.

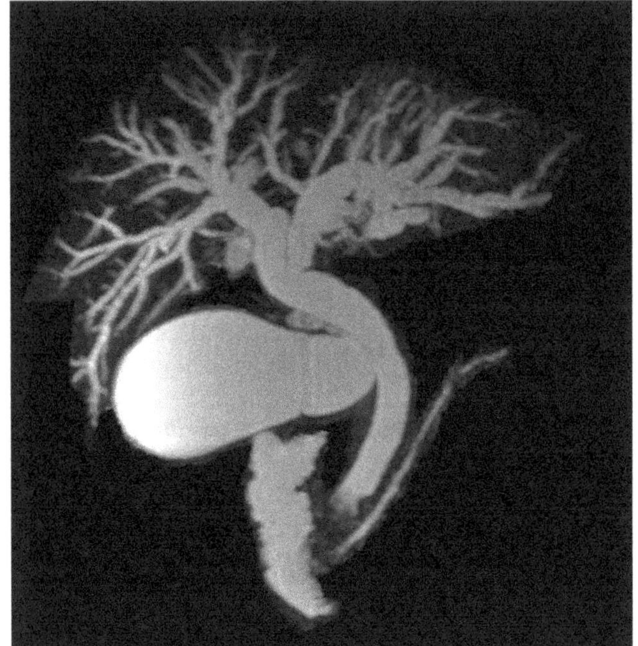

Figure 4.25.1

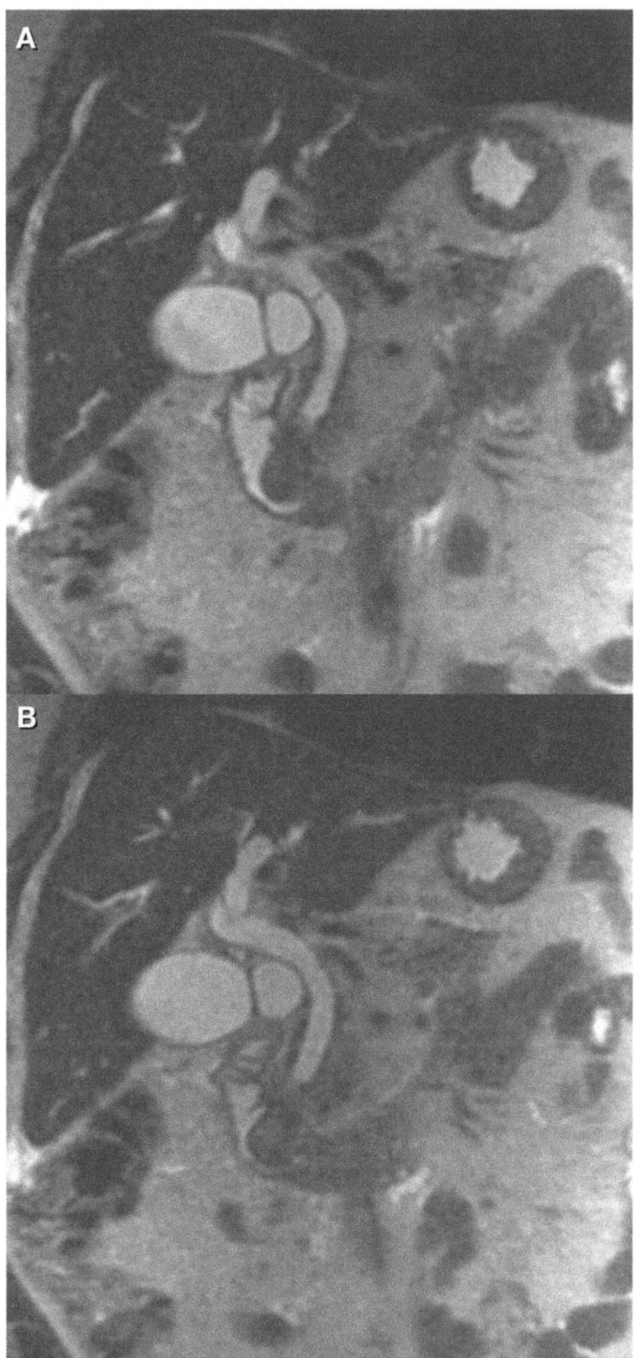

Figure 4.25.2

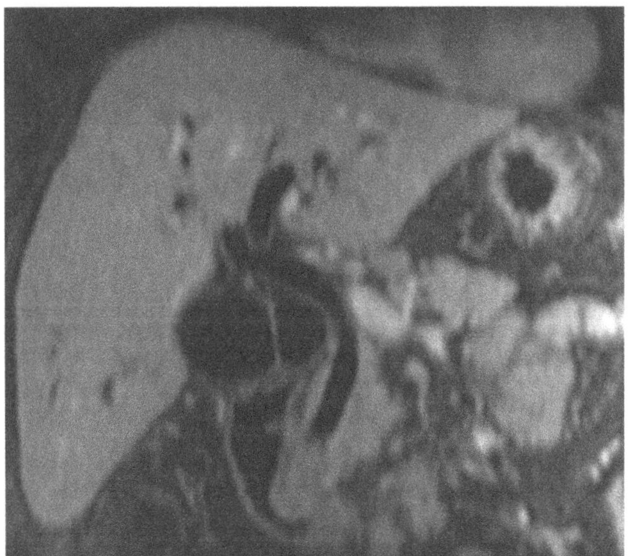

Figure 4.25.3

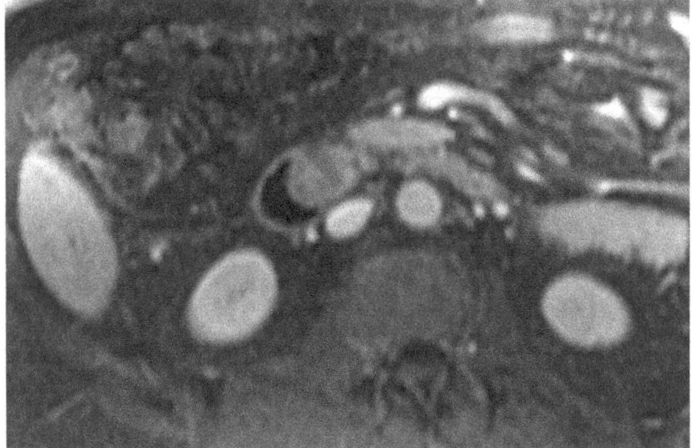

Figure 4.25.4

HISTORY: 64-year-old man with elevated liver function tests

IMAGING FINDINGS: MIP image from 3D FRFSE MRCP (Figure 4.25.1) reveals a filling defect in the distal common bile duct, diffuse intrahepatic biliary dilatation, and mild dilatation of the pancreatic duct. Coronal oblique SSFSE images (Figure 4.25.2) demonstrate an ovoid ampullary mass projecting into the duodenum with obstruction of the common bile duct. Portal venous phase 3D SPGR images in coronal oblique (Figure 4.25.3) and axial oblique (Figure 4.25.4) reformations show mild heterogeneous enhancement of the ampullary lesion.

DIAGNOSIS: Ampullary carcinoma

COMMENT: Ampullary carcinoma arises from the epithelial lining of the ampulla of Vater, where the common bile duct and the pancreatic duct drain into the second portion of the duodenum at the duodenal papilla. This rare disease accounts for 0.2% of all gastrointestinal tract cancer; however, if all periampullary tumors are included (ie, pancreatic carcinoma, cholangiocarcinoma, and duodenal carcinoma occurring within 2 cm of the ampulla), the percentage increases to 5%.

Pathologists have identified 2 distinct types of ampullary carcinomas that are distinguished by their epithelium of origin: intestinal and pancreaticobiliary. Intestinal tumors originate from the intestinal epithelium overlying the ampulla, and pancreaticobiliary tumors arise from the lining of the distal common duct and pancreatic duct. Most authors believe that intestinal ampullary tumors carry a more favorable prognosis than pancreaticobiliary lesions, although this has not been demonstrated in large series.

Ampullary carcinomas typically occur in older patients (more often men) and more frequently in patients with familial polyposis syndromes. Biliary obstruction causes symptoms at an early stage, which probably leads to early detection and an improved prognosis; however, this also means that often the lesions are small and difficult to detect on MRI. For this reason, it is important to perform a complete examination and not just MRCP. MRCP sequences (ie, 2D SSFSE and 3D FSE or FRFSE sequences with very long TEs) are designed to image fluid and suppress signal from anything with a shorter T2 relaxation time (like solid tissue). Therefore, MRCP images will effectively localize the site of obstruction but often don't provide much information about the underlying cause. Dynamic contrast-enhanced 3D SPGR images, T2-weighted images, and diffusion-weighted images are often helpful in visualizing and characterizing these lesions.

Several findings have been described in patients with ampullary carcinoma, the most common of which are probably ampullary bulging and a nodular ampullary mass projecting into the duodenum, as seen in this case. Irregular narrowing of the distal common bile duct or pancreatic duct (or both), according to 1 paper, is seen almost exclusively in pancreaticobiliary tumors.

Even with a complete examination with good images, it is not always possible to make a definitive diagnosis. Other possibilities include papillary edema or stenosis, a stone in the distal common bile duct (sometimes harder to sort out than you might think), ampullary adenoma, cholangiocarcinoma, pancreatic carcinoma, and duodenal carcinoma. A small obstructive lesion centered at the ampulla with mild enhancement less than in adjacent pancreas should raise the possibility of an ampullary carcinoma. The ampullary region is an unusual location for cholangiocarcinoma, and most of these lesions have involvement of a longer segment of the common bile duct. Pancreatic carcinoma is usually larger at diagnosis and might have a more eccentric origin. Impacted stones or debris can sometimes be difficult to distinguish from a small mass, especially if they are not outlined by fluid. Precontrast fat-saturated SPGR images may be helpful if they reveal high-signal-intensity material in the distal common bile duct (this is more likely debris or stones than neoplasm, and, of course, stones or debris should not enhance after contrast administration).

Patients with ampullary carcinoma have a better prognosis than those with pancreatic adenocarcinoma. Surgical resection is the preferred treatment, and 5-year survival rates are 35% to 65%.

CASE 4.26

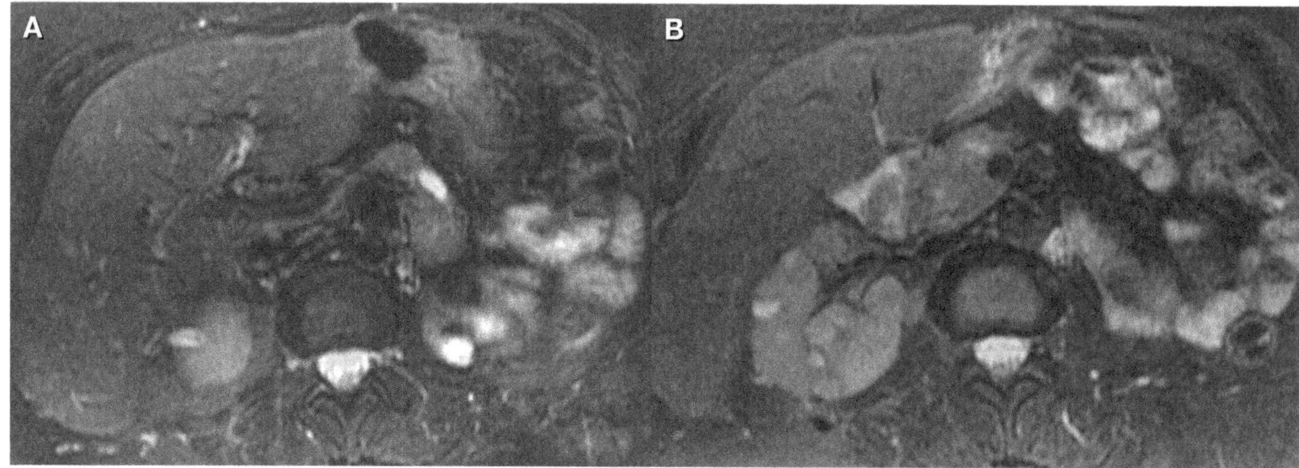

Figure 4.26.1

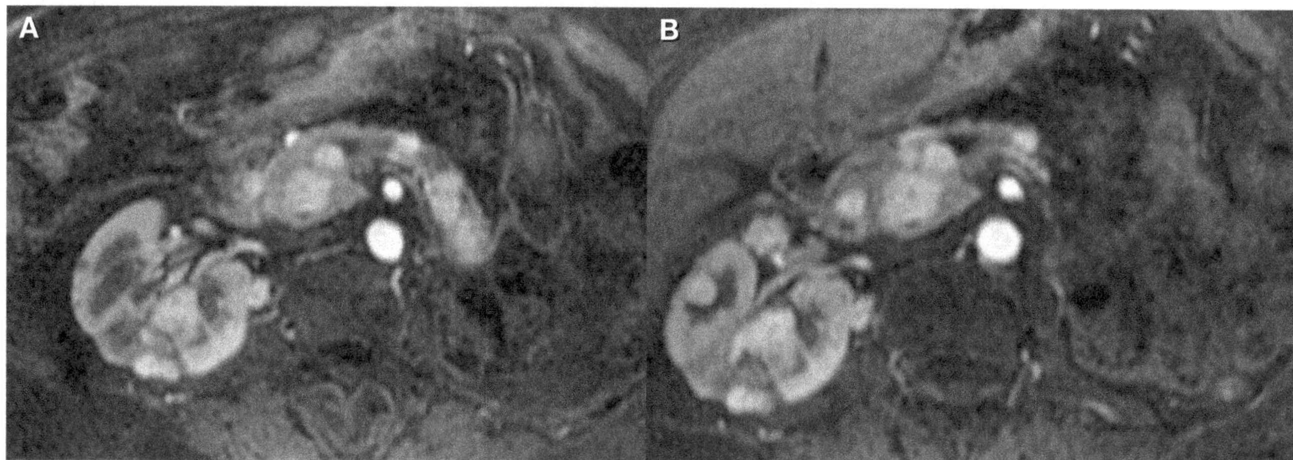

Figure 4.26.2

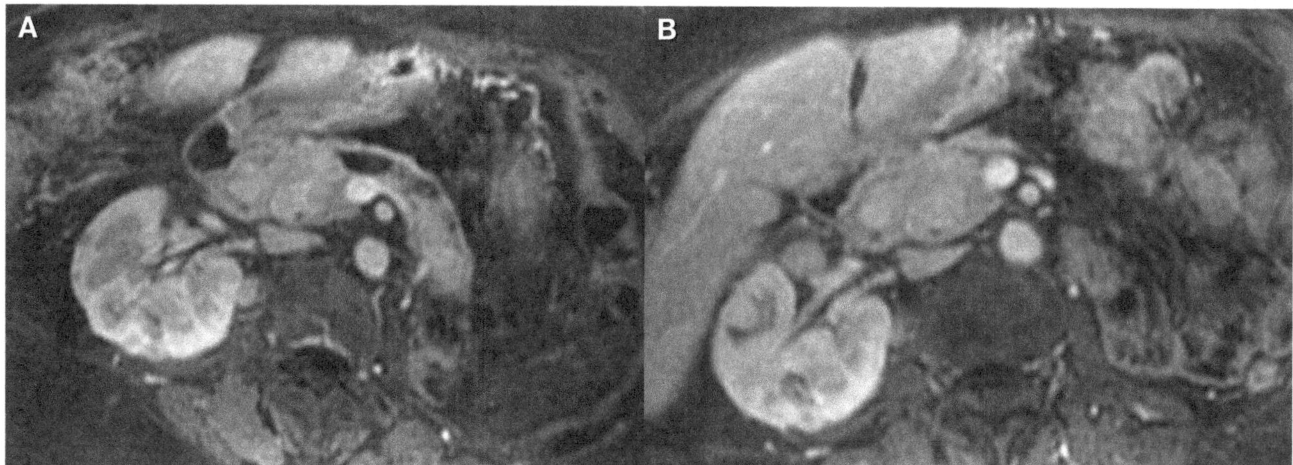

Figure 4.26.3

HISTORY: 78-year-old man with a history of renal cell carcinoma

IMAGING FINDINGS: Axial fat-suppressed FRFSE T2-weighted images (Figure 4.26.1) reveal multiple mildly hyperintense lesions in the pancreatic body and head. Arterial phase (Figure 4.26.2) and venous phase (Figure 4.26.3) post-gadolinium 3D SPGR images also demonstrate multiple hypervascular pancreatic lesions. Notice also the absent left kidney (from a nephrectomy) and multiple solid enhancing lesions in the right kidney.

DIAGNOSIS: Pancreatic metastases from renal cell carcinoma

COMMENT: Metastatic involvement of the pancreas by renal cell carcinoma is less common than metastasis to the liver and lungs and is often overlooked. Pancreatic metastases are relatively rare. The reported incidence for patients with advanced cancers is 1% to 11%, and these account for 2% to 5% of all pancreatic malignant tumors. Renal cell carcinoma is the most common tumor that metastasizes to the pancreas, and pancreatic metastases are found synchronously in 12% of patients presenting with widespread metastatic disease. Numerous case reports have also described isolated pancreatic metastases occurring in asymptomatic patients as many as 20 to 30 years after the initial nephrectomy. Whether renal cell carcinoma cells truly have an affinity for the pancreas is a matter of debate in the literature, and the value of surgical resection of the isolated pancreatic metastasis is also not well established.

This case emphasizes the importance of obtaining good arterial phase postgadolinium images that include the pancreas (and liver) when performing surveillance imaging of patients who have had resection of renal cell carcinoma. The lesions are faintly visible on T2-weighted images if you look carefully, but they and the multiple recurrent lesions in the right kidney are much more obvious on the arterial phase 3D SPGR acquisition (before becoming inconspicuous again on the portal venous phase images). For this reason, we always perform multiphase dynamic imaging with a test bolus to optimize the arterial phase acquisition in patients with renal cell carcinoma. We also find that the axial plane rather than the coronal plane (favored by some for renal imaging) is more conducive to actually looking at the pancreas and is probably more accurate for preoperative staging of tumor thrombus in the renal vein and inferior vena cava.

The imaging characteristics of the pancreatic lesions are nonspecific. NETs could have an identical appearance, as could other hypervascular metastases such as melanoma or breast carcinoma. However, since the left kidney is absent and the right kidney has multiple solid lesions, the odds of an additional diagnosis are fairly low. The 1 instance when the differential diagnosis is more than an academic exercise is VHL syndrome, in which both renal cell carcinoma metastases and NET are very real possibilities for an enhancing pancreatic mass.

Precontrast series should not be overlooked when assessing for pancreatic lesions. Many years ago, a somewhat arcane discussion in the literature considered whether contrast was really necessary to identify pancreatic masses. Some authors believed that noncontrast T1-weighted (and T2-weighted) images were sufficient. This is undoubtedly true some of the time, and occasionally lesions are actually less conspicuous on postgadolinium images (this is much more likely to occur if you're not performing 3D dynamic imaging), but it is not really a serious issue today. Nearly everyone gives contrast if possible, and everyone should perform precontrast T1-weighted imaging. DWI can also be helpful in identifying pancreatic lesions. There are almost no published data on optimal b values for detection of pancreatic metastases, but generally DWI tends to increase lesion conspicuity compared with conventional T2-weighted FSE imaging at a cost in the signal to noise ratio.

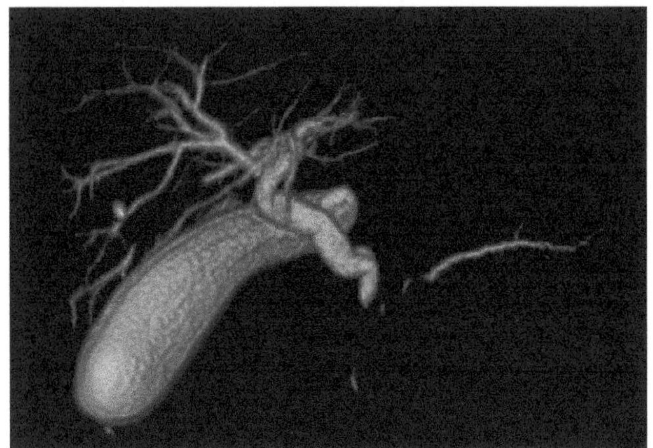

Figure 4.27.1

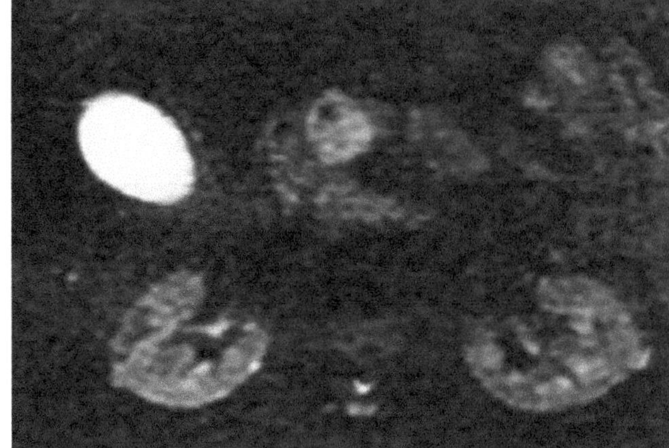

Figure 4.27.3

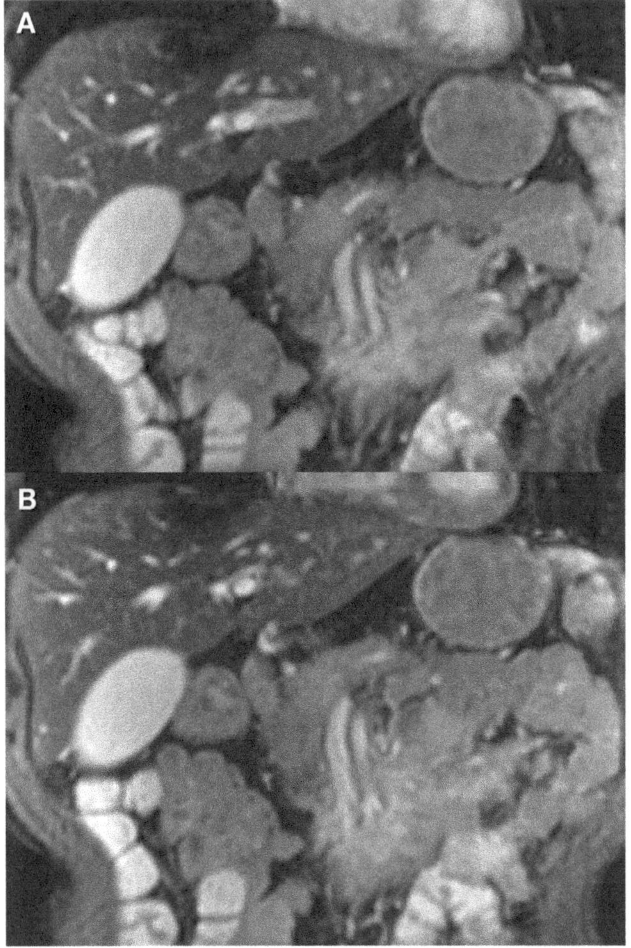

Figure 4.27.2

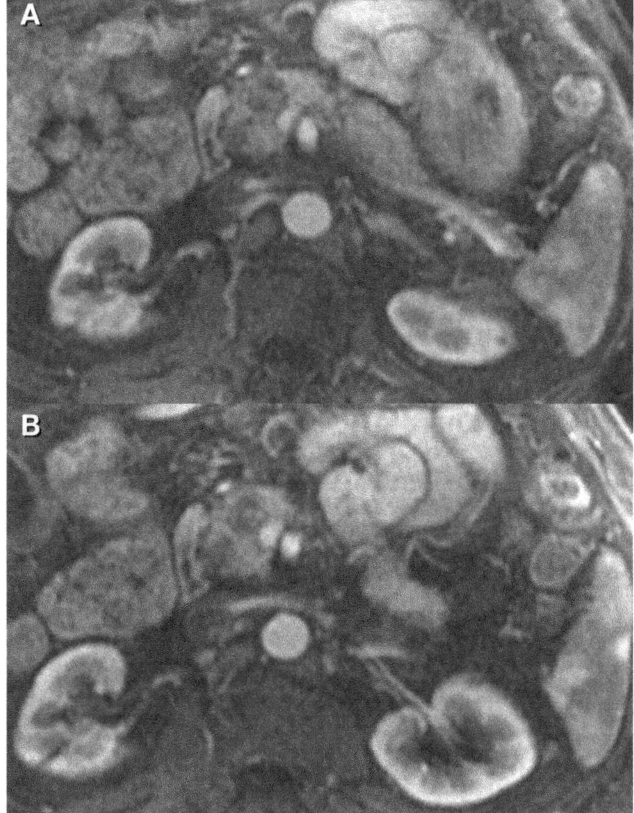

Figure 4.27.4

HISTORY: 67-year-old man with dilated bile ducts and a pancreatic mass on US

IMAGING FINDINGS: VR image from 3D FRFSE MRCP (Figure 4.27.1) reveals obstruction of the common bile duct and the pancreatic duct at the level of the pancreatic head. Coronal fat-suppressed 2D SSFP images (Figure 4.27.2) demonstrate the dilated pancreatic duct extending to an ill-defined mass in the pancreatic head slightly hyperintense to adjacent pancreas. Conglomerate mesenteric adenopathy is seen inferior to the pancreas. Axial diffusion-weighted image (b=300 s/mm^2) (Figure 4.27.3) also shows a hyperintense mass in the pancreatic head. Arterial phase postgadolinium 3D SPGR images in axial oblique reformatted views (Figure 4.27.4) demonstrate a corresponding hypoenhancing mass as well as a smaller lesion posteriorly in the pancreatic head.

DIAGNOSIS: Pancreatic lymphoma (secondary)

COMMENT: Pancreatic lymphoma, either primary or secondary, is usually B-cell non-Hodgkin lymphoma, which frequently arises in extranodal sites. Approximately 40% to 50% of patients have extranodal involvement at diagnosis, most commonly in the stomach and small bowel. Primary pancreatic non-Hodgkin lymphoma is rare and accounts for less than 0.5% of all pancreatic malignancies and 1% of extranodal lymphomas. Secondary involvement of the pancreas is more common. Although only 1% to 2% of patients have obvious pancreatic disease at presentation, autopsy studies have shown pancreatic involvement in 30% of patients who died of disseminated lymphoma.

Presenting symptoms of patients who have pancreatic lymphoma are typically nonspecific and include abdominal pain, weight loss, a palpable mass, and, less commonly, jaundice and acute pancreatitis. Focal and diffuse forms of pancreatic involvement have been described in the radiology literature. The focal presentation, shown in this case, may be difficult to distinguish from ductal adenocarcinoma and most commonly occurs in the pancreatic head, with a variable size at presentation. Lesions usually show decreased T1-signal intensity relative to normal pancreas, mildly increased T2-signal intensity, and moderately increased signal intensity on diffusion-weighted images, with relatively homogeneous hypoenhancement relative to pancreas on all phases of dynamic postgadolinium acquisitions.

A few imaging features may help to distinguish pancreatic lymphoma from adenocarcinoma. A large tumor with relatively little biliary or pancreatic ductal dilatation is more likely a lymphoma. This case shows mild dilatation of the pancreatic duct in the tail, and one could argue that an adenocarcinoma of similar size would likely have resulted in more severe ductal obstruction. Enlarged lymph nodes below the level of the renal vein are more commonly seen in lymphoma, as are prominent conglomerate mesenteric nodes, bulky retroperitoneal nodes, and splenomegaly. Vascular invasion is also much less frequent in lymphoma than in adenocarcinoma.

The diffuse form of pancreatic lymphoma is infiltrative and leads to diffuse enlargement of the pancreas with poorly defined margins, an appearance that occasionally can be confused with acute pancreatitis or autoimmune pancreatitis (in fact, diffuse pancreatic lymphoma may cause pancreatitis). The pancreas generally has low signal intensity on T1-weighted images and normal or mildly reduced signal intensity on T2-weighted images, with a variable appearance on postgadolinium images.

Treatment of pancreatic lymphoma usually consists of chemotherapy or radiotherapy (or both), which is different from adenocarcinoma, where surgical excision is the treatment of choice, so a tissue diagnosis is important for confirming the diagnosis. A study of 42 cases of hematologic malignancies involving the pancreas found that in 36% of the cases a hematologic diagnosis was not suspected before the tissue diagnosis, and this resulted in 4 resections for presumed pancreatic adenocarcinoma. Patients with secondary pancreatic lymphoma have a more favorable prognosis (5-year survival rates, 30%-35%) than patients with adenocarcinoma. The limited statistics for primary pancreatic lymphoma are somewhat less encouraging, with 12-month survival of 33% in 1 series.

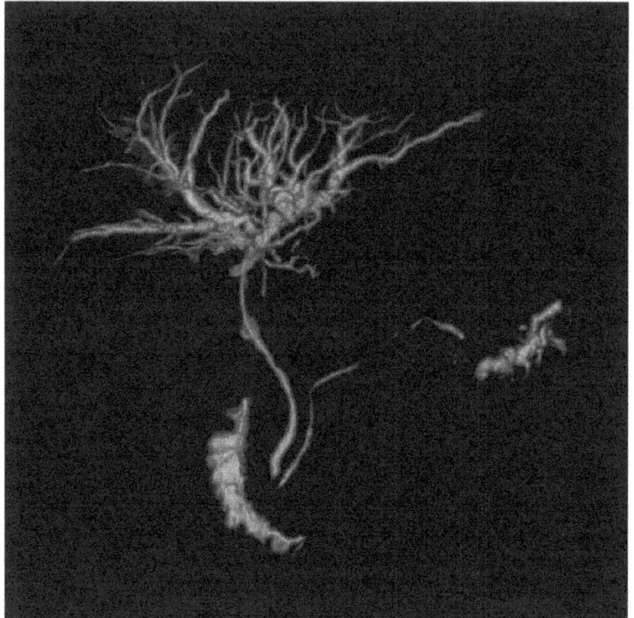

Figure 4.28.1

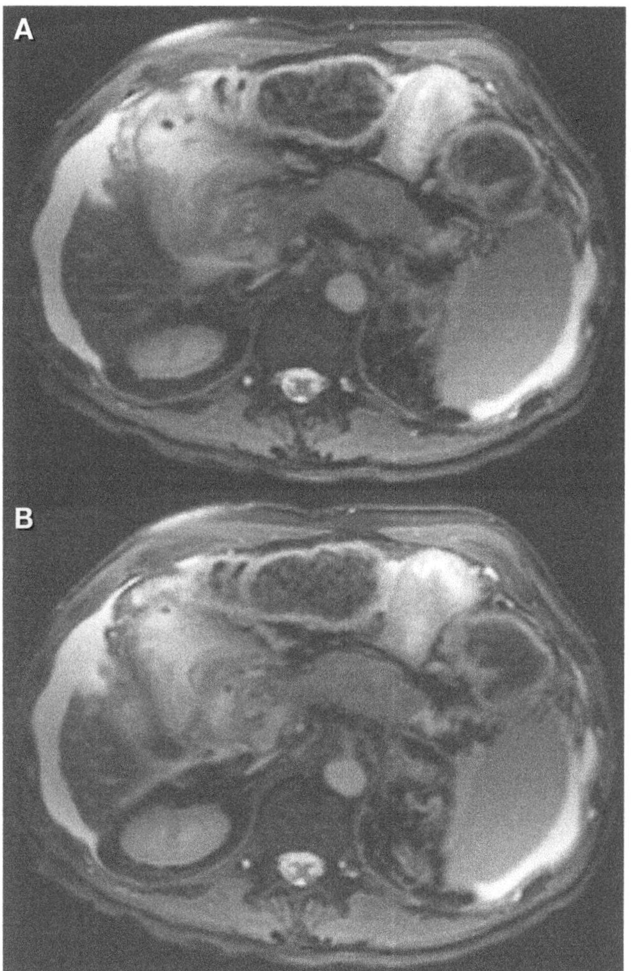

Figure 4.28.2

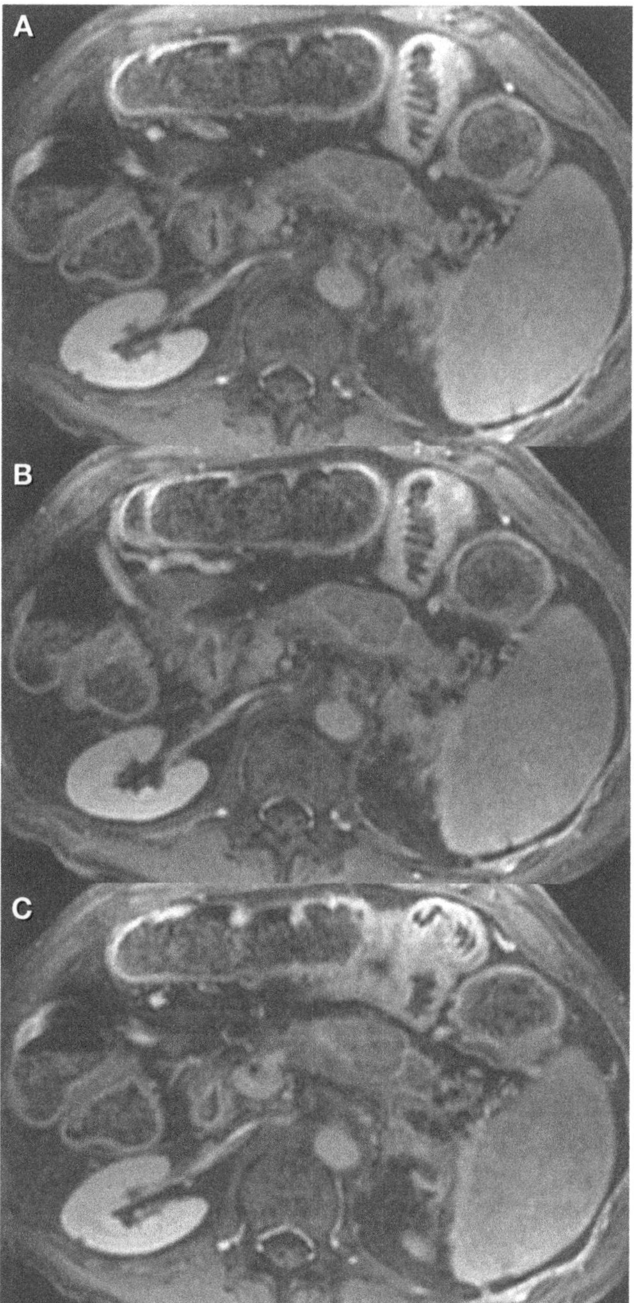

Figure 4.28.3

HISTORY: 63-year-old man with abdominal pain

IMAGING FINDINGS: VR image from 3D FRFSE MRCP (Figure 4.28.1) demonstrates focal dilatation of the pancreatic duct in the tail of the pancreas. Note also moderate diffuse intrahepatic biliary dilatation. Axial fat-suppressed SSFP images (Figure 4.28.2) reveal a mass enlarging the pancreatic body, dilatation of the pancreatic duct proximally in the tail, and atrophy of the pancreatic tail. Axial equilibrium phase postgadolinium 3D SPGR images (Figure 4.28.3) demonstrate a corresponding hypoenhancing mass with a hyperintense rim in the body of the pancreas. The splenic vein is absent, and there is ill-defined enhancing soft tissue adjacent to the splenic hilum.

DIAGNOSIS: Acinar cell carcinoma

COMMENT: ACC is a rare neoplasm that arises from the acinar cells of the pancreas, typically in patients who are older (aged 50-70 years) and male. Even though pancreatic tissue consists of more than 80% acinar cells (vs 4% ductal epithelial cells), ACC occurs much less frequently than ductal adenocarcinoma and comprises approximately 1% of pancreatic neoplasms.

Presenting symptoms are typically vague, consisting of abdominal pain, weight loss, chronic anemia, and pancreatitis. Jaundice is a relatively infrequent manifestation. Two features are especially interesting: 1) ACC is unique among pancreatic tumors in that it can be associated with elevated α-fetoprotein levels, and 2) some reports have linked ACC with lipase hypersecretion syndrome, which is characterized by fevers, arthralgias, skin rashes, and fat necrosis.

Histologic examination of ACC has revealed 2 distinct growth patterns: 1) an acinar organization (ie, the berry-shaped terminus of an exocrine gland) and 2) cells in solid sheets or cords. Immunohistochemical staining is strongly positive for the digestive enzymes of the exocrine pancreas (eg, trypsin, chymotrypsin, lipase, and phospholipase).

The MRI appearance of ACC has not been well characterized. The largest MRI series consists of 4 cases; the CT experience is slightly larger. In general, ACCs tend to be larger than most adenocarcinomas at diagnosis, and a sizable percentage contain cystic or necrotic components. Lesions are frequently well marginated, in contrast to the infiltrative appearance of adenocarcinoma, and an enhancing capsule has been identified in 50% to 60% of cases (including this case). On dynamic postgadolinium images, ACC is generally hypointense relative to adjacent pancreas on all phases. Pancreatic or biliary ductal obstruction is thought to occur less frequently in ACC than in ductal adenocarcinoma, although this case has a prominent obstruction of the pancreatic duct in the tail of the pancreas.

Prospective ACC diagnosis based on imaging findings alone is unlikely; however, in an older patient, the presence of a large hypoenhancing pancreatic mass with well-defined margins, an enhancing capsule, and cystic or necrotic components could suggest something other than the garden-variety ductal adenocarcinoma. The differential diagnosis also includes NET, which is not always a hyperenhancing tumor, and cystadenoma or cystadenocarcinoma if lesions have prominent cystic or necrotic components.

The prognosis with ACC is thought to be relatively poor, although given the rarity of the disease, these statistics are of uncertain value. In 1 series of 39 patients with ACC, median survival was 19 months, with longer survival among patients who had localized disease; recurrence was frequent after surgical resection.

CASE 4.29

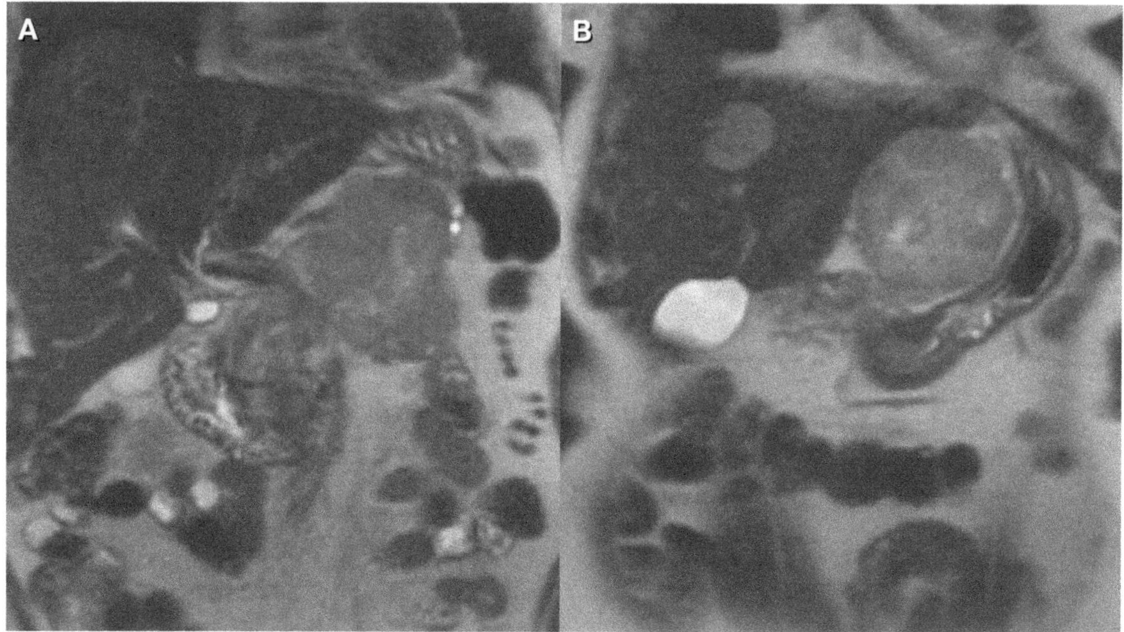

Figure 4.29.1

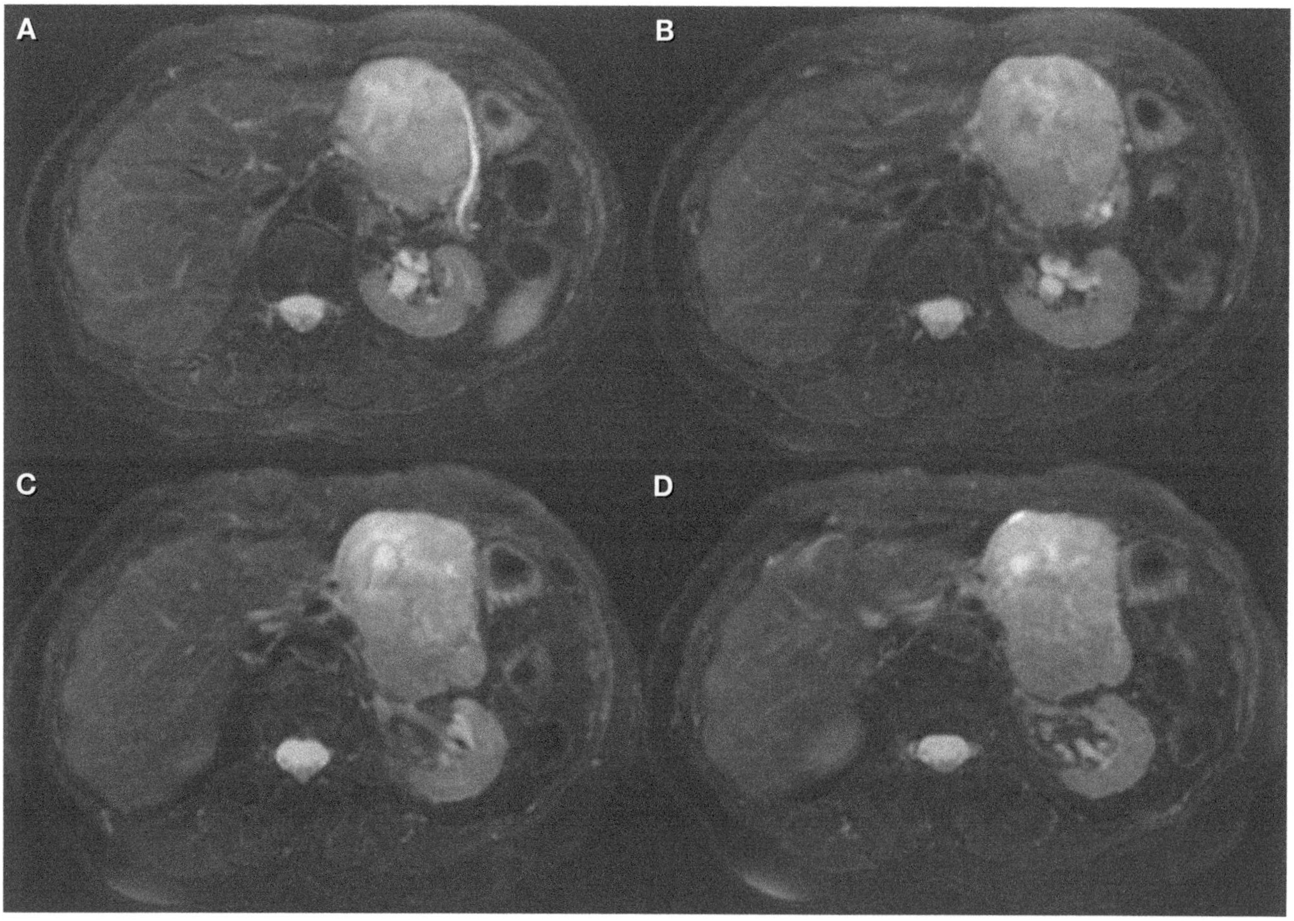

Figure 4.29.2

HISTORY: 84-year-old woman who palpated a mass in her upper abdomen

IMAGING FINDINGS: Coronal SSFSE images (Figure 4.29.1) demonstrate a large heterogeneous mass in the gastrohepatic ligament originating from the pancreas and displacing the stomach to the left. Note the high-signal-intensity lesion in the anterior left hepatic lobe. Axial fat-suppressed FSE T2-weighted images (Figure 4.29.2) reveal a heterogeneous mass with moderately increased signal intensity that appears intimately associated with the pancreas. The pancreatic duct is mildly dilated in Figure 4.29.2A.

DIAGNOSIS: Pancreatic leiomyosarcoma with hepatic metastasis

COMMENT: Primary leiomyosarcomas of the pancreas are extremely rare. They account for approximately 0.1% of pancreatic malignancies, and fewer than 50 cases have been described. The presenting symptoms are nonspecific and most commonly include abdominal pain, weight loss, epigastric tenderness, and a palpable mass. The age at presentation is variable, ranging from 14 to 84 years (the patient in this case is apparently the oldest), and males are affected more frequently.

MRI typically demonstrates a large mass (average diameter in reported cases, approximately 10 cm) with heterogeneous high signal intensity on T2-weighted images and heterogeneous enhancement. Cystic or necrotic components are frequently present, and some lesions have been described as predominantly cystic. A definitive organ of origin is often difficult to ascertain for large upper abdominal tumors; however, in this case, the mass encircles the pancreatic body and does not clearly invade the adjacent stomach or liver.

The pathologic diagnosis relies primarily on immunohistochemical characteristics, including the presence of desmin or smooth muscle actin. Most lesions show features typical of aggressive tumors (eg, high cellularity, pleomorphism, and high mitotic counts). The clinical behavior often reflects this aggressiveness, with frequent local invasion, hematogenous metastasis, and nodal metastatic disease. The prognosis is generally considered to be poor; however, long-term survival has been described for a few patients after surgical resection of localized disease.

The differential diagnosis includes metastatic or locally invasive leiomyosarcoma originating from another organ as well as atypical presentations of more common lesions such as adenocarcinoma or NETs. A large gastrointestinal stromal tumor could have a similar appearance.

ABBREVIATIONS

ACC acinar cell carcinoma
ADC apparent diffusion coefficient
AIP autoimmune pancreatitis
CF cystic fibrosis
CP chronic pancreatitis
CT computed tomography
DWI diffusion-weighted imaging
FRFSE fast-recovery fast-spin echo
FSE fast-spin echo
IgG4 immunoglobulin G4
IPAS intrapancreatic accessory spleen
IPMN intraductal papillary mucinous neoplasm
MCN mucinous cystic neoplasm
MIP maximum intensity projection
MRA magnetic resonance angiography
MRCP magnetic resonance cholangiopancreatography
MRI magnetic resonance imaging
NET neuroendocrine tumor
SCN serous cystic neoplasm
SPGR spoiled gradient recalled
SPIO superparamagnetic iron oxide
SPN solid pseudopapillary neoplasm
SSFP steady-state free precession
SSFSE single-shot fast-spin echo
TE echo time
3D 3-dimensional
2D 2-dimensional
US ultrasonography
VHL von Hippel-Lindau
VR volume-rendered
WHO World Health Organization

5.

SPLEEN

CASE 5.1

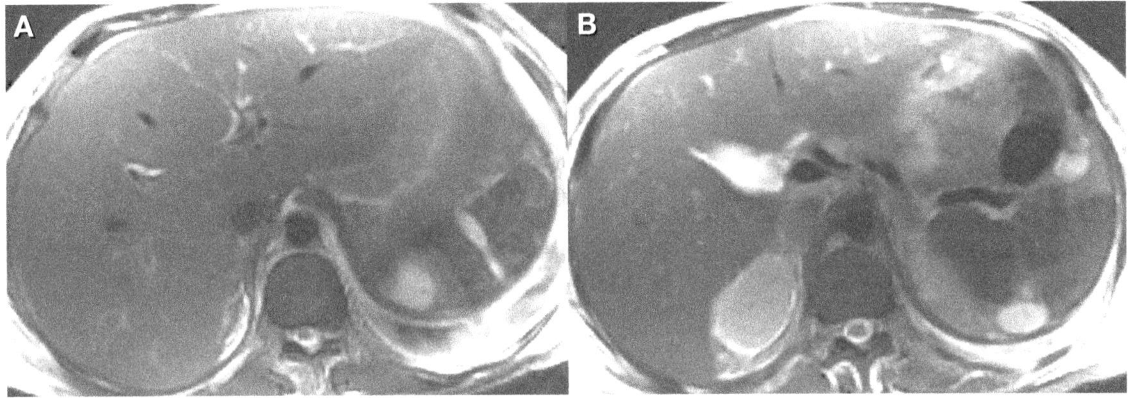

Figure 5.1.1

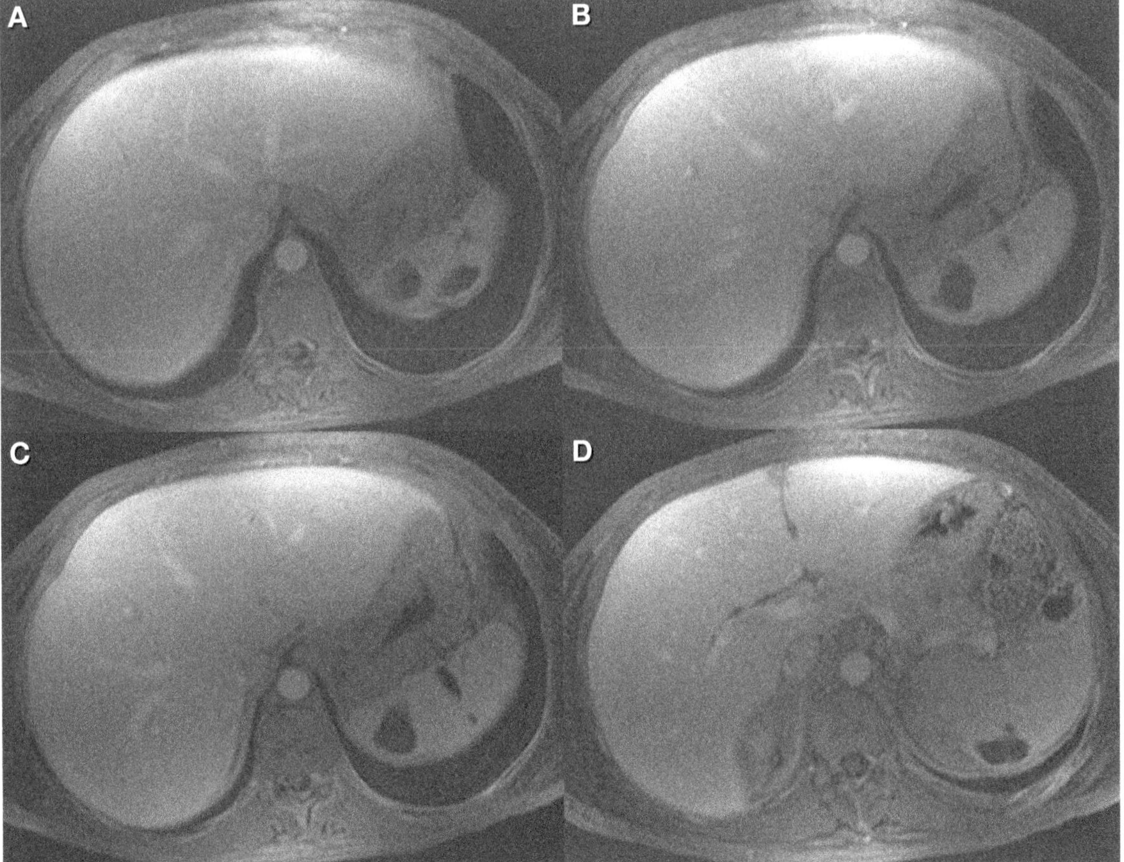

Figure 5.1.2

HISTORY: 35-year-old man with a long history of diabetes mellitus and recent episode of peritonitis now presents with recurrent abdominal pain and fever

IMAGING FINDINGS: Axial fat-suppressed FSE T2-weighted images (Figure 5.1.1) show multiple hyperintense lesions in the spleen. The diffuse, decreased signal intensity throughout the remainder of the spleen is due to hemosiderosis and iron deposition. Gadolinium-enhanced axial 3D SPGR images (Figure 5.1.2) show multiple hypoenhancing lesions in the spleen, most with subtle ring enhancement.

DIAGNOSIS: Splenic abscesses

COMMENT: The spleen is relatively resistant to infection: Abscesses in the spleen are rare compared to abscesses in other organs, with autopsy studies suggesting an incidence of 0.14% to 0.7%. Risk factors for developing a splenic abscess include immunodeficiency (accounting for as many as 28% of cases), neoplasia, trauma, metastatic infection, splenic infarct, and diabetes mellitus. The clinical presentation is often nonspecific, and the most frequently reported symptoms are fever, nausea, weight loss, malaise, and abdominal pain.

The most common organisms responsible for splenic abscesses reported in large series include aerobic microbes such as streptococci and *Escherichia coli*. Fungal organisms also have a prominent role, and fungal abscesses more commonly manifest as multiple small lesions. Abscesses in the spleen have a similar appearance to abscesses in any other organ. Fluid collections are bright on T2-weighted images and dark on T1-weighted images, with rim enhancement after gadolinium administration. Rim enhancement is somewhat more variable in the spleen than in the liver, probably because of the more heterogeneous enhancement of the background spleen.

Treatment of splenic abscesses is somewhat controversial. Standard therapy includes intravenous antibiotics or antifungal agents with or without splenectomy. The role of percutaneous aspiration or drainage is unclear. Most studies have shown a lower success rate compared with surgery; however, percutaneous methods can be useful in patients who are not surgical candidates.

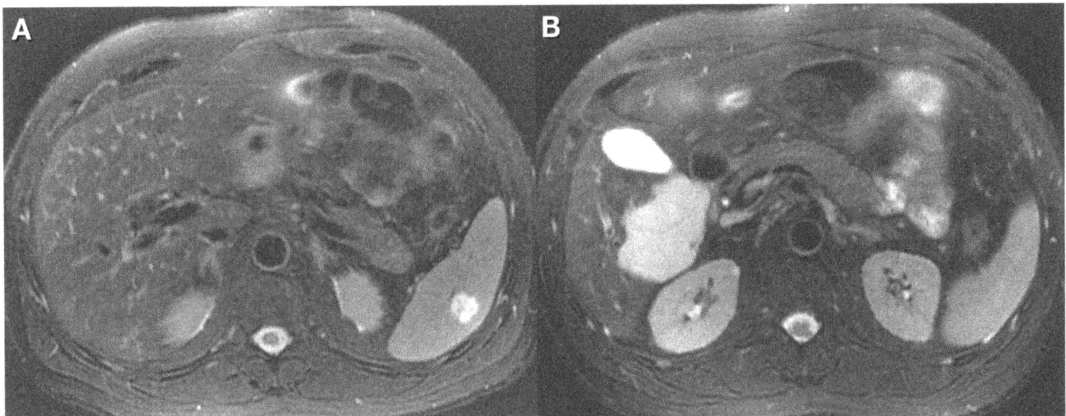

Figure 5.2.1

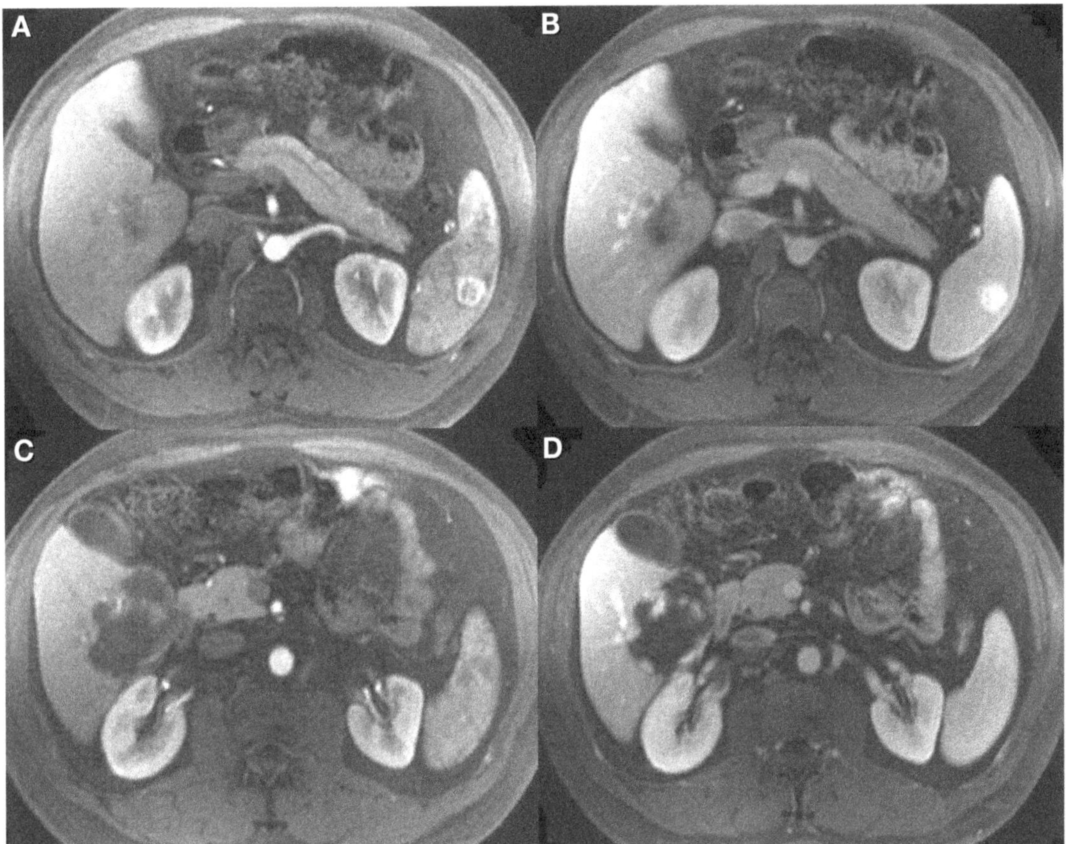

Figure 5.2.2

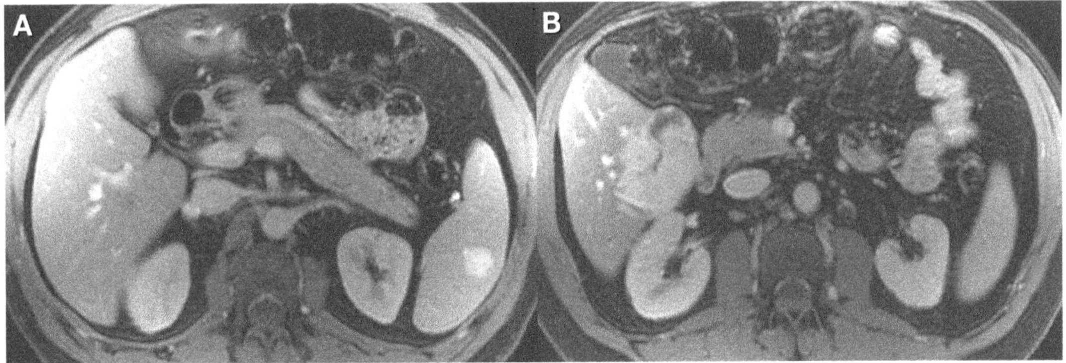

Figure 5.2.3

HISTORY: 51-year-old man with a hepatic mass detected on US at another medical facility

IMAGING FINDINGS: Axial fat-suppressed FSE T2-weighted images (Figure 5.2.1) show markedly hyperintense lesions in the spleen and inferior right hepatic lobe. There is early enhancement of the splenic lesion on an arterial phase postgadolinium 3D SPGR image (Figure 5.2.2A), and the lesion becomes uniformly hyperenhancing compared to the spleen on a portal venous phase image (Figure 5.2.2B). The hepatic lesion shows nodular peripheral enhancement on arterial phase (Figure 5.2.2C) and portal venous phase (Figure 5.2.2D) images. The splenic lesion retains persistent hyperenhancement compared to the spleen on a 5-minute delayed postgadolinium 2D SPGR image (Figure 5.2.3A), while the hepatic lesion has almost completely filled in (Figure 5.2.3B).

DIAGNOSIS: Splenic and hepatic hemangiomas

COMMENT: Hemangiomas are the most common benign primary neoplasm of the spleen, with the prevalence at autopsy ranging from 0.3% to 14%. They are generally asymptomatic and are detected as incidental findings. Multiple splenic hemangiomas have been reported in association with KTS. Complications are rare and include rupture and Kasabach-Merritt syndrome (anemia, thrombocytopenia, and coagulopathy).

Splenic hemangiomas are considered to be congenital lesions arising from the sinusoidal epithelium as nonencapsulated proliferations of vascular channels of variable size lined with a single layer of endothelium.

Early reports on the CT and MRI features of splenic hemangiomas tended to conclude that they looked just like hepatic hemangiomas, with high T2-signal intensity and nodular peripheral enhancement on postcontrast arterial phase images with centripetal progression and persistent enhancement. Others have noted that nodular peripheral enhancement is a relatively uncommon feature of splenic hemangiomas, possibly because the rapid and heterogeneous enhancement of splenic pulp makes this feature difficult to discern. Likewise, the high T2-signal intensity may be somewhat less apparent when compared with the higher baseline T2 signal of the spleen compared to the liver. In any event, a splenic lesion with early and persistent enhancement and T2 hyperintensity is likely a hemangioma, even if it doesn't strictly meet all the criteria for a hepatic hemangioma.

CASE 5.3

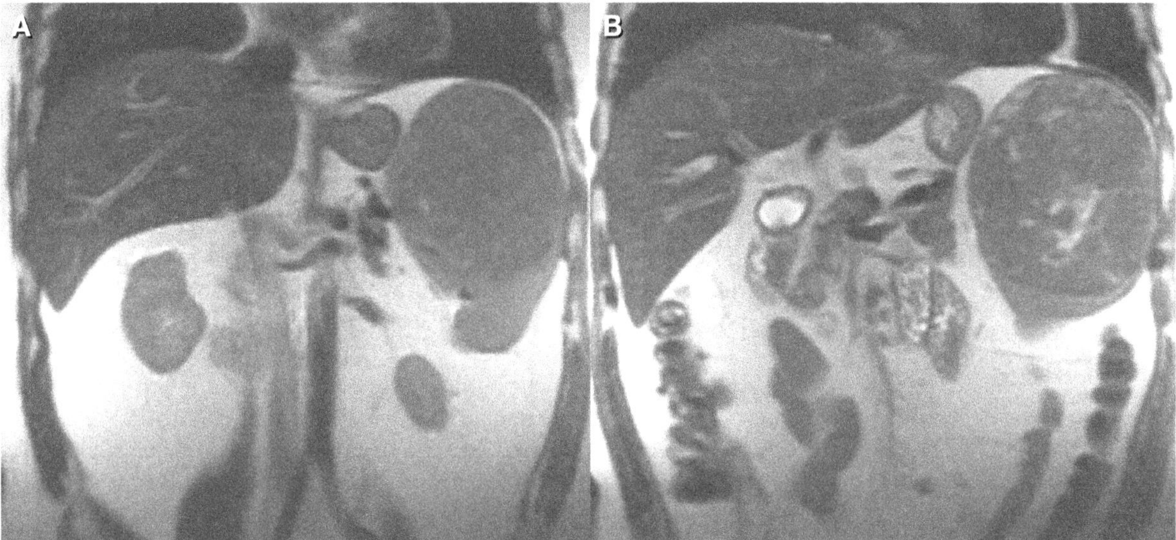

Figure 5.3.1

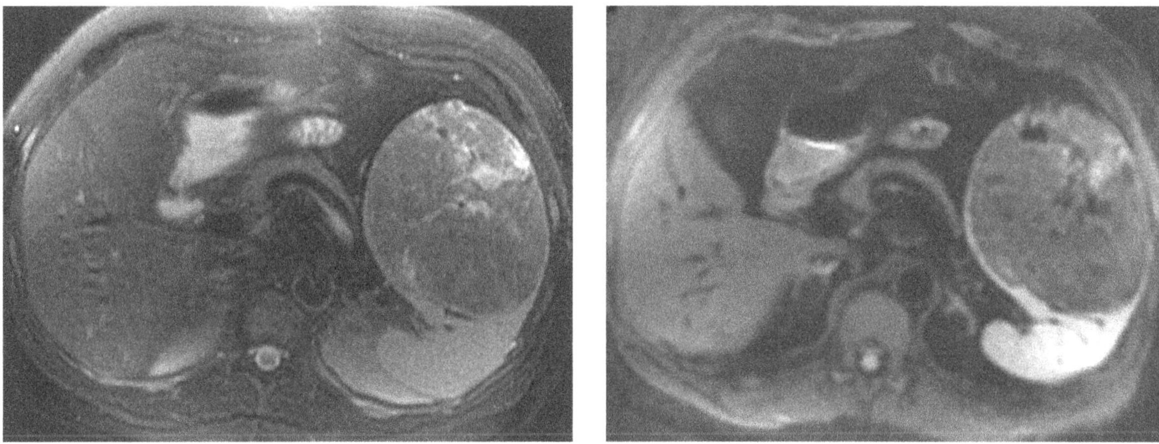

Figure 5.3.2

Figure 5.3.3

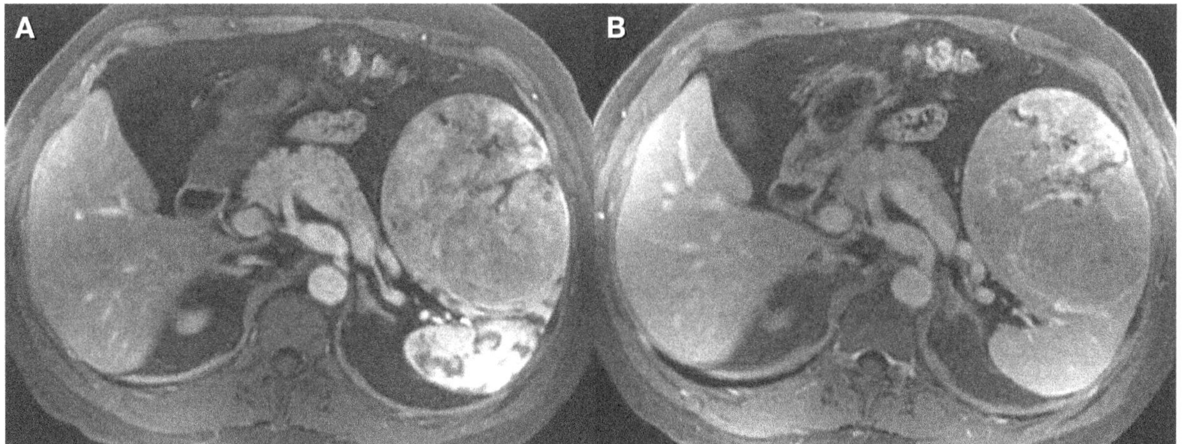

Figure 5.3.4

HISTORY: 53-year-old man with a history of idiopathic thrombocytopenic purpura, elevated liver function tests, and splenomegaly and abdominal CT that showed a focal splenic mass

IMAGING FINDINGS: Coronal SSFSE images (Figure 5.3.1) show a large, mildly heterogeneous mass in the spleen. The mass is hypointense compared to the spleen on axial fat-suppressed FRFSE T2-weighted image (Figure 5.3.2) and on low b-value diffusion-weighted image (b=100 s/mm^2) (Figure 5.3.3). Arterial phase (Figure 5.3.4A) and equilibrium phase (Figure 5.3.4B) postgadolinium 3D SPGR images show mild hypoenhancement of the mass compared to the spleen.

DIAGNOSIS: Splenic hamartoma

COMMENT: The tried-and-true method of dealing with splenic masses ("I don't know what it is, but it's probably benign") has been remarkably successful for many years and across multiple modalities, but occasionally you'll encounter a mass so large that even clinicians will notice it and begin to ask inconvenient questions. This case fits into that category. The presence of a large mass, and probably an ambiguous report ("the lesion could represent a primary or secondary splenic neoplasm"), eventually led to a splenectomy.

Splenic hamartomas are rare lesions first described by Rokitansky in 1861; 150 to 200 cases have been published. The true incidence is unknown, but autopsy studies have suggested a prevalence of 0.024% to 0.13%. Most patients are asymptomatic, and the lesion is typically discovered as an incidental finding. Splenic hamartomas have been reported in association with tuberous sclerosis and Wiskott-Aldrich syndrome.

Some controversy in the pathology literature exists concerning whether a hamartoma is a true neoplasm, a posttraumatic lesion, or a congenital abnormality. Hamartomas are composed of a mixture of unorganized vascular channels surrounded by fibrotic cords of red pulp with or without lymphoid white pulp. Distinguishing a hamartoma from a hemangioma may be difficult, although usually immunohistochemical analysis is helpful; endothelial cells from hamartomas are CD8$^+$, whereas those from hemangiomas are not.

Hamartomas are typically large solitary lesions that have mildly decreased or increased T2-signal intensity relative to the adjacent normal spleen, mild T1 hypointensity, and mild heterogeneous enhancement after gadolinium administration. The differential diagnosis includes hemangioma, lymphoma, metastasis, and other rarer splenic tumors.

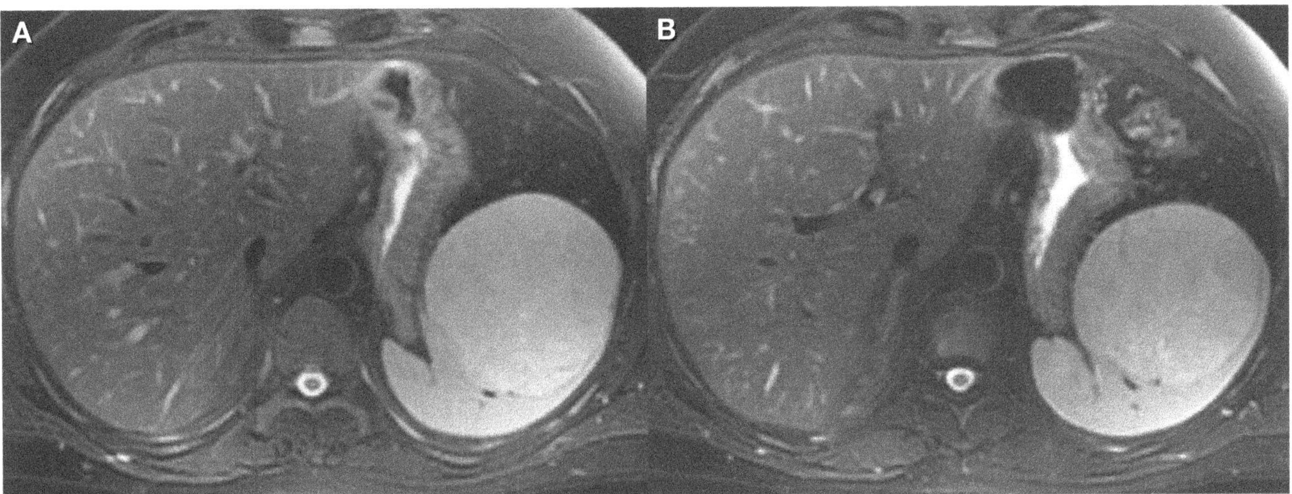

Figure 5.4.1

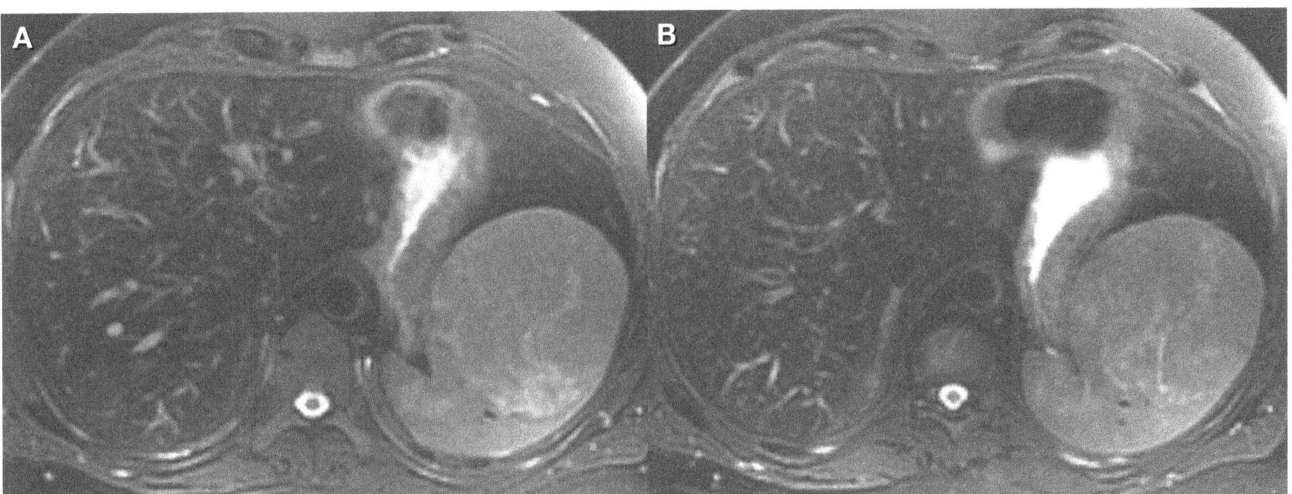

Figure 5.4.2

HISTORY: 59-year-old man with a recent diagnosis of renal cell carcinoma and CT that showed an incidental splenic lesion

IMAGING FINDINGS: Axial fat-suppressed FSE T2-weighted images before (Figure 5.4.1A) and after (Figure 5.4.1B) administration of ferumoxides (Feridex) show a large mass in the anterior spleen with mild heterogeneity and signal intensity similar to that of the adjacent spleen. Postcontrast images (Figure 5.4.2) show signal dropout in the liver and spleen as well as in the splenic mass.

DIAGNOSIS: Splenic hamartoma

COMMENT: An SPIO contrast agent (Feridex) was used in this case to help confirm that the lesion was benign, since renal cell carcinoma had just been diagnosed and metastasis was a consideration. The hamartoma takes up Feridex in essentially the same manner as adjacent spleen and liver, losing signal intensity on the postcontrast FSE images and indicating the presence of functional reticuloendothelial cells. This essentially excluded the diagnosis of metastasis and provided enough assurance to the oncologists and surgeons to save the patient's spleen. The mass remained stable after 4 years of follow-up examinations. SPIO agents are no longer commercially available, but if they are reintroduced with a more successful marketing campaign, keep this application in mind.

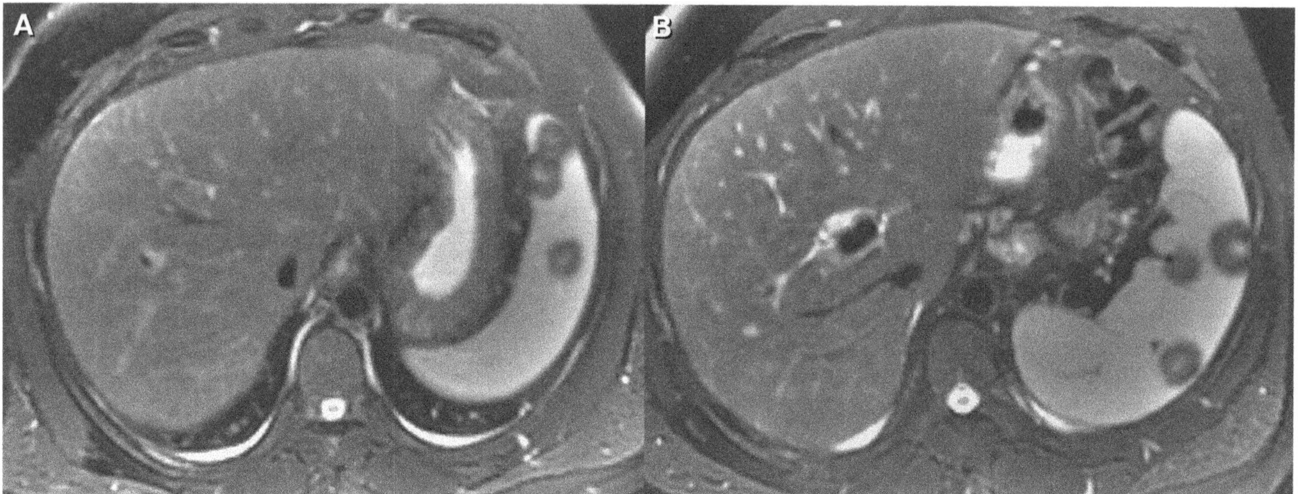

Figure 5.5.1

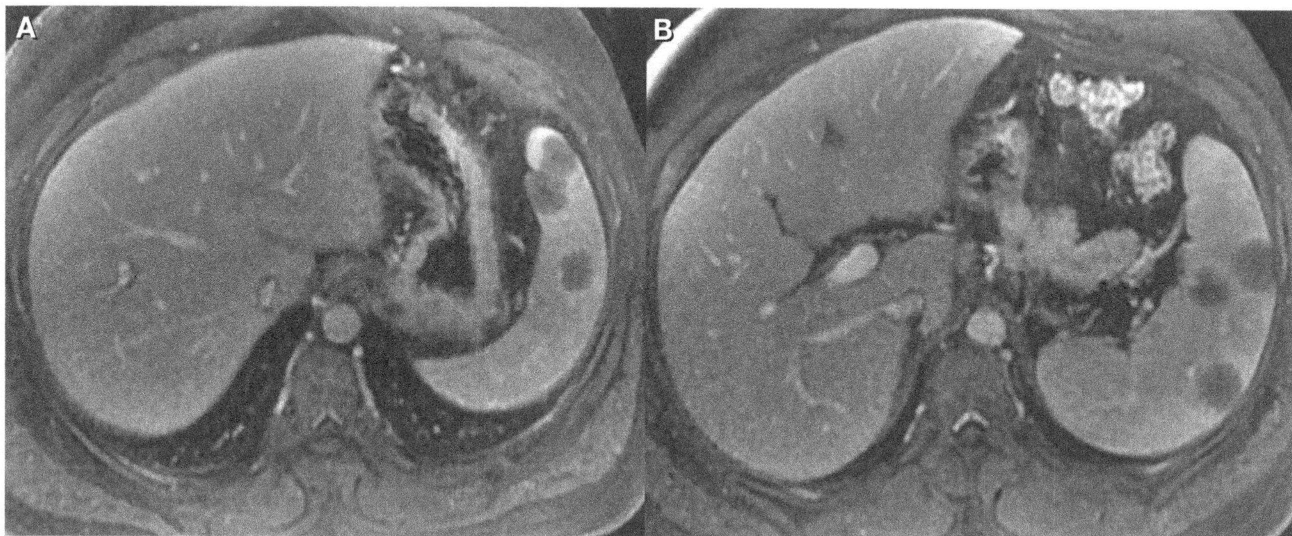

Figure 5.5.2

HISTORY: 42-year-old man with abdominal pain and elevated liver enzymes

IMAGING FINDINGS: Axial fat-suppressed FSE T2-weighted images (Figure 5.5.1) show multiple round splenic lesions that are predominantly hypointense compared to normal spleen, with small hyperintense centers. On equilibrium phase postgadolinium 3D SPGR images (Figure 5.5.2), the lesions are hypoenhancing compared to normal spleen.

DIAGNOSIS: Splenic sarcoid

COMMENT: Sarcoidosis is a multisystem disease characterized by proliferation of noncaseating granulomas containing epithelioid cells and large multinucleated giant cells. Most frequently, sarcoidosis involves the lungs, lymph nodes, eyes, spleen, liver, and skin. The cause is unknown, but current theories favor autoimmune and genetic causes. Peak incidence occurs between 20 and 40 years, with a female predominance. The lungs and the hilar and mediastinal lymph nodes are most frequently affected (90%), with splenic involvement reported in 40% to 60% of patients.

The most common appearance of splenic sarcoid is the least exciting (ie, splenomegaly), but focal involvement (occurring in 6%-30% of patients) is also seen with regularity. Splenic lesions in sarcoid are not absolutely distinctive and have an appearance similar to that of other fungal or granulomatous diseases—decreased signal intensity on T1- and T2-weighted images, sometimes with central T2 hyperintensity as in this case. The classic fungal infection in an immunocompromised patient more often has smaller lesions with more prominent T2 hyperintensity. Sarcoid lesions in the spleen usually do not show early enhancement and are generally hypoenhancing compared with spleen on 1 or more phases of dynamic postgadolinium images. An interesting feature we have seen in a few cases is a tendency to gradually accumulate contrast medium over time, becoming hyperintense on delayed images (as in Case 5.6).

Sarcoid is an unusual disease in that most patients improve without therapy. Symptomatic patients are often treated with corticosteroids or immunosuppressive drugs.

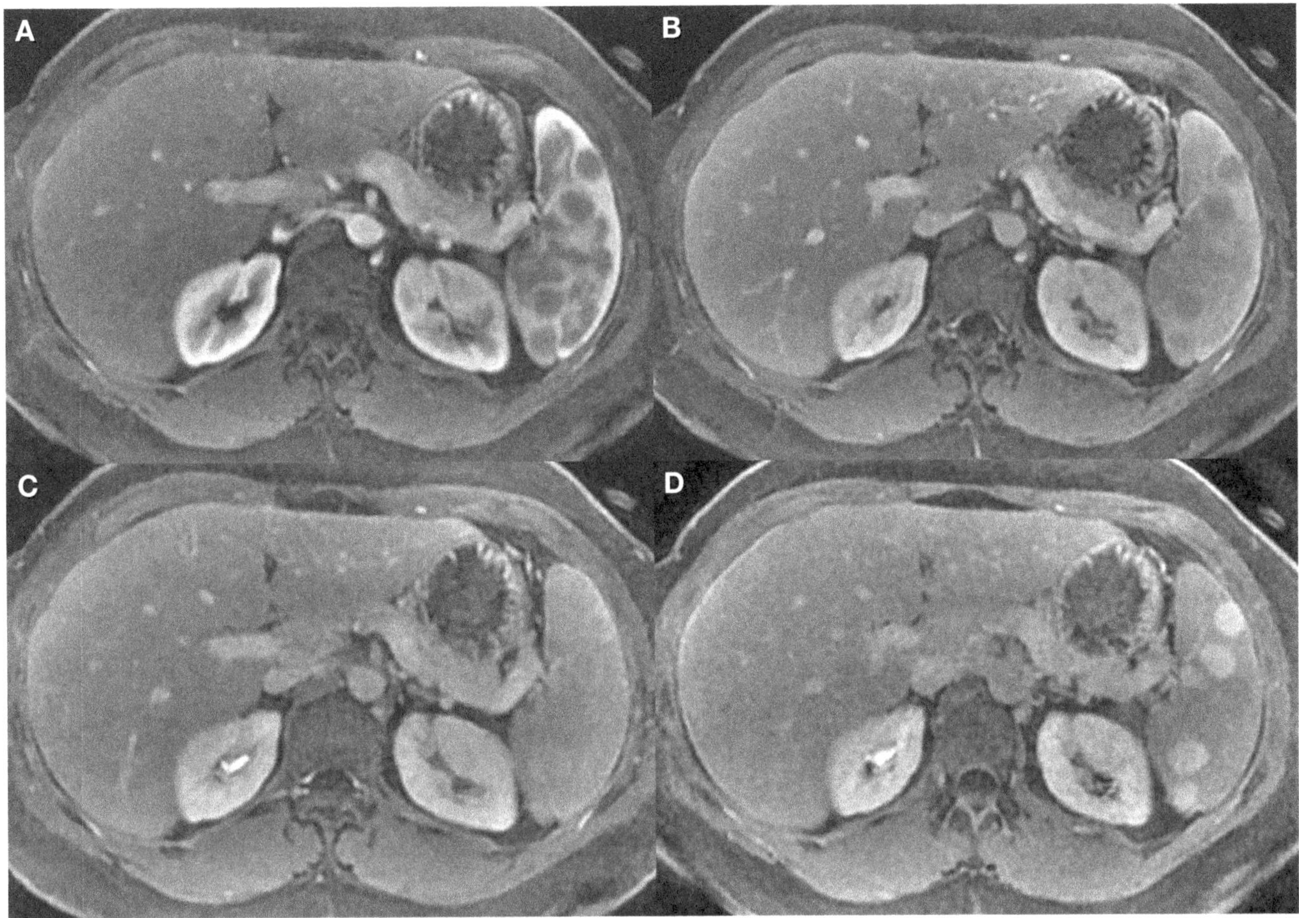

Figure 5.6.1

HISTORY: 37-year-old woman with a history of recurrent pancreatitis and abdominal pain

IMAGING FINDINGS: Arterial phase (Figure 5.6.1A), portal venous phase (Figure 5.6.1B), equilibrium phase (Figure 5.6.1C), and 8-minute delayed phase (Figure 5.6.1D) postgadolinium 3D SPGR images show multiple splenic lesions that are initially hypoenhancing relative to adjacent spleen and become hyperintense on delayed images.

DIAGNOSIS: Splenic sarcoid

COMMENT: This case is another example of focal splenic sarcoid. The enhancement pattern is similar but not identical to that in Case 5.5: The lesions show initial hypoenhancement relative to the adjacent spleen on arterial and portal venous phase images but are then nearly isointense to the spleen on the equilibrium phase image. With an additional delay, the lesions become hyperintense. We have seen this pattern of hyperenhancing splenic lesions on delayed images in a few cases of sarcoidosis, most often on examinations performed to assess for cardiac involvement, where late gadolinium enhancement images are always obtained 10 to 20 minutes after the initial contrast injection.

CASE 5.7

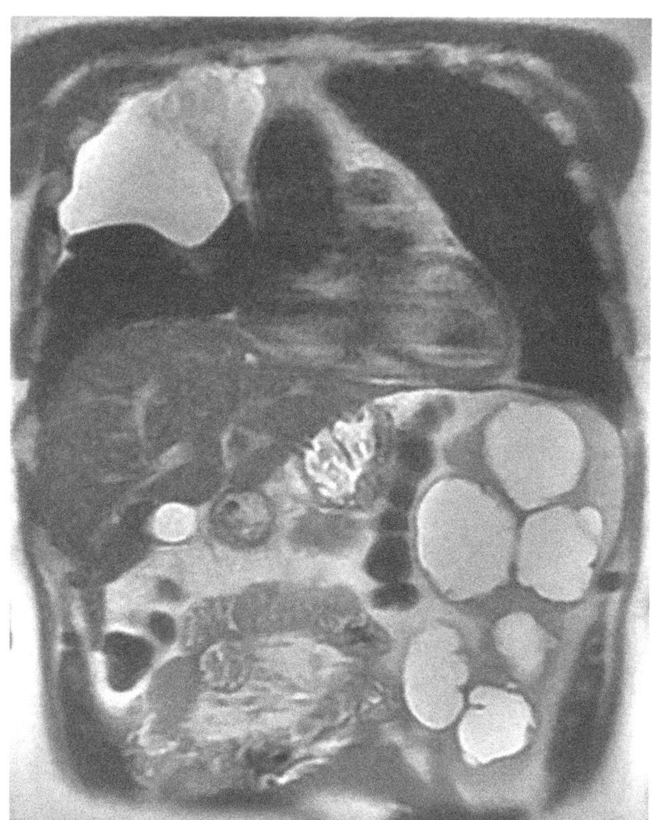

Figure 5.7.1

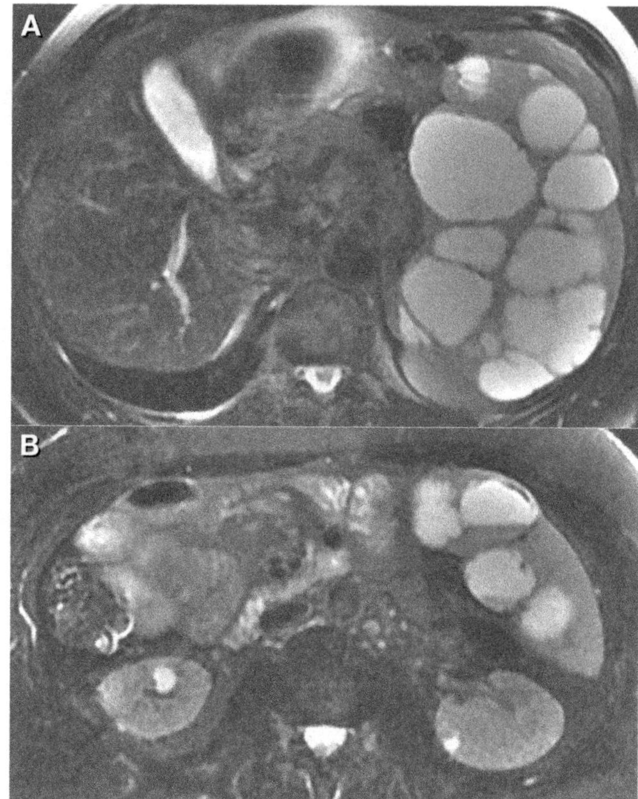

Figure 5.7.2

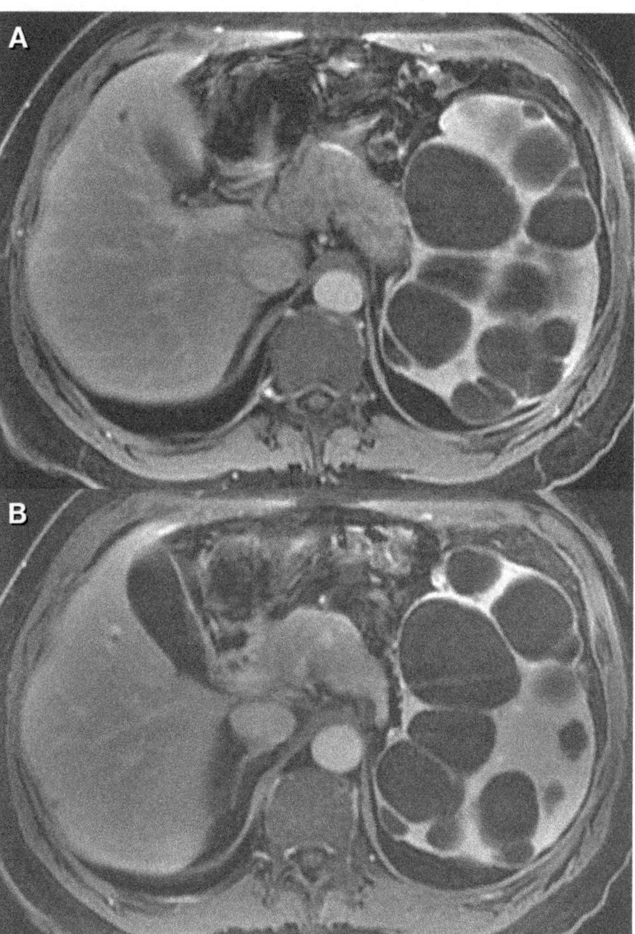

Figure 5.7.3

HISTORY: 38-year-old man with a history of a benign asymptomatic chest mass and mild thrombocytopenia

IMAGING FINDINGS: Coronal SSFSE (Figure 5.7.1) and axial fat-suppressed FSE T2-weighted images (Figure 5.7.2) show multiple large cystic lesions throughout the spleen. Note the fluid-fluid levels in the inferior FSE image as well as the cystic mass in the right upper chest on the SSFSE image. Axial postgadolinium equilibrium phase 3D SPGR images (Figure 5.7.3) show no significant enhancement of the splenic lesions.

DIAGNOSIS: Splenic and thoracic lymphangiomas

COMMENT: Lymphangiomas are benign neoplasms or malformations of the lymphatic system that are usually diagnosed in children. Splenic lymphangiomas are typically asymptomatic, but mass effect on adjacent organs can cause symptoms, including left upper quadrant pain, nausea, and abdominal distention. Lymphangiomatosis is a syndrome in which multiple organs are involved. The mediastinum, retroperitoneum, axilla, and neck are common locations. Multiple splenic lymphangiomas or hemangiomas have also been associated with KTS (an example is shown in Case 5.8).

Classified as capillary, cavernous, or cystic on the basis of the size and location of the vascular channels, lymphangiomas consist of a single layer of endothelium-lined spaces filled with eosinophilic proteinaceous material (rather than blood as seen in hemangiomas).

Splenic lymphangiomas appear as cystic lesions with high T2-signal intensity and low T1-signal intensity relative to adjacent spleen and have thin septations that may show mild enhancement or calcification (better appreciated on CT). The presence of fluid-fluid levels in cystic lesions has been considered a hallmark of lymphangiomas; however, it is not a universal finding and can occur in association with many other entities. The differential diagnosis includes cyst, pseudocyst, and hydatid cyst. The presence of multiple cystic lesions throughout the spleen and the concurrent mediastinal lesion in this case are highly suggestive of lymphangiomatosis.

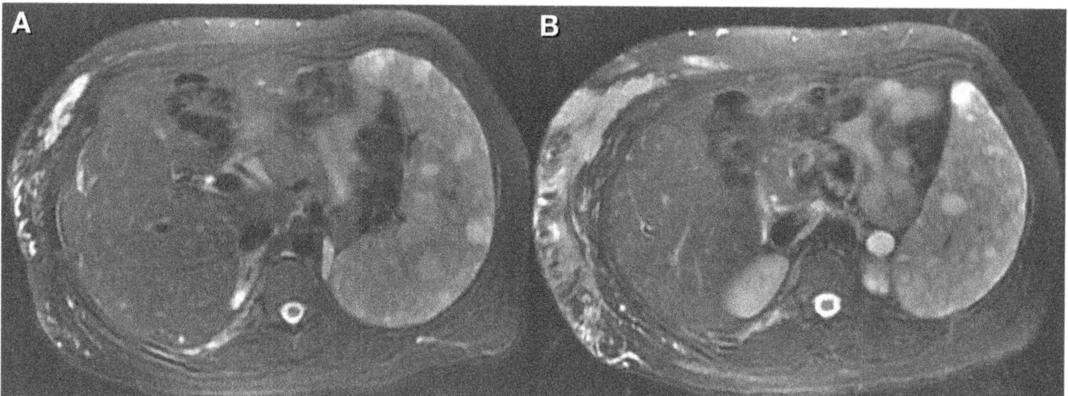

Figure 5.8.1

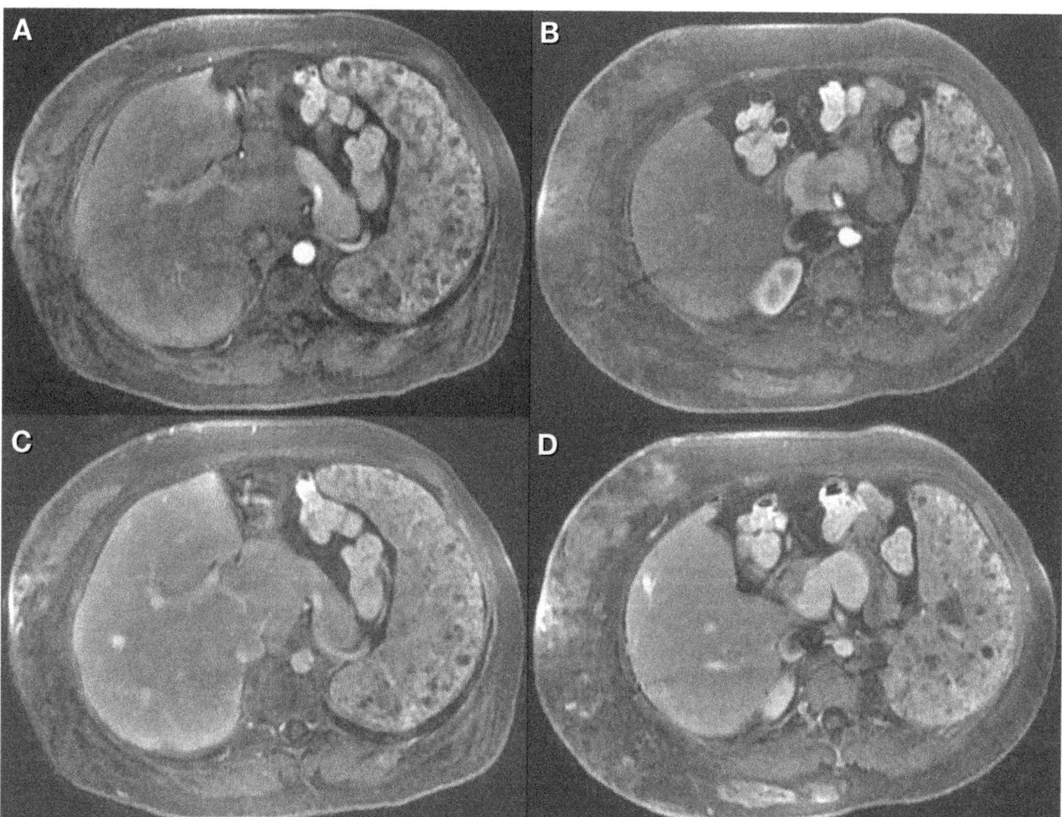

Figure 5.8.2

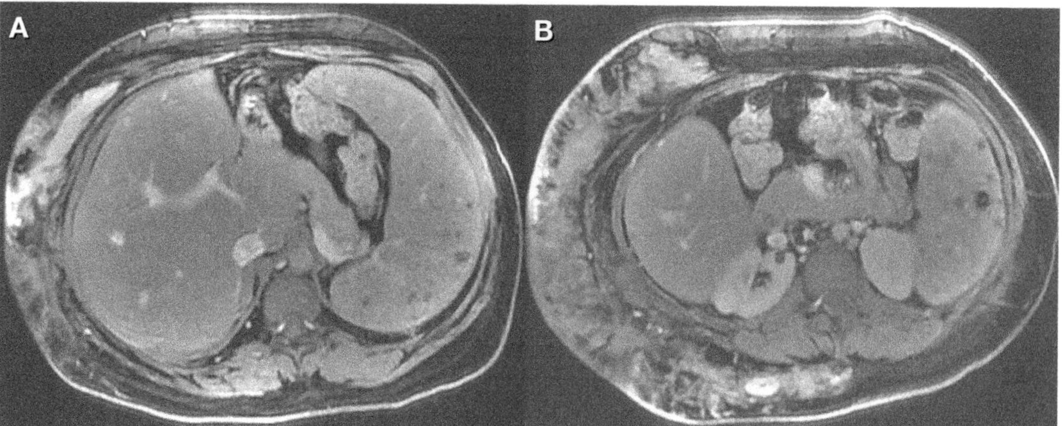

Figure 5.8.3

HISTORY: 31-year-old woman with a venous malformation of the right lower extremity

IMAGING FINDINGS: Axial fat-suppressed FSE T2-weighted images (Figure 5.8.1) show multiple small hyperintense splenic lesions; several appear cystic. Note also the markedly hyperintense, poorly defined lesion in the right lateral subcutaneous tissues. Arterial phase (Figure 5.8.2A and 5.8.2B) and equilibrium phase (Figure 5.8.2C and 5.8.2D) 3D SPGR images show heterogeneous enhancement of the spleen with multiple small lesions; some of the lesions fill in on the equilibrium phase images and some remain hypointense. Axial 6-minute delayed phase postgadolinium 2D SPGR images (Figure 5.8.3) show that most of the splenic lesions have filled in; a few persistent cystic foci remain. The right lateral subcutaneous soft tissue lesion also shows diffuse enhancement.

DIAGNOSIS: KTS with splenic involvement and subcutaneous hemangioma in the right abdominal wall

COMMENT: KTS is a rare congenital disorder characterized by the clinical triad of 1) bony and soft tissue hypertrophy that usually affects 1 extremity, 2) cutaneous hemangiomas, and 3) varicosities or venous malformations. All these features are not universally present. About two-thirds of KTS patients have all 3 features, and one-third have 2 of the 3 features. First described by Klippel and Trénaunay in 1900, KTS is considered to be a combined capillary, lymphatic, and venous malformation (an additional example is Case 16.15 in Chapter 16).

Unilateral lower limb involvement is seen in 95% of patients. Limb hypertrophy affects both length and circumference, with prominent subcutaneous fat in the involved extremity.

Once thought to be uncommon, involvement of the gastrointestinal and genitourinary tracts is increasingly recognized and may occasionally cause significant morbidity and mortality, generally from massive bleeding. Vascular or lymphatic malformations may affect the gastrointestinal tract, liver, spleen, bladder, kidney, lung, heart, penis, scrotum, and vagina. Most reports of splenic involvement describe either hemangiomas or lymphangiomas, with a mixture of both lesions occasionally reported. This case is probably a hemangioma/lymphangioma mixture—some lesions are clearly cystic and show no enhancement, while others fill in on delayed postgadolinium images. A second example (Case 5.9) illustrates more uniform involvement of the spleen by cystic lymphangiomas.

Reports of complications related to splenic involvement in KTS are extremely rare; however, spontaneous rupture of large lesions, hypersplenism, and Kasabach-Merritt syndrome have been reported to occur in patients with large splenic hemangiomas and lymphangiomas.

CASE 5.9

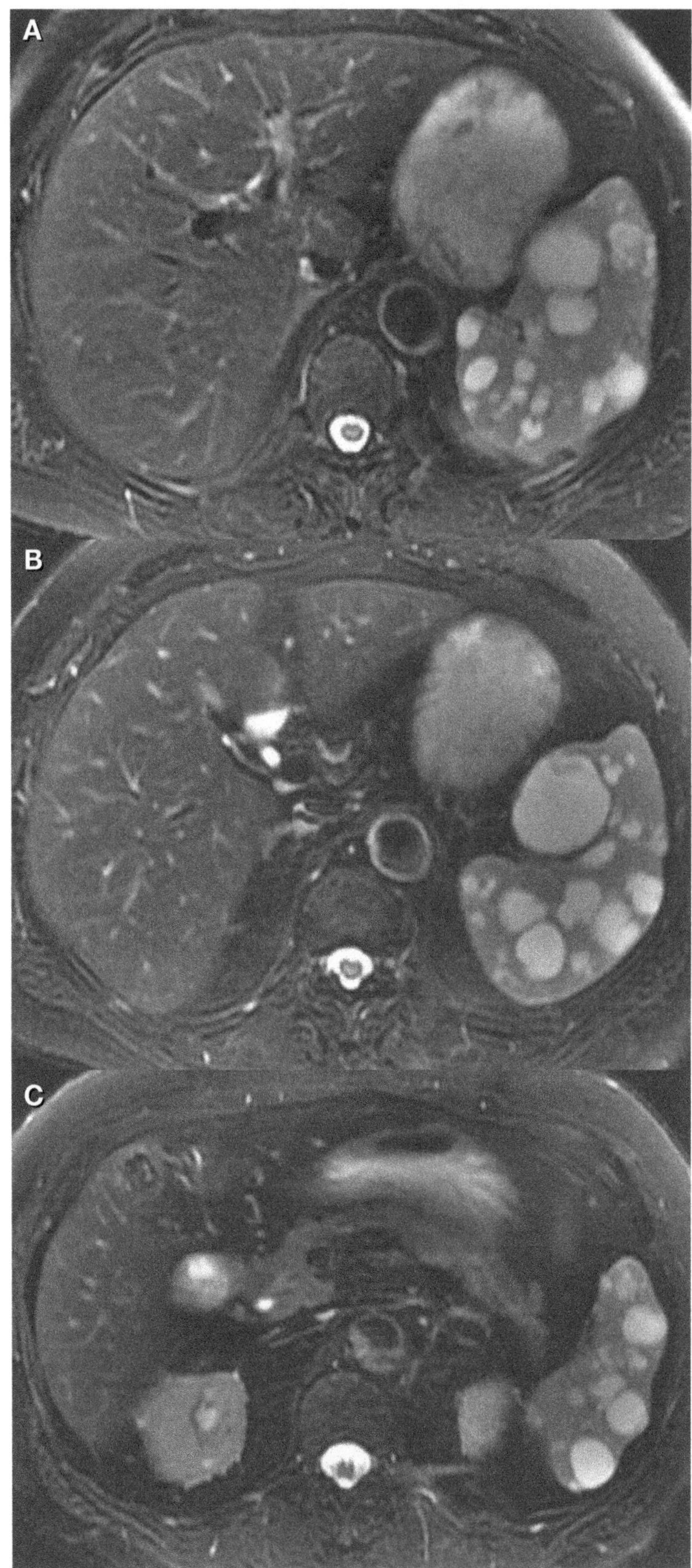

Figure 5.9.1

HISTORY: 72-year-old woman with KTS affecting her right lower extremity

IMAGING FINDINGS: Axial fat-suppressed FSE T2-weighted images (Figure 5.9.1) show multiple cystic lesions throughout the spleen.

DIAGNOSIS: KTS with splenic lymphangiomatosis

COMMENT: The differential diagnosis for multiple splenic cystic lesions also includes infectious and posttraumatic etiologies; however, the large number of lesions and their simple appearance in combination with the history of KTS makes splenic lymphangiomatosis the best choice.

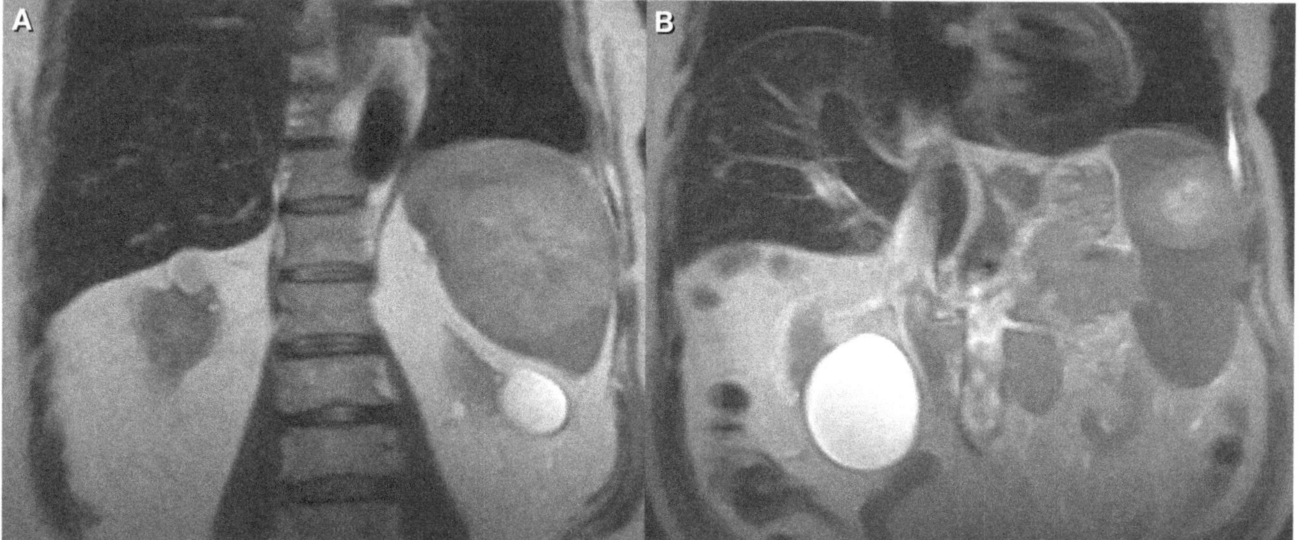

Figure 5.10.1

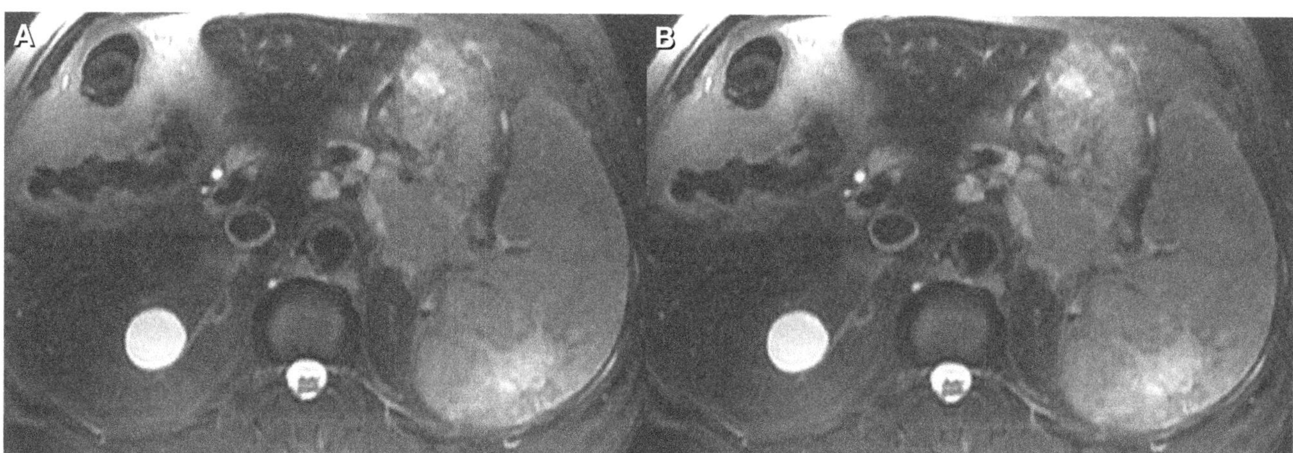

Figure 5.10.2

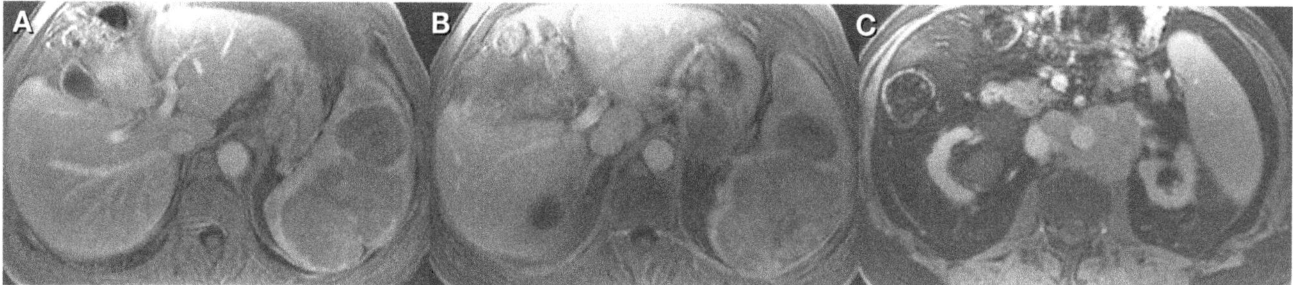

Figure 5.10.3

HISTORY: 77-year-old man with a history of renal insufficiency and weight loss

IMAGING FINDINGS: Coronal SSFSE (Figure 5.10.1) and axial fat-suppressed FRFSE images (Figure 5.10.2) show large mildly hyperintense masses in the spleen. These are hypovascular on portal venous phase 3D SPGR images (Figure 5.10.3A and 5.10.3B), and a more inferior image (Figure 5.10.3C) shows extensive retroperitoneal adenopathy. Adenopathy is also apparent in the splenic hilum on SSFSE and T2-weighted images.

DIAGNOSIS: NHL with splenic and nodal involvement

COMMENT: Lymphoma, the most common malignancy affecting the spleen, may be primary or secondary, although most patients have secondary disease. Splenic involvement is common in both HD and NHL and is apparent in approximately 40% of patients at presentation.

In the past, assessment for splenic disease had much greater urgency for HD patients. Approximately 85% present with apparently localized supradiaphragmatic disease; however, the spleen is affected by occult disease as the only infradiaphragmatic site of involvement in as many as 10%. This distinction had significant implications in staging and prognosis, but advances in chemotherapeutic regimens have improved overall survival to the extent that failure to detect splenic involvement at presentation no longer alters the overall prognosis. Advanced disease is much more common at presentation among patients who have NHL (80%), for which systemic chemotherapy is the mainstay of treatment regardless of whether the spleen is affected.

The imaging appearance of splenic lymphoma has been divided into 3 categories: normal, splenomegaly without focal lesions, and focal lesions. Splenomegaly alone is not a reliable indicator of lymphomatous infiltration. Although massive splenomegaly is almost always predictive of splenic involvement, mild to moderate splenomegaly has been reported in 30% of HD patients and 70% of NHL patients who do not have splenic disease. In these patients, splenomegaly is thought to result from inflammation or congestion. Conversely, the spleen is involved in up to one-third of lymphoma patients without splenomegaly.

Some evidence suggests that MRI is more successful than CT in detecting focal lymphomatous lesions in the spleen (a specific example of a more general truth). Small lesions (<1 cm) are more common in HD; larger lesions are more often seen in NHL. Lesions typically show mild T2 hyperintensity and are hypovascular relative to normal spleen on dynamic postgadolinium 3D SPGR images. In this case, the lesions are most apparent on portal venous phase postgadolinium images, but it is not uncommon to see them best on T2- or diffusion-weighted images. The differential diagnosis for lymphoma with multiple focal lesions includes metastases, infection, and sarcoid. The extensive retroperitoneal and perisplenic adenopathy in this case is typical of NHL and is a reminder to include the entire abdomen (not just the liver and spleen) in the examination.

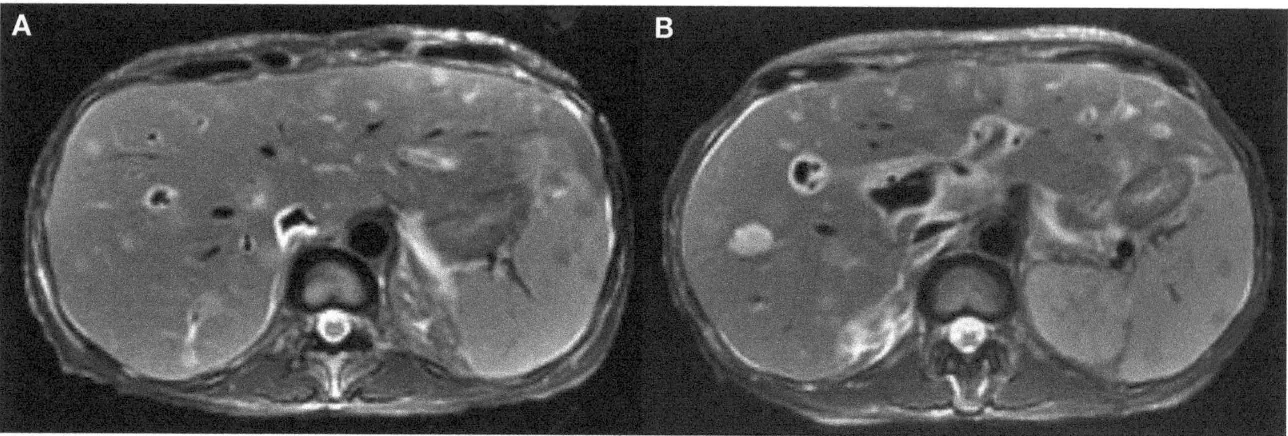

Figure 5.11.1

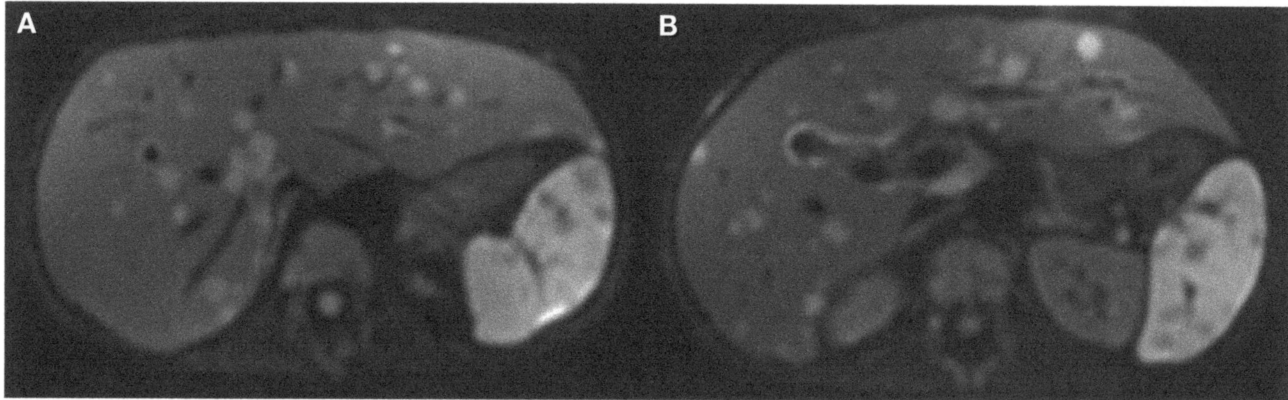

Figure 5.11.2

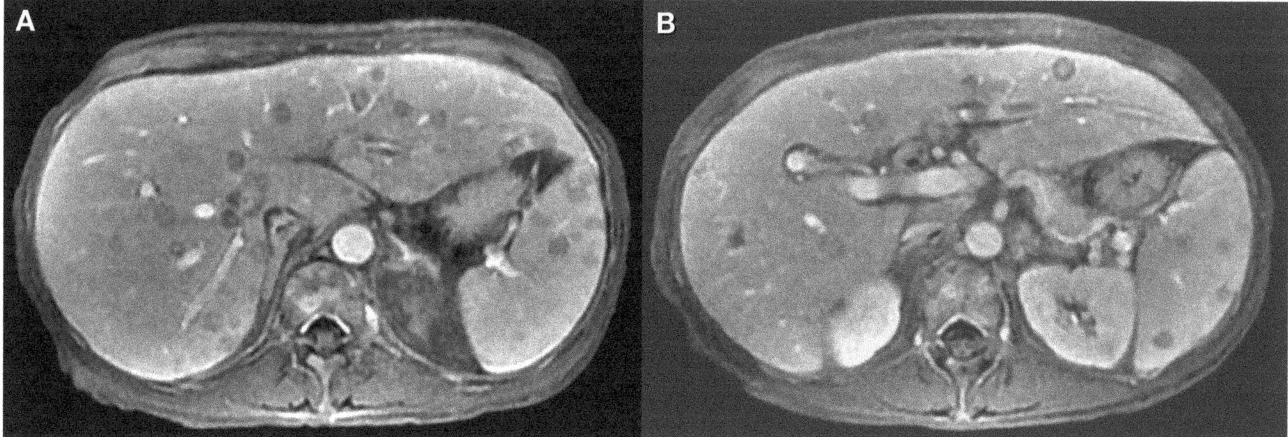

Figure 5.11.3

HISTORY: 51-year-old woman with a history of breast cancer

IMAGING FINDINGS: Axial fat-suppressed FSE T2-weighted images (Figure 5.11.1), axial diffusion-weighted images (b=100 s/mm^2) (Figure 5.11.2), and axial portal venous phase postgadolinium 3D SPGR images (Figure 5.11.3) show multiple nodules in the liver and spleen. Hepatic lesions have increased signal intensity relative to liver, while the splenic lesions show decreased signal intensity compared with normal spleen on T2- and diffusion-weighted images. Most lesions show hypoenhancement compared with liver and spleen, although several hepatic lesions have central enhancement. Note also small enhancing lesions in an upper lumbar vertebral body.

DIAGNOSIS: Breast cancer with hepatic, splenic, and bone metastases

COMMENT: This case is unusual in that the splenic metastases have a different appearance compared to the hepatic lesions. The splenic metastases are hypointense rather than hyperintense compared with adjacent normal parenchyma on T2- and diffusion-weighted images. This is an occupational hazard of splenic lesions given the high baseline T2-signal intensity of the spleen and should not dissuade anyone from suggesting the correct diagnosis.

Splenic metastases are relatively uncommon. Autopsy studies have shown a prevalence of 2.3% to 7%, with an increasing incidence among patients who have widespread metastatic disease (50% in patients who also had metastases in ≥5 other organs). The most common primary tumors are breast, lung, ovarian, colorectal, gastric, and melanoma. Melanoma has the highest rate of splenic metastases per primary tumor (approximately 30%). Solitary splenic metastases are rare, with fewer than 100 published cases.

The differential diagnosis for multiple hypoenhancing splenic masses includes lymphoma, sarcoid, fungal infection, littoral cell angioma, and Gaucher disease; however, with the evidence of widespread metastases, this case is not a diagnostic dilemma.

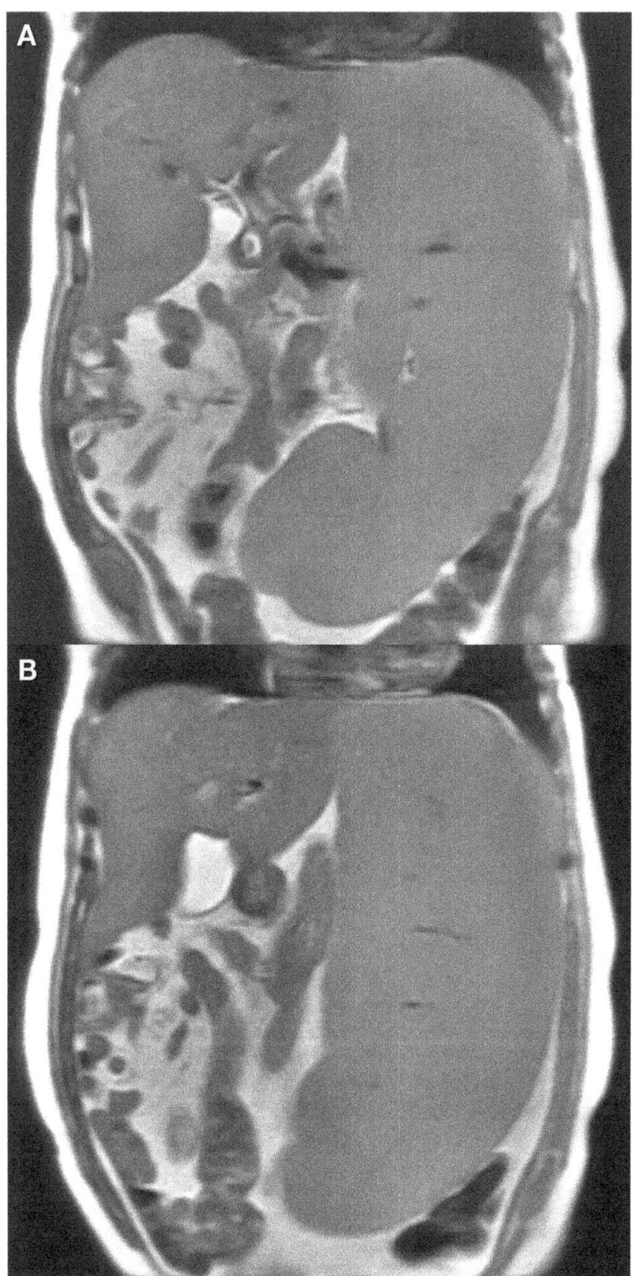

Figure 5.12.1

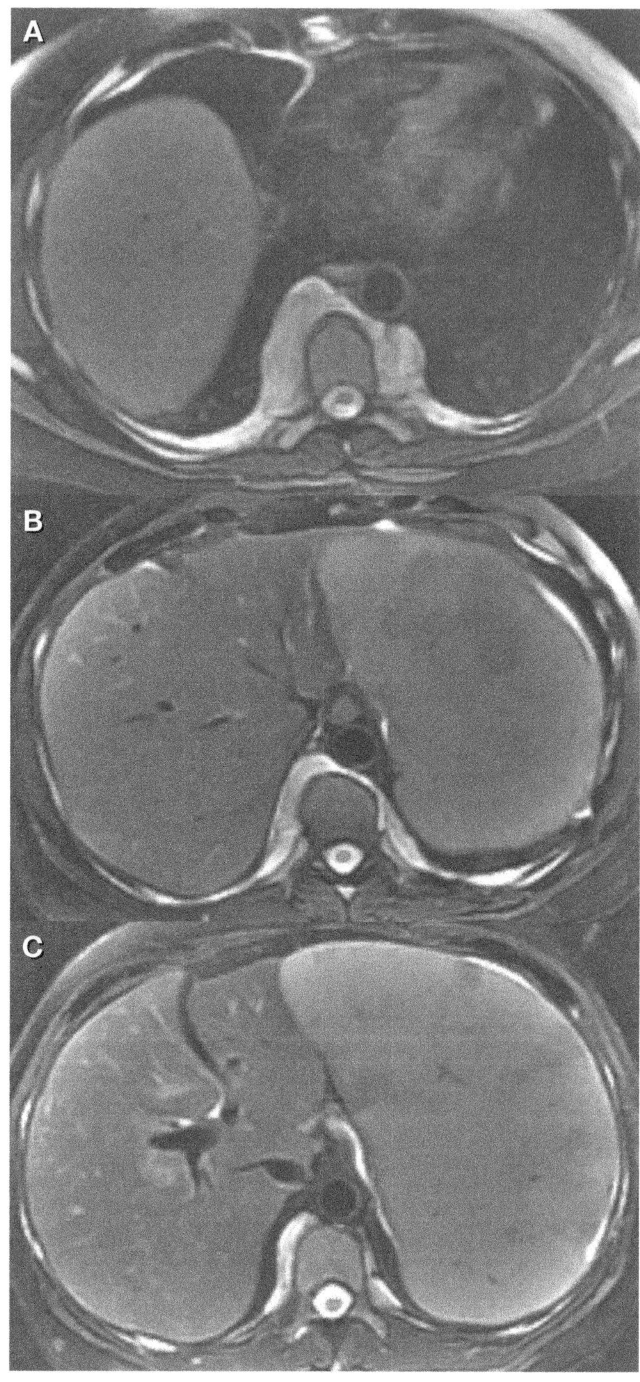

Figure 5.12.2

HISTORY: 60-year-old woman with a chronic hematologic disorder

IMAGING FINDINGS: Coronal SSFSE images (Figure 5.12.1) show massive splenomegaly. Axial fat-suppressed FSE T2-weighted images (Figure 5.12.2) show splenomegaly and prominent high-signal soft tissue adjacent to the lower thoracic vertebral bodies.

DIAGNOSIS: Myelofibrosis with massive splenomegaly and extramedullary hematopoiesis

COMMENT: Primary myelofibrosis is categorized by the World Health Organization in a group of myeloid malignancies that include polycythemia vera, essential thrombocythemia, and chronic myelogenous leukemia. It is characterized by bone marrow fibrosis, splenomegaly with extramedullary hematopoiesis, and peripheral blood leukoerythroblastosis; 50% to 60% of patients with primary myelofibrosis (and 95% of patients with polycythemia vera) share a common mutation in the *JAK2* gene involved in erythroid, myeloid, and megakaryocytic development. Patients typically present with anemia and massive splenomegaly and have characteristic results on peripheral blood smears.

Patients with primary myelofibrosis have a relatively poor prognosis, with a median survival of 6 years; however, there is wide variation among patients, and several prognostic scoring systems have been developed to better categorize newly diagnosed disease. The International Prognostic Scoring System uses 5 risk factors and defines 4 categories from low risk to high risk; mean survival is 17.5 years for low-risk patients and 1.8 years for high-risk patients.

The differential diagnosis for massive splenomegaly (craniocaudal diameter >20 cm) is fairly broad and includes leukemia, lymphoma, hemolytic anemia, polycythemia vera, portal hypertension, and storage diseases. In this case, the relatively normal appearance of the liver helps to eliminate causes related to portal hypertension, and the absence of significant abdominal adenopathy makes lymphoma less likely. Myelofibrosis is a primary consideration because of the truly massive splenic enlargement along with prominent extramedullary hematopoiesis.

Extramedullary hematopoiesis can occur in chronic anemias and hematologic malignancies. The liver, spleen, and lymph nodes are the most common sites of involvement, and the splenomegaly in primary myelofibrosis is partially a consequence of splenic extramedullary hematopoiesis. Paraspinous extramedullary hematopoiesis is less common but well described, and the appearance of lobulated paraspinous soft tissue with moderately increased T2-signal intensity is characteristic, particularly in a patient who has a history of myelofibrosis as in this case. A few case reports have described epidural extramedullary hematopoiesis resulting in symptomatic spinal cord compression, which is exceedingly rare.

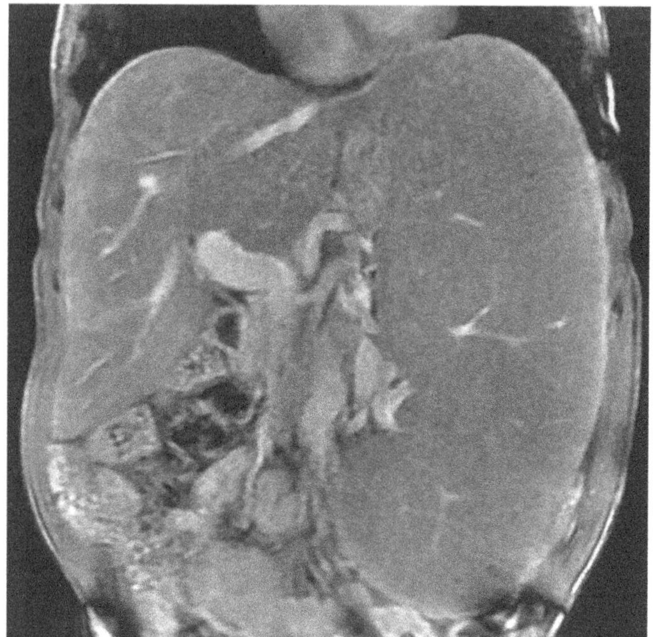

Figure 5.13.1

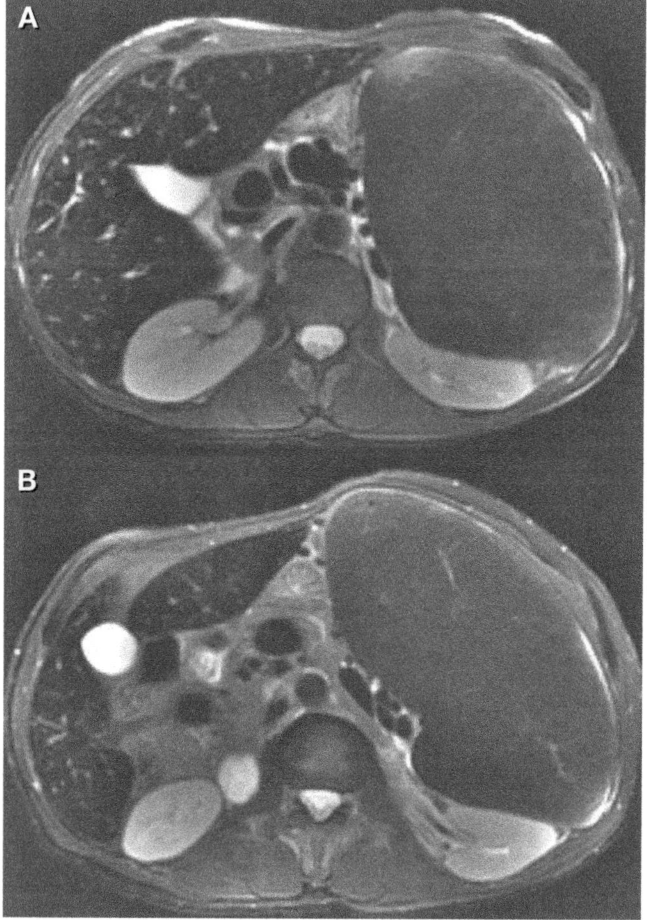

Figure 5.13.2

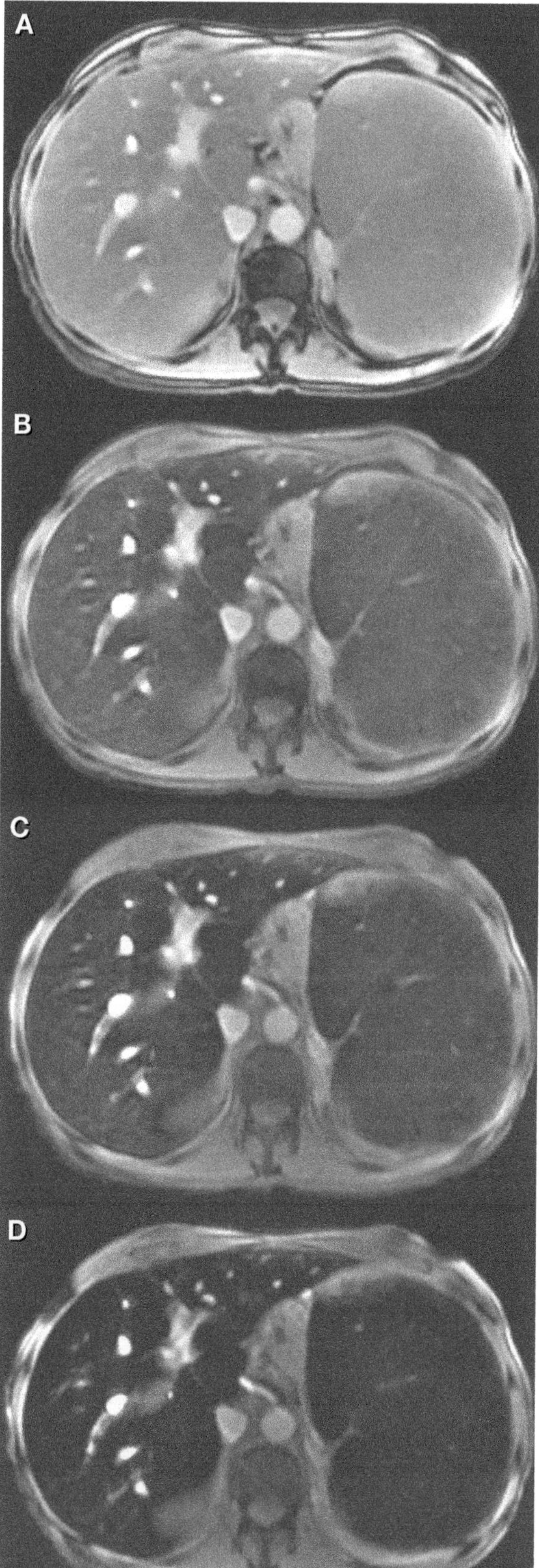

Figure 5.13.3

HISTORY: 63-year-old man with a chronic hematologic disorder

IMAGING FINDINGS: Coronal postgadolinium 3D SPGR image (Figure 5.13.1) shows massive splenomegaly. Axial fat-suppressed FSE T2-weighted images (Figure 5.13.2) show splenomegaly and markedly decreased signal intensity in the liver and spleen. Axial images at the same location from a multiple-echo GRE sequence (TE = 2.5, 6.5, 10.5, and 14.5 ms in panels A, B, C, and D, respectively, of Figure 5.13.3) show rapid signal loss in the liver and spleen as TE increases.

DIAGNOSIS: Myelofibrosis with massive splenomegaly and splenic and hepatic hemosiderosis secondary to multiple transfusions

COMMENT: The "Comment" section for Case 5.12 discusses myelofibrosis in greater detail. This case illustrates the typical appearance of hemosiderosis caused by iron deposition within the reticuloendothelial cells of the liver and spleen. Iron particles cause T2 and T2* shortening on T2- and T2*-weighted images and amplify the effect of T2* relaxation in what are normally considered T1-weighted images; this accounts for the signal loss from out-of-phase to in-phase images corresponding to a small change in TE of 2.3 ms at 1.5T. This effect can also be seen in the multiple-echo GRE sequence shown in Figure 5.13.3, with an impressive decline in signal with each increment of TE. This pulse sequence can be used to measure T2* or R2* (the relaxivity or inverse of T2*), and these values, with the aid of a calibration curve, can predict the tissue iron concentration, a technique more often employed for the liver and heart to diagnose iron overload and monitor the response to chelation therapy.

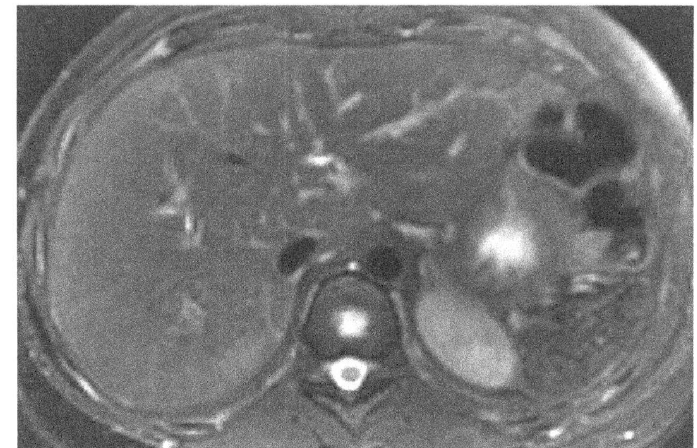

Figure 5.14.1

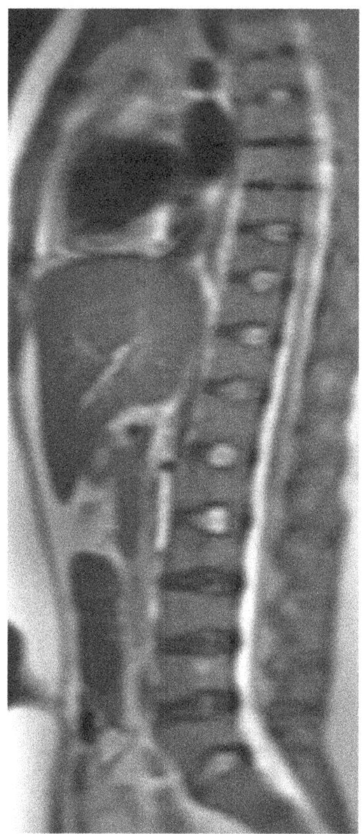

Figure 5.14.4

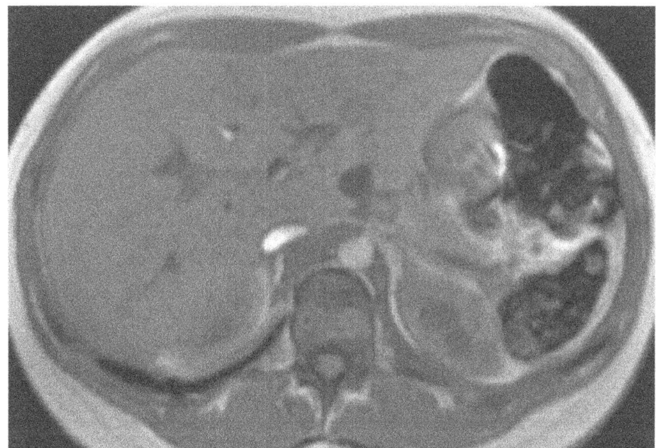

Figure 5.14.2

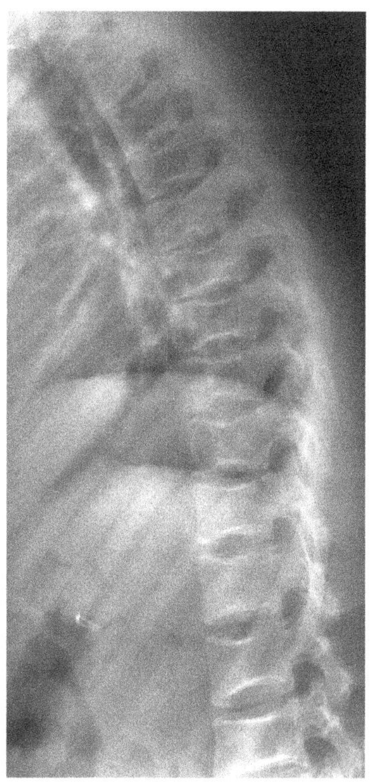

Figure 5.14.5

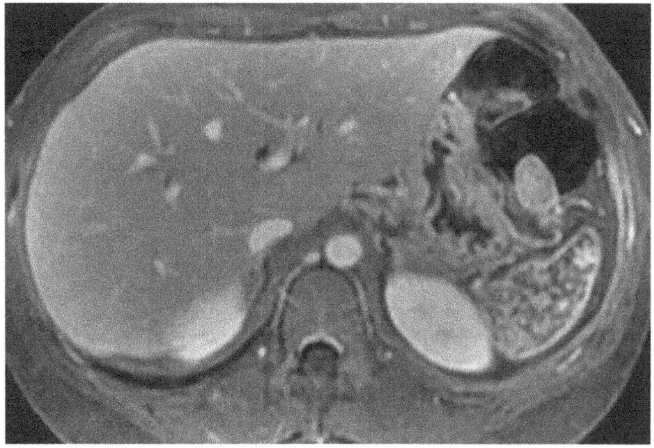

Figure 5.14.3

HISTORY: 20-year-old woman with a history of hemoglobinopathy

IMAGING FINDINGS: Axial fat-suppressed FSE T2-weighted image (Figure 5.14.1) and axial in-phase SPGR image (Figure 5.14.2) show a small spleen with decreased T2-signal intensity and markedly decreased signal on the in-phase image. Axial postgadolinium 2D SPGR image (Figure 5.14.3) shows generalized hypoenhancement with innumerable siderotic nodules (Gamna-Gandy bodies). Sagittal scout view of the thoracolumbar spine (Figure 5.14.4) and lateral plain radiograph of the spine (Figure 5.14.5) show central end-plate deformities in multiple vertebral bodies.

DIAGNOSIS: Sickle cell disease with autoinfarction of the spleen

COMMENT: Sickle cell anemia was first described in 1910 by Herrick after his intern, Irons (not a coauthor), noted elongated, sickle-shaped red blood cells in a patient with anemia. Linus Pauling and colleagues in 1949 reported that the disease occurs as a result of an alteration in the hemoglobin molecule. Sickle cell disease is caused by a mutation in the β-globin gene. The single amino acid switch results in the formation of hemoglobin S, which polymerizes when deoxygenated to generate a gelatinous network of polymers. This network stiffens the erythrocyte membrane and increases membrane viscosity, leading to the characteristic sickle shape of the erythrocyte and causing erythrocytes to lose the pliability needed to traverse small capillary networks. The resulting episodic microvascular occlusions and premature erythrocyte destruction (hemolytic anemia) cause the clinical manifestations of sickle cell disease.

Sickle cell disease is the most common structural hemoglobinopathy; the heterozygous form (ie, the sickle cell trait) occurs in 8% of the United States African American population and the homozygous form in 0.25%.

The spleen is a frequent target in sickle cell disease. It is often enlarged during the first decade of life but then undergoes progressive atrophy as a result of repeated vasoocclusive episodes and multiple infarctions (ie, autoinfarction). The resulting atrophic, nonfunctional, densely calcified spleen is a classic finding in sickle cell disease on plain radiographs and abdominal CT. The appearance on MRI results from the accumulated iron stores in the spleen and is characterized by low signal intensity on virtually all pulse sequences. Iron quantification can be performed in the spleen with the same spin echo or gradient echo techniques applied in the liver and heart, but the clinical utility is not certain. An interesting bit of physics trivia to emerge from articles on iron quantification is that the correlation between spin echo and gradient echo methods (R2 vs R2*) is less for the spleen than for the liver and heart because the mean effective diameter of the iron deposits in the spleen is much larger. The resulting magnetic disturbances are larger in scale and cause static refocusing in spin echo experiments and lead to lower R2 values.

Autoinfarction is by far the most common fate of the spleen in sickle cell disease; however, a few additional complications can occur, including acute splenic sequestration crisis, hypersplenism, splenic abscess, and massive infarction. Acute splenic sequestration crisis usually occurs in patients younger than 2 years, is a significant cause of death, and results from rapid sequestration of erythrocytes in the spleen. *Hypersplenism* is defined as splenomegaly with significant anemia or thrombocytopenia (or both) and is occasionally an indication for splenectomy in sickle cell patients.

End-plate deformities in thoracic and lumbar vertebral bodies ("*H*-shaped" or "Lincoln Log" are the usual descriptors) also indicate vasoocclusive episodes and infarction. They serve as a reminder to 1) obtain scout images that are diagnostically useful (ie, SSFSE or SSFP rather than SPGR pulse sequences), 2) look at the scout images, and 3) recognize that musculoskeletal and nervous system anatomy is included in every abdominal MRI examination and does need to be inspected.

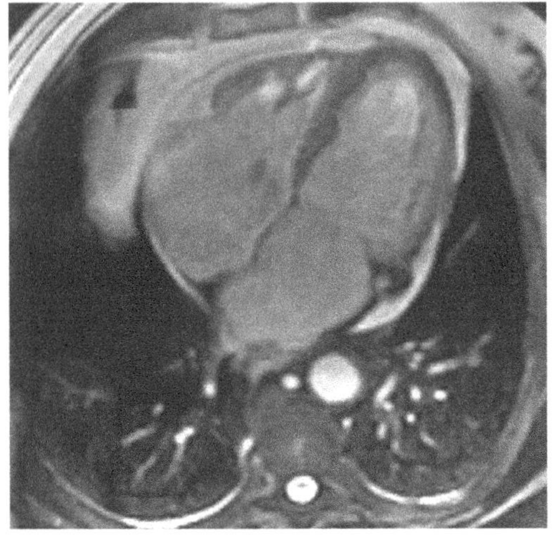

Figure 5.15.1

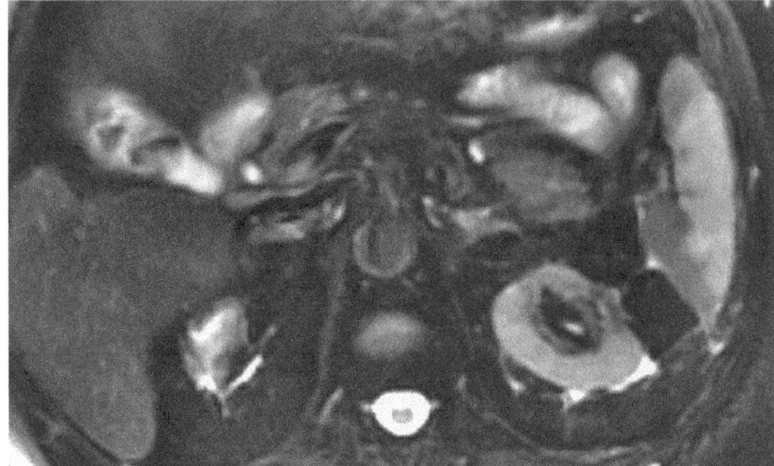

Figure 5.15.2

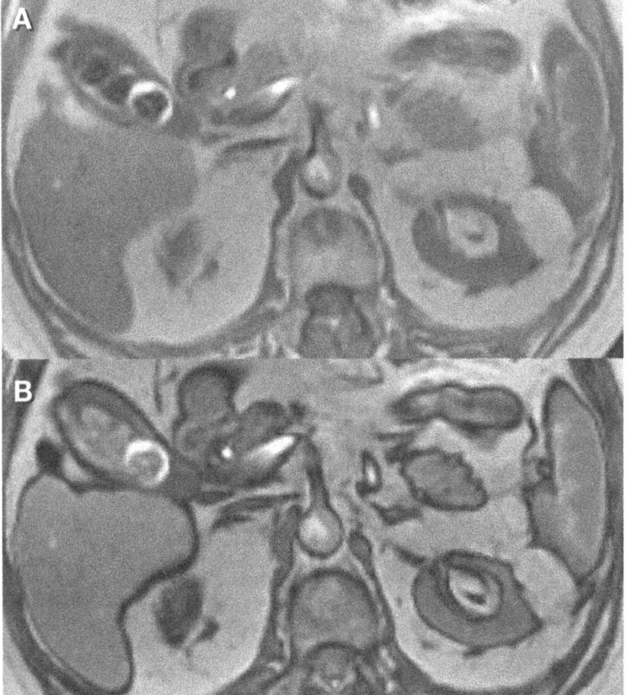

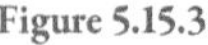

Figure 5.15.3

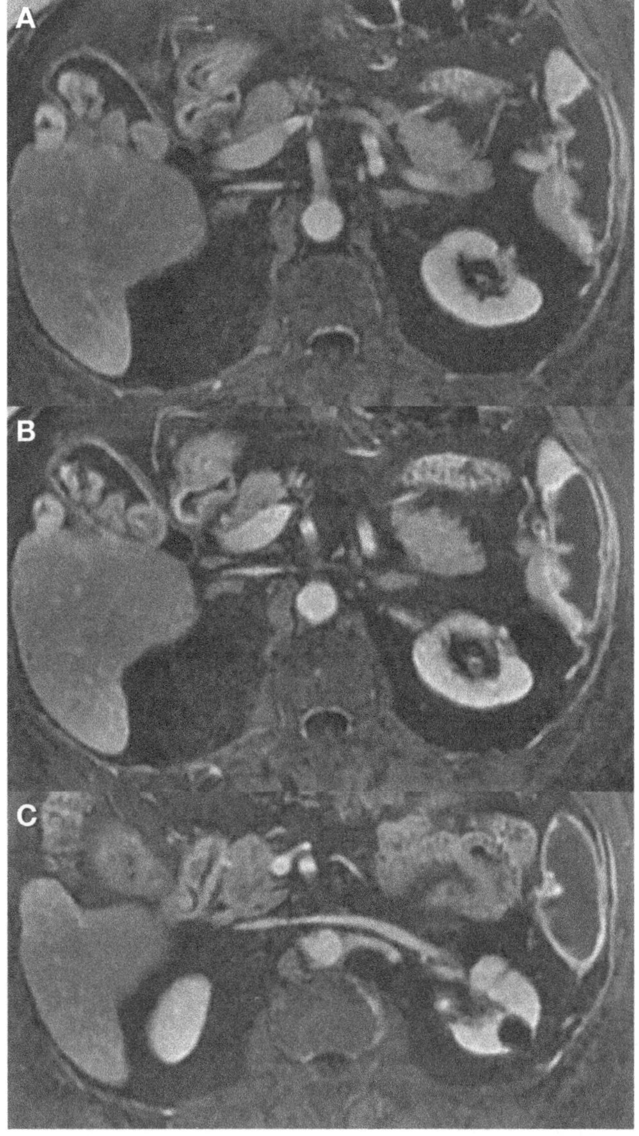

Figure 5.15.4

HISTORY: 75-year-old man with a history of hepatocellular carcinoma

IMAGING FINDINGS: Axial fat-suppressed SSFP-weighted image shows cardiomegaly with biatrial enlargement (Figure 5.15.1). Fat-suppressed FSE T2-weighted image shows a wedge-shaped region of increased signal within the spleen (Figure 5.15.2). Axial in-phase and out-of-phase SPGR images (Figure 5.15.3) show a hyperintense rim surrounding the splenic lesion with a more hypointense center. Portal venous phase postgadolinium 3D SPGR images (Figure 5.15.4) show no enhancement of the splenic lesion. Cholelithiasis is incidentally noted on nearly all images.

DIAGNOSIS: Splenic infarct in a patient with uncontrolled atrial fibrillation

COMMENT: This patient had at least 2 risk factors for splenic infarction: malignancy with its potential hypercoagulable state and atrial fibrillation with an increased incidence of atrial thrombus. Subsequent echocardiography showed a left atrial appendage thrombus, and therefore atrial fibrillation is the most likely cause of the infarction.

Splenic infarction is most often embolic, but it can be thrombotic, particularly in younger patients, with causes that include vasculitis, hematologic disorders, and splenic neoplasms.

Splenic infarcts are usually easy to recognize as wedge-shaped regions of nonenhancing parenchyma, often with a rim of spared capsular enhancement as seen in this case. Signal intensity on T1- and T2-weighted precontrast images is variable and depends on the age of the infarct and the age of the blood products within the infarct. As with hematomas in other organs, the presence of a serpiginous rim of increased signal intensity on T1-weighted images is a good indication of a hematoma or infarct rather than a neoplasm or abscess. Splenic infarcts tend to shrink as they age (just like people), and fairly large infarcts may become virtually undetectable except for a small contour deformity and minimal residual parenchymal scarring.

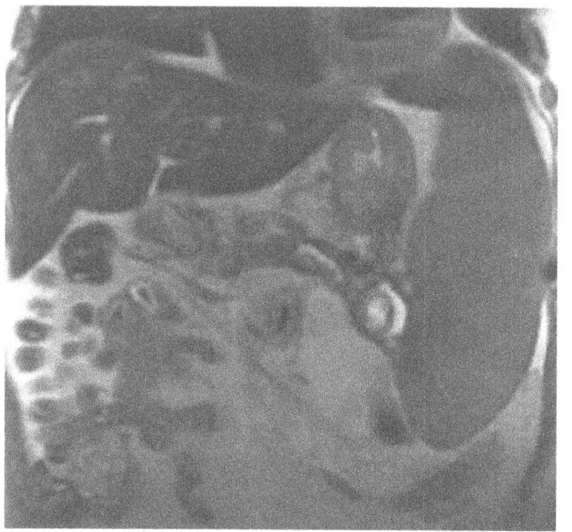

Figure 5.16.1

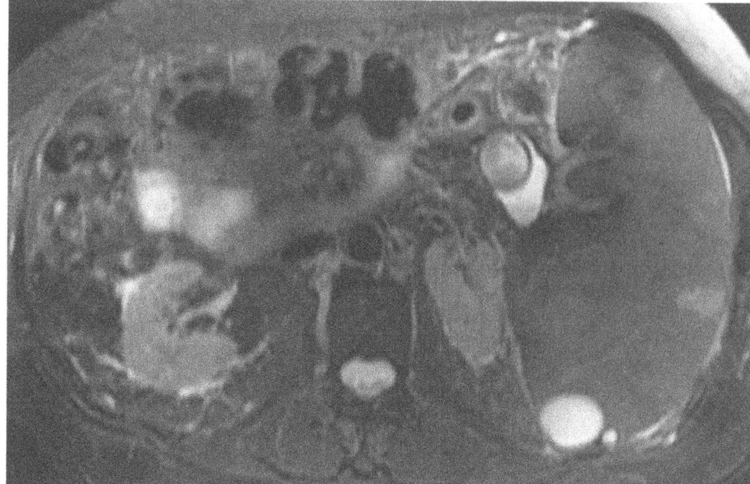

Figure 5.16.2

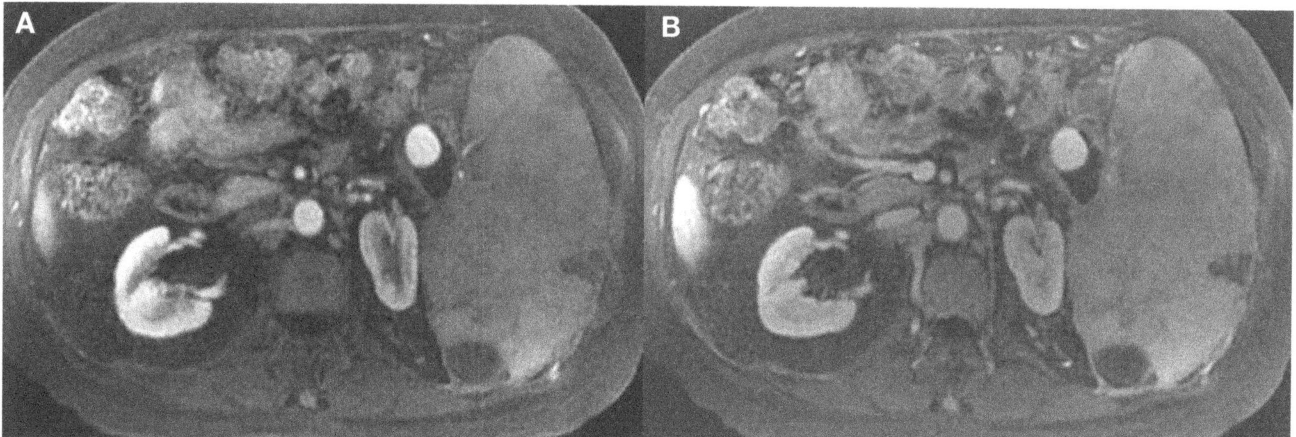

Figure 5.16.3

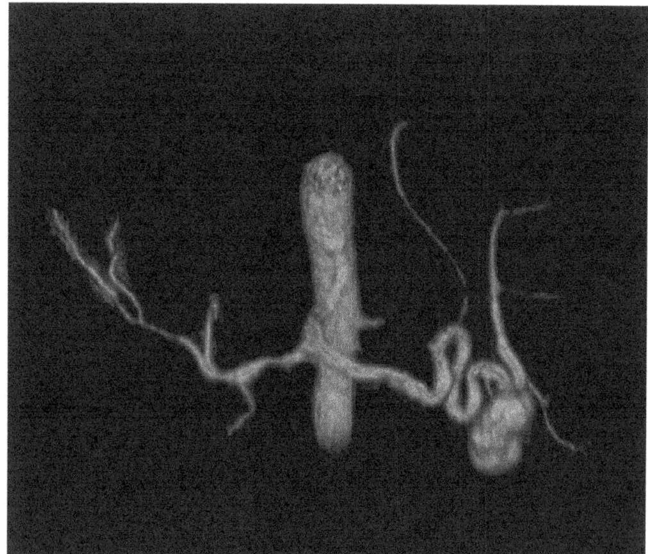

Figure 5.16.4

HISTORY: 68-year-old man with a history of polycythemia vera and a recent episode of pancreatitis, which required endoscopic drainage of a pancreatic pseudocyst with a cystogastrostomy tube

IMAGING FINDINGS: Coronal SSFSE (Figure 5.16.1) and axial fat-suppressed FSE T2-weighted (Figure 5.16.2) images show splenomegaly with a cyst in the posterior spleen. Note also the decreased signal intensity in the liver and spleen due to hemosiderosis from multiple blood transfusions. A round structure in the splenic hilum is bright on T2-weighted images and is surrounded by a small amount of fluid containing a fluid-fluid level. Axial arterial phase and portal venous phase postgadolinium 3D SPGR images (Figure 5.16.3) show intense enhancement of the hilar structure. A small peripheral infarct is seen laterally in the spleen on portal venous phase image and FSE image. VR image reconstructed from arterial phase 3D SPGR source data (Figure 5.16.4) shows focal enlargement of the splenic artery in the splenic hilum.

DIAGNOSIS: Splenic artery pseudoaneurysm secondary to cystogastrostomy tube placement

COMMENT: Splenic artery pseudoaneurysms are rare, with fewer than 200 published cases. Most occur in association with pancreatitis, and the mechanism is thought to be digestion of the arterial wall by pancreatic enzymes. This case could be attributed indirectly to pancreatitis, since the transgastric drainage was performed in response to an episode of pancreatitis with formation of a lesser sac pseudocyst, but it is better classified as posttraumatic, which is another mechanism documented in the literature although never in this fashion.

In our experience, MRI is rarely performed specifically to assess for a visceral artery pseudoaneurysm. In this case, the examination was performed to look for additional peripancreatic fluid collections since the patient was not doing well. CT angiography might be a better first step because it provides higher spatial resolution and requires shorter examination times, but even if the MRI is not optimized for vascular imaging, visualization of a large pseudoaneurysm should be possible. Alternatively, conventional angiography could be performed first, particularly if embolization is a consideration.

This case has multiple abnormalities: splenomegaly secondary to polycythemia vera, a splenic cyst, a small splenic infarction, hemosiderosis from prior blood transfusions, a dilated pancreatic duct, and splenic vein thrombosis (not shown). Even so, the pseudoaneurysm is an obvious finding, appearing as a round structure with arterial phase enhancement contiguous with the splenic artery and surrounded by nonenhancing thrombus. Notice that it is often possible to generate perfectly acceptable 3D reconstructions of arterial anatomy from arterial phase axial 3D SPGR images; although not necessary to make the diagnosis, they can be helpful in convincing skeptical clinical colleagues.

The distinction between a splenic artery aneurysm and a pseudoaneurysm is not trivial but is often aided by the clinical history. An aneurysm is usually atherosclerotic, occasionally secondary to vasculitis or portal hypertension, and tends to appear as a symmetrical enlargement of the vessel compared with the more eccentric dilatation of a pseudoaneurysm. The risk of rupture of a splenic artery aneurysm increases with the diameter of the aneurysm; the risk of rupture of a pseudoaneurysm, however, does not seem to correlate with size.

In general, all splenic artery pseudoaneurysms should be treated, either with surgical resection and splenectomy or with transcatheter embolization.

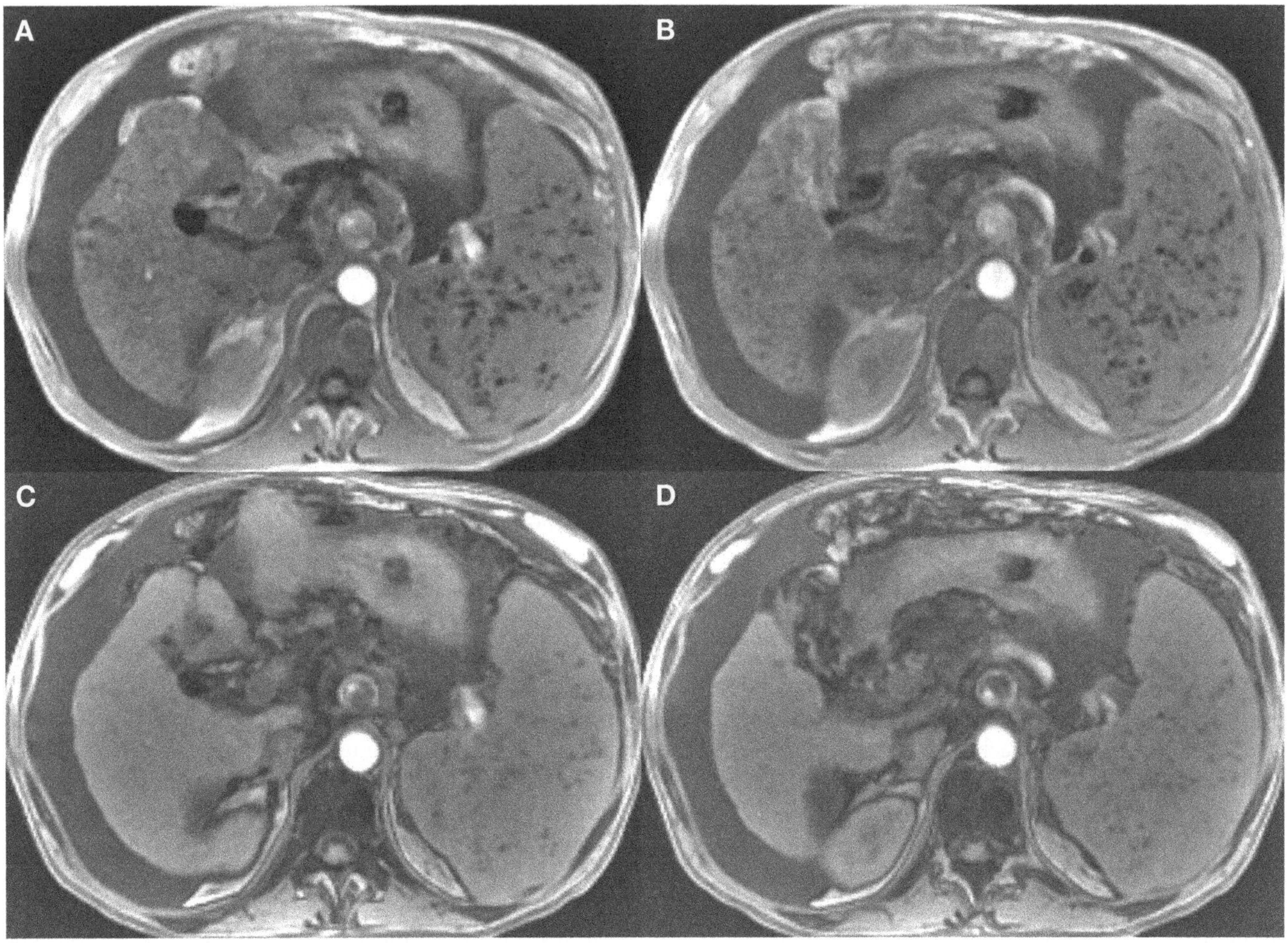

Figure 5.17.1

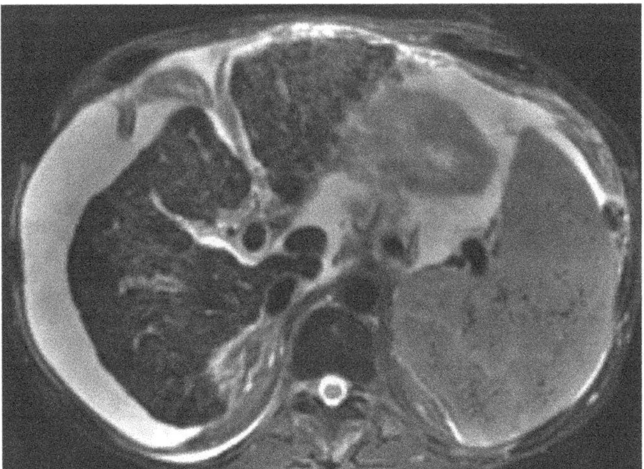

Figure 5.17.2

HISTORY: 50-year-old man with a history of hepatitis C and cirrhosis

IMAGING FINDINGS: Axial in-phase and out-of-phase 2D SPGR images (Figure 5.17.1) show a cirrhotic liver with moderate splenomegaly. The spleen contains multiple hypointense nodules that show signal loss on in-phase images relative to out-of-phase images. The low-signal-intensity lesions are also seen on axial fat-suppressed FSE T2-weighted image (Figure 5.17.2) but are much less prominent.

DIAGNOSIS: Cirrhosis with splenomegaly and splenic Gamna-Gandy bodies

COMMENT: Gamna-Gandy bodies, or siderotic nodules, are caused by small focal hemorrhages in the red pulp of the spleen, and are thought to result from hypertension in the splenic vein, sinusoidal dilatation, and coagulation abnormalities. Gamna-Gandy bodies have been identified in patients who have portal or splenic vein thrombosis, hemolytic anemia, leukemia or lymphoma, hemochromatosis, or paroxysmal nocturnal hemoglobinuria and in patients receiving multiple blood transfusions.

Gamna-Gandy bodies are much easier to see on MRI than on CT by virtue of the susceptibility (or T2*) effects of hemosiderin. The nodules appear hypointense on all imaging sequences but are particularly prominent on gradient echo images with long TEs. The lesions are more conspicuous on in-phase images than on out-of-phase images; the more prominent blooming artifact on the in-phase acquisition is a consequence of a TE that is 2.3 ms longer than the out-of-phase TE. The Gamna-Gandy bodies are least prominent on the FSE images, which are T2-weighted rather than T2*-weighted acquisitions.

There really isn't a differential diagnosis for this entity other than multiple splenic granulomas, which are usually not as numerous and tend not to have such a uniform appearance. In general, Gamna-Gandy bodies are not visualized before overt manifestations of cirrhosis and portal hypertension, so they're rarely useful as early markers of cirrhosis.

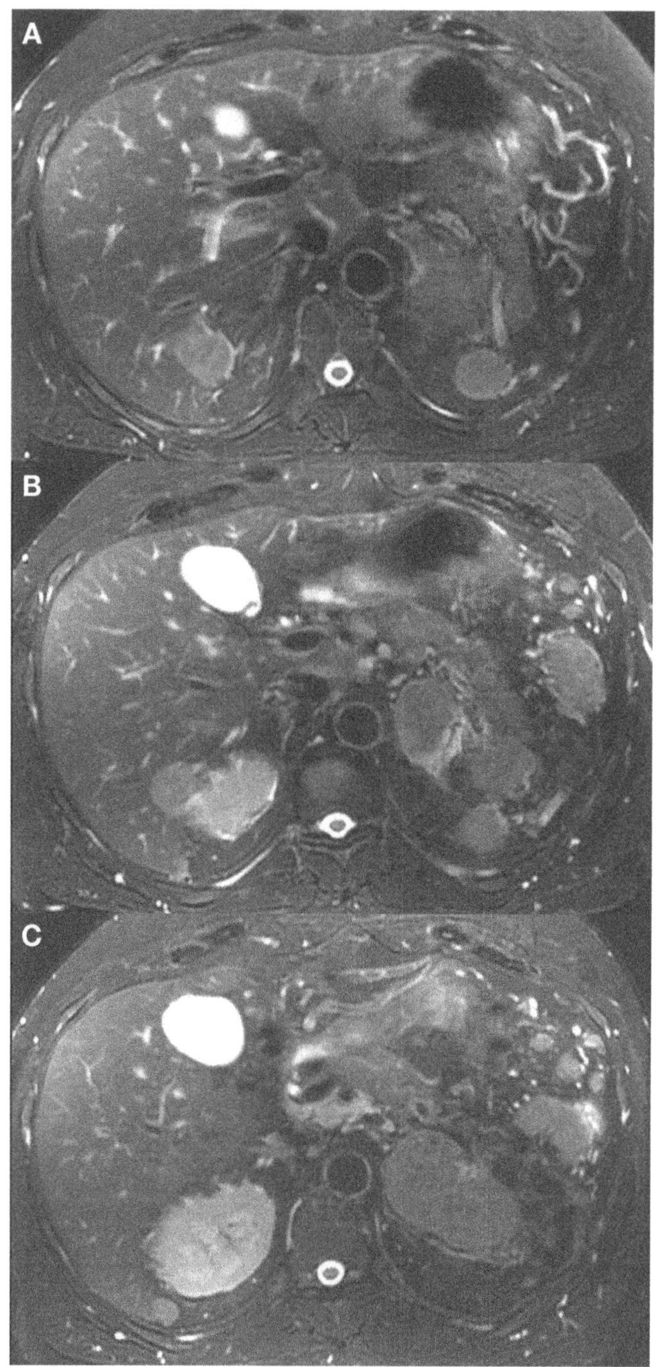

Figure 5.18.1

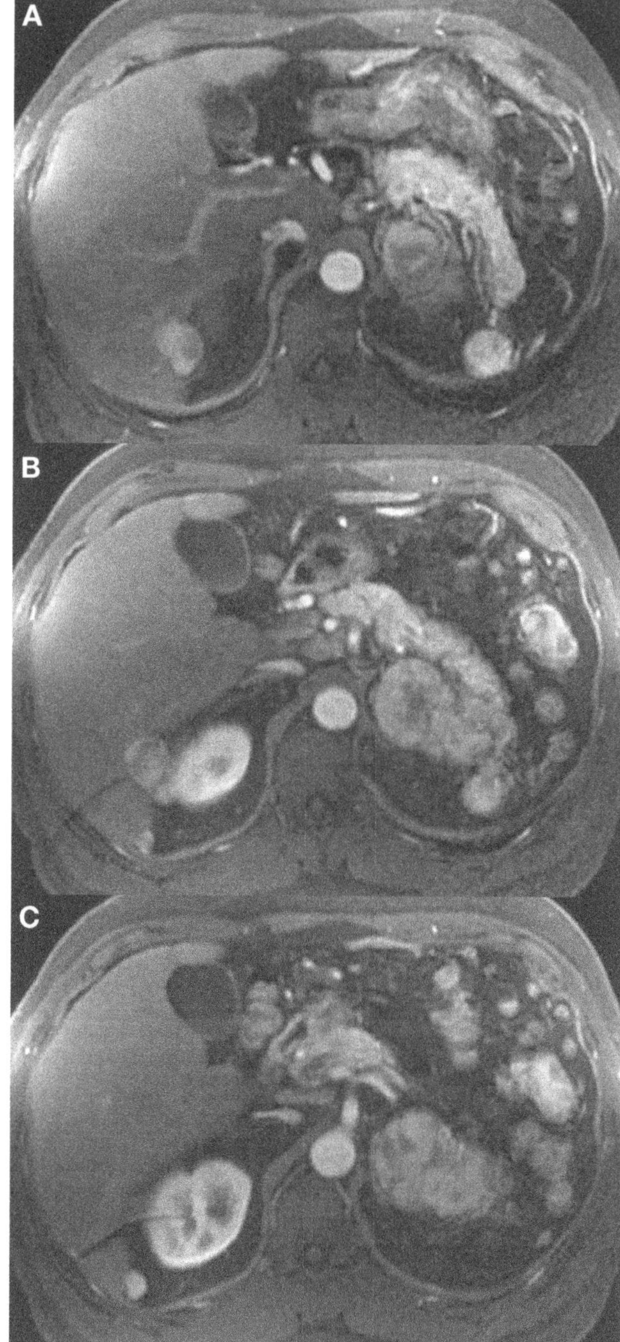

Figure 5.18.2

HISTORY: 49-year-old man with hepatitis C and a remote history of splenectomy after trauma

IMAGING FINDINGS: Axial fat-suppressed FSE T2-weighted images (Figure 5.18.1) show multiple hypointense masses in the left upper quadrant and the right pararenal space. Axial arterial phase postgadolinium 3D SPGR images (Figure 5.18.2) show heterogeneous enhancement of the lesions. No normal spleen is identified.

DIAGNOSIS: Splenosis

COMMENT: *Splenosis* is defined as autotransplantation of splenic tissue onto vascularized intraperitoneal or extraperitoneal surfaces after splenic injury. This usually occurs in the setting of splenic trauma followed by elective splenectomy, although it has occasionally been reported after splenectomy alone. The presumed mechanism is spillage and seeding of damaged splenic pulp onto various surfaces with an adequate blood supply, although a few reports have suggested an additional hematogenous mechanism. Once considered a relatively rare occurrence, abdominal pelvic splenosis is now thought to occur with nearly two-thirds of splenic ruptures. Thoracic splenosis is less common and requires concurrent diaphragmatic rupture.

Most histologic reports describe the ectopic splenic tissue as lacking the normal trabecular structure of the spleen, with absent or poorly formed white pulp. Nevertheless, it can perform normal splenic functions; therefore, Howell-Jolly and Heinz bodies may not be present in a peripheral blood smear as would be expected after splenectomy.

Most splenosis patients are asymptomatic; however, complications have been reported, including gastrointestinal tract bleeding, bowel obstruction, and pain related to infarction of the ectopic tissue.

The diagnosis of splenosis is usually straightforward if you recognize that the spleen is absent (a fact rarely included in the clinical history) and that the multiple abdominal masses or pelvic masses (or both), which may be located far from the splenic bed, look like little spleens. Problems arise when there is another potential explanation for the presence of peritoneal nodules, such as a primary malignancy. In particularly challenging cases, a nuclear medicine liver-spleen scan may be needed to resolve lingering doubts. In the days when SPIO contrast agents were available, pre- and post-SPIO T2- or T2*-weighted images could show signal loss in the masses, indicating the presence of functional reticulocytes and, therefore, ectopic splenic tissue. This case looks like an example of this signal loss, since the ectopic spleen has low signal intensity on the T2-weighted images. This abnormality is likely explained by hemosiderosis resulting from multiple transfusions at the time of the initial trauma. DWI is helpful for visualizing all the splenic foci, since they have very high signal intensity against a relatively dark background; however, they are not particularly useful for distinguishing splenosis from intraperitoneal metastases.

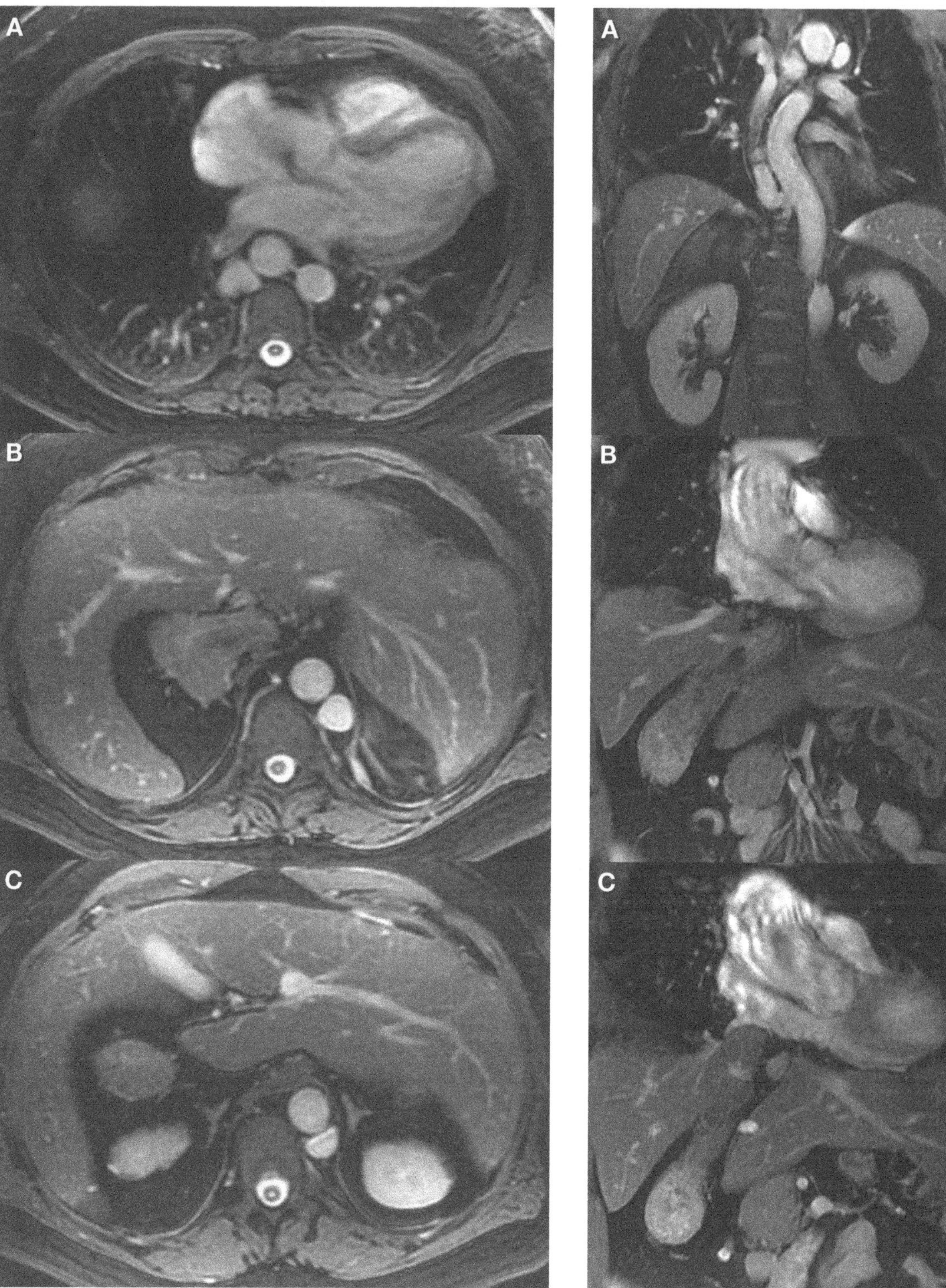

Figure 5.19.1

Figure 5.19.2

HISTORY: 67-year-old woman with a history of bicuspid aortic valve and ascending aortic aneurysm

IMAGING FINDINGS: Axial (Figure 5.19.1) and coronal (Figure 5.19.2) fat-suppressed SSFP images show midline orientation of the liver and the absence of a spleen. The IVC is also absent, with a prominent hemiazygos vein in the abdomen and azygos and hemiazygos veins in the lower chest. The aortic root and ascending aorta are dilated.

DIAGNOSIS: Asplenia syndrome

COMMENT: Asplenia and polysplenia (an example is shown in Case 5.20) represent 2 points on the spectrum of situs anomalies. The term *situs* refers to position and is used to describe the position of the heart and viscera in relation to the midline. *Situs solitus* is the normal state, with the cardiac apex, spleen, stomach, and aorta located on the left and the liver and IVC on the right. *Situs inversus* is a mirror-image reflection of *situs solitus* (although there is a rare subcategory of *situs inversus* with levocardia). *Situs ambiguus*, or *heterotaxia*, is a spectrum of abnormal arrangements of the organs and vessels that are neither situs solitus nor situs inversus. Although patients with situs solitus (<1%) or situs inversus (3%-5%) have a low incidence of congenital heart disease, patients with situs ambiguus have a much higher incidence (50%-100%).

Situs ambiguus with asplenia, also known as right isomerism or bilateral right-sidedness, is characterized by male predominance (66%), ambiguous locations of the abdominal organs, and an absence of the spleen. Nearly 100% of affected patients have congenital heart disease, which is generally more severe than that occurring with polysplenia and other situs abnormalities. Adults with polysplenia are rarely encountered since as many as 95% die within the first year of life, usually as a consequence of severe congenital heart disease or overwhelming infection related to an absent spleen.

A midline location of the liver is common in asplenia, and other associated anomalies may include an atretic pancreas and variable forms of malrotation. Interruption of the IVC with azygos continuation (as in this case) is rarely described in asplenia and is much more common in patients with polysplenia.

In adults, incidental detection of situs abnormalities is important because their presence can cause confusion when patients have common diseases such as appendicitis or cholecystitis and their pain does not correspond to the expected location of the organ in question.

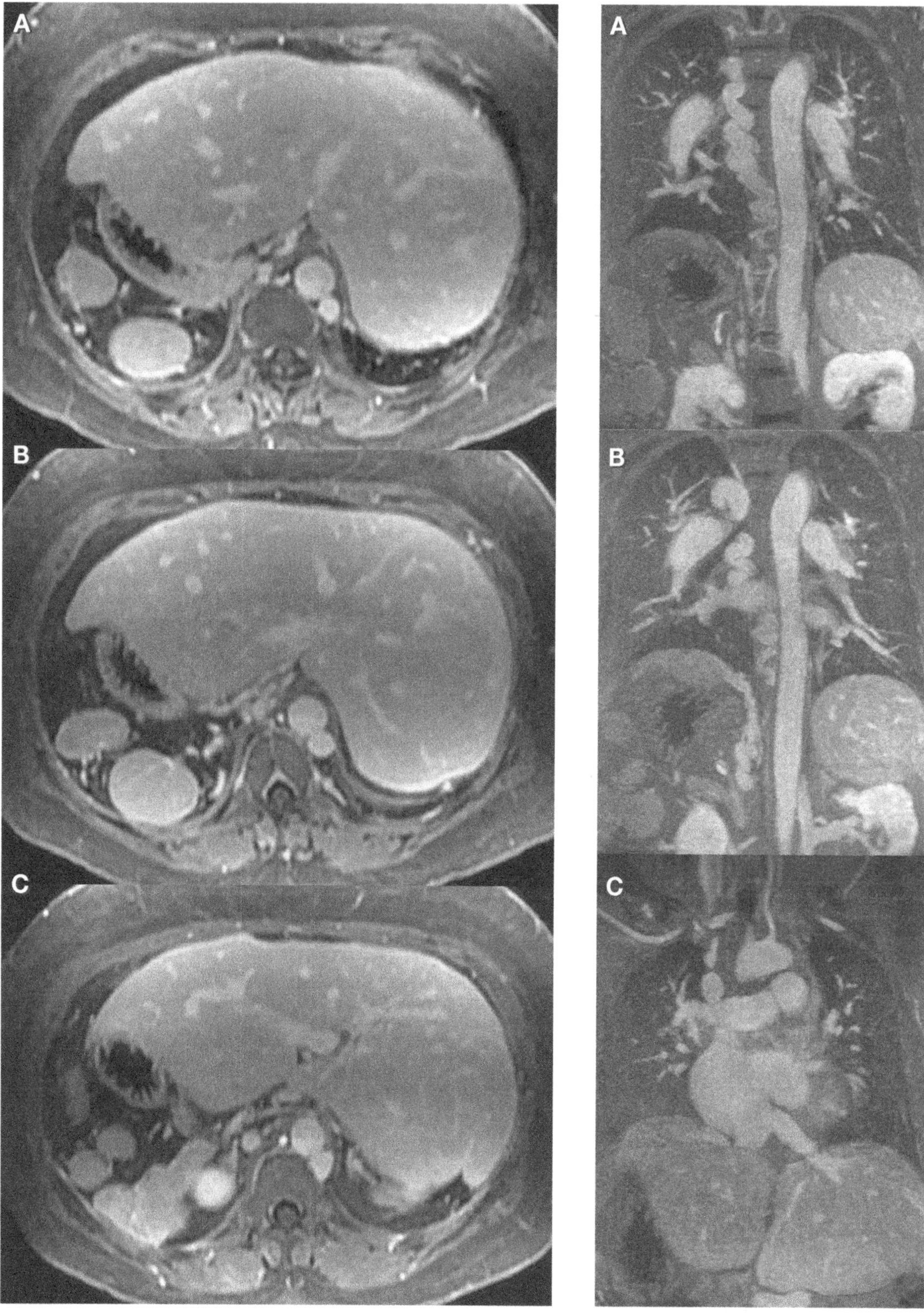

Figure 5.20.1

Figure 5.20.2

HISTORY: 55-year-old woman with a history of complex congenital heart disease

IMAGING FINDINGS: Axial postgadolinium 3D SPGR images (Figure 5.20.1) show a left-sided liver, right-sided stomach, and multiple small accessory spleens in the right upper quadrant. The IVC is absent, and the azygos and hemiazygos veins are prominent. Coronal postgadolinium 3D SPGR images (Figure 5.20.2) show prominent collateral veins in the posterior abdomen and thorax and drainage of the left hepatic vein directly into the right side of a common atrium.

DIAGNOSIS: Polysplenia

COMMENT: By definition, patients with polysplenia have multiple spleens (an average of 6 was reported in 1 series), which may be on the right or the left. As in this case, the stomach is almost always located on the same side as the spleens. Midline orientation of the liver is the most common position; a right-sided location is slightly less frequent, and a left-sided orientation is rare. An atretic or truncated pancreas and rotational abnormalities of the bowel are frequent findings in polysplenia. Interruption of the IVC with azygos continuation, in contrast to asplenia, is common in patients with polysplenia and is seen in this case.

ABBREVIATIONS

CT	computed tomography
DWI	diffusion-weighted imaging
FRFSE	fast-recovery fast-spin echo
FSE	fast-spin echo
GRE	gradient-recalled echo
HD	Hodgkin disease
IVC	inferior vena cava
JAK2	Janus kinase 2
KTS	Klippel-Trénaunay syndrome
MRI	magnetic resonance imaging
NHL	non-Hodgkin lymphoma
SPGR	spoiled gradient recalled
SPIO	superparamagnetic iron oxide
SSFP	steady-state free precession
SSFSE	single-shot fast-spin echo
TE	echo time
3D	3-dimensional
2D	2-dimensional
US	ultrasonography
VR	volume-rendered

6.

ADRENAL GLANDS

CASE 6.1

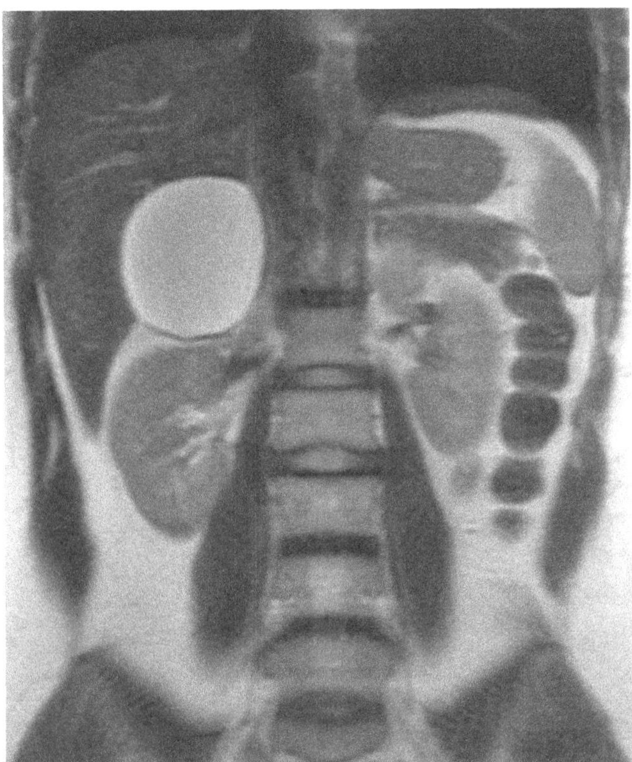

Figure 6.1.1

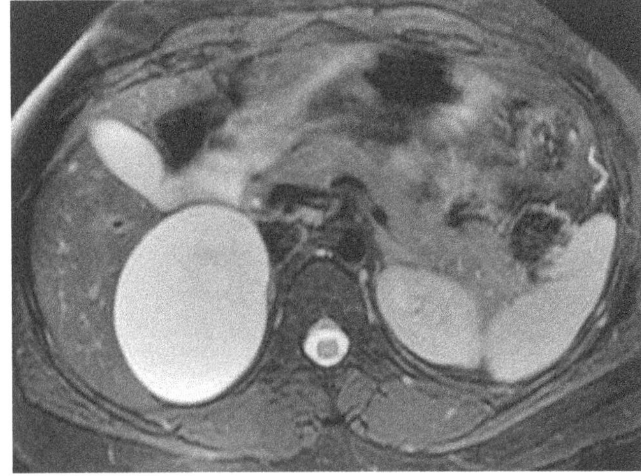

Figure 6.1.2

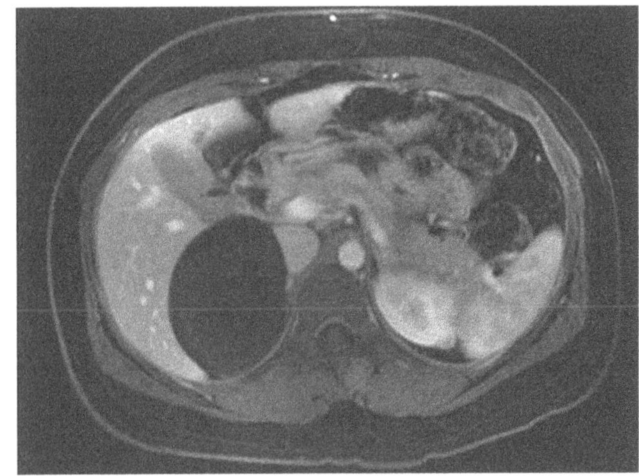

Figure 6.1.3

HISTORY: 24-year-old postpartum woman with right-sided pelvic discomfort, fever, and elevated white blood cell count several days after normal vaginal delivery; abdominal pelvic noncontrast CT showed a right adrenal mass, and MRI was performed for further characterization

IMAGING FINDINGS: Coronal SSFSE image (Figure 6.1.1) demonstrates a large right adrenal cystic lesion with imperceptible margins and no nodules or septations. Axial fat-suppressed FSE T2-weighted image (Figure 6.1.2) shows similar findings. Axial portal venous phase postgadolinium 3D SPGR image (Figure 6.1.3) reveals no significant enhancement of the lesion.

DIAGNOSIS: Adrenal cyst

COMMENT: Adrenal cysts are rare lesions that ambitious pathologists have classified into 4 histologic subtypes: endothelialized (endothelial) cysts, pseudocysts, parasitic cysts, and epithelial cysts. Endothelial cysts are the most common subtype, accounting for 45% of adrenal cysts. Pseudocysts lack an epithelial lining and probably arise from prior episodes of hemorrhage. Most cysts do not cause symptoms and are incidentally detected. Larger cysts, which may cause symptoms from the mass effect, have been treated by aspiration or laparoscopic removal.

The appearance of adrenal cysts is identical to the appearance of cysts in the liver, kidneys, and pancreas—fluid-filled structures with thin walls and without significant enhancement after administration of gadolinium. Complex adrenal cysts can contain proteinaceous fluid, blood products, debris, and septations. These are more likely to occur in pseudocysts. The differential diagnosis for a complex adrenal cyst includes abscess, necrotic primary or metastatic tumor, and cystic pheochromocytoma.

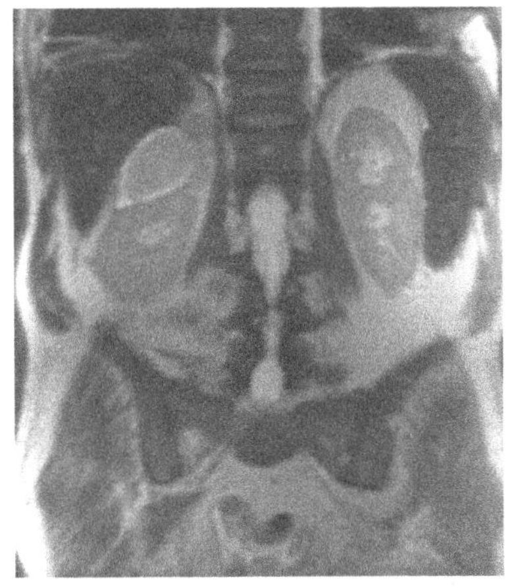

Figure 6.2.1

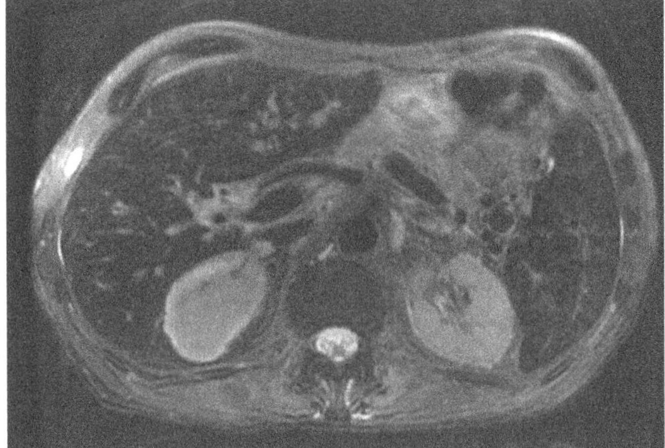

Figure 6.2.2

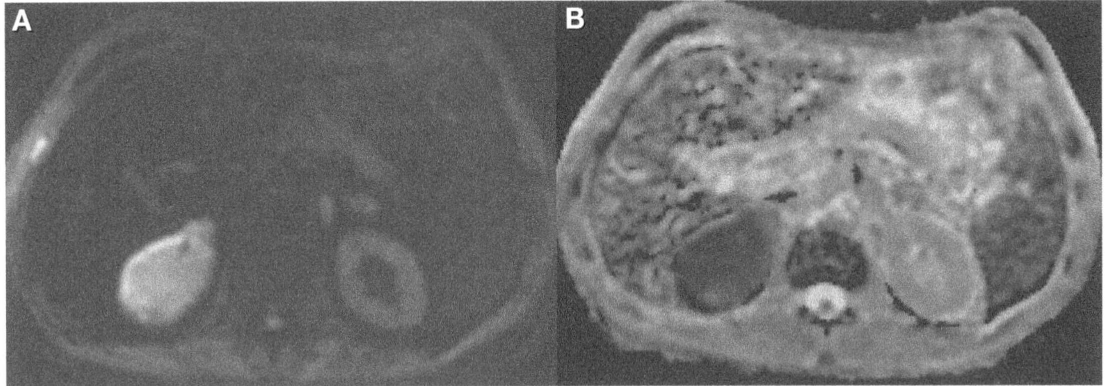

Figure 6.2.3

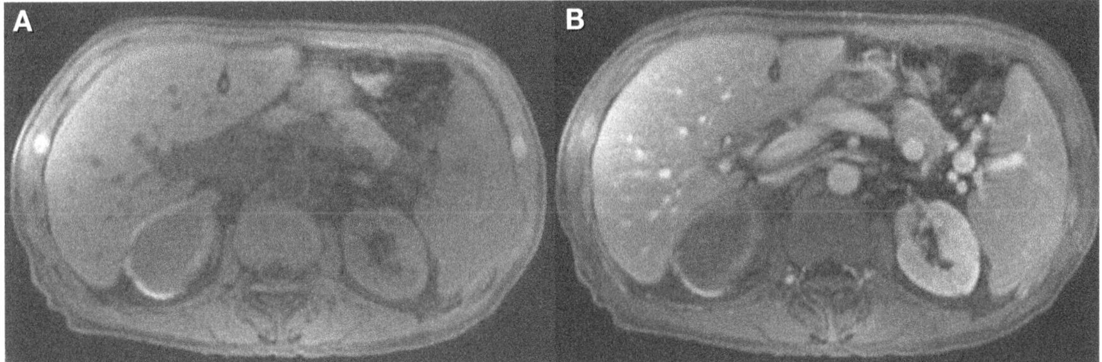

Figure 6.2.4

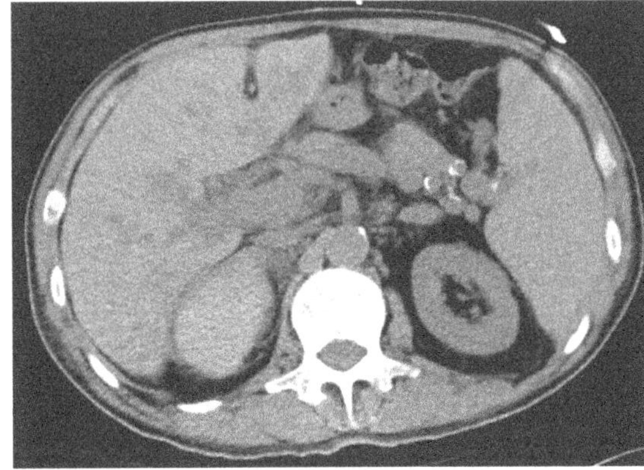

Figure 6.2.5

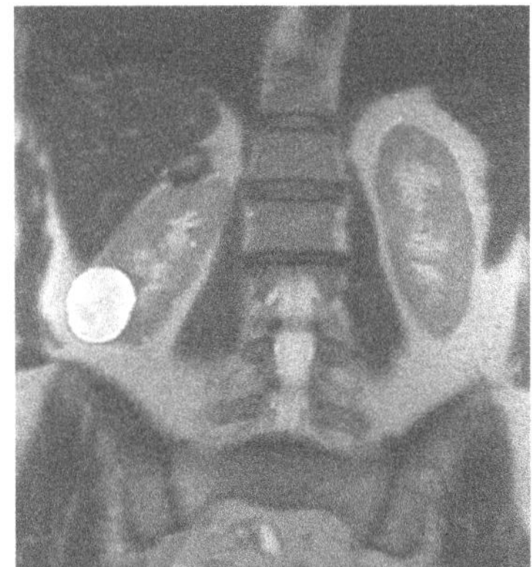

Figure 6.2.6

HISTORY: 72-year-old man with a history of autoimmune hemolytic anemia and recurrent fevers of unknown origin presenting with new right flank pain

IMAGING FINDINGS: Coronal SSFSE (Figure 6.2.1) and axial fat-suppressed T2-weighted FSE images (Figure 6.2.2) demonstrate a lenticular right adrenal lesion with a hyperintense outer margin. Diffusion-weighted image (b=600 s/mm^2) (Figure 6.2.3A) and corresponding ADC map (Figure 6.2.3B) show that the lesion has a diffuse high signal intensity and restricted diffusion. Precontrast fat-suppressed 3D SPGR image (Figure 6.2.4A) demonstrates a hyperintense outer rim. The lesion shows no significant enhancement on postcontrast 3D SPGR image (Figure 6.2.4B). The adrenal mass has diffuse high attenuation on an axial image from noncontrast CT performed 3 days earlier (Figure 6.2.5). Coronal SSFSE image from a follow-up examination 6 months later (Figure 6.2.6) reveals that the lesion is considerably smaller and has a hypointense rim. A simple cyst is seen in the lower pole of the right kidney.

DIAGNOSIS: Adrenal hematoma

COMMENT: Adrenal hemorrhage can result from physiologic stress, trauma, or coagulopathy or from bleeding into an existing adrenal neoplasm. Most adrenal hematomas are unilateral, and most unilateral hematomas occur on the right side. Bilateral hematomas, which are more common in patients who have coagulopathies, can result in Addison disease. The classic appearance of a subacute hematoma in the adrenal gland or elsewhere (and most hematomas imaged with MRI are subacute) is that of a T1- and T2-hyperintense rim, indicating the presence of methemoglobin. When methemoglobin is converted into hemosiderin in the chronic state, the rim becomes dark on both T1- and T2-weighted images, as seen in the SSFSE image from the follow-up examination (Figure 6.2.6). In our experience, the T1-bright rim is the most specific finding and is best appreciated on noncontrast (or precontrast) fat-suppressed 2D or 3D SPGR images. It's worth noting that, as in this case, hematomas frequently show high signal intensity on diffusion-weighted images and restricted diffusion on ADC maps. This illustrates the general principle that basing your decisions about whether a lesion is benign or malignant on ADC values alone is almost never a good idea. Notice also the diffuse, decreased signal intensity in the liver, spleen, and bone marrow on the T2-weighted images, a consequence of the patient's hemolytic anemia and the resulting iron deposition in the reticuloendothelial system. The diagnosis in this case is obvious from the high-attenuation adrenal mass that is apparent with the noncontrast CT performed a few days earlier. The MRI was requested to search for an intra-abdominal abscess as a possible source for the patient's fever of unknown origin.

As for most hematomas in body imaging, a simple hematoma must be distinguished from one containing a hemorrhagic lesion. Usually, this distinction is fairly easy: Simple hematomas tend to be simple and hemorrhagic masses tend to be complex, and most patients with uncomplicated hematomas have an underlying cause that can be identified if you're willing to spend some time reading the medical record. Dynamic contrast-enhanced images can be helpful in making this distinction—you shouldn't see anything enhancing in a hematoma except possibly mild rim enhancement from inflammation or granulation tissue. An adrenal mass, however, will enhance unless it is completely necrotic. Since adrenal hematomas often contain components with high T1-signal intensity, postcontrast minus precontrast subtraction images may help to visualize an enhancing mass or, conversely, to demonstrate the absence of enhancement; of course, the utility of these images relies on good source data without motion or misregistration artifact. From a practical standpoint, to resolve any doubt, a follow-up examination performed a few months later will show that the hematoma has either resolved or significantly decreased in size and continues to show no enhancement or minimal enhancement. Adrenal lesions that are especially prone to hemorrhage include pheochromocytoma, myelolipoma, hemangioma, and adrenal cortical carcinoma.

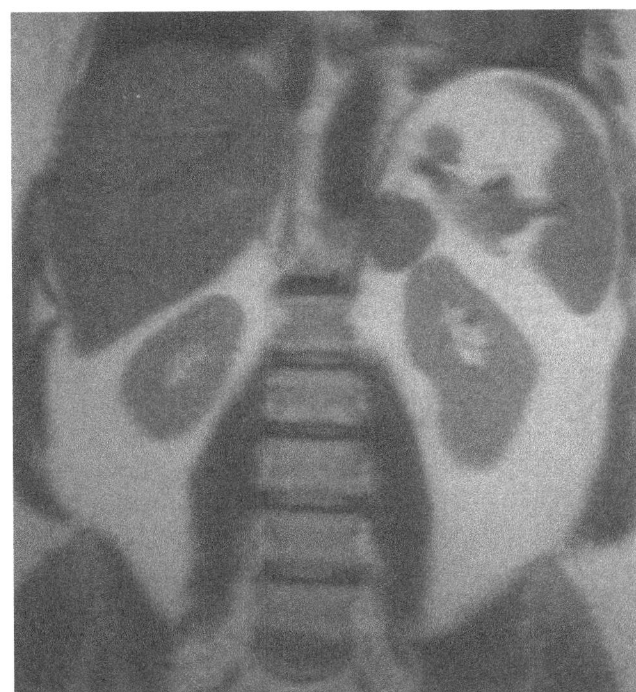

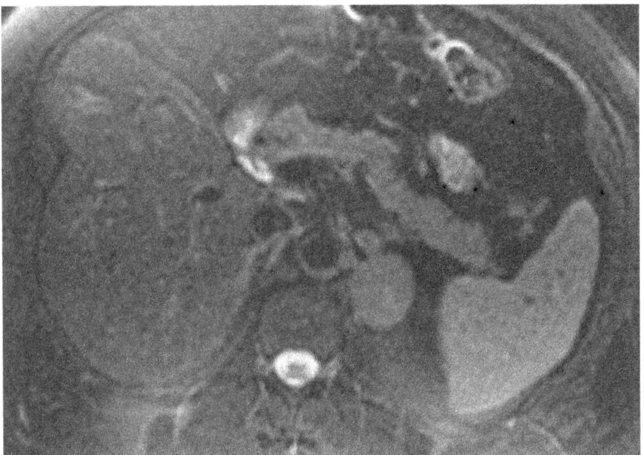

Figure 6.3.2

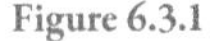

Figure 6.3.1

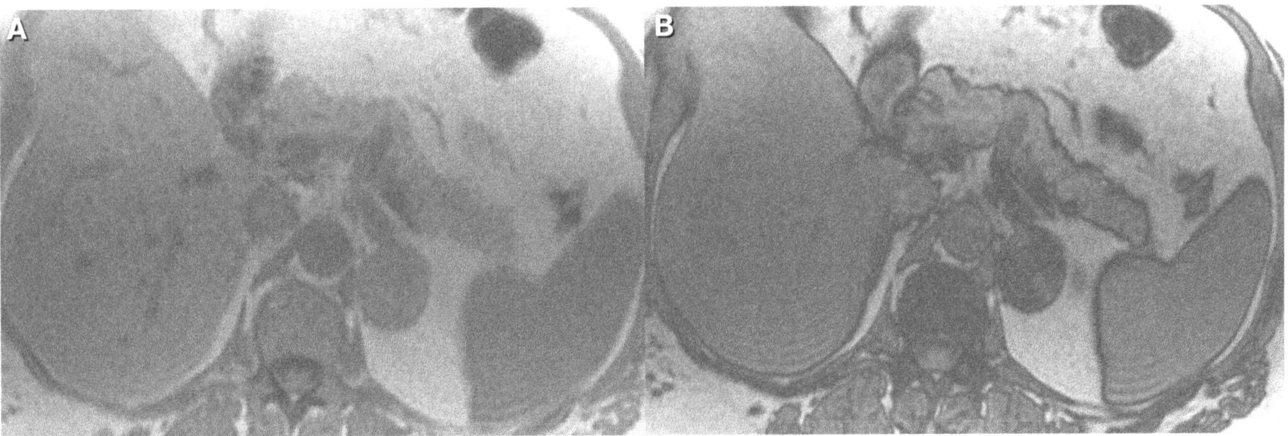

Figure 6.3.3

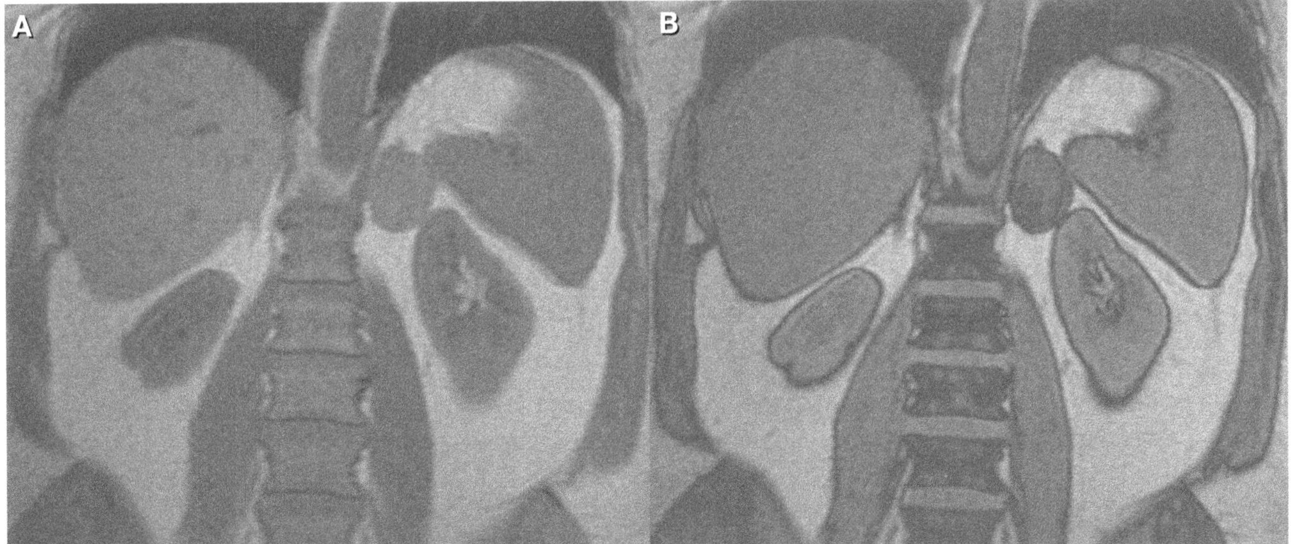

Figure 6.3.4

HISTORY: 52-year-old woman with chest discomfort; chest CT showed an indeterminate adrenal lesion

IMAGING FINDINGS: A well-circumscribed left adrenal mass shows signal intensity similar to that of the normal adrenal gland on coronal SSFSE (Figure 6.3.1) and axial fat-suppressed FSE T2-weighted (Figure 6.3.2) images. Notice the extensive signal loss within the lesion between IP (Figure 6.3.3A) and OP (Figure 6.3.3B) axial images and between IP (Figure 6.3.4A) and OP (Figure 6.3.4B) coronal images. The OP images also show mild signal loss in the liver, indicating the presence of hepatic steatosis.

DIAGNOSIS: Adrenal adenoma

COMMENT: Adrenal adenomas are very common—autopsy series have reported an 8% incidence—and generally easy to diagnose. Usually they are incidental findings on an examination performed for another indication. Adenomas are characterized by the presence of intracellular lipid, as shown by significant signal dropout between IP and OP images.

Adenomas generally are small (<3 cm), have similar signal intensity or mild hyperintensity relative to the normal adrenal gland on T2-weighted images, and show arterial phase enhancement with relatively rapid washout on dynamic contrast-enhanced images. Adrenal hyperplasia also sometimes manifests as diffuse fatty infiltration, and the distinction is relatively unimportant, although adenomas are usually discrete masses. Over 90% of adenomas reliably show signal dropout on OP images; however, a small subset of lipid-poor adenomas do not have enough fat to show signal loss. In theory, one can apply the same sorts of criteria for rapid contrast washout described for CT (ie, >50% washout on 10- to 15-minute delayed images), but the supporting MRI literature is relatively sparse.

The question inevitably arises: How large a difference on IP-OP images is required to reach significance and make the diagnosis of an adenoma? We have a couple of rules that keep us out of trouble most of the time: 1) If you can see an obvious signal intensity difference with the same window and level settings, it's an adenoma. 2) If you think there's fat but aren't sure, place a region of interest in the lesion, copy it to the other view, and then look at the average signal intensity. If the difference is higher than the standard deviation of the measurement, it's an adenoma. If you're still not sure, try another acquisition plane or thinner sections (adenomas are often small, and volume averaging can be problematic).

Several early publications on chemical shift imaging of adrenal adenomas discussed quantification of signal dropout, and many authors favored the use of internal reference standards such as liver, spleen, and skeletal muscle (ie, the ratio of adrenal tissue to liver tissue on IP-OP images). Internal references for imaging quantification are usually a bad idea simply because the reference tissue may also have something wrong with it and thereby lead to an abnormal ratio and an erroneous diagnosis. In chemical shift imaging, the liver (fatty infiltration and iron deposition), skeletal muscle (fatty infiltration), and spleen (iron deposition) all have obvious potential flaws, which could lead to large signal intensity changes in the reference between IP and OP images.

Probably the most important thing to remember about adenomas is that you should put yourself in a position to make the diagnosis even when you're not necessarily looking for one. This opportunity often arises with renal MRAs. Adrenal adenomas can cause hypertension, and we believe that it's well worth the extra minute to add an IP-OP series to your renal MRA protocol to characterize an incidental adrenal lesion.

Mild heterogeneity within an adenoma is not unheard of and should not preclude making a confident diagnosis. We remember a case of a nearly classic adenoma with a small amount of modestly increased T2-signal intensity in the periphery. We discussed the case with a resident, decided that the lesion was an adenoma, glanced briefly at the conclusion of the resident's dictation, which said "consistent with adenoma," and signed the report. A couple of months later, we needed images of an adenoma for a talk. When we retrieved the case, we noticed that the patient had had an adrenalectomy to remove what the endocrinologist described as an indeterminate adrenal lesion (which turned out to be an adenoma). We reread the resident's report more carefully and saw that in the body of the report, he had stated that the appearance was not classic for adenoma and that sometimes collision lesions have a similar appearance, but this lesion was somewhat more likely to be an adenoma than a collision lesion. Lessons learned from this case include 1) either read everything in residents' reports carefully or delete everything but the conclusion, and 2) remember that not everyone handles uncertainty in the same way. Collision lesions, by the way, describe a usually malignant lesion that partially or completely engulfs an adenoma, so that part of the lesion looks like an adenoma (which it is), but the rest of the lesion does not. Collision lesions are very rare and should not cause anyone to lose sleep over the possibility of a misdiagnosis.

Most adrenal adenomas are nonfunctional (which is why they are often incidental findings), but hypersecreting adenomas can cause Cushing syndrome or Conn syndrome (primary aldosteronism, the most common cause of secondary renal hypertension). No MRI criteria can reliably distinguish functional adenomas from nonfunctional adenomas.

The most important differential diagnosis for adenoma is metastasis. At our institution, an adrenal-specific MRI is probably requested most often to decide whether an adrenal lesion seen on CT in a patient with a known malignancy is an adenoma or metastasis. Metastases should not have enough lipid to show signal dropout on OP images, so the distinction is usually fairly easy, but some caution is warranted if patients have fat-containing primary tumors such as hepatocellular carcinoma or clear cell RCC. Adrenal metastases with OP signal dropout are very rare—we haven't seen any in our practice (or perhaps have just missed all of them), but we have been shown a few examples with actual pathologic correlation. The distinction between a lipid-poor adenoma and metastasis is difficult and might be resolved by interval growth, activity on PET, or biopsy.

While IP-OP imaging is the most important technique for distinguishing adenomas from metastases, more complete protocols with T2- and diffusion-weighted images and dynamic contrast-enhanced acquisitions may provide useful information, even though there is considerable overlap between features of benign and malignant adrenal lesions on all of these pulse sequences. In our experience, these techniques are most helpful for identifying additional lesions outside the adrenal glands.

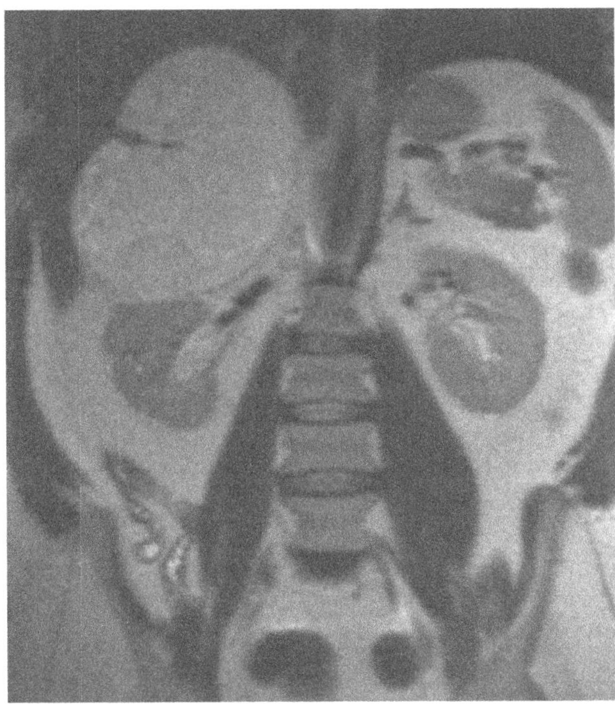

Figure 6.4.1

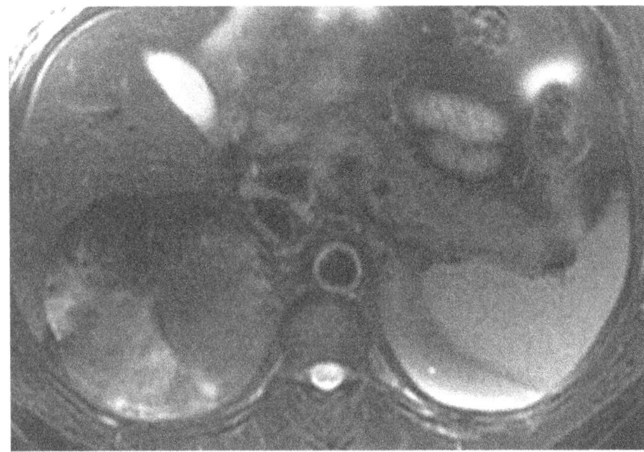

Figure 6.4.2

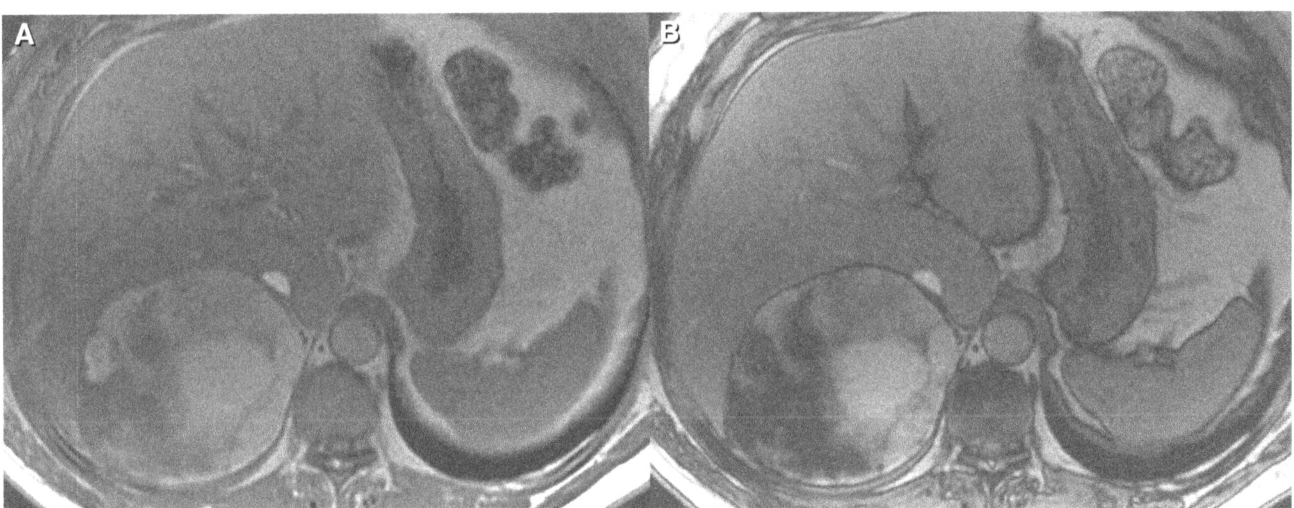

Figure 6.4.3

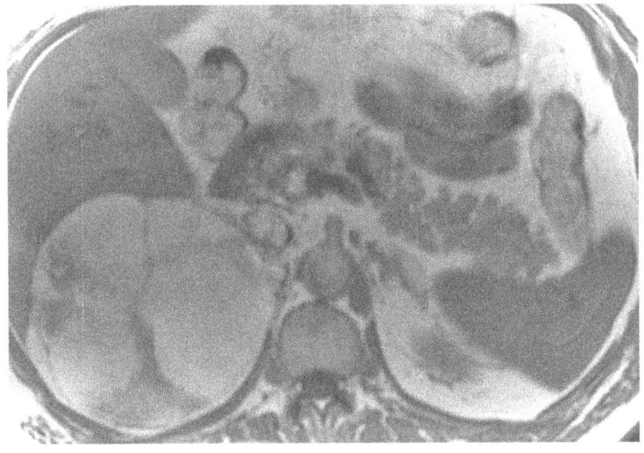

Figure 6.4.4

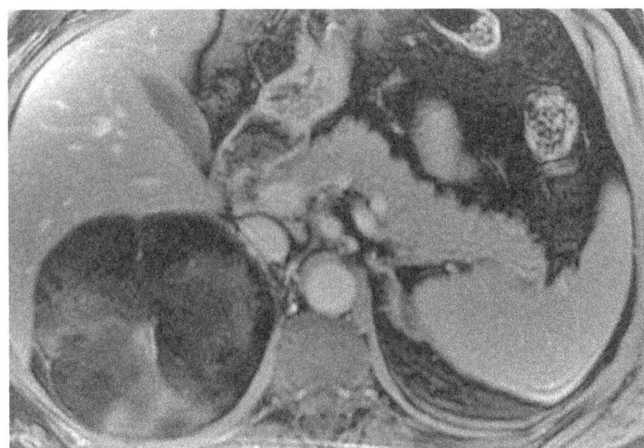

Figure 6.4.5

HISTORY: 51-year-old man with a history of right flank discomfort and renal stones; a large renal mass was detected on renal stone CT at another medical facility

IMAGING FINDINGS: Coronal SSFSE image (Figure 6.4.1) reveals a large hyperintense right adrenal lesion. Axial fat-suppressed FRFSE image (Figure 6.4.2) demonstrates that much of the lesion has very low signal intensity. Axial IP (Figure 6.4.3A) and OP (Figure 6.4.3B) images show that the medial portion of the lesion has high signal intensity without much change in signal between the 2 views, while the lateral part of the lesion shows significant signal dropout on the OP image. Axial FSE T1-weighted image (Figure 6.4.4) also demonstrates diffuse high signal intensity within the lesion with scattered regions of lower signal intensity. Axial postgadolinium SPGR image (Figure 6.4.5) reveals a predominantly hypointense mass with regions of mild hyperenhancement.

DIAGNOSIS: Adrenal myelolipoma

COMMENT: Adrenal myelolipomas are usually easy to detect and characterize because the presence of macroscopic fat is essentially diagnostic. You may not always see signal dropout within a myelolipoma on OP images (in contrast to an adenoma) because the internal water content is so small that the signal intensity differences between IP and OP fat and water are minimal. In this case, the myelolipoma is somewhat heterogeneous and contains regions without signal dropout (which have nearly 100% fat) and regions with significant signal dropout (which have fat and water components).

An efficient technique for clinching the diagnosis in a single breath-hold is a Dixon 2D or 3D SPGR pulse sequence, which acquires images with 2 or more TEs and then uses some clever math to reconstruct IP, OP, fat, and water images. The fat images are often ignored but can be helpful in several situations, including quantifying fat in the liver, visualizing hepatic adenomas and ovarian dermoids, detecting marrow-replacing lesions in bones, and documenting macroscopic fat in adrenal myelolipomas.

Myelolipomas are uncommon benign lesions composed of mature adipose and hematopoietic tissues. Most lesions do not cause symptoms, and nearly all are hormonally inactive. Symptomatic lesions usually occur as a result of local mass effect or hemorrhage. Myelolipomas can become large, and occasionally the appearance is heterogeneous, particularly in hemorrhagic lesions, but the presence of macroscopic fat establishes the diagnosis.

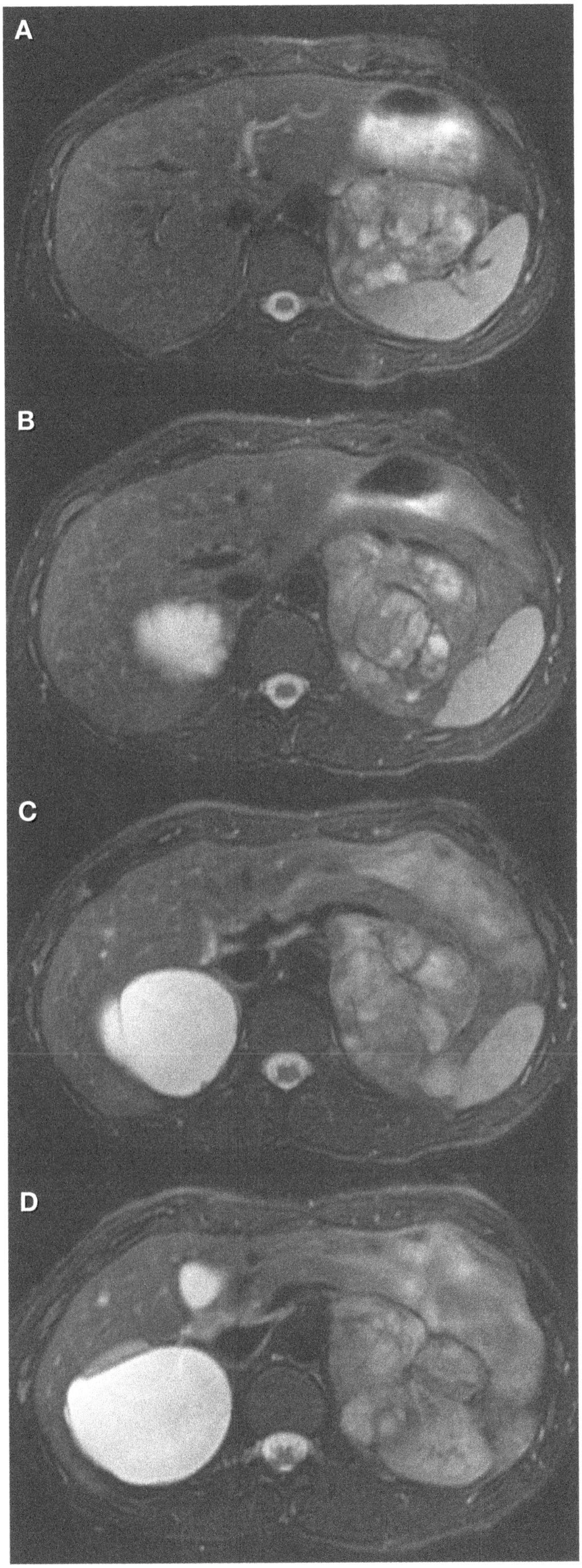

Figure 6.5.1

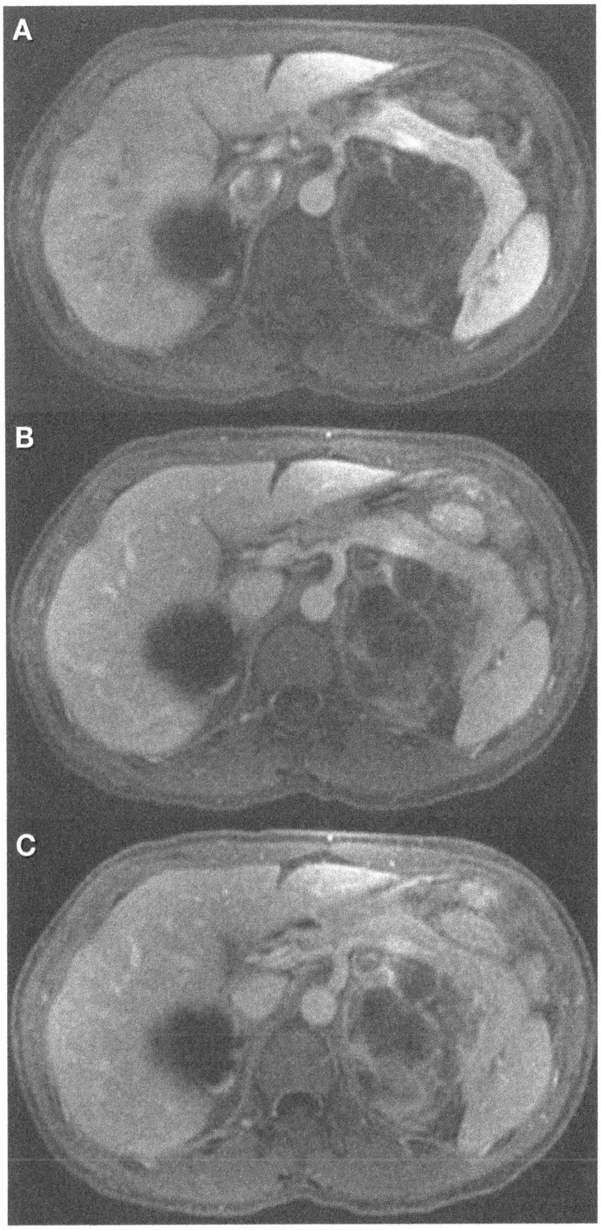

Figure 6.5.2

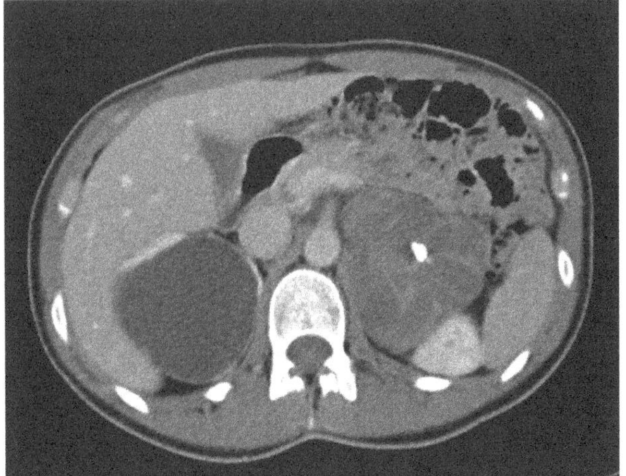

Figure 6.5.3

HISTORY: 33-year-old woman with infertility and hydronephrosis; an adrenal lesion was incidentally noted on a CT urogram

IMAGING FINDINGS: Axial fat-suppressed FSE T2-weighted images (Figure 6.5.1) reveal a large left adrenal mass with heterogeneous increased T2-signal intensity. Arterial (Figure 6.5.2A), portal venous (Figure 6.5.2B), and equilibrium phase (Figure 6.5.2C) postgadolinium 3D SPGR images demonstrate initial hypoenhancement with increasing mild enhancement on equilibrium phase images. Axial postcontrast CT image (Figure 6.5.3) demonstrates central calcification within the heterogeneous low-attenuation lesion. A large right renal cyst can be seen in multiple images.

DIAGNOSIS: Ganglioneuroma

COMMENT: The patient's infertility and hydronephrosis are red herrings in this case—this is a true incidentaloma. Adrenal ganglioneuromas are uncommon tumors of neural crest origin that occur most often in children and young adults. Since they are not hormonally active, they can be fairly large at presentation. The differential diagnosis includes pheochromocytoma, adrenal carcinoma, and metastasis. Ganglioneuromas usually contain abundant myxoid tissue, which has high signal intensity on T2-weighted images and is responsible for the slow enhancement after gadolinium administration. Case series have reported the presence of focal calcification in some of these lesions, which is an obvious finding on CT but difficult to visualize on MRI. This case was initially read as a probable adrenal lymphangioma, an equally rare lesion, although it more frequently has clearly cystic components.

The appearance of ganglioneuroma or ganglioneuroblastoma is probably not characterized well enough to allow prospective diagnosis in most cases, but the presence of whorled, high T2-signal intensity regions with gradual enhancement may suggest a neurogenic cause. For practical purposes, if you see one of these lesions, hopefully you'll notice that it doesn't have the small size and uniform signal dropout on OP images that are characteristic of an adenoma. That leaves the other classic adrenal lesions to consider: adrenal carcinoma, pheochromocytoma, and metastasis. Adrenal carcinomas may have central areas of necrosis and nonenhancement and often have venous tumor extension, a phenomenon never reported in ganglioneuromas. Pheochromocytomas tend to have fairly brisk arterial phase enhancement and washout. Metastatic disease is more difficult to exclude since the appearance of adrenal metastases is quite variable; however, the relatively young age and lack of a known primary malignancy may be clues that the lesion in this case is not a run-of-the-mill adrenal mass.

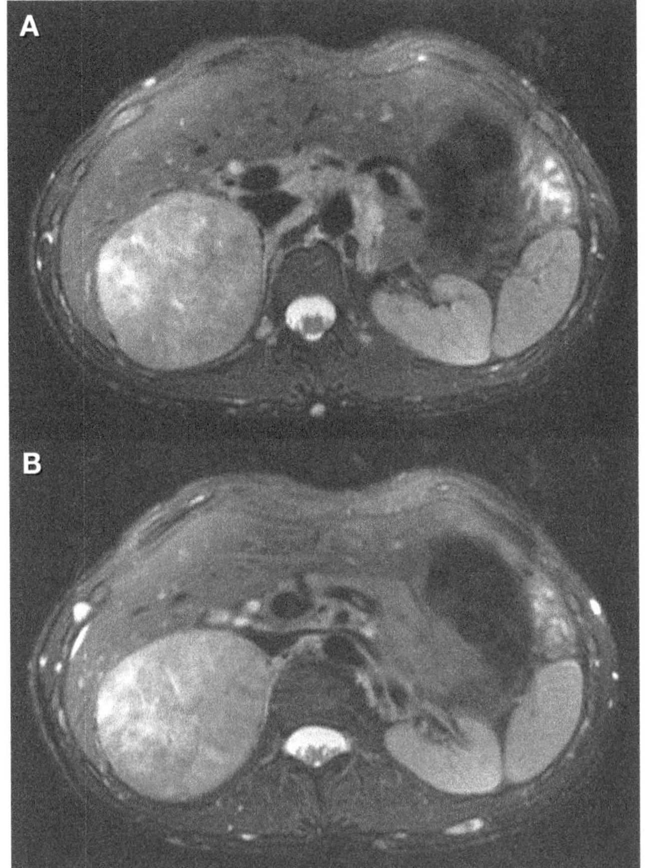

Figure 6.6.1

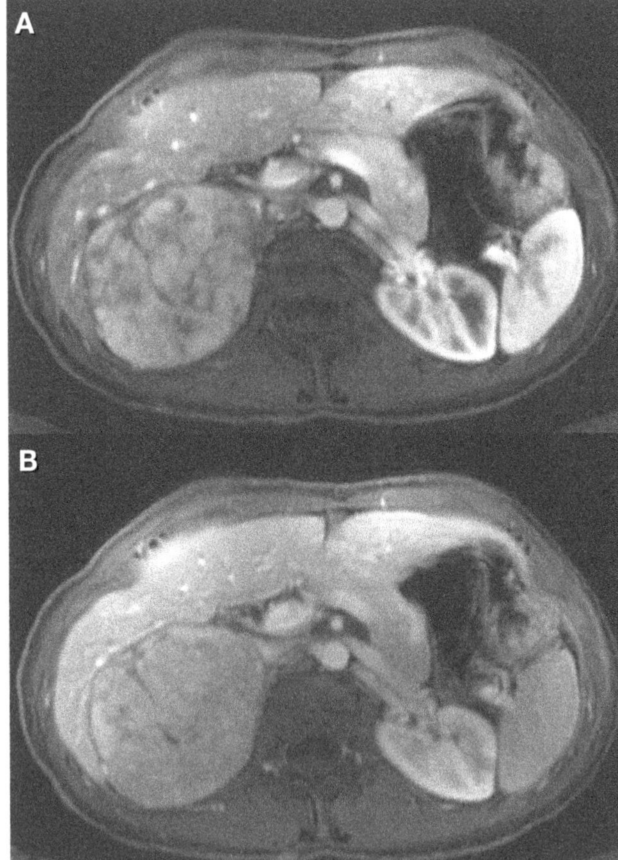

Figure 6.6.3

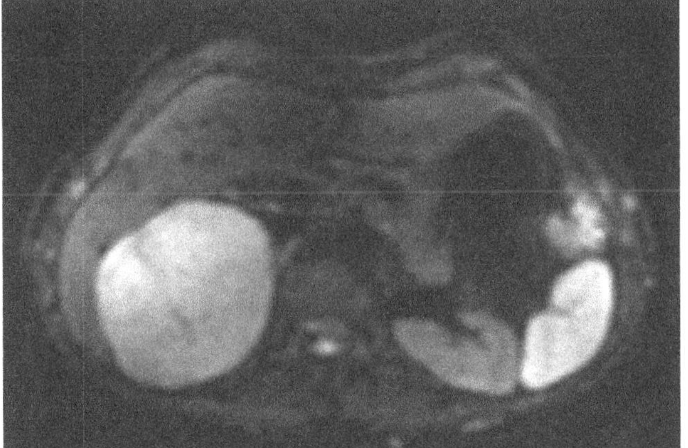

Figure 6.6.2

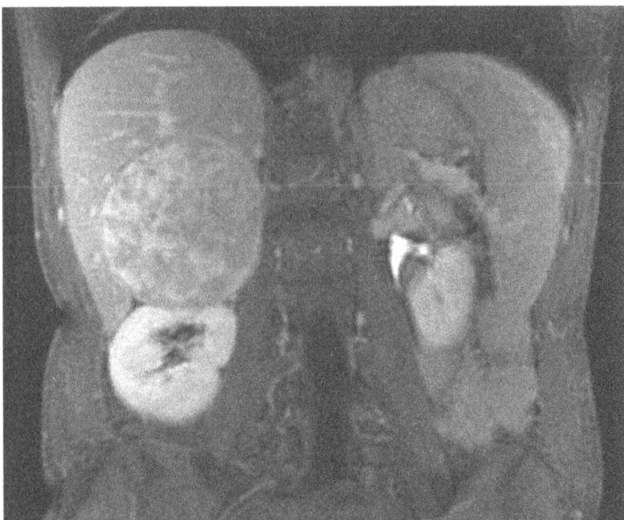

Figure 6.6.4

HISTORY: 35-year-old woman with a genetic disease

IMAGING FINDINGS: Axial fat-suppressed FSE T2-weighted images (Figure 6.6.1) demonstrate a large right adrenal mass with scattered regions of high T2-signal intensity. The lesion shows moderately high signal intensity on diffusion-weighted image (b=600 s/mm^2) (Figure 6.6.2) and heterogeneous enhancement on axial arterial phase postgadolinium 3D SPGR image (Figure 6.6.3A). Enhancement increases gradually on portal venous image (Figure 6.6.3B) and coronal equilibrium phase image (Figure 6.6.4). The T2-weighted images also show multiple cutaneous and subcutaneous hyperintense nodules and diffuse increased signal intensity surrounding the celiac axis.

DIAGNOSIS: Suprarenal neurofibroma in a patient with neurofibromatosis type 1

COMMENT: This lesion somewhat resembles the ganglioneuroma shown in Case 6.5, another tumor of neural crest origin, but the real key to the diagnosis is the cutaneous neurofibromas. Once you have identified them, the diagnosis of neurofibromatosis can be made; then you have to decide whether the patient has both neurofibromatosis and an unusual (nonadenomatous) adrenal lesion. (The high T2-signal intensity surrounding the celiac axis on the FSE T2-weighted images represents a small plexiform neurofibroma.) Patients with neurofibromatosis type 1 have an increased incidence of pheochromocytoma; however, an adrenal lesion with this appearance is more likely a neurofibroma. Classic pheochromocytomas are markedly hyperintense on T2-weighted images (although this is somewhat more myth than reality), but pheochromocytomas usually show intense arterial phase enhancement with rapid washout on postgadolinium images, which is definitely not seen in this case. The presence of a dominant mass in a patient with neurofibromatosis always raises the possibility of sarcomatous degeneration of a neurofibroma. Often the distinction between neurofibroma and neurofibrosarcoma cannot be made with MRI, although the presence of marked internal heterogeneity, local invasion, and metastases is suggestive.

CASE 6.7

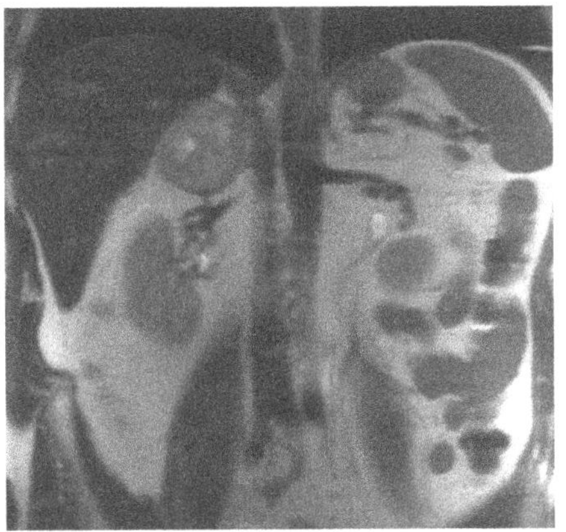

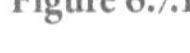

Figure 6.7.1

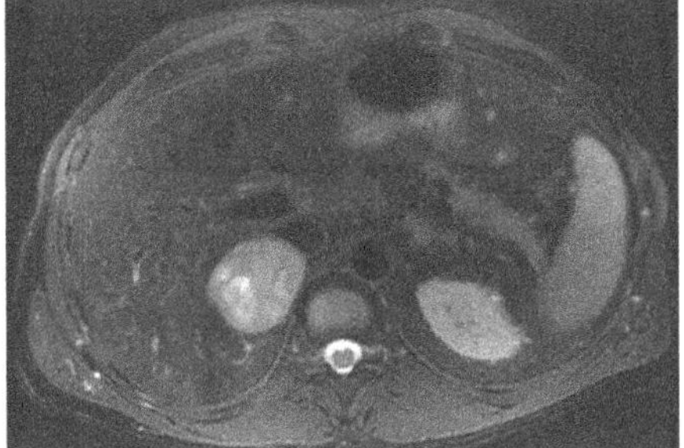

Figure 6.7.2

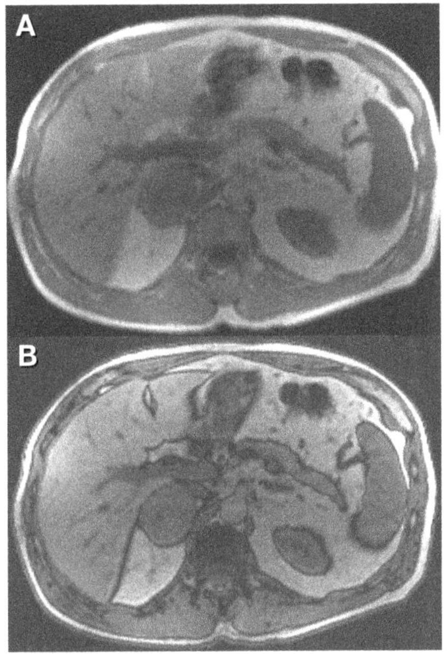

Figure 6.7.3

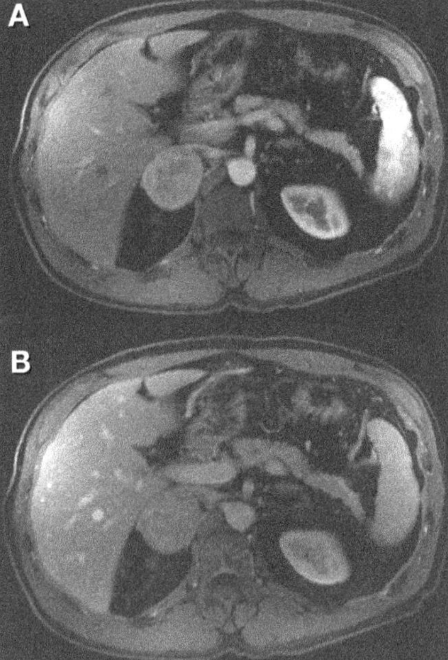

Figure 6.7.4

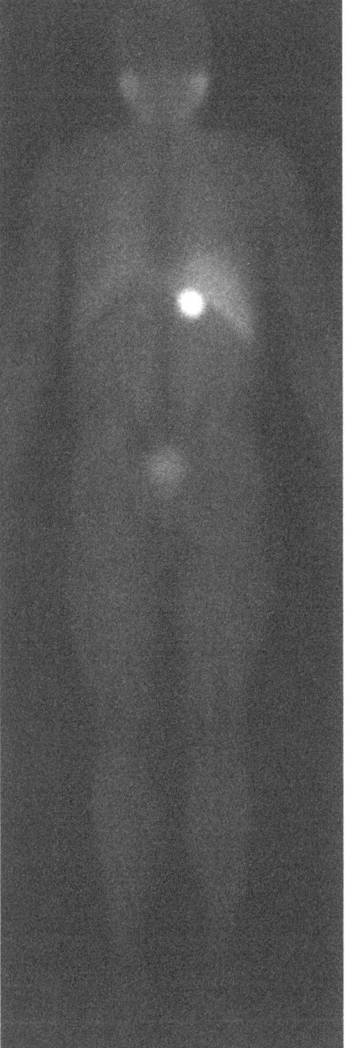

Figure 6.7.5

HISTORY: 53-year-old man with a 4-year history of spells consisting of palpitations, sweating, shortness of breath, and hypertension and 1 episode in which he fainted and was admitted to the hospital with mildly elevated troponin levels and electrocardiographic changes; an incidental adrenal mass was noted on cardiac MRI

IMAGING FINDINGS: Coronal SSFSE image (Figure 6.7.1) demonstrates a large heterogeneous right adrenal mass. Axial fat-suppressed T2-weighted FSE image (Figure 6.7.2) shows heterogeneous regions of increased signal intensity within the mass. Axial IP (Figure 6.7.3A) and OP (Figure 6.7.3B) 2D SPGR images reveal no signal dropout on the OP image to suggest the presence of intracellular fat. Axial arterial phase (Figure 6.7.4A) and portal venous phase (Figure 6.7.4B) postgadolinium 3D SPGR images show mild arterial phase enhancement of the lesion with washout on the portal venous phase image. Posterior image from ^{123}I-MIBG scan (Figure 6.7.5) demonstrates intense radiotracer activity corresponding to the right adrenal mass.

DIAGNOSIS: Pheochromocytoma

COMMENT: Pheochromocytomas are catecholamine-producing tumors originating from the sympathetic nervous system, most commonly the adrenal medulla. This case illustrates some of the classic symptoms, including paroxysmal hypertension, flushing, tachycardia, headaches, diaphoresis, and chest pain. Pheochromocytomas are estimated to cause 0.1% to 0.5% of all cases of newly diagnosed hypertension, but they can also be completely asymptomatic and detected as incidental findings on abdominal imaging (a Mayo Clinic review found that 50% of pheochromocytomas were detected at autopsy). The peak incidence of pheochromocytoma is in the third and fourth decades, and it occurs with equal frequency in women and men. Initial evaluation for pheochromocytoma includes screening for plasma metanephrine (99% sensitive) or urinary vanillylmandelic acid (95% sensitive).

The 10% rule for pheochromocytomas is widely quoted: 10% are bilateral, 10% are extra-adrenal, 10% are malignant, 10% are familial, and 10% are in children; it could also be added that 10% are detected serendipitously. The incidence of malignancy is higher with extra-adrenal lesions and with larger lesions. Hereditary syndromes associated with pheochromocytoma include neurofibromatosis, von Hippel-Lindau disease, multiple endocrine neoplasia type 2A (medullary thyroid cancer, hyperparathyroidism, and pheochromocytoma), and familial pheochromocytoma. von Hippel-Lindau disease is associated with pheochromocytoma, cerebellar hemangioblastoma, RCC, renal and pancreatic cysts, and epididymal cystadenomas. One study found that von Hippel-Lindau disease accounted for nearly 20% of patients with pheochromocytomas. Neurofibromatosis is characterized by multiple neurofibromas involving the skin, nervous system, bones, and endocrine glands. Only 1% of patients with neurofibromatosis have pheochromocytomas, but as many as 5% of patients with pheochromocytomas also carry a diagnosis of neurofibromatosis.

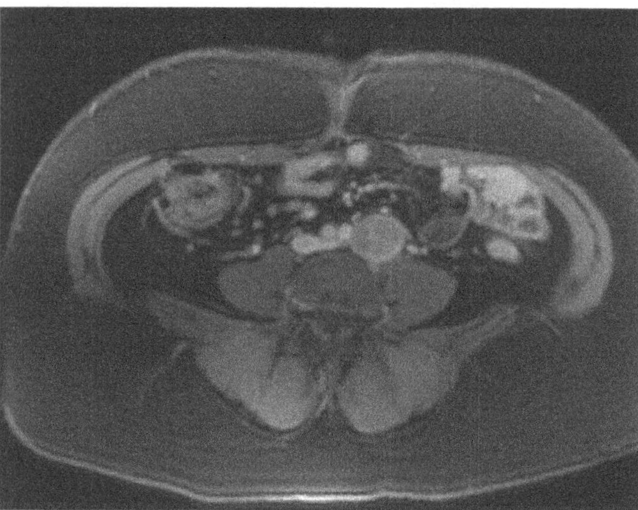

Figure 6.7.6

The role of MRI in patients with elevated metanephrine levels and suspected pheochromocytoma is to find the lesion. The classic teaching is that if you don't find an adrenal mass (and even if you do, since multiple lesions are possible), the abdomen should be covered through the organs of Zuckerkandl. These are the chromaffin bodies adjacent to the abdominal sympathetic plexus, extending from above the inferior mesenteric artery origin through the aortic bifurcation, and the most common site of extra-adrenal pheochromocytomas (accounting for about 75%). Remaining sites include the bladder (10%), thorax (10%), and skull base and neck (5%). Complete abdominal coverage on at least 1 or 2 sequences is almost always a good idea: Figure 6.7.6 shows an extra-adrenal pheochromocytoma (or paraganglioma), at the aortic bifurcation. The hypoenhancing mass was detected on the inferiormost image of a postcontrast 2D SPGR acquisition from a renal MRA performed in a patient with medication-resistant hypertension. Paravesicular pheochromocytoma is a rare but classic lesion, and an example is included in Chapter 8 ("Ureters and Bladder").

The imaging appearance of adrenal pheochromocytoma is often nonspecific. The concept of the "light bulb" pheochromocytoma (markedly hyperintense on T2-weighted images and distinguishable from other lesions on this basis) has lost credence over the years; however, we still occasionally encounter a resident or fellow who is reluctant to include pheochromocytoma in the differential for an indeterminate adrenal lesion because it's not bright enough on T2-weighted images. Figure 6.7.7 illustrates the classic light bulb appearance of a pheochromocytoma in the right adrenal gland, with markedly hyperintense signal intensity on fat-suppressed FSE T2-weighted images. Remember that this appearance may be the result of cystic or necrotic degeneration.

This case illustrates a pheochromocytoma that is not particularly bright on T2-weighted images, although it does have a few foci of moderately increased signal intensity. The most useful feature to discriminate a pheochromocytoma from an adenoma is the absence of signal dropout from IP to OP images. A few case reports describe pheochromocytomas containing lipid; however, this is so rare that it's probably best to forget that you ever heard about it. Pheochromocytomas generally show arterial phase hyperenhancement and often rapid washout (similar to adenomas). They tend to be more heterogeneous than adenomas and are typically smaller than adrenal carcinomas since they usually cause symptoms while still fairly small.

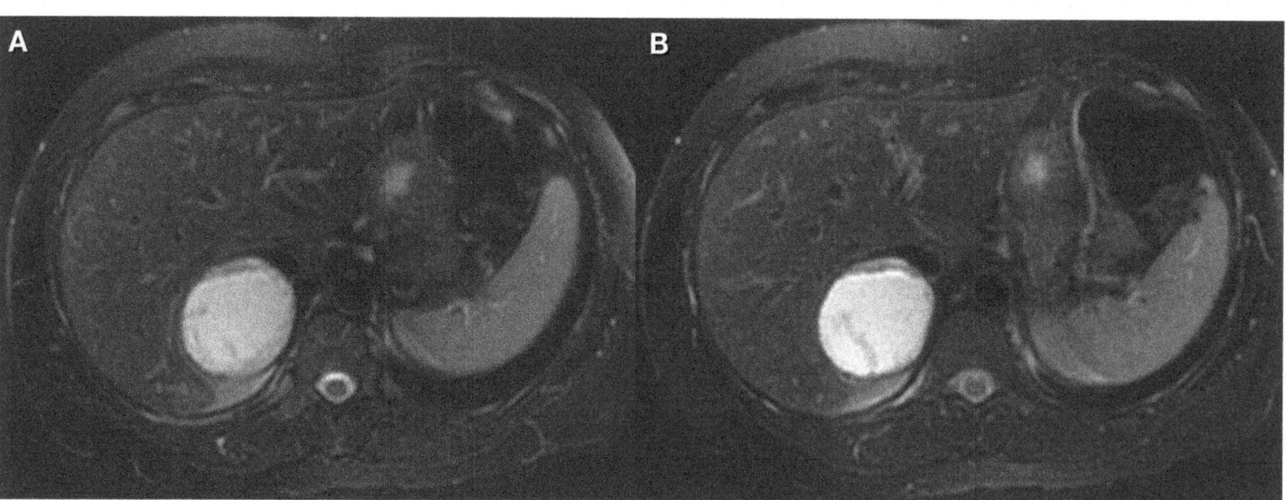

Figure 6.7.7

CASE 6.8

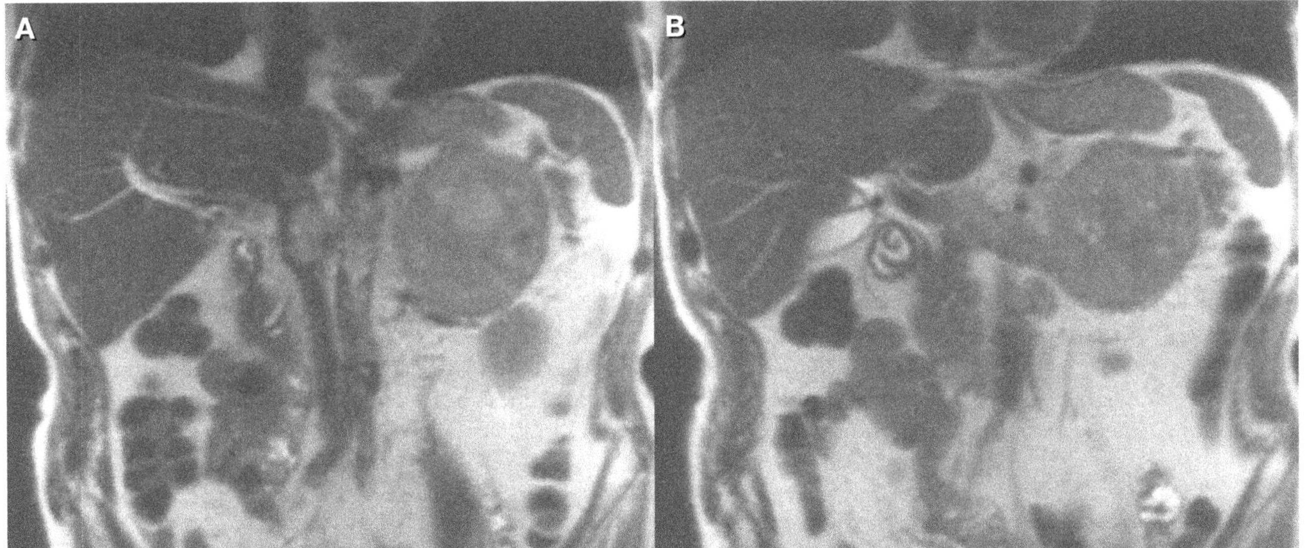

Figure 6.8.1

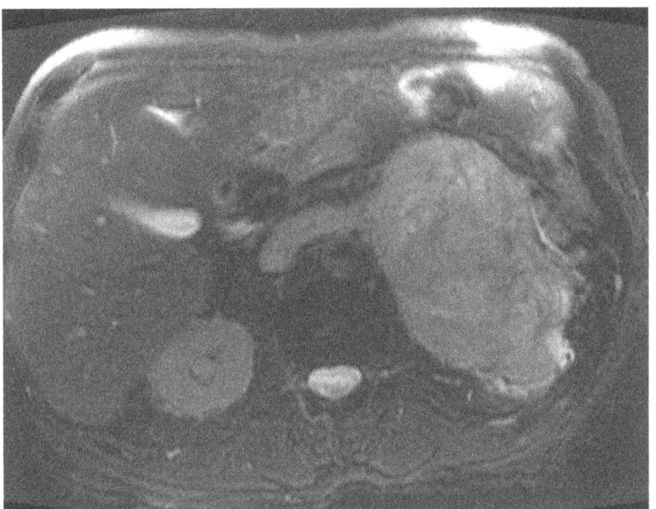

Figure 6.8.2

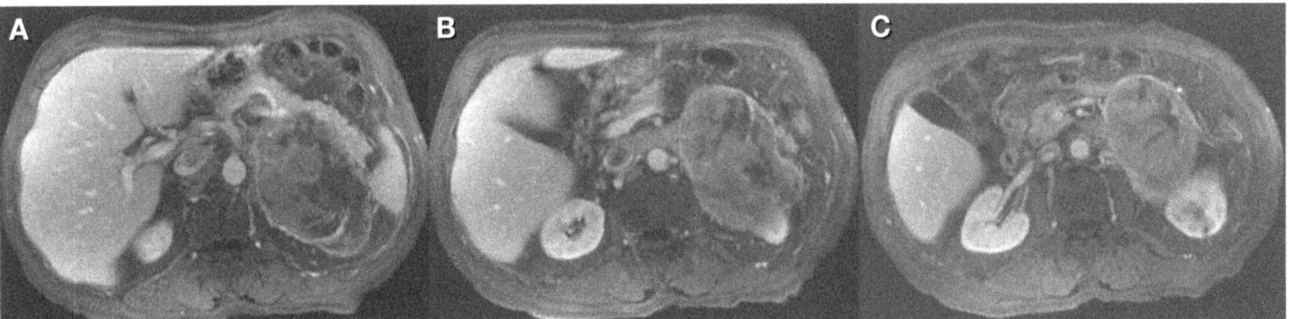

Figure 6.8.3

HISTORY: 76-year-old man with weight loss and progressive weakness

IMAGING FINDINGS: Coronal SSFSE images (Figure 6.8.1) reveal a large heterogeneous left adrenal mass and expansion of the adrenal vein. Axial fat-suppressed T2-weighted FRFSE image (Figure 6.8.2) demonstrates similar findings. Venous phase axial postgadolinium 3D SPGR images (Figure 6.8.3) show a heterogeneous hypoenhancing left adrenal mass with tumor thrombus expanding the adrenal vein and extending into the IVC.

DIAGNOSIS: Adrenal carcinoma

COMMENT: Adrenal carcinoma is a rare malignancy with an estimated annual incidence of 1 per million and a bimodal age distribution, with peaks for children and adults in the fourth and fifth decades of life. Adrenal carcinomas arise from the cortex, and most produce hormones (cortisol most commonly), which are often not fully functional. These lesions are usually large (>5 cm) at presentation and are often accompanied by metastatic disease. Venous extension is a common feature of adrenal carcinoma that is rarely seen in other adrenal lesions, so the presence of adrenal vein and IVC tumor thrombus is highly suggestive of the diagnosis.

The imaging appearance is that of a heterogeneous aggressive mass, often with central necrosis. A few case reports have described focal regions of signal dropout on OP images in adrenal carcinomas; however, distinction from adenomas is usually straightforward on the basis of the large size and heterogeneous, aggressive appearance of adrenal carcinoma. Differential diagnostic considerations include metastasis and pheochromocytoma.

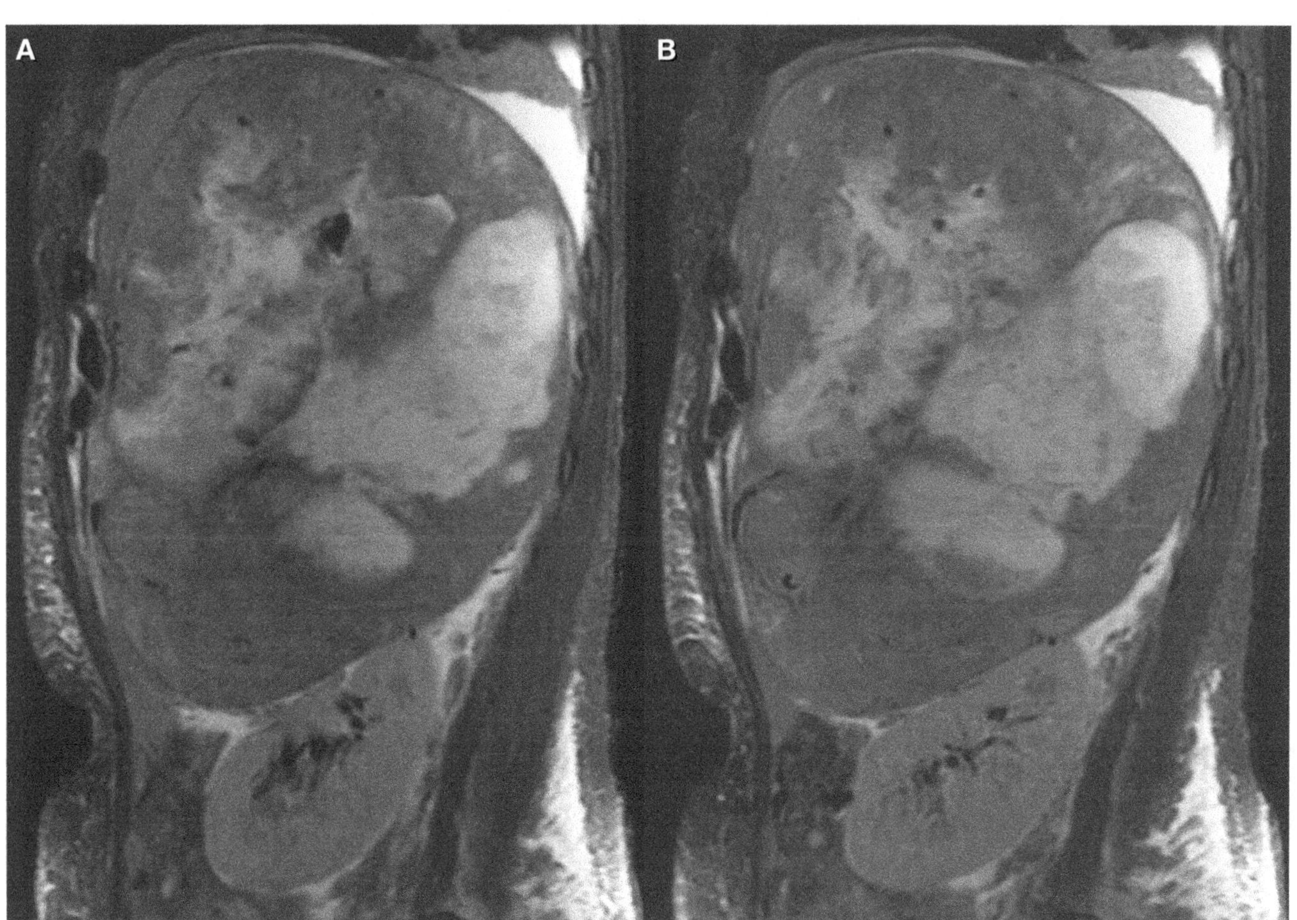

Figure 6.8.4

The sagittal plane, in our opinion, is often neglected in MRI, but it is well suited for adrenal imaging. Distinguishing between adrenal and renal origins can be difficult on axial images alone and sometimes even when coronal images are included. This is especially true with large masses. The sagittal plane almost always answers the question and is also a great way to evaluate the IVC. Figure 6.8.4 shows another large adrenal carcinoma, where the sagittal fat-suppressed FSE T2-weighted images clearly demonstrate the suprarenal origin of the large heterogeneous mass with central necrosis.

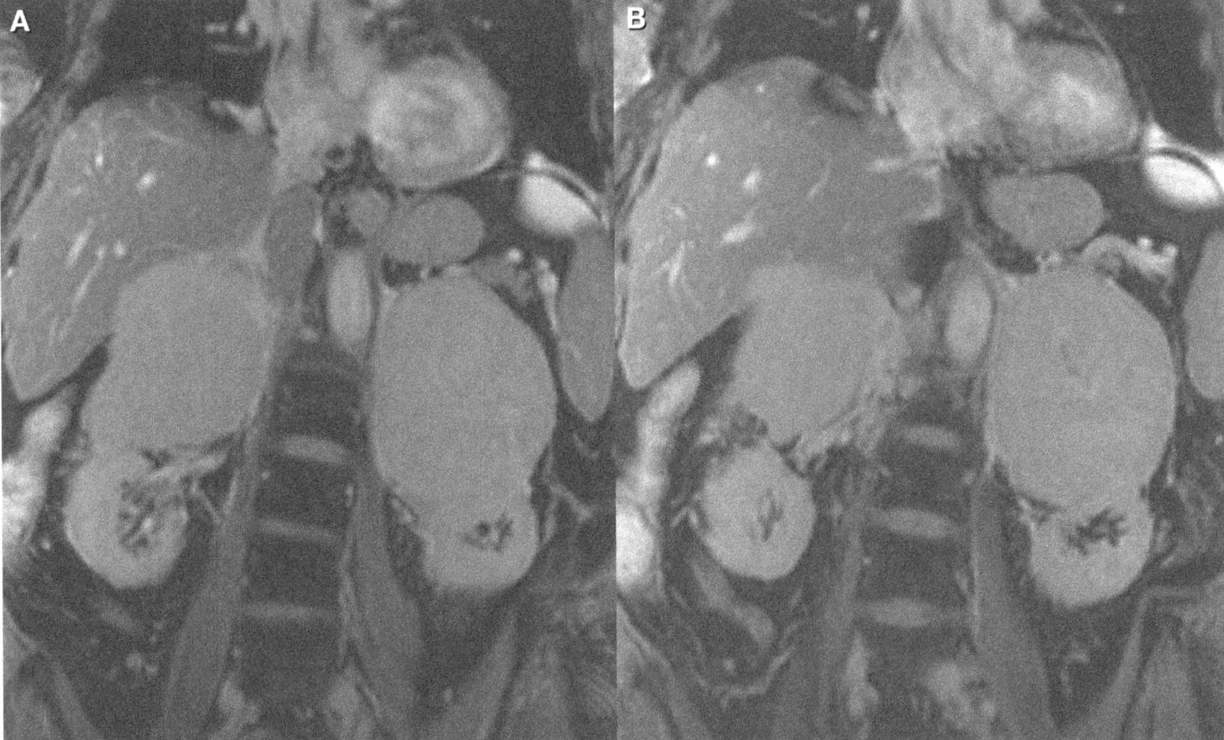

Figure 6.9.1

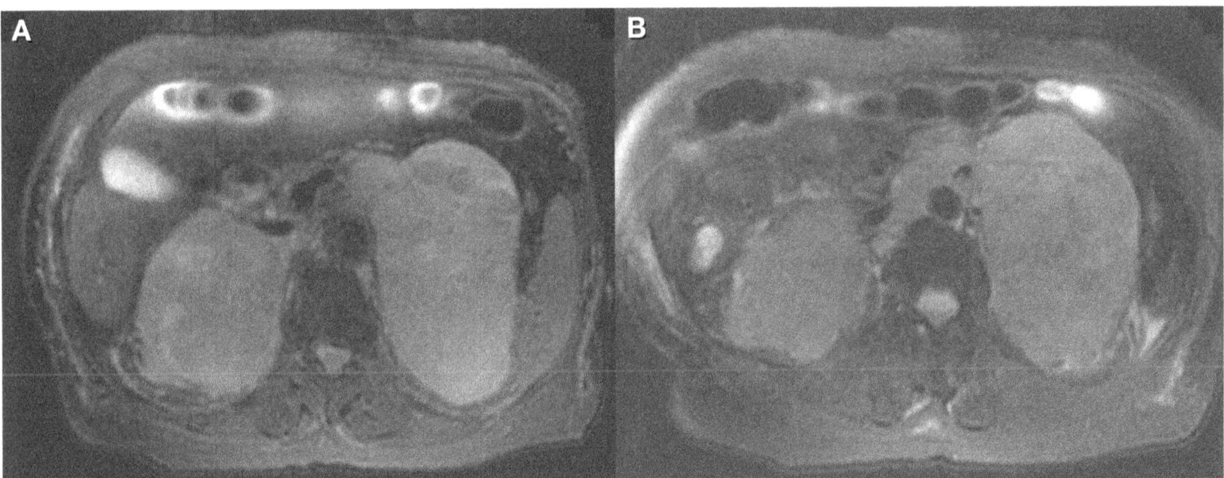

Figure 6.9.2

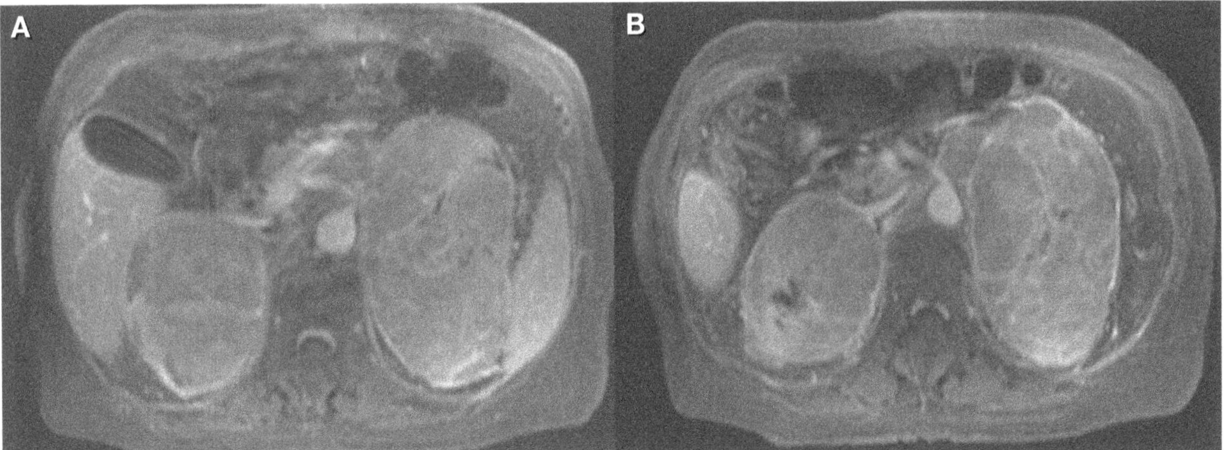

Figure 6.9.3

HISTORY: 68-year-old woman with back pain, leg weakness, and new-onset renal failure; renal US at another medical facility showed bilateral renal masses

IMAGING FINDINGS: Coronal fat-suppressed SSFSE images (Figure 6.9.1) demonstrate large bilateral hypointense adrenal masses. The lesions show uniform, moderate signal intensity on axial fat-suppressed FRFSE images (Figure 6.9.2) and heterogeneous hypoenhancement on portal venous phase postgadolinium 3D SPGR images (Figure 6.9.3). Mild para-aortic adenopathy is noted in the upper abdomen.

DIAGNOSIS: Adrenal lymphoma

COMMENT: Lymphoma occasionally involves the adrenal glands, most often in patients with advanced disseminated disease and usually of the non-Hodgkin type. Several case reports describe the much less common primary adrenal lymphoma in which the only manifestation of disease at diagnosis is involvement of the adrenal glands. Adrenal insufficiency and immunodeficiency have been reported in patients with primary adrenal lymphoma.

The imaging appearance of lymphoma in the adrenal glands is similar to the appearance of lymphoma anywhere else: Lesions tend to be uniform, mildly hypointense on T2-weighted images, and relatively hypoenhancing compared with most other adrenal masses. While the appearance of adrenal lymphoma is somewhat nonspecific, and this entity is rare, the diagnosis was suggested on the basis of the MRI findings. Probably the main differential diagnosis in this case is bilateral adrenal metastases, although the patient had no known primary malignancy.

Additional findings that may suggest lymphoma as a diagnosis include extensive adenopathy or splenomegaly (ie, extra-adrenal involvement) in a more typical pattern of lymphoma. Adrenal lymphoma tends to cause diffuse enlargement of the gland rather than a focal mass, although the distinction is somewhat moot in this case.

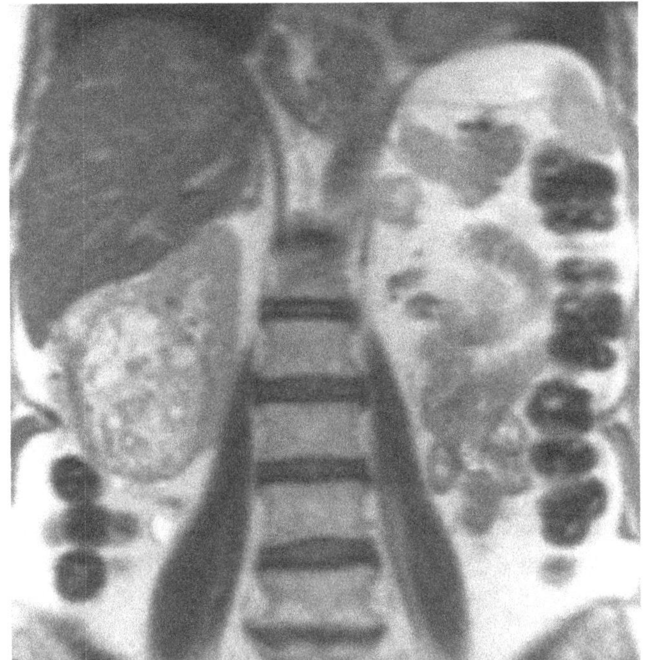

Figure 6.10.1

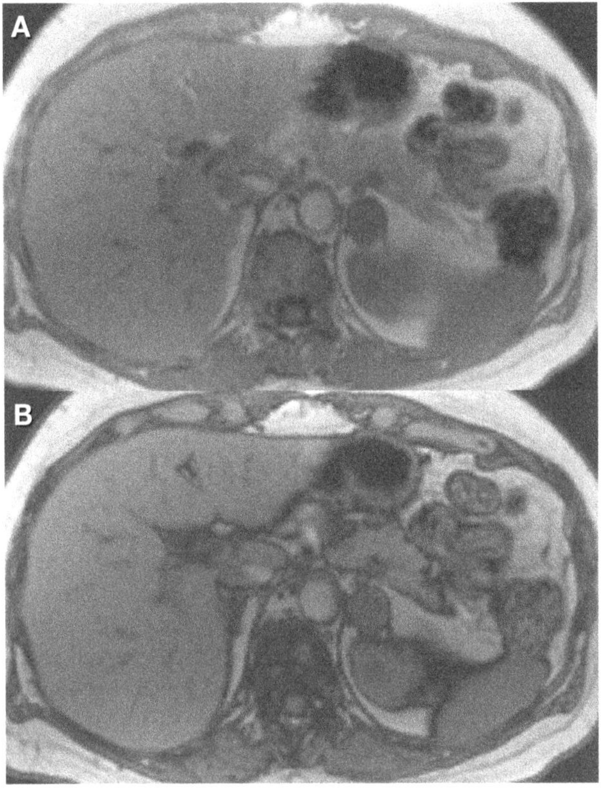

Figure 6.10.3

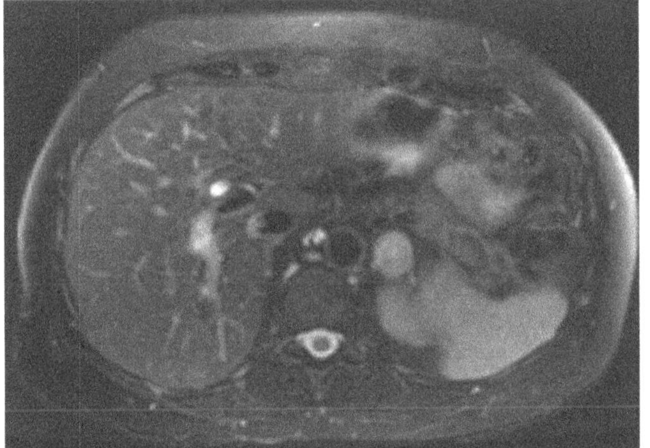

Figure 6.10.2

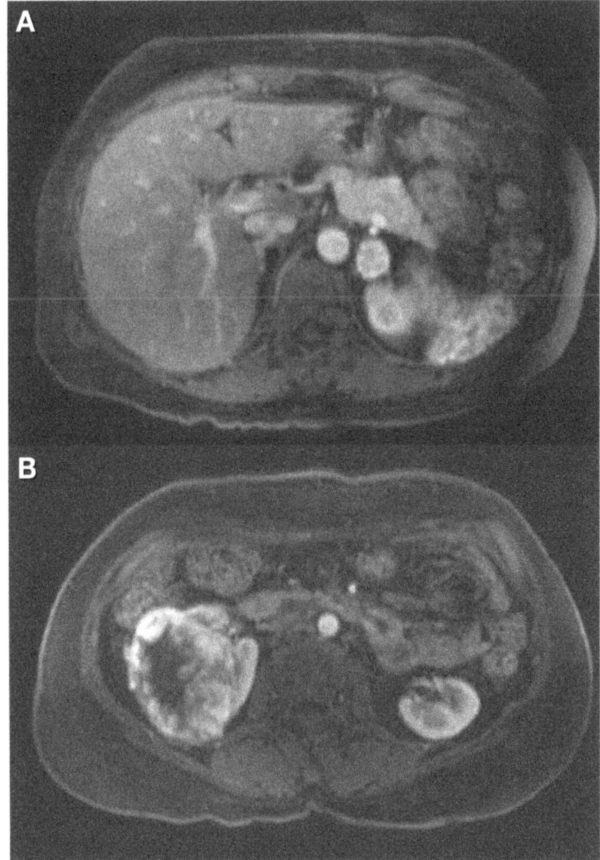

Figure 6.10.4

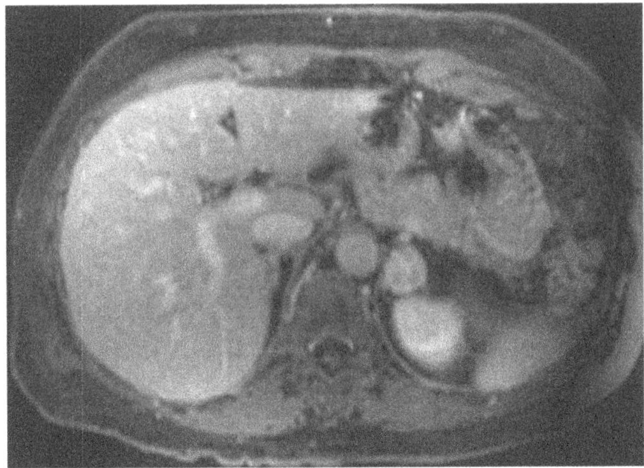

Figure 6.10.5

HISTORY: 56-year-old woman with abdominal pain and a renal mass, which was found on CT at another medical facility

IMAGING FINDINGS: Coronal SSFSE image (Figure 6.10.1) demonstrates a small left adrenal lesion and a large heterogeneous mass in the right kidney. Axial fat-suppressed T2-weighted FSE image (Figure 6.10.2) shows that the adrenal mass has mildly increased signal intensity. IP (Figure 6.10.3A) and OP (Figure 6.10.3B) axial 2D SPGR images reveal no signal dropout within the lesion on the OP image. Arterial phase postgadolinium 3D SPGR images (Figure 6.10.4) demonstrate hyperenhancement of the left adrenal and right renal masses. Equilibrium phase postgadolinium 3D SPGR image (Figure 6.10.5) shows washout of the left adrenal lesion.

DIAGNOSIS: RCC with contralateral adrenal metastasis

COMMENT: The adrenal glands are a common site for metastatic disease, a fact well known by virtually every radiologist, and the reason why our technologists are trained to extend all chest CT scans inferiorly to include the adrenal glands, so that the presence or absence of adrenal masses can be noted when staging lung cancer. Common primary tumors that metastasize to the adrenal glands include lung, breast, RCC, and melanoma, but many additional malignancies may also spread to the adrenals. However, the presence of an adrenal mass in a patient with a known primary malignancy does not automatically indicate a metastasis: Adrenal masses found in patients undergoing lung cancer staging, for example, are metastases less than half the time. The main differential diagnosis is adenoma, by far the most common adrenal lesion; in nearly all cases, IP-OP images should allow you to make the distinction with a high level of confidence.

Let's take a brief physics detour: IP-OP pulse sequences acquire 2D or 3D SPGR images in which the TE is adjusted so that the signal from water and fat within each voxel is either in phase (ie, additive) or out of phase (ie, subtractive). This is possible because water and fat have slightly different resonant frequencies; therefore, when the radiofrequency (B_1) pulse excites the nuclear spins into the transverse plane, they precess at different speeds. This transverse signal can be measured at any point, determined by the TE, and it can occur when the signals are in phase, out of phase, or any phase in between. At 1.5T, the first out-of-phase (180° apart) TE occurs at 2.1 ms, and the first in-phase TE at 4.2 ms (these values are different at 3T, since the resonant frequencies are different). Other factors being equal, if an image voxel contains a significant amount of fat, there will be a noticeable difference in signal intensity between the IP and OP images. Keep in mind that this works only if both fat and water are present within the same voxel, and this is why you often won't see this effect in myelolipomas (which contain macroscopic fat and not much water) or in subcutaneous fat.

Another effect of the different resonant frequencies of fat and water is the India ink artifact seen on OP images along the frequency-encoding direction. This occurs because the spatial location of the signal in MRI is mapped by spatially dependent changes in resonance frequency caused by the small gradients applied on top of the large static magnetic field. Since the baseline frequencies of fat and water are slightly different, they are mapped to slightly different locations along the frequency-encoding axis (usually 1 or 2 pixels apart). This is a relatively minor effect, but it is noticeable at fat-water boundaries, such as those in abdominal organs surrounded by mesenteric fat. The location of the fat signal is shifted slightly in the same direction along the frequency-encoding axis, so that a relative signal void is created at an edge of the fat-organ interface (fat pixels are shifted onto the edge of the water-containing organ, but they're out of phase so the signal subtracts). This effect is absent when fat and water signals are in phase or when fat suppression is applied, so that all fat is dark. The India ink effect can be accentuated with a low receiver bandwidth: This determines the range of frequencies sampled across the image; the lower the bandwidth, the larger the relative pixel shift between fat and water-containing elements.

In this case, the adrenal lesion is fairly small, but not small enough so that the India ink effect becomes problematic in distinguishing real internal signal dropout in the lesion. If it does become an issue for very small lesions, potential solutions include increasing the spatial resolution of the acquisition (ie, use a higher imaging matrix for a given field of view) or increasing the receiver bandwidth (or both). Don't be fooled by the presence of a contralateral adrenal metastasis in RCC. Although it is less common than metastatic disease to the same side, it does occur, and after the possibility of an adenoma (or at least a lipid-rich adenoma) has been eliminated, a contralateral adrenal metastasis becomes the most likely alternative.

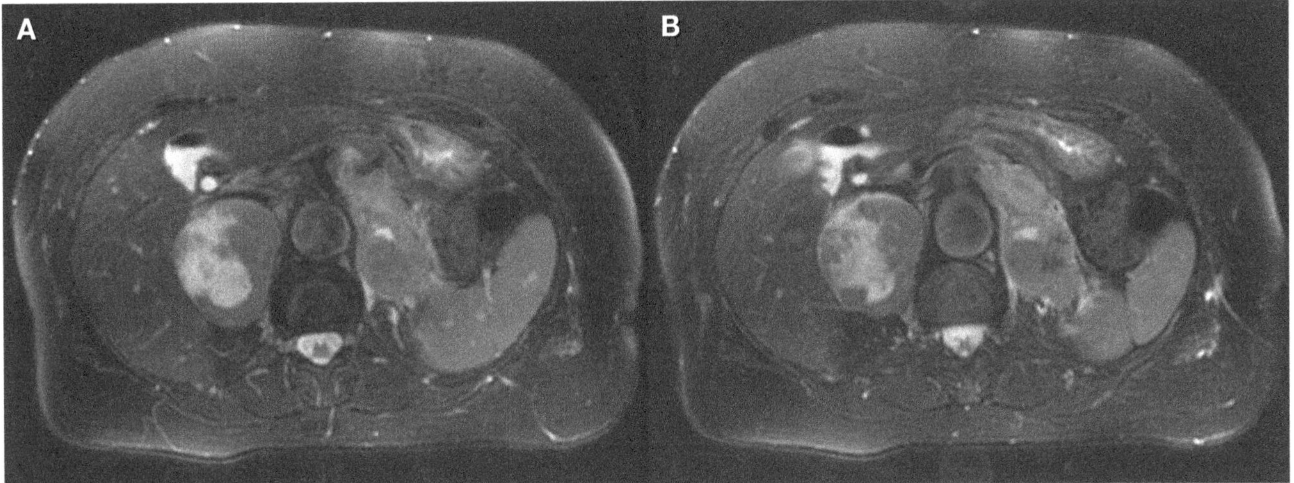

Figure 6.10.6

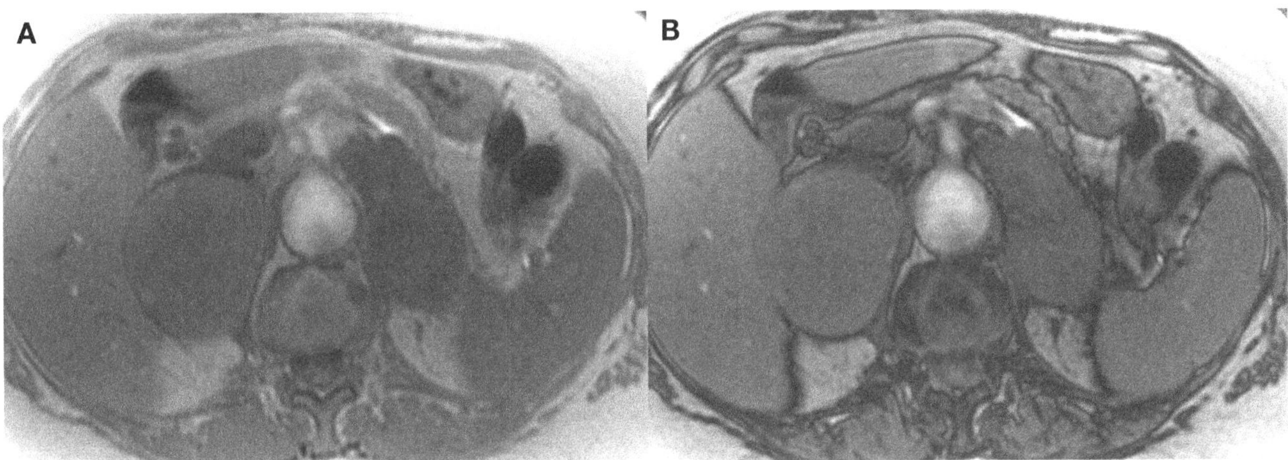

Figure 6.10.7

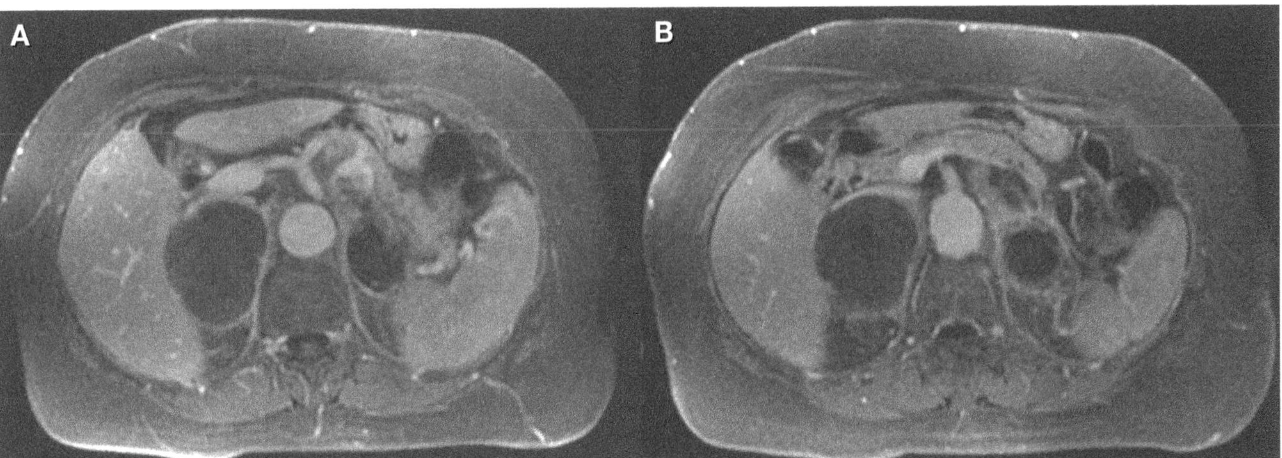

Figure 6.10.8

Most adrenal metastases don't look anything like adenomas—they tend to be larger and more heterogeneous, and they have different enhancement characteristics, as seen in images from a patient with non-small cell lung carcinoma. Axial fat-suppressed FSE T2-weighted images (Figure 6.10.6) demonstrate large bilateral adrenal masses with heterogeneous signal intensity. Axial IP (Figure 6.10.7A) and OP (Figure 6.10.7B) 2D SPGR images reveal no significant signal dropout on the OP image. Postgadolinium portal venous phase 3D SPGR images (Figure 6.10.8) show only minimal rim enhancement of the adrenal lesions.

The differential diagnosis for adrenal metastasis includes adrenal carcinoma and pheochromocytoma, but remember that these are very rare lesions. If a patient has a known primary malignancy, the odds are in your favor if you say that an adrenal lesion without the imaging characteristics of an adenoma is a metastasis.

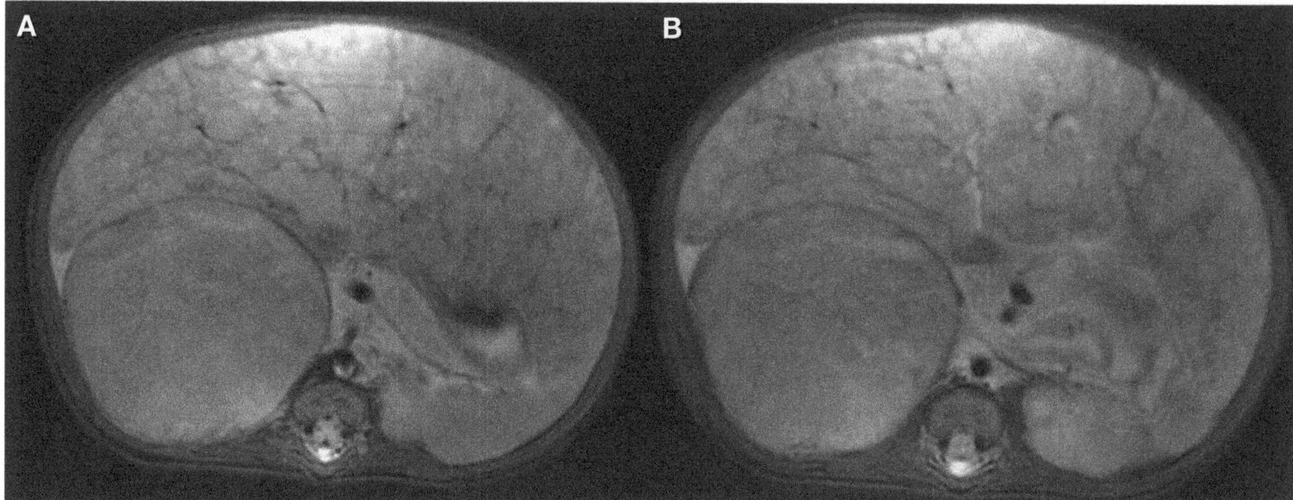

Figure 6.11.1

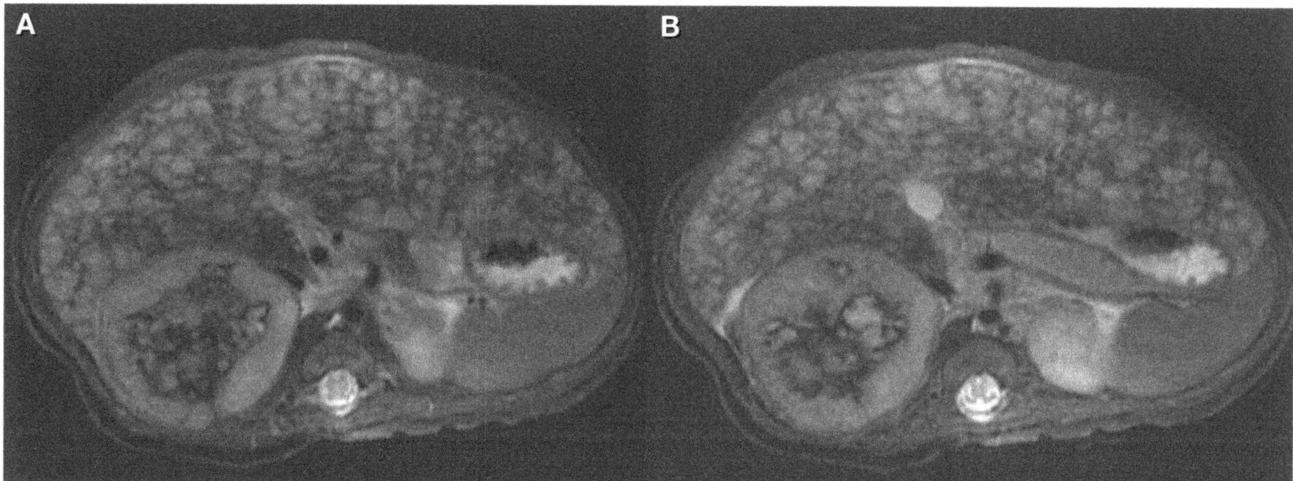

Figure 6.11.2

HISTORY: 1-month-old female infant with a renal or adrenal mass

IMAGING FINDINGS: Axial fat-suppressed FSE T2-weighted images (Figure 6.11.1) reveal a large mass originating from the right adrenal gland with heterogeneously increased signal intensity. Extensive small hyperintense metastases essentially replace the visualized hepatic parenchyma. Axial fat-suppressed FSE images from the 6-week follow-up examination (Figure 6.11.2) demonstrate that the adrenal mass has decreased in size, with central fibrosis or calcification and some improvement in the hepatic metastases.

DIAGNOSIS: Neuroblastoma with hepatic metastases

COMMENT: Neuroblastoma is the most common extracranial pediatric neoplasm and the third most common pediatric malignancy after leukemia and central nervous system tumors. In the first year of life, neuroblastoma accounts for 50% of neoplasms: 25% of neuroblastomas are detected in the first year, and up to 60% in the first 2 years. Like ganglioneuromas and ganglioneuroblastomas, neuroblastomas arise from neural crest cells, which are responsible for generating the adrenal medulla and sympathetic nervous system. These tumors can arise from any location along the sympathetic chain, although an adrenal origin is the most common. Metastases occur in one-half to two-thirds of cases, most often to the liver, bones, and lymph nodes. Direct extension into the neural canal is a frequent feature of these lesions and is easily seen on T2-weighted images. Neuroblastomas generally show mild enhancement after gadolinium administration. Calcifications are seen in up to 50% of neuroblastomas, generally appearing as a signal void on MRI.

Neuroblastoma is usually not a diagnostic dilemma, and it should be the first consideration in the differential diagnosis for a large adrenal mass in an infant. MRI is generally requested to confirm the diagnosis and stage the lesion, so adequate coverage must be provided to assess not only the adrenal mass but also the liver, bone marrow, and lymph nodes.

Body MRI in the pediatric population is not always straightforward, and discussion of the most effective (and ineffective) techniques is relatively limited in the imaging literature. If your practice generally performs intubation and full anesthesia (as is most often the case at Mayo Clinic), pediatric patients can generally be treated as little adults, with respiratory-gated sequences triggered by the respirator and breath-held sequences when the respirator is turned off (but not for too long). It is important, however, to modify the slice thickness and matrix to achieve a higher spatial resolution than is routinely acquired for adults and to choose a smaller coil to optimize the signal to noise ratio. For neonates and infants, the number of signals acquired may need to be increased to maintain an adequate signal to noise ratio. Scanning these patients during conscious sedation (ie, while asleep but not intubated) is much more difficult. Image quality is usually acceptable with fast sequential acquisitions, such as SSFSE and SSFP, since they can be performed with acquisition times of less than 1 second per slice. Respiratory gating is often problematic because respiratory excursions are small, irregular, and difficult to monitor. Dynamic contrast-enhanced imaging is also difficult because the gadolinium doses are small and generally cannot be injected quickly and because patients are unlikely to hold their breath in this situation. An alternative is to run a set of sequential 2D SPGR images during and after gadolinium injection for about 1 to 2 minutes with the minimum available TR and relatively low spatial resolution. (*Sequential* means that the slices are acquired 1 slice at a time. Traditional SPGR acquisitions are obtained with longer TRs and with multiple slices excited simultaneously—this is more efficient, but a longer percentage of the total acquisition time is spent acquiring data for any given slice, which in turn greatly increases the opportunity for motion artifact.) Changing the acquisition order to sequential and minimizing TR effectively creates a perfusion sequence (this can be done by using a cardiac perfusion sequence and turning off electrocardiographic gating). Image quality is not ideal, but motion artifact is minimized and dynamic contrast-enhanced images can be acquired, usually with good visualization of lesions with at least moderate enhancement.

ABBREVIATIONS

ADC	apparent diffusion coefficient
CT	computed tomography
FRFSE	fast-recovery fast-spin echo
FSE	fast-spin echo
IP	in-phase
^{123}I-MIBG	iodine-123 metaiodobenzylguanidine
IVC	inferior vena cava
MRA	magnetic resonance angiography
MRI	magnetic resonance imaging
OP	out-of-phase
PET	positron emission tomography
RCC	renal cell carcinoma
SPGR	spoiled gradient recalled
SSFP	steady-state free precession
SSFSE	single-shot fast-spin echo
TE	echo time
3D	3-dimensional
TR	repetition time
2D	2-dimensional
US	ultrasonography

7.

KIDNEYS

CASE 7.1

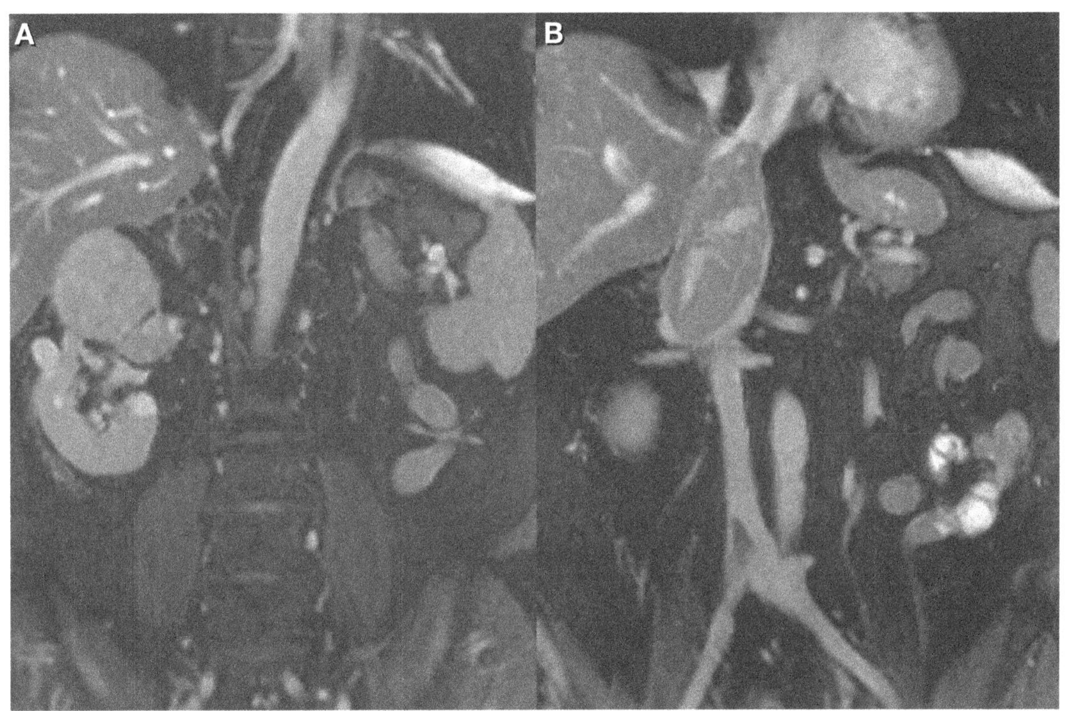

Figure 7.1.1

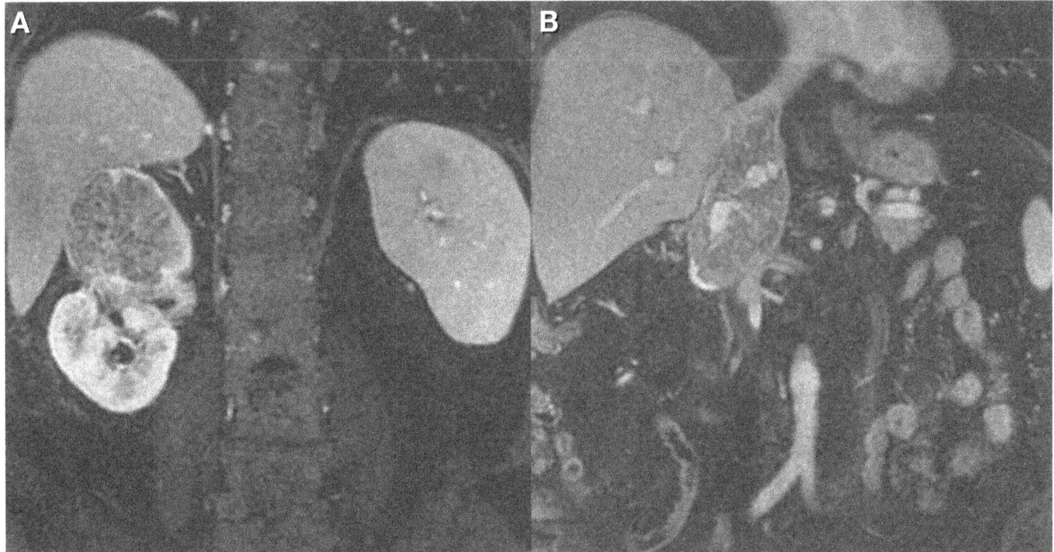

Figure 7.1.2

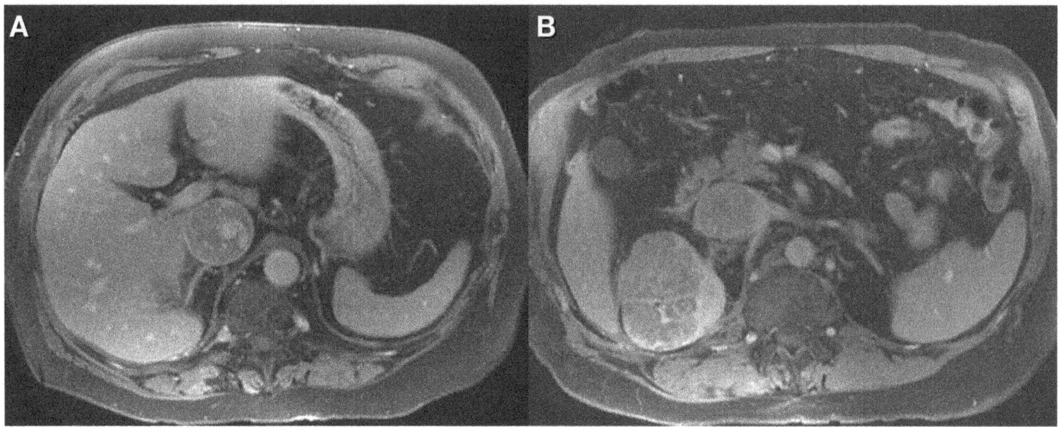

Figure 7.1.3

HISTORY: 74-year-old man with a solitary kidney and new microscopic hematuria

IMAGING FINDINGS: Coronal 2D fat-suppressed SSFP images (Figure 7.1.1) reveal a mass in the upper pole of the right kidney with heterogeneous expansile thrombus in the subhepatic and intrahepatic IVC. Note also the small, more hypointense filling defect in the IVC inferiorly just above the bifurcation, representing bland thrombus. Coronal venous phase 3D SPGR images (Figure 7.1.2) and axial nephrogenic phase 2D SPGR images (Figure 7.1.3) also demonstrate a heterogeneously hypoenhancing mass in the right kidney with expansile IVC thrombus. Note the prominent neovascularity within the IVC tumor thrombus.

DIAGNOSIS: Renal cell carcinoma (clear cell)

COMMENT: RCC accounts for about 3% of all cancer deaths and 3% of all cancer cases in the United States, with an incidence estimated at 12 per 100,000 persons. The overall 5-year survival rate for all RCCs is 65%. RCC is twice as common in men as in women, with median age at diagnosis between 50 and 60 years. Risk factors include smoking; unopposed estrogen exposure; toxic exposure to petroleum products, heavy metals, or asbestos; and acquired cystic disease of dialysis. Common presenting signs and symptoms include hematuria and flank pain or mass; however, an increasing number of cases are detected incidentally at cross-sectional imaging performed for a different indication.

RCCs are divided into 3 histologic subtypes: clear cell RCC (75% of cases), papillary RCC (10%), and chromophobe RCC (5%). (Additional uncommon lesions are collecting duct and unclassified RCCs.) The 3 subtypes have different imaging characteristics, as well as different prognoses. Clear cell RCCs have the greatest metastatic potential and the lowest survival rates (5-year survival, 50%-60% vs 80%-90% for papillary and chromophobe variants). Multifocal tumors are relatively uncommon but do occur in approximately 5% of patients with sporadic RCC and are much more common in patients with hereditary syndromes, such as VHL disease.

Imaging of patients with known or suspected RCC should focus on identifying the lesion, determining whether it is suspicious, and staging the disease if it is present. In general, a solid renal mass (except for an AML) is a suspicious lesion, and there are no universally effective criteria on MRI or any other imaging modality to reliably distinguish benign from malignant solid lesions. Cystic lesions exist along a spectrum from obviously benign simple cysts to mildly suspicious lesions with septations or minimal wall thickening to clearly worrisome lesions with solid nodules. The Bosniak criteria are widely applied in the assessment of cystic renal lesions, and new subcategories are added with alarming regularity. However, these rules essentially can be summarized as follows: 1) leave benign lesions alone, 2) follow mildly suspicious lesions, and 3) remove moderately and highly suspicious lesions. Staging of RCCs should include assessment for extracapsular extension, venous invasion with tumor thrombus (and, often, bland thrombus) in the renal vein and IVC, enlarged lymph nodes, and metastatic lesions involving the adrenals, contralateral kidney, liver, bones, lungs (better assessed with CT), and pancreas.

Clear cell RCCs are more likely than papillary or chromophobe RCCs to be hypervascular and to show extracapsular extension or metastatic disease. Another interesting characteristic of clear cell RCCs is their propensity to contain intracellular lipid and therefore to show signal dropout between IP and OP SPGR images (Figure 7.1.4). This is the reason why it's not a good idea to base your diagnosis of AML on this finding—look for macroscopic fat instead.

This case illustrates a clear cell RCC that isn't terribly hypervascular (not all lesions follow the rules) but is an excellent example of venous tumor extension. Tumor thrombus in the IVC is easy to identify in this case; it expands the lumen, which is an unusual occurrence with bland thrombus, and it shows heterogeneous enhancement with internal neovascularity. The distinction between tumor thrombus and bland thrombus is sometimes trickier when contrast cannot be administered; however, both FSE and diffusion-weighted images generally show heterogeneous increased signal intensity relative to bland thrombus. SSFP images are ideal for identifying venous thrombus, but they do not always allow a clear distinction between tumor thrombus and bland thrombus, although in this case, there's a distinct difference between the tumor thrombus extending into the IVC from the left renal vein and the focal bland thrombus in the IVC just above the bifurcation. As a general rule, tumor thrombus travels upward, and it's uncommon to see tumor thrombus extending below the level of the renal veins.

Describing the extent of thrombus in the IVC is helpful to the surgeons. If it is below the level of the liver, they generally can clamp the IVC and remove the thrombus from below; if it involves the intrahepatic IVC, they'll have to make other arrangements. When thrombus reaches the right atrium, it sometimes can be detected initially on echocardiography and mistaken for an intracardiac mass, in which case the patient may have an extensive (and expensive) work-up before someone thinks about scanning the abdomen.

The optimal plane for acquiring 3D dynamic SPGR images in patients with RCC is somewhat controversial in our practice. Coronal acquisition can generate beautiful images of renal vein and IVC thrombus (as illustrated in this case), particularly if the patient can lift his arms above the head to minimize wrap-around artifact. There are some limitations to consider, however, including the following: 1) it's generally less efficient than an axial acquisition (ie, more sections needed and less likely to be able to use a partial phase field of view) and therefore requires a longer acquisition time to completely cover the kidneys, pancreas, and liver; 2) phase ghosting artifact from aortic pulsation is often more annoying in the coronal plane than the axial plane; 3) you're probably more likely to miss subtle lesions in the liver and pancreas; and 4) coronal acquisitions can be surprisingly unhelpful when trying to sort out whether the IVC is compressed by large nodes or invaded by tumor thrombus.

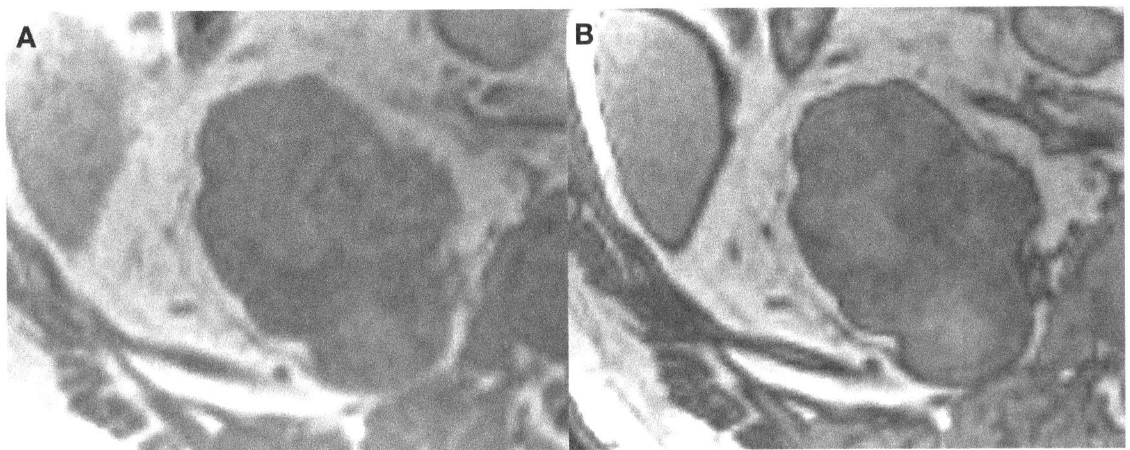

Figure 7.1.4

Axial IP (Figure 7.1.4A) and OP (Figure 7.1.4B) 2D SPGR images in a patient with clear cell RCC in the right kidney demonstrate relatively subtle signal dropout in the center of the mass on the OP image, indicating the presence of intracellular lipid.

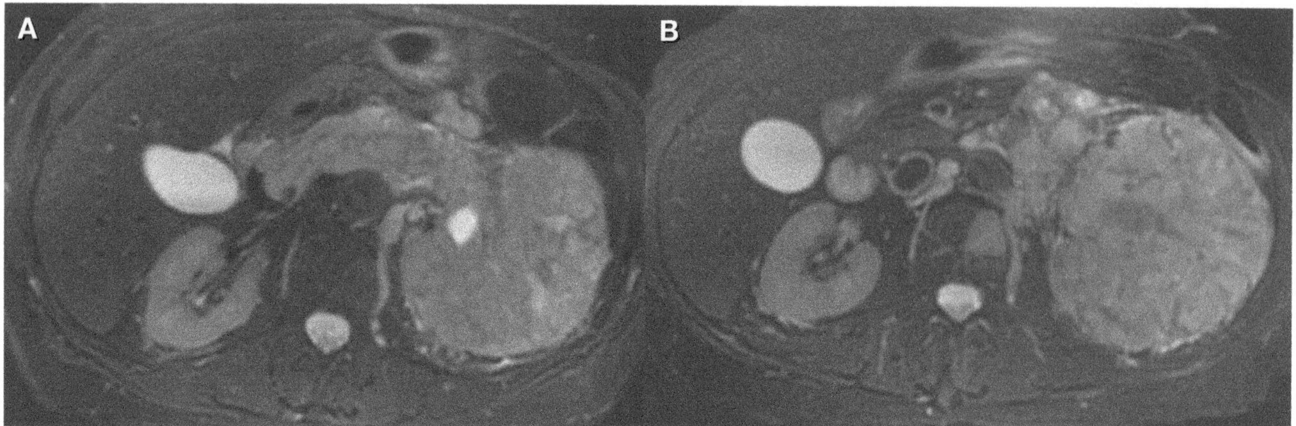

Figure 7.2.1

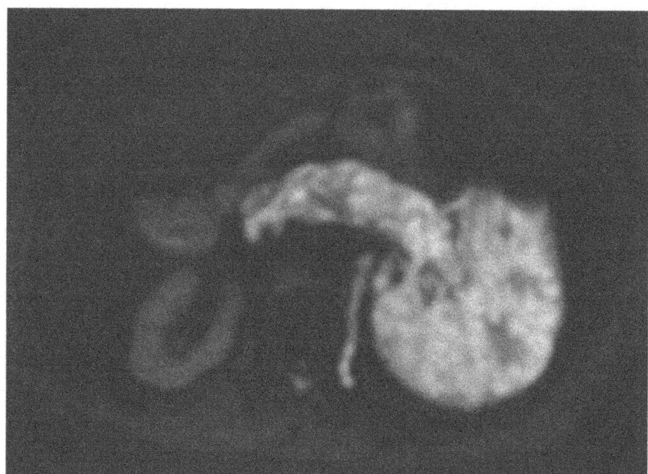

Figure 7.2.2

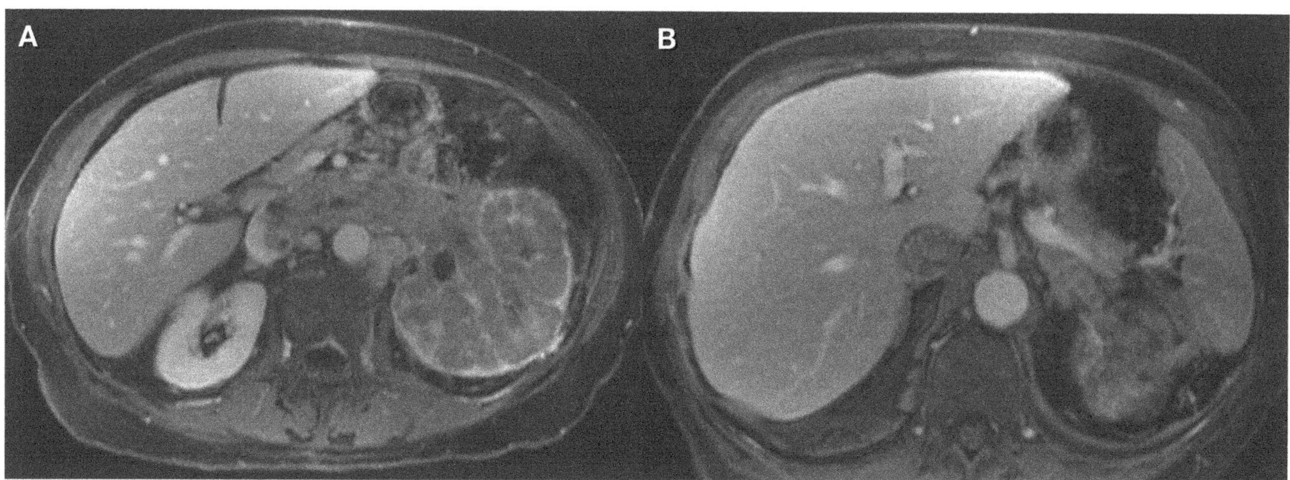

Figure 7.2.3

HISTORY: 71-year-old woman with gradual onset of early satiety and minimal left flank pain; CT at an outside institution demonstrated a large left renal mass

IMAGING FINDINGS: Axial fat-suppressed FSE T2-weighted images (Figure 7.2.1) reveal complete replacement of the left kidney with high-signal-intensity tumor and expansion of the left renal vein with tumor thrombus. Note the metastatic lesion in a lumbar vertebral body. Diffusion-weighted image (b=800 s/mm^2) (Figure 7.2.2) shows diffuse high signal intensity throughout the left kidney and renal vein. Notice also the slight prominence of the left-sided lumbar vein and its high signal intensity, indicating tumor thrombus. Axial venous phase postgadolinium 3D SPGR images (Figure 7.2.3) show heterogeneous enhancement of the infiltrative left renal mass and renal vein thrombus. An image superior to the left hilum (Figure 7.2.3B) shows extension of tumor thrombus into the intrahepatic IVC.

DIAGNOSIS: Poorly differentiated carcinoma with neuroendocrine characteristics replacing the left kidney and expanding the left renal vein and IVC with tumor thrombus

COMMENT: We originally chose this case as a typical example of venous extension in RCC, but this is not a classic RCC. Instead, it is a poorly differentiated carcinoma with neuroendocrine characteristics. Neuroendocrine carcinoma of the kidney has been described in a few case reports in the medical literature; however, since there are no neuroendocrine cells in the normal adult renal parenchyma, this neoplasm is very rare. The aggressive invasion of the renal vein and extension into the IVC are typical of RCCs and are most often seen in clear cell RCC, particularly in those with sarcomatoid differentiation.

MRI is an ideal technique for identifying and characterizing renal vein and IVC tumor thrombus. If you look at the literature comparing CT to MRI in this regard, CT probably comes off a little worse than it should. With today's multidetector technology and the ability to obtain high spatial resolution with isotropic voxels, images can be reformatted in any plane to optimize visualization of venous tumor extension (the multiplanar capabilities of MRI used to be its ultimate trump card). Even so, it's still true that CT often requires multiple acquisitions to obtain optimal visualization of the IVC in a patient with extensive thrombus, and at some point, most of us feel ethically obligated to stop radiating the patient. The end result, on occasion, is CT images with marginal venous contrast, and delineating tumor thrombus extension in these cases can require an active imagination. And, of course, if you can't give contrast, then most of the time you can't say anything at all.

MRI without intravenous contrast is nearly as effective as contrast-enhanced MRI. We find overlapping fat-suppressed 2D SSFP images particularly useful. FSE images often show a flow void in patent veins compared with high-signal-intensity tumor thrombus and, generally, lower-signal-intensity bland thrombus. But remember that the presence of flow voids has a complex dependence on the interplay between phasic venous flow patterns and the acquisition of the central lines of k-space, and these considerations are responsible for the intermittent high-signal-intensity, slow-flow artifacts occasionally seen within veins. DWI is also useful for visualization of tumor thrombus. Diffusion gradients provide natural blood suppression (ie, the signal from moving objects disappears), and tumor thrombus is generally seen with high signal intensity and high contrast against the dark background of normal tissue and blood vessels (note the superb visualization of lumbar vein tumor thrombus in this case).

Dynamic contrast-enhanced 3D SPGR images continue to be the workhorse for detecting and staging tumor thrombus. Some of the same limitations noted earlier for CT also apply. In the presence of significant IVC thrombus, slow filling of the IVC from below often occurs, which can create artifacts and generally reduces the ability to detect thrombus. However, you can run this sequence as many times as desired until the venous enhancement is optimal without worrying about radiation burns.

Long-term survival can be achieved in about half of patients with tumor extension into the IVC. The prognosis of these patients is influenced primarily by other staging considerations, such as capsular invasion, nodal disease, and distant metastases, rather than by venous extension itself. However, the extent of venous involvement has an important role in surgical planning and thus is important to describe.

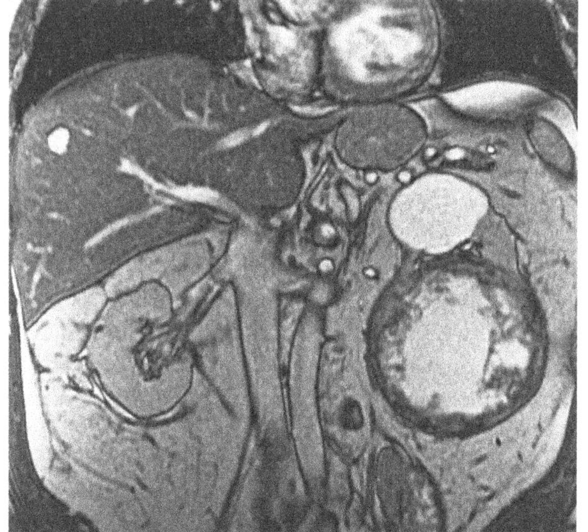

Figure 7.3.1

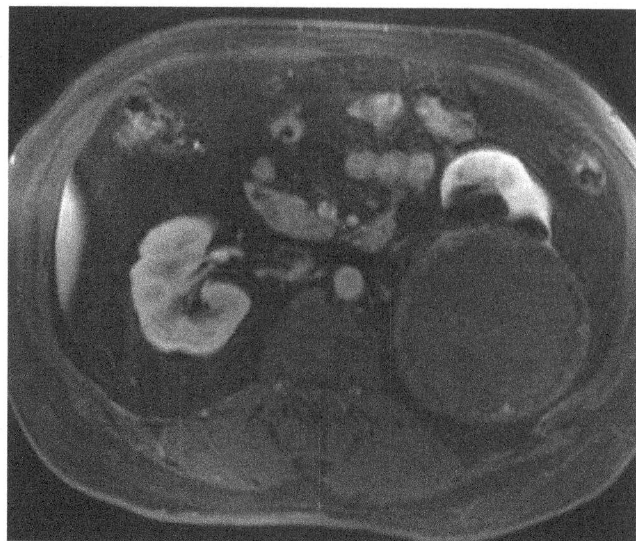

Figure 7.3.3

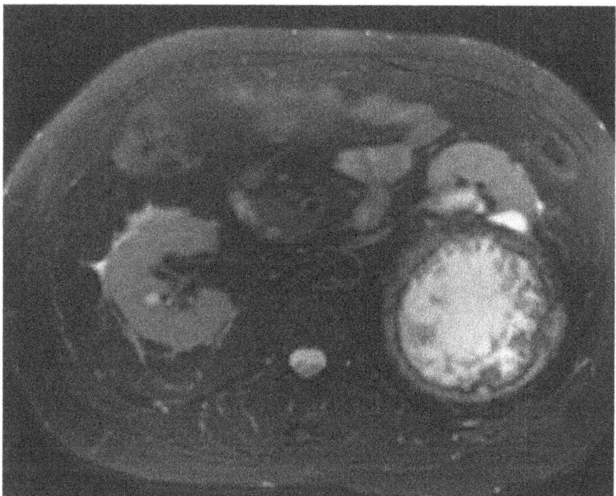

Figure 7.3.2

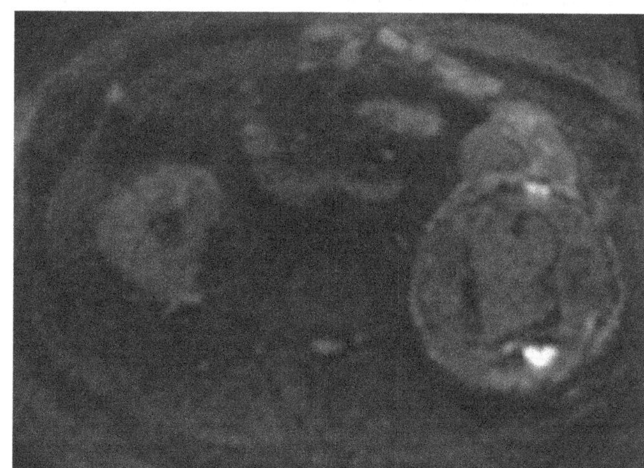

Figure 7.3.4

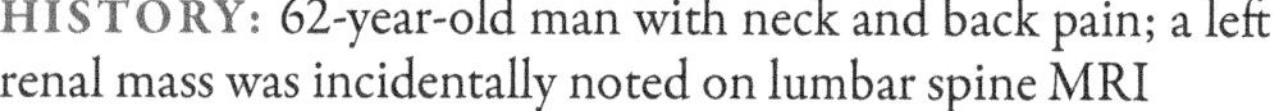

HISTORY: 62-year-old man with neck and back pain; a left renal mass was incidentally noted on lumbar spine MRI

IMAGING FINDINGS: Coronal SSFP image (Figure 7.3.1) and axial fat-suppressed FSE image (Figure 7.3.2) reveal a large, complex cystic mass with a thick wall projecting from the lower pole of the left kidney (and a simple cyst in the upper pole). Axial arterial phase 3D SPGR image (Figure 7.3.3) shows almost no enhancement of the lesion except for a small nodular focus in the posterior wall. Axial diffusion-weighted image (b=800 s/mm^2) (Figure 7.3.4) demonstrates marked hyperintensity in this same region, as well as a smaller focus of restricted diffusion in the anterior wall of the cystic mass.

DIAGNOSIS: Cystic renal cell carcinoma (papillary)

COMMENT: This case is a better example of a cystic RCC than a papillary RCC. At first glance, this is the kind of lesion that doesn't really leave any doubts about its nature: The rim is thick and irregular and multiple nodular septations extend into the center of the mass. For this lesion, there is no need to invoke Bosniak criteria; simply take it out. But after gadolinium is injected, the situation can become a little more confusing, with virtually no enhancement except for the tiny focus seen posteriorly. Although uncommon, it is not unheard of for a lesion like this to turn out to be a complex hemorrhagic cyst. In this case, diffusion-weighted images were helpful in removing any lingering doubts, because the high-signal-intensity focus posteriorly matches the small region of enhancement and another suspicious region can be seen anteriorly.

Since DWI is the latest fashionable new technique in body MRI, it isn't surprising that many papers have evaluated the utility of DWI in assessing renal lesions. The general consensus (although it's still very early) seems to be the following:

1) ADC measurements can be helpful in distinguishing clear cell RCC (higher ADC) from papillary and chromophobe RCC (lower ADC)

2) DWI with relatively high b values (600-800 s/mm^2) can be useful in imaging complex cystic renal lesions, especially when intravenous contrast cannot be given, again looking for regions of relative restricted diffusion
3) It would be very foolish to read one of these papers and then use the authors' criteria for matching ADC values to malignant vs nonmalignant lesions or to RCC subtypes, since there is enormous variation in the published ADC values. This variation is probably related to differences in vendors, field strengths, b values, and imaging parameters
4) Exceptions to these general rules are not hard to find (see Case 7.29 of perinephric hematoma with restricted diffusion, for example)

A few authors have suggested that hemorrhagic cysts with a uniform, markedly hyperintense appearance on pre-contrast-enhanced T1-weighted images are almost always benign. Authors of another paper have invoked the angular interface sign: Exophytic lesions that have an angular, triangular interface with the parenchyma, as opposed to a uniform, rounded interface, are almost always benign. These signs are occasionally helpful and usually true, but not always.

Subtraction of dynamic contrast-enhanced images from precontrast images is a common practice and has many advocates. Subtraction images can clearly demonstrate mild, diffuse enhancement within a heterogeneous lesion and sometimes are effective at showing focal enhancement in the rim of a complex cystic lesion. Remember, however, that subtracted images are only as good as the input data. If there is substantial motion artifact on 1 or both sequences or if there is significant misregistration between the 2 acquisitions, it's possible to generate spurious and, at times, very convincing regions of pseudoenhancement. The bottom line for subtracted images is that you always must return to the source data and convince yourself that what you're seeing is real.

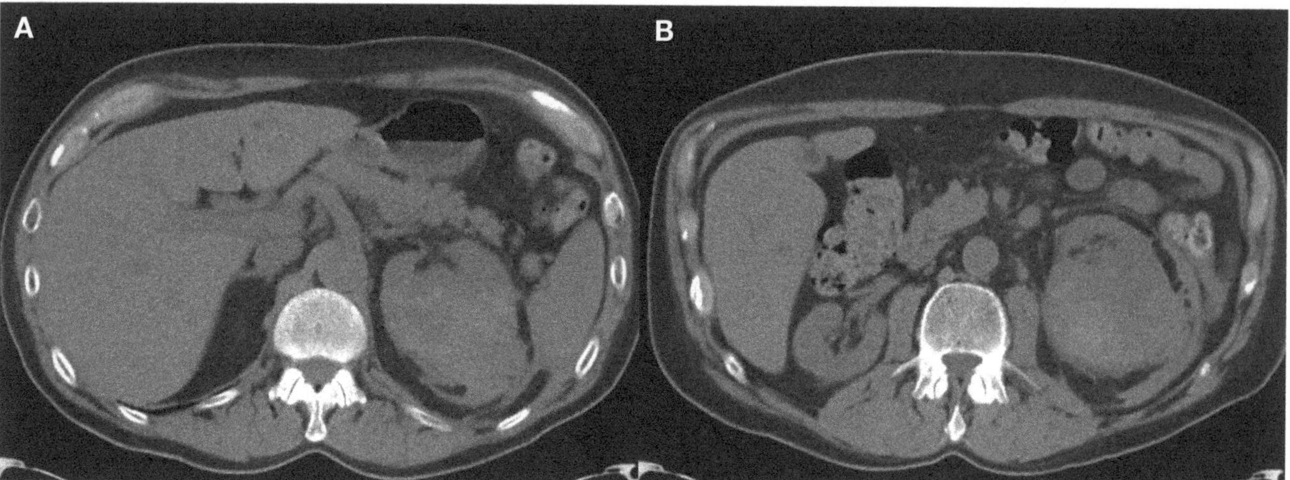

Figure 7.4.1

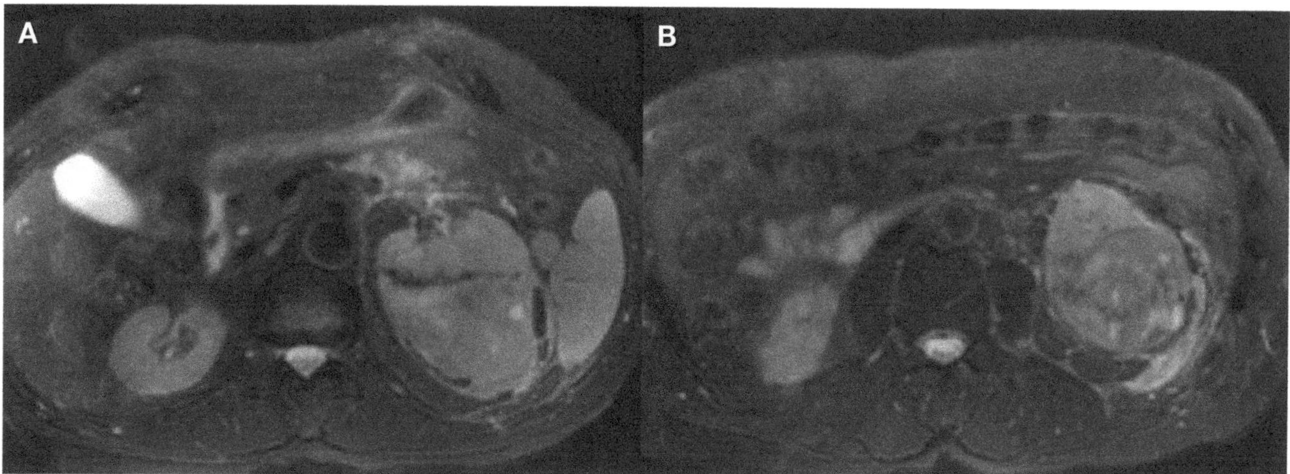

Figure 7.4.2

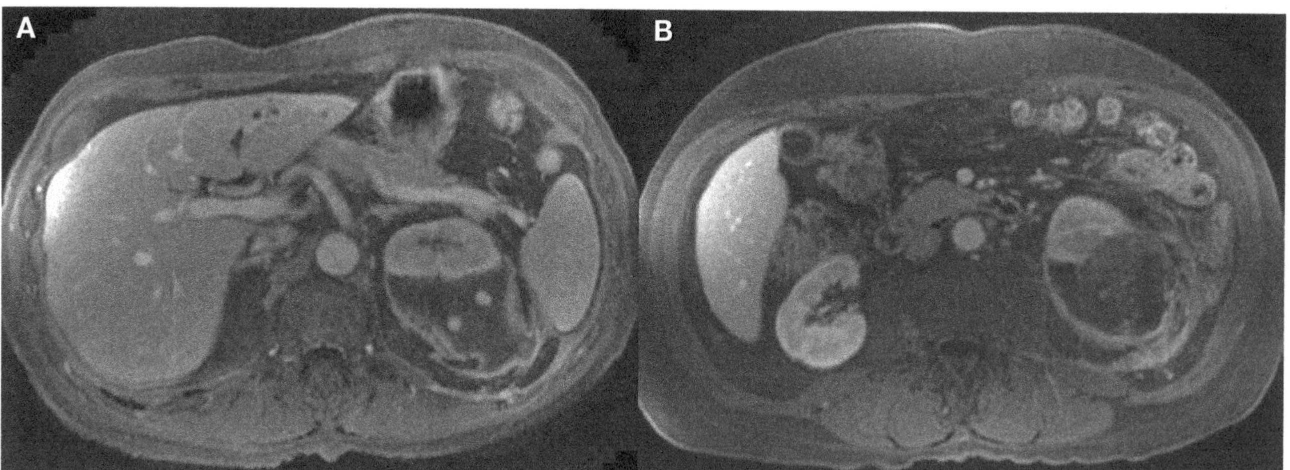

Figure 7.4.3

HISTORY: 64-year-old man with a history of necrotizing glomerulonephritis who has new-onset left flank pain

IMAGING FINDINGS: Axial images from noncontrast-enhanced renal stone protocol CT (Figure 7.4.1) show hyperdense subcapsular material along the posterior margin of the left kidney. Axial fat-suppressed FSE T2-weighted images (Figure 7.4.2) from a follow-up MRI obtained 1 week later demonstrate the same process along the posterior superior margin of the kidney. The inferior-most image (Figure 7.4.2B) shows a more well-defined mass projecting from the lower pole parenchyma. Axial postgadolinium 3D SPGR images (Figure 7.4.3) again demonstrate a heterogeneous hypoenhancing mass projecting from the lower pole of the left kidney. The superior image (Figure 7.4.3A) shows 2 enhancing nodules in a nonenhancing hematoma, with enhancement of the surrounding rim.

DIAGNOSIS: Ruptured renal cell carcinoma (clear cell)

COMMENT: This case and a subsequent case (see Case 7.29) illustrate some of the difficulties of imaging patients with perirenal hematomas. You always have to be vigilant about looking for an underlying cause of the hemorrhage, and it may not be easy to distinguish a small mass within a complex hematoma. This dilemma is less problematic if you can give gadolinium since, as a general rule, RCCs enhance and hematomas don't. Again, subtracted images can be useful in this situation, provided the patient is cooperative and holds his breath at the same location for the pre- and postcontrast acquisitions.

One could argue that the diagnosis could be suggested even on noncontrast-enhanced CT because the inferior image (Figure 7.4.1B) shows a more rounded contour to the hematoma, implying the presence of a mass. And if intravenous contrast had been given, the mass in all likelihood would have been appreciated. But the mass is easier to see even on the precontrast T2-weighted images, and small, enhancing tumor nodules within the hematoma are easily visualized on the dynamic postgadolinium 3D SPGR images.

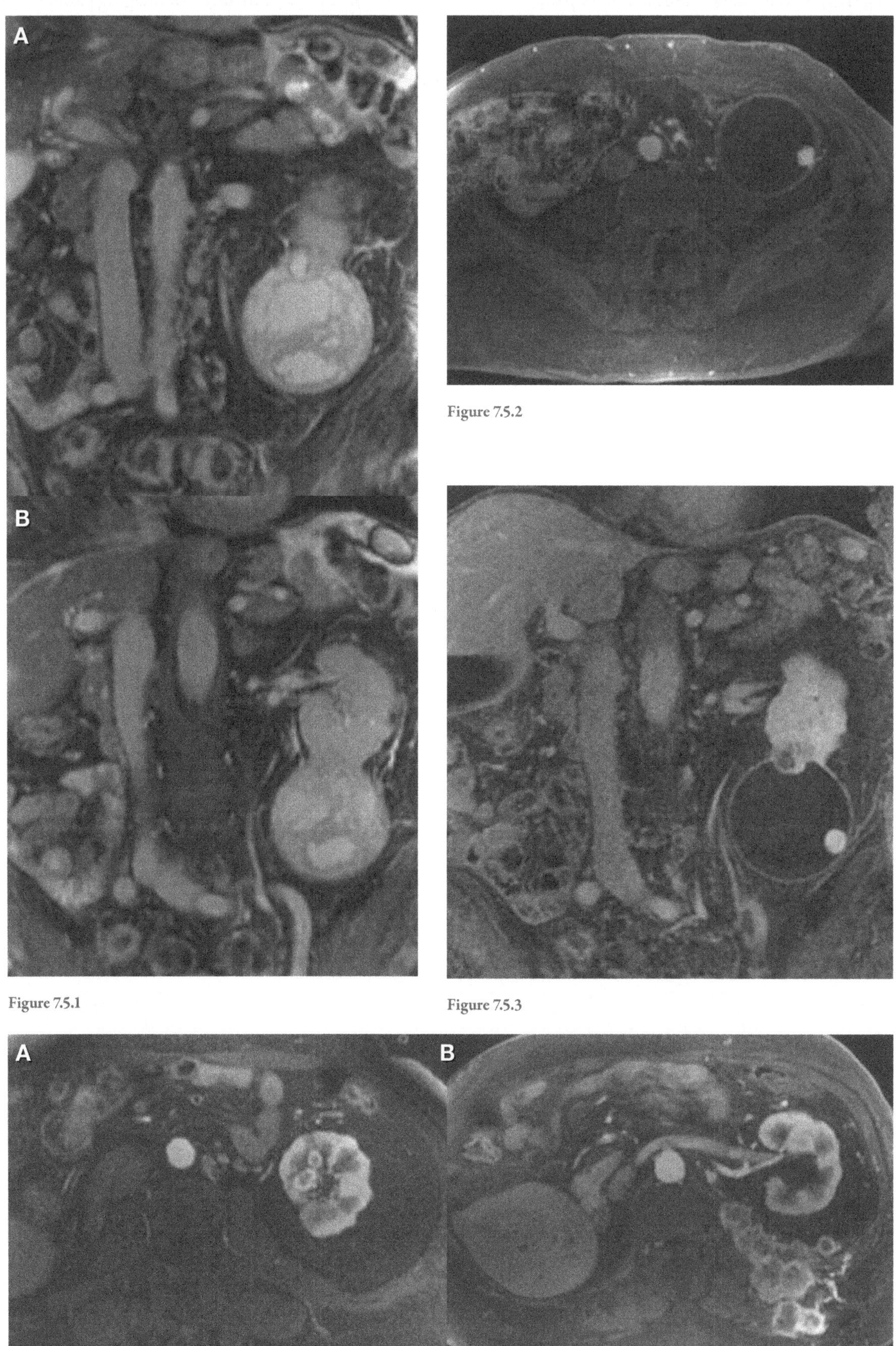

Figure 7.5.1

Figure 7.5.2

Figure 7.5.3

Figure 7.5.4

HISTORY: 68-year-old man with new-onset anuria and a remote right nephrectomy; an obstructing left ureteral stone was found on CT, as well as a cystic left renal mass

IMAGING FINDINGS: Coronal SSFP images (Figure 7.5.1) reveal a complex, septated cystic mass projecting from the lower pole of the left kidney. Axial arterial phase (Figure 7.5.2) and coronal nephrogenic phase (Figure 7.5.3) postgadolinium 3D SPGR images demonstrate a predominantly cystic lesion with enhancing mural nodules. Axial arterial phase, postgadolinium 3D SPGR images (Figure 7.5.4) from the first follow-up examination after partial left nephrectomy show small enhancing lesions in the lower pole of the left kidney near the surgical margin, as well as multiple ring-enhancing metastases in the posterior left abdominal wall.

DIAGNOSIS: Sarcomatoid renal cell carcinoma (clear cell)

COMMENT: Clear cell RCC is the most common subtype, accounting for roughly 75% of RCCs. Of all RCCs at histologic examination, 8% to 10% have foci of spindle-shaped, eosinophilic, and fibroblastoid cells resembling malignant fibrous histiocytoma or fibrosarcoma. This appearance has been designated *sarcomatoid RCC* and predicts more aggressive tumor behavior and a worse prognosis—sarcomatoid RCC is much more likely to metastasize and to spread to adjacent organs. Median survival of patients with sarcomatoid RCC is 3 to 10 months at diagnosis.

This case illustrates the classic cystic RCC with an enhancing mural nodule on the dynamic contrast-enhanced 3D SPGR images. The appearance on precontrast SSFP images is much more complex and again emphasizes how much easier it is to sort out lesions if you can give intravenous contrast. The extensive metastatic disease at the initial 3-month follow-up examination is unusual but should not be unexpected in a patient with sarcomatoid RCC. RCC can spread to a wide range of abdominal organs, as well as bone, muscle, and lymph nodes, so a vigilant search and a protocol that provides adequate anatomic coverage are important elements of the post-nephrectomy examination.

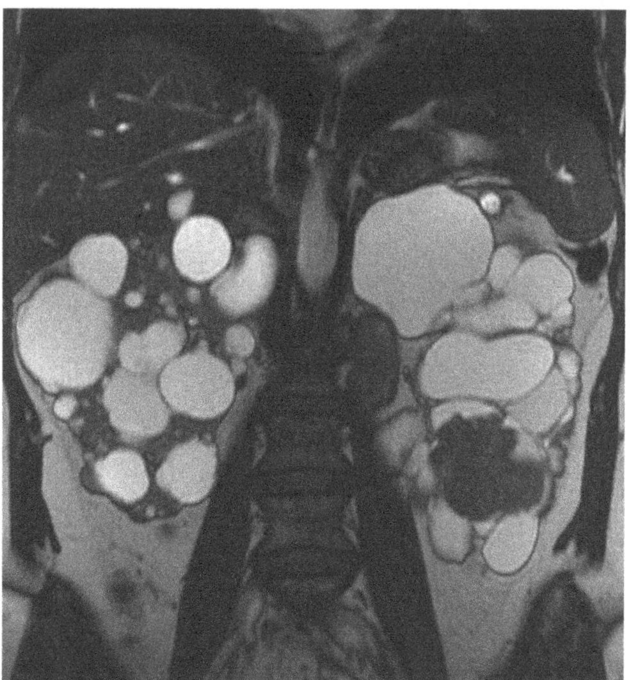

Figure 7.6.1

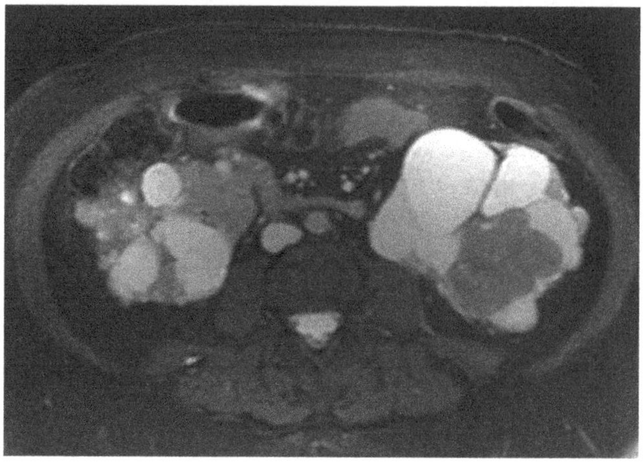

Figure 7.6.2

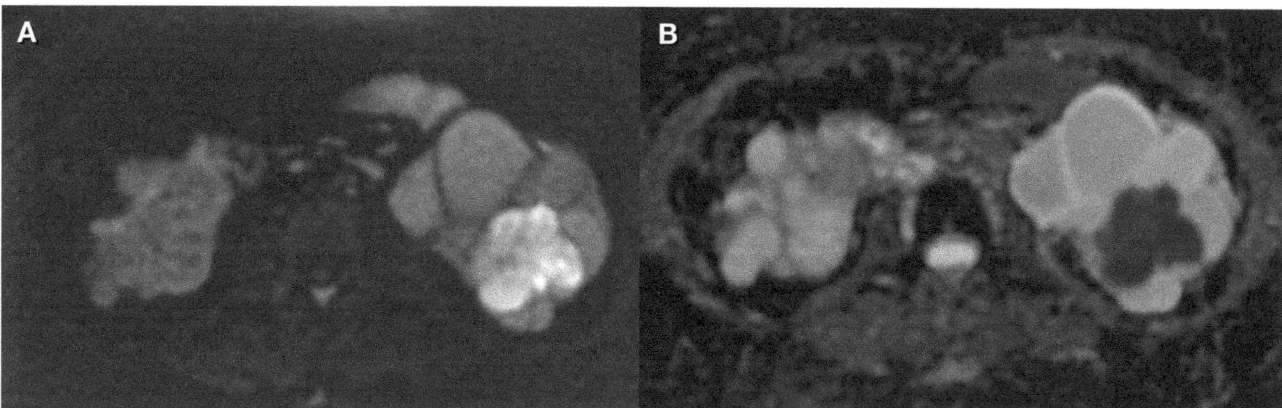

Figure 7.6.3

HISTORY: 62-year-old woman with ADPKD and new onset anorexia, weight loss, night sweats, and fever

IMAGING FINDINGS: Coronal SSFP (Figure 7.6.1) and axial fat-suppressed SSFP (Figure 7.6.2) images reveal enlarged, polycystic kidneys. There is a relatively hypointense mass in the lower pole of the left kidney. Axial diffusion-weighted image (b=800 s/mm^2) and the corresponding ADC map (Figure 7.6.3) demonstrate that the lesion has high signal intensity and a low ADC value, suspicious for RCC.

DIAGNOSIS: Renal cell carcinoma in polycystic kidneys (clear cell sarcomatoid)

COMMENT: Evaluating ADPKD patients for a renal mass can be very challenging. There are hundreds of cysts, many of which are hemorrhagic, and quite often, you cannot use gadolinium-based contrast agents because renal function is compromised. (But if you can, subtraction imaging may be useful.)

In this case, it requires no great brilliance to identify the mass: It's a large solid lesion that doesn't look like the small amount of normal renal parenchyma remaining, and it is fairly easy to identify on conventional SSFP images. However, this case is a nice example of the utility of DWI in patients with ADPKD. Diffusion-weighted images with a relatively high b value (800 s/mm^2 in this case) have enough diffusion weighting to overcome the T2 shine-through effect of renal cysts. Therefore, the cysts are only mildly hyperintense, and the solid lesion with restricted diffusion is markedly hyperintense and demonstrates excellent contrast in comparison to the adjacent cysts. The ADC map isn't really necessary in this case (or in most other cases), but again it illustrates the mass with low ADC values (ie, low signal intensity) surrounded by fluid-filled cysts with high ADC values and high signal intensity.

Keep in mind that although this method is not foolproof, it can be helpful in PKD patients and can simplify the search for the small mass among the "haystack" of cysts.

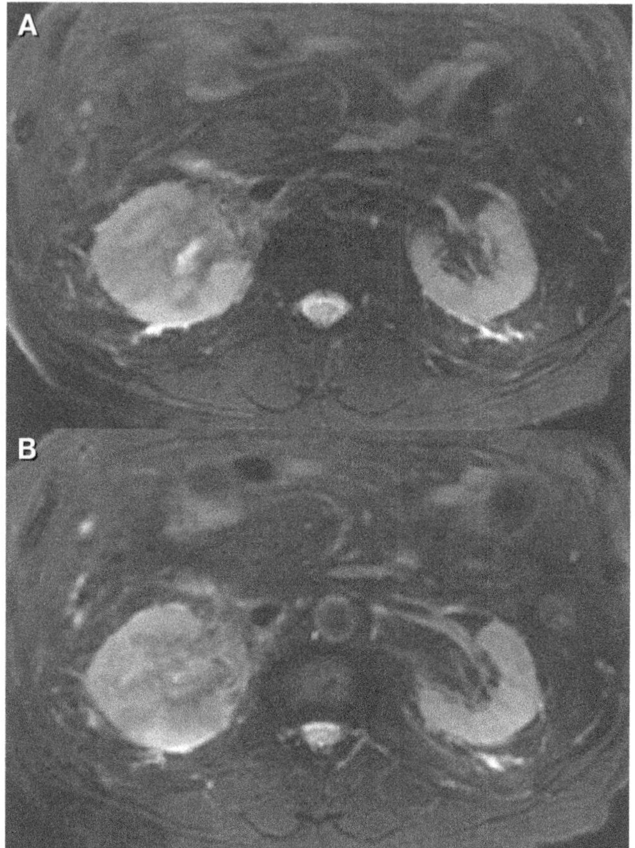

Figure 7.7.1

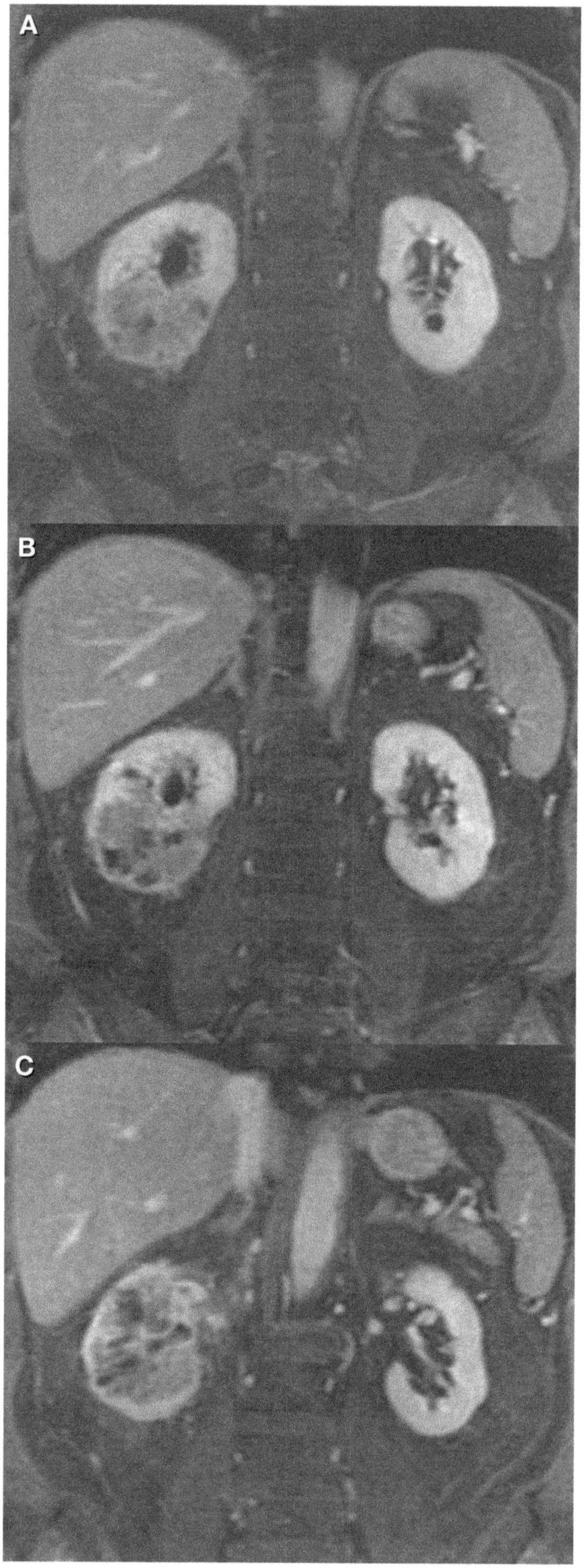

Figure 7.7.2

HISTORY: 72-year-old man with hematuria, right flank pain, and weight loss

IMAGING FINDINGS: Axial fat-suppressed FSE T2-weighted images (Figure 7.7.1) and coronal nephrogenic phase postgadolinium 3D SPGR images (Figure 7.7.2) reveal an infiltrative hypoenhancing and mildly T2 hypointense mass in the lower pole of the right kidney.

DIAGNOSIS: Renal urothelial cell carcinoma (transitional cell carcinoma)

COMMENT: Five percent of urothelial tumors arise from the ureter, renal pelvis, or calyces, and these account for approximately 10% of upper tract neoplasms. *Urothelial cell carcinoma* is probably the preferred term among pathologists currently, although *transitional cell carcinoma* is used at least as often. Upper tract TCC typically occurs in the sixth or seventh decade of life, with men affected 3 times as frequently as women. Other risk factors include smoking, chemical exposures, and, possibly, heavy caffeine consumption. Patients may present with hematuria, flank pain, or renal colic. Upper tract TCCs are characterized by multiplicity and a high incidence of recurrent and metachronous tumors. Among patients initially presenting with upper tract TCCs, 50% will develop metachronous tumors in the bladder, and so frequent surveillance is required after initial surgery in these patients. Conversely, upper tract tumors occur in 2% to 4% of patients with bladder cancer.

Eighty-five percent of upper tract TCCs are low-stage, superficial papillary neoplasms that usually are small at diagnosis, grow slowly, and follow a relatively benign course. Infiltrating tumors are less common, accounting for approximately 15% of upper tract TCCs, and are more aggressive and further advanced at diagnosis. Infiltrating TCCs involving the renal pelvis frequently invade the kidney.

Small TCCs in the renal pelvis appear as a filling defect, pelvicaliceal irregularity or thickening, or a focal or diffuse obstruction of the calyces or renal pelvis. Advanced TCC extends into the renal parenchyma in an infiltrative pattern that often preserves the kidney's reniform shape but distorts the renal architecture. By comparison, RCCs tend to be more exophytic and have more clearly defined margins (ie, the ball vs bean analogy, which is actually true on occasion). TCCs are usually hypoenhancing relative to renal parenchyma after gadolinium administration and typically are less vascular than RCCs (particularly the clear cell subtype). Hydronephrosis is a common finding in upper tract TCC, but it can also be seen in RCC. Vascular invasion is much more common in RCC but does occasionally occur in upper tract TCC.

As noted earlier, certain characteristics of renal lesions on MRI favor TCC over RCC and vice versa, but these features are by no means absolutely definitive. If your evaluation is not a work-up of an unknown renal mass, but instead surveillance imaging of a patient with a history of TCC, an MRU protocol is probably a better choice than a standard renal mass protocol.

Our MRU protocol consists of coronal oblique 3D SPGR images covering the kidneys, ureters, and bladder after administration of gadolinium, as well as a small amount of furosemide to dilute the gadolinium in the collecting system and prevent significant susceptibility artifact. This acquisition is repeated as many times as necessary to visualize excreted contrast in the calyces, renal pelvis, ureters, and bladder. Small tumors appear as either hyperenhancing lesions on arterial phase images or filling defects on excretory phase images.

Additional T2-weighted images (FSE and SSFP) are acquired before gadolinium administration. The sensitivity for detection of small upper tract lesions with MRU is lower than CT urography in most studies, probably because of the lower spatial resolution. In obstructed systems, injection of gadolinium is not a particularly good idea, and generally you're better off running your MRCP sequence (respiratory-triggered 3D FRFSE) centered over the urinary tract. DWI has been advocated recently for imaging TCCs in both the upper and lower tracts; in theory, small lesions can be detected with high contrast (and without gadolinium). It's important to choose a relatively high b value (typically, 800-1,000 s/mm^2) to adequately suppress the signal from fluid and minimize the T2 shine-through of urine.

CASE 7.8

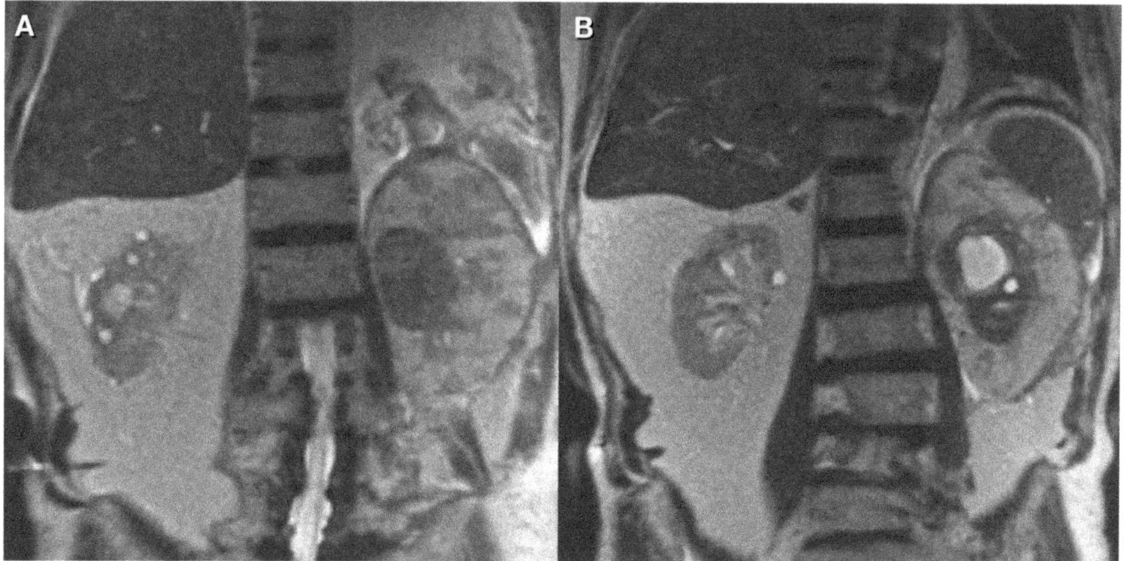

Figure 7.8.1

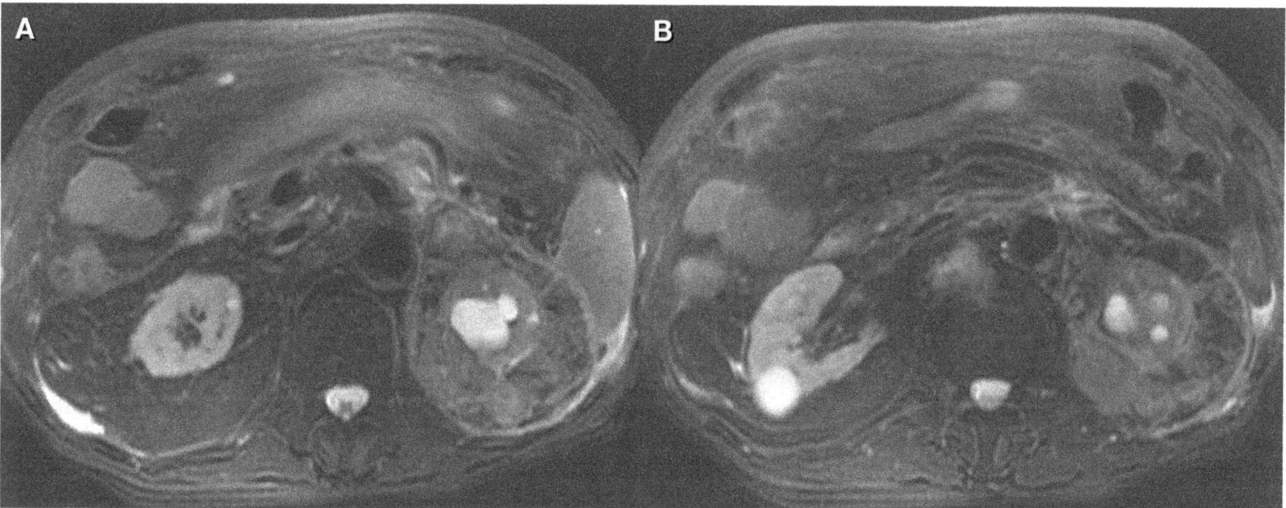

Figure 7.8.2

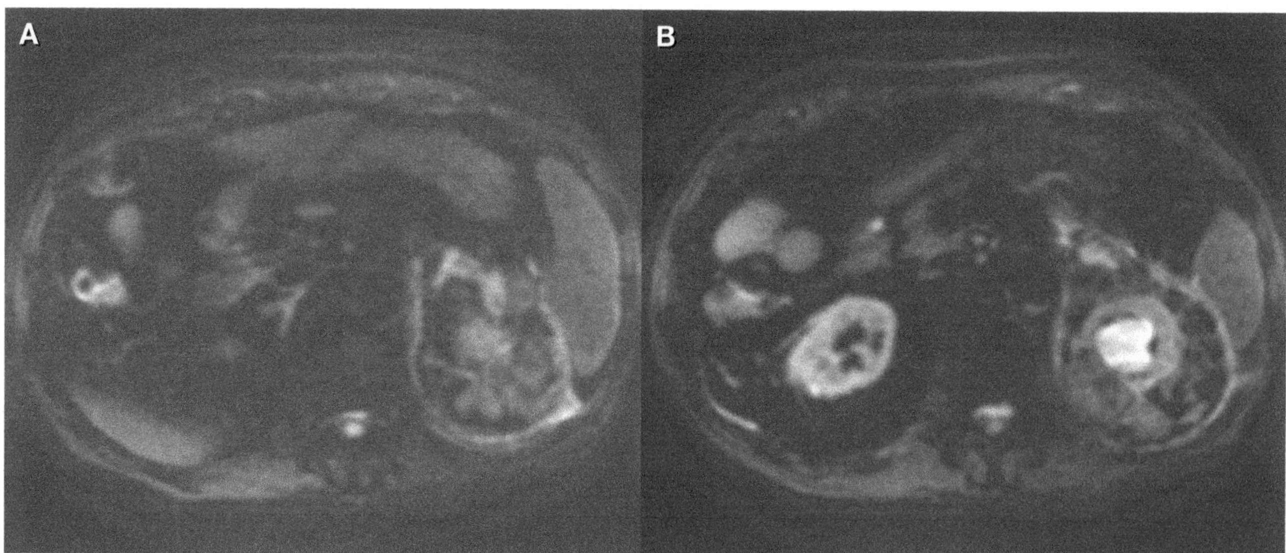

Figure 7.8.3

HISTORY: 85-year-old man with acute on chronic renal failure

IMAGING FINDINGS: Coronal SSFSE (Figure 7.8.1), axial FSE (Figure 7.8.2), and axial diffusion-weighted (b=100 s/mm^2) (Figure 7.8.3) images reveal a small left kidney with hydronephrosis of upper pole calyces. Nodular thickening involves the renal capsule and Gerota fascia, with larger nodules adjacent to the renal hilum and within the perinephric fat. Note also the right-sided renal cysts.

DIAGNOSIS: Urothelial cell carcinoma of the renal pelvis with extension to the perinephric fat and Gerota fascia

COMMENT: This appearance is unusual for renal urothelial cell carcinoma. The renal pelvis mass was probably the incident lesion, with slow growth and development of hydronephrosis and renal atrophy followed by infiltrative growth through the urothelium and spread through the renal capsule and into the pararenal space. The nodular appearance of the renal capsule and perinephric lesions should help you avoid a diagnosis of retroperitoneal fibrosis.

CASE 7.9

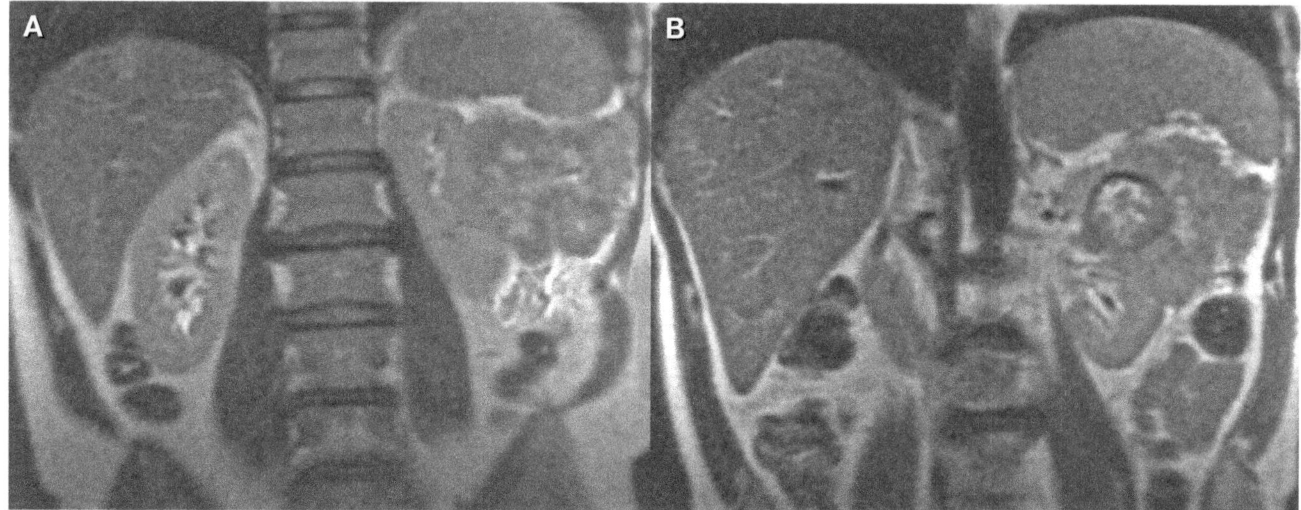

Figure 7.9.1

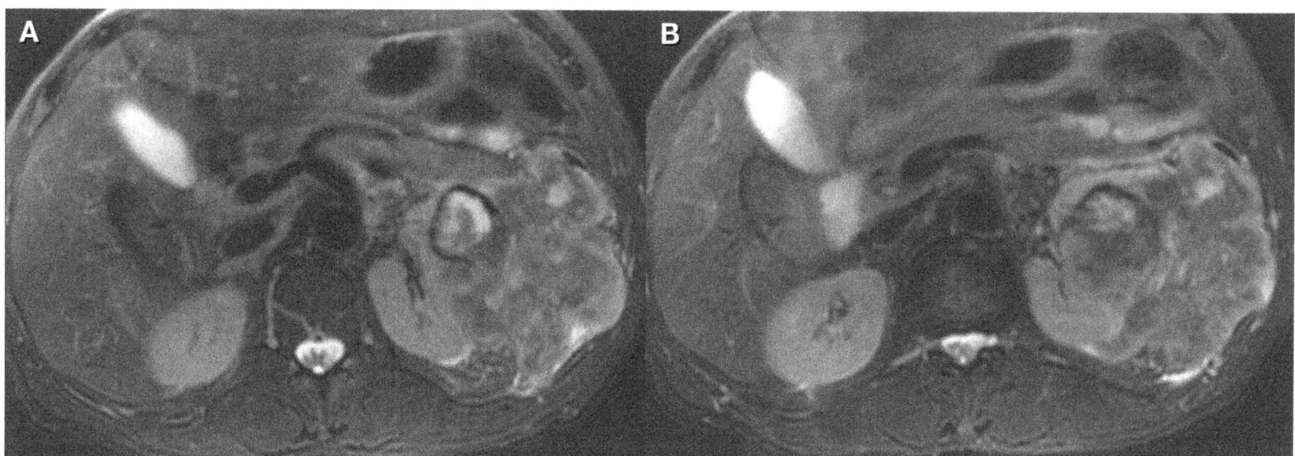

Figure 7.9.2

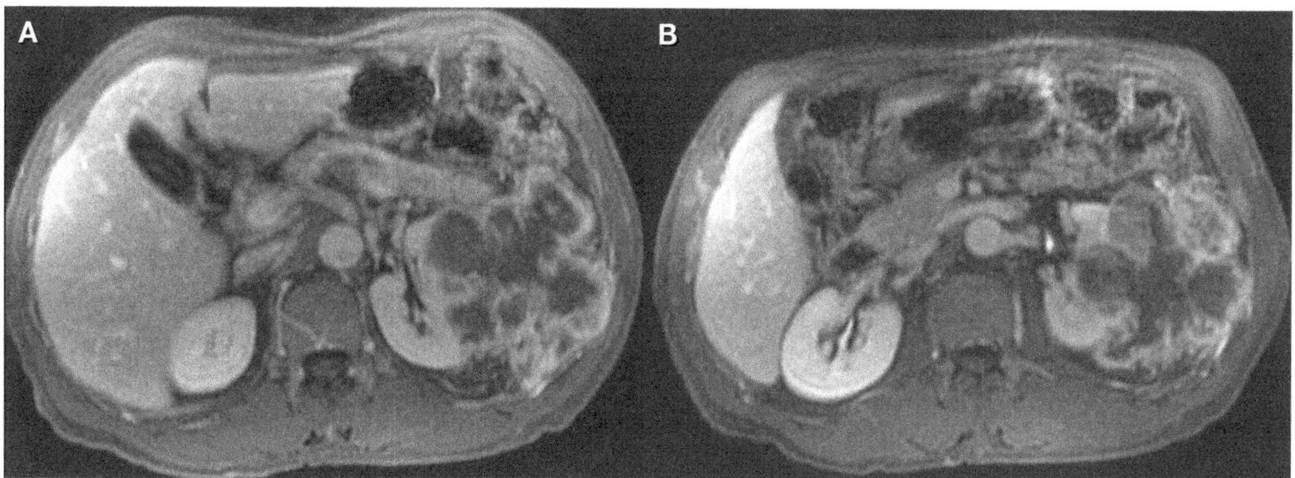

Figure 7.9.3

HISTORY: 57-year-old man with a 2-month history of fatigue, weight loss, and left-sided flank pain

IMAGING FINDINGS: Coronal SSFSE images (Figure 7.9.1), axial fat-suppressed FSE T2-weighted images (Figure 7.9.2), and axial venous phase postgadolinium 3D SPGR images (Figure 7.9.3) demonstrate a large, heterogeneously enhancing exophytic mass in the left kidney abutting and possibly invading the left lateral abdominal wall.

DIAGNOSIS: Renal leiomyosarcoma

COMMENT: Leiomyosarcoma is the most common primary sarcoma of the kidney, accounting for 50% to 60% of renal sarcomas. Leiomyosarcomas can arise from the renal capsule, parenchyma, renal pelvis, or renal vein, and most occur in patients between ages 40 and 70 years. Histologic examination reveals tumors composed of spindle cells interspersed with connective tissue. The presence of nuclear pleomorphism, mitoses, and necrosis differentiates leiomyosarcoma from a benign leiomyoma.

Leiomyosarcomas typically are large at presentation and show heterogeneous T1- and T2-signal intensity and heterogeneous enhancement. Regions of fibrotic tissue may have decreased T1- and T2-signal intensity, with gradual enhancement after contrast administration. No reliable criteria are available for distinguishing renal sarcomas from RCC; however, sarcomas generally are larger and more heterogeneous at presentation. A large heterogeneous and aggressive renal mass such as this one is still statistically more likely to be RCC (or sarcomatoid RCC), but including sarcoma in the differential diagnosis is not unreasonable, and once in a while you might even be right.

Nephrectomy is the standard treatment for leiomyosarcoma, followed by radiotherapy and chemotherapy. These tumors have a poor prognosis, with 5-year survival rates between 29% and 36%.

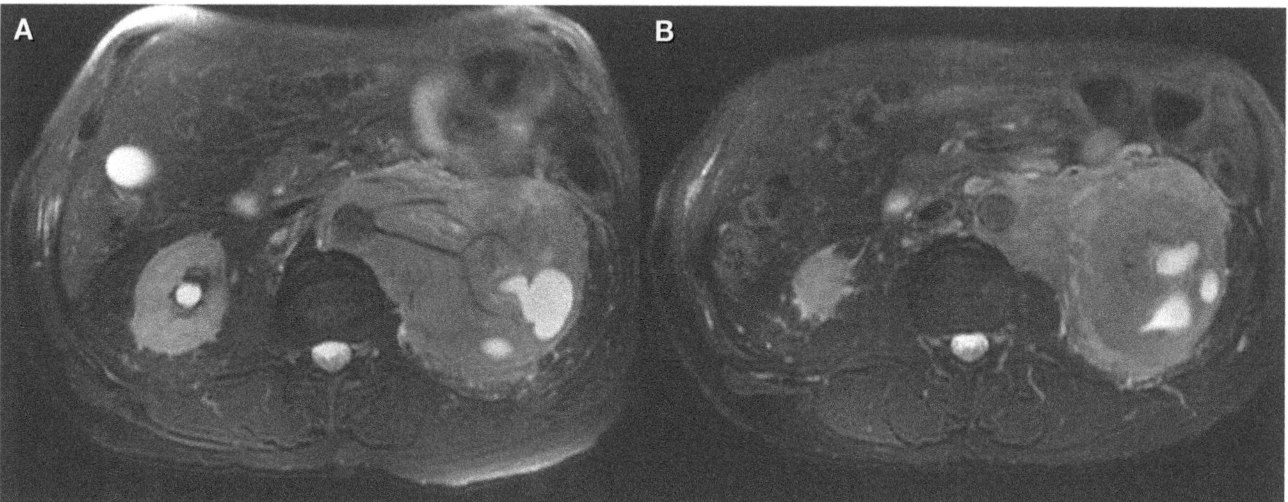

Figure 7.10.1

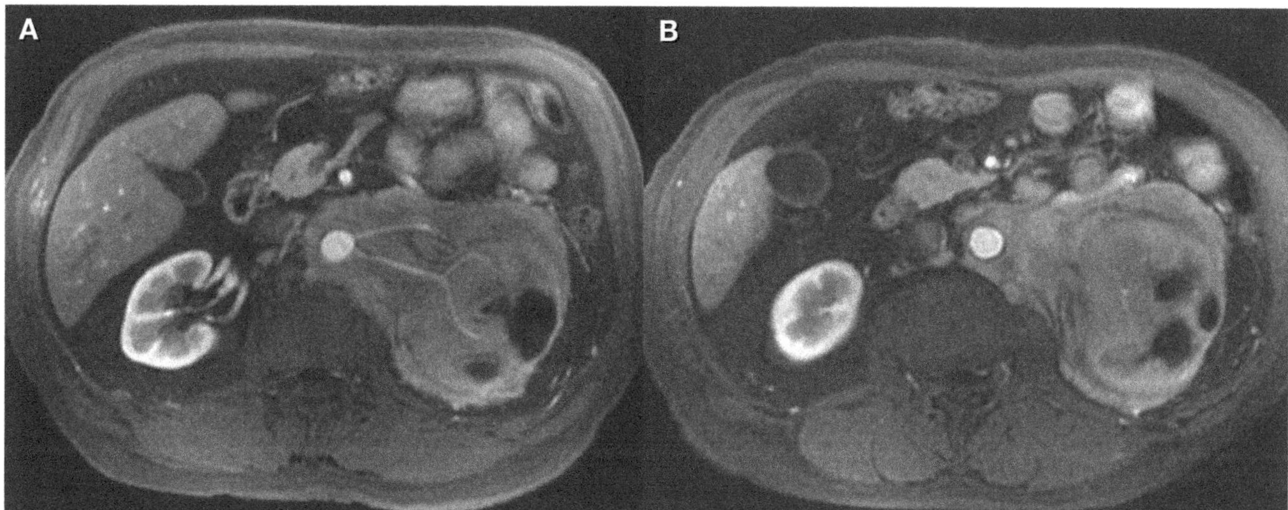

Figure 7.10.2

HISTORY: 70-year-old man with recent hematuria; varicocele was noted on physical examination

IMAGING FINDINGS: Axial fat-suppressed FSE T2-weighted images (Figure 7.10.1) and axial arterial phase postgadolinium 3D SPGR images (Figure 7.10.2) show a homogeneous mass surrounding the left kidney, as well as the aorta and left renal artery. Note the moderate left hydronephrosis.

DIAGNOSIS: Renal lymphoma

COMMENT: The GU system is frequently affected by extranodal spread of lymphoma, almost always of the non-Hodgkin type (intermediate- and high-grade B-cell lymphoma and Burkitt lymphoma). In 1 autopsy study, renal involvement in lymphoma was detected in 37% of patients. However, as an imaging finding, it is much less commonly reported, with most series describing evidence of renal involvement in 3% to 8% of patients. Renal lymphoma is generally asymptomatic, and imaging detection seldom affects staging and treatment.

As is the general rule with lymphoma, renal involvement can have many different manifestations. Because lymphoid tissue is normally absent in the kidney, primary renal lymphoma is thought to be extremely rare, with most cases occurring by direct extension or hematogenous spread. Direct extension can occur when retroperitoneal tumor invades the renal capsule or infiltrates the renal sinus and encases the renal pelvis and vessels. Involvement of renal parenchyma can occur by direct extension or hematogenous spread—this initially involves the interstitium, with the vessels, collecting ducts, and nephrons used as scaffolding for further growth.

The MRI patterns seen in renal lymphoma reflect these mechanisms of renal involvement and growth. The most common appearance is multiple, usually bilateral renal masses (in 50%-60% of cases). Differential diagnosis for this appearance includes multifocal RCC, oncocytosis, and infection. The presence of bulky retroperitoneal and mesenteric adenopathy is not a universal finding, but when seen, is a useful clue to the diagnosis.

Renal lymphoma appearing as a solitary mass is less common (in 10%-25% of cases) but represents a more difficult diagnostic challenge (see the example in the final paragraph of this case). Lymphoma classically has lower signal intensity on T2-weighted images than RCC and is generally hypoenhancing relative to the kidney following gadolinium administration, but chromophobe and papillary RCCs can have an identical appearance. Vascular invasion is uncommon with renal lymphoma, and its presence should suggest an alternative diagnosis. Likewise, cystic masses are not likely to be lymphoma, although necrotic regions can occur, particularly after chemotherapy. Diffuse nephromegaly may occur with relatively little mass effect or distortion of the collecting system or renal contour.

Contiguous extension to the kidneys from the retroperitoneum occurs in 25% to 30% of cases and is probably the most easily recognizable form of renal lymphoma, typically appearing as large lesions surrounding the renal capsule or renal sinus, or both. Although hydronephrosis resulting from renal sinus or ureteral compression is not uncommon (as in this case), vascular invasion is rare. Most commonly, perinephric extension is associated with bulky retroperitoneal masses. This case is somewhat unusual in that there are no large retroperitoneal nodes distinct from the mass encasing the aorta and left kidney. Nevertheless, the appearance is so characteristic that the correct diagnosis should be made without hesitation. Differential diagnosis for the perinephric forms includes metastases to the perinephric space, sarcomas involving the renal capsule, perinephric hematoma, and retroperitoneal fibrosis.

The potential diagnosis of renal lymphoma is useful to keep in mind when reviewing examinations with renal masses. The treatment of renal lymphoma is medical—vs partial or complete nephrectomy for nonmetastatic RCC. It's a good thing to be able to suggest the diagnosis prospectively and then perhaps confirm it with a percutaneous biopsy, to spare the patient unnecessary surgery.

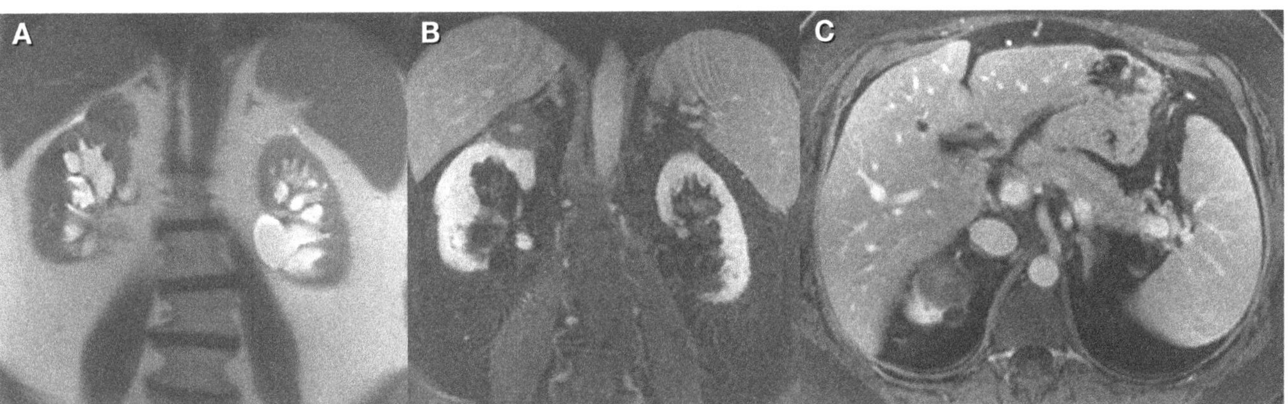

Figure 7.10.3

This companion case is an example of renal lymphoma appearing as a focal mass. Coronal SSFSE image (Figure 7.10.3A) and coronal (Figure 7.10.3B) and axial (Figure 7.10.3C) postgadolinium 3D SPGR images demonstrate a T2 hypointense, hypoenhancing focal mass projecting from the upper pole of the right kidney.

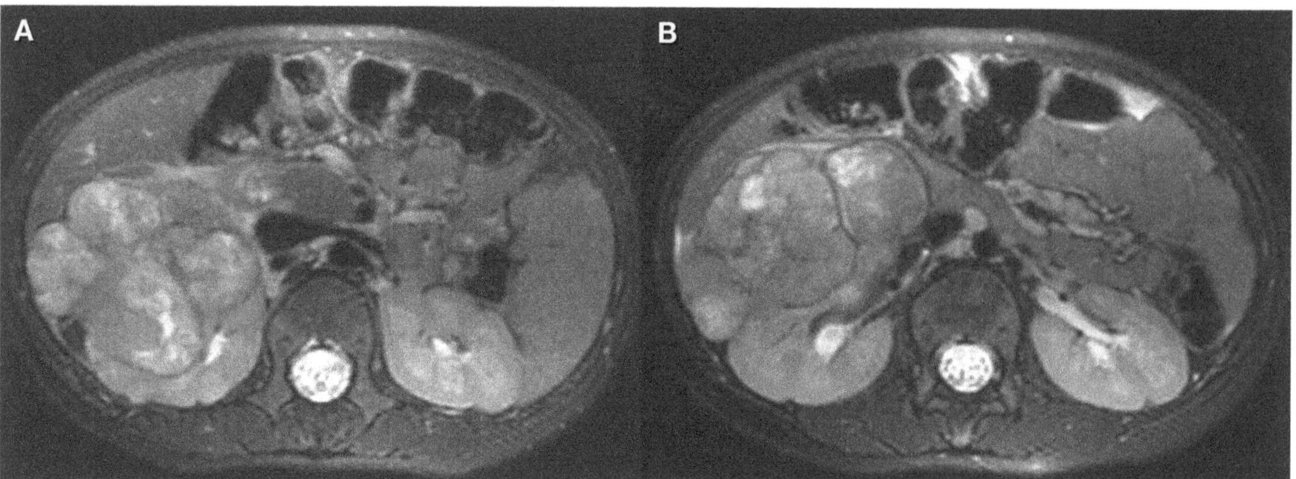

Figure 7.11.1

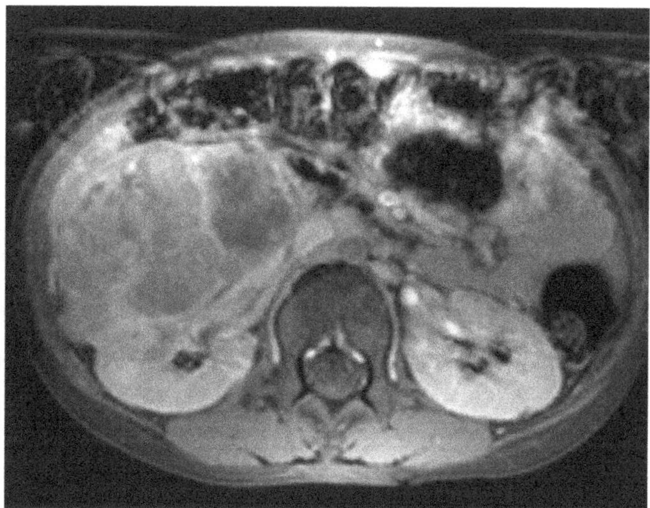

Figure 7.11.2

HISTORY: 4-year-old girl with vomiting, diarrhea, fever, and a palpable abdominal mass

IMAGING FINDINGS: Axial fat-suppressed FSE (Figure 7.11.1) and axial postgadolinium 3D SPGR (Figure 7.11.2) images show a large heterogeneous mass originating from the anterior right kidney.

DIAGNOSIS: Wilms tumor

COMMENT: Wilms tumor is the most common abdominal malignancy in children, with an annual incidence of 8 cases per 1 million persons. Most patients (80%) present between ages 1 and 5 years, usually with an incidentally discovered abdominal mass. Bilateral tumors are found in 5% of cases, and these are associated with an earlier presentation, a higher incidence of associated congenital abnormalities, and a higher incidence of nephroblastomatosis (multiple rests of persistent embryonic renal parenchyma). Among children with Wilms tumor, 12% have associated congenital abnormalities, including GU abnormalities (5%), hemihypertrophy (2%), and aniridia (1%). Syndromes associated with Wilms tumor include Beckwith-Wiedemann (macroglossia, exomphalos, and gigantism), Denys-Drash (male pseudohermaphroditism and glomerular disease), WAGR (Wilms tumor, aniridia, GU abnormalities, and mental retardation), Sotos (cerebral gigantism), and Bloom (immunodeficiency and facial telangiectasia).

Wilms tumor arises in persistent embryonic tissue, and the classic tumor shows triphasic histology, containing epithelial, blastemal, and stromal cell lines. Prognosis depends on the presence and degree of anaplasia (nuclear and mitotic atypia), and approximately 90% of Wilms tumors show favorable histology.

Wilms tumors are solid heterogeneous lesions that favor the periphery of the kidneys. Regions of hemorrhage, necrosis, and cystic change are fairly common, and fat also can be seen within these lesions. Regional lymphadenopathy is not uncommon, and metastatic disease most frequently involves the lungs and liver. Tumor extension into the renal veins and IVC may occur; approximately 4% of patients have IVC or right atrial thrombus at presentation.

Treatment consists of nephrectomy followed by adjuvant chemotherapy. The prognosis for most patients is excellent, with 4-year survival rates of 85% to 95% for stages I through III and up to 70% for widespread metastases or bilateral involvement (stages IV and V). Prognosis for the 4% of patients with anaplastic histology is much less favorable, with 4-year survival rates of 45% for stage III disease and 7% for stage IV disease.

The list of differential diagnoses for a solid renal mass in a young child is relatively short. Nephroblastomatosis may be seen in 1 or both kidneys and typically appears as more uniform regions of hypoenhancement, often in the periphery of the kidneys. These lesions can be precursors of Wilms tumors. Mesoblastic nephroma is a benign neoplasm with an earlier presentation in the neonatal period (mean age at presentation, 3 months) that may have a similar appearance to Wilms tumor, although vascular invasion is not seen. Clear cell sarcoma is less common than Wilms tumor, but it presents at a similar age and has a similar appearance. The presence of a lytic bone lesion in a patient with presumed Wilms tumor might suggest the alternative diagnosis of clear cell sarcoma. Rhabdoid tumor of the kidney is a rare and aggressive childhood renal neoplasm and usually is diagnosed in the first year of life.

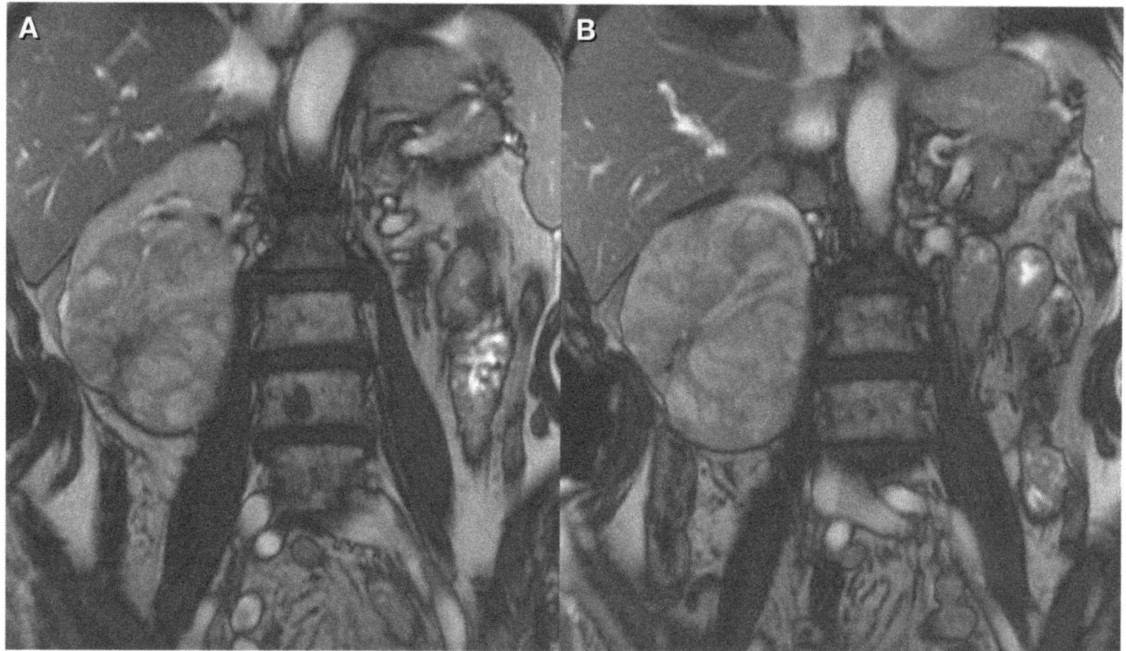

Figure 7.12.1

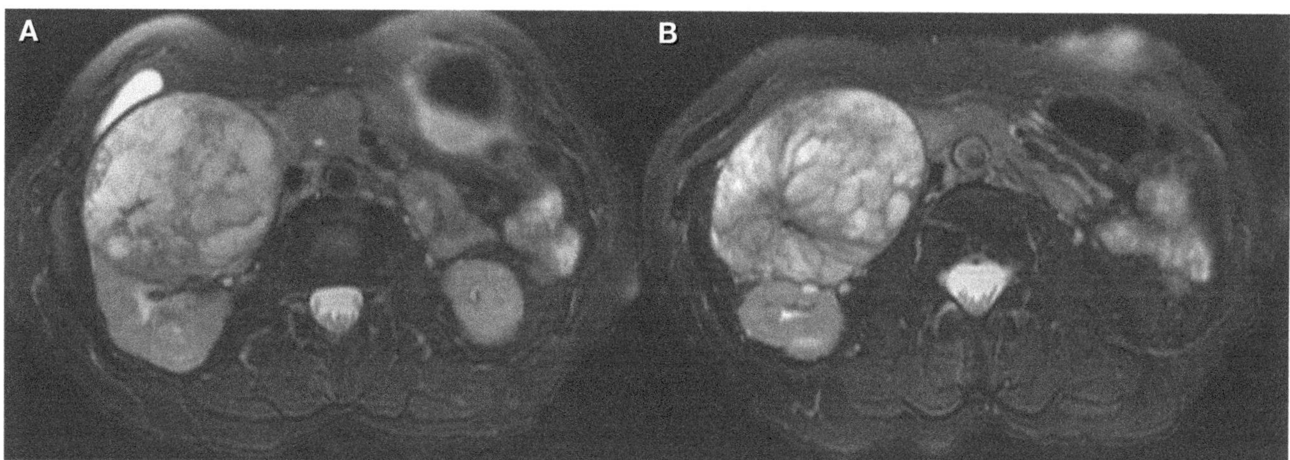

Figure 7.12.2

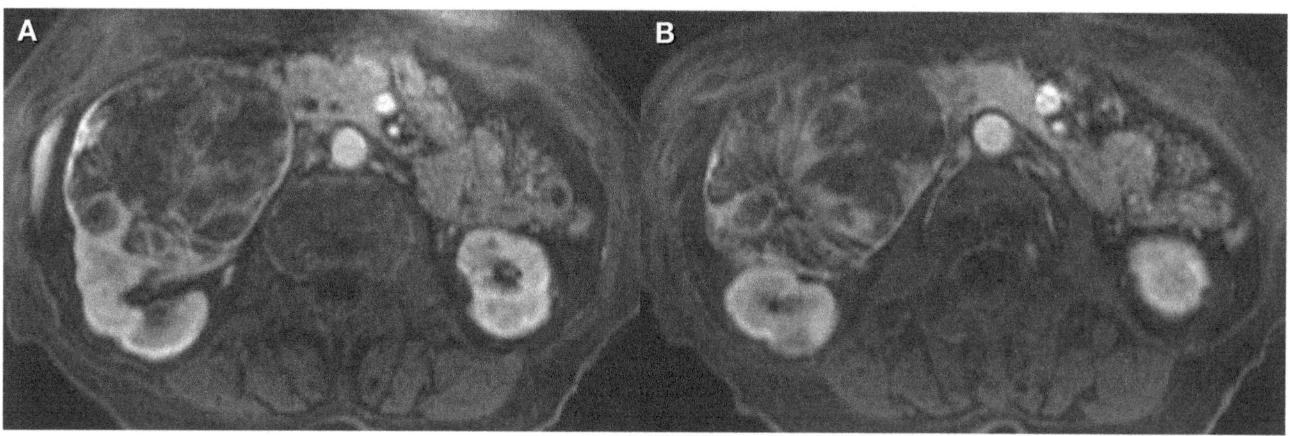

Figure 7.12.3

HISTORY: 85-year-old woman with nausea; CT performed in the emergency department revealed a large right renal mass

IMAGING FINDINGS: Coronal SSFP (Figure 7.12.1), axial fat-suppressed FSE (Figure 7.12.2), and axial postgadolinium 3D SPGR (Figure 7.12.3) images show a heterogeneous mass in the upper pole of the right kidney, with the suggestion of a central scar.

DIAGNOSIS: Oncocytoma

COMMENT: Oncocytoma is a benign neoplasm accounting for approximately 5% of all renal tumors and is thought to originate from type A intercalated cells of the cortical collecting ducts. Oncocytomas usually are detected in asymptomatic older patients, with the peak age of incidence in the seventh decade. They typically are solitary, well-demarcated lesions. Often described as homogeneous, they nevertheless can have widely varying appearances, with larger lesions tending to be less uniform.

The classic central stellate fibrotic scar described in most textbooks is seen in about one-third of oncocytomas and is arguably present in this case. However, this finding is nonspecific; a recent paper comparing oncocytomas to chromophobe RCCs found no difference in the detection of a central scar. The central scar probably represents the first attempt to distinguish benign oncocytomas from RCCs with imaging. Segmental enhancement inversion also has been described, in which corticomedullary phase images show components of relatively greater and lesser enhancement in a renal mass, and early excretory phase images show inversion of these relative signal intensities. These findings have proved no more specific than the central scar.

More recently, DWI and ADC measurements have been claimed to reliably distinguish oncocytoma from RCC. This conclusion was based on measurements in 6 oncocytomas, and only a single chromophobe RCC (the RCC subtype that most resembles oncocytoma) was included in the study, so the odds seem fairly long that ADC measurements will ever become a fail-safe method for distinguishing benign from malignant solid renal masses.

The close pathologic resemblance between oncocytoma and RCC, particularly chromophobe RCC, has meant that percutaneous biopsy did not always yield accurate results. However, the combined use of Hale colloidal iron stain and cytokeratin 7 stains greatly improves the specificity of the pathologic diagnosis.

CASE 7.13

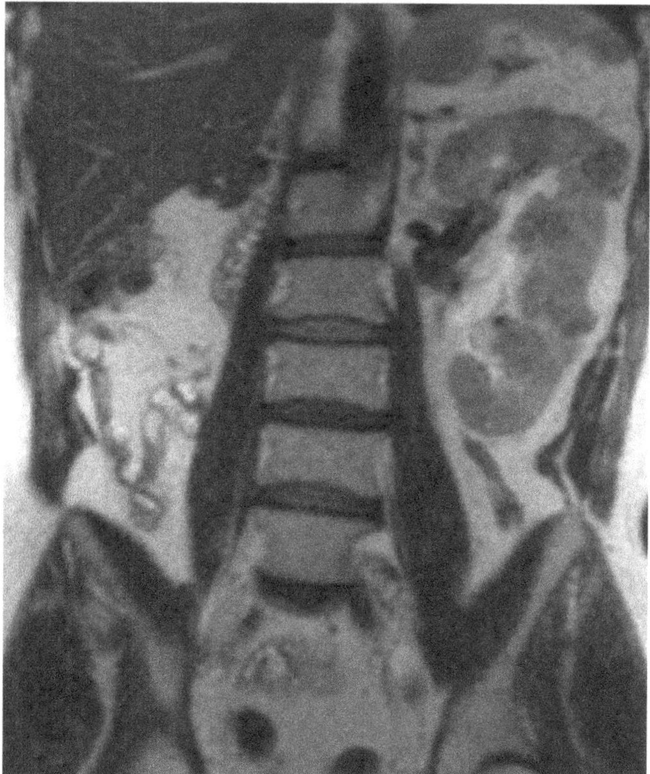

Figure 7.13.1

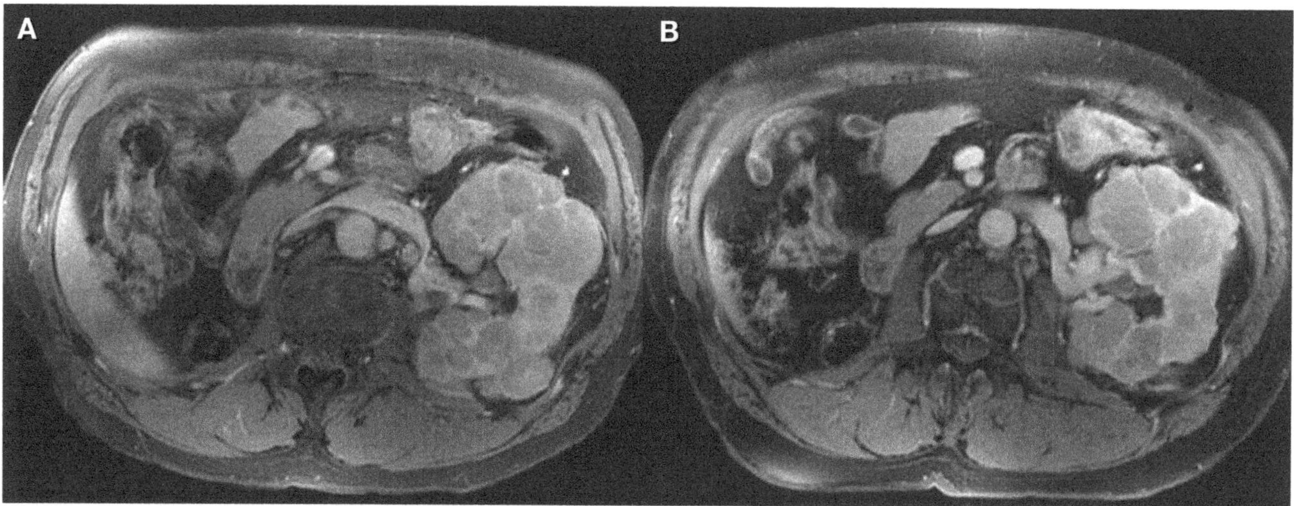

Figure 7.13.2

HISTORY: 61-year-old man presents for routine surveillance after right nephrectomy

IMAGING FINDINGS: Coronal SSFSE (Figure 7.13.1) and axial postgadolinium 2D SPGR (Figure 7.13.2) images show a prior right nephrectomy and multiple hypoenhancing left renal masses, which are also mildly hypointense on the SSFSE image.

DIAGNOSIS: Oncocytosis

COMMENT: Renal oncocytosis is a rare condition in which the renal parenchyma is diffusely involved with oncocytic nodules. The nodules typically show a wide spectrum of oncocytic changes, rather than simply the presence of oncocytomas, including oncocytic cysts, dispersed oncocytic cells infiltrating between benign nephrons, and oncocytic changes in nonneoplastic tubules. The presence of these more diffuse changes prompted the name change to *oncocytosis* from the more specific *oncocytomatosis*.

The largest series of oncocytosis (20 patients) was reported recently by a group at Memorial Sloan-Kettering Cancer Center. Most patients (85%) were asymptomatic at presentation and had multiple solid tumors detected incidentally; 75% had bilateral renal masses, and most of the others had had a prior nephrectomy. Interestingly, the most common dominant tumor histology was a hybrid tumor (with pathologic features intermediate between oncocytoma and chromophobe RCC), followed by chromophobe RCC and oncocytoma. In most patients, the renal masses have various pathologies; only 15% had oncocytomas alone.

Even though most patients with oncocytosis probably have chromophobe RCC in 1 or both kidneys, oncocytosis seems fairly benign from the oncologic standpoint. Metastatic disease has rarely been reported, and no patients in the largest published series died of causes related to malignant disease. Chromophobe RCC as an isolated lesion is associated with the least malignant potential and the best prognosis compared with other RCC subtypes. Preservation of renal function is a significant problem in these patients, who develop renal insufficiency both as a consequence of nephrectomies or partial nephrectomies and by replacement of normal parenchyma with oncocytic nodules. The use of percutaneous biopsy to verify the diagnosis is controversial, since the various histologies encountered in these patients can be confusing.

Oncocytosis should be considered in any patient with multiple solid renal masses. The differential diagnosis includes VHL disease and TS, although the association with AMLs in the case of TS and with renal or pancreatic cystic disease, or both, in the case of VHL disease, as well as the extrarenal manifestations of both entities, usually makes the distinction straightforward. By comparison, Birt-Hogg-Dube syndrome is a more difficult differential diagnosis. This is an autosomal dominant inherited syndrome that predisposes patients to skin lesions (fibrofolliculomas), renal tumors, lung cysts, and spontaneous pneumothoraces. Patients with Birt-Hogg-Dube syndrome present with various renal tumor histologic subtypes, including hybrid oncocytic tumors, chromophobe RCC, and clear cell RCC. More than half of patients with Birt-Hogg-Dube syndrome also show features of renal oncocytosis. Additional considerations in a patient with multiple solid nodules include lymphoma, multifocal RCC, metastatic disease, and infection.

CASE 7.14

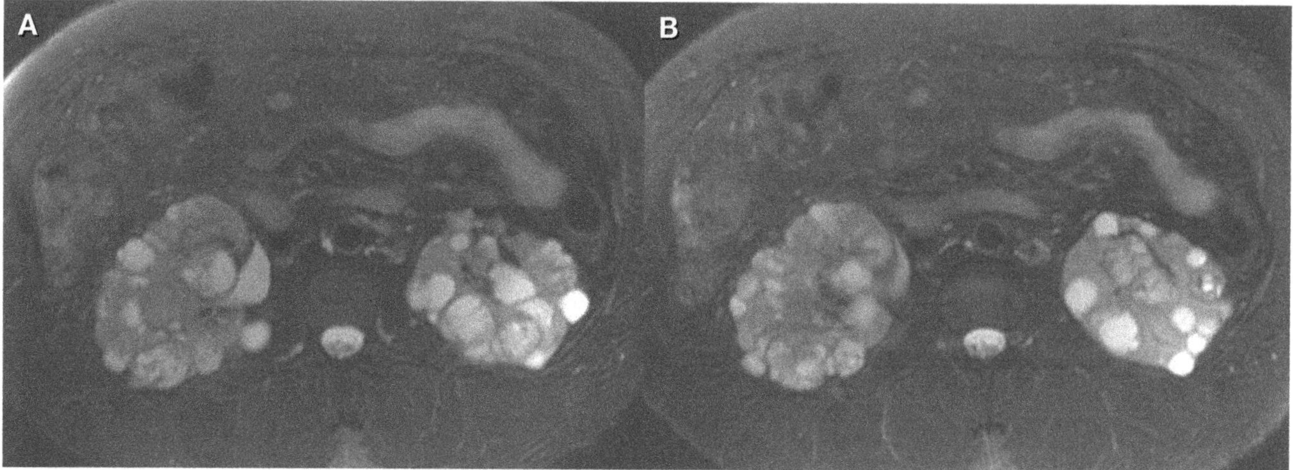

Figure 7.14.1

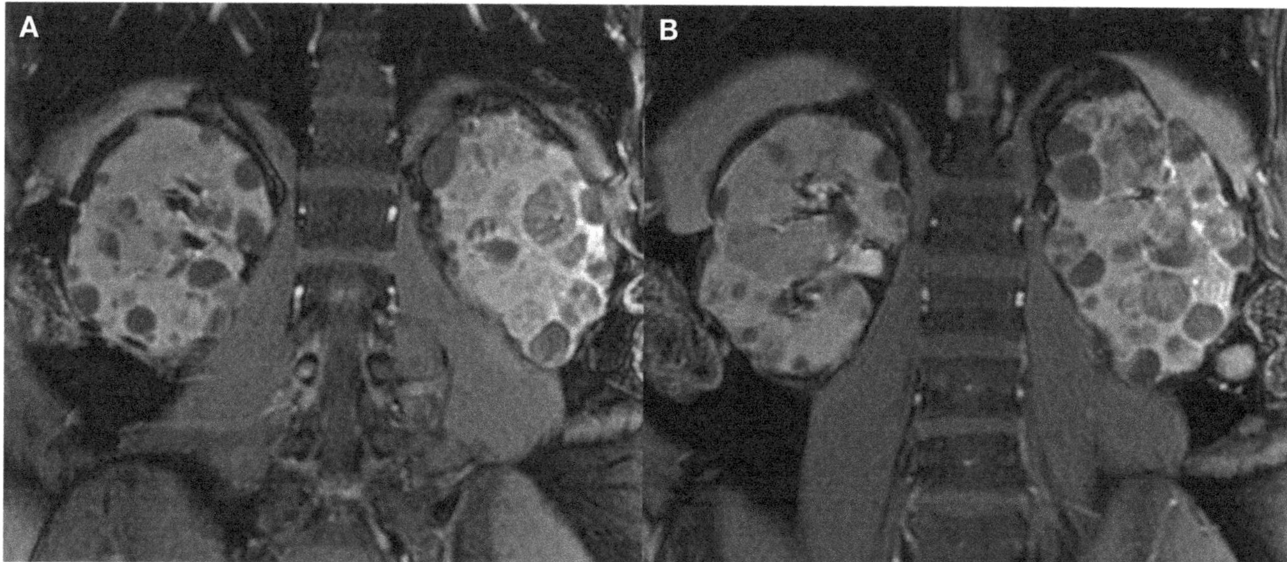

Figure 7.14.2

HISTORY: 43-year-old man with a systemic disorder

IMAGING FINDINGS: Axial fat-suppressed FSE T2-weighted images (Figure 7.14.1) show multiple cysts and solid masses in the kidneys bilaterally. Coronal postgadolinium 2D SPGR images (Figure 7.14.2) show similar findings.

DIAGNOSIS: von Hippel-Lindau disease with bilateral renal cysts and bilateral renal cell carcinomas

COMMENT: VHL disease is an autosomal dominant inherited disorder resulting from mutations in the VHL tumor suppressor gene located on the short arm of chromosome 3. The estimated prevalence is 1 in 35,000 to 55,000 live births, with 20% of cases arising sporadically.

VHL disease is characterized by the appearance of multiple neoplasms, including central nervous system hemangioblastomas, which occur in 60% to 80% of patients and are a presenting feature in 40%. Retinal angiomas are the most common presenting feature of VHL disease and are multiple and bilateral in about half of the cases. Pheochromocytomas can occur in both adrenal and extra-adrenal locations, as well as pancreatic islet cell tumors, serous cystadenomas, and endolymphatic sac tumors.

Renal involvement is characterized by development of clear cell RCC, often with multiple and bilateral lesions. Although the risk of RCC varies in different subtypes of VHL disease, in the most common forms the lifetime risk is approximately 70%. Frequent surveillance of the central nervous system and abdomen is required for these patients and MRI is a good choice to avoid the high cumulative radiation doses associated with CT. Renal and pancreatic cysts are frequent manifestations of VHL disease and can sometimes complicate the assessment of the kidneys for solid lesions.

Differential diagnosis for multiple solid renal masses includes metastases, infection, lymphoma, and oncocytosis, although the presence of multiple cysts in this case makes VHL disease the best diagnostic option.

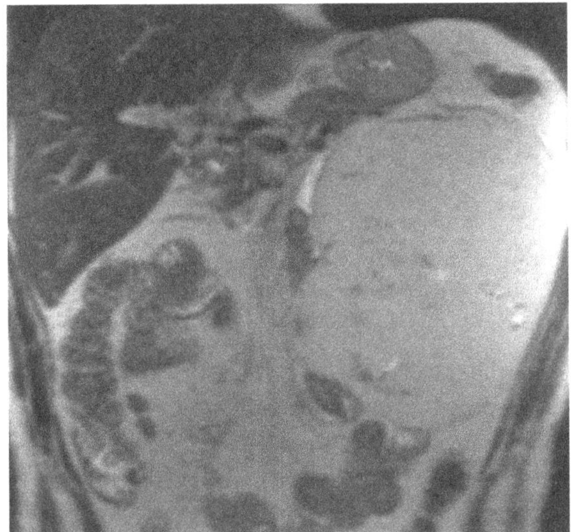

Figure 7.15.1

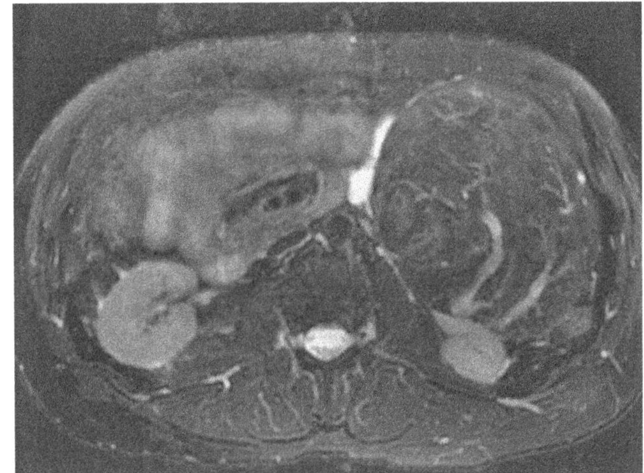

Figure 7.15.2

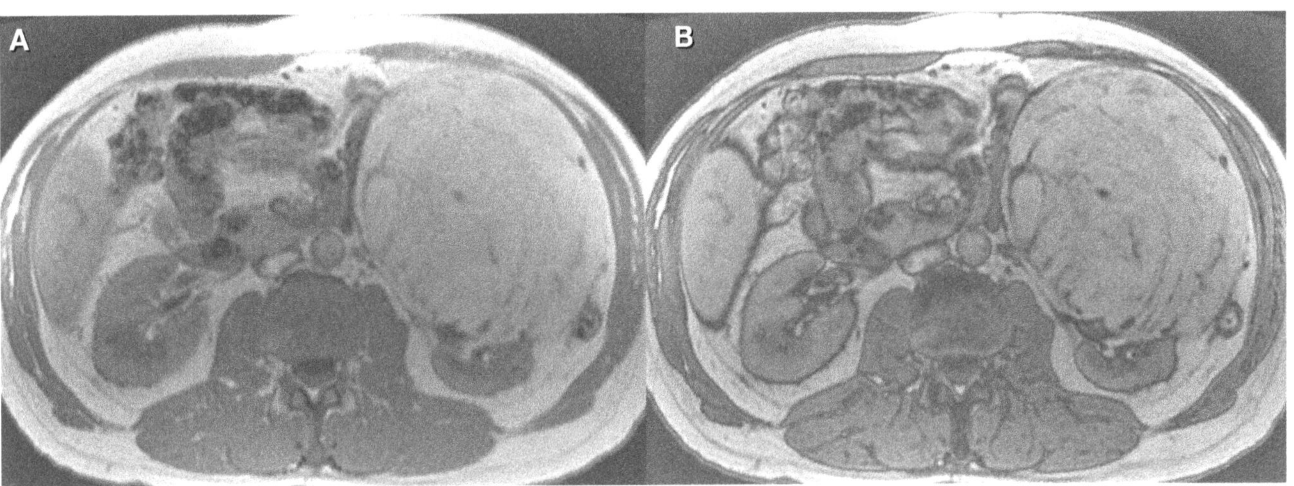

Figure 7.15.3

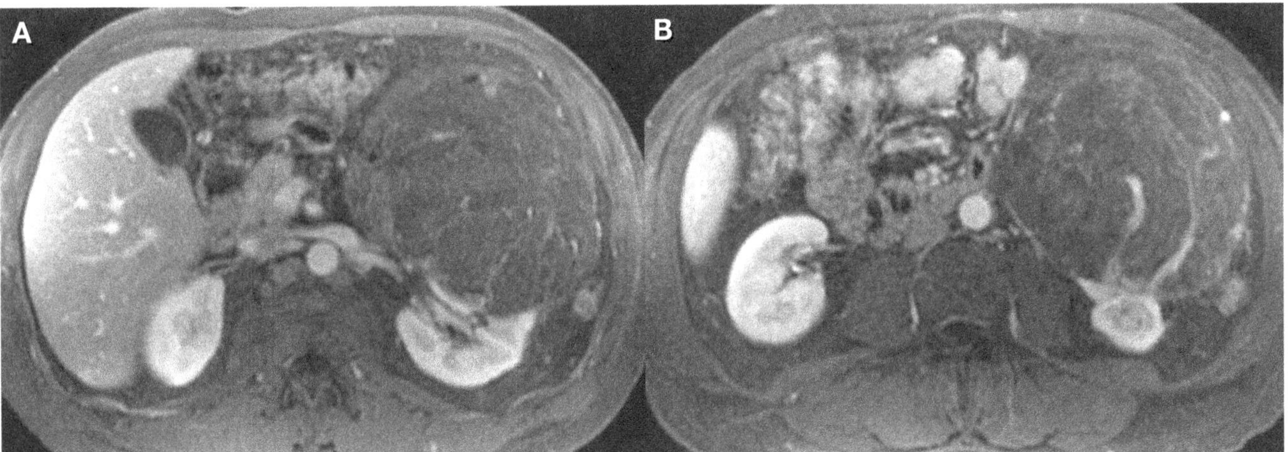

Figure 7.15.4

HISTORY: 51-year-old man with a palpable left abdominal mass

IMAGING FINDINGS: Coronal SSFSE (Figure 7.15.1), axial fat-suppressed T2-weighted FSE (Figure 7.15.2), axial IP-OP 2D SPGR (Figure 7.15.3), and axial postgadolinium 3D SPGR (Figure 7.15.4) images reveal a large exophytic mass originating from the left kidney. The mass is composed almost entirely of fat, interspersed with prominent vessels.

DIAGNOSIS: Large renal angiomyolipoma

COMMENT: AML is the most common benign mesenchymal tumor of the kidney and is composed of mature adipose tissue, dysmorphic blood vessels, and smooth muscle in varying proportions. Renal AMLs are included under the more general category of neoplasms of perivascular epithelioid cells, or PEComas, and are divided into 2 histologic subtypes: classic triphasic and monotypic epithelioid. Epithelioid AML is relatively uncommon, and this entity is discussed separately (see Case 7.16).

AMLs may develop sporadically or in association with TS. Sporadic AMLs account for 50% to 70% of cases, are typically solitary, and generally develop during the fourth to sixth decades with a 4:1 female preponderance. Larger lesions can be symptomatic and present with flank pain, hematuria, or a palpable mass. The most serious complication of renal AML is hemorrhage; this occurs more frequently in larger lesions (>4 cm) and in lesions with prominent aneurysmal (>5 mm) blood vessels.

The diagnosis of AML is usually straightforward. Any lesion in the kidney with macroscopic fat should be an AML, with a few rare exceptions, including the following:

1) Liposarcoma involving the kidney (usually not a difficult distinction, but a renal parenchymal defect where the lesion arises is a distinguishing feature of AML, whereas the presence of calcium should lead to consideration of liposarcoma)
2) Renal lipoma (an extremely rare lesion and one for which the distinction probably is not all that important)
3) The widely described and almost never encountered RCC engulfing perirenal or renal sinus fat

However, other lesions may contain intracellular fat, including oncocytomas and clear cell RCC. For this reason, it's not a good idea to equate signal dropout from IP to OP SPGR images with AMLs. Instead, look for obvious macroscopic fat on T1- or T2-weighted images that shows complete or near complete signal loss when fat suppression is added. (Dixon FSE or SPGR acquisitions are also useful in this regard, allowing simultaneous reconstruction of fat and water images.)

Nevertheless, a small percentage (<5%) of AMLs have no detectable macroscopic fat, with the epithelioid variant heavily represented. In such cases, no reliable MRI method is available for distinguishing these lesions from other solid renal masses.

CASE 7.16

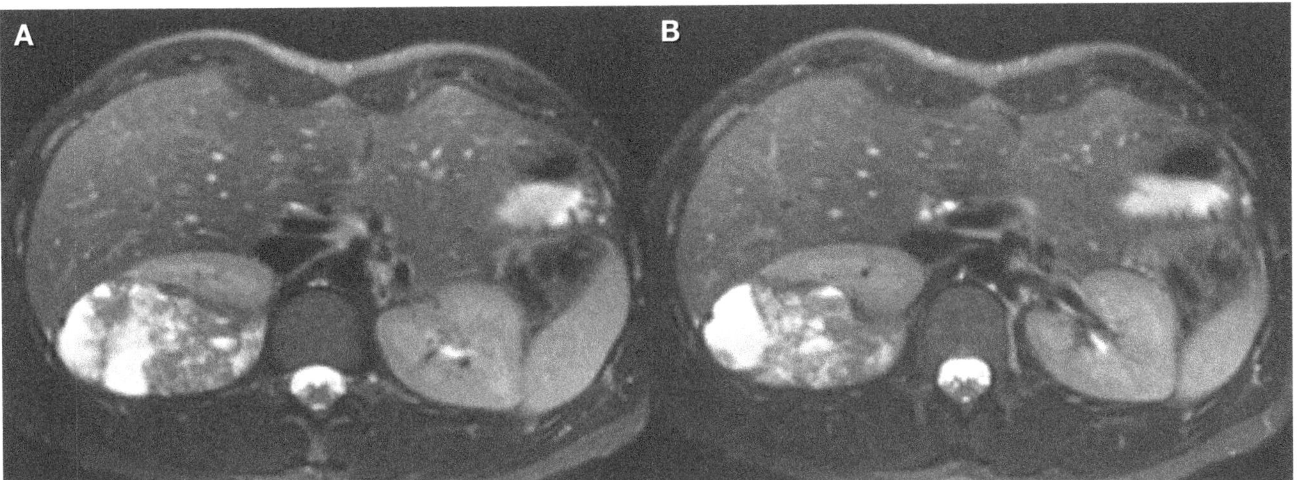

Figure 7.16.1

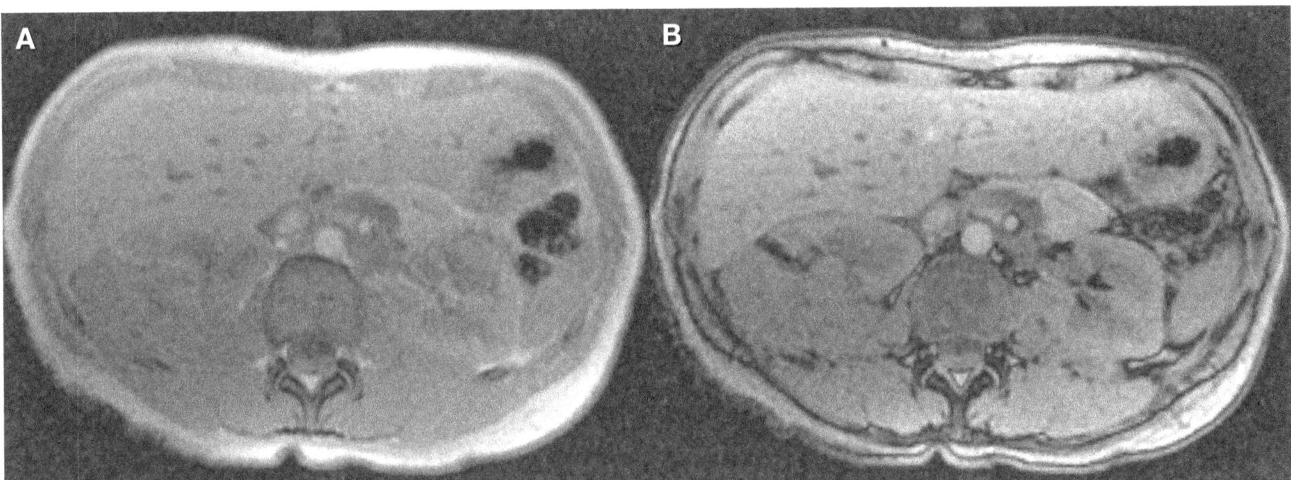

Figure 7.16.2

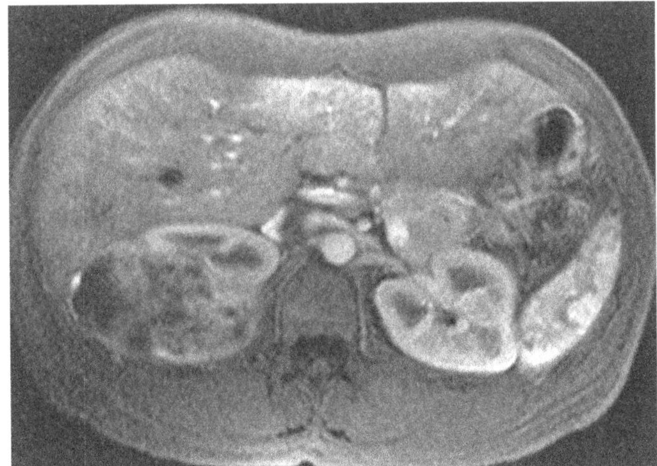

Figure 7.16.3

HISTORY: 31-year-old woman with epigastric discomfort found to have a renal mass on CT at an outside institution

IMAGING FINDINGS: Axial fat-suppressed T2-weighted FSE (Figure 7.16.1), axial IP-OP 2D SPGR (Figure 7.16.2), and axial postgadolinium 3D SPGR (Figure 7.16.3) images show a mass originating from the posterior right kidney with heterogeneous increased T2-signal intensity and irregular enhancement. No definite fat content is identified.

DIAGNOSIS: Malignant epithelioid angiomyolipoma

COMMENT: Renal AML is a mesenchymal neoplasm composed of variable portions of adipose tissue, spindle cells, epithelioid smooth muscle cells, and abnormal thick-walled blood vessels. AMLs are by definition benign tumors. However, 10 to 15 years ago a few reports emerged describing variants of AML with worrisome pathologic features and an often aggressive clinical course characterized by recurrence, distant metastases, and death. These lesions were described initially as atypical AMLs; later, the term *epithelioid AML* was adopted in 2004 by the World Health Organization Classification of Tumors. This terminology is somewhat confusing, since epithelioid morphology of smooth muscle–like cells can occur in regular AMLs.

One of the largest case series (40 patients), published by a group from Johns Hopkins Hospital, denoted all AMLs with epithelioid morphologic characteristics as *epithelioid AMLs* and then divided these AMLs into groups with and without cellular atypia. The category with atypia corresponds to the lesions with malignant potential described in the literature. Among the patients who had epithelioid AML with atypia, 26% had malignant features and showed evidence of recurrence or metastases, or both, although other series have reported both higher and lower numbers. The presence of at least 3 of the following histologic features is correlated with aggressive clinical behavior: nuclear atypia in more than 70% of epithelioid cells, mitotic count greater than 2 per 10 high-power fields, presence of atypical mitotic figures, and necrosis. Epithelioid AML has some characteristic immunohistochemical properties, including markers for melanocytes and smooth muscle cells and negativity for epithelial markers.

The clinical and imaging features of epithelioid AML are not well understood. Some lesions have a growth pattern similar to AML, but others are more invasive and may metastasize. Imaging features are nonspecific, and epithelioid AML may be difficult to distinguish from a high-grade RCC or renal sarcoma. This case illustrates such a dilemma—a heterogeneous lesion with regions of markedly increased T2-signal intensity and irregular enhancement that was presumed to represent RCC or renal sarcoma. Macroscopic fat may or may not be present, but in the perspective of the case report literature, it seems to be fairly uncommon in the malignant lesions. Since few conventional-appearing AMLs are surgically resected, it is not clear how many of these cases are actually epithelioid AMLs. Solid lesions indistinguishable from RCC or renal sarcoma are often resected, and treatment of these patients is controversial. Some authors have advocated chemotherapy, with reports of both successful and unsuccessful outcomes.

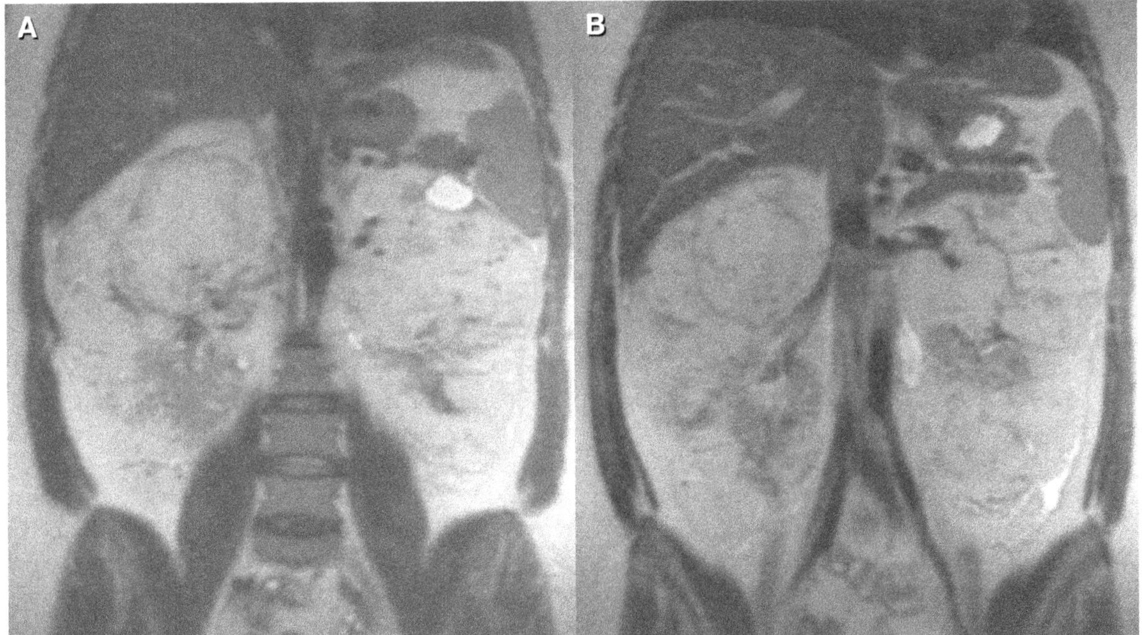

Figure 7.17.1

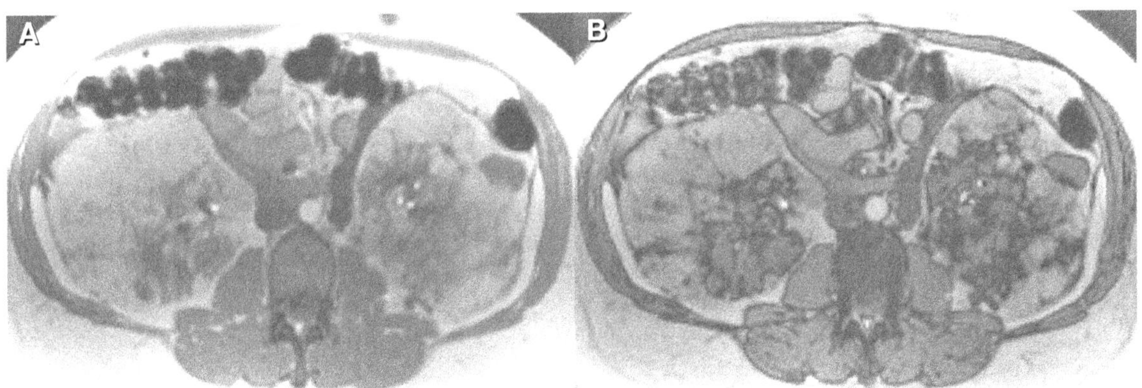

Figure 7.17.2

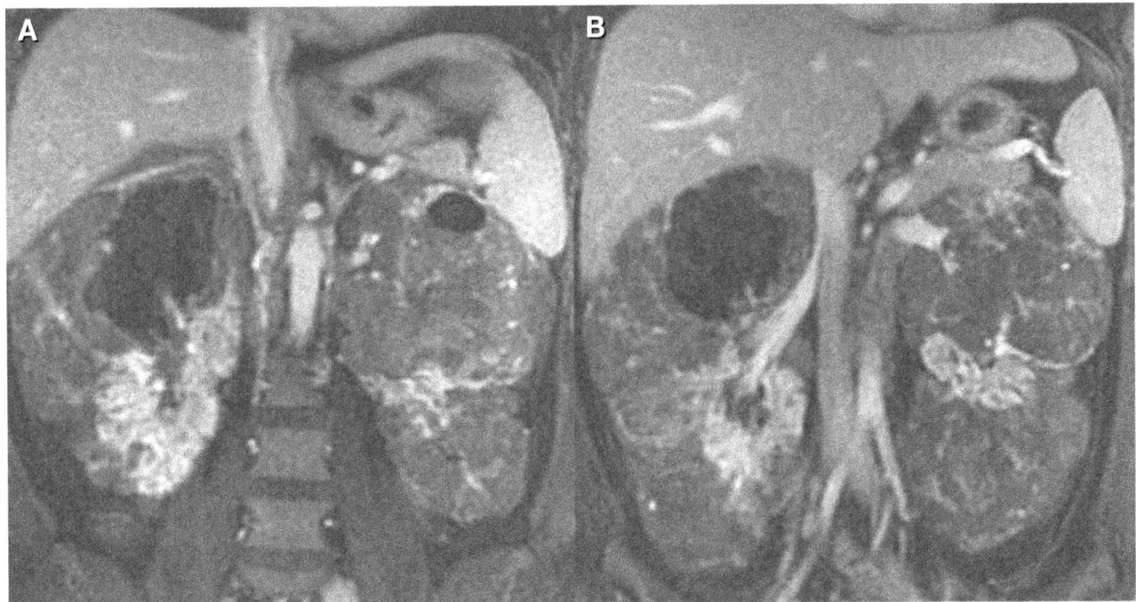

Figure 7.17.3

HISTORY: 42-year-old woman with a long-standing multisystemic disorder

IMAGING FINDINGS: Coronal SSFSE images (Figure 7.17.1) show massive bilateral renal enlargement and replacement of renal parenchyma. Axial IP-OP 2D SPGR images (Figure 7.17.2) demonstrate fatty replacement of much of the renal parenchyma. Coronal postgadolinium 3D SPGR images (Figure 7.17.3) again show massive bilateral renal enlargement and fatty replacement.

DIAGNOSIS: Tuberous sclerosis with bilateral angiomyolipomas

COMMENT: TS is a neurocutaneous syndrome with autosomal dominant inheritance characterized by hamartomatous lesions in multiple organ systems. The estimated prevalence is between 1 in 6,000 and 1 in 12,000, and approximately two-thirds of cases are sporadic. The classically described clinical triad of mental retardation, epilepsy, and adenoma sebaceum is somewhat misleading, since half of TS patients have normal intelligence and 25% do not have epilepsy.

TS is caused by mutations of the *TSC1* and *TSC2* genes, located on chromosomes 9 and 16, respectively, and encoding the proteins hamartin and tuberin, which are involved in the regulation of cell growth and differentiation and are found in various organs. The *TSC2* gene locus is contiguous with the *PKD1* gene, which probably accounts for the occasional occurrence of renal cystic disease in patients with TS.

The manifestations of TS are numerous and difficult for most radiologists to store beyond short-term memory. Skin lesions include hypopigmented macules (ash leaf spots) in more than 90% of patients, facial angiofibromas (adenoma sebaceum) in 75%, shagreen patches (grayish/light brown pigmentation in the lumbosacral region) in 20% to 30%, and ungual fibromas beneath fingernails and toenails in 20%. Neurologic involvement includes cortical tubers or subependymal nodules, or both, in 95% to 100% of cases, white-matter abnormalities in 40% to 90%, and subependymal giant cell astrocytomas in 2% to 25%. Cardiac rhabdomyomas occur in 50% to 65% of TS patients, and 40% to 80% of patients with rhabdomyomas have TS. These are interesting lesions that generally appear very early in life or in utero, favor the interventricular septum, and spontaneously regress in 70% of patients without causing clinical symptoms. LAM is the most common pulmonary manifestation, occurring almost exclusively in female patients and characterized by pulmonary cystic disease, recurrent spontaneous pneumothorax, and chylous pleural effusion or ascites.

Renal involvement is a common feature, and renal AMLs are found in 55% to 75% of TS patients. As in this case, renal AMLs in TS are more frequently multiple, larger, and bilateral; exhibit more rapid growth; and appear at a younger age. We have seen the massive enlargement of the kidneys bilaterally with AMLs illustrated in this case in several TS patients and never in a patient without TS. (Of course, it's also true that we have never made a spontaneous diagnosis of TS in a patient referred for abdominal MRI.) The AMLs in TS are often symptomatic, causing abdominal pain, nausea, vomiting, hematuria, anemia, and hypertension. The most serious complication is rupture and hemorrhage (a not-infrequent occurrence since these tumors are vascular), sometimes termed *Wunderlich syndrome*.

Diagnosis is straightforward in these cases, once you recognize what you're looking at and appreciate that the kidneys are replaced predominantly by fat. Renal cysts may be seen less commonly in TS patients and should not present a diagnostic dilemma. In addition, there is an association with RCC; although meta-analysis has shown that the overall incidence of RCC is no greater in TS patients than in the general population, RCCs tend to occur in younger patients and to grow more slowly in the clinical setting of TS.

TS is not a benign disease. Although recent advances in treatment have improved morbidity rates, the lifespan of most patients continues to be relatively short, with more than 40% of patients dying by age 35 years of renal failure, LAM, status epilepticus, and other causes.

CASE 7.18

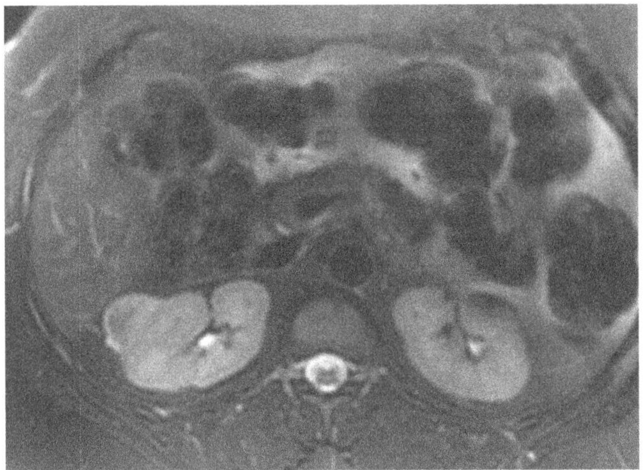

Figure 7.18.1

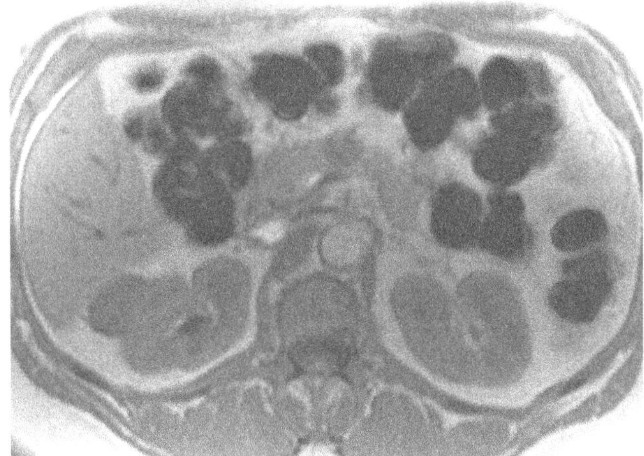

Figure 7.18.2

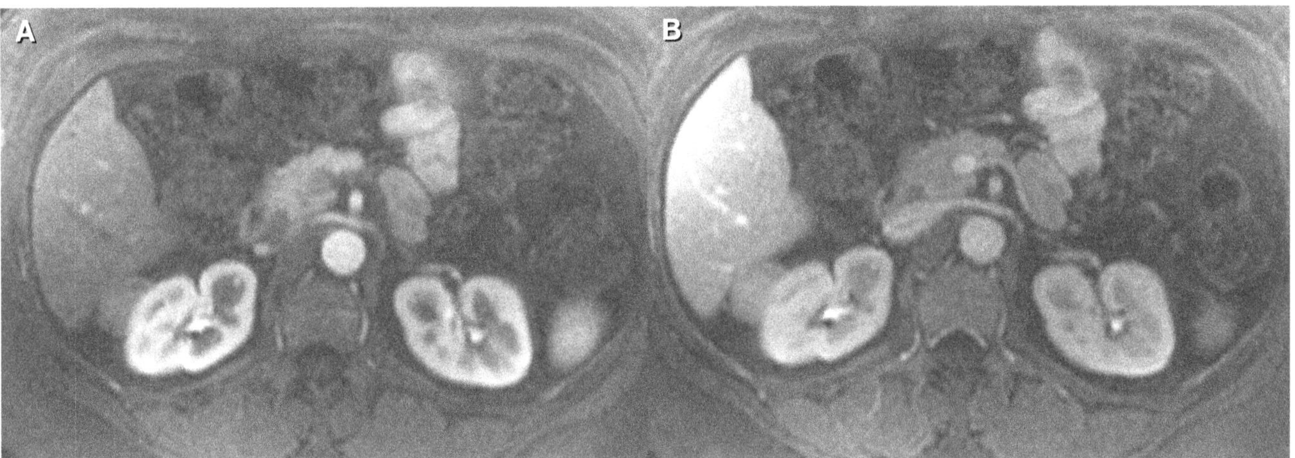

Figure 7.18.3

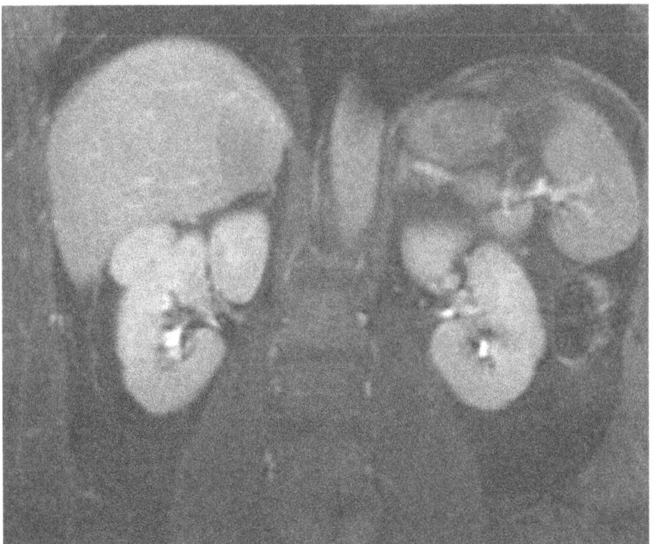

Figure 7.18.4

HISTORY: 49-year-old woman with intermittent right upper quadrant pain; an incidental right renal mass was noted on CT

IMAGING FINDINGS: Axial fat-suppressed T2-weighted FSE image (Figure 7.18.1) demonstrates an exophytic mass with predominantly low signal intensity projecting from the upper pole of the right kidney. Axial IP 2D SPGR image (Figure 7.18.2) at the same level shows the mass to have T1-signal intensity slightly hypointense to the kidney. Axial arterial and venous phase postgadolinium 3D SPGR images (Figure 7.18.3) and an equilibrium phase coronal 3D SPGR image (Figure 7.18.4) show gradual enhancement of the mass, which becomes hyperintense to the kidney on equilibrium phase images.

DIAGNOSIS: Renal leiomyoma

COMMENT: Renal leiomyomas are either a rare neoplasm, with fewer than 40 reported cases in the literature, or a common tumor, with a reported incidence of 5% in 1 autopsy study. We tend to favor the rare narrative. An ever-increasing amount of abdominal MRI and CT is performed for both renal and nonrenal applications, and since these lesions don't really have specific imaging signs to indicate their benign nature, they should be resected at a fairly high rate, and yet, this is the only path-proven case we have seen.

Renal leiomyomas can appear in all structures containing smooth muscle, with 90% originating in the renal capsule, as in this case, and the other 10% in the renal pelvis and renal vessels. These lesions probably occur more frequently in whites, have a female predominance, and typically occur in the second to fifth decades. Most lesions are asymptomatic and are detected incidentally; however, large lesions may present with a palpable mass or flank pain.

The imaging characteristics are fairly typical of what you would expect a leiomyoma to look like—T2 and T1 mild hypointensity with gradual enhancement after contrast administration. But this appearance is by no means diagnostic and could be consistent with a papillary or chromophobe RCC.

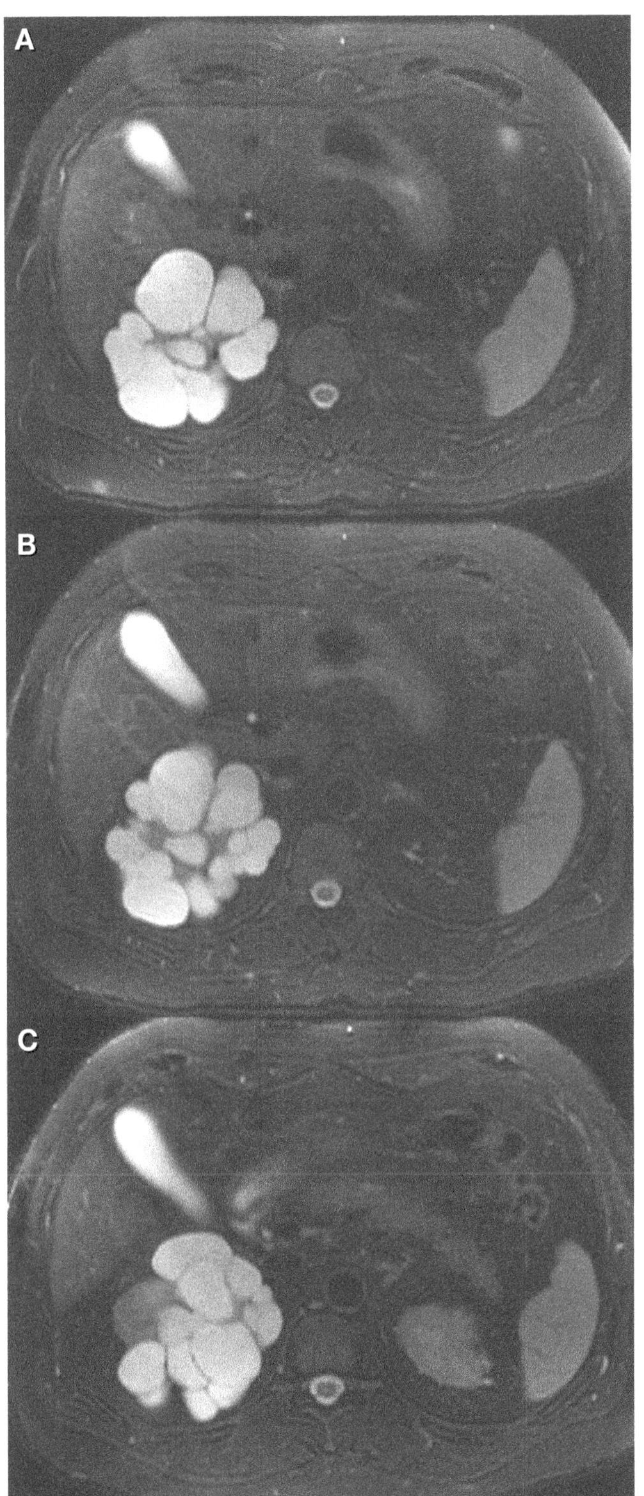

Figure 7.19.1

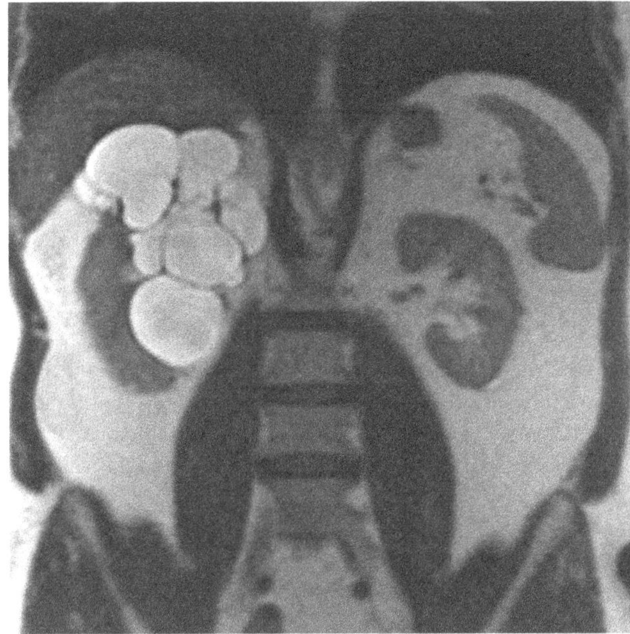
Figure 7.19.2

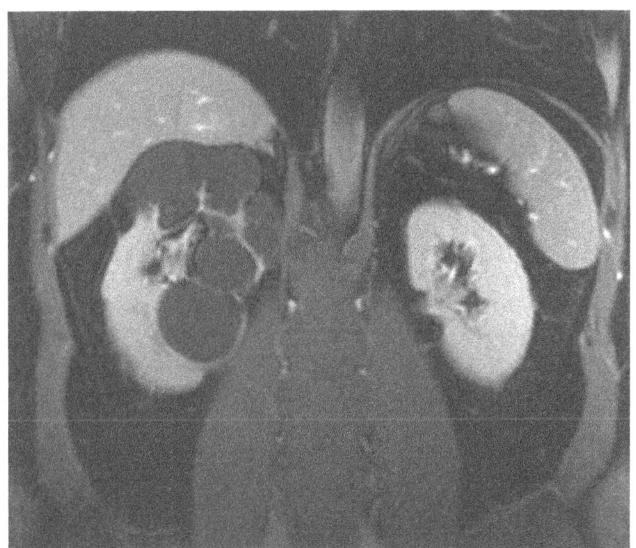
Figure 7.19.3

HISTORY: 50-year-old man with Crohn disease and urinary frequency and urgency; a cystic renal mass was found at renal sonography

IMAGING FINDINGS: Axial fat-suppressed T2-weighted FSE (Figure 7.19.1), coronal SSFSE (Figure 7.19.2), and coronal postgadolinium 2D SPGR (Figure 7.19.3) images show multiple small cystic lesions without significant enhancement clustered in the upper pole of the right kidney.

DIAGNOSIS: Multilocular cystic renal tumor

COMMENT: Multilocular cystic renal tumor represents a spectrum of disease, including cystic nephroma, where multiple cystic lesions are lined by an epithelium and fibrous septa containing mature tubules, and cystic partially differentiated nephroblastoma, where the septa contain foci of blastemal cells. No reliable imaging criteria are available for distinguishing the 2 lesions. Multilocular cystic renal tumor has had many previous names, most notably *multilocular cystic nephroma*.

Multilocular cystic renal tumor has a bimodal age and sex distribution, with a peak incidence in boys aged 3 months to 4 years (mostly cystic partially differentiated nephroblastoma) and in women aged 40 to 60 years. Lesions usually are solitary, although bilateral cases have been reported. Some evidence suggests that the tumors in adults actually may represent a distinct entity. Clinical manifestations are variable. Most frequently, multilocular cystic renal tumor presents in children as a painless abdominal mass, while in adults it presents more often with abdominal pain or hematuria.

The imaging appearance is that of a well-circumscribed, encapsulated multicystic lesion with variably enhancing septa. No solid components should be visualized in multilocular cystic renal tumor, and no contrast should be excreted into the cystic components. As is true of most cystic lesions, the signal intensity of the cysts on T1- and T2-weighted imaging is variable, reflecting the presence of proteinaceous material or hemorrhage, or both. Differential diagnosis includes cystic Wilms tumor, cystic RCC, clear cell sarcoma, cystic variants of mesoblastic nephroma, and multicystic dysplastic kidney. In the adult patient, the differential of complex cyst can be added, depending on the size and complexity of the lesion. Treatment usually consists of nephrectomy or partial nephrectomy, although in some adult cases, the lesions are simply monitored.

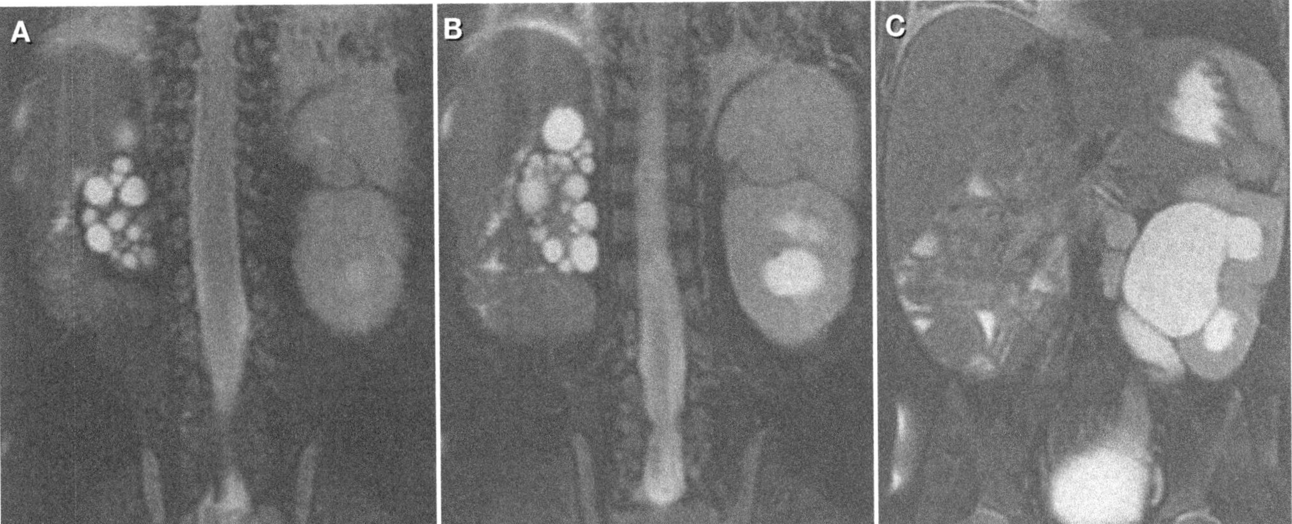

Figure 7.20.1

HISTORY: 2-year-old boy with a history of anorectal malformation and imperforate anus, status post surgical repair

IMAGING FINDINGS: Coronal fat-suppressed T2-weighted FRFSE images (Figure 7.20.1) reveal an atrophic right kidney replaced by cysts of various sizes. Also note hydronephrosis and hydroureter of the left kidney.

DIAGNOSIS: Right multicystic dysplastic kidney, with left hydronephrosis and hydroureter resulting from an ectopic ureterocele

COMMENT: Multicystic dysplastic kidney is a common cause of renal masses in infants, and the diagnosis often is made on prenatal sonography. It occurs with an incidence of approximately 1 in 4,000 live births and generally is attributed to a failure of differentiation of the mesenchymal metanephros and the epithelial cells of the ureteral bud, leading to obstruction and dysregulation of the developing kidney. Multicystic dysplastic kidney has been divided into 2 subtypes on the basis of gross appearance: a solid cystic dysplasia and a hydronephrotic form. The fate of the affected kidney is variable; 60% to 90% involute or decrease in size, while the remainder may not change or may increase in size.

Probably the most important consideration when multicystic dysplastic kidney is diagnosed is assessment of the contralateral kidney: There is a high incidence (25%) of urinary tract abnormalities, including vesicoureteral reflux in approximately 15% and ureteropelvic junction obstruction in 5%. The patient in this case had an ectopic ureterocele, which accounted for the dilated left ureter and collecting system.

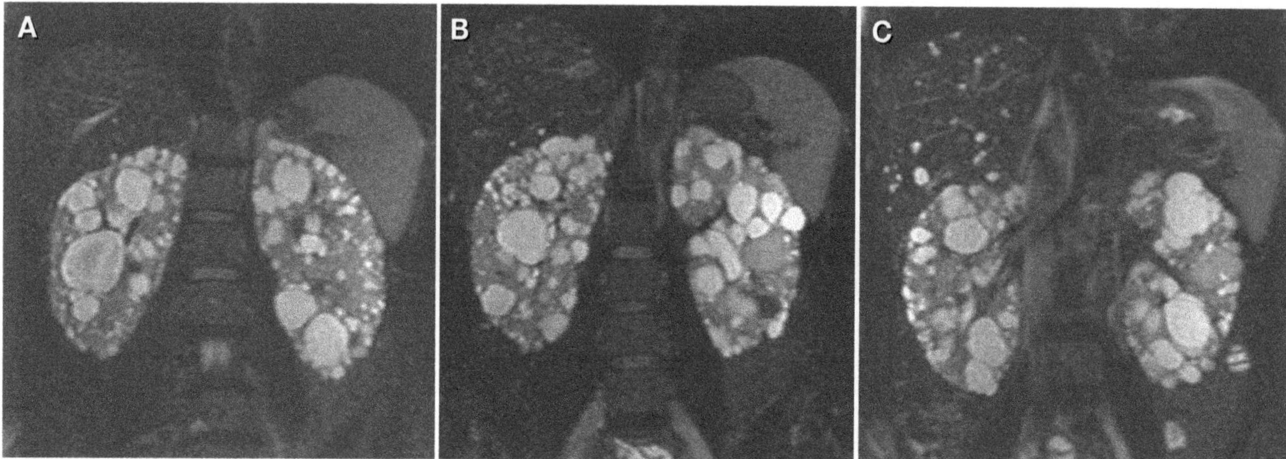

Figure 7.21.1

HISTORY: 40-year-old woman with chronic disease

IMAGING FINDINGS: Coronal SSFSE images (Figure 7.21.1) reveal bilateral enlarged kidneys containing innumerable cysts of various sizes, including some with hemorrhagic debris. Note also the multiple small hepatic cysts.

DIAGNOSIS: Autosomal dominant polycystic kidney disease

COMMENT: ADPKD is one of the most common hereditary renal disorders, with an estimated prevalence between 1 in 300 and 1 in 1,000 persons. It accounts for approximately 8% to 10% of patients with end-stage renal disease in the United States and Europe. ADPKD has autosomal dominant inheritance in 90% of cases; 10% occur sporadically. Two separate genetic mutations are responsible for most cases of ADPKD: the *PKD1* gene on chromosome 16 (80%-85%) and the *PKD2* gene on chromosome 4 (15%-20%). Patients with a mutation in the *PKD1* gene have more severe renal disease, and the onset of end-stage renal disease occurs 15 to 20 years earlier than for patients with a mutation in the *PKD2* gene. *PKD1* and *PKD2* encode proteins called *polycystin-1* and *polycystin-2*. Polycystin-1 is a membrane protein localized at sites of cyst formation, including renal tubular epithelial cells and hepatobiliary ductules. Polycystin-2 is expressed primarily in the distal tubules, collecting ducts, and thick ascending limb.

ADPKD is characterized by progressive cyst formation and renal enlargement—renal and cyst volumes typically increase at an annual growth rate of about 5%. As cysts develop and grow, renal parenchyma is destroyed and the normal architecture disrupted. Symptoms arise in late adulthood and may include flank pain, hematuria, hypertension, and recurrent urinary tract infections. Despite progressive cyst growth, renal function is well preserved as nephrons undergo compensatory hypertrophy. This compensation is maintained until the fourth to sixth decades, when a rapid decline in renal function occurs. Chronic renal failure is present in about 50% of ADPKD patients by age 60 years.

More than 90% of the MRIs performed in our practice on patients with ADPKD are research protocols; however, we occasionally screen family members with MRI or assess patients with known ADPKD for such complications as an infected or rapidly growing cyst, potential solid renal mass, or compression of the IVC.

The diagnosis of ADPKD is usually trivial—enlarged kidneys with cysts of various sizes. Nearly all ADPKD patients have 1 or more hemorrhagic renal cysts, and about 90% of patients also have hepatic cysts. Pancreatic cysts may occur but are much less common. An additional important association is intracranial aneurysms, for which all ADPKD patients should be screened. In a small percentage of patients, the primary manifestation is hepatic cystic disease, but in general, renal cysts predominate and renal function is more severely affected than hepatic function. Differentiating ADPKD from the recessive variant or other renal cystic disease is usually possible from the clinical history alone; however, if that isn't provided, distinction is often possible on the basis of the appearance of the cysts, which are generally smaller in ARPKD and manifest at an earlier age. Kidney size in ARPKD is also typically smaller in comparison to ADPKD. The cysts in ARPKD are generally smaller and appear at an earlier age. Cystic renal disease of dialysis most often has fewer cysts in atrophic or more normal-sized kidneys.

ADPKD patients sometimes cannot receive gadolinium contrast because of renal insufficiency. In these cases, diffusion-weighted images are useful to help identify solid lesions, as well as detect infected cysts.

CASE 7.22

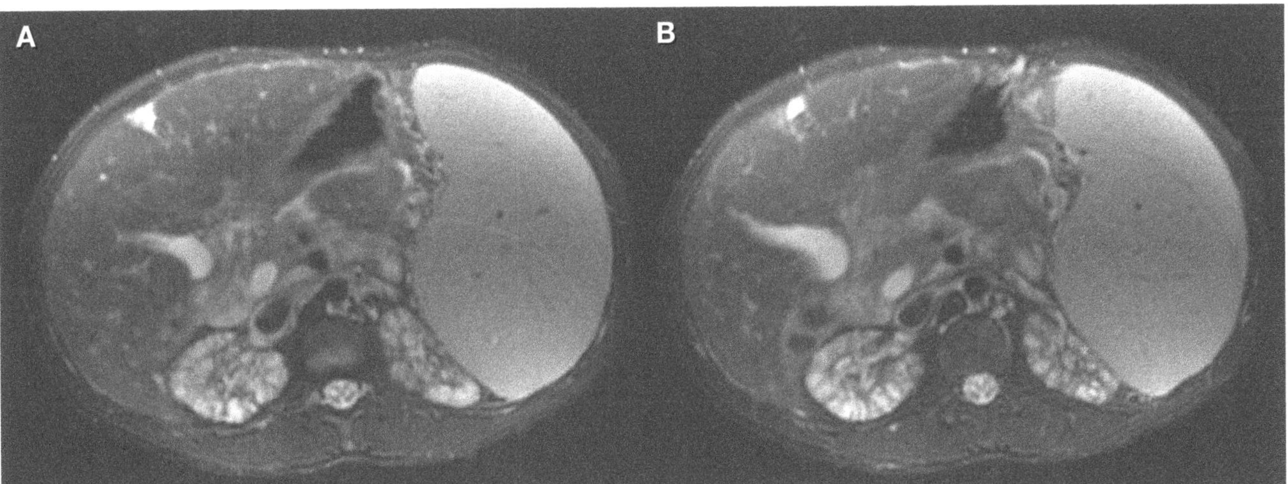

Figure 7.22.1

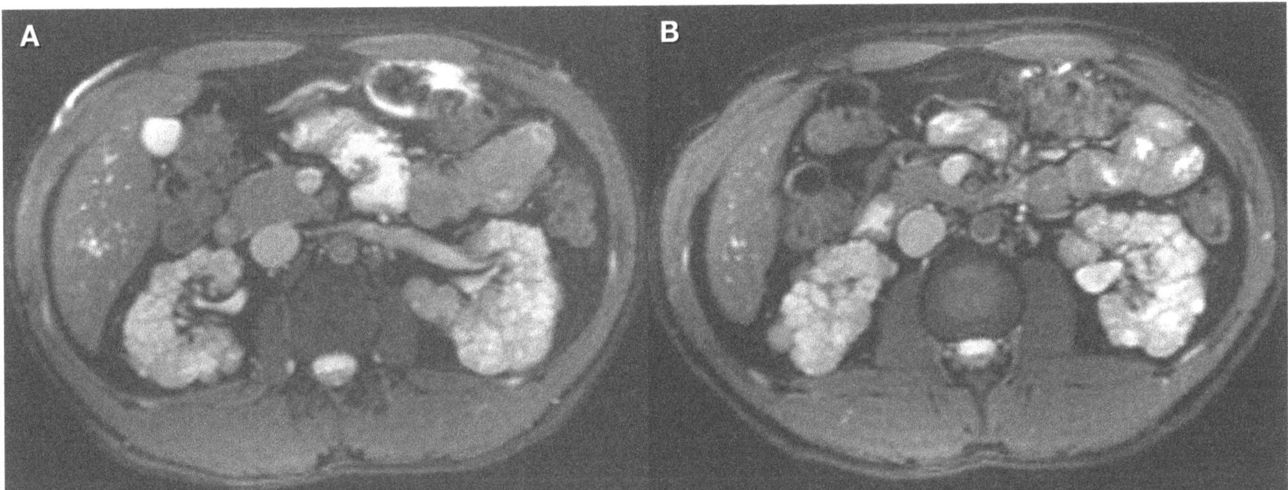

Figure 7.22.2

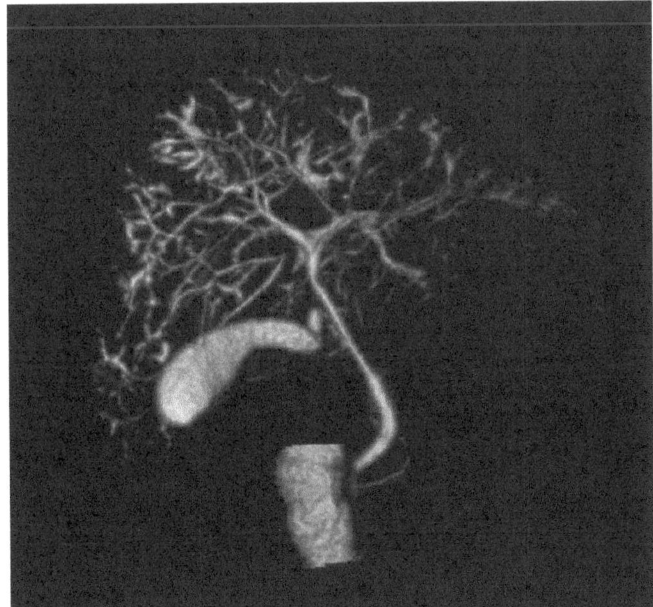

Figure 7.22.3

HISTORY: 8-year-old girl with chronic kidney disease, hypertension, and growth delay; a dilated common bile duct was noted incidentally at renal sonography

IMAGING FINDINGS: Axial fat-suppressed FSE T2-weighted images (Figure 7.22.1) demonstrate replacement of much of the renal parenchyma with small, fairly uniform cysts. The common bile duct is dilated, the liver has a mildly cirrhotic appearance, and the spleen is markedly enlarged. Axial fat-suppressed SSFP images (Figure 7.22.2) from a second patient also show extensive cystic disease involving both kidneys. A volume-rendered image from 3D FRFSE MRCP (Figure 7.22.3) shows numerous mildly dilated peripheral biliary ducts.

DIAGNOSIS: Autosomal recessive polycystic kidney disease with congenital hepatic fibrosis and Caroli disease

COMMENT: ARPKD is an inherited disorder characterized by nonobstructive fusiform dilatation of the renal tubules. It causes enlarged spongiform kidneys and ductal plate malformation of the liver, leading to congenital hepatic fibrosis and Caroli disease. ARPKD occurs with an estimated frequency of 1 in 20,000 live births, and approximately 20% of cases occur in persons with a documented family history of ARPKD. Most patients are identified perinatally with oligohydramnios caused by decreased fetal urine output and hypoplastic lungs; other patients present later in life with clinical symptoms predominantly related to either renal failure or hepatic dysfunction, or both.

ARPKD is caused by mutations in the *PKHD1* gene located on chromosome 6p12. This gene codes for the protein fibrocystin, which is present on the primary cilia of renal and biliary epithelial cells. Dysfunctional fibrocystin leads to abnormal regulation of proliferation and differentiation of renal and biliary epithelium.

Cystic kidneys in ARPKD result from dilated collecting ducts, some of which become enclosed cysts. Generally, the cysts in ARPKD are smaller than those seen in ADPKD and are less prone to hemorrhage or infection. Another distinction is that in ARPKD, kidney growth plateaus in the first 2 or 3 years of life; in ADPKD, kidneys show progressive enlargement throughout life.

Hepatic abnormalities are present in all patients with ARPKD, to varying degrees, but often are clinically apparent much later than the renal manifestations and may not be detectable until adulthood. Hepatic fibrosis with hepatosplenomegaly, portal hypertension, cirrhosis, and prominent varices are predominant features in some patients; macrocystic dilatation of peripheral or central biliary ducts may be more apparent in other patients. The simultaneous presence of congenital hepatic fibrosis with Caroli disease is termed *Caroli syndrome*. The appearance of the liver in ARPKD can vary substantially, and additional examples are included in the biliary chapter.

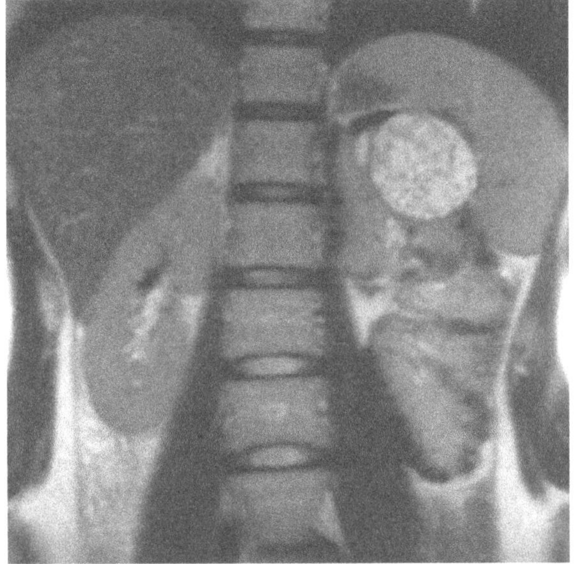

Figure 7.23.1

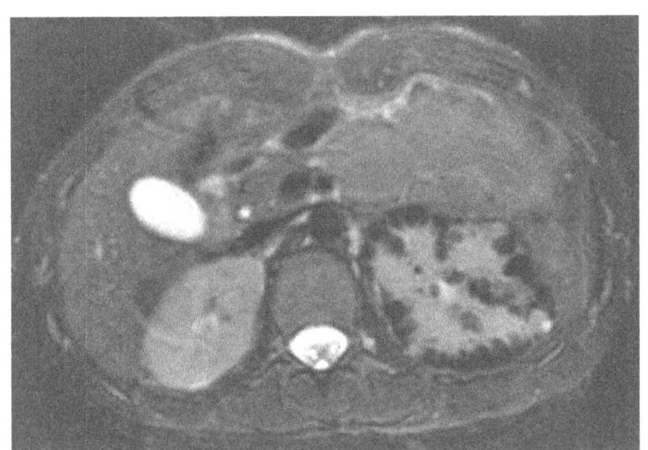

Figure 7.23.2

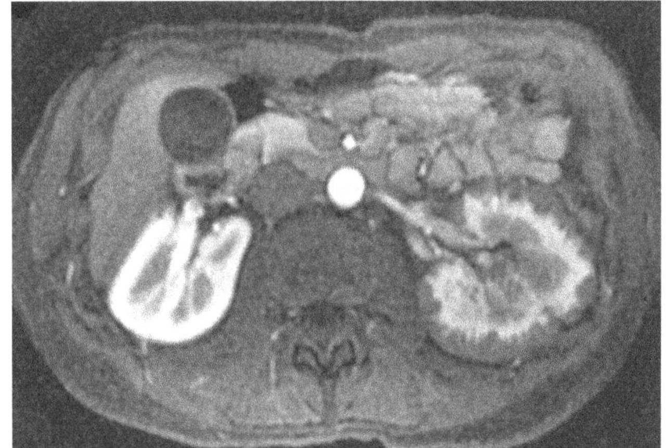

Figure 7.23.3

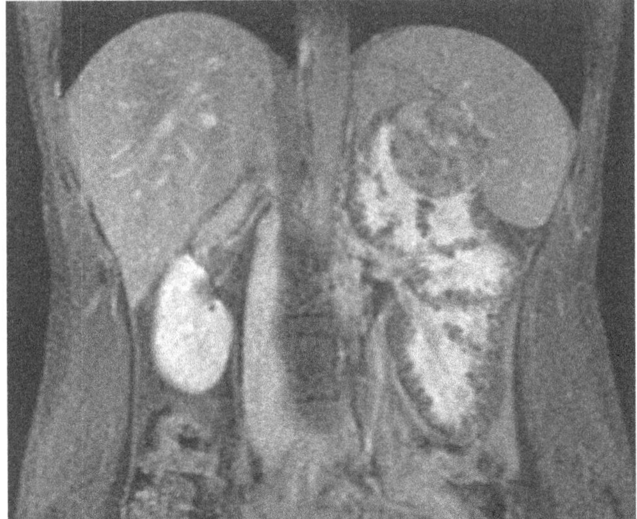

Figure 7.23.4

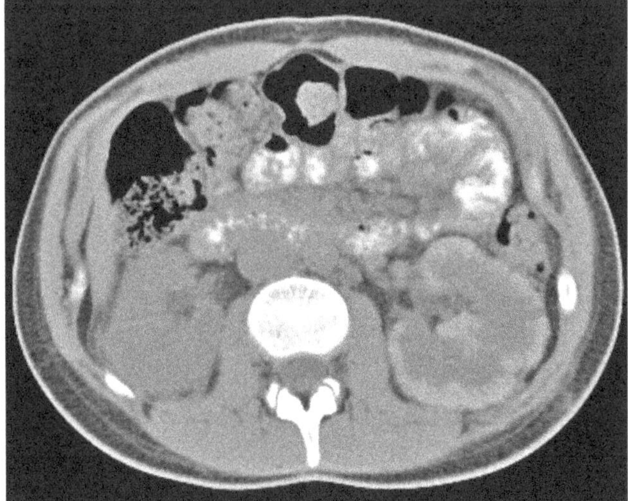

Figure 7.23.5

HISTORY: 21-year-old woman with chronic abdominal pain; CT revealed an incidental left renal mass

IMAGING FINDINGS: Coronal SSFSE (Figure 7.23.1) and axial fat-suppressed FSE T2-weighted (Figure 7.23.2) images show a complex cystic lesion in the upper pole of the left kidney. Note also innumerable round lesions throughout the cortex of the left kidney showing markedly decreased T2-signal intensity. Axial arterial phase (Figure 7.23.3) and coronal nephrogenic phase (Figure 7.23.4) postgadolinium 3D SPGR images again demonstrate the hypoenhancing mass in the upper pole of the left kidney and the numerous left-sided hypoenhancing cortical cysts. Non–contrast-enhanced CT image (Figure 7.23.5) demonstrates that the cortical cysts are hyperintense relative to the rest of the kidney.

DIAGNOSIS: Unilateral glomerulocystic kidney with papillary renal cell carcinoma

COMMENT: This case is very unusual, but we included it because it beautifully illustrates the cyst distribution in GCK, even though it has many atypical elements: It is unilateral, the cysts have diffusely decreased T2-signal intensity, and a papillary RCC is also present.

GCK is a rare form of cystic renal disease characterized histologically by cystic dilatation of the Bowman capsule. The cysts are located predominantly in the subcapsular region of the renal cortex and spare the tubular portions of the nephron. This cortical distribution of cysts distinguishes GCK from the more common ADPKD and ARPKD, as well as multicystic dysplastic kidney and cystic disease of dialysis.

A recently published summary of more than 200 cases noted that patients were predominantly male (62%) and children (72%). Of these cases, 10 were identified with asymmetrical, unilateral, or segmental involvement. Both sporadic and inherited cases have been reported, and GCK has been associated with a large number of syndromes, most frequently TS and Zellweger syndrome (ie, white-matter leukodystrophy). GCK also has been associated with both ADPKD and ARPKD, as well as biliary ductal abnormalities. Patients with GCK may have early renal insufficiency that progresses to end-stage renal disease; however, some patients may have only minimal renal impairment. Groups of patients with autosomal dominant GCK have been described, some with enlarged kidneys and some with hypoplastic kidneys.

The patient in this case had no renal dysfunction, and a renal DMSA scan performed preoperatively revealed only mildly reduced tracer uptake in the left kidney. Genetic screening was negative and screening of first-degree relatives revealed no additional cases. The abnormally low signal intensity in the cortical cysts presumably represents old blood products, but we have no good explanation for it.

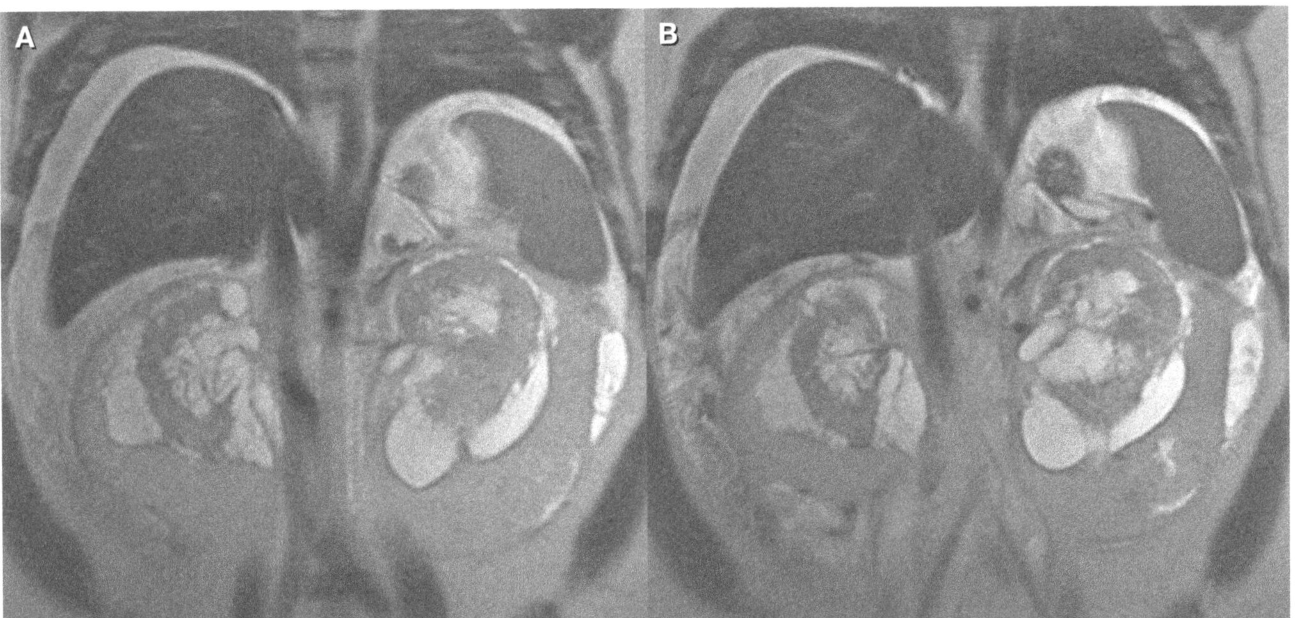

Figure 7.24.1

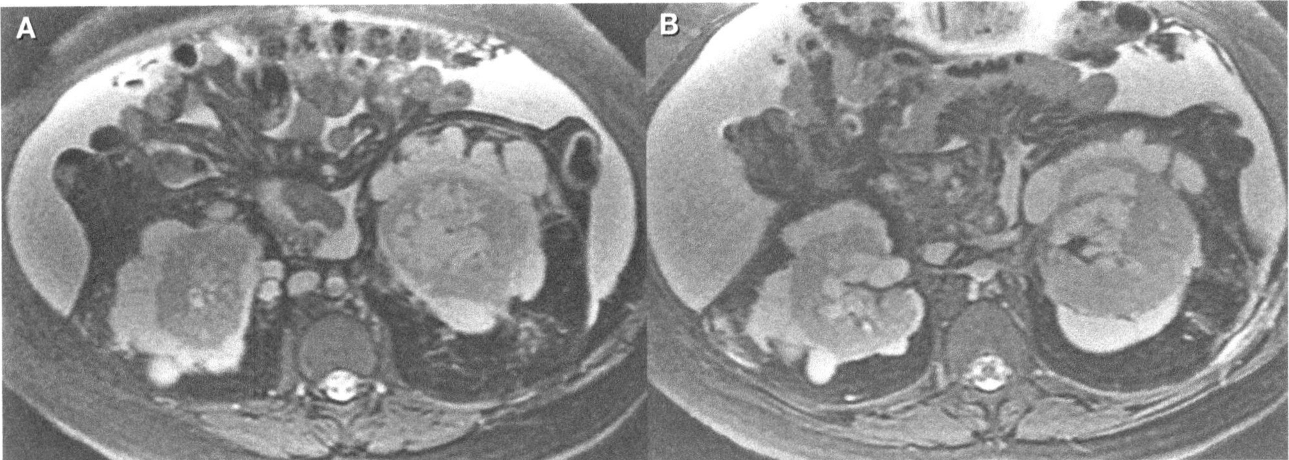

Figure 7.24.2

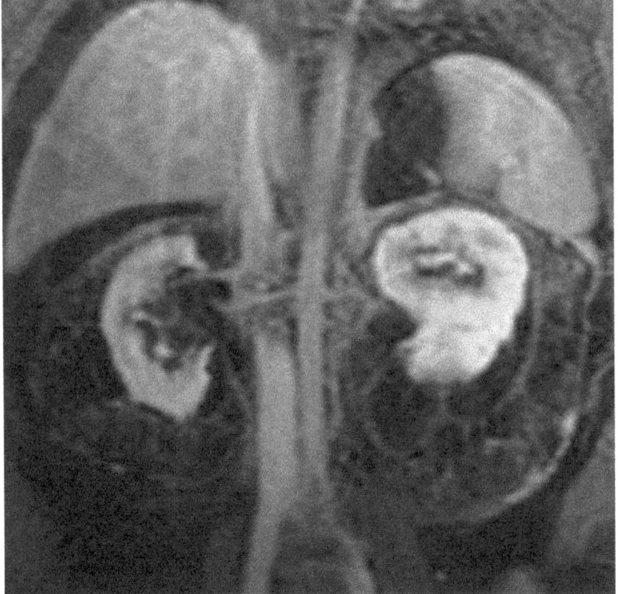

Figure 7.24.3

HISTORY: 10-year-old boy with a history of chronic ascites

IMAGING FINDINGS: Coronal SSFSE (Figure 7.24.1) and axial fat-suppressed SSFP (Figure 7.24.2) images show cystic lesions surrounding the renal contours bilaterally, as well as prominent abdominal ascites. Coronal postgadolinium 3D SPGR image (Figure 7.24.3) shows minimal septal enhancement of the perirenal cystic lesions.

DIAGNOSIS: Renal lymphangiomatosis

COMMENT: Renal lymphangiomatosis is a rare developmental disorder of the lymphatic system. Lymphangiomatosis in itself is rare and most often occurs in the head and neck (75%) and the axilla (20%), with the other 5% of cases occurring in all other locations. Lymphangiomas are thought to occur because the involved lymphatics fail to develop appropriate drainage into the normal lymphatic system. They are classified as capillary or cavernous according to the size of the lymphatic spaces. In the case of renal lymphangiomatosis, the obstruction is thought to occur at the renal pedicle.

Renal lymphangiomas may be asymptomatic and incidentally detected or present with flank pain, abdominal distention, ascites, hematuria, hypertension, or, rarely, impaired renal function. In general, this condition presents sporadically, although familial associations have been described.

MRI is a great technique for imaging patients with lymphangiomas, which appear as thin-walled nonenhancing cystic lesions surrounding the renal capsule and, sometimes, the parapelvic space. Coronal and axial T2-weighted images should confirm the diagnosis, and this is one of the rare instances where faster sequences (SSFSE and SSFP) are actually preferable to longer breath-held or respiratory-triggered FSE images, since motion artifact is minimized and the fluid-filled lesions are well seen. Exclusive parapelvic involvement has been reported, in which case it might be difficult to distinguish this entity from the far more common parapelvic cysts. The differential diagnosis for lesions surrounding the kidneys includes retroperitoneal fibrosis, Erdheim-Chester disease, and lymphoma—but none of these disorders look at all like renal lymphangiomatosis (ie, they're solid, not cystic).

Treatment of symptomatic renal lymphangiomatosis should be approached with great caution and is probably best left to tertiary centers that have experience with this condition. Percutaneous aspiration or sclerotherapy almost always results in reaccumulation of fluid in the lymphangiomas and may result in communication with the peritoneal cavity and development of intractable ascites.

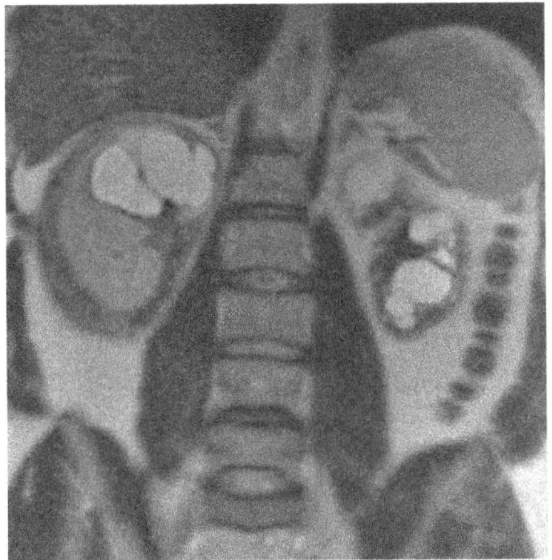

Figure 7.25.1

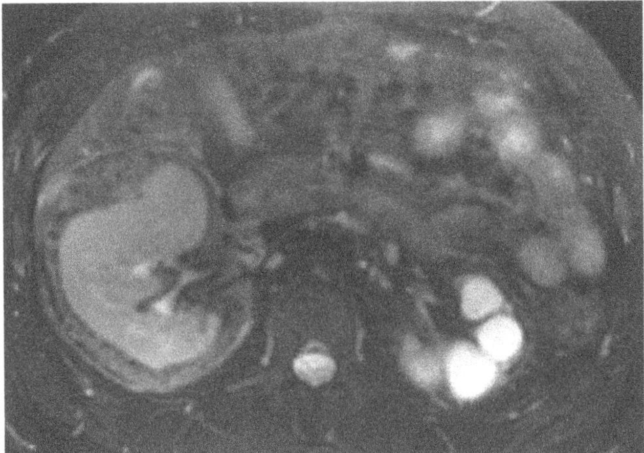

Figure 7.25.2

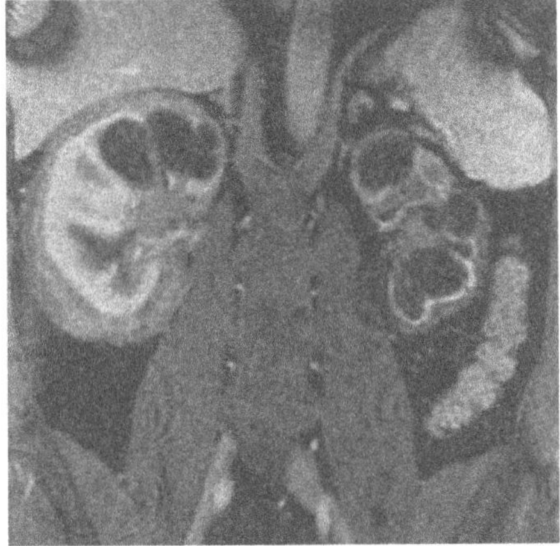

Figure 7.25.3

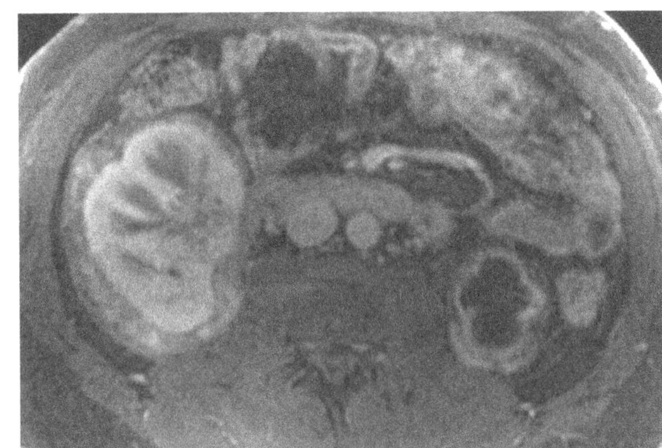

Figure 7.25.4

HISTORY: 30-year-old man with decreased renal function

IMAGING FINDINGS: Coronal SSFSE (Figure 7.25.1) and axial fat-suppressed T2-weighted FSE (Figure 7.25.2) images reveal hydronephrosis in the upper pole of the right kidney and an atrophic left kidney with hydronephrosis. Note the rind of hypointense soft tissue surrounding both kidneys. Coronal (Figure 7.25.3) and axial (Figure 7.25.4) postgadolinium 3D SPGR images show diffuse enhancement of the perinephric soft tissue.

DIAGNOSIS: Perirenal retroperitoneal fibrosis

COMMENT: RPF is an uncommon condition, with an estimated prevalence of 1.4 per 100,000 persons. It is characterized by fibroinflammatory tissue surrounding the aorta and iliac arteries. The soft tissue infiltration can extend into the retroperitoneum to encase adjacent structures, most often the ureters. Renal involvement is less common, and the isolated involvement of the kidneys with sparing of the periaortic region seen in this case is fairly unusual, although we have seen a few additional examples.

A Mayo Clinic review of RPF in 185 patients found a male predominance (61%) and frequent renal insufficiency (42%) in patients with newly diagnosed RPF. Location of the primary retroperitoneal mass was periaortic or periureteral in 90% of patients, with various additional locations (including perirenal) accounting for the other 10%. Although this condition traditionally has been considered an inflammatory process, elevated levels of inflammatory markers are not universal and nearly half of presenting patients have a normal erythrocyte sedimentation rate or a normal C-reactive protein level. Treatment of RPF consists of administration of corticosteroids and other anti-inflammatory medications and interventional therapy for patients with hydronephrosis from ureteral or renal involvement. Most patients respond to therapy; stabilization occurs in approximately one-third of patients and improvement in 50%.

The typical imaging appearance of RPF is an infiltrative soft tissue mass surrounding the aorta, classically with relatively low signal intensity on T2-weighted images and with gradual, persistent enhancement following gadolinium administration. Isolated renal involvement, although rare, has a relatively short list of differential diagnoses, which includes lymphoma and Erdheim-Chester disease. Lymphoma can have bilateral soft tissue infiltration of the kidneys and may be associated with retroperitoneal disease as well, but it is typically more bulky and heterogeneous in its distribution and is more likely to have associated adenopathy. Erdheim-Chester disease is a rare form of non–Langerhans cell histiocytosis characterized by infiltration of the skeleton and viscera by foamy histiocytes. The perirenal soft tissue infiltration can have an appearance identical to RPF, and some authors have suggested that a percentage of the noninflammatory RPF cases might in fact be misdiagnosed Erdheim-Chester disease. Erdheim-Chester disease has different clinical characteristics (bone pain, diabetes insipidus, and exophthalmus) and usually can be distinguished from RPF through the classic appearance of skeletal involvement—bilateral patchy or diffuse symmetrical sclerosis of the medullary cavity of the major long bones, with relative epiphyseal sparing.

This case was performed before the era of NSF. Today, we would be reluctant to give gadolinium to anyone with kidneys that look as bad as in this case (although it might be reasonable to use one of the more stable gadolinium agents if the eGFR were >30 mL/minute/m^2). Although post-gadolinium images are helpful, they weren't absolutely necessary to make the diagnosis. T1- and T2-weighted images demonstrating the rind of perinephric soft tissue with a typical fibrotic appearance are sufficient, given such a classic appearance.

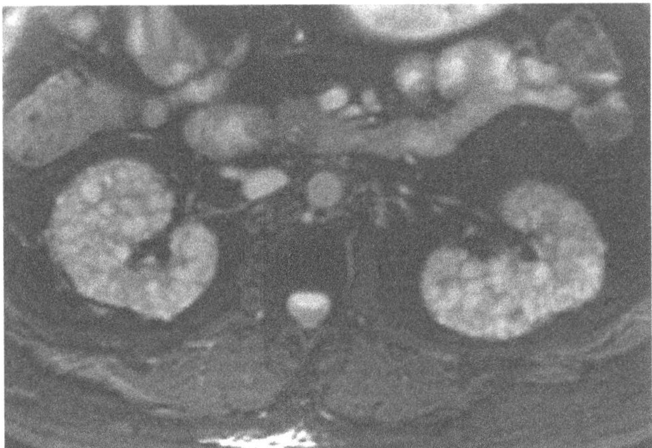

Figure 7.26.1

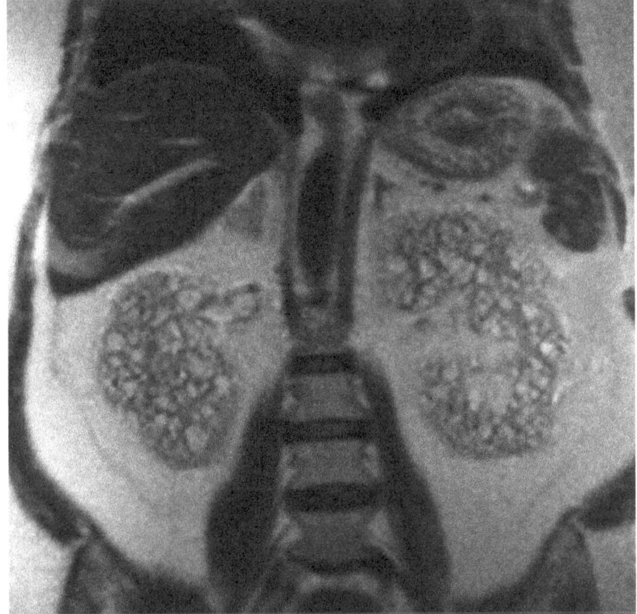

Figure 7.26.2

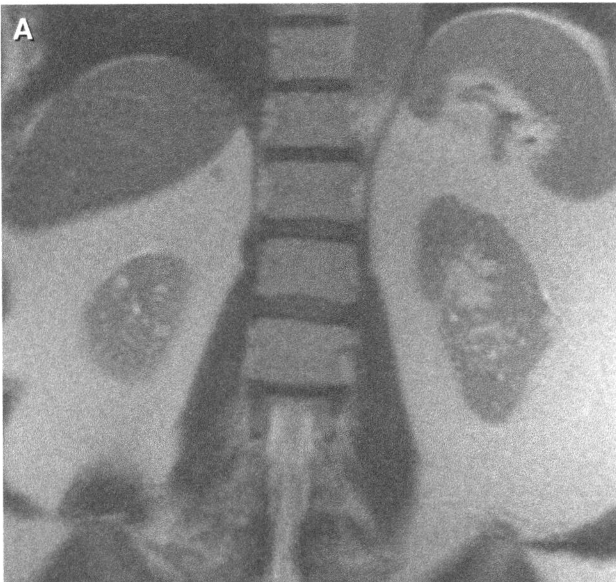

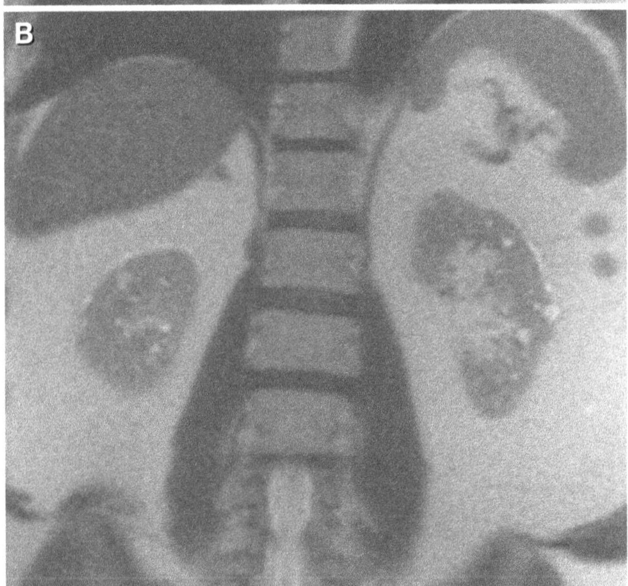

Figure 7.26.3

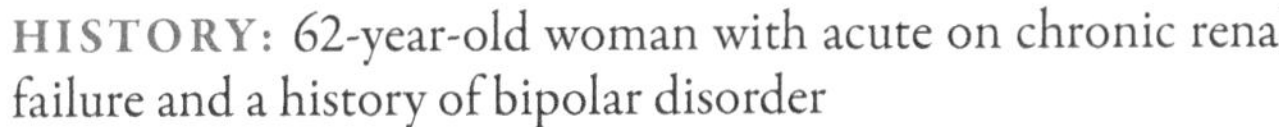

HISTORY: 62-year-old woman with acute on chronic renal failure and a history of bipolar disorder

IMAGING FINDINGS: Axial fat-suppressed SSFP (Figure 7.26.1) and coronal SSFSE (Figure 7.26.2) images reveal innumerable small cysts throughout both kidneys. Coronal SSFSE images (Figure 7.26.3) of a second patient with less severe disease demonstrate multiple small cysts involving both kidneys.

DIAGNOSIS: Renal lithium toxicity

COMMENT: Lithium has been applied therapeutically for more than 150 years, although its use as an effective drug spans a far shorter period. Cade in 1949 observed the calming effect of lithium on guinea pigs and then tested it in 10 manic patients, with highly successful results. Initial enthusiasm was dimmed by the death of several patients due to lithium intoxication, after which the Food and Drug Administration withdrew the drug from the market in the United States. Lithium was reintroduced in 1970 and has been a mainstay in the treatment of bipolar disorder ever since, with symptomatic improvement reported in 70% to 80% of patients.

Despite its success in treating mood disorders, lithium has a relatively narrow therapeutic window and can cause a number of adverse effects, of which tremor is the most common, affecting 25% to 50% of patients. Renal complications include impairment of tubular function and development of diabetes insipidus and renal tubular acidosis. Reduced urinary concentrating ability occurs in more than half of patients. The tubular dysfunction is initially reversible with cessation of lithium, but with continued use, eventually irreversible polyuria and polydipsia (diabetes insipidus) appear in 20% to 40% of patients. Progressive chronic kidney disease develops secondary to lithium-induced tubulointerstitial nephritis, characterized by cortical and medullary interstitial fibrosis and tubular atrophy, cortical and medullary tubular cysts, and tubular dilatation.

The cysts and dilated tubules can be seen with MRI. On a few occasions, nephrologists in our practice have found a noncontrast examination useful to identify the presence or absence of cysts in a patient with reduced renal function who is taking lithium but also has other risk factors for renal disease. In general, the cysts in lithium toxicity are smaller and more uniform than those seen in ADPKD, but differentiating early or less severe cases from other causes of renal cystic disease is probably difficult when based on imaging findings alone. Fortunately, the clinical history is helpful when the examination is performed specifically with this question in mind.

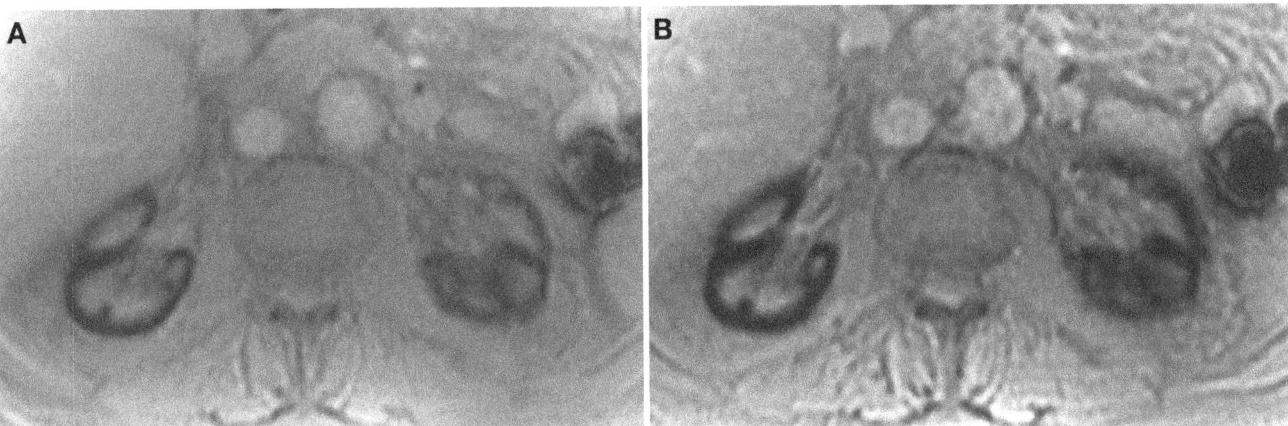

Figure 7.27.1

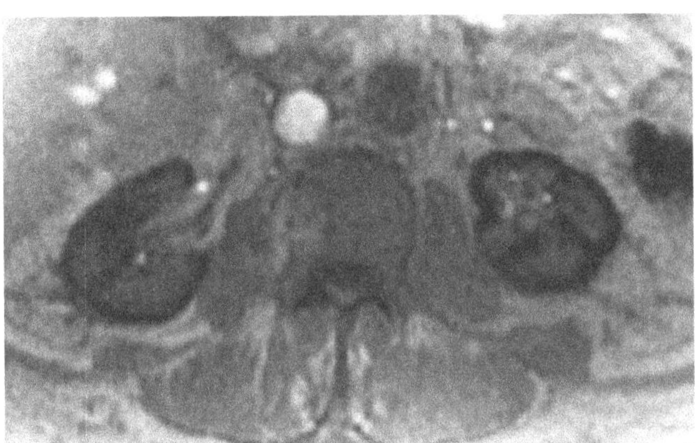

Figure 7.27.2

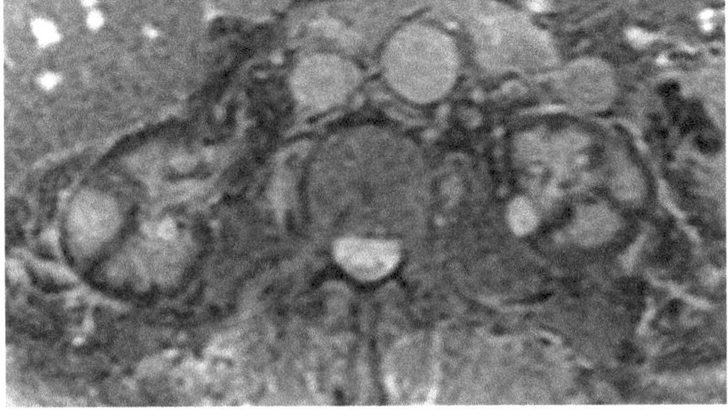

Figure 7.27.3

HISTORY: 72-year-old man with aortic dissection who underwent aortic root replacement and prosthetic aortic valve replacement 14 years ago; the patient has had worsening periprosthetic regurgitation and cardiac failure and has required multiple transfusions

IMAGING FINDINGS: Two axial GRE images from a BOLD acquisition (Figure 7.27.1) show markedly decreased signal intensity within the renal cortex that becomes more pronounced with increasing TE (Figure 7.27.1B has a longer TE). Axial IP 2D SPGR image (Figure 7.27.2) and axial fat-suppressed 2D SSFP image (Figure 7.27.3) also demonstrate diffuse signal loss throughout the renal cortex. Notice that there is no corresponding signal abnormality in the liver, spleen, or pancreas.

DIAGNOSIS: Renal cortical siderosis secondary to mechanical intravascular hemolysis from a prosthetic valve

COMMENT: Paroxysmal nocturnal hemoglobinuria is the classic differential diagnosis for renal cortical iron deposition, but this appearance also can be seen (as in this case) in patients with mechanical damage from prosthetic heart valves, resulting in intravascular hemolysis. Both of these conditions result in intravascular hemolysis sufficient to saturate plasma haptoglobin with iron. The residual free hemoglobin is filtered by the glomeruli and partially reabsorbed in the proximal tubules, where part of the iron is incorporated into hemosiderin deposits and the rest is excreted in urine. The intravascular hemolysis seen in these disorders does not result in hemosiderin accumulation in the liver and spleen. This is in contradistinction to other hemolytic anemias, such as sickle cell disease, hereditary spherocytosis, and autoimmune hemolytic anemia, which have extravascular hemolysis and subsequent iron deposition in the liver, spleen, and bone marrow.

Paroxysmal nocturnal hemoglobinuria is a myelodysplastic hematopoietic stem cell disorder caused by an increased sensitivity to complement, resulting in acute and chronic intravascular hemolysis. Hemolysis may be precipitated by various factors, including infections, drugs, exercise, surgery, and transfusions. Paroxysmal nocturnal hemoglobinuria may produce chronic renal failure as a result of hemosiderin deposition in the proximal convoluted tubules in the renal cortex that, in turn, causes cellular damage through repeated microinfarctions or the direct nephrotoxic effect of iron.

The MRI appearance of renal cortical siderosis is similar to that of iron deposition in other, more familiar places (ie, the liver and spleen)—diffuse decreased signal intensity on

T2- and T2*-weighted images. Usually, there is decreased T1-signal intensity as well, which occurs because of the overwhelming T2* effect on T1-weighted images. Small concentrations of hemosiderin, however, can actually result in higher signal intensity because of the paramagnetic T1-shortening effect. If you acquire IP and OP images through the kidneys, you will see signal dropout on IP images of patients with cortical siderosis because the 2-ms difference in echo time (2 ms OP echo time vs 4 ms IP echo time at 1.5 T) is large enough to cause significant signal loss. Gradient echo images are much more sensitive to iron than conventional spin echo or FSE sequences, and the most impressive images in this case are from a BOLD acquisition, which is just a multi-echo GRE sequence that acquires multiple images with increasing echo times. This technique can be used to quantify R2* or T2*, and if a tissue calibration curve is available, these values can be related to the tissue iron content.

In healthy kidneys, the renal cortex has a shorter T1 than the medulla and therefore is hyperintense relative to the medulla on T1-weighted images. This is the normal corticomedullary differentiation, which is lost in various conditions resulting in reduced renal function and is reversed in cortical hemosiderosis.

Low renal cortical signal intensity can be seen also in renal cortical necrosis, which can occur in utero or in association with severe traumatic or septic shock, severe dehydration, transfusion reaction, or hemolytic uremic syndrome or as a posttransplantation complication. Renal vein thrombosis and renal artery thrombosis can both lead to decreased cortical signal intensity, but these conditions also affect the renal medulla, in distinction with cortical siderosis. Renal siderosis can occur with sickle cell disease, in which intravascular hemolysis occurs in acute hemolytic crises; however, there is usually considerably greater iron deposition in the liver and spleen.

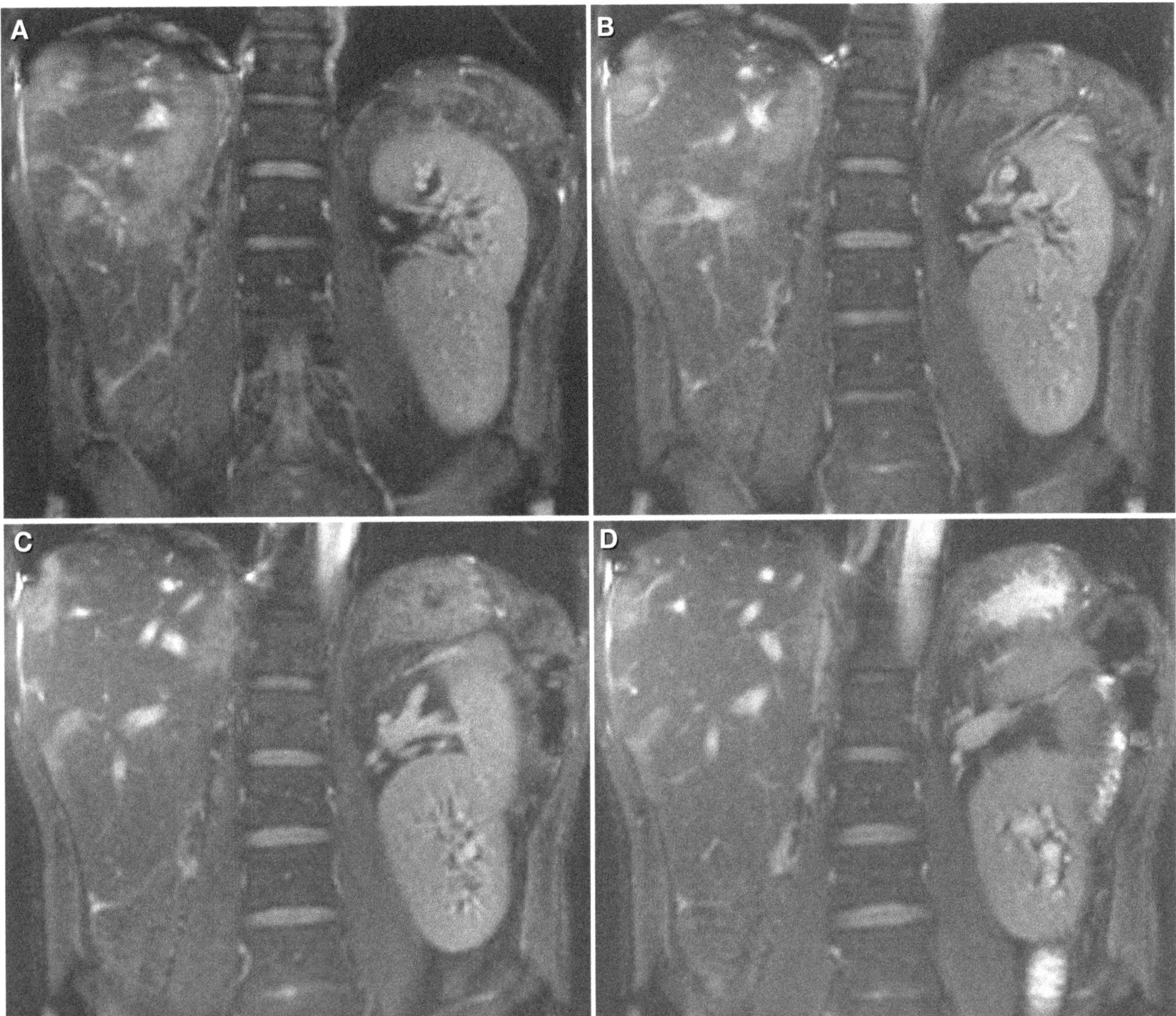

Figure 7.28.1

HISTORY: 39-year-old man with complications following hepatic transplantation

IMAGING FINDINGS: Coronal fat-suppressed SSFP images (Figure 7.28.1) show 2 kidneys fused in the left abdomen, with absence of a kidney in the right renal fossa. Note also heterogeneous increased signal intensity in the transplant liver secondary to ischemic injury.

DIAGNOSIS: Cross-fused ectopia

COMMENT: Cross-fused ectopia is the second most frequent fusion anomaly of the urinary tract (horseshoe kidney ranks first) and is thought to result from abnormal development of the ureteric bud and metanephric blastema during the fourth to eighth weeks of gestation, leading to fusion of the kidneys on the same side. Two separate ureters arise from the respective kidneys, and the ureter arising from the ectopic kidney travels back to the opposite side to insert into the bladder. Blood supply to the kidneys in cross-fused ectopia is often atypical and arises from the lower abdominal aorta or iliac arteries in a majority of cases.

The estimated prevalence of cross-fused ectopia ranges from 1 in 1,300 to 1 in 7,500, with a slight male predominance. It has been associated with an increased incidence of urinary tract infections, ureteropelvic junction obstruction, hydronephrosis, reflux, ectopic ureteroceles, nephrolithiasis, and uroepithelial tumors, and so life-long surveillance has been advocated by some authors. Additional congenital anomalies may be seen in association with cross-fused ectopia, including skeletal, cardiovascular, and GU anomalies. Crossed-fused ectopic kidneys have been further classified into 4 or 6 subcategories, although these divisions are controversial and their practical value is unclear.

Horseshoe kidney (Figure 7.28.2) is more common (estimated incidence, 1 in 400) and accounts for 90% of renal fusion abnormalities. The lower poles are typically fused, with the isthmus lying anterior to the aorta. Blood supply to horseshoe kidneys is also highly variable and should be sorted out before renal surgery or intervention is undertaken. The abnormal orientation of the horseshoe kidney means that the ureters are somewhat angulated and therefore are more prone to obstruction, infection, and stone formation. Horseshoe kidneys are detected as an incidental finding in one-third of cases. Symptomatic patients generally have hydronephrosis, infection, or renal stone disease.

As with cross-fused ectopia, associated GU anomalies are common with horseshoe kidney, occurring in as many as two-thirds of patients and including vesicoureteral reflux, ureteral duplication, ectopic ureterocele, cystic disease, hypospadias, bicornuate uterus, undescended testes, and septate vagina. Nongenitourinary anomalies are also associated and include skeletal, cardiovascular, gastrointestinal, and central nervous system abnormalities.

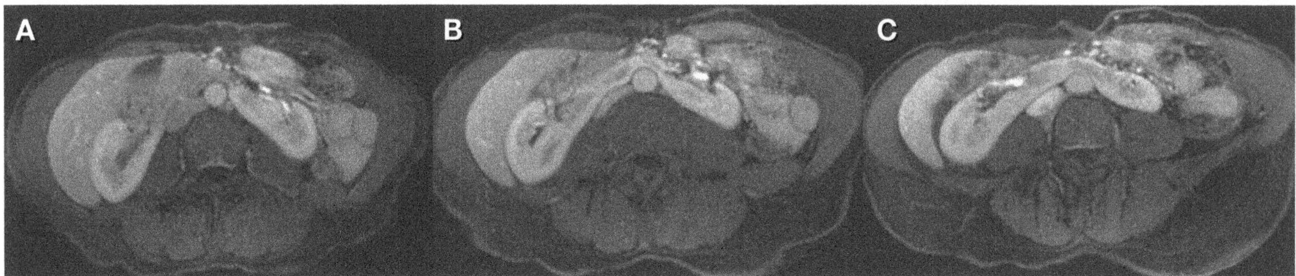

Figure 7.28.2

Axial postgadolinium 3D SPGR images show horseshoe kidneys with abnormally oriented right and left kidneys that are fused centrally, overlying the aorta.

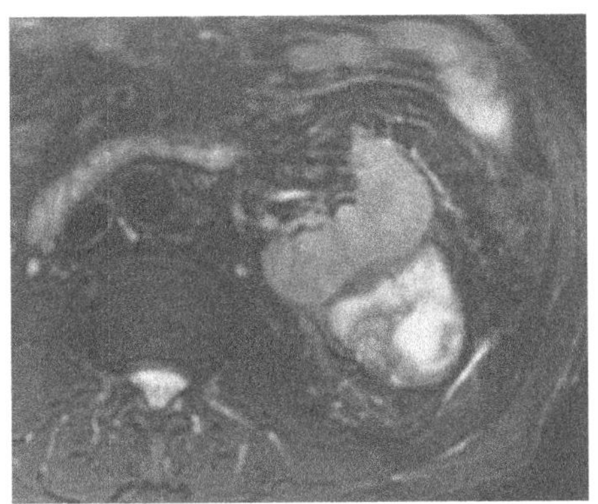

Figure 7.29.1

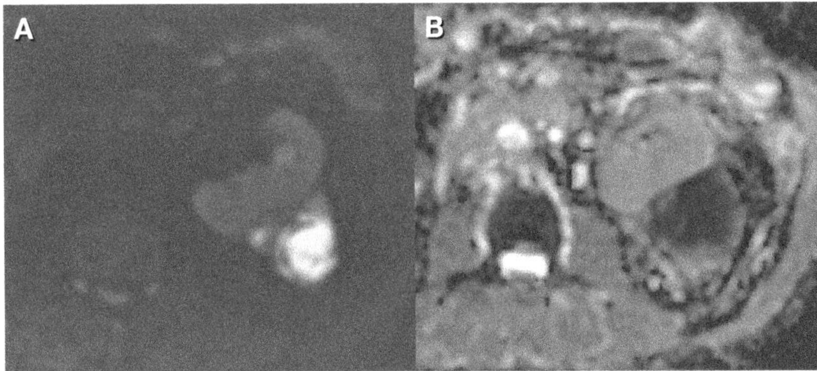

Figure 7.29.2

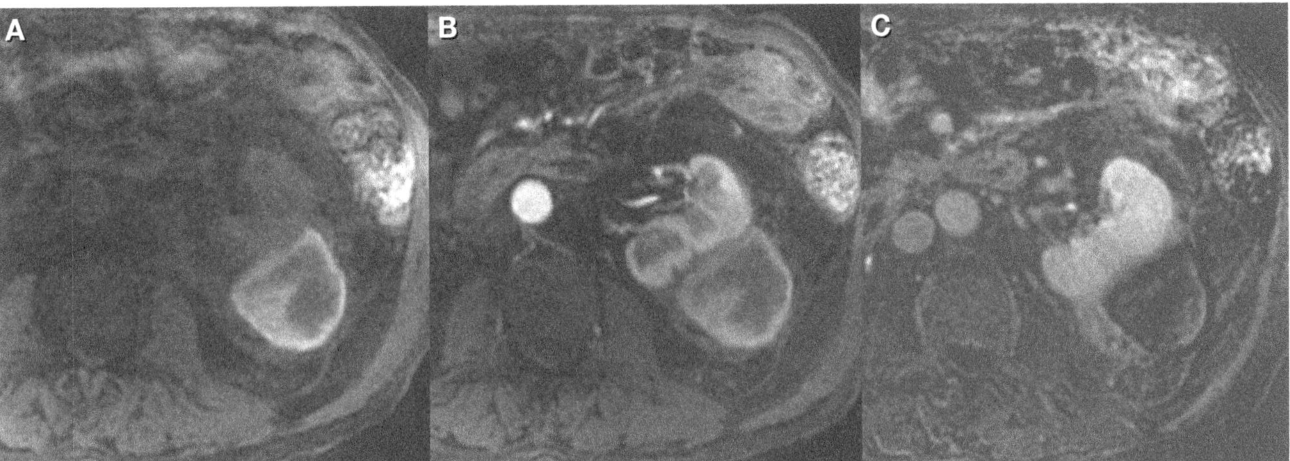

Figure 7.29.3

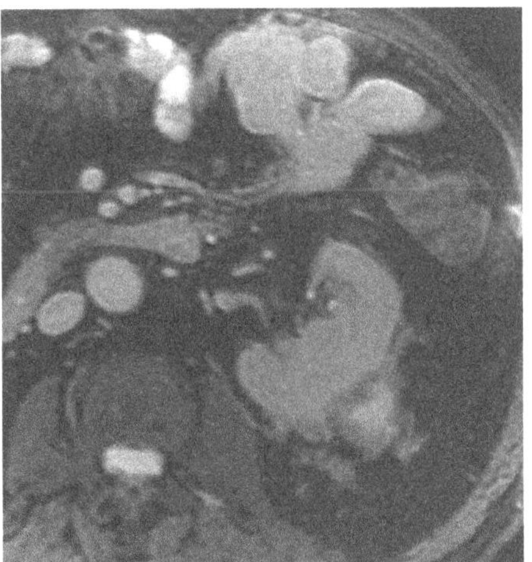

Figure 7.29.4

HISTORY: 72-year-old man with left flank pain and a history of bleeding diathesis, for which he takes warfarin

IMAGING FINDINGS: Axial FSE T2-weighted image (Figure 7.29.1) reveals a posterior left perinephric mass with heterogeneous increased signal intensity. Axial diffusion-weighted image (b=800 s/mm^2) and the corresponding ADC map (Figure 7.29.2) show the lesion to have high signal intensity and correspondingly low ADC values. Precontrast, arterial phase postgadolinium, and subtracted (nephrogenic phase minus precontrast) 3D SPGR images (Figure 7.29.3) demonstrate that this lesion has a rim of high T1-signal intensity with questionable rim enhancement on subtracted images. An axial fat-suppressed SSFP image from a 3-month follow-up examination (Figure 7.29.4) shows that the perinephric process has markedly decreased in size.

DIAGNOSIS: Perinephric hematoma

COMMENT: This is a companion case to the ruptured RCC (Case 7.4) and illustrates some of the pitfalls of DWI. By any published criteria in the literature, the ADC values measured in this perinephric hematoma fall into the category of suspicious for neoplasm, and yet the hematoma has a fairly classic lentiform shape, has the typical rim of increased T1-signal intensity of a hematoma, and doesn't enhance after contrast administration. (It's useful to remember that DWI is a reflection of the physical microenvironment of water molecules but not always of the histology.) The subtracted image is somewhat problematic because it shows the suggestion of a thicker rind of enhancing tissue posteriorly; however, this could not be verified on the source images and most likely results from misregistration artifact due to inconsistent breath-holding. The single SSFP image from the 3-month follow-up examination shows that the hematoma is much smaller and, in fact, it wasn't identifiable on a CT scan performed 6 months after that.

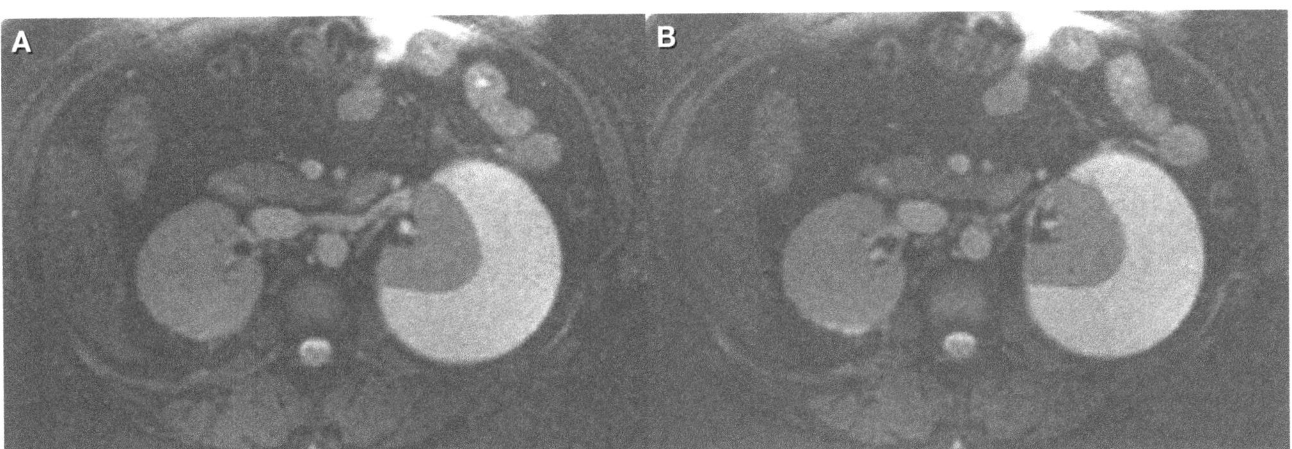

Figure 7.30.1

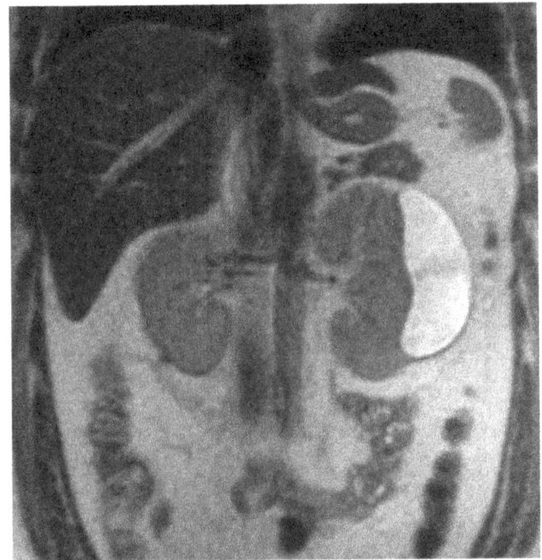

Figure 7.30.2

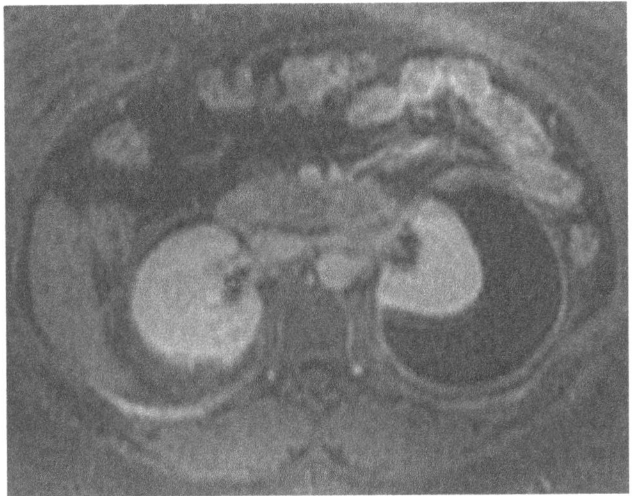

Figure 7.30.3

HISTORY: 32-year-old woman with a history of bilateral perinephric hematomas approximately 4 months ago that resulted in acute renal failure and new onset of hypertension; renal failure has resolved, but she has persistent hypertension

IMAGING FINDINGS: Axial fat-suppressed SSFP images (Figure 7.30.1) and a coronal SSFSE image (Figure 7.30.2) reveal a subcapsular fluid collection along the lateral border of the left kidney. Axial postgadolinium 3D SPGR image (Figure 7.30.3) shows minimal rim enhancement of the fluid collection. Note the small remnant subcapsular hematoma in the posterior right kidney.

DIAGNOSIS: Subcapsular hematoma and Page kidney

COMMENT: *Page kidney* refers to the development of hypertension in response to extrinsic compression of 1 or both kidneys, usually by a hematoma or mass, presumably through activation of the renin-angiotensin-aldosterone system. The phenomenon was first described in 1939 by Page, who compressed canine kidneys by wrapping them with cellophane and observed a hypertensive response.

The diagnosis of Page kidney cannot be made on imaging findings alone, but the presence of a subcapsular hematoma with compression or mass effect on the associated renal parenchyma in a patient with new hypertension should suggest the diagnosis. In this case, the mass effect is somewhat subtle, probably most easily appreciated on the coronal image and also by noting that the left kidney appears slightly smaller than the right one on all axial images.

The initial clinical description of Page kidney was of a football player whose blunt trauma resulted in a perirenal hematoma and hypertension. Most of the initial cases described in the literature had a similar history of trauma. However, a majority of recent reports have described Page kidney occurring in renal transplant recipients, usually after biopsy.

Treatment of Page kidney includes evacuation of the hematoma, nephrectomy, or medical antihypertensive therapy.

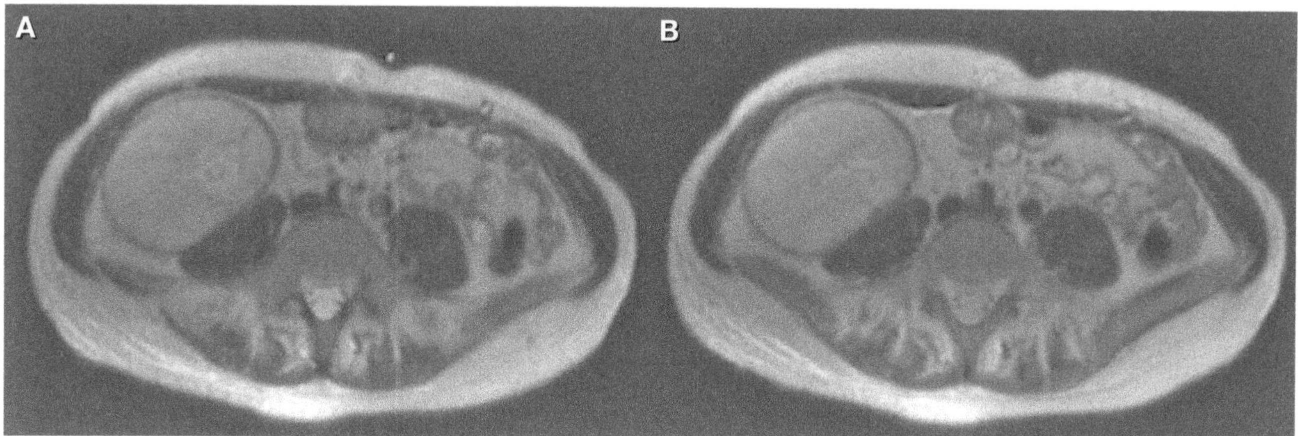

Figure 7.31.1

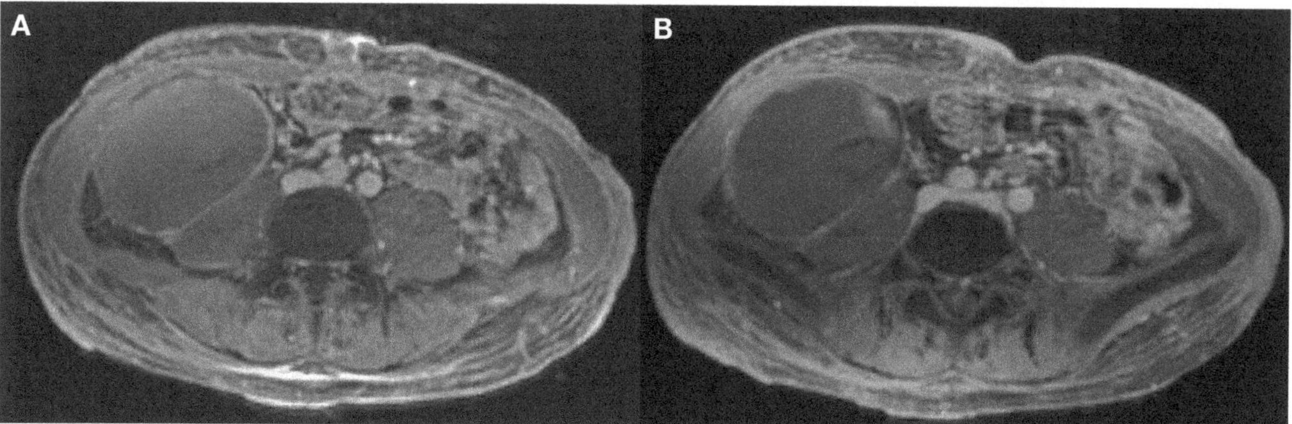

Figure 7.31.2

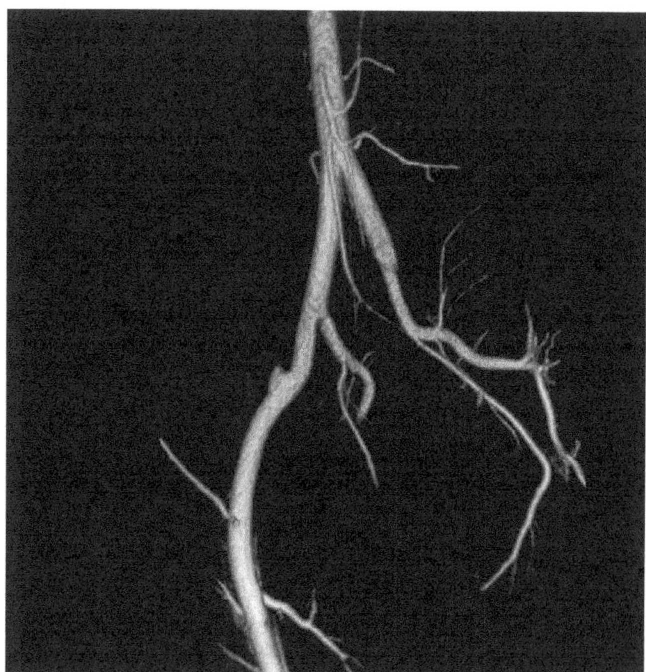

Figure 7.31.3

HISTORY: 19-year-old man with recent renal transplantation for focal segmental glomerulosclerosis who now has declining renal function and new-onset diffuse alveolar hemorrhage and reduced cardiac function

IMAGING FINDINGS: Axial SSFSE images (Figure 7.31.1) reveal diffuse increased signal intensity throughout the featureless right lower quadrant renal transplant. Axial postgadolinium 2D SPGR images (Figure 7.31.2) show no enhancement of the renal transplant except for a thin capsular rim. A volume-rendered image from 3D contrast-enhanced MRA (Figure 7.31.3) demonstrates a stub of the transplant renal artery origin from the right external iliac artery, with thrombosis distal to the origin.

DIAGNOSIS: Renal transplant artery thrombosis with infarcted transplant kidney

COMMENT: Renal transplantation is the treatment of choice for most cases of chronic renal failure, but transplanted kidneys are susceptible to a large number of acute and chronic complications. It is difficult to sort out clinically which particular problem is responsible for the pain, fever, hypertension, reduced renal function, and other symptoms, and so imaging has an important role in evaluating these patients. US usually is the test of choice, but occasionally it is inconclusive—particularly in the assessment of vascular stenosis or occlusion—and MRI can be a useful confirmatory examination in these cases. (It's worth noting that MRI is a recent entrant into the acute tubular necrosis vs rejection sweepstakes, with both perfusion and DWI used to distinguish between the two. This research has not yet seen widespread clinical application, however, and there is reluctance to use even the small amounts of gadolinium required for standard perfusion imaging.)

Vascular complications are relatively infrequent, occurring in less than 10% of these cases, but they can be significant, as in this case. Vascular anastomoses vary depending on the transplant type. In cadaveric transplants, the donor kidney is usually transplanted with the entire renal artery and a piece of the donor aorta, known as a *Carrel patch*, which then is attached to the recipient iliac artery. This procedure is not a good idea in a living donor, for which an end-to-side anastomosis is made between the donor renal artery and the recipient external iliac artery or an end-to-end anastomosis from the donor renal artery to the recipient internal iliac artery. Renal veins are typically harvested in both cadaveric and living donors without an attached piece of the IVC, with end-to-end anastomosis to the external iliac vein.

Renal vein complications occur less frequently than arterial problems and usually in the early postoperative period. Renal vein thrombosis or stenosis can occur as a result of surgical complications, hypovolemia, and compression from adjacent fluid collections.

Renal artery stenosis is the most common vascular complication, with an incidence of approximately 10%. It occurs more commonly in cadaveric transplants and usually appears within the first 3 months after transplantation, presenting with hypertension. Remember to evaluate the entire scope of the arterial inflow and transplant renal artery and not just the anastomosis. Stenosis can occur in the donor iliac artery, at the anastomosis (end-to-end anastomosis has the highest risk), or distal to the anastomosis in the donor renal artery.

Renal artery thrombosis, seen in this case, is much less common, occurring in less than 1% of cases and most often in the early postoperative period. The most common cause is acute or hyperacute rejection, with additional etiologies that include surgical misadventures, acute tubular necrosis, and hypercoagulable states. The diagnosis is relatively easy to make with MRI: The renal artery is not seen, and the complete infarction of the transplant kidney is an indication that salvage is unlikely.

This case is an older one and occurred before the era of NSF. However, it still would be reasonable to perform a gadolinium-enhanced 3D MRA in a transplant patient with mild to moderately reduced renal function, using one of the more stable gadolinium agents. The patient in this case probably had very poor renal function and a low eGFR, so today contrast would not be given. Instead, a noncontrast MRA would be performed with a 3D SSFP acquisition with inflow enhancement and fat suppression (see Chapter 17 for a brief description). This technique is nearly identical to 3D contrast-enhanced MRA (in the literature anyway) in its ability to identify significant renal artery stenosis or thrombosis. These noncontrast techniques are generally not designed for venography acquisitions, but most of the time you can adequately visualize the transplant renal vein and iliac vein with overlapping 2D or 3D SSFP images. If you are performing 3D contrast-enhanced MRA, it's important to verify that your technologist knows exactly what to cover: We have seen a few unfortunate cases where the wrong side of the pelvis was initially imaged (in the setting of multiple or older nonfunctional transplants) or the native kidneys were initially imaged.

CASE 7.32

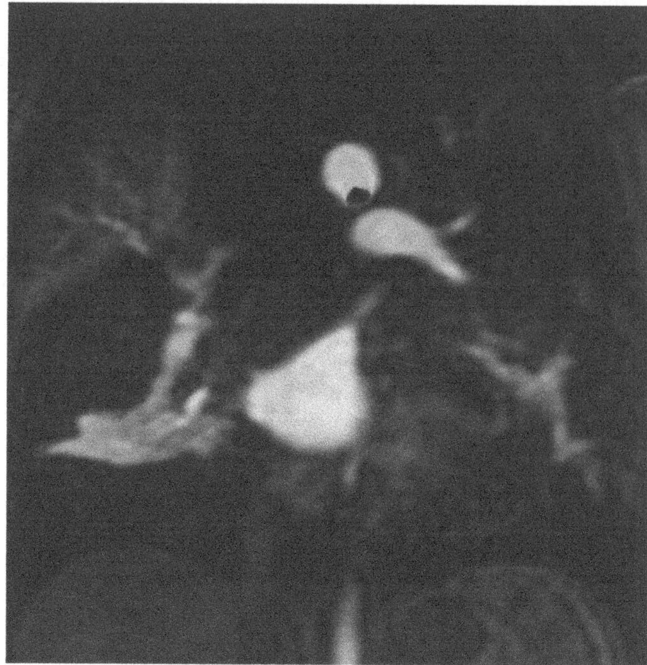

Figure 7.32.1

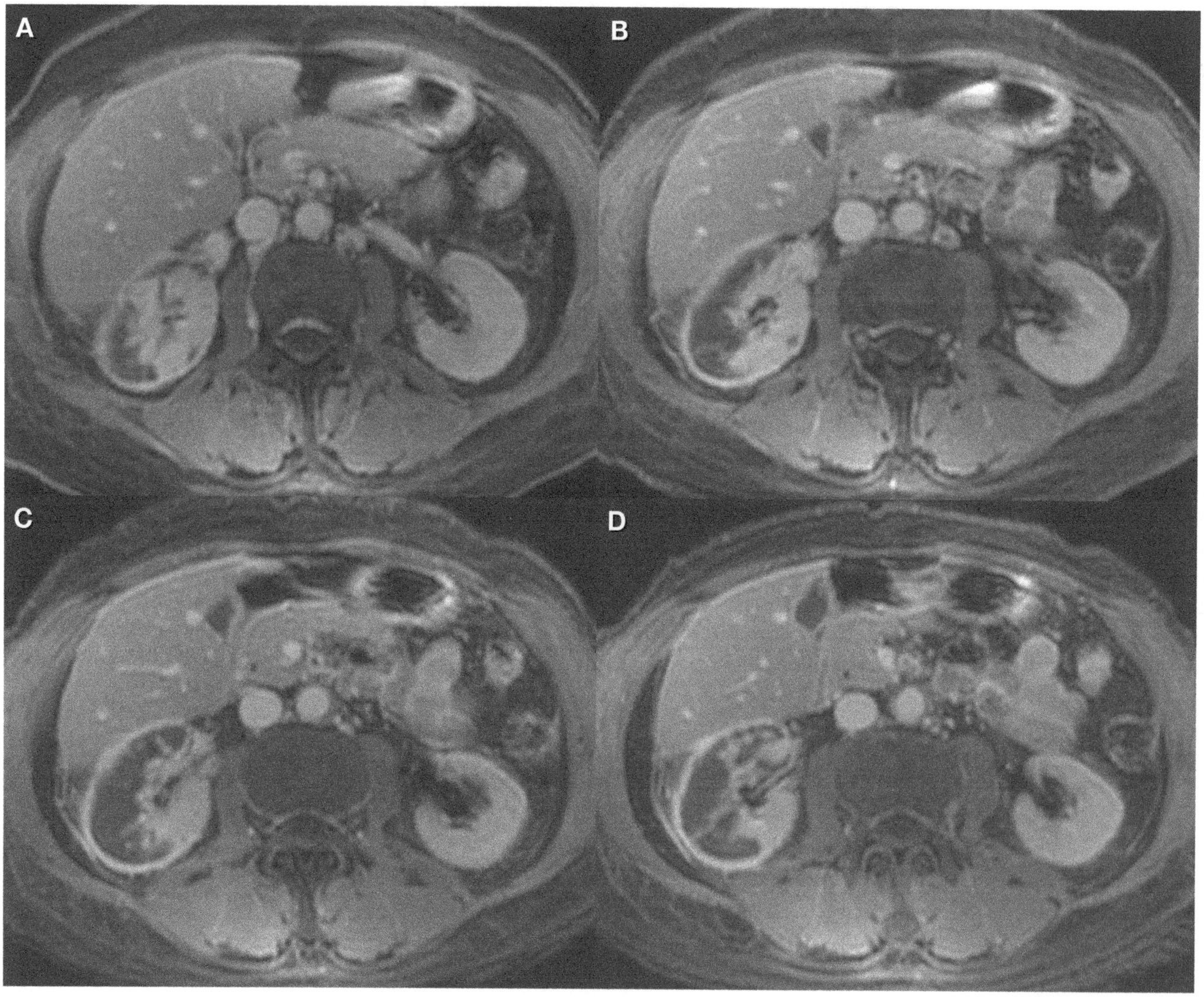

Figure 7.32.2

HISTORY: 62-year-old woman with chest discomfort and right upper quadrant pain

IMAGING FINDINGS: Coronal source image from 3D contrast-enhanced MRA (Figure 7.32.1) shows a prominent eccentric thrombus in the lumen of the posterior aortic arch. Post-MRA, 2D SPGR axial images (Figure 7.32.2) through the upper abdomen demonstrate a large region of absent perfusion in the right kidney, with preserved capsular enhancement.

DIAGNOSIS: Embolic renal infarct

COMMENT: Small renal infarcts typically appear wedge shaped and become more confluent as the infarct size increases. All infarcts are characterized in the acute and subacute state by an absence of enhancement after contrast administration, often with variable increased T2-signal intensity. As the infarct ages, progressive scarring reduces the size of the initial lesion, eventually leaving a cortical defect, sometimes with a barely perceptible perfusion abnormality.

Thrombotic renal infarcts can occur in the clinical setting of trauma or dissection, but embolic infarcts are more common. In this case, the source of the renal infarct was the large irregular plaque in the aortic arch. Notice the preserved enhancement of the renal capsule, which has a different blood supply. In addition, note the small thrombus in the superior mesenteric artery.

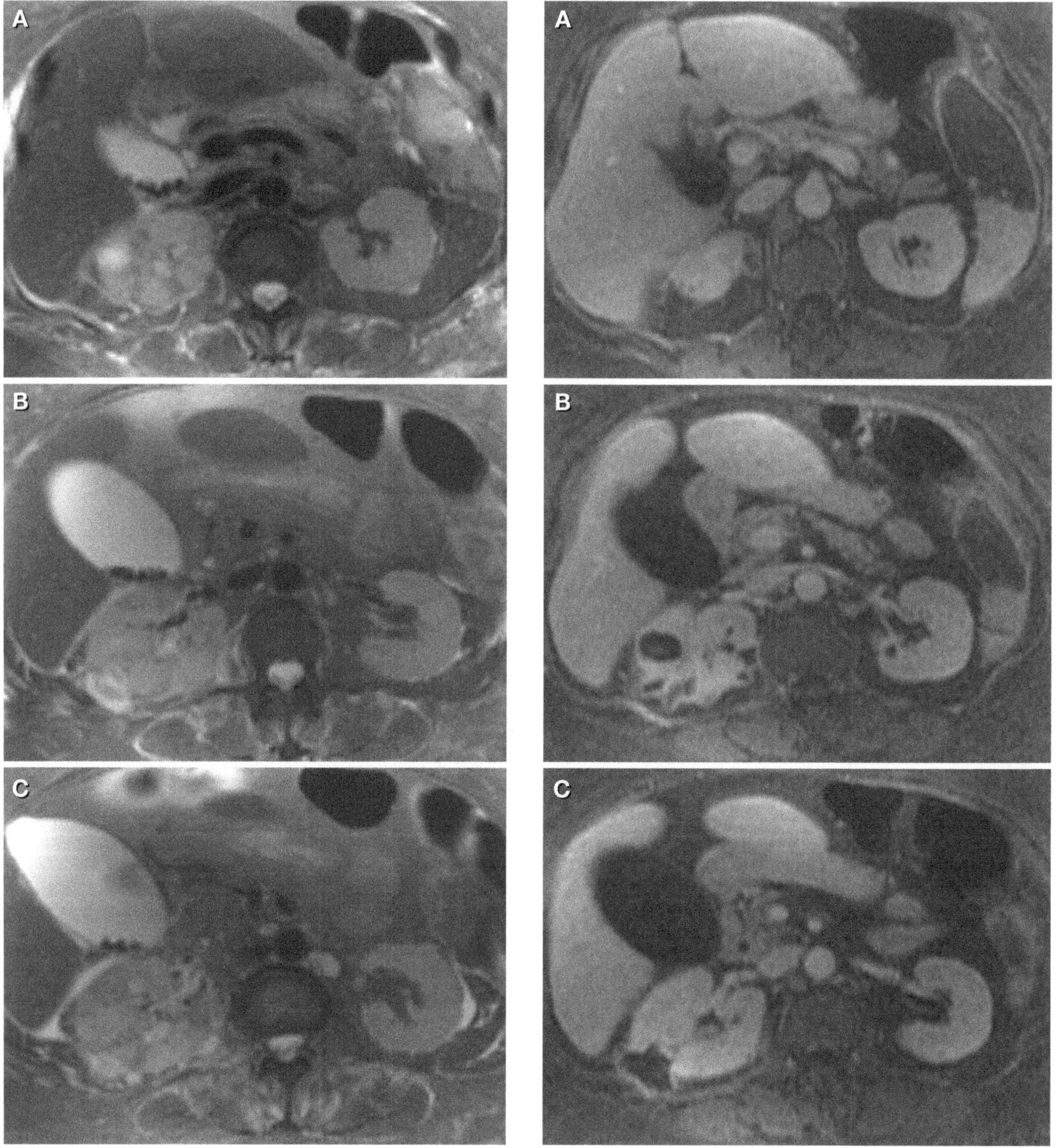

Figure 7.33.1

Figure 7.33.2

HISTORY: 63-year-old woman with mitral valve vegetations, septicemia, and new left upper quadrant pain

IMAGING FINDINGS: Axial breath-hold T2-weighted FRFSE images (Figure 7.33.1) show mild soft tissue stranding around the right kidney, as well as several small, T2-hyperintense lesions throughout the right kidney. Axial nephrogenic phase postgadolinium 3D SPGR images (Figure 7.33.2) reveal multiple cystic lesions in both kidneys, some with prominent walls and rim enhancement. Note the large acute infarct in the anterior spleen, with heterogeneous, increased T2-signal intensity and absent enhancement.

DIAGNOSIS: Renal abscesses

COMMENT: Renal abscesses probably occur most often in untreated or incompletely treated pyelonephritis but can also result from hematogenous spread, as in this case, or extension from an adjacent extrarenal inflammatory process. Immunocompromised patients, diabetic patients, and patients with urinary obstruction are at increased risk for developing renal abscesses. Ascending infections more often result in solitary abscesses, whereas hematogenous abscesses are commonly multiple and bilateral. In addition, ascending infections are usually caused by gram-negative organisms, while gram-positive organisms suggest a hematogenous route.

The cystic appearance of the lesions, along with prominent rim enhancement, helps distinguish these lesions from solid masses and, given the clinical history and the impressive splenic infarction in this case, the diagnosis is fairly obvious.

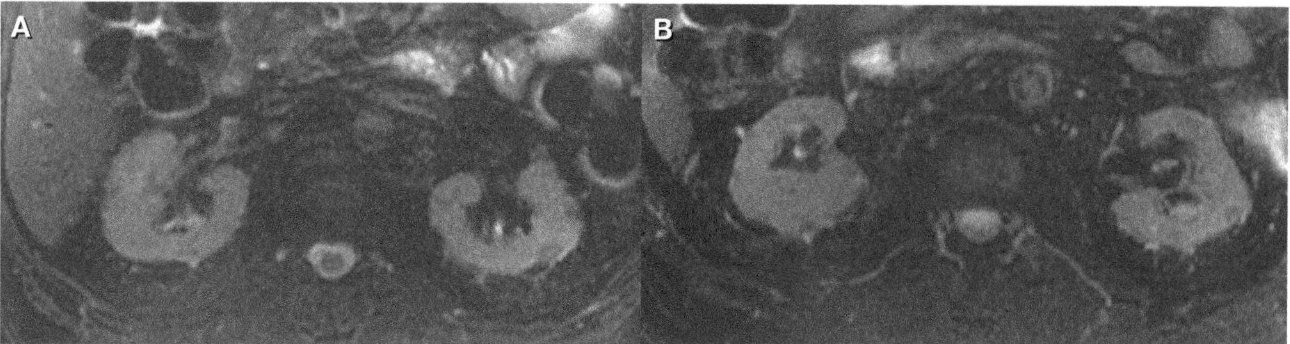

Figure 7.34.1

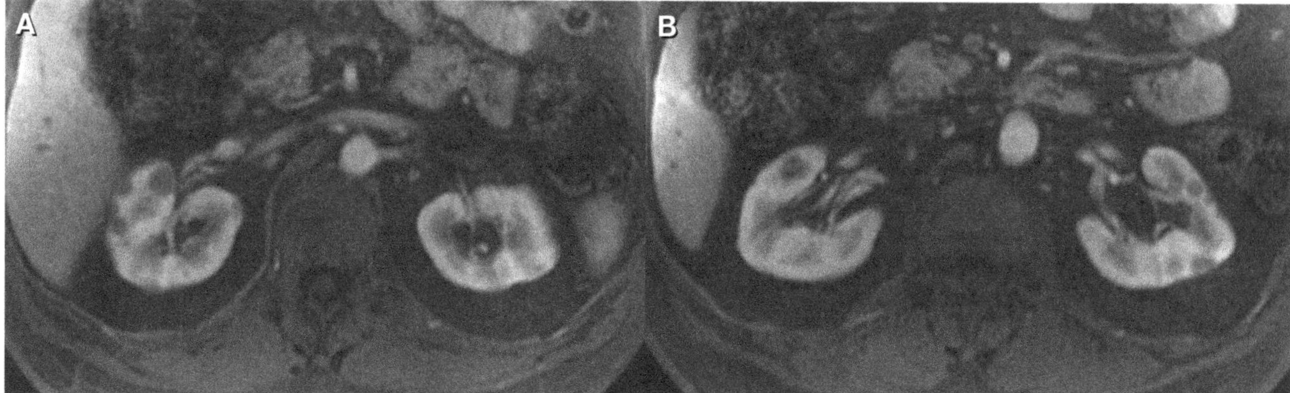

Figure 7.34.2

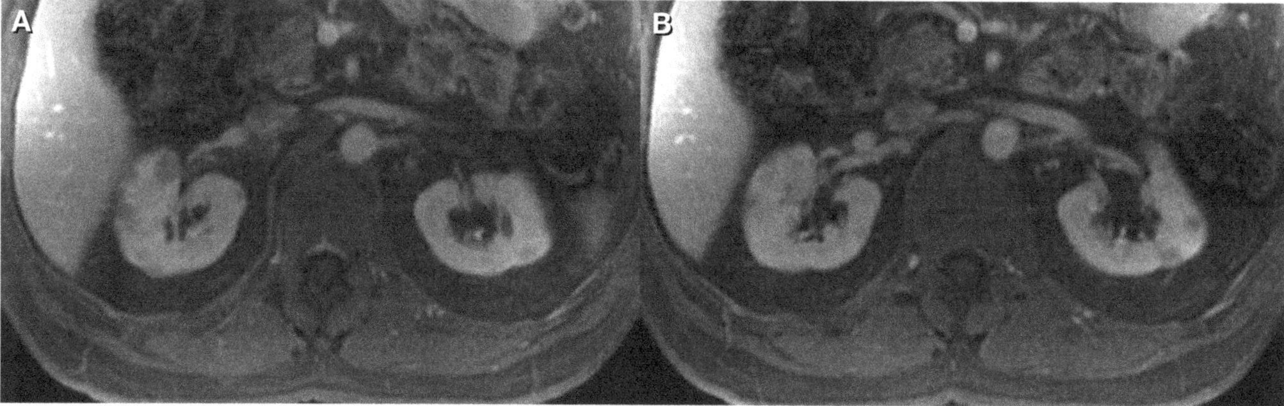

Figure 7.34.3

HISTORY: 66-year-old man with a recent episode of meningitis; hypointense lesions in the liver and kidneys were noted on a recent non–contrast-enhanced CT

IMAGING FINDINGS: Axial fat-suppressed T2-weighted FRFSE images (Figure 7.34.1) show subtle hypointense nodules in the kidneys bilaterally. Axial arterial phase (Figure 7.34.2) and venous phase (Figure 7.34.3) postgadolinium 3D SPGR images show multiple hypoenhancing cortical nodules in the kidneys bilaterally.

DIAGNOSIS: Renal histoplasmosis

COMMENT: Renal fungal infections are described in the recent literature as occurring almost exclusively in renal transplants, but they can occur in native kidneys, most often in immunocompromised patients. In this case, meningitis was caused by disseminated histoplasmosis, which reached the kidneys through hematogenous spread. The appearance of multiple bilateral, hypoenhancing lesions is classic for fungal infection but is also nonspecific; the differential diagnosis includes lymphoma and bilateral RCCs or oncocytomas.

Histoplasma is found worldwide and is particularly common in the Midwest and Southwest regions of the United States, where a high percentage of the population has been exposed, usually through bird droppings. More than 90% of these exposures are clinically silent or result in mild respiratory infections, while a small percentage of patients have serious pulmonary or disseminated infection. Renal involvement in disseminated histoplasmosis was estimated to occur in approximately 20% of cases in 1 study.

ABBREVIATIONS

ADC	apparent diffusion coefficient
ADPKD	autosomal dominant polycystic kidney disease
AML	angiomyolipoma
ARPKD	autosomal recessive polycystic kidney disease
BOLD	blood oxygen level–dependent
CT	computed tomography, computed tomographic
DMSA	dimercaptosuccinic acid
DWI	diffusion-weighted imaging
eGFR	estimated glomerular filtration rate
FRFSE	fast-recovery fast-spin echo
FSE	fast-spin echo
GCK	glomerulocystic kidney
GRE	gradient-recalled echo
GU	genitourinary
IP	in-phase
IP-OP	in-phase and out-of-phase
IVC	inferior vena cava
LAM	lymphangioleiomyomatosis
MRA	magnetic resonance angiography
MRCP	magnetic resonance cholangiopancreatography
MRI	magnetic resonance imaging
MRU	magnetic resonance urography
NSF	nephrogenic systemic fibrosis
OP	out-of-phase
PKD	polycystic kidney disease
RCC	renal cell carcinoma
RPF	retroperitoneal fibrosis
SPGR	spoiled gradient-recalled echo
SSFP	steady-state free precession
SSFSE	single-shot fast-spin echo
TCC	transitional cell carcinoma
TE	echo time
3D	3-dimensional
TS	tuberous sclerosis
2D	2-dimensional
US	ultrasonography
VHL	von Hippel-Lindau

8.

URETERS AND BLADDER

CASE 8.1

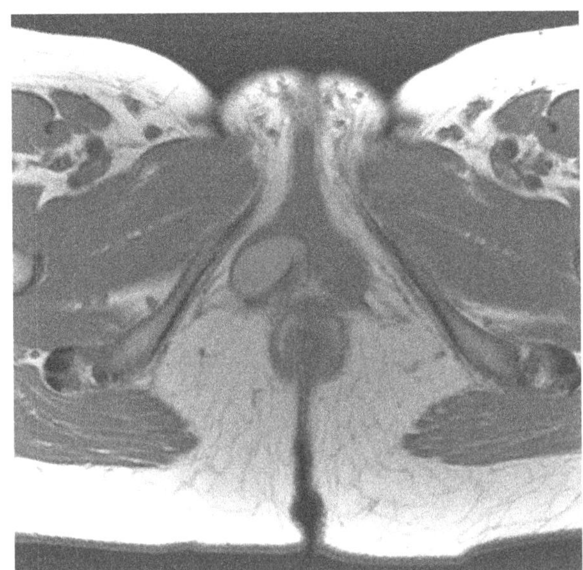

Figure 8.1.1

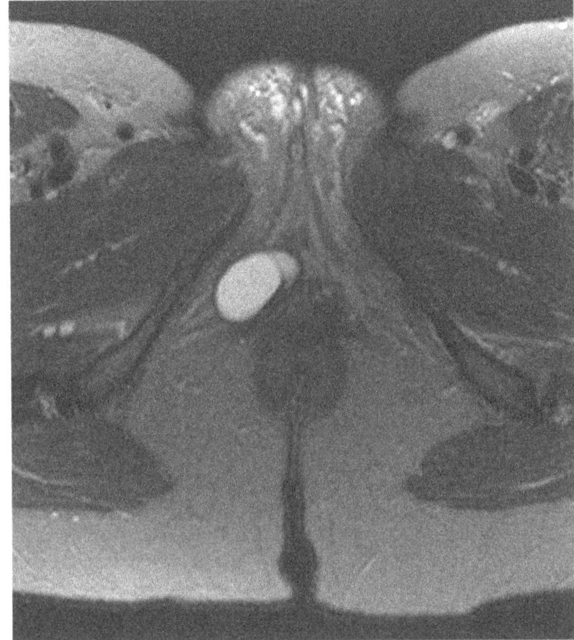

Figure 8.1.2

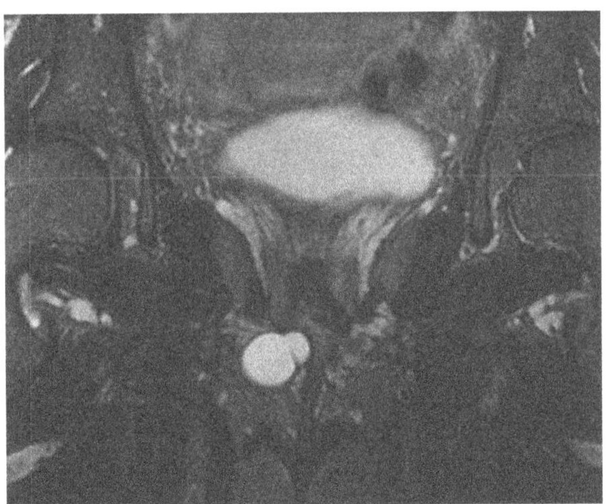

Figure 8.1.3

HISTORY: 51-year-old woman with dysuria and sensation of a mass in the region of the urethra

IMAGING FINDINGS: Axial FSE T1-weighted image (Figure 8.1.1) and axial (Figure 8.1.2) and coronal (Figure 8.1.3) FSE T2-weighted images demonstrate a lobular cystic structure immediately adjacent to the urethral orifice in the perineum.

DIAGNOSIS: Skene duct cyst

COMMENT: There are many glands in the female pelvis, all with different names and slightly different locations. Recognizing a cyst or abscess in one of these glands is usually straightforward by virtue of their characteristic appearance; the main problem is remembering the name of the specific gland involved so you do not appear ignorant to the referring clinician. (Although the alternative method of calling everything a perivaginal or periurethral cyst is also widely employed.)

Skene glands are multiple (6-30) paraurethral glands that are somewhat similar in function to the male prostate and secrete mucus to provide urethral lubrication. Most of these glands are in the mid-distal urethra near the lateral margins.

Skene duct cysts are retention cysts lined with stratified squamous epithelium and caused by inflammatory obstruction of the paraurethral ducts. Symptomatic cysts may be treated by surgical excision or marsupialization.

Differential diagnosis includes urethral diverticulum (more commonly located in the middle third of the urethra and closely opposed to the margin of the urethra), Bartholin duct cyst (cyst in glands along the posterolateral margins of the inferior third of the vagina and derived from the urogenital sinus), Gartner duct cyst (embryologic secretory retention cysts arising from residual wolffian duct remnants located along the anterolateral vagina above the level of the inferior margin of the pubic symphysis), and epidermal inclusion cysts (located at sites of prior trauma or surgery in the posterior or lateral vagina).

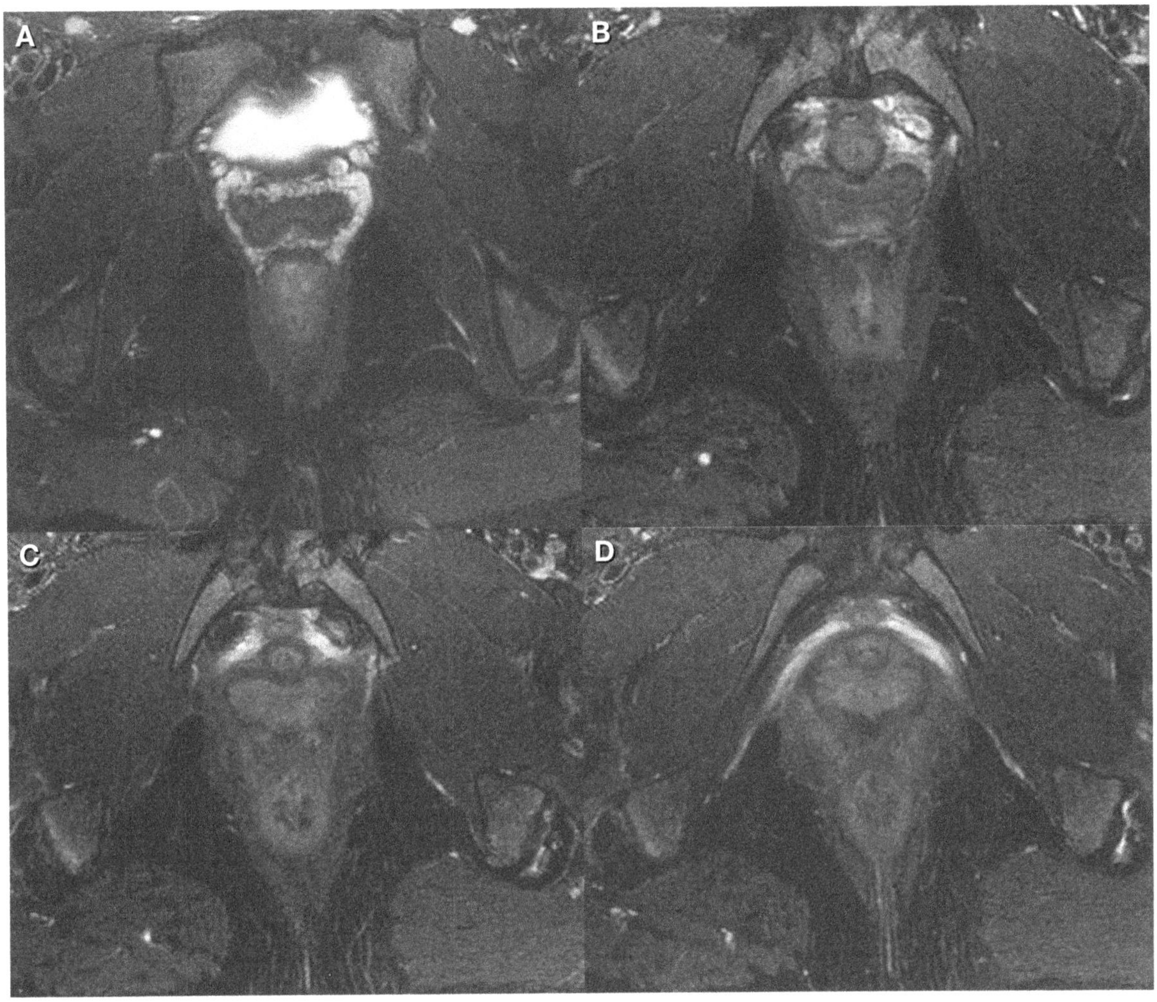

Figure 8.2.1

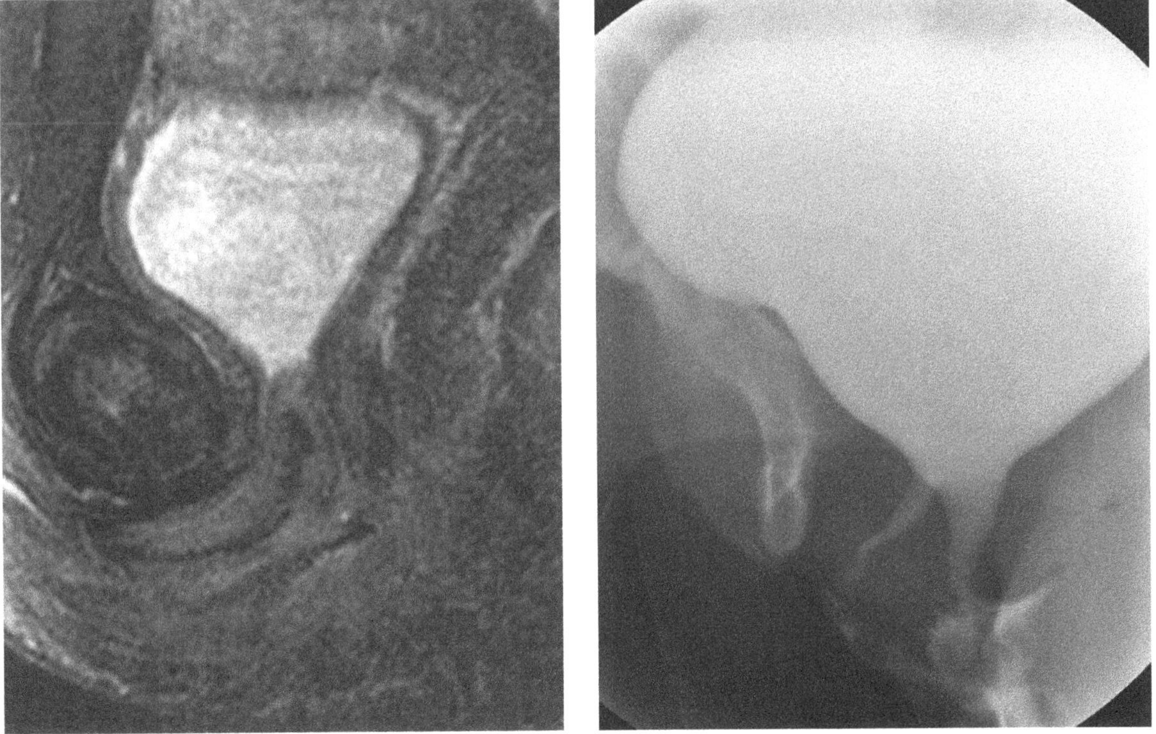

Figure 8.2.2

Figure 8.2.3

HISTORY: 31-year-old woman with stress urinary incontinence

IMAGING FINDINGS: Axial fat-suppressed FSE T2-weighted images (Figure 8.2.1) demonstrate a small round structure anterior to the urethra emerging from the bladder base. A sagittal FSE T2-weighted image (Figure 8.2.2) shows 2 urethras extending from the base of the bladder, and a similar appearance is shown on an image from a voiding cystourethrogram (Figure 8.2.3).

DIAGNOSIS: Duplicated urethra

COMMENT: Urethral duplication is a rare anomaly that occurs most frequently in men and is often associated with other GU and gastrointestinal tract abnormalities. Explanations for urethral duplication include persistence of the cloacal membrane that causes posterior displacement of the mesoderm of the urogenital tubercle and division of the urethral plate, as well as injury during urethral development, resulting in urethral plate division and subsequent duplication.

Reports of women with duplicated urethra are rare and include cases of double urethra and double bladder, double proximal urethra and single distal urethra, accessory urethra posterior to the normal channel, and single proximal urethra with duplicated distal urethra. The most common presenting symptom is incontinence, as in this case, although recurrent UTIs and bladder outlet obstruction have also been reported, and some patients are asymptomatic.

MRI is a good technique for demonstration of GU tract anomalies, and this includes the urethra. Soft tissue contrast is more than adequate to provide excellent visualization of most normal and abnormal anatomy, and sufficient spatial resolution can usually be obtained to visualize small structures like a duplicated urethra. Remember that it's always worthwhile at some point in an examination of anomalous pelvic anatomy to perform a large field-of-view coronal acquisition to document the presence of both kidneys.

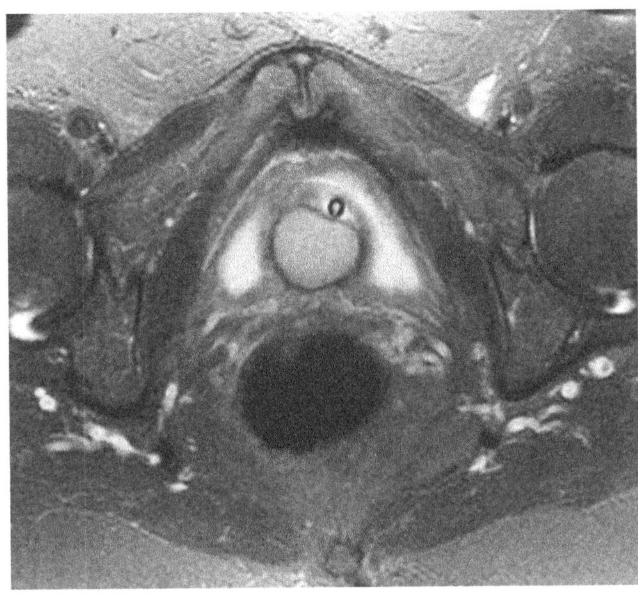

Figure 8.3.1

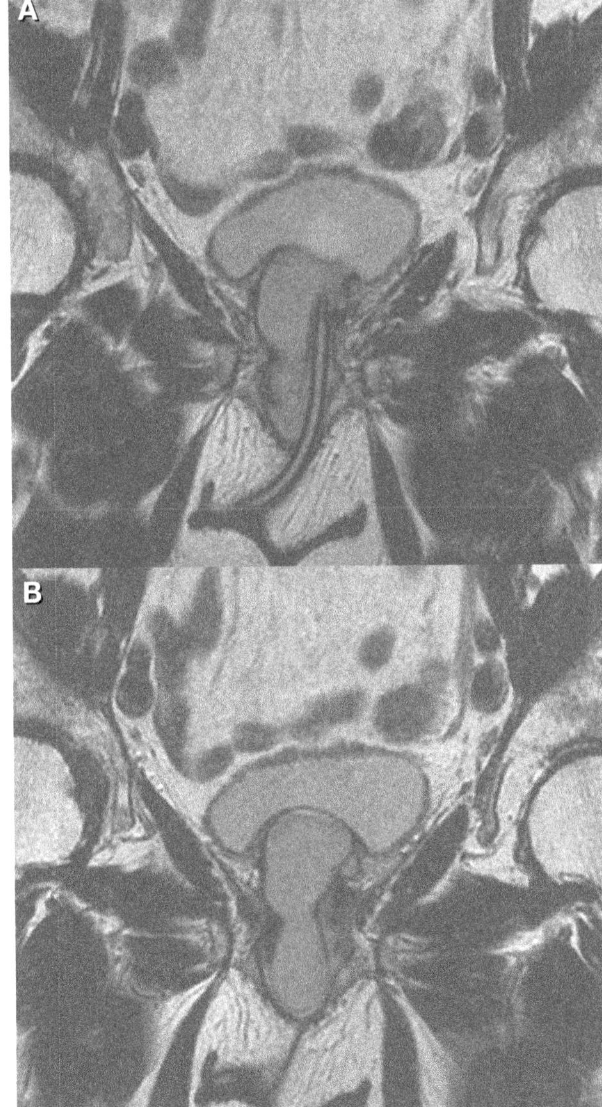

Figure 8.3.2

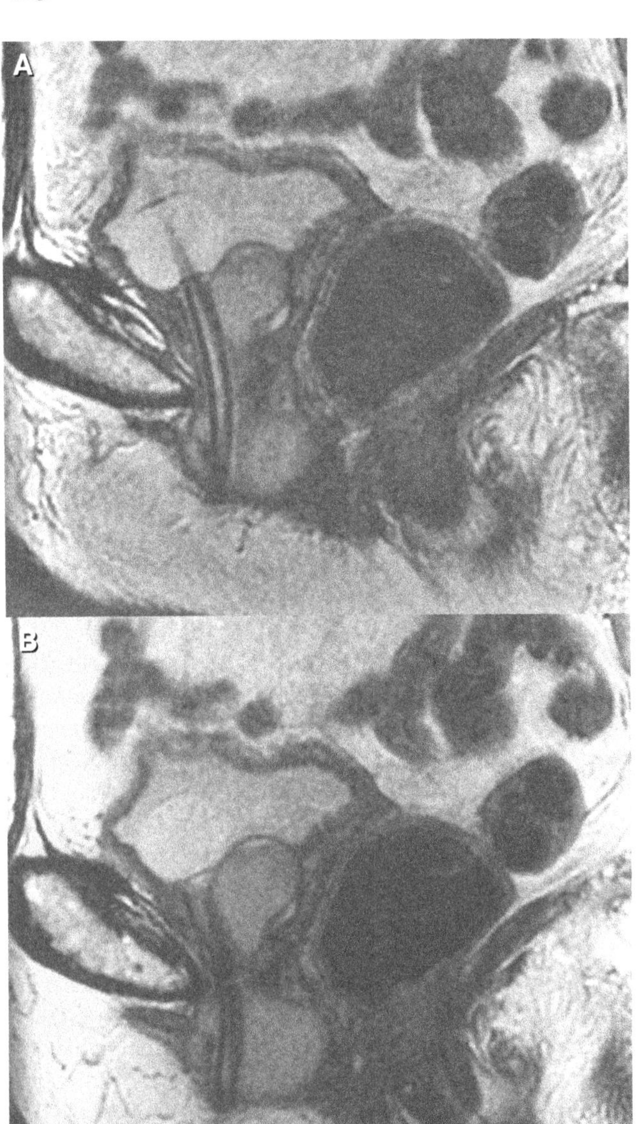

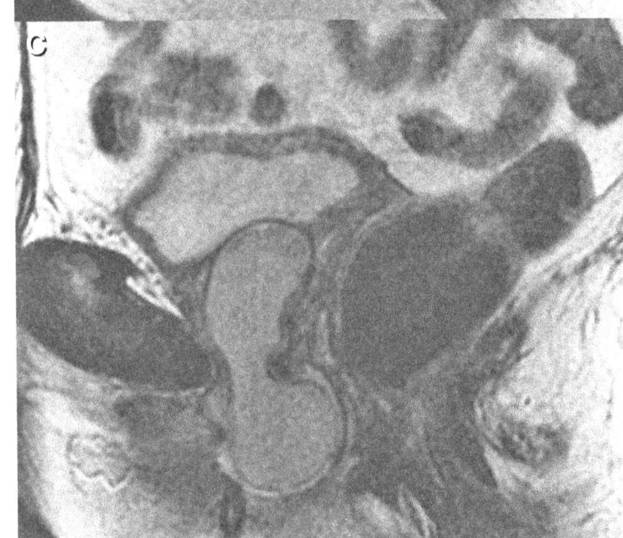

Figure 8.3.3

HISTORY: 80-year-old woman with dysuria and urinary retention

IMAGING FINDINGS: Axial fat-suppressed FSE T2-weighted image (Figure 8.3.1) and coronal (Figure 8.3.2) and sagittal (Figure 8.3.3) FSE T2-weighted images demonstrate a large, lobulated periurethral cystic lesion adjacent to the posterior lateral margin of the urethra and slightly displacing the course of the urethra. Note the Foley catheter in the urethra and bladder.

DIAGNOSIS: Large urethral diverticulum

COMMENT: Urethral diverticuli are protrusions of the urethra into the periurethral fascia lined by epithelium and communicating with the urethra. The prevalence of urethral diverticuli in women is estimated to be 0.6% to 6%, although some authors consider this an underestimation, given a subpopulation with asymptomatic diverticuli who rarely undergo diagnostic imaging. Patients with urethral diverticuli usually present between the ages of 30 and 60 years with repeated lower UTIs, urinary incontinence, dysuria, urgency, urethral pain, or dyspareunia. The classic finding on physical examination is a tender lesion in the anterior vaginal vault, encountered in approximately 50% of cases.

The vast majority of diverticuli are acquired and are thought to arise from rupture of a chronically obstructed and infected paraurethral gland into the urethral lumen. The ruptured gland eventually epithelializes and becomes a true diverticulum. Most diverticuli are located in the middle third of the urethra and involve the posterolateral wall. Approximately one-third of patients have multiple or compound diverticuli.

Although traditional methods for diagnosing urethral diverticuli include voiding cystourethrogram, double-balloon urethrography, or fiberoptic urethroscopy, MRI is now widely recognized as a sensitive and specific technique for identifying these lesions. Optimal MRI protocols should include small field-of-view, high spatial resolution, T2-weighted images with and without fat suppression in axial and sagittal planes, as well as axial T1-weighted images before and after gadolinium administration. 3D FSE sequences are often helpful, and use of a 3-T system with improved SNR is a good idea when available.

Some authors have advocated the use of endovaginal coils and have demonstrated an improved ability to identify the diverticular ostium, but this technique is probably not necessary in all patients. Postgadolinium images are usually not necessary to identify the diverticulum, but the presence of significant rim enhancement can suggest active inflammation or infection. The availability of a fast 10- to 20-second acquisition sometimes saves the day in restless patients whose T2-weighted images are overwhelmed by motion artifact (SSFP or SSFSE images are also helpful in this situation).

Diverticuli on MRI appear as cystic lesions, usually along the posterior and lateral margins of the middle urethra and occasionally with proteinaceous or complex fluid showing high signal intensity on T1-weighted images. Infection and calculus formation are the most common complications of urethral diverticuli and, in most patients, are easily demonstrated on MRI. Neoplasms can arise within diverticuli, most often adenocarcinoma, and the presence of nodular enhancing soft tissue within a diverticulum should raise suspicion of this rare complication.

This case represents a large diverticulum and should be nearly impossible to miss on any cross-sectional modality (although even large lesions can be overlooked on voiding cystourethrography, which depends on adequate filling of the diverticulum with contrast). Case 8.4 shows a more typical example, with a small cystic lesion demonstrating minimal rim enhancement surrounding the posterior and left lateral margins of the urethra.

Differential diagnosis includes cystic lesions of the vagina and perineum: Gartner duct cyst and Bartholin gland cyst (anterior upper vagina and posterolateral lower vagina, respectively), as well as Skene duct cyst (lateral margins of the urethral meatus [see Case 8.1]).

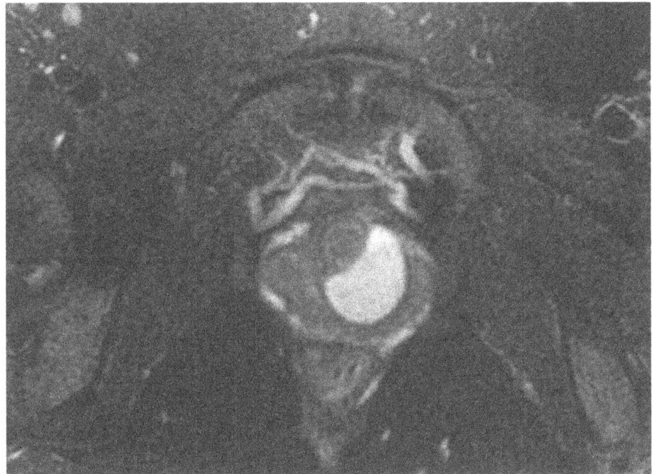

Figure 8.4.1

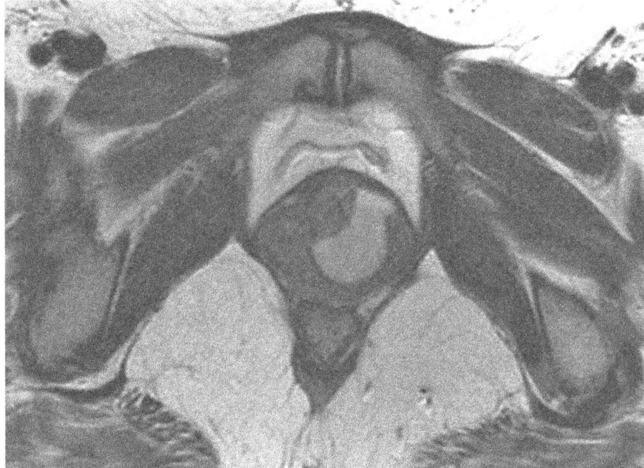

Figure 8.4.2

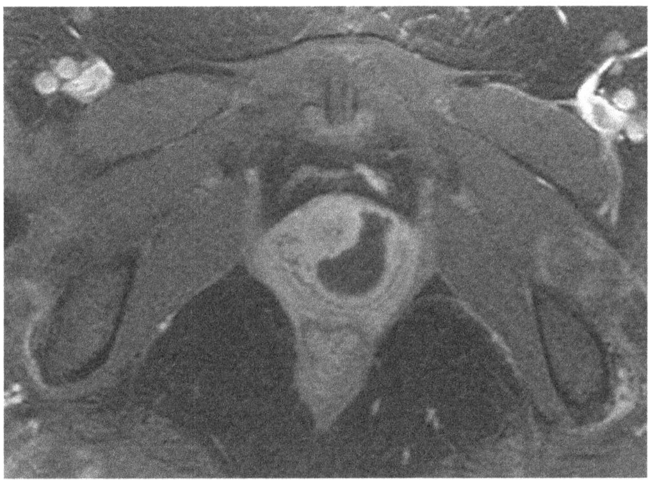

Figure 8.4.3

HISTORY: 35-year-old woman with urge and stress incontinence

IMAGING FINDINGS: Axial FSE T2-weighted images with (Figure 8.4.1) and without (Figure 8.4.2) fat suppression demonstrate a crescentic cystic lesion wrapping around the posterolateral margin of the urethra. Axial postgadolinium 2D SPGR image (Figure 8.4.3) demonstrates mild thickening of the wall and mild rim enhancement of the lesion.

DIAGNOSIS: Urethral diverticulum with mild inflammation or infection

COMMENT: This companion case to Case 8.3 shows the more typical appearance of a urethral diverticulum. The lesion is small and wraps around the posterior lateral margin of the middle urethra. The mild rim enhancement after gadolinium administration could indicate inflammation or infection.

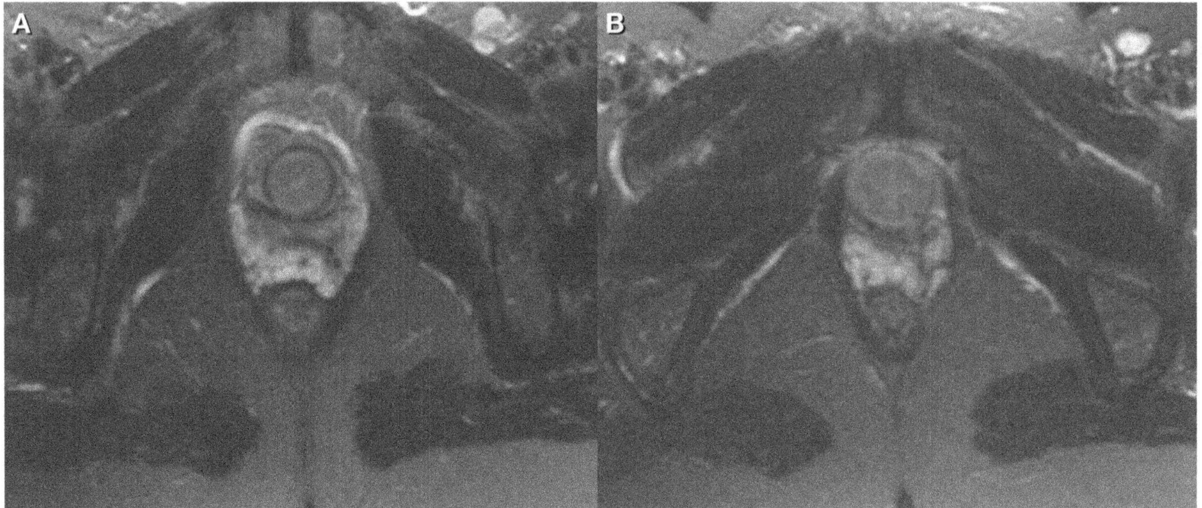

Figure 8.5.1

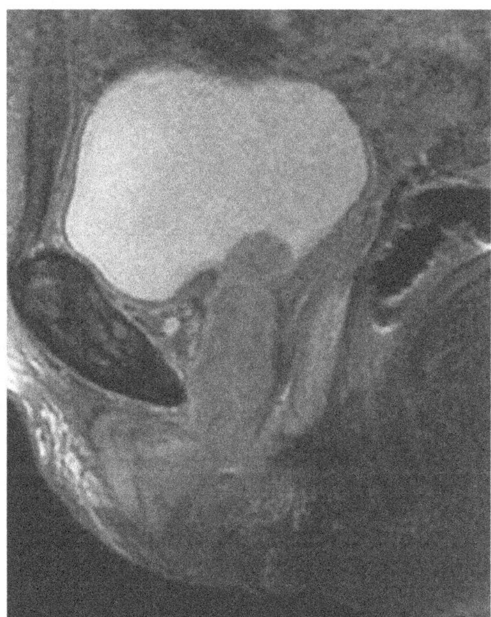

Figure 8.5.2

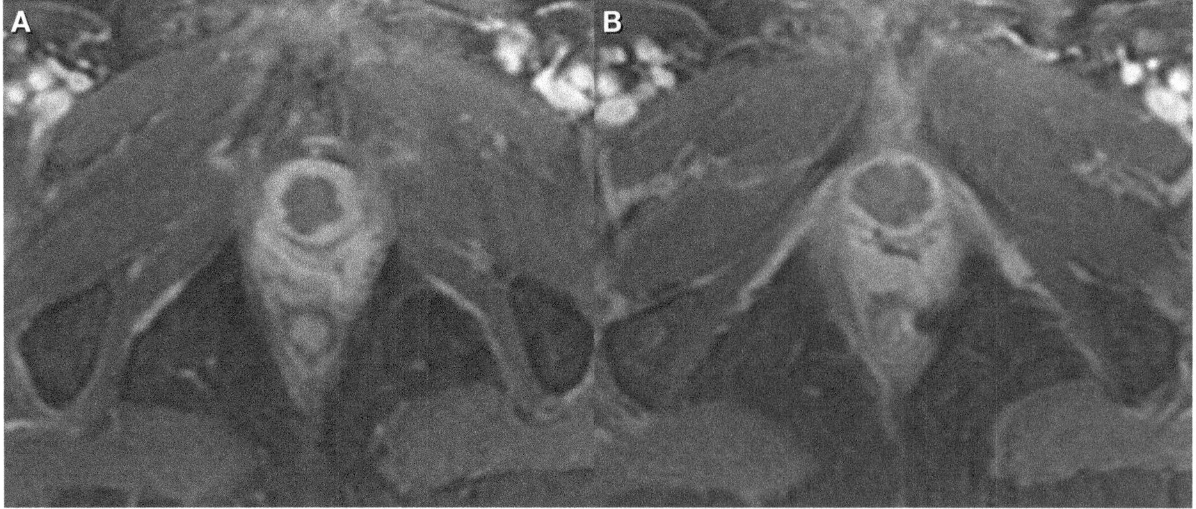

Figure 8.5.3

HISTORY: 56-year-old woman with hematuria

IMAGING FINDINGS: Axial (Figure 8.5.1) and sagittal (Figure 8.5.2) fat-suppressed FSE T2-weighted images demonstrate diffuse soft tissue infiltration of the urethra that protrudes into the bladder base on the sagittal image. Axial postgadolinium 3D SPGR images (Figure 8.5.3) show a rim-enhancing lesion replacing the urethra.

DIAGNOSIS: Urethral squamous cell carcinoma

COMMENT: Urethral carcinoma is an uncommon neoplasm, accounting for 1% of GU cancers. Risk factors include chronic UTIs, urethral diverticuli, human papillomavirus infection, and urethral caruncles, adenomas, polyps, and leukoplakia. SCC is the most common subtype, occurring in 70% of cases and generally involving the distal urethra and external meatus. Transitional cell carcinoma (20%) and adenocarcinoma (10%) usually occur in the proximal urethra.

Urethral tumors involving only the distal third of the urethra are known as *anterior tumors*, have a better prognosis, and are treated with local excision. Lesions involving the proximal urethra usually require a combination of surgery, radiation therapy, and chemotherapy.

Presenting symptoms are nonspecific and include dysuria, urinary frequency, incontinence, and urinary retention.

MRI reveals urethral carcinomas as soft tissue masses that replace the urethra. The normal target appearance of the urethra on T2-weighted images is lost, and extension beyond the outer muscular layer with invasion of adjacent structures can generally be detected with high accuracy. As with imaging of any urethral abnormality, the key to a good examination is obtaining images with high spatial resolution and an adequate SNR—which means a small field of view and multiple signal averages. Using a 3-T system is probably a good idea, with the goal of improving the SNR of the required high-spatial-resolution acquisitions, provided that a 3-T magnet is available and that the patient's urethra isn't encompassed within the dark zone of a shading artifact. An example of carcinoma involving the penile urethra is shown in Case 12.9.

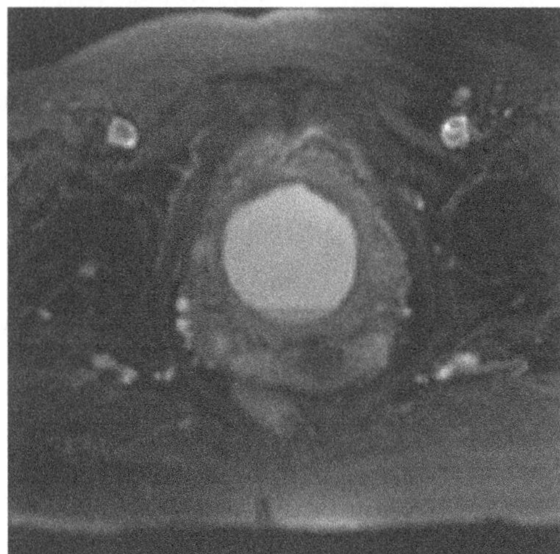

Figure 8.6.1

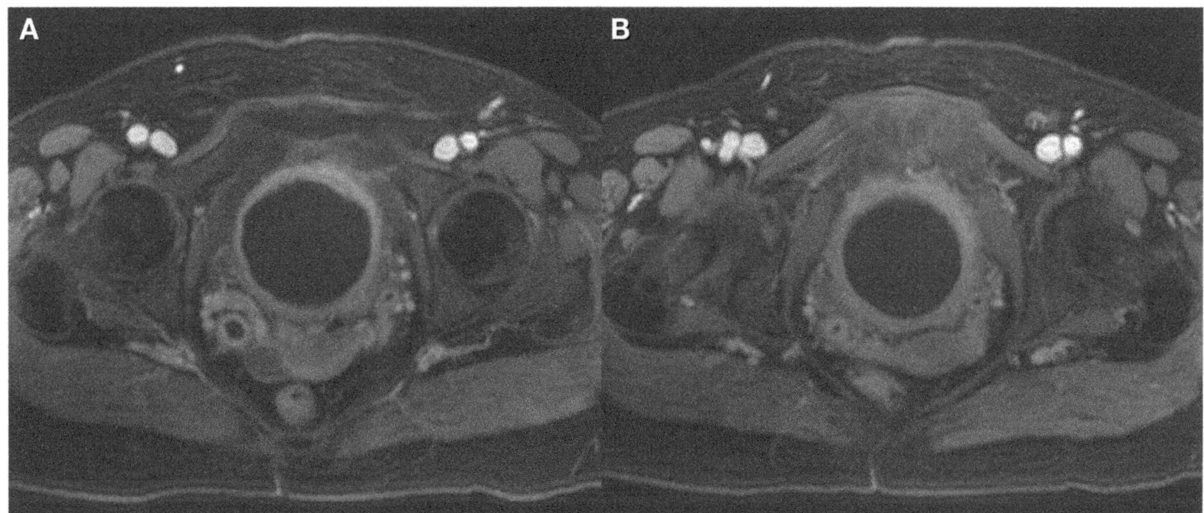

Figure 8.6.2

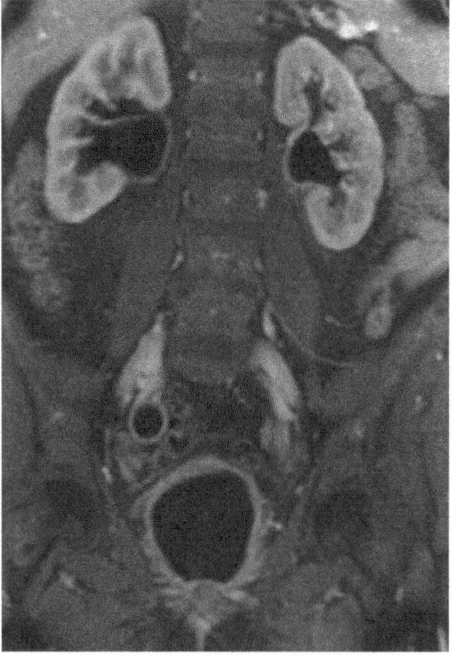

Figure 8.6.3

HISTORY: 64-year-old woman with severe pelvic pain, dysuria and urinary frequency, and gross hematuria

IMAGING FINDINGS: Axial fat-suppressed FSE T2-weighted image (Figure 8.6.1) shows prominent, diffuse bladder wall thickening. Note the fluid-fluid level in the bladder. Axial (Figure 8.6.2) and coronal (Figure 8.6.3) postgadolinium 3D SPGR images again show diffuse bladder wall thickening and enhancement. Note also the dilated and thickened distal ureters, as well as the mild bilateral hydronephrosis.

DIAGNOSIS: Interstitial cystitis

COMMENT: Interstitial cystitis is a chronic syndrome characterized by symptoms of urinary frequency or urgency (or both) and pelvic pain in the absence of bacterial infection or other identifiable pathologic factors. The term *interstitial cystitis* is becoming synonymous with another vaguely defined disorder called *painful bladder syndrome*. Interstitial cystitis was previously considered a rare diagnosis, but recent studies have suggested the diagnosis in as many as 2% of women.

The pathogenesis of interstitial cystitis is not well understood and is probably multifactorial. A prominent theory invokes dysfunction of the normally impermeable bladder urothelium, allowing passage of urinary toxins and irritants, such as potassium, into the bladder wall.

The differential diagnosis of urgency, frequency, and pelvic pain is broad and includes UTI, endometriosis, pelvic inflammatory disease, and vulvovaginitis. Cystoscopy and ureteroscopy were indicated in this patient with gross hematuria, to exclude a malignancy.

The role of imaging and of MRI in particular is unclear in this disorder. MRI was ordered in this case to evaluate the bladder, as well as to survey the pelvis for any additional source of pelvic pain. The appearance of a diffusely thickened bladder wall with mildly increased T2-signal intensity and diffuse enhancement is more suggestive of an inflammatory process than a neoplasm, with involvement of the distal ureters and ureterovesical junctions and subsequent obstruction. Chronic cystitis can lead to an end-stage bladder with reduced capacity and poor function.

Although diffuse involvement of the bladder is probably the most common presentation of cystitis, there are rare varieties, including eosinophilic cystitis and cystitis glandularis, that may occasionally present as focal masses indistinguishable from a neoplasm.

Cystitis has been subjected to several different classification schemes, none of which is completely satisfactory or comprehensive, mainly depending on the limited interests of the specialty involved. Some of these classifications include infectious (bacterial, viral, protozoal, and fungal) vs noninfectious (irritative, toxic, radiation related, and allergic) and acute vs chronic. Clinical or pathologic descriptors of cystitis include *hemorrhagic, bullous* (fluid-filled collections in the bladder submucosa), and *emphysematous*. Cystitis cystica and cystitis glandularis are inflammatory disorders that occur in the clinical setting of chronic irritation and reactive metaplasia of the urothelium. The urothelium proliferates into buds, which grow into the connective tissue of the lamina propria and subsequently differentiate into cystic deposits (cystitis cystica) or mucin-secreting glands (cystitis glandularis). It is much more common for both of these histologic features to be present than to have either one in its pure form.

The ability to distinguish a particular type of cystitis with MRI is probably limited, although when they are large enough, the cysts of cystitis cystica can be visualized. Otherwise, diffuse bladder wall thickening and enhancement are common features.

CASE 8.7

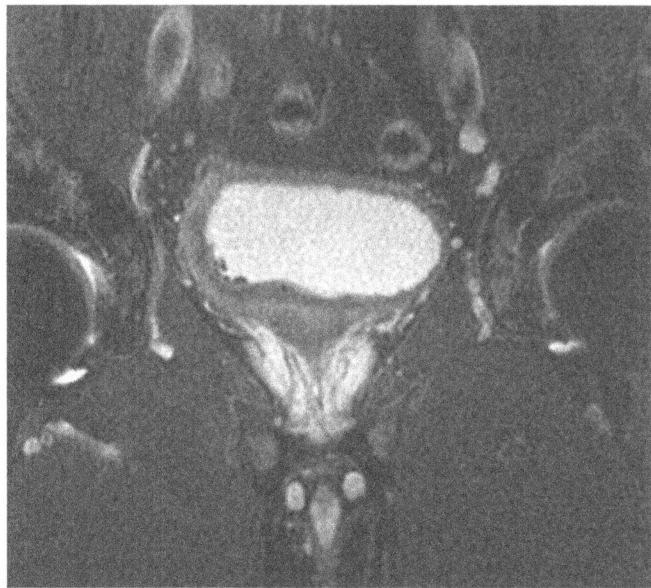

Figure 8.7.1

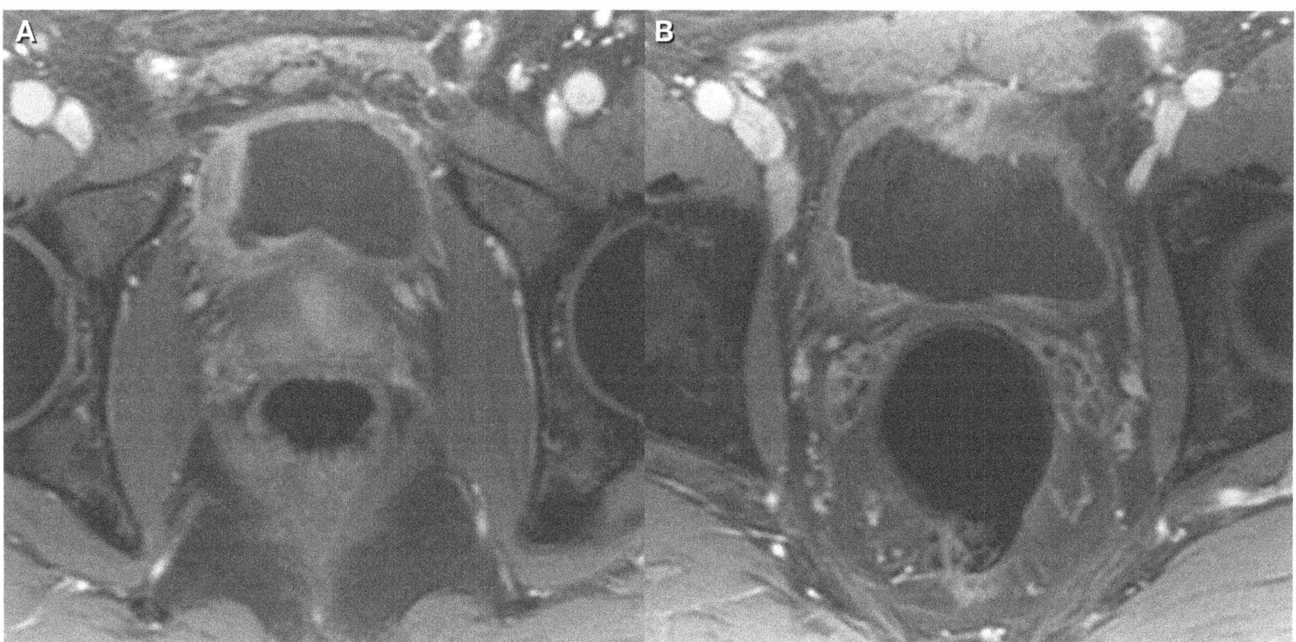

Figure 8.7.2

HISTORY: 52-year-old man with an episode of gross hematuria

IMAGING FINDINGS: Coronal fat-suppressed FSE T2-weighted image (Figure 8.7.1) demonstrates moderate thickening of the right lateral and inferior bladder wall. Axial postgadolinium 2D SPGR images (Figure 8.7.2) again show thickening and mild enhancement of the right bladder wall, as well as focal thickening and enhancement of the anterior wall.

DIAGNOSIS: Bladder amyloid

COMMENT: Just as the state bird of Maryland is the Baltimore oriole, the unofficial house disease of the Johns Hopkins Hospital radiology department is amyloidosis (at least, it was when I was a resident). This situation had the beneficial effect of heightening awareness of the numerous manifestations of a rare disease, but it did tend to skew the residents' perspectives to the extent that it was not uncommon in case conferences to hear *amyloid* mentioned as the second or third differential diagnosis in a patient with cirrhosis, interstitial lung disease, or small bowel fold thickening (and not uncommonly, that was the correct answer).

Amyloidosis represents a heterogeneous group of diseases characterized by deposition of amyloid proteins into the extracellular matrix of 1 or more organs. A number of different misfolded proteins have been identified in amyloid deposits. These proteins are arranged in a β-pleated sheet configuration, and groups of β-pleated sheets constitute insoluble amyloid fibrils that resist proteolysis, cause mechanical disruption, and generate local oxidative stress in various organs. Amyloid deposits, regardless of their composition, all have a characteristic appearance on light microscopy, staining pink with Congo red dye and exhibiting apple-green birefringence under polarized light.

Amyloidosis can be classified by the protein precursors as primary or secondary, with a few additional, much less common forms. Primary amyloidosis (abbreviated *AL* and also called *light chain amyloidosis*) is caused by abnormal plasma cells that produce amyloidogenic immunoglobulin light chain proteins. Secondary amyloidosis (abbreviated *AA*) results from accumulation of fibrils formed from an acute-phase reactant, serum amyloid A protein, and may be associated with rheumatoid arthritis, chronic infections, and inflammatory bowel disease.

Amyloidosis is most commonly systemic, progressive, and fatal, with death resulting from renal or cardiac failure. Localized amyloidosis (usually primary) is seen in 10% to 20% of patients and has a more benign prognosis. Amyloidosis of the urinary tract is most often localized and the bladder is the most common location.

Patients with localized bladder amyloidosis may present with painless hematuria or irritative symptoms. Involvement of the posterior and posterolateral walls is the most common presentation and is seen in this case; however, focal masses projecting into the lumen of the bladder have also been described. Most authors have described the relatively low signal intensity on T2-weighted images as a feature distinguishing amyloid from the main differential diagnosis of urothelial carcinoma. This is a somewhat helpful sign, but remember that many urothelial carcinomas have only mildly increased T2-signal intensity relative to the bladder wall, and this distinction can be particularly difficult to make when the T2-weighted images are acquired without fat suppression. Heterogeneous enhancement is often present and is nonspecific. Early enhancement may reflect underlying inflammation, and its presence may help to identify the lesion but not to distinguish it from urothelial carcinoma. Linear submucosal or mural calcification (best seen on CT) is characteristic of amyloidosis and is rarely seen in untreated urothelial carcinoma.

Treatment of localized bladder amyloidosis usually consists of fulguration or laser therapy, with transurethral resection or partial cystectomy reserved for larger lesions.

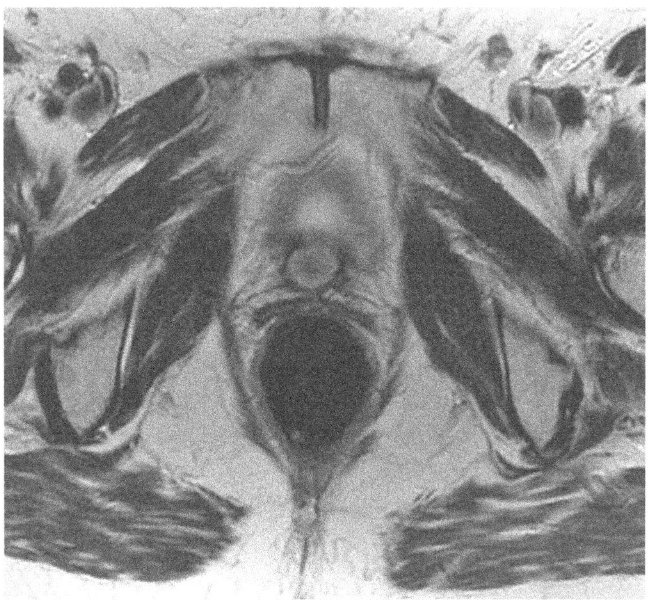

Figure 8.8.1

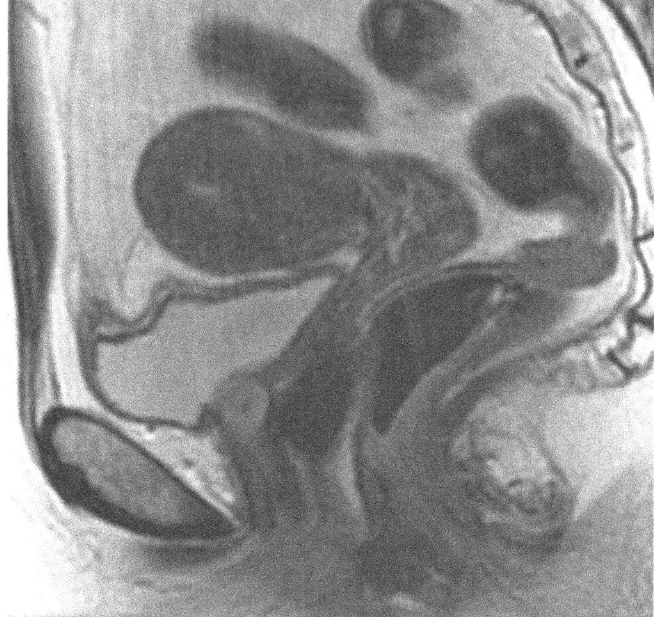

Figure 8.8.2

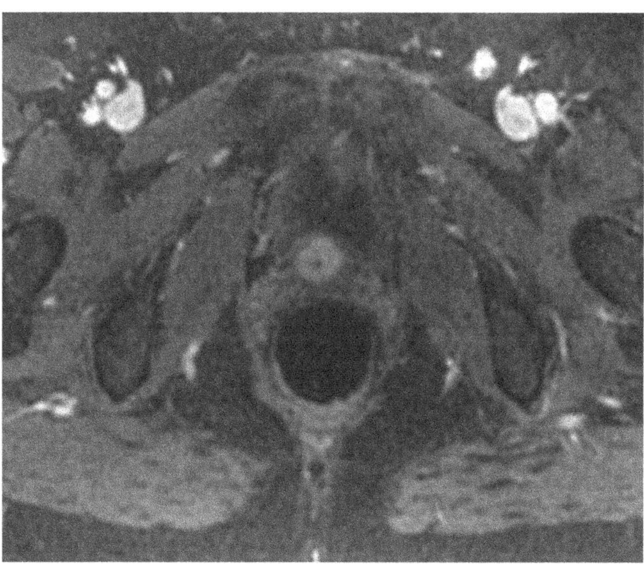

Figure 8.8.3

HISTORY: 48-year-old woman who has dysfunctional uterine bleeding and cyclic bladder irritation; pelvic US revealed a bladder mass

IMAGING FINDINGS: Axial (Figure 8.8.1) and sagittal (Figure 8.8.2) FSE T2-weighted images demonstrate a hyperintense mass near the ureterovesical junction. Venous phase postgadolinium 3D SPGR image (Figure 8.8.3) shows uniform enhancement of the lesion.

DIAGNOSIS: Perivesical and periureteral endometriosis

COMMENT: Endometriosis occurs when endometrial tissue, glands, or stroma are found outside the myometrium or uterine cavity. This common disorder most often occurs in young women aged 25 to 35 years and has been estimated to affect 4% to 15% of all women of child-bearing age. The most common locations for endometrial implants include the ovaries in 54%, broad ligament, pouch of Douglas, and uterosacral ligament. Urinary tract endometriosis is uncommon, but when it occurs, the bladder is the most frequent location (85%), with an estimated prevalence of 1% to 15% of all women with endometriosis.

Symptoms of perivesical and periureteral endometriosis are often nonspecific. Cyclic hematuria is highly suggestive of the diagnosis but is documented in only 20% of cases. Cyclic pain, dysuria, urinary urgency, and pelvic pain are more common symptoms—and are much less specific.

Theories regarding the cause of bladder endometriosis include retrograde menstruation seeding the bladder serosa surface. Endometrial tissue also may be spread to the surface of the bladder during surgery, such as caesarean section. Metaplasia of müllerian remnants has also been invoked, and some authors regard the disease as a true neoplastic process.

Most bladder implants occur along the posterior margin at the vesicouterine pouch. Lesions may present as serosal masses or grow into bladder wall muscle and submucosa, resulting in a mural or submucosal mass. Less frequently, polypoid lesions are seen projecting into the bladder lumen. Typical features of bladder endometriosis include hemorrhagic foci with high T1-signal intensity on precontrast images. This is the classic MRI description of endometriosis, but it was not seen in our patient (which is why there is no precontrast T1-weighted image). Endometrial implants are often heterogeneous and may contain regions with low signal intensity on T1- and T2-weighted images, likely representing fibrosis or hemosiderin, or focal high T2-signal intensity, which may reflect functional endometrial glandular tissue. Most lesions (at least the nonhemorrhagic components) show impressive enhancement after gadolinium administration.

This case has a somewhat atypical lesion located posteriorly just above the vesicourethral junction. The urethra is difficult to visualize on the images provided but was not directly involved.

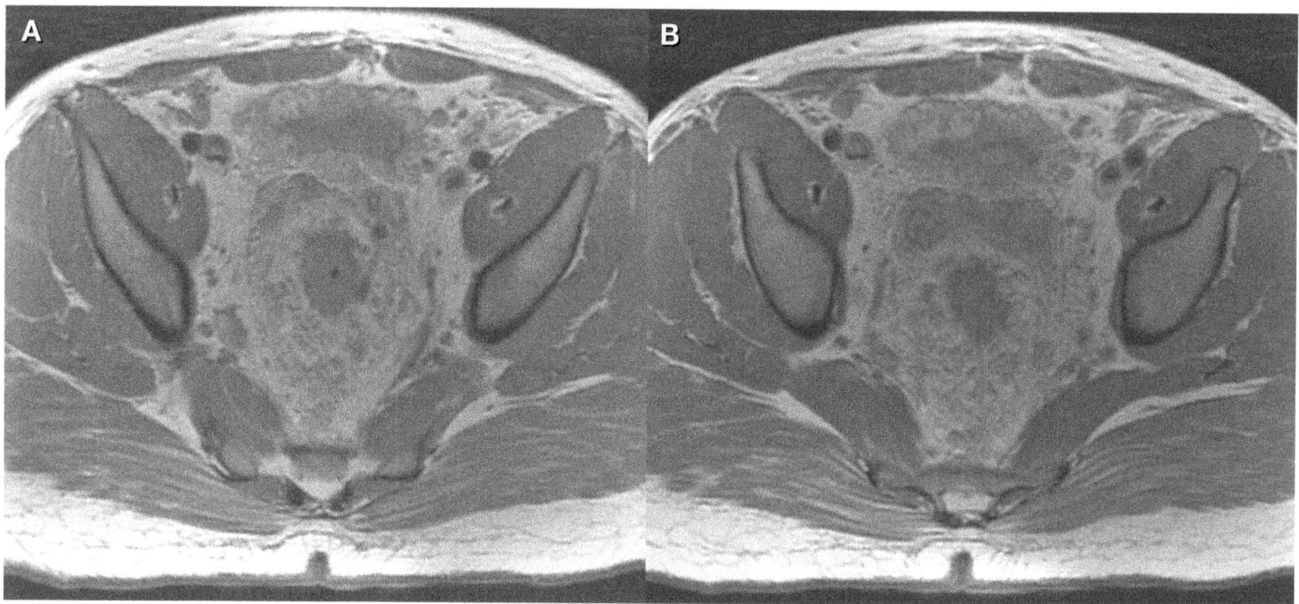

Figure 8.9.1

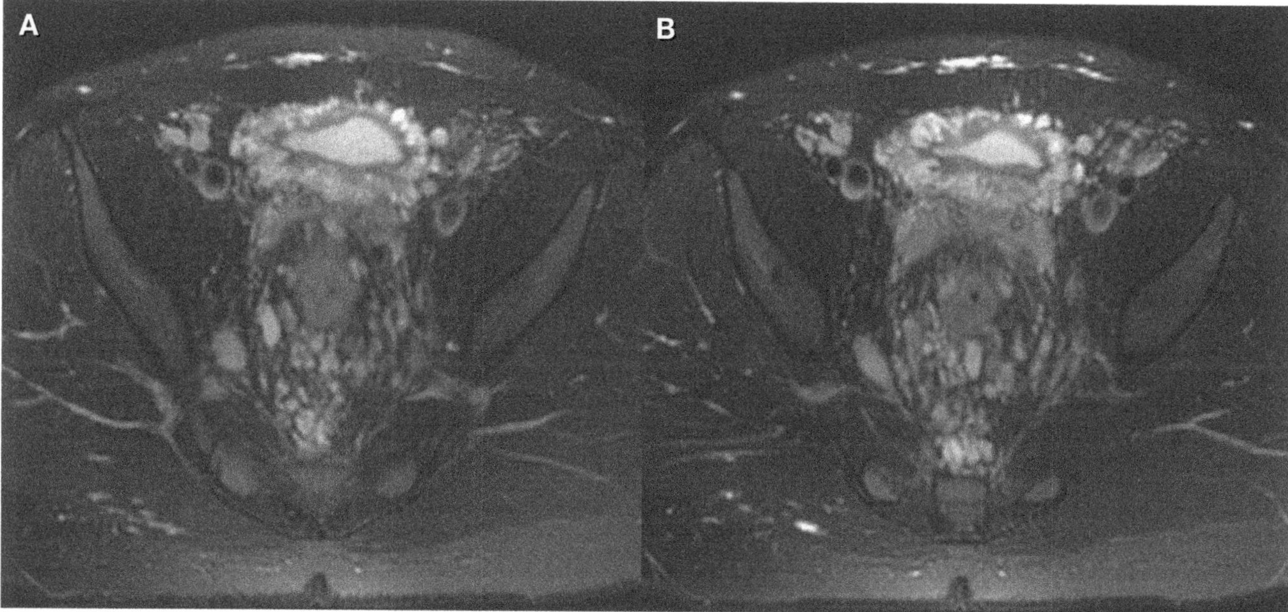

Figure 8.9.2

HISTORY: 20-year-old man with intermittent rectal bleeding

IMAGING FINDINGS: Axial T1-weighted (Figure 8.9.1) and fat-suppressed T2-weighted (Figure 8.9.2) FSE images demonstrate infiltration of the bladder wall by innumerable small, cystic lesions. Note infiltration of the mesorectal fat by nodular serpiginous structures also bright on T2-weighted images.

DIAGNOSIS: Lymphangiomatosis involving the bladder and rectosigmoid colon

COMMENT: Lymphangiomatosis is a rare developmental disorder of the lymphatic system, with 95% of cases occurring in the head, neck, and axilla. The other 5% develop in various locations, and involvement of the GU system occurs most frequently in the kidneys. Renal lymphangiomatosis, although rare, has a striking and classic appearance that has been well described in the literature (and also in Case 7.24 of this book). Lymphangiomatosis affecting the bladder is less common.

This case shows the expected cystic lesions with markedly hyperintense signal on T2-weighted images and circumferential infiltration of the bladder wall. This patient also had diffuse involvement of his mesentery, with lesions extending inferiorly to encompass the mesorectal fat and rectum. He had no symptoms attributable to the bladder involvement, but he did report intermittent rectal bleeding, which undoubtedly was related to the rectal lymphangiomas.

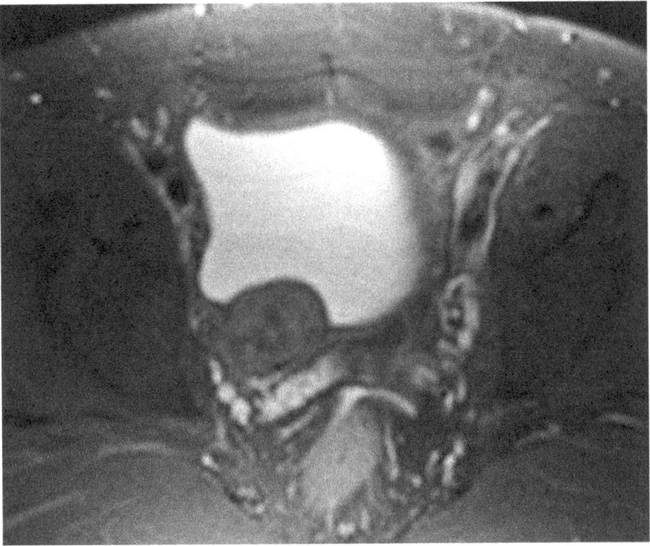

Figure 8.10.1

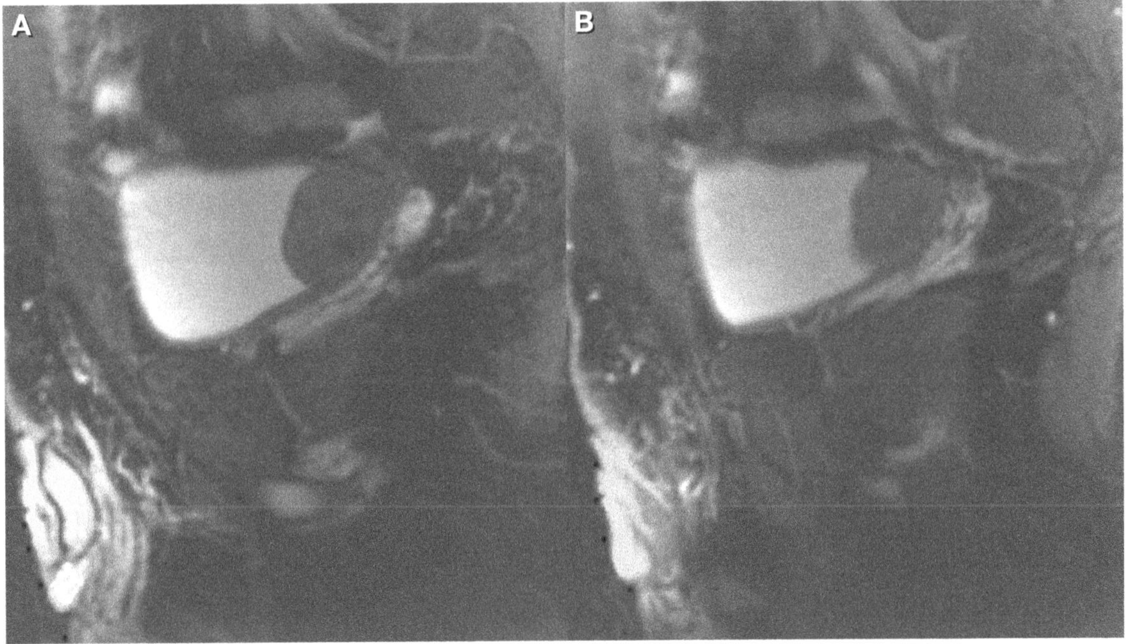

Figure 8.10.2

HISTORY: 40-year-old man with hypertension and hyperaldosteronism; a CT performed at an outside institution demonstrated an incidental bladder mass

IMAGING FINDINGS: Axial (Figure 8.10.1) and sagittal (Figure 8.10.2) fat-suppressed FSE T2-weighted images show a round, well-circumscribed mass in the posterior wall of the bladder with uniformly low T2-signal intensity.

DIAGNOSIS: Bladder leiomyoma

COMMENT: Bladder leiomyomas are rare lesions, accounting for 0.4% of all bladder tumors. However, they are the most common benign bladder neoplasm and the most common bladder tumor of mesenchymal origin. They probably have a female predilection, and most patients present between 40 and 60 years of age. Leiomyomas may be asymptomatic, but more commonly they present with obstructive or irritative symptoms or with hematuria.

Leiomyomas arise in the submucosa of the bladder and may have submucosal (7%), intravesical (63%), or extravesical

(30%) growth patterns. They are composed of smooth muscle cells lacking mitotic activity, cellular atypia, and necrosis. Lesions generally are well defined with smooth margins. The classic description of leiomyomas outside of the uterus is that they look like uterine fibroids, with low signal intensity on T1- and T2-weighted images and variable enhancement after gadolinium administration.

This case fits this pattern, and the relatively low T2-signal intensity and smooth margins suggest the diagnosis. But remember that not all uterine fibroids have this appearance, and it seems unreasonable to expect any more consistent behavior from extrauterine leiomyomas. Solitary fibrous tumors of the bladder (we don't have an example) also have low T2-signal intensity, but fortunately they are also benign lesions with a similar presentation and similar excellent prognosis following surgical resection.

CASE 8.11

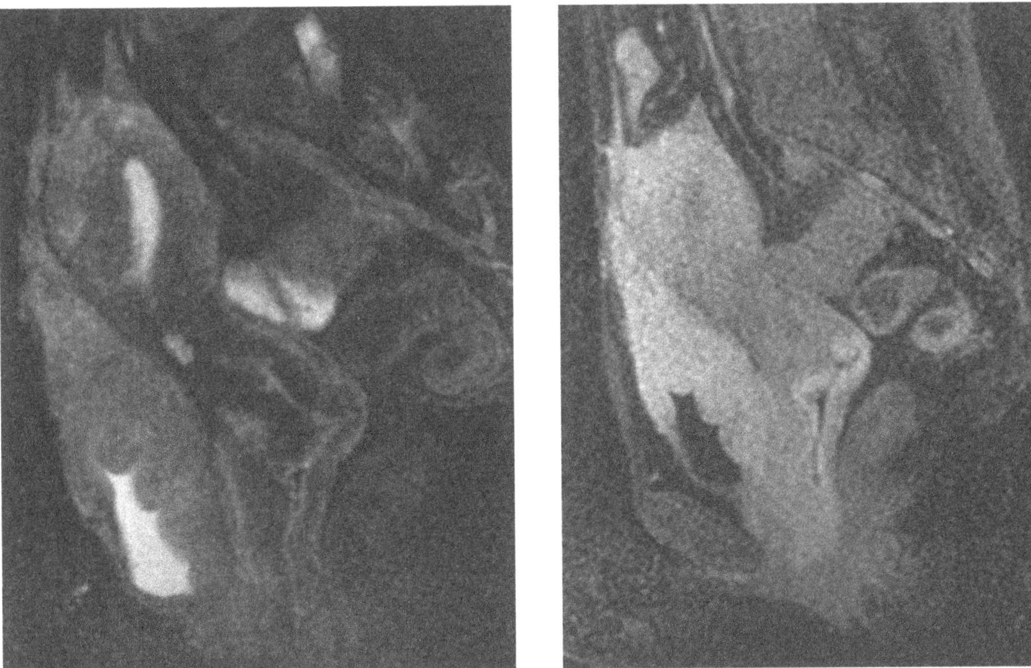

Figure 8.11.1

Figure 8.11.3

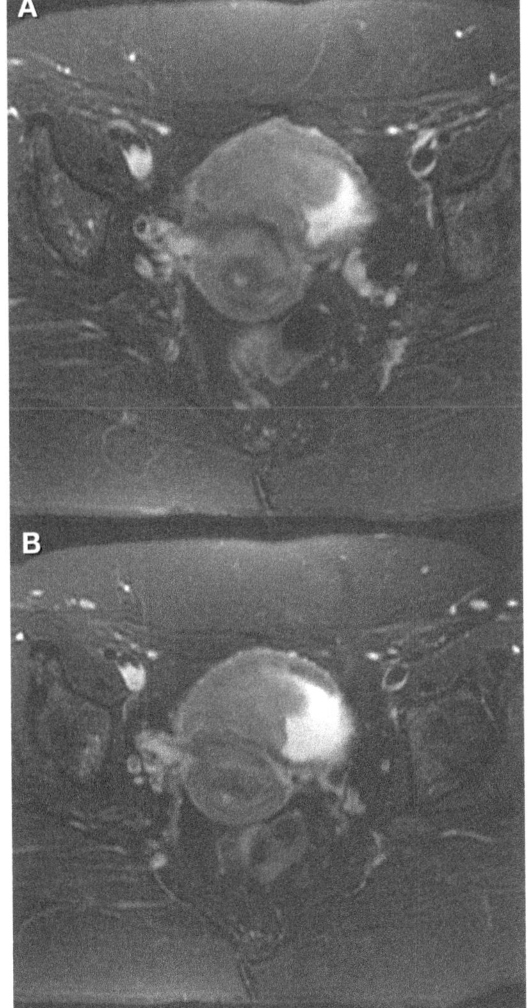

Figure 8.11.2

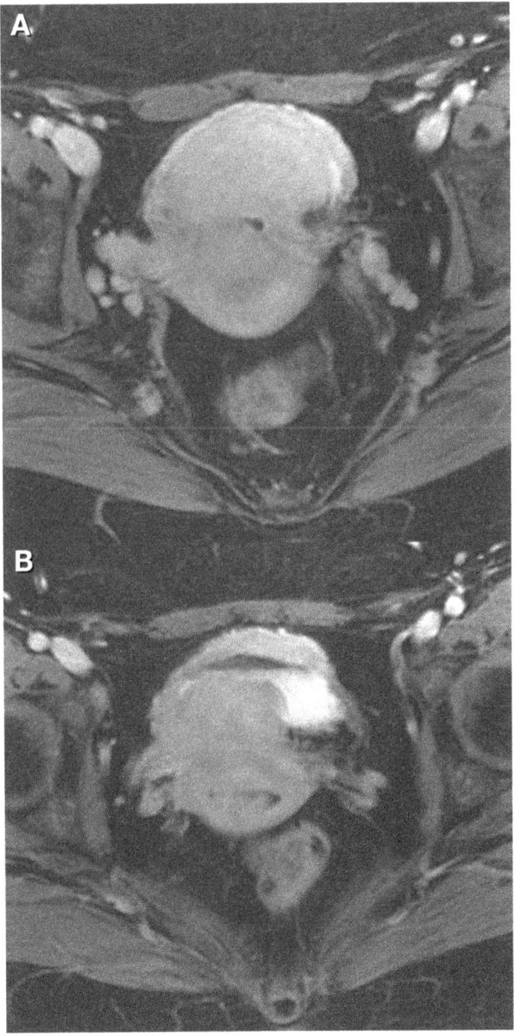

Figure 8.11.4

HISTORY: 37-year-old woman with a history of neurofibromatosis and menometrorrhagia

IMAGING FINDINGS: Sagittal fat-suppressed 3D FSE T2-weighted image (Figure 8.11.1) and axial 2D fat-suppressed FSE images (Figure 8.11.2) reveal masslike thickening of the posterior and superior bladder walls, with relatively low signal intensity. Sagittal arterial phase postgadolinium 3D SPGR image (Figure 8.11.3) demonstrates early uniform enhancement of the lesion. Axial delayed postgadolinium 3D SPGR images (Figure 8.11.4) show moderate diffuse, persistent enhancement of the mass.

DIAGNOSIS: Bladder ganglioneuroma

COMMENT: Neurogenic tumors of the bladder are rare, and bladder ganglioneuromas have been reported only a few times in the literature, including 1 case in a Labrador retriever. The history of neurofibromatosis in this case suggests that this might be a neurogenic lesion. (Menometrorrhagia is not a particularly helpful symptom for a bladder mass, except possibly in endometriosis, which typically has a more focal appearance often accompanied by hemorrhagic foci with increased T1-signal intensity.) The smooth, lobulated appearance of the lesion is nonspecific, and so are the relatively low T2-signal intensity and the moderate arterial and late phase enhancement; this would be somewhat atypical for a neurofibroma. Plexiform neurofibromas can have an infiltrative appearance, but often they are more heterogeneous on T2-weighted images, with regions of focally high signal intensity (ie, a target appearance). Urothelial carcinoma should probably be included in the differential diagnosis for completeness, mostly on the basis of its relatively high prevalence, and lymphoma could also be a consideration (see Case 8.14 for an example).

Ganglioneuromas are classified among the neuroblastic tumors, which include neuroblastoma, ganglioneuroblastoma, and ganglioneuroma. The distinction between the different lesions depends on the degree of maturation of the neoplastic neuroblasts and development of schwannian stroma. Ganglioneuromas usually have at least modestly increased T2-signal intensity relative to adjacent parenchyma—not really seen in this case—but the infiltrative nature of the mass and the moderate diffuse enhancement are typical features.

Considered benign tumors, ganglioneuromas nevertheless have potential for malignant degeneration. Because of the diffuse involvement of the bladder in this case, surgery was not considered a good option. This patient has been monitored for 8 years without a significant change in the appearance of the mass.

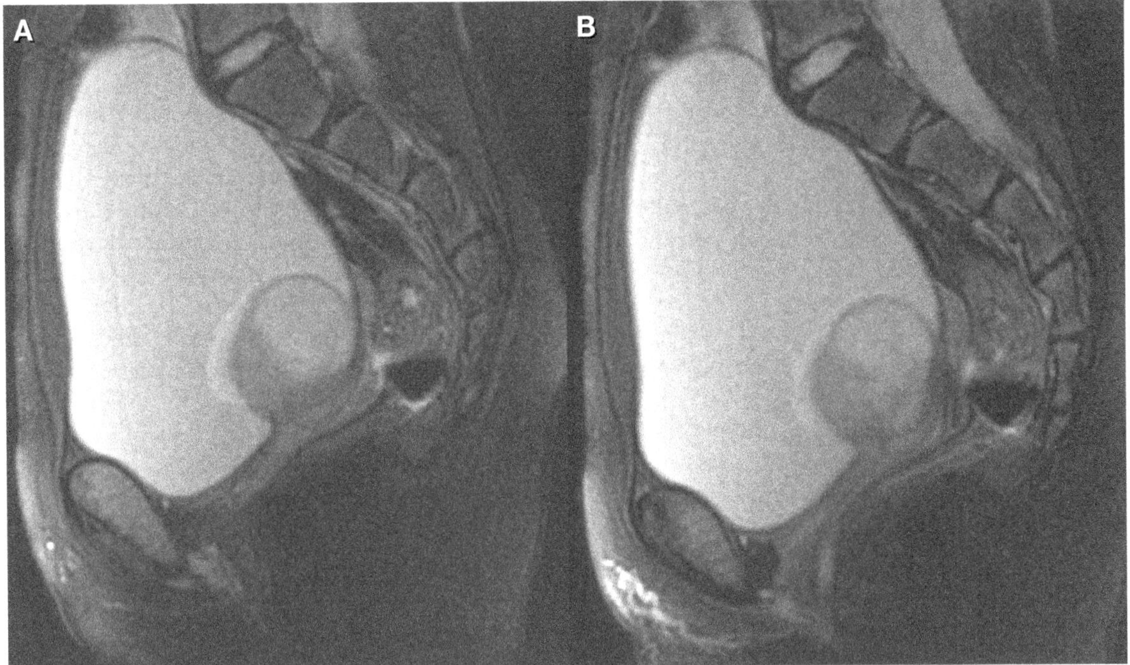

Figure 8.12.1

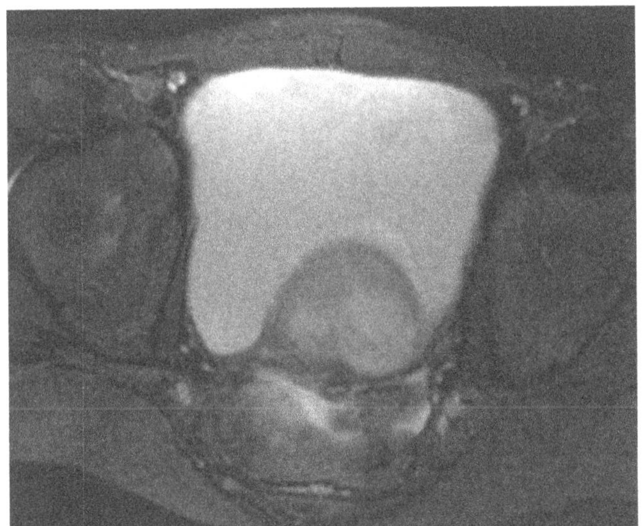

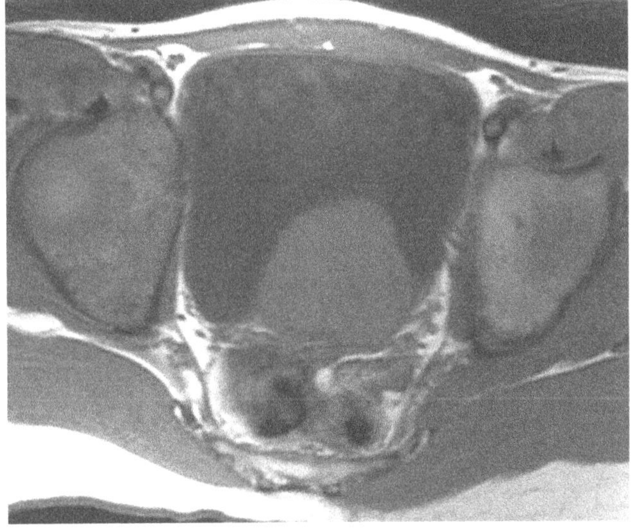

Figure 8.12.2

Figure 8.12.3

HISTORY: 10-year-old girl with urinary frequency and urgency and dysuria

IMAGING FINDINGS: Sagittal (Figure 8.12.1) and axial (Figure 8.12.2) fat-suppressed FSE T2-weighted images demonstrate a heterogeneous mass with cystic components in the posterior bladder. An axial T1-weighted FSE image (Figure 8.12.3) shows uniform moderate signal intensity throughout the bladder mass.

DIAGNOSIS: Inflammatory myofibroblastic tumor

COMMENT: IMT represents a rare benign lesion with a variable histologic appearance that usually includes myofibroblast and fibroblast spindle cells, a collagenous or myxoid matrix, and inflammatory cells consisting of plasma cells, lymphocytes, and eosinophils. This appearance can mimic sarcomas and spindle cell carcinomas; however, IMT is distinguished by lack of marked cytologic atypia and atypical mitotic figures. Rhabdomyosarcoma is the usual differential diagnosis in the pediatric setting and can be excluded if immunohistochemical staining for MyoD1 or myogen is negative.

The cause of IMT is uncertain. The prevailing view is that IMT represents a reactive inflammatory lesion, while others believe it more likely to be a low-grade mesenchymal malignancy. IMTs have been found in children, as well as in adults after bladder instrumentation or surgery. Some authors make a distinction between the 2 lesions—the adult postinstrumentation lesion is termed *inflammatory pseudotumor* and is considered nonneoplastic.

IMTs are slow-growing tumors that follow a benign course. Most patients present with hematuria, although pain and dysuria have also been reported. A conservative surgical approach with partial cystectomy or local excision usually has excellent results. Recurrence of IMT has been reported in adults after resection but not in children, and there are no reports of malignant degeneration or metastatic disease.

The appearance of IMT on MRI is nonspecific, typically consisting of heterogeneous polypoid lesions with regions of increased T2-signal intensity and heterogeneous enhancement. In children, the major differential diagnosis is rhabdomyosarcoma, and the lesions are often indistinguishable on the basis of imaging appearance. In adults, IMT (or inflammatory pseudotumor) may have an appearance similar to a papillary urothelial carcinoma or other, less common bladder tumors.

As an unrelated technical issue, notice the signal nonuniformity on the axial T1-weighted image. Signal intensity and SNR are much lower on the left side than on the right side, and this usually occurs because of a failure of left-sided phased array coil elements (it's much more difficult to appreciate this characteristic on the fat-suppressed T2-weighted images). Sometimes, the fix is as simple as making sure the coil is completely plugged in, but repair or replacement of the affected coil may be required. Both technologists and radiologists should inspect all clinical images for quality control issues. It's surprising how often problems like this one are initially ignored or forgotten, and eventually, everyone becomes accustomed to looking at bad images.

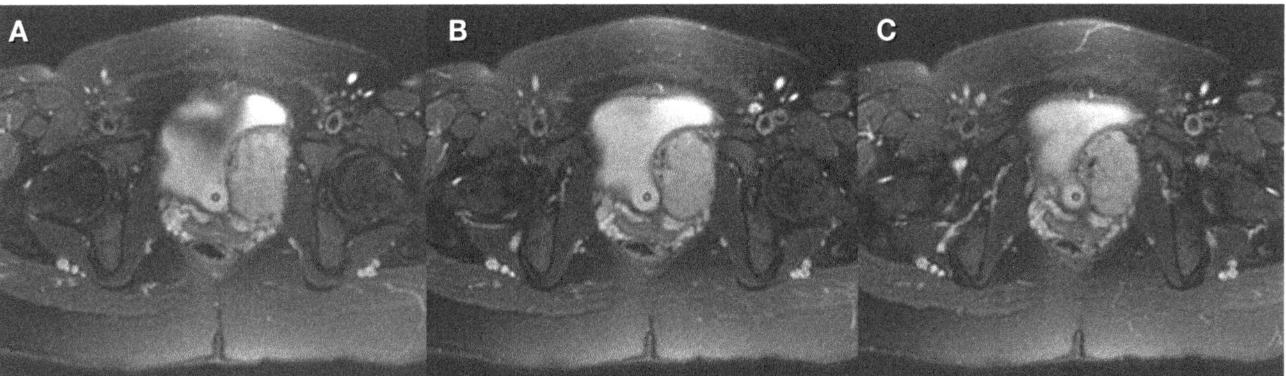

Figure 8.13.1

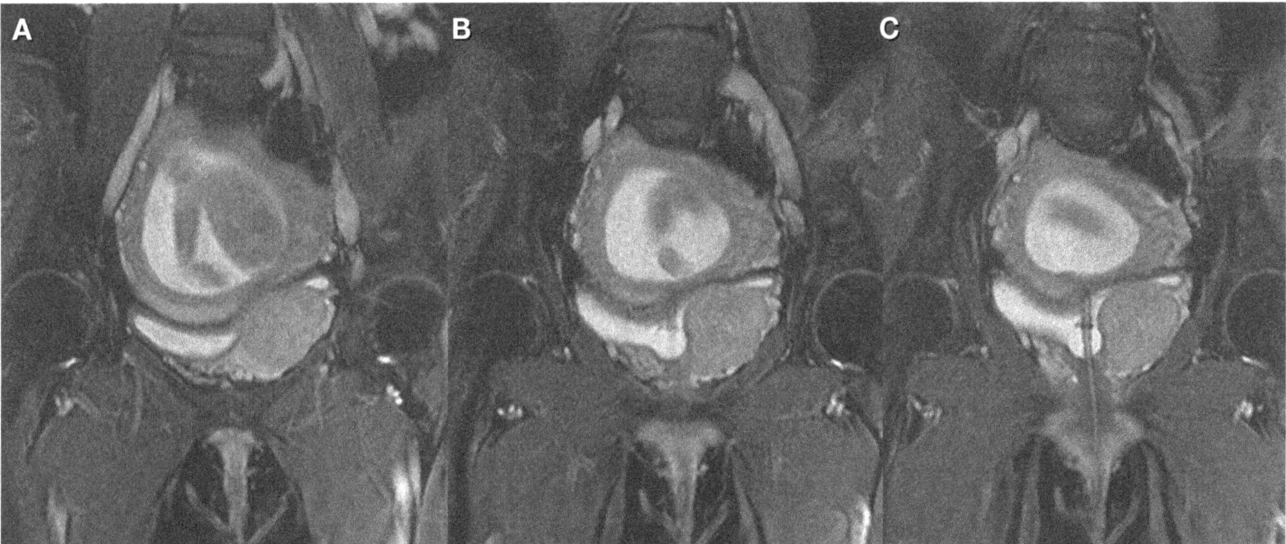

Figure 8.13.2

HISTORY: 37-year-old pregnant woman with episodes of shortness of breath, headache, visual changes, and palpitations occurring with urination

IMAGING FINDINGS: Axial fat-suppressed FSE T2-weighted images (Figure 8.13.1) and coronal fat-suppressed SSFP images (Figure 8.13.2) demonstrate a well-defined mass with high T2-signal intensity adjacent to or originating from the left bladder wall. Note also the vascular flow voids near the inferior medial margin of the mass on the axial images, as well as the gravid uterus, on the coronal images.

DIAGNOSIS: Paravesicular paraganglioma (pheochromocytoma)

COMMENT: Pheochromocytomas are catecholamine-secreting tumors derived from mature chromaffin cells of the sympathetic nervous system. Most extra-adrenal pheochromocytomas (about 10% of all lesions) occur in sympathetic ganglia and paraganglia and are therefore termed *paragangliomas*. Bladder paragangliomas are rare, accounting for 6% of paragangliomas and less than 1% of all bladder tumors, but the classic clinical presentation is so memorable that these lesions are almost always included in any review of bladder tumors.

Classic symptoms occur in 65% to 85% of patients and include headaches, hypertension, palpitations, and sweating in association with bladder contraction during micturition. Hypertensive crises have also been triggered by defecation, sexual intercourse, and bladder instrumentation. Most patients are fairly young at diagnosis, with an average age of 40 years, and men and women are affected equally. Urinary and plasma catecholamine levels are elevated in nearly all patients. Hematuria, a much less distinctive sign, is present in a majority of patients.

Bladder paragangliomas often have an appearance similar to paragangliomas in other locations: well-demarcated, fairly homogeneous lesions when small, with moderate to high signal intensity on T2-weighted images and intense early enhancement following gadolinium administration and with rapid washout on venous and equilibrium phase images. Ring calcification was described as a distinctive feature in a CT case series but has not been widely reported, and in any event would be difficult to delineate with MRI. One small series noted the unusual finding of high signal intensity on precontrast T1-weighted images, although we have not seen this feature in the few cases we have encountered.

Treatment of bladder paragangliomas is surgical, consisting of local excision following adrenergic blockade.

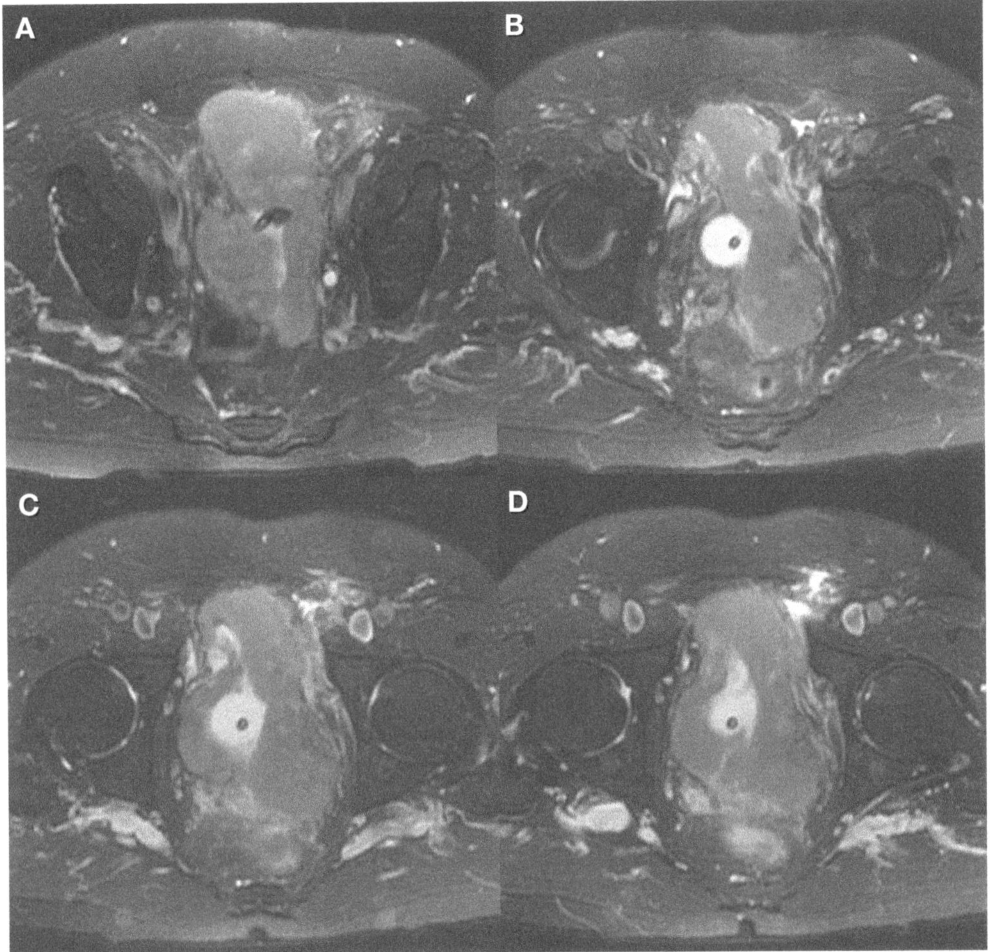

Figure 8.14.1

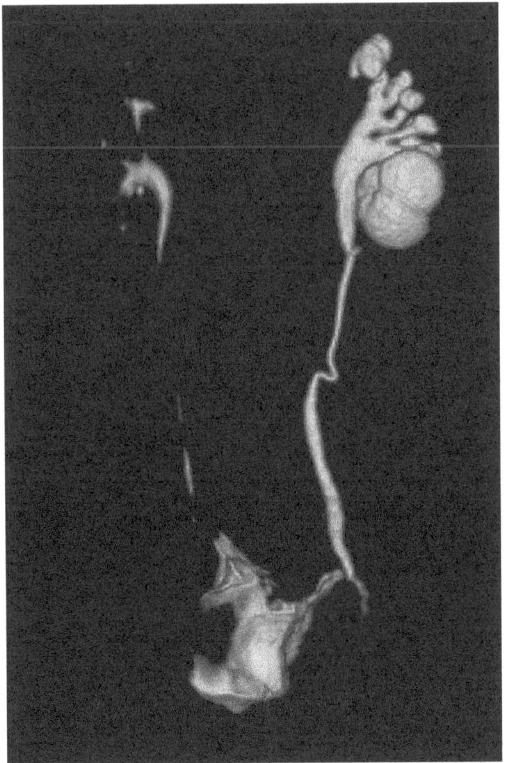

Figure 8.14.2

HISTORY: 77-year-old man with intermittent, increasing gross hematuria

IMAGING FINDINGS: Axial fat-suppressed T2-weighted FSE images (Figure 8.14.1) show marked diffuse thickening of the bladder wall, with relatively low mural signal intensity. A volume-rendered image from 3D FRFSE noncontrast MR urography (Figure 8.14.2) reveals mild left hydronephrosis and hydroureter with severe distortion of the bladder lumen by the thickened walls (note also the left renal cyst).

DIAGNOSIS: Bladder lymphoma

COMMENT: This case is an example of primary bladder lymphoma, a rare diagnosis accounting for less than 1% of bladder neoplasms and 0.2% of all lymphomas. Secondary bladder involvement is more common and is seen in 10% to 20% of terminal non-Hodgkin lymphoma cases. The most common cell types are mucosa-associated lymphoid tissue (abbreviated *MALT*) and diffuse large B-cell lymphoma. Common presenting symptoms include intermittent hematuria, dysuria, and urinary frequency. Primary bladder lymphoma has a female predilection, occurring 6.5 times more frequently in women than men.

The prognosis of primary bladder lymphoma is uncertain given the relative rarity of the disease, but it is thought to be favorable in most cases. Primary bladder lymphoma can be treated with chemotherapy, irradiation, or surgery, or a combination.

The appearance at MRI is nonspecific and can be similar to urothelial carcinoma and other bladder neoplasms. Both diffuse infiltration of the bladder wall (as seen in this case) and 1 or more focal masses have been described.

At our institution, when an MRI is ordered to evaluate a suspected bladder mass, the examinations requested are about equally divided between MR urograms, which include upper-tract imaging, and pelvic MRIs, which do not. If you're not able to check the images before the patient leaves, it's probably a good idea to include in your protocol at least 1 or 2 large field-of-view acquisitions covering the kidneys and ureters. This step may prevent the patient from returning for an additional examination that may or may not be paid for by insurance, and it may even occasionally yield useful diagnostic information.

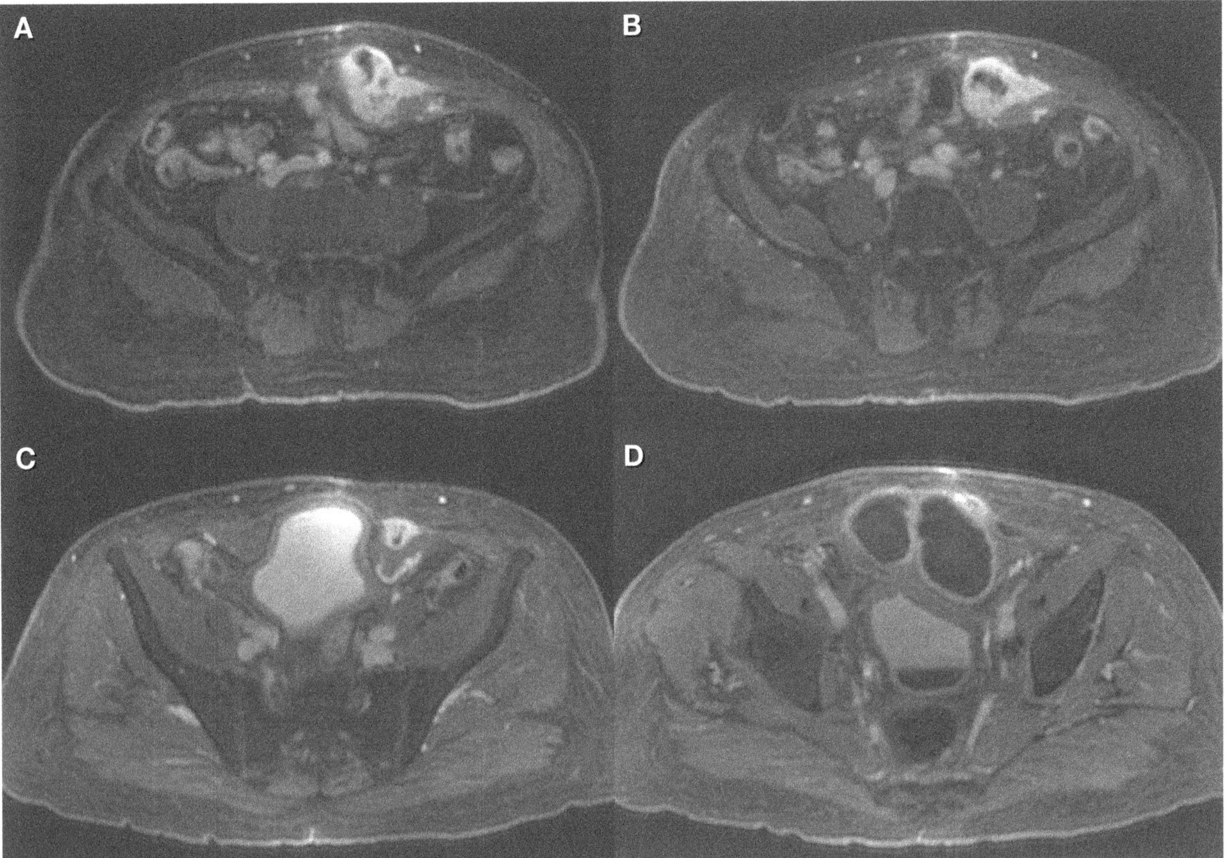

Figure 8.15.1

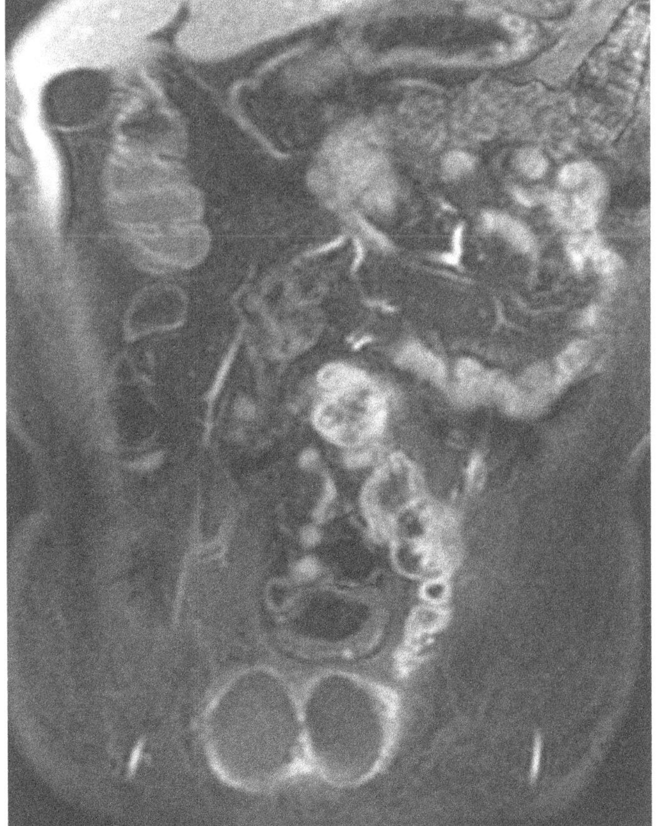

Figure 8.15.2

HISTORY: 59-year-old man with voiding dysfunction; a bladder mass was found at cystoscopy

IMAGING FINDINGS: Axial (Figure 8.15.1) and coronal (Figure 8.15.2) postgadolinium 3D SPGR images show a complex, partially cystic or necrotic mass extending from the bladder superiorly along the anterior abdominal wall toward the umbilicus.

DIAGNOSIS: Urachal carcinoma

COMMENT: The urachus is a structure connecting the bladder to the allantois during early embryologic development and usually regresses in late fetal life to form the median umbilical ligament extending from the dome of the bladder to the umbilicus. Incomplete regression can lead to anomalies, including patent urachus, urachal cyst, and umbilical urachal fistula. Urachal remnants are surprisingly common and usually asymptomatic; they have been identified in one-third of patients in autopsy studies.

Although the urachus is lined by transitional epithelium, adenocarcinomas comprise 90% of urachal tumors. Adenocarcinomas represent 2% of all bladder neoplasms, and urachal adenocarcinoma accounts for one-third of these. Urachal carcinoma has a male predilection, with most patients presenting between age 40 and age 70 years with symptoms that include hematuria, dysuria, suprapubic mass, abdominal pain, mucosuria, and discharge of blood, mucus, or pus from the umbilicus.

Urachal carcinomas can be identified by their characteristic location near the dome of the bladder, often extending into the abdominal wall along the course of the urachus. Of these lesions, 90% occur near the bladder rather than the umbilicus, and the prominent extravesical component is atypical of most other bladder neoplasms. Urachal carcinomas usually are large at diagnosis and have solid components, as well as prominent cystic, mucin-containing elements showing high signal intensity on T2-weighted images. Peripheral stippled calcification is present in 70% of cases and is uncommon in most other bladder neoplasms.

This case shows many of the classic features of urachal carcinoma on MRI, with large, predominantly cystic lesions adjacent to the bladder (albeit at the inferior margin) and extensive nodular tumor growth along the urachus to the umbilicus. The anterior bladder wall was involved in this case but without a large intravesical component.

Most tumors are locally invasive at diagnosis, and approximately 50% of patients present with metastatic disease. The overall prognosis is relatively poor, with 5-year survival rates of 20% to 40%. Surgery, when feasible, usually consists of cystectomy with en bloc resection of the urachal mass, posterior rectus fascia, peritoneum, and abdominal wall.

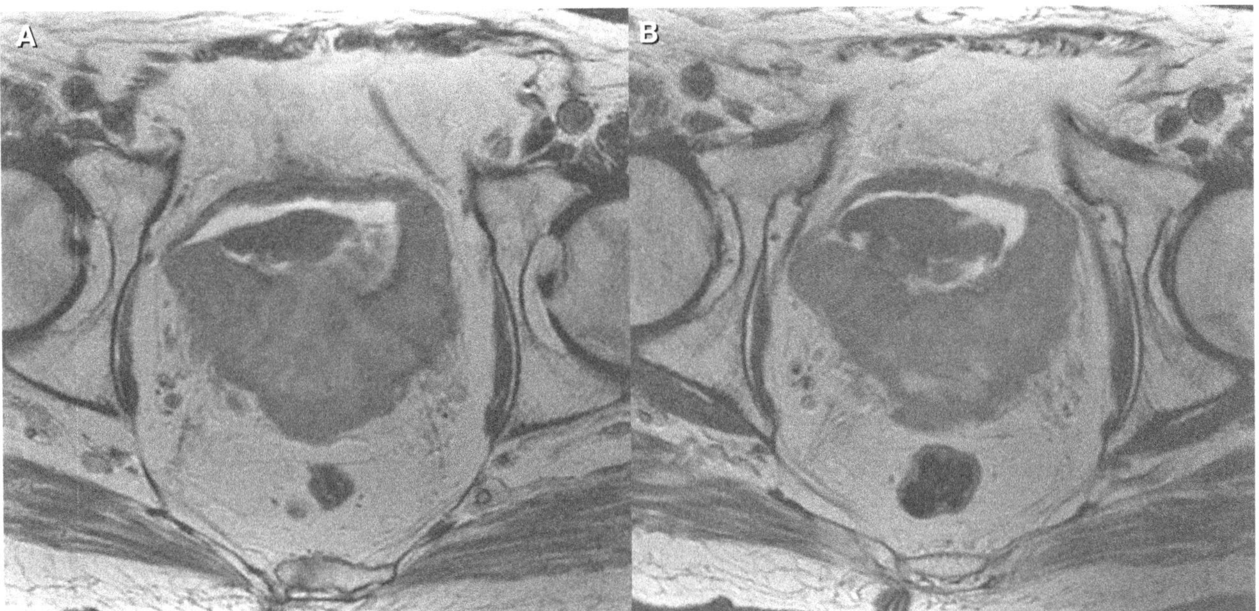

Figure 8.16.1

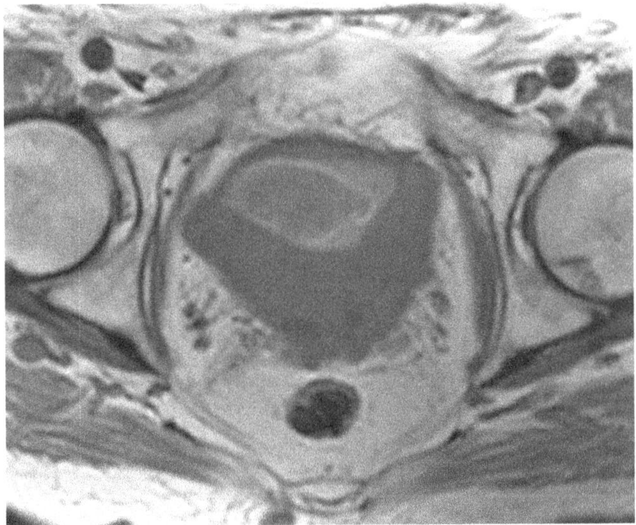

Figure 8.16.2

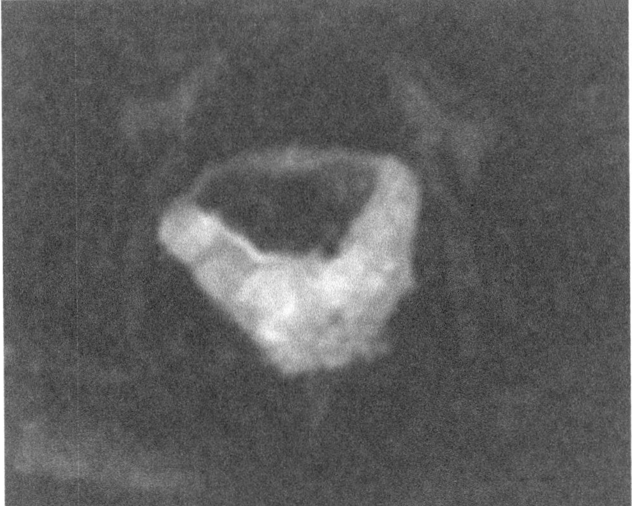

Figure 8.16.3

Figure 8.16.4

HISTORY: 68-year-old man with hematuria

IMAGING FINDINGS: Axial T2-weighted (Figure 8.16.1) and T1-weighted (Figure 8.16.2) FSE images, axial diffusion-weighted image (b=800 s/mm^2) (Figure 8.16.3), and sagittal T2-weighted FSE image (Figure 8.16.4) demonstrate marked heterogeneous thickening of the posterior and lateral bladder walls, with high signal intensity on the diffusion-weighted image. The mass has extended posteriorly to invade and encase the seminal vesicles and prostate. Note also a large filling defect present in the bladder lumen, with a hyperintense rim on the T1-weighted image.

DIAGNOSIS: Squamous cell carcinoma of the bladder, with a large clot in the bladder lumen

COMMENT: The vast majority of bladder tumors in the United States are urothelial carcinomas, with SCC accounting for less than 5%. This isn't true in other parts of the world where schistosomiasis is endemic; in these regions, SCC is the dominant tumor and represents more than 50% of bladder cancers.

Risk factors for SCC in the schistosomiasis-free population include chronic irritation and inflammation from indwelling catheters, bladder calculi, or chronic infection. Patients usually present after age 60 years, in contrast to the earlier presentation in patients with schistosomiasis.

SCC usually has a sessile growth pattern, as in this case, in contrast to the high percentage of papillary urothelial carcinomas. There are very few other features that can be used to distinguish SCC from other types of bladder cancer. The prognosis of bladder SCC is generally poor since these tumors are often high grade and locally aggressive, and most patients have extravesical extension at the time of diagnosis.

Nearly all forms of bladder cancer show high signal intensity on DWI, and a few investigators have demonstrated that this technique can identify very small tumors without the need for gadolinium administration. It's important to use a relatively high b value in this setting (our default value is 800 s/mm^2) in order to completely eliminate the fluid signal from the bladder so that the high signal intensity from a bladder wall lesion is not masked by urine. The high b value eliminates the T2 shine-through effect of urine, and the corresponding loss in SNR can be compensated by increasing the number of excitations.

Bladder clots or hematomas are not uncommon in patients with bladder carcinoma. They usually are easy to identify by their high T1-signal intensity on precontrast images and their lack of enhancement after gadolinium administration.

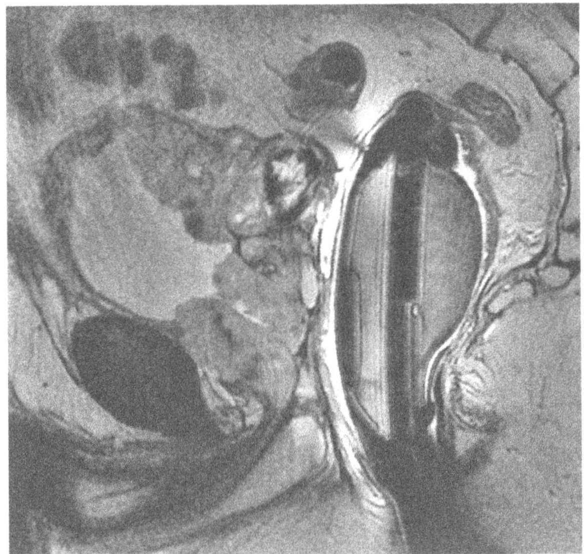

Figure 8.17.1

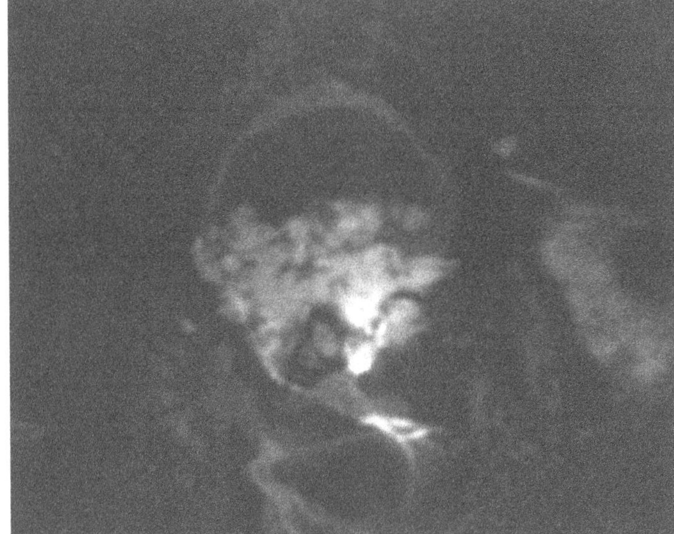

Figure 8.17.2

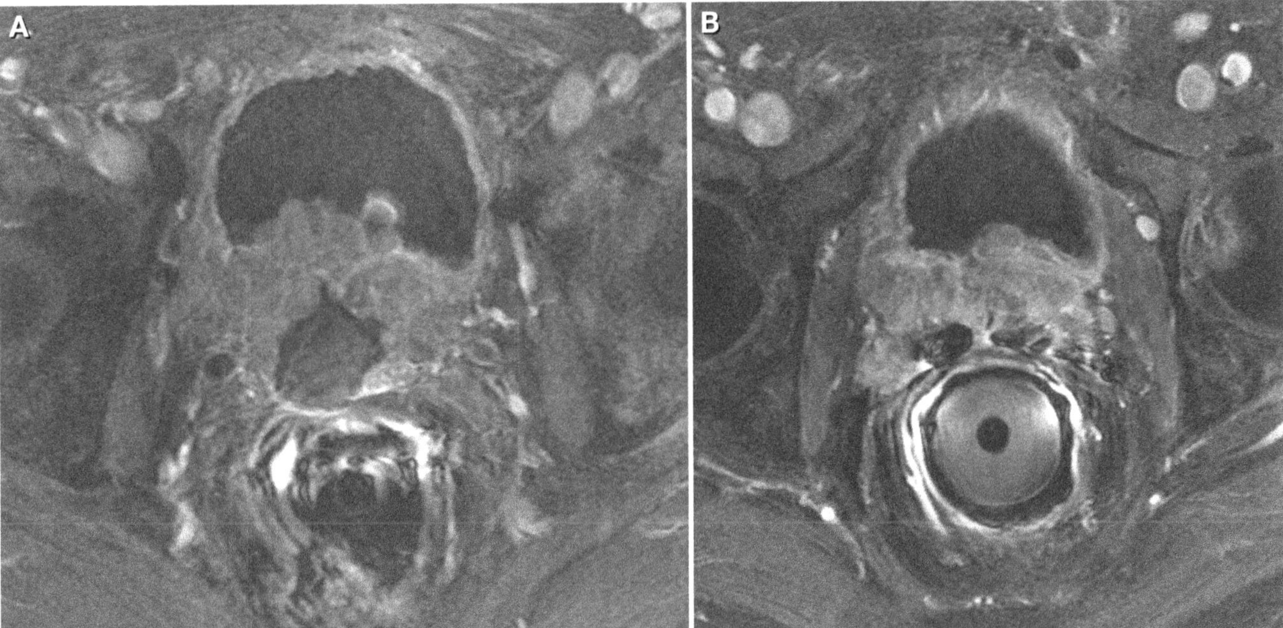

Figure 8.17.3

HISTORY: 68-year-old man with a history of prostatectomy for prostate adenocarcinoma, increasing nocturnal urinary frequency, and rising PSA level

IMAGING FINDINGS: Sagittal FSE T2-weighted image (Figure 8.17.1) obtained using an endorectal coil shows a large lobulated mass in the posterior bladder wall extending superiorly to the dome and inferiorly to the vesicourethral junction. The mass has high signal intensity on an axial diffusion-weighted image (b=1,000 s/mm^2) (Figure 8.17.2). Notice also the increased signal intensity within the left acetabulum. Axial postgadolinium 3D SPGR images (Figure 8.17.3) demonstrate mild heterogeneous enhancement of the mass, with a prominent cystic or necrotic region centrally and with mild enhancement of the left acetabulum.

DIAGNOSIS: Prostate carcinoma metastasis to the bladder with left acetabulum bone metastasis

COMMENT: Prostate cancer is the most common solid malignancy in men and is the second leading cause of cancer death. Bladder involvement by a secondary tumor can occur as a result of hematogenous metastasis or direct extension, and these lesions account for approximately 15% of malignant bladder tumors. Prostate carcinoma invading the bladder is the second most frequent bladder metastasis, with colorectal cancer ranking first.

The posterior location of the lesion in this case is suggestive of direct involvement of the bladder by the prostate cancer. Also suggestive of a prostatic etiology is the presence of the endorectal coil (rarely used for other pathologies). MRI is a well-accepted technique for identification of small, recurrent lesions in the prostate bed following prostatectomy in patients with elevated PSA levels. The endorectal coil enables small field-of-view acquisitions with preserved SNRs, and generally, dynamic gadolinium-enhanced 3D SPGR images are the most sensitive for detection of small enhancing lesions. There is some controversy regarding whether endorectal coils are really necessary in the era of 3-T magnets; however, it probably is true that even at 3 T, they do provide an incremental improvement in image quality, albeit at a cost in patient comfort.

An endorectal coil was certainly not necessary to detect the large bladder lesion in this case and was not used during a follow-up examination. The appearance of the lesion is nonspecific without the clinical context and could represent a primary bladder malignancy.

The diffusion-weighted image is not very pretty, with distortion and susceptibility artifact in the region of the endorectal coil (a common problem); however, it shows the acetabular metastasis more clearly than any other sequence in the examination.

CASE 8.18

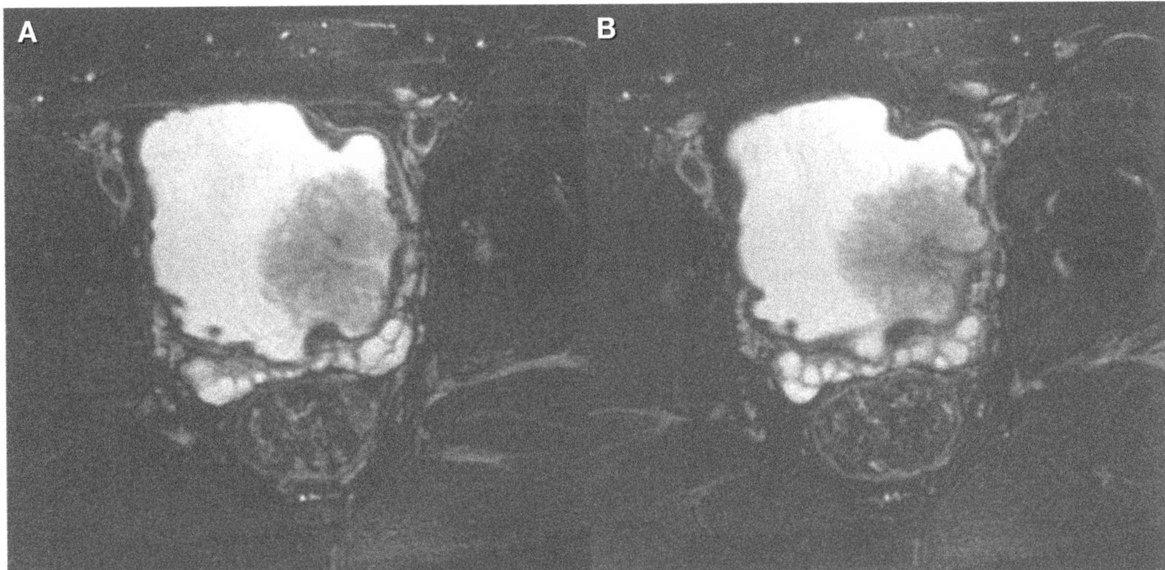

Figure 8.18.1

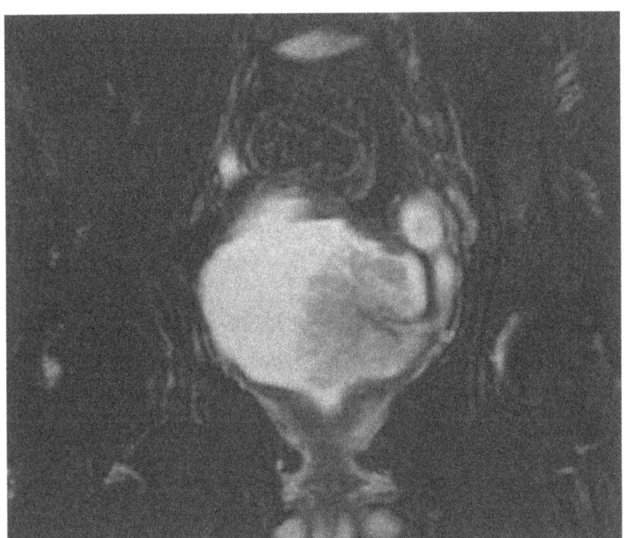

Figure 8.18.2

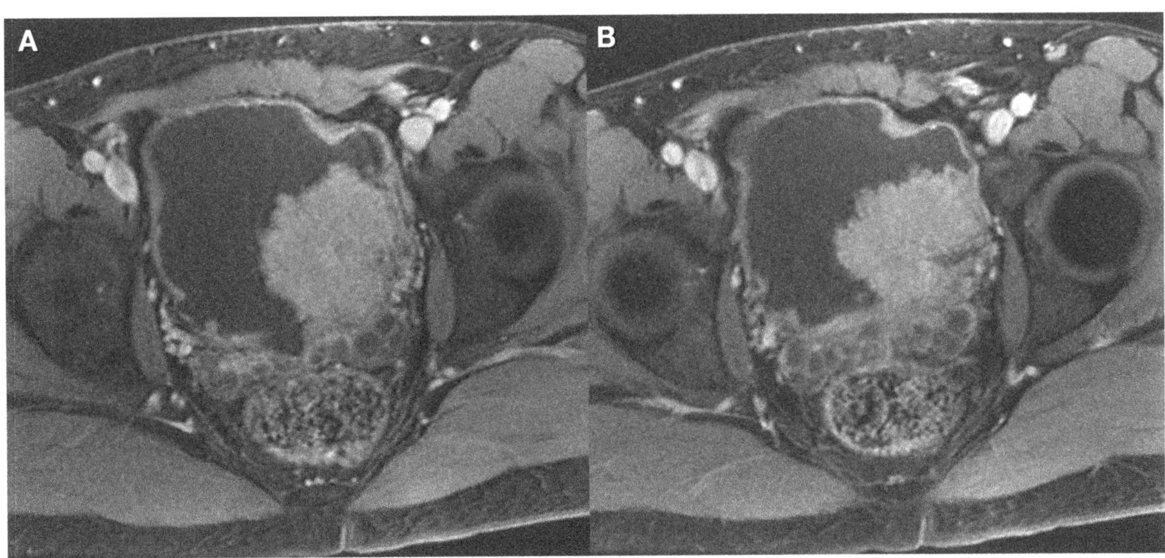

Figure 8.18.3

HISTORY: 25-year-old man with 3-year history of gross hematuria

IMAGING FINDINGS: Axial (Figure 8.18.1) and coronal (Figure 8.18.2) fat-suppressed FSE T2-weighted images show a large frondlike mass in the posterior left bladder. Note the dilated distal left ureter on the coronal image. Axial postgadolinium 2D SPGR images (Figure 8.18.3) demonstrate mild diffuse enhancement of the lesion.

DIAGNOSIS: Bladder urothelial carcinoma

COMMENT: Bladder urothelial carcinoma is the most common tumor of the urinary system, with an estimated lifetime risk of 3.4% in men and 1.2% in women. Incidence peaks in the sixth and seventh decades of life, and women tend to present with more advanced disease at diagnosis and have a higher mortality rate. A number of risk factors have been identified, and the most significant is smoking, which increases risk by a factor of 5. Cigarette smoking is thought to account for one-third to one-half of all cases of bladder cancer. Additional risk factors include exposure to β-naphthylamines, phenacetin, and cyclophosphamide.

Bladder urothelial carcinoma is generally classified as *superficial* (stages T0-T1) or *invasive* (stage T2 or higher). Superficial tumors account for 70% to 80% of bladder cancers and are limited to the mucosa and lamina propria (layers of the bladder wall from inside to outside include the urothelium, lamina propria, muscularis propria [or detrusor muscle], and adventitia). These lesions have an excellent prognosis, with little metastatic potential; however, they have a high rate of recurrence (70% at 3 years). In fact, urothelial carcinoma has the highest recurrence rate of any cancer, necessitating rigorous surveillance protocols. Approximately 2% to 4% of patients with bladder cancer will develop an upper-tract urothelial carcinoma. Conversely, approximately 40% of patients with an upper-tract urothelial carcinoma will develop a tumor in the lower tract. Most superficial tumors (70%) are papillary, with the remainder being flat carcinoma in situ lesions. Carcinoma in situ is more common in men and has a higher rate of recurrence.

Invasive lesions have a worse prognosis than superficial lesions, and mortality is strongly correlated with the pathologic stage. Patients with superficial tumors have a 5-year survival rate of approximately 80%; this rate drops to 40% for tumors invading the muscular layer, 20% for invasion of the perivesical fat, and 6% for metastatic disease.

MRI has not proved particularly accurate in staging bladder neoplasms: Distinguishing between superficial and muscle invasive tumors with high accuracy is difficult. The distinction between superficial and invasive tumors can usually be made at biopsy, but the endoscopic and clinical staging methods are not good at determining local tumor extension or metastatic disease—a strength of MRI.

DWI of bladder neoplasms has stimulated many recent papers. This technique is excellent for identifying even small, flat lesions, provided your b value is high enough to eliminate the fluid signal from the bladder and allow identification of high-signal-intensity masses against a uniformly dark background (b values of 800-1,000 s/mm^2 are recommended). Some authors have even claimed high staging accuracy with DWI, although skepticism is probably warranted given the intrinsically low spatial resolution of this technique and the small number of patients studied. Dynamic gadolinium-enhanced 3D SPGR images are also useful for identifying small lesions, which generally show early enhancement above the level of the normal mucosa.

This case is not a diagnostic dilemma; the large lesion is a classic frondlike papillary tumor. There is no obvious mural involvement (and the lesion was superficial at surgery), but even on these limited images it's easy to appreciate how difficult the staging of muscle invasion might be. An interesting feature of this case is obstruction of the distal left ureter. A classic teaching is that ureteral obstruction is highly associated with invasive tumors. However, a papillary tumor as large as this one can easily obstruct 1 or more ureteral orifices.

CASE 8.19

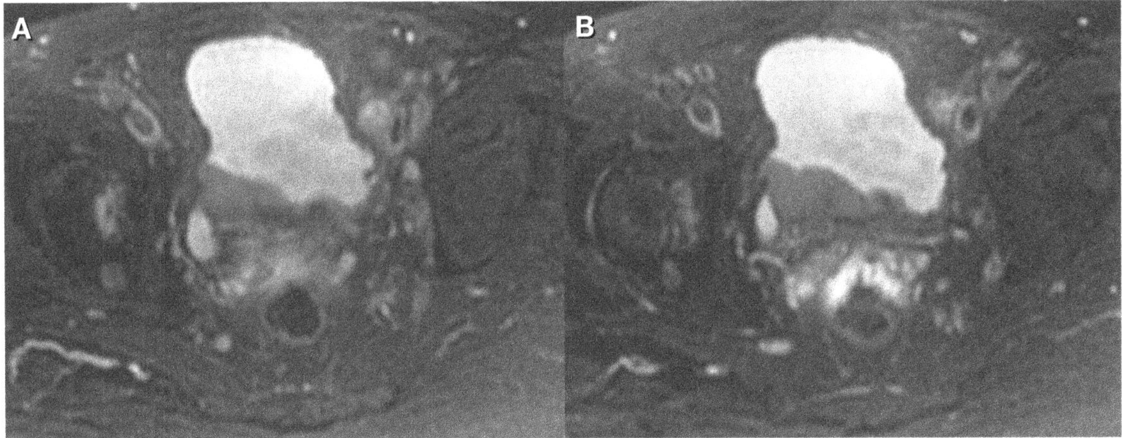

Figure 8.19.1

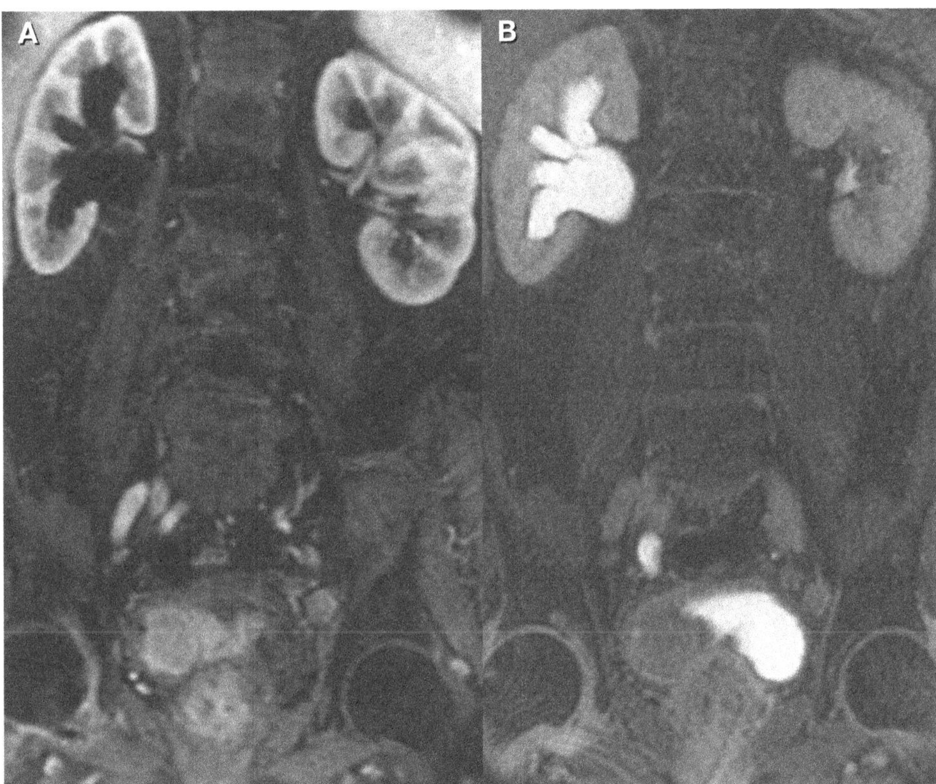

Figure 8.19.2

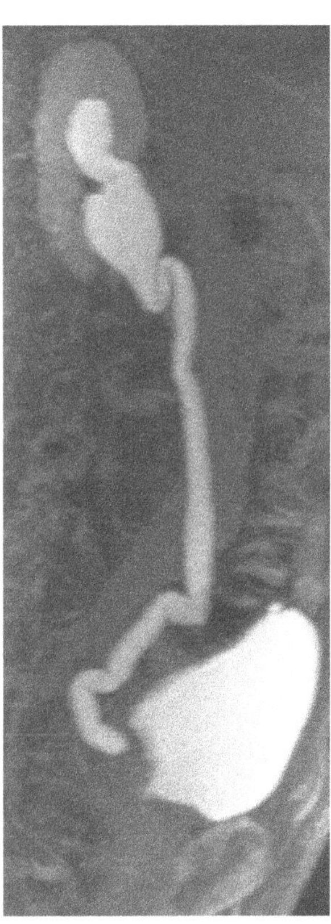

Figure 8.19.3

HISTORY: 75-year-old man with history of gross hematuria

IMAGING FINDINGS: Axial fat-suppressed FSE T2-weighted images (Figure 8.19.1) show a mass in the bladder posteriorly near the right ureterovesical junction with mild increased signal intensity obstructing the distal right ureter. Arterial phase and 10-minute delayed postgadolinium coronal 3D SPGR images from an MR urogram (Figure 8.19.2) reveal intense arterial phase enhancement of the mass, which becomes hypointense on the delayed image. Maximum intensity projection image (Figure 8.19.3) from 10-minute delayed acquisition shows a filling defect in the bladder and distal right ureter corresponding to the mass.

DIAGNOSIS: Bladder urothelial carcinoma

COMMENT: This case illustrates an invasive urothelial carcinoma causing ureteral obstruction, the more typical scenario in comparison to Case 8.18, where a large superficial carcinoma caused ureterovesical junction obstruction. The tumor is a flat lesion involving the posterior bladder, with mildly increased T2-signal intensity relative to the normal bladder wall. Notice the intense enhancement of the mass on the coronal arterial phase MR urogram image, which then becomes a filling defect on the delayed urographic images. This enhancement pattern is fairly typical for urothelial carcinoma, and dynamic contrast-enhanced images are often useful for detecting small lesions, particularly during the arterial phase.

MR urography was initially developed with the idea that it would be a useful adjunct technique in patients with renal insufficiency who needed CT urography. Needless to say, this was before the era of nephrogenic systemic fibrosis, and the arguments in favor of MR urography are now less compelling. It is probably true that MRI does a better job than CT at local staging of bladder cancers, but CT urography, by virtue of its superior spatial resolution, is more accurate in detecting small upper-tract lesions, an important consideration given the high incidence of synchronous and metachronous lesions. MR urography can also be helpful in patients with high-grade obstruction, where 2D and 3D T2-weighted images can be performed instead of or in addition to the traditional gadolinium-enhanced 3D SPGR technique. Even though the patient in this case had distal ureteral obstruction, there was enough gadolinium excretion to generate diagnostic excretory phase images.

Most sequences in typical MR urography protocols are oriented in the coronal oblique plane to capture the kidneys, ureters, and bladder in a single breath-hold. This case illustrates the importance of obtaining axial images for staging bladder neoplasms. It's very difficult to figure out whether the tumor extends beyond the margin of the bladder wall on coronal views alone, and the same principle applies for urothelial tumors in the renal pelvis. In this case, the lesion invaded muscle but had not extended beyond the bladder.

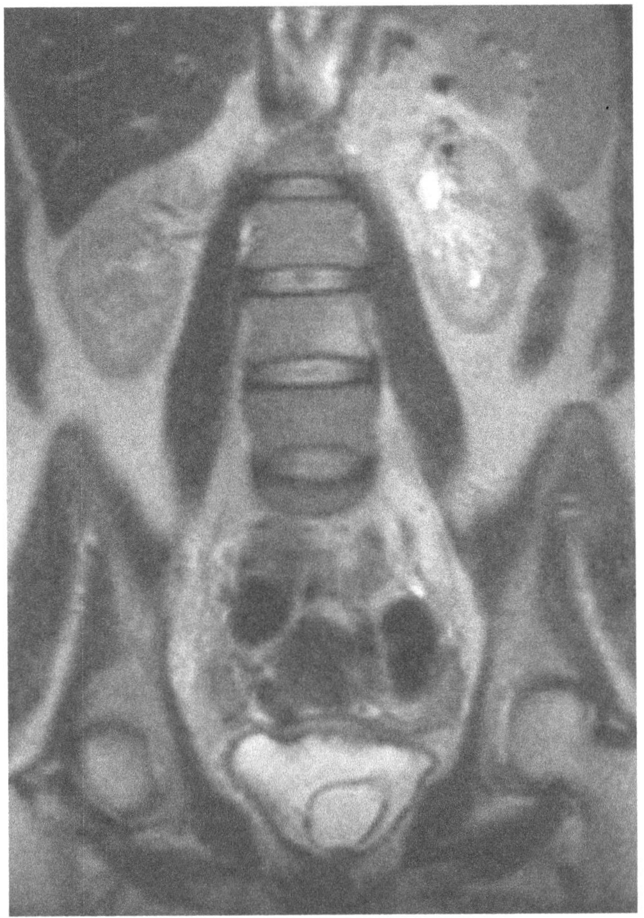

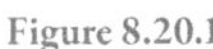

Figure 8.20.1

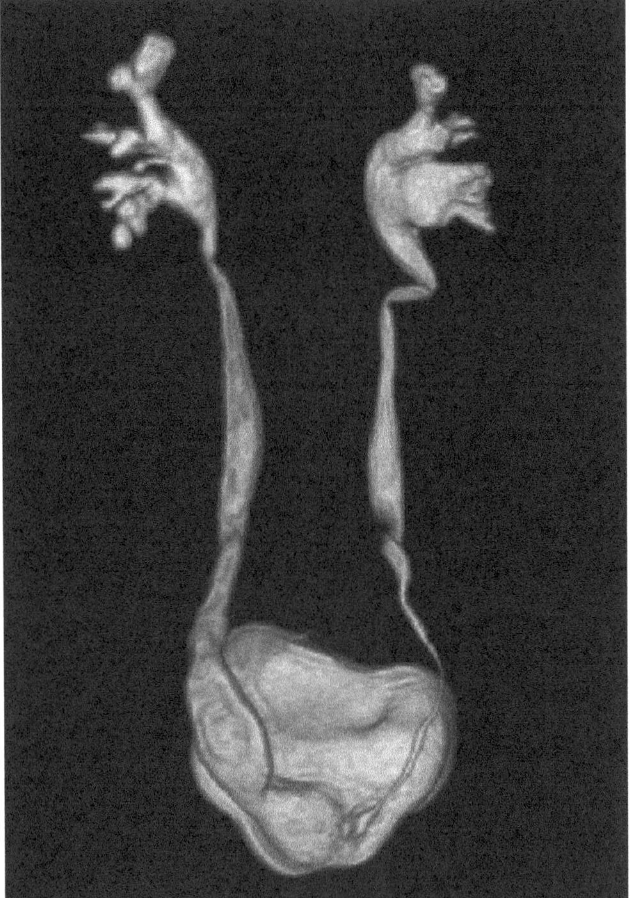

Figure 8.20.2

HISTORY: 51-year-old woman with chronic UTIs

IMAGING FINDINGS: Coronal SSFSE image (Figure 8.20.1) shows a cystic filling defect centrally in the bladder. A much smaller ovoid cystic structure is faintly visible on the right side of the bladder. Posterior volume-rendered image from a 3D FRFSE MR urogram (Figure 8.20.2) reveals focal dilatation of the distal ureters, which protrude into the bladder.

DIAGNOSIS: Bilateral ureteroceles (orthotopic)

COMMENT: Ureteroceles represent a congenital stenosis of the ureteral orifice, resulting in cystic dilatation of the submucosal ureter, which then prolapses into the bladder lumen. This is thought to occur when the epithelial membrane between the bladder and ureter (Chwalla membrane) fails to recanalize. Ureterocele is one of the most common congenital urogenital malformations, with an estimated incidence of 1 in 500 persons, and occurs 4 to 6 times more frequently in women than men. Ureteroceles are commonly associated with a duplicated collecting system (80% of cases) and may insert into the bladder (orthotopic location) or into an ectopic site, such as the bladder neck, urethra, or vagina. Ectopic ureteroceles are 4 times more common than the orthotopic type and are usually associated with ureteral duplication.

Orthotopic ureteroceles may be detected as an incidental finding or may be associated with urinary tract obstruction, urosepsis, hematuria, urinary retention, and stone disease. Larger ureteroceles (>2 cm at greatest diameter) are more likely to be associated with ureteral obstruction and stone formation within the ureterocele.

The classic cobra-head appearance of the ureterocele described on intravenous urography applies equally well to MRI and represents the fluid-filled ureterocele lumen projecting into the fluid-filled bladder, with the 2 spaces separated by the thin, dark wall of the ureterocele. This can be seen on either T2-weighted images (ideally a 3D FSE acquisition acquired with the same technique used for MR cholangiopancreatography, as in this case), 2D or 3D SSFP images (with pseudo T2 weighting), or delayed images from 3D SPGR gadolinium MR urograms, in which both the bladder and the ureters are filled with gadolinium.

The treatment of orthotopic ureteroceles has evolved over the past 10 to 15 years, from complicated major surgery to minimally invasive endoscopic treatment—namely, endoscopic puncture. The reoperation rate following endoscopic puncture of orthotopic ureteroceles (usually related to reflux) ranges from 7% to 23%; however, additional surgery is much more frequent in the clinical setting of ectopic ureteroceles.

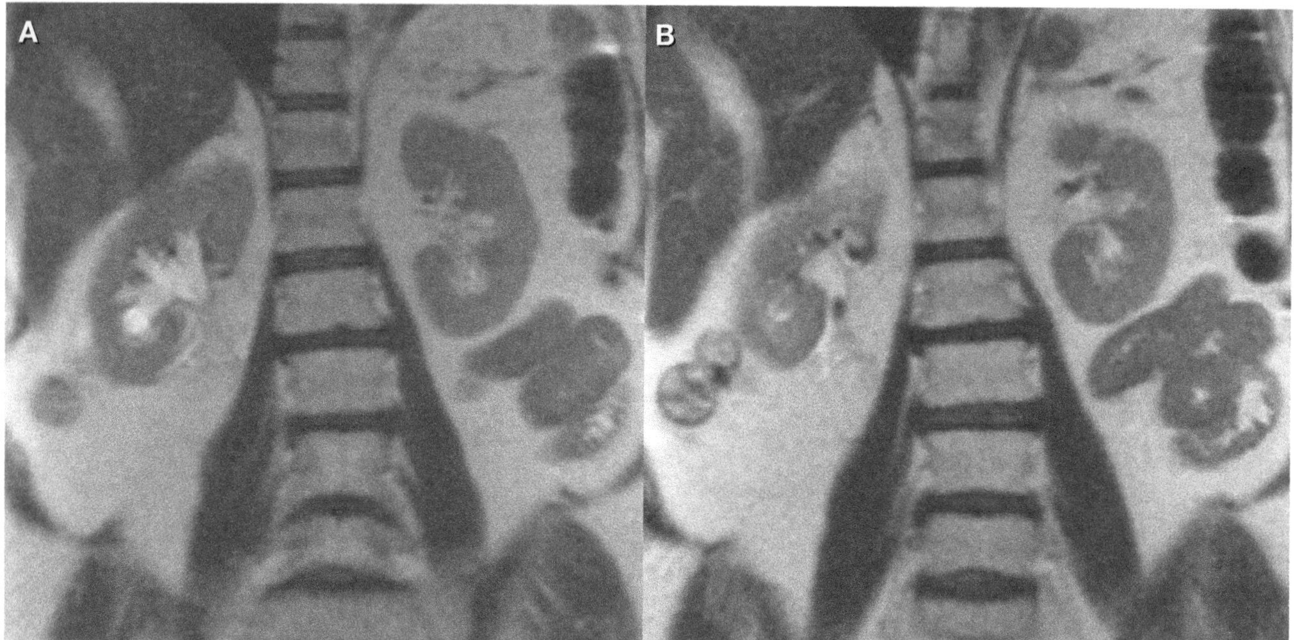

Figure 8.21.1

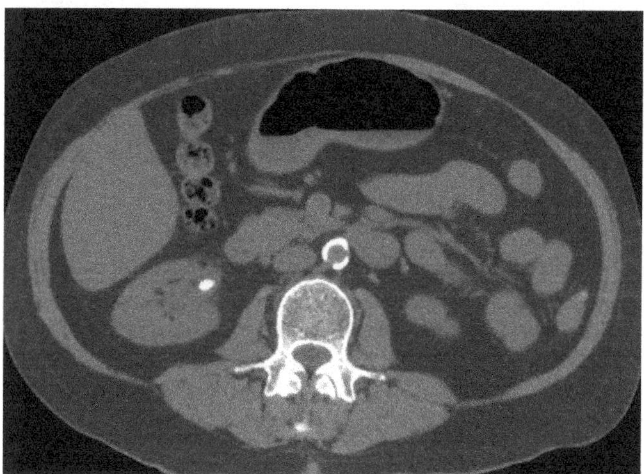

Figure 8.21.2

HISTORY: 68-year-old woman with severe intermittent right abdominal pain; MRA was performed for suspected mesenteric ischemia

IMAGING FINDINGS: Coronal SSFSE images (Figure 8.21.1) demonstrate mild hydronephrosis of the right kidney with a small, hypointense filling defect in the ureteropelvic junction. Note also mild right-sided perinephric soft tissue stranding. Axial image from noncontrast CT (Figure 8.21.2) shows a prominent calculus corresponding to the filling defect on MRI.

DIAGNOSIS: Obstructing ureteropelvic junction calculus

COMMENT: MR urography is not particularly well suited for identification of small renal or ureteral stones in patients with (or, even worse, without) acute obstructive symptoms. Noncontrast CT is nearly ideal for this indication, as you can realize by asking yourself which images in this case you would rather look at to identify the renal pelvis calculus. This isn't really a fair comparison—the clinical examination was an MRA, and the coronal SSFSE images were from a large field-of-view acquisition performed to visualize bowel and help plan for the MRA prescription. Nevertheless, it is true that renal stones are notoriously difficult to visualize on MRI.

Renal and ureteral stones present an interesting contrast to cholelithiasis and choledocholithiasis, where MRI is without question far superior to CT and is considered the noninvasive gold standard for diagnosis. There are a few reasons for this distinction: Gallstones and renal stones have different compositions and gallstones are more likely to be invisible or nearly invisible on CT. Remember that the gallbladder and, to some extent, even the biliary tree are more reliably fluid filled, and it's much easier to spot a small, dark filling defect against a very bright background of fluid on T2-weighted images than to identify the defect adjacent to renal parenchyma with only slightly higher signal intensity. In addition, the renal collecting system and ureters extend over a much larger volume, and therefore achieving motion-free images with high spatial resolution is more challenging, even before you consider ureteral peristalsis.

A few investigators have actually achieved excellent results (sensitivities of 95%-100% for detection of ureteral calculi) using gadolinium MR urography with low-dose diuretic administration and have showed that this technique is more effective than noncontrast, static fluid T2-weighted methods. There is some understandable reluctance to administer diuretics in the clinical setting of acute obstructive symptoms, even though few patients actually experience any worsening of their pain. However, this point again emphasizes the relative ease of performing noncontrast CT in this patient population. Limitations of gadolinium urography include use in patients with high-grade obstruction, where waiting for the gadolinium to arrive in the distal ureter can be a long proposition, and the occasional problems with concentrated gadolinium in the calyces and renal pelvis (exacerbated when obstruction is present). As the concentration of gadolinium increases, its predominant relaxation mechanism becomes T2*, leading to the appearance of signal voids on 3D SPGR images that can look very much like calculi.

The well-known limitation of noncontrast CT for ureteral stones is that if you don't see a stone, it may then be difficult to identify an alternative explanation involving the GU tract unless you repeat the examination using intravenous contrast. Here, MRI has the advantage because you're much more likely to pick up small renal, ureteral, or bladder soft tissue masses with MRI than with CT, and if you use gadolinium, you don't have to worry about doubling the radiation dose.

In our practice, we have performed only a handful of examinations specifically to look for ureteral stones, mainly in pregnant patients. Identification of renal and ureteral calculi occurs more frequently as an incidental finding (or a missed incidental finding). Keep this potential diagnosis in mind when you see unilateral perinephric or periureteral stranding or focal ureteral thickening and enhancement on an examination almost invariably not optimized for visualization of the GU tract.

CASE 8.22

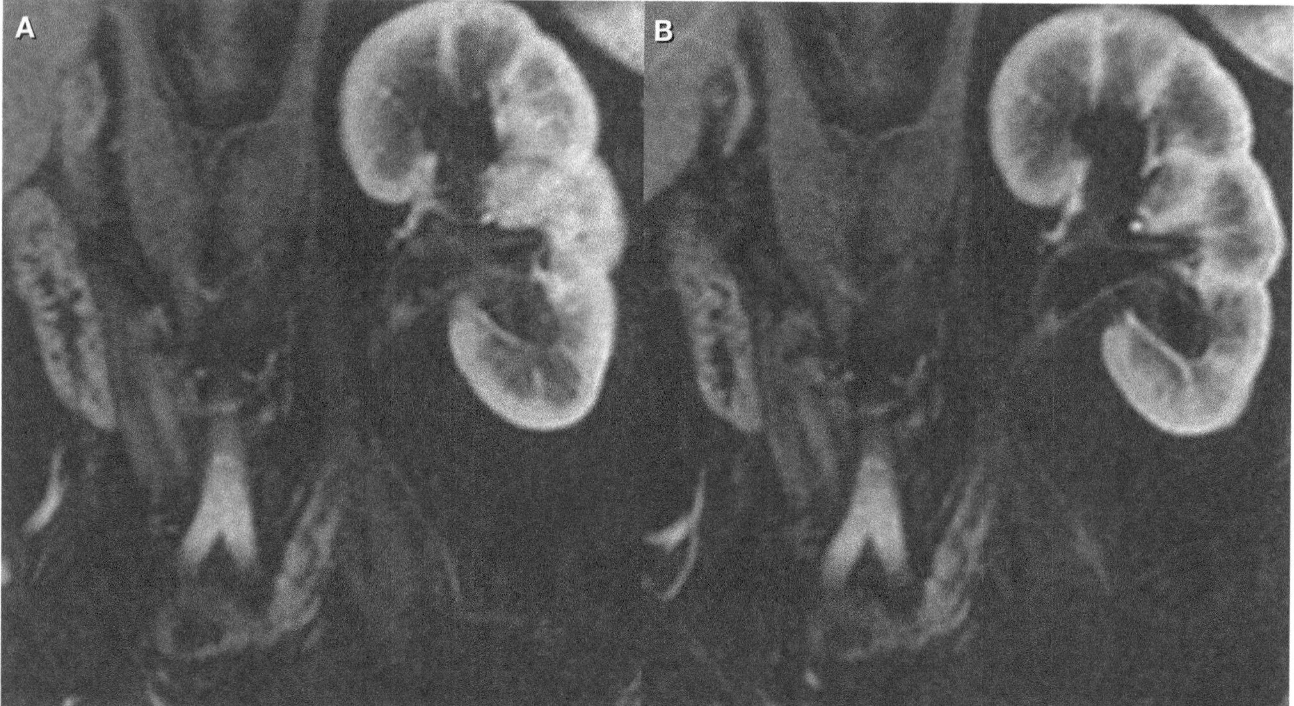

Figure 8.22.1

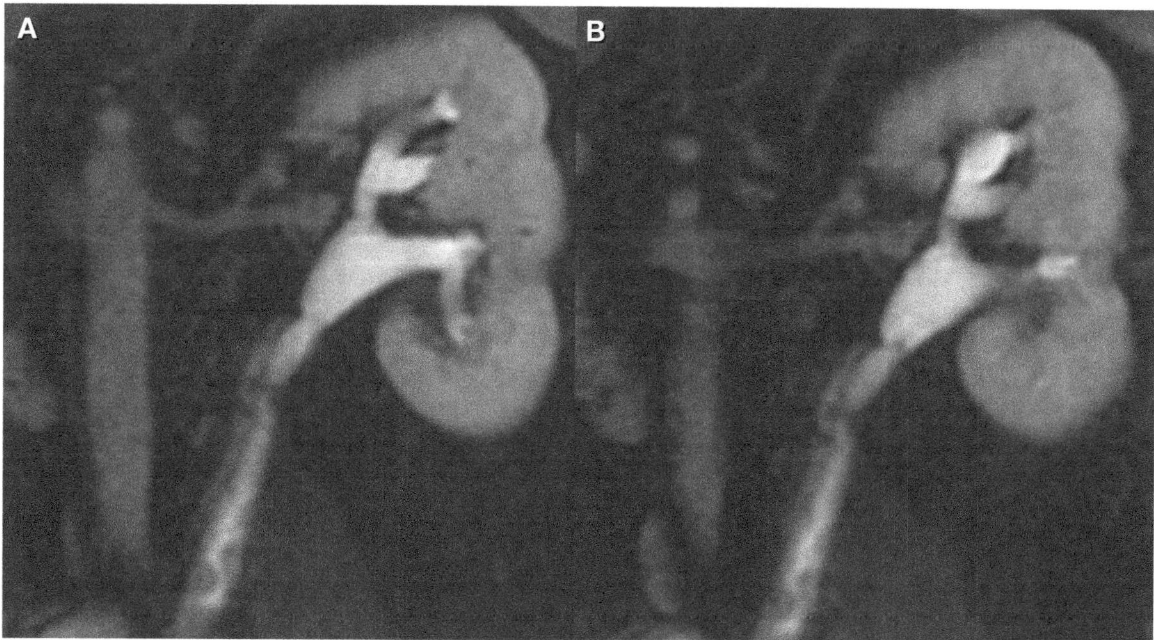

Figure 8.22.2

HISTORY: 62-year-old man with previous radical cystectomy and neobladder formation for urothelial cell carcinoma

IMAGING FINDINGS: Coronal oblique arterial phase 3D SPGR images from gadolinium MR urography (Figure 8.22.1) demonstrate multiple enhancing nodules in the distal ureter, as well as a small nodule in the renal pelvis. These lesions appear as filling defects on 10-minute delayed images (Figure 8.22.2).

DIAGNOSIS: Ureteral recurrence of bladder urothelial cell carcinoma

COMMENT: As noted in discussion of Case 8.18, bladder tumors have a recurrence rate of 2% to 4% in the upper tract, and so frequent surveillance is mandatory after cystectomy. This case is a good example of this principle. These lesions were found on the third surveillance examination after cystectomy.

Also noted previously (Case 8.21) is the relative disadvantage of MR urography with respect to CT urography in detecting very small ureteral, renal pelvis, or calyceal lesions by virtue of its lower spatial resolution.

Nevertheless, with optimal technique, MR urography should detect most lesions larger than 1 cm and a substantial proportion of smaller lesions. Gadolinium-enhanced MR urography is in general preferable to static fluid, heavily T2-weighted techniques for detection of small tumors since they appear initially as enhancing lesions and later as filling defects, which helps to distinguish them from small stones or clot, another dilemma that is generally easier to resolve with CT than MRI.

Urothelial tumors arise from the ureter, renal pelvis, or calyces in 5% of cases, and these account for approximately 10% of upper-tract neoplasms (RCC is the leader in this category). In as many as 40% of patients who present with an upper-tract urothelial tumor, metachronous bladder tumors will develop, usually within 2 years of the initial diagnosis. Upper-tract urothelial carcinoma is histologically similar to bladder urothelial tumors: 85% are low-stage superficial papillary neoplasms that usually are small at presentation, grow slowly, and have a benign prognosis. Infiltrative lesions, as in the bladder, behave more aggressively and have a worse prognosis. These tumors may appear as focal thickening of the ureteral wall, with or without soft tissue extension into the kidney or periureteral fat.

On the first few examinations following cystectomy, there often is prominent inflammatory thickening of the ureters, particularly when ureteral stents have been placed. This is frequently bilateral and symmetrical and may be difficult to distinguish from recurrent tumor. Conversely, extensive ureteral or periureteral thickening may occasionally hide small nodular recurrent lesions. Case 8.23 shows an example of an extensive inflammatory response to cystectomy and ureteral stents. It's easy to appreciate how problematic this appearance can be when trying to detect recurrent disease in the ureters. Diffuse thickening was not a problem in this patient, and the multiple enhancing nodules projecting into the distal ureteral lumen (as well as the smaller renal pelvis lesion, best seen on the arterial phase images) are much more characteristic of tumor than inflammation.

A small amount of phase ghosting artifact can be seen adjacent to the ureters on both the arterial phase and excretory phase images. This artifact could result from either poor breath-holding or ureteral peristalsis and illustrates one of the technical problems of MR urography—namely, that it can be difficult to find the optimal balance between complete volumetric coverage with high spatial resolution and an acceptable breath-hold for the individual patient.

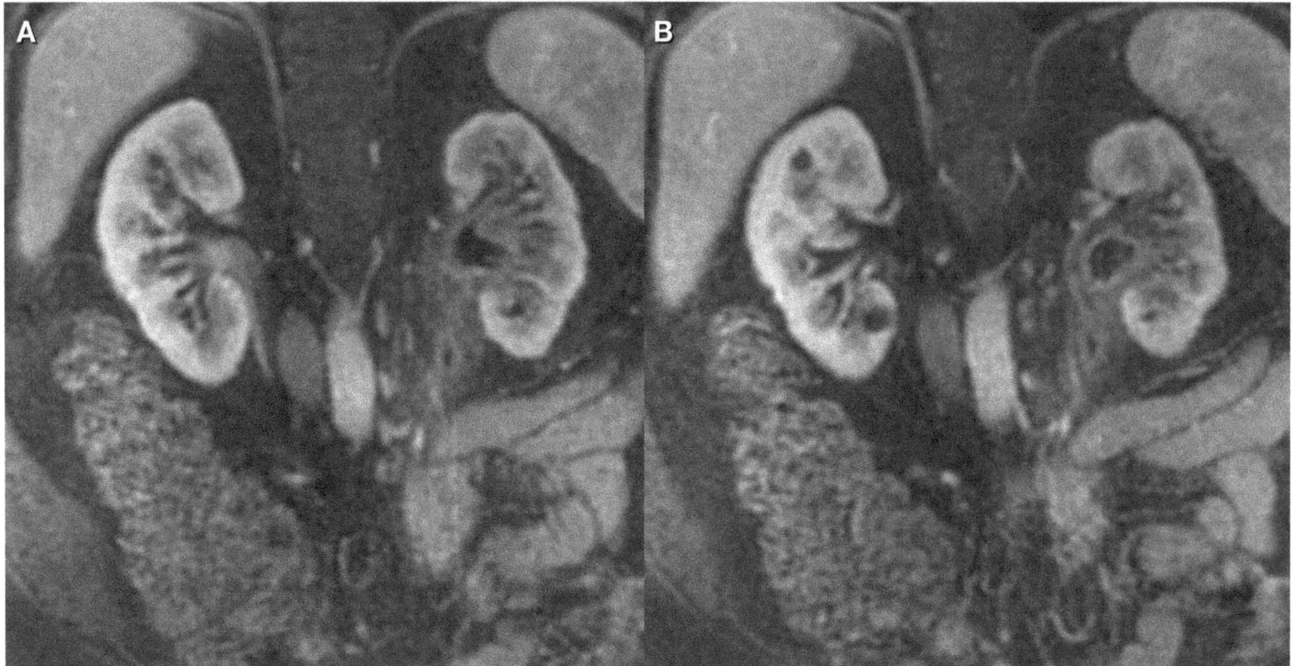

Figure 8.23.1

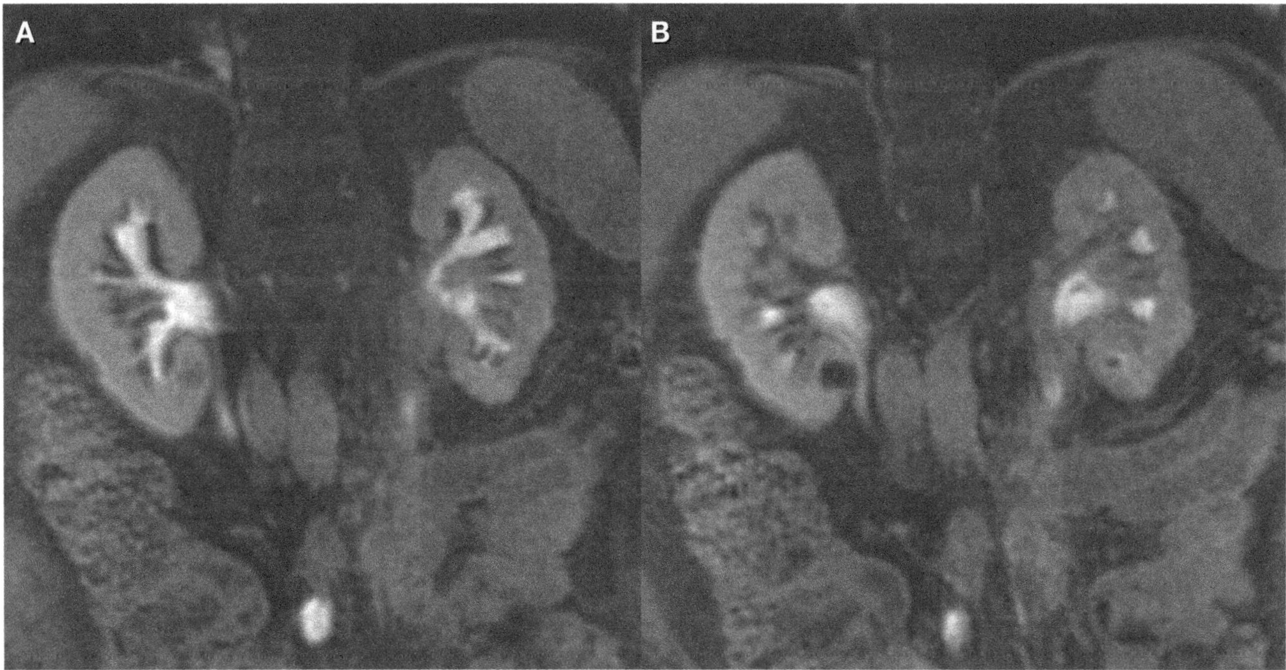

Figure 8.23.2

HISTORY: 73-year-old man presenting for surveillance examination 9 months following cystectomy for an invasive urothelial tumor

IMAGING FINDINGS: Coronal oblique arterial phase (Figure 8.23.1) and excretory phase (Figure 8.23.2) postgadolinium 3D SPGR images from gadolinium MR urography show marked periureteral peripelvic soft tissue thickening and mild enhancement involving the left kidney and proximal ureter, with mild associated hydronephrosis. Bilateral nephroureteral stents are present and can be perceived faintly on the excretory phase image. Note also the right renal cysts and a small filling defect in a left lower pole calyx; this was a small calculus.

DIAGNOSIS: Inflammatory changes following cystectomy and ureteral stent placement

COMMENT: This case illustrates a severe (and asymmetrical) inflammatory response in the renal pelvis and ureter following cystectomy and ureteral stent placement. Initial readings raised concern for possible recurrent malignancy. However, follow-up examinations showed gradual resolution of this process, and results on urine cytology continued to be negative for malignancy.

Uniform thickening of the ureter or renal pelvis is a less common manifestation of recurrent disease than a focal mass or nodularity, but this appearance does occur and can also be seen in rare diseases such as periureteral lymphoma (Case 8.25). In general, symmetrical uniform involvement is less concerning than unilateral heterogeneous thickening, and the inflammatory changes should slowly resolve on follow-up examinations. Even so, inflammation can mask a small underlying recurrent tumor, and frequent follow-up examinations, as well as examination of urine cytology and even biopsy, may be necessary to exclude recurrent disease.

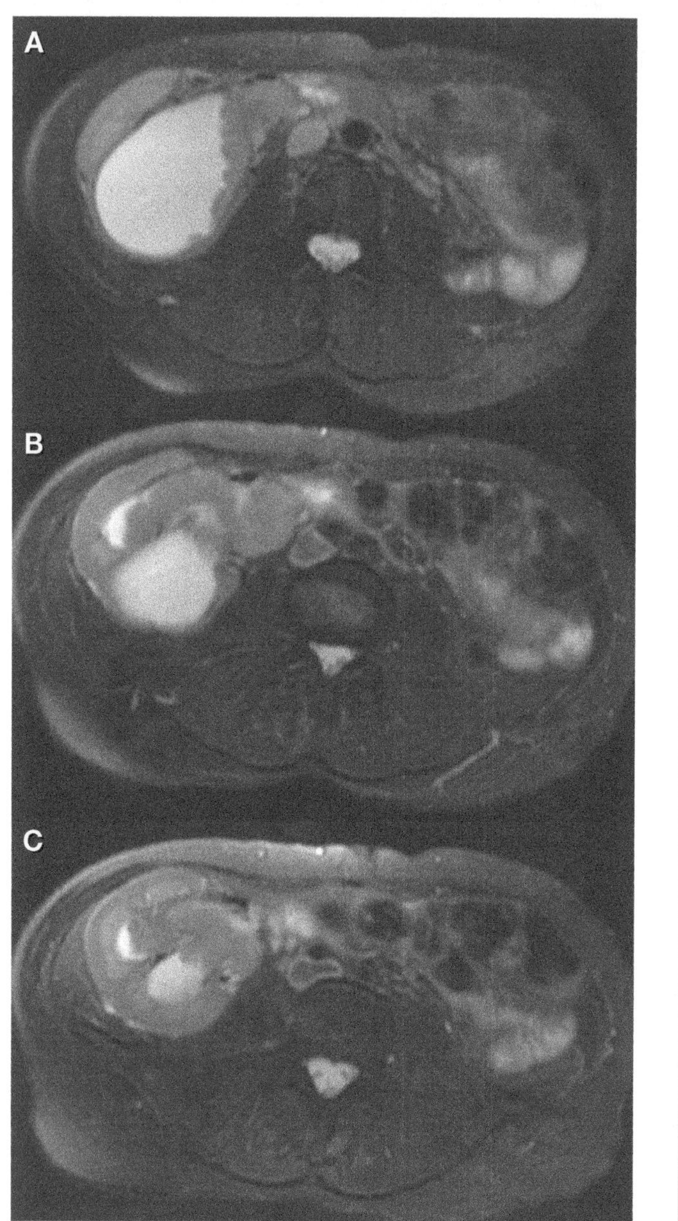

Figure 8.24.1

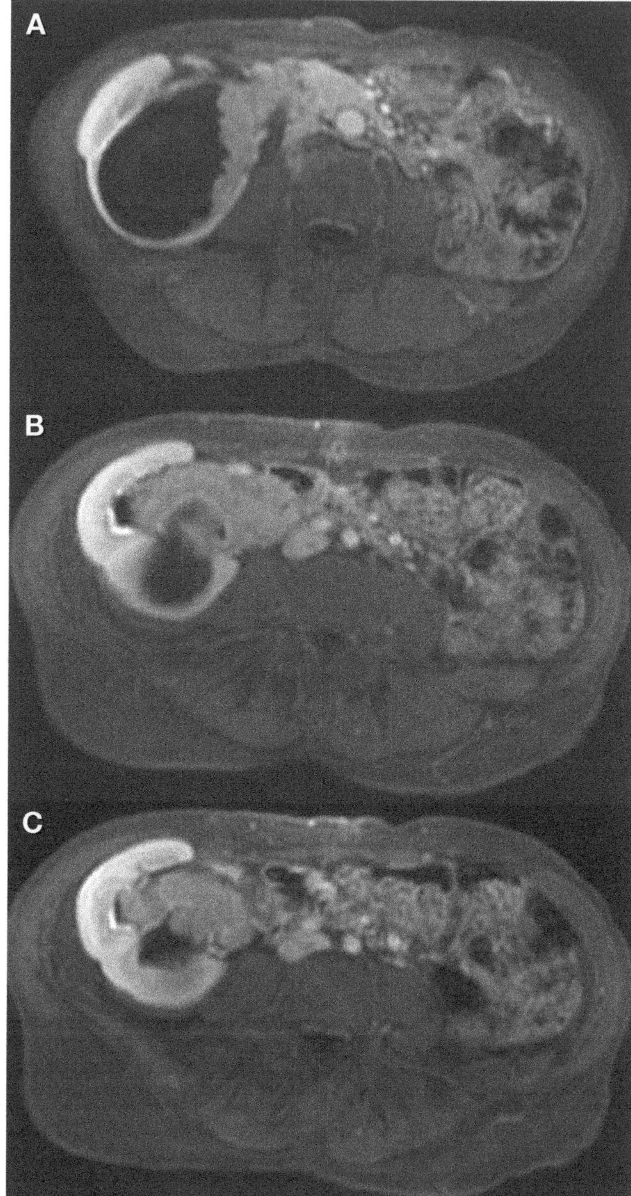

Figure 8.24.2

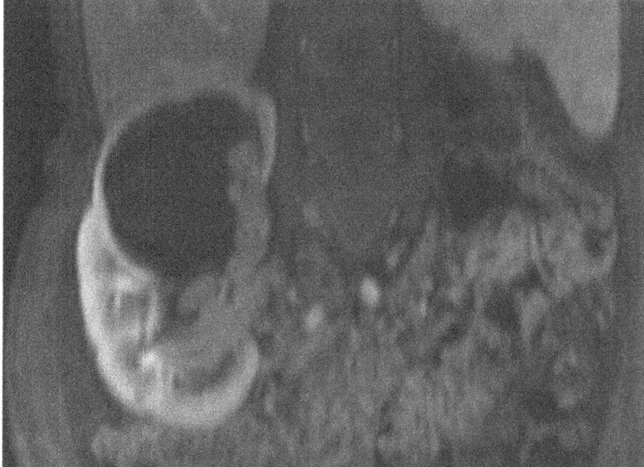

Figure 8.24.3

HISTORY: 65-year-old woman with a congenitally absent left kidney and hematuria

IMAGING FINDINGS: Axial fat-suppressed FSE T2-weighted images (Figure 8.24.1) show a soft tissue mass involving much of the renal pelvis and causing hydronephrosis, most marked in the upper pole. Axial postgadolinium 3D SPGR images (Figure 8.24.2), as well as a coronal reformatted image (Figure 8.24.3), demonstrate similar findings, with mild enhancement of the infiltrative soft tissue mass.

DIAGNOSIS: Renal pelvis urothelial cell carcinoma

COMMENT: Urothelial carcinoma accounts for approximately 10% of upper-tract neoplasms, and it has been estimated that up to 15% of renal tumors are renal pelvis urothelial carcinomas. Low-stage superficial tumors comprise 85% of upper-tract lesions, while the remainder are infiltrating or invasive lesions. Invasive upper-tract tumors are generally more aggressive than invasive bladder neoplasms, possibly a consequence of the thinner walls of the calyces, renal pelvis, and ureters. The invasive renal pelvis urothelial carcinoma growing into the kidney and causing diffuse enlargement gives rise to the ball (RCC) vs bean (urothelial carcinoma) mnemonic.

This case is not a diagnostic dilemma, but it illustrates many features of renal pelvis urothelial carcinoma: extensive soft tissue growth along the renal pelvis and into the calyces, with marked obstruction of an upper pole calyx. As with urothelial tumors in other locations, this lesion has mildly hyperintense signal on T2-weighted images and mild enhancement following gadolinium administration. Although urothelial tumors often show hyperenhancement on arterial phase images (a particularly useful characteristic in bladder and ureteral tumors), infiltrative tumors invading the kidney generally show less arterial phase enhancement than RCCs (with the exception of papillary and chromophobe RCC variants).

Venous invasion is another feature often used to help distinguish RCC from urothelial carcinoma; it is much more common in RCC but can be seen infrequently with urothelial carcinoma. Hydronephrosis or a focally dilated calyx is a classic finding of renal urothelial carcinoma since these lesions originate in the collecting system, and even relatively small masses can cause high-grade obstruction. But again, this is not a universal truth, and large or strategically located RCCs may cause significant hydronephrosis.

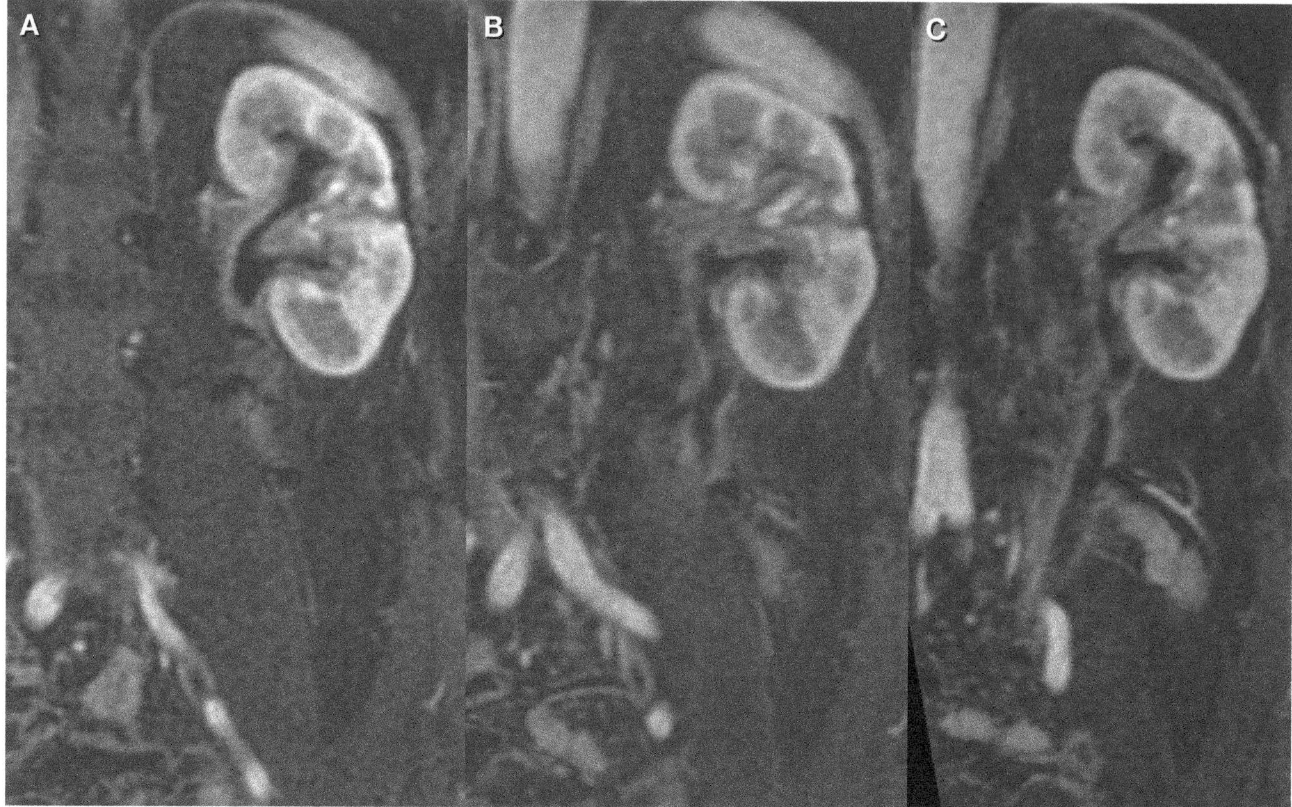

Figure 8.25.1

HISTORY: 68-year-old woman with microhematuria

IMAGING FINDINGS: Coronal oblique arterial phase 3D SPGR images from MR urography (Figure 8.25.1) demonstrate soft tissue thickening surrounding the renal pelvis and proximal ureter, with mild hydronephrosis and hydroureter.

DIAGNOSIS: Periureteral lymphoma

COMMENT: Involvement of the GU system by non-Hodgkin lymphoma is not infrequent, and the kidneys are most often affected. Ureteral lymphoma generally occurs as a result of contiguous spread from adjacent retroperitoneal nodes or from the kidney. This case is unusual in that ureteral involvement was the primary manifestation of the disease.

The diffuse soft tissue thickening surrounding the renal pelvis and proximal ureter would be a somewhat unusual appearance for urothelial carcinoma, with primarily extraureteral involvement and only mild hydronephrosis. However, urothelial cell carcinoma should be a major consideration in the differential diagnosis since it is by far the most common neoplasm in this location. Retroperitoneal fibrosis would be another reasonable possibility; periureteral fibrosis sparing the kidneys and periaortic region is an atypical, but not unheard of, presentation.

Inflammatory or infectious causes should also be considered, although the extensive soft tissue thickening seen in this case is not often encountered in these situations. Ureteral or periureteral thickening is particularly common in the clinical setting of cystectomy with neobladder formation or diverting urostomy (see Case 8.23) and can be difficult to distinguish from recurrent urothelial carcinoma (the usual indication for cystectomy), although a bilateral presentation without focal dominant thickening is probably more suggestive of an inflammatory process.

This patient was treated successfully with chemotherapy and has had no recurrence in 6 years of follow-up examinations.

ABBREVIATIONS

CT computed tomography
DWI diffusion-weighted imaging
FRFSE fast-recovery fast-spin echo
FSE fast-spin echo
GU genitourinary
IMT inflammatory myofibroblastic tumor
MR magnetic resonance
MRA magnetic resonance angiography
MRI magnetic resonance imaging
PSA prostate-specific antigen
RCC renal cell carcinoma
SCC squamous cell carcinoma
SNR signal to noise ratio
SPGR spoiled gradient-recalled echo
SSFP steady-state free precession
SSFSE single-shot fast-spin echo
3D 3-dimensional
2D 2-dimensional
US ultrasonography
UTI urinary tract infection

9.

BOWEL

CASE 9.1

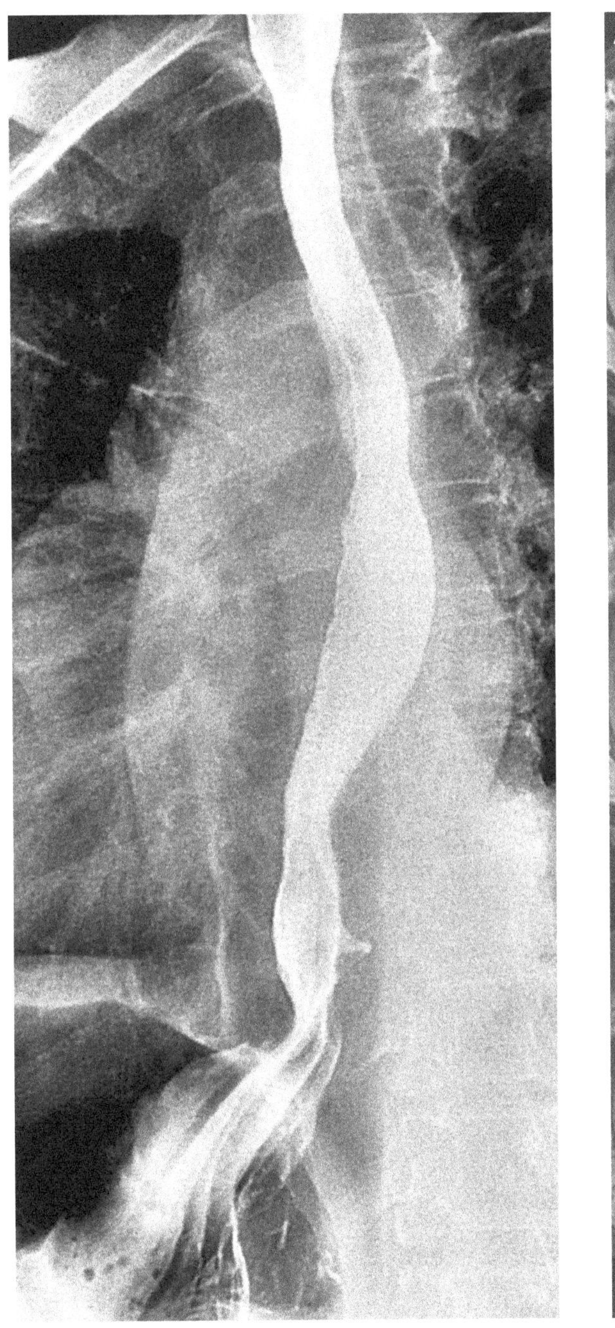

Figure 9.1.1

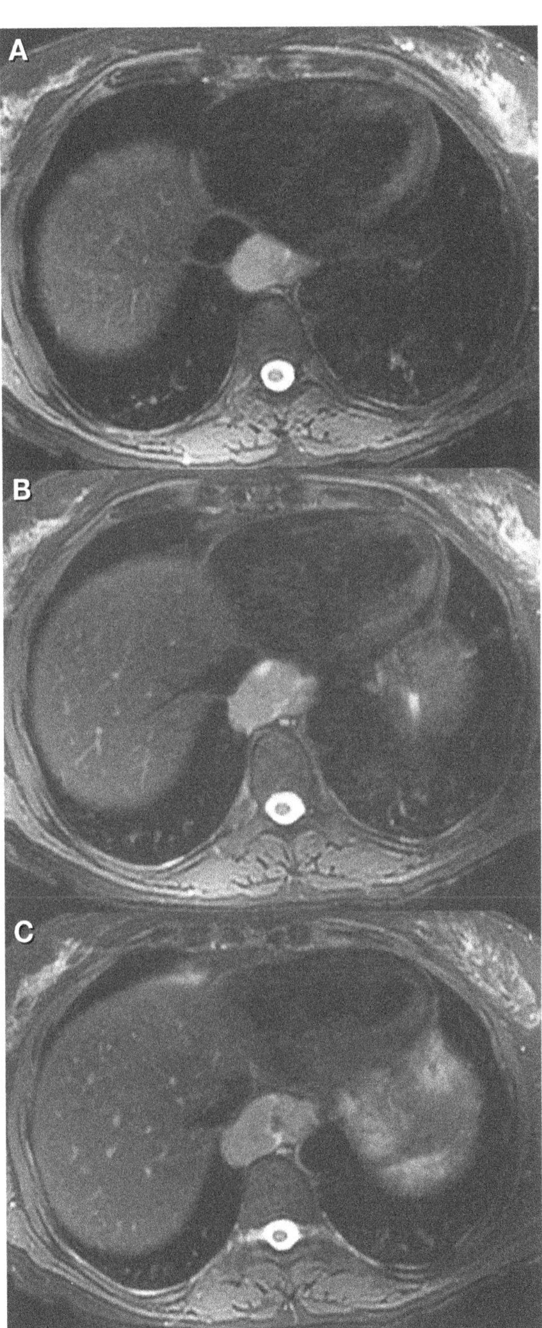

Figure 9.1.2

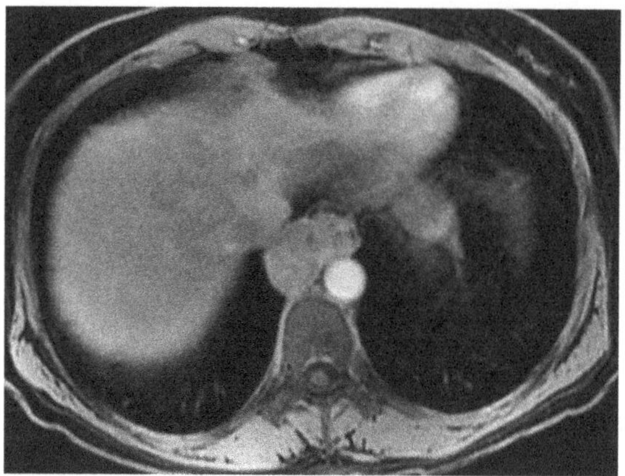

Figure 9.1.3

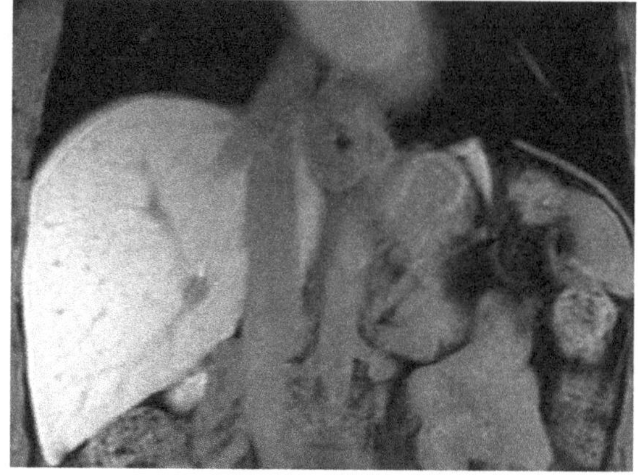

Figure 9.1.4

HISTORY: 56-year-old asymptomatic woman with liver mass thought to be focal nodular hyperplasia on CT

IMAGING FINDINGS: Image from a double-contrast esophagram (Figure 9.1.1) demonstrates a relatively subtle mural lesion in the distal esophagus with a small central ulceration. Axial fat-suppressed T2-weighted FSE images (Figure 9.1.2) show a moderate-sized homogeneous lesion in the wall of the distal esophagus with mild hyperintensity relative to liver and paraspinous skeletal muscle. Axial arterial phase (Figure 9.1.3) and coronal hepatobiliary phase (Figure 9.1.4) images reveal only mild enhancement of the lesion.

DIAGNOSIS: Esophageal leiomyoma

COMMENT: Benign tumors of the esophagus are uncommon. A large autopsy study from the 1940s, for example, found that only 0.4% of esophageal tumors were benign. Leiomyoma, however, is by far the most common benign esophageal tumor, accounting for 75% to 80% of lesions. The appearance on barium studies (accounting for the bulk of the radiology literature) is a smooth, round or lobulated intramural lesion with sharply demarcated margins between the lesion and uninvolved esophagus. About 60% of leiomyomas occur in the distal third of the esophagus; 33%, the middle third; and 7%, the upper third. Ulceration of esophageal leiomyomas, as seen in this case, is rare, in contrast to gastric leiomyomas, in which it is more common.

The few case reports in the literature describing the MRI appearance of leiomyomas emphasize uniform, well-defined lesions with isointense to mildly hyperintense T2-signal intensity relative to normal esophagus and mild enhancement after gadolinium administration. The smooth margins and mildly increased T2-signal intensity of this lesion are suggestive, but probably not diagnostic, of leiomyoma, and the differential diagnosis includes esophageal carcinoma and other, less common esophageal masses. This patient had laparoscopic resection of the mass without complication.

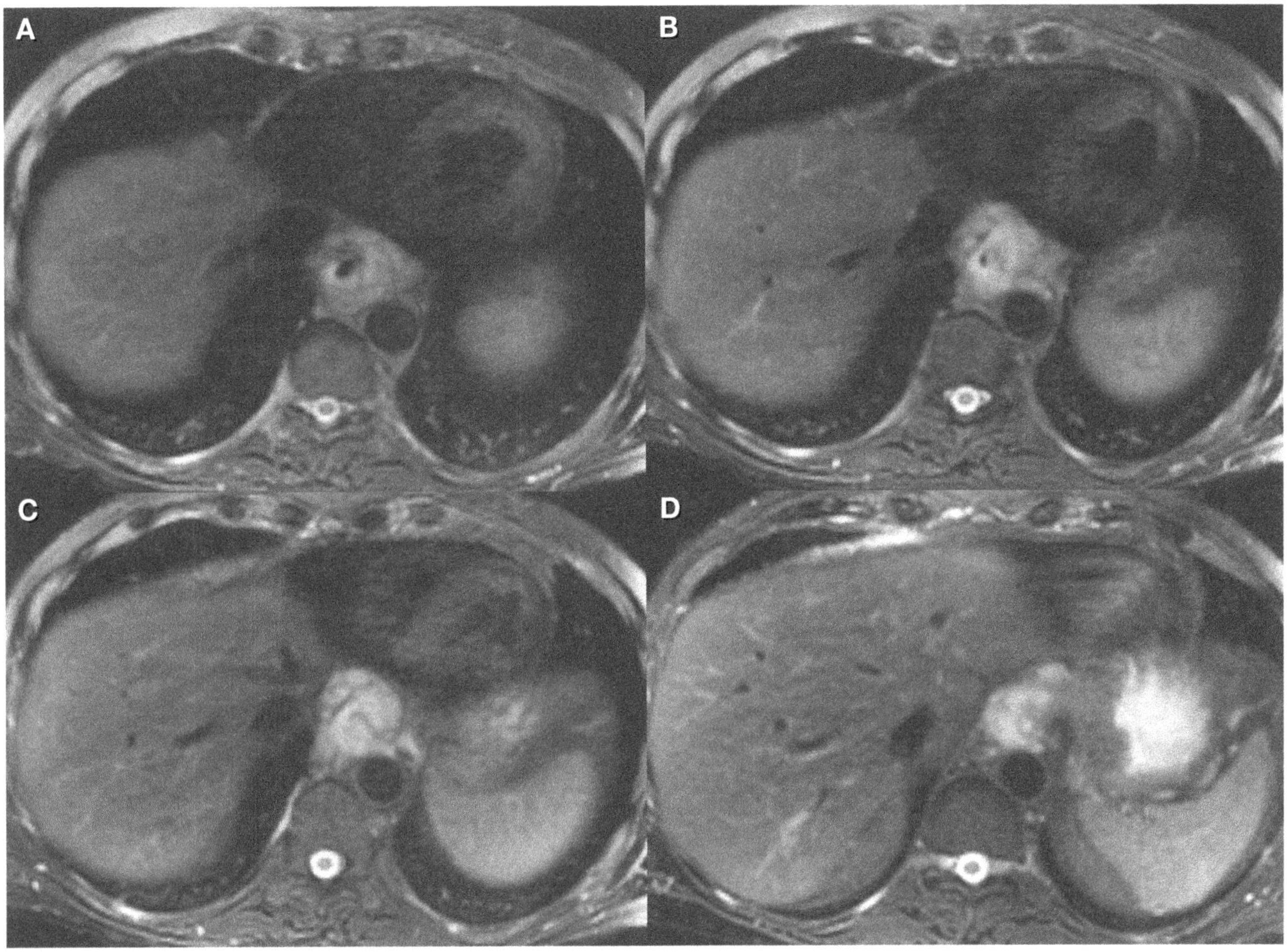

Figure 9.2.1

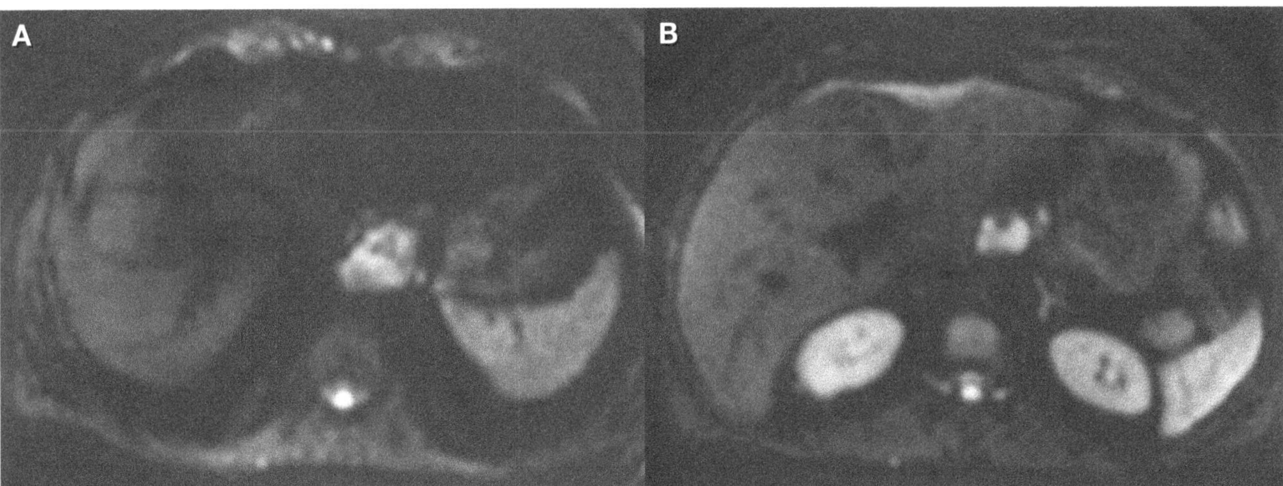

Figure 9.2.2

HISTORY: 56-year-old man with progressive solid-food dysphagia and a 15-lb weight loss over the past 3 months

IMAGING FINDINGS: Axial fat-suppressed FSE T2-weighted images (Figure 9.2.1) show circumferential thickening and mildly increased signal intensity in the distal esophagus. Axial diffusion-weighted images with a b value of 600 s/mm^2 (Figure 9.2.2) also show increased signal intensity in the distal esophagus, as well as hyperintense lymph nodes in the gastrohepatic ligament.

DIAGNOSIS: Esophageal adenocarcinoma

COMMENT: Esophageal adenocarcinoma is an uncommon indication for abdominal MRI and is, in our experience, either an incidental finding or a known primary lesion in an examination performed to assess for metastatic disease. These tumors generally have increased T2-signal intensity, high signal intensity on diffusion-weighted images, and mild enhancement following gadolinium administration and may cause obstruction, with associated proximal esophageal dilatation. Ulceration is a common characteristic.

Although esophageal carcinoma is relatively rare in the United States, it is the seventh leading cause of cancer death worldwide, with the highest incidence in northern Iran, southern Russia, and northern China. Squamous cell carcinoma accounts for 95% of esophageal cancers; however, adenocarcinoma is increasing in incidence in the Western world and in fact now exceeds the incidence of squamous cell carcinoma in the United States. Squamous cell carcinoma is strongly associated with smoking and alcohol consumption, while adenocarcinomas arise in the distal esophagus in the presence of chronic gastroesophageal reflux and gastric metaplasia of the epithelium (Barrett esophagus).

Most patients are 50 to 70 years old at diagnosis and present with symptoms of dysphagia and weight loss. Since the esophagus lacks a serosal layer, local spread to the pericardium, trachea, lung, and vertebrae is common, and more than 75% of patients have nodal involvement at diagnosis. The prognosis is poor for both squamous cell carcinoma and adenocarcinoma, with an overall 5-year survival rate of approximately 5%.

Initial staging is performed with endoscopic US, which allows determination of the depth of invasion, as well as the sampling of regional nodes. CT, MRI, and positron emission tomography are all useful for evaluating patients with suspected metastatic disease.

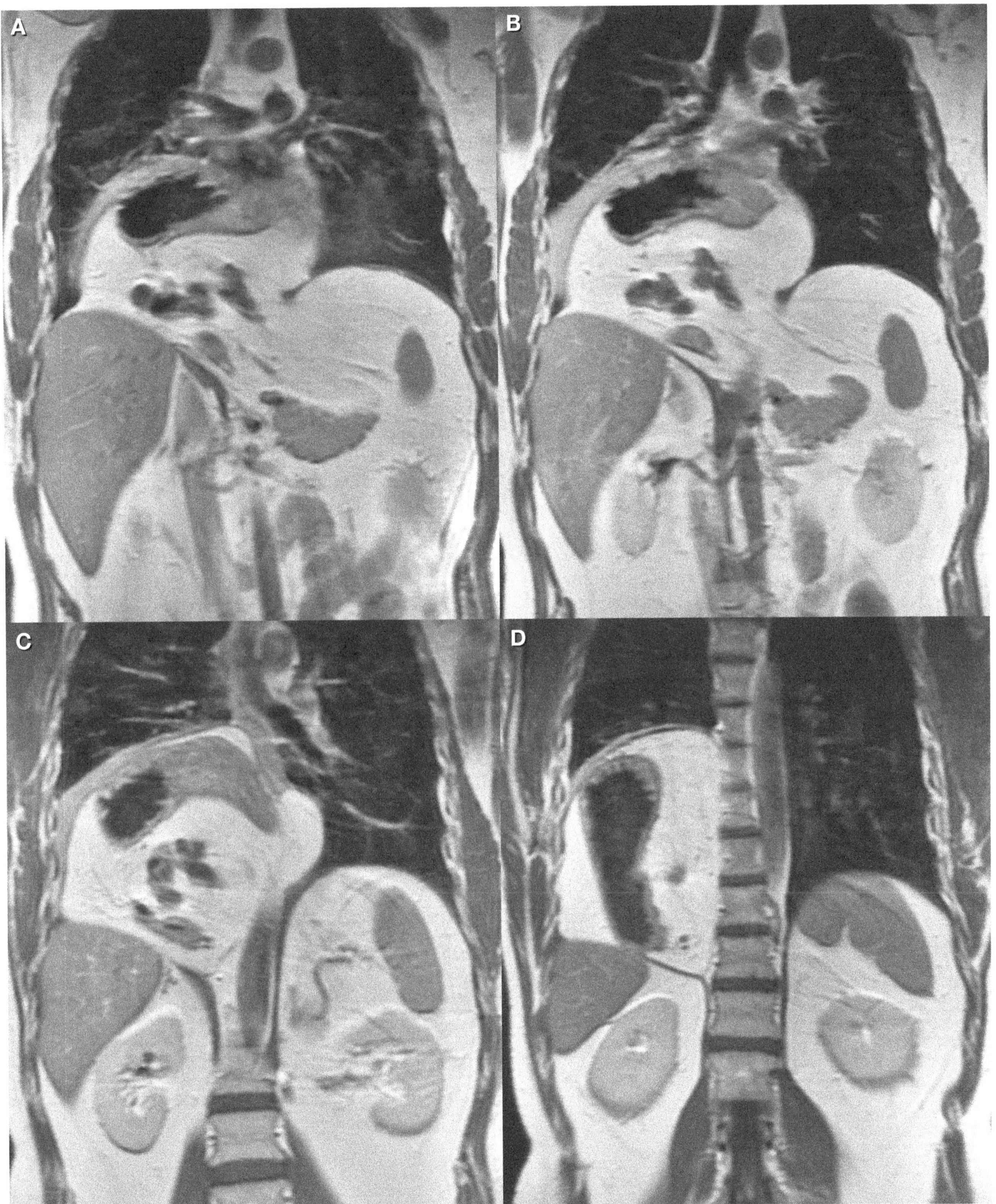

Figure 9.3.1

HISTORY: 39-year-old man with early satiety and postprandial discomfort

IMAGING FINDINGS: Coronal T1-weighted FSE images (Figure 9.3.1) show herniation of the stomach through the diaphragmatic hiatus, as well as a large quantity of peritoneal fat and a portion of the transverse colon.

DIAGNOSIS: Large hiatal hernia with intrathoracic stomach

COMMENT: This diagnosis is not easy to miss and, in fact, had already been made on a previous chest radiograph. But MRI is an excellent technique for characterizing hernias, including their location and contents, and determining whether they are obstructive or nonobstructive.

Hiatal hernias are extremely common, but even so, they are probably overreported, providing the opportunity to make a positive diagnosis in an otherwise negative examination and implying that since you found the hernia, you probably spent at least a few minutes looking at the images. When residents, we once briefly tracked the diagnosis of hiatal hernias made by staff radiologists in abdominal CT, with the winner achieving a rate of nearly 80%. A hernia this large, though, is noteworthy, especially in a patient with an intrathoracic stomach.

Diaphragmatic defects can be classified as *congenital* or *acquired*. Bochdalek and Morgagni hernias are congenital; hiatal hernias and diaphragmatic rupture are acquired. The diaphragm is a complex, musculotendinous structure separating the thorax from the abdominal cavity. Three muscle groups converge to form the central tendon, and gaps separating the muscle groups covered by pleura, peritoneum, and fascial layers represent potential sites of Bochdalek and Morgagni hernias posteriorly and anteriorly, respectively.

Herniation of the stomach through the esophageal hiatus constitutes a hiatal hernia and is due to stretching, tearing, or weakening of the phrenoesophageal membrane, which normally covers the esophageal hiatus. There are 2 types of hiatal hernia. The sliding hernia, where the gastroesophageal junction is displaced above the hiatus, is most common and is seen in this case. The less common paraesophageal hernia occurs when all or part of the stomach enters the thorax through a defect in the phrenoesophageal membrane adjacent to the esophagus, but the gastroesophageal junction remains below the diaphragm within the peritoneal cavity. Distinguishing between the 2 types is important, since gastric volvulus is much more common with paraesophageal hernias. Our residents are always very concerned about the difference between organoaxial volvulus (twisting around the long axis of the stomach) and mesenteroaxial volvulus (around the short axis), probably because this question occasionally appears on board exams. Regardless of the type, gastric volvulus is a serious condition that may lead to bowel ischemia. Sometimes, a combination of the sliding and paraesophageal hiatal hernias occurs and is called a *mixed hiatal hernia*.

Before the advent of multidetector CT, the diaphragm was a structure beloved by MRI experts, who never failed to point out that the optimal coronal and sagittal planes could be obtained through MRI, but CT only allowed axial acquisitions. This is no longer a compelling argument in the age of multidetector CT with isotropic submillimeter spatial resolution, allowing data to be reconstructed in any plane, but it is true that occasionally, the superior soft tissue contrast of MRI is useful for visualizing relatively subtle diaphragmatic tears or hernias. T1- or T2-weighted images without fat suppression are generally best for these indications, to highlight the distinction between diaphragmatic muscle with relatively low signal intensity and the high signal of peritoneal fat.

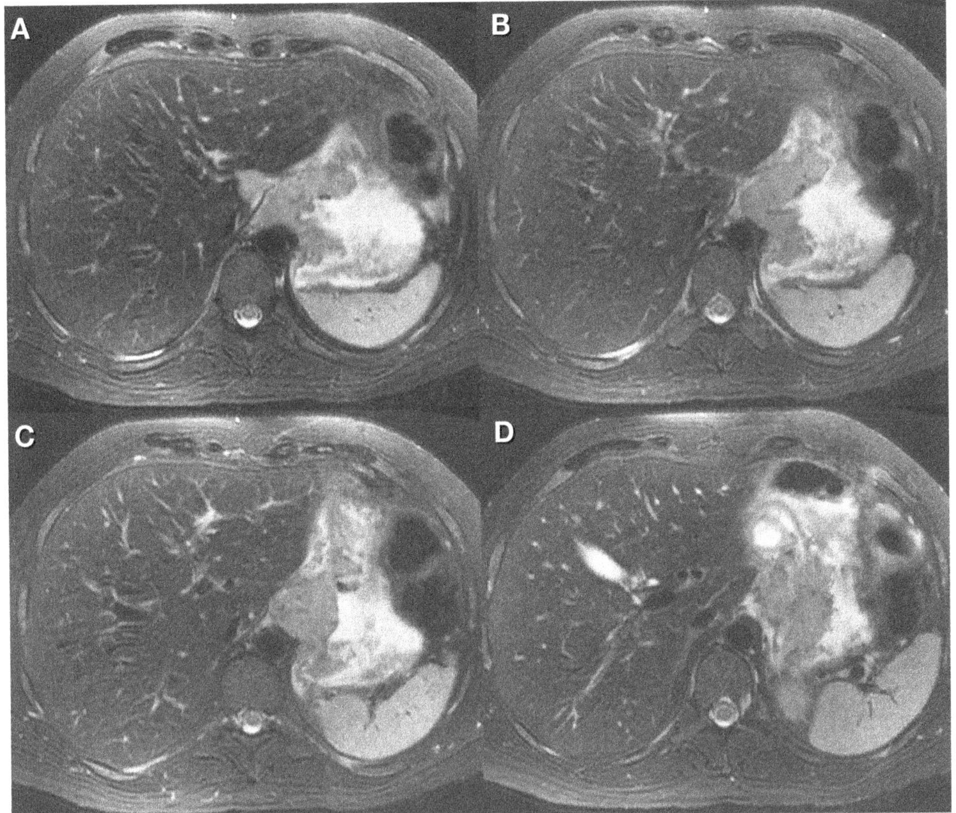

Figure 9.4.1

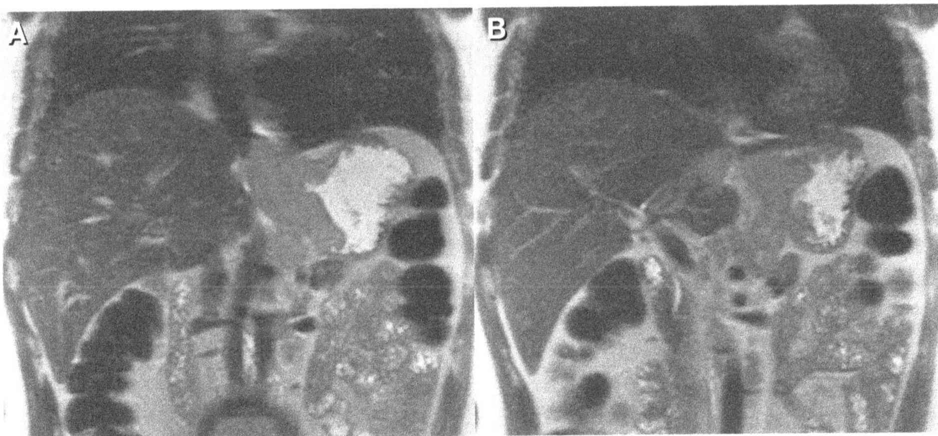

Figure 9.4.2

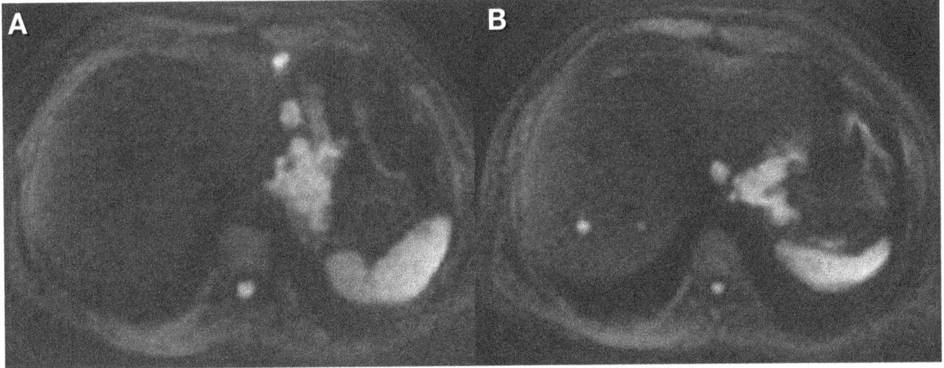

Figure 9.4.3

HISTORY: 34-year-old man with a history of gastroesophageal reflux and recent solid food dysphagia

IMAGING FINDINGS: Axial fat-suppressed FSE T2-weighted images (Figure 9.4.1) and coronal SSFSE images (Figure 9.4.2) demonstrate an infiltrative mass in the gastric cardia and fundus with marked mural thickening and slight hyperintensity relative to normal stomach. Axial diffusion-weighted images with a b value of 600 s/mm^2 (Figure 9.4.3) show restricted diffusion and markedly increased signal intensity within the lesion. Note the easily visualized hepatic metastases; they are much more difficult to appreciate on FSE T2-weighted images.

DIAGNOSIS: Gastric carcinoma

COMMENT: Visualization of the primary gastric carcinoma is generally not the indication for abdominal MRI in these patients, at least in our practice. We are usually asked to look for hepatic metastases and nodal disease or to distinguish benign from malignant hepatic lesions, often for patients with a contraindication to CT, although MRI is probably more sensitive than CT for both of these tasks. Notice, for example, how easily the hepatic lesions and gastrohepatic ligament nodes are seen on diffusion-weighted images.

Characterization of the gastric tumor is often hit or miss, in large part because few body MRI protocols (besides enterography) use the oral contrast agents routinely employed in CT and, therefore, it is somewhat unusual to distend the stomach enough to clearly visualize a mass. This patient had a glass of water before his examination, which, while not ideal, provided adequate distention of the lumen. Masslike thickening of the gastric cardia and fundus can be seen, with effacement of folds, mildly increased T2-signal intensity relative to the adjacent stomach wall (although this wall is so thin that the comparison is fairly hard to make), and increased signal intensity on diffusion-weighted images, reflecting both restricted diffusion and T2 shine-through.

Our residents love to say "restricted diffusion" in their reports. Experts in diffusion-weighted imaging often discuss T2 shine-through as a confounding factor and then describe at great length how this effect can be eliminated by generating ADC maps. But in the vast majority of cases, T2 shine-through is your friend. It increases the contrast between the lesion and normal tissue, and the relative contribution of each effect is generally of academic interest only.

Gastric cancer incidence and mortality rates have sharply declined over the past 70 years in the United States (death due to gastric cancer in men, for instance, has decreased from 28 per 100,000 to 5 per 100,000). The incidence of gastric cancer remains high in Japan, China, Chile, and Iceland. Risk factors include dietary carcinogens, including nitrates in dried, smoked, and salted foods.

Of gastric neoplasms, 85% are adenocarcinomas, with the other 15% mainly accounted for by lymphoma and GISTs. Gastric adenocarcinomas can be divided into focal and diffuse forms. In the diffuse form, cell cohesion is poor, and therefore the neoplastic cells infiltrate throughout the gastric wall without forming a discrete mass—this is known as *linitis plastica*. Masslike lesions, as seen in this case, are easier to identify. They are most common in the lesser curvature and antrum and frequently have ulcerations.

Presenting signs and symptoms of gastric cancer are often vague, with epigastric pain, nausea and vomiting, and weight loss all common. Prognosis depends heavily on staging. Early-stage lesions limited to the mucosa or lamina propria have 5-year survival rates of 60% to 90%; however, these represent only 8% of lesions. Stage III and stage IV lesions (node positive or extension through the gastric wall, or both) account for 65% of lesions and have 5-year survival rates ranging from 3% to 15%.

The MR literature is limited on the subject of gastric carcinoma, although, interestingly, a number of studies have been published evaluating ex vivo staging of resected gastric carcinoma specimens, likely a reflection of the well-documented shortcomings of most other staging techniques. Not surprisingly, it turns out that if you perform high-resolution imaging on motionless specimens at high field strengths, your results are good, but there has been little successful work so far in translating these techniques to real patients with partially gas-filled stomachs and prominent peristalsis. A good analogy can be made to rectal carcinoma staging, where MRI is becoming a common (and useful) examination. In the rectum, however, the anatomic target is smaller, less prone to motion, and more reliably distensible, either with endorectal US gel or an endorectal coil.

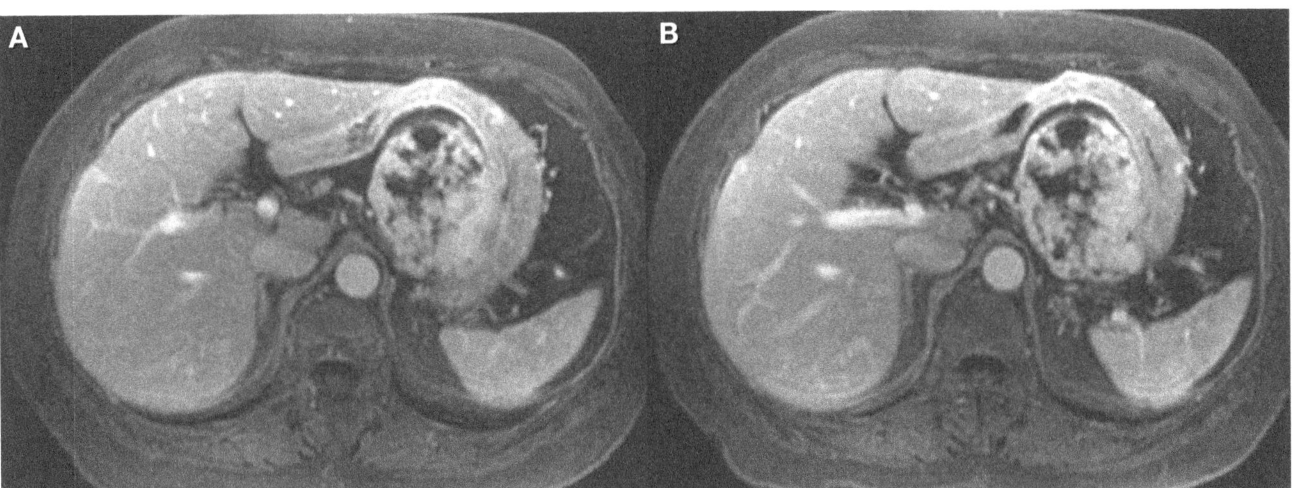

Figure 9.5.1

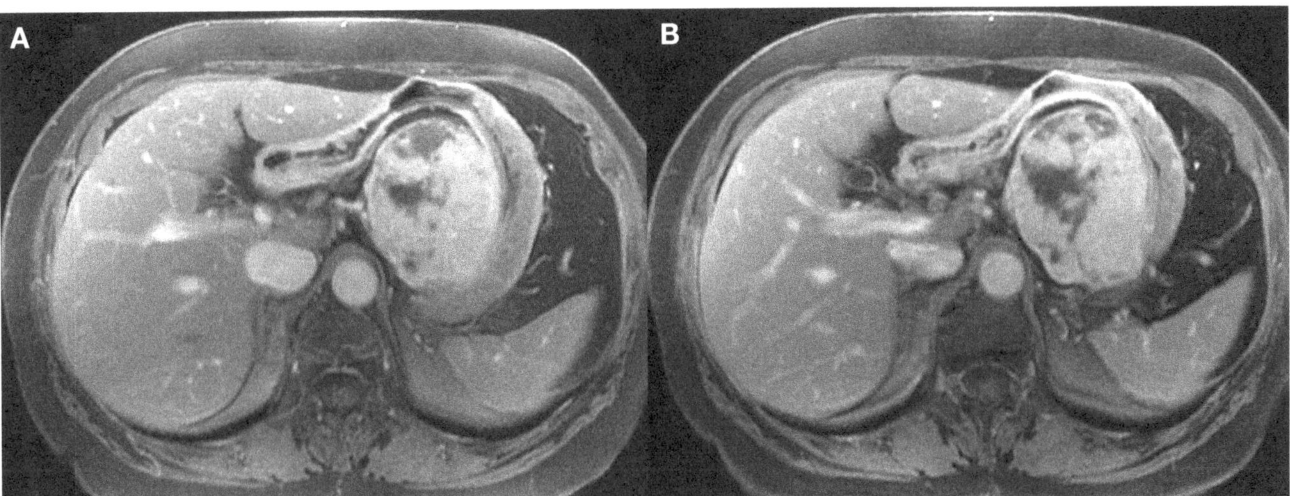

Figure 9.5.2

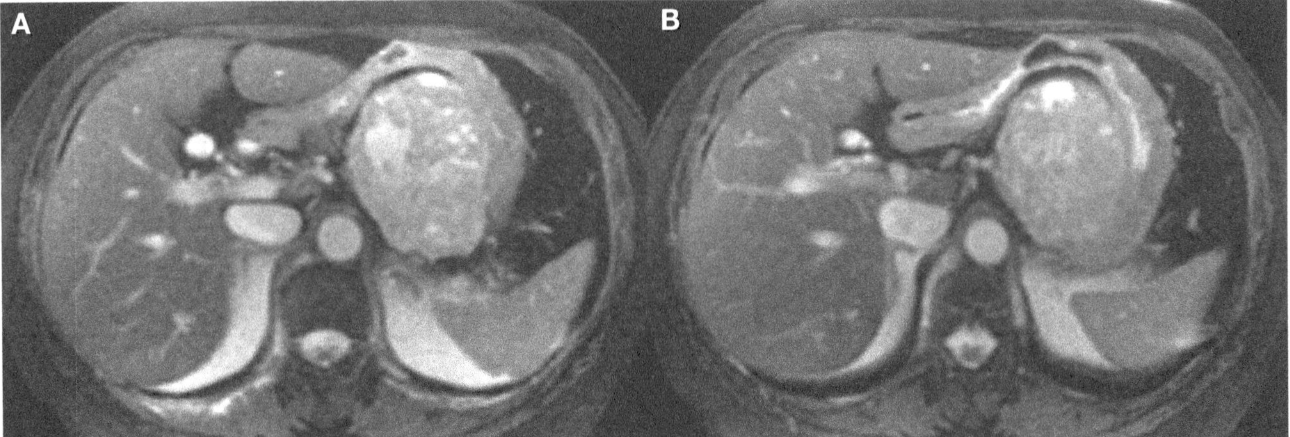

Figure 9.5.3

HISTORY: 75-year-old woman with abdominal cramping and diarrhea; CT at an outside institution found an indeterminate mass, possibly an exophytic hepatic hemangioma

IMAGING FINDINGS: Axial arterial phase (Figure 9.5.1) and equilibrium phase (Figure 9.5.2.) 3D SPGR images reveal a heterogeneously enhancing mass in the gastrohepatic ligament originating from the lesser curvature of the stomach. Equilibrium phase images show some accumulation of contrast agent within the lesion. Axial fat-suppressed 2D SSFP images (Figure 9.5.3) show a heterogeneous appearance with regions of cystic or necrotic degeneration.

DIAGNOSIS: Gastric gastrointestinal stromal tumor

COMMENT: GISTs are a relatively recent development in the pathology literature. Mesenchymal tumors of the GI tract were generally classified as leiomyomas or leiomyosarcomas until the 1980s, when it was discovered that a number of these tumors lacked features of smooth muscle and expressed antigens related to neural crest cells. More specifically, GISTs are defined as cellular spindle cell, epithelioid, pleomorphic mesenchymal tumors that express the Kit protein. Kit is a stem cell factor receptor protein, and activation of the receptor leads to unchecked cell growth and resistance to apoptosis.

GISTs are relatively rare tumors, accounting for 1% to 3% of all GI tract neoplasms, with approximately 2,000 new cases diagnosed annually in the United States, but they are the most common GI mesenchymal tumor. The peak age of incidence is 50 to 60 years, with a slight male predominance. Most tumors (60%-70%) arise in the stomach; 20% to 30% arise in the small intestine, with less frequent lesions in the esophagus, mesentery, colon, and rectum. Approximately 20% to 30% are malignant, and the liver and peritoneal cavity are the most common sites of metastases.

The appearance on MRI has not been well documented in the literature. In our experience, the larger lesions tend to look like sarcomas—heterogeneous enhancement that persists on venous and equilibrium phase images and multiple regions of cystic degeneration or necrosis with high T2-signal intensity. Lesion growth can be exophytic or intraluminal, and exophytic lesions are often large by the time they become symptomatic. Small lesions may have a more uniform appearance, although ulceration has been observed in intraluminal gastric GISTs. This case has a typical appearance for an exophytic lesion: a large mass in a patient presenting with relatively nonspecific symptoms and typical heterogeneous T2-signal intensity and enhancement. Following is an example of a smaller intraluminal mass with a central ulceration.

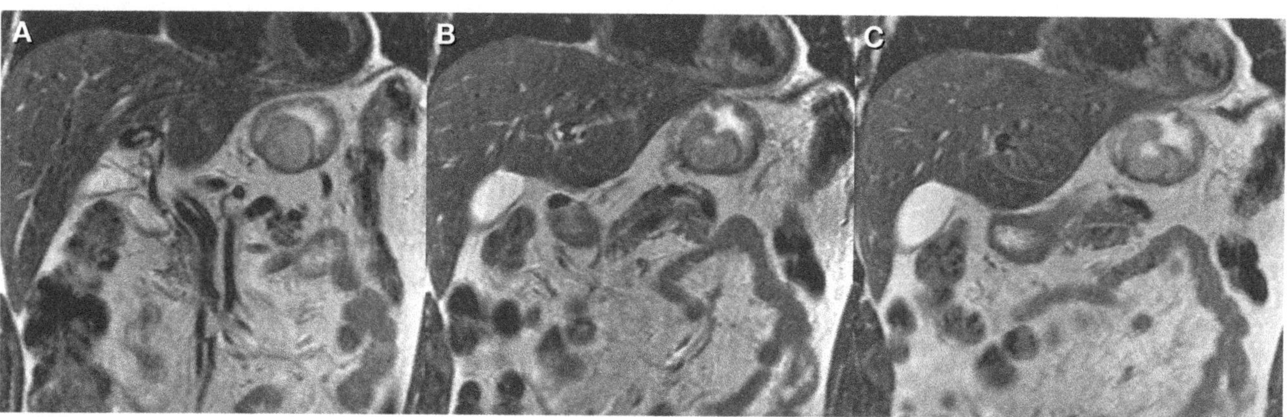

Figure 9.5.4

In this example of intraluminal gastric GIST, coronal FSE T2-weighted images (Figure 9.5.4) of a 56-year-old man with epigastric pain show a well-defined round mass in the gastric body with a central ulceration.

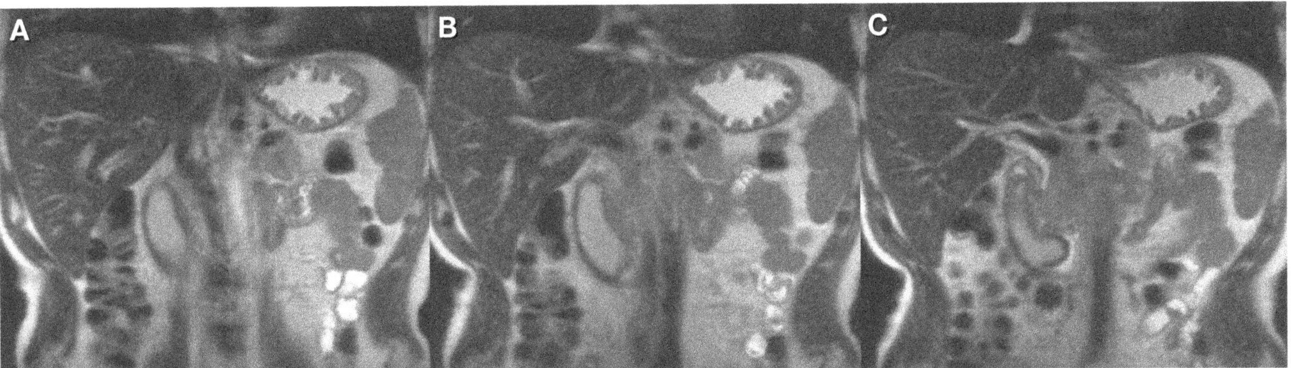

Figure 9.6.1

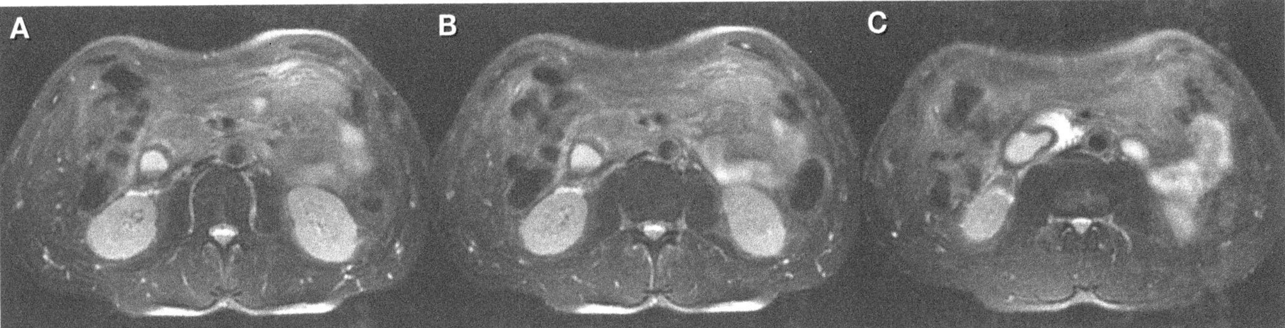

Figure 9.6.2

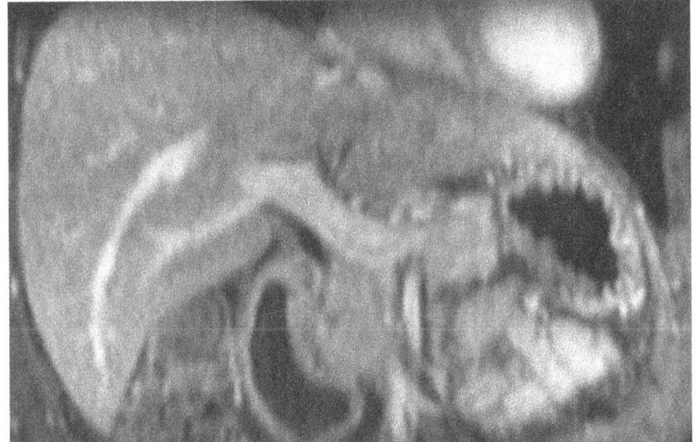

Figure 9.6.3

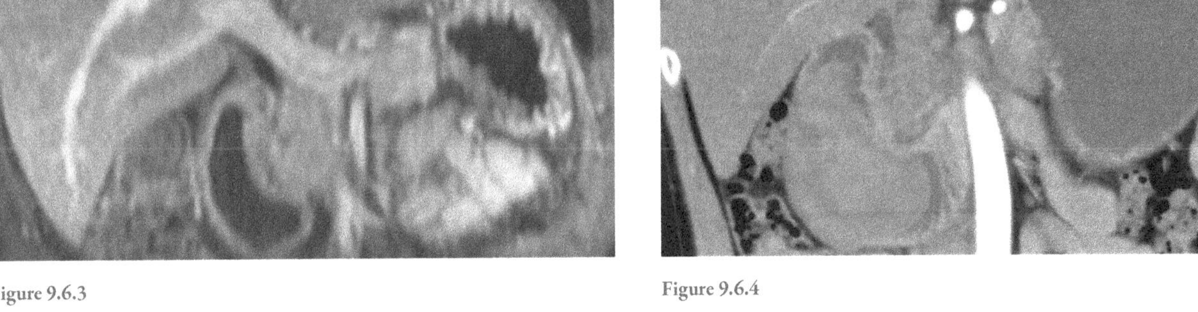

Figure 9.6.4

HISTORY: 35-year-old man admitted to an outside hospital 3 weeks previously with pancreatitis; he was treated and dismissed but returned a few days later with nausea and vomiting; endoscopy demonstrated a complex lesion in the duodenum

IMAGING FINDINGS: Coronal SSFSE (Figure 9.6.1) and axial fat-suppressed FSE T2-weighted (Figure 9.6.2) images show a crescentic lesion with increased signal intensity surrounded by a dark rim. A small fluid-fluid level is noted on the axial images. Coronal reformatted image from a postgadolinium 3D SPGR acquisition (Figure 9.6.3) shows no enhancement of the central component of the lesion. A corresponding coronal reformatted image from an arterial phase CT (Figure 9.6.4) demonstrates high attenuation of the lesion.

DIAGNOSIS: Intramural duodenal hematoma

COMMENT: IDHs are uncommon lesions that are rarely imaged with MRI. First described by MacLauchan as an autopsy finding in 1838, most IDHs (70%-75%) occur following blunt abdominal trauma and are often the result of physical abuse in young children. Nontraumatic IDH can occur in the clinical setting of anticoagulant therapy or bleeding disorders, and several cases have been reported following endoscopy with biopsy, sclerotherapy, or other intervention. A few case reports also have described IDH in the clinical setting of pancreatitis, either as an inciting event (ie, the hematoma obstructs the pancreatic duct, resulting in pancreatitis) or as a complication (vascular damage and bleeding resulting from release of pancreatic enzymes).

Traumatic IDH usually occurs at the subserosal layer of the duodenum, whereas nontraumatic IDH is most commonly located in the submucosa, sometimes dissecting into the muscular layer of the duodenum. Nontraumatic IDH is thought to more likely result in obstruction of the pancreatic and biliary ducts.

IDH has a classic appearance on upper GI barium studies: a threadlike lumen with a coiled-spring appearance. As barium studies slowly (or not so slowly) go the way of pneumoencephalograms, it is now probably more common to see an IDH on CT, where it appears as a nonenhancing duodenal mass, often with increased attenuation on noncontrast acquisitions. The appearance on MRI can be more complex, reflecting the age of the hematoma and the constituent blood products. Since MRI is generally not performed immediately after blunt abdominal trauma (or even in the nontraumatic clinical setting of a rapidly decreasing hematocrit), IDHs probably will be seen, as in this case, in the subacute to chronic clinical setting. The classic appearance is then a mural lesion that is hyperintense on T1-weighted images without enhancement. This case was not hyperintense on precontrast 3D SPGR images (it might have been slightly too old) but, given the clinical history and appearance of the prior CT, is not a diagnostic dilemma. Differential diagnosis includes other duodenal masses such as duodenal adenocarcinoma, metastasis, ampullary carcinoma, pancreatic adenocarcinoma, or IBD. The high precontrast T1-signal intensity (if present) and lack of enhancement, usually coupled with a compelling clinical history, should be more than enough to yield the correct diagnosis in most cases.

Most IDHs are treated conservatively and resolve with time; however, complications occasionally develop, including bowel ischemia and perforation, obstruction, and severe pancreatitis. Bypass surgery or resection of the affected duodenum has been performed in severe cases.

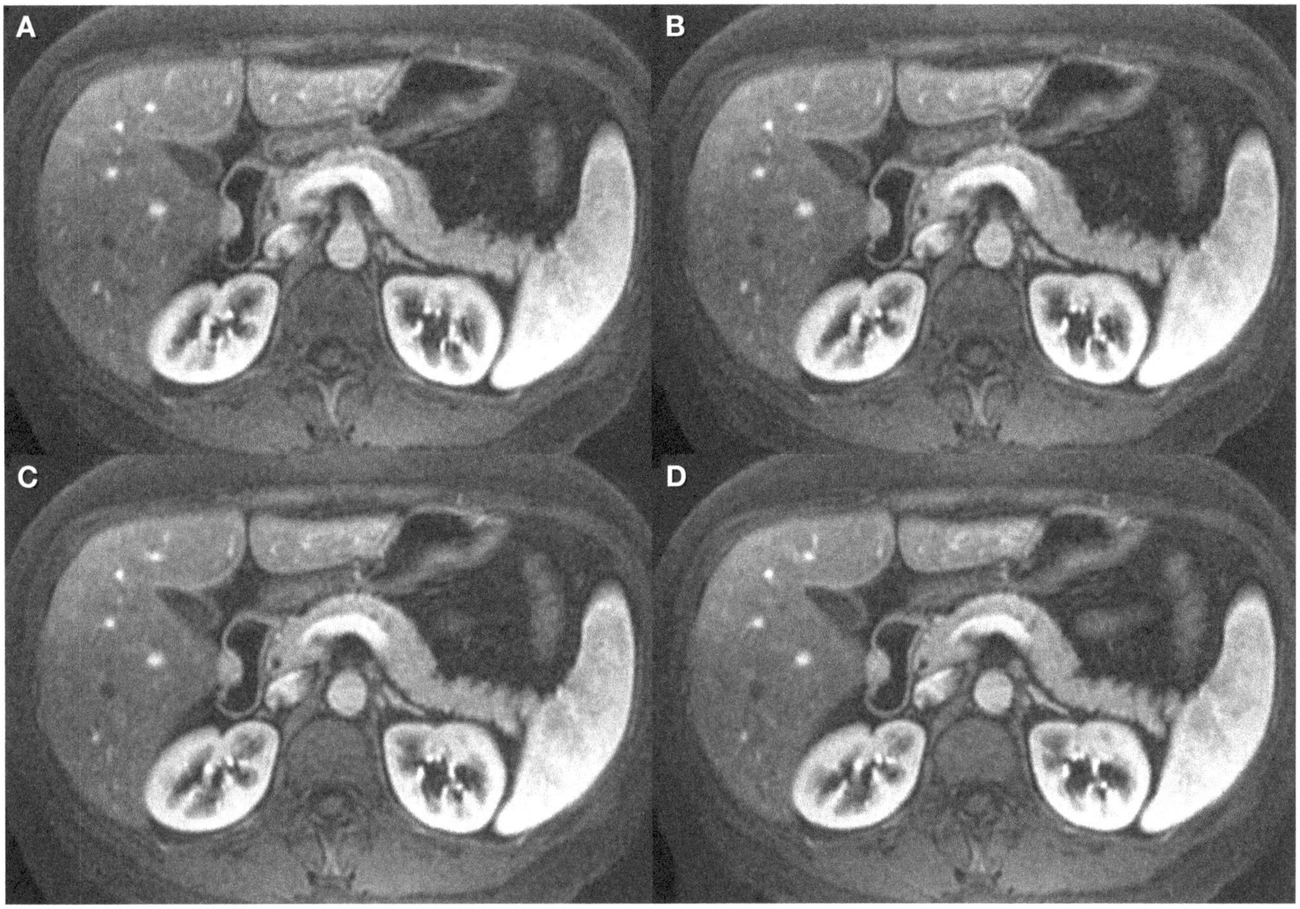

Figure 9.7.1

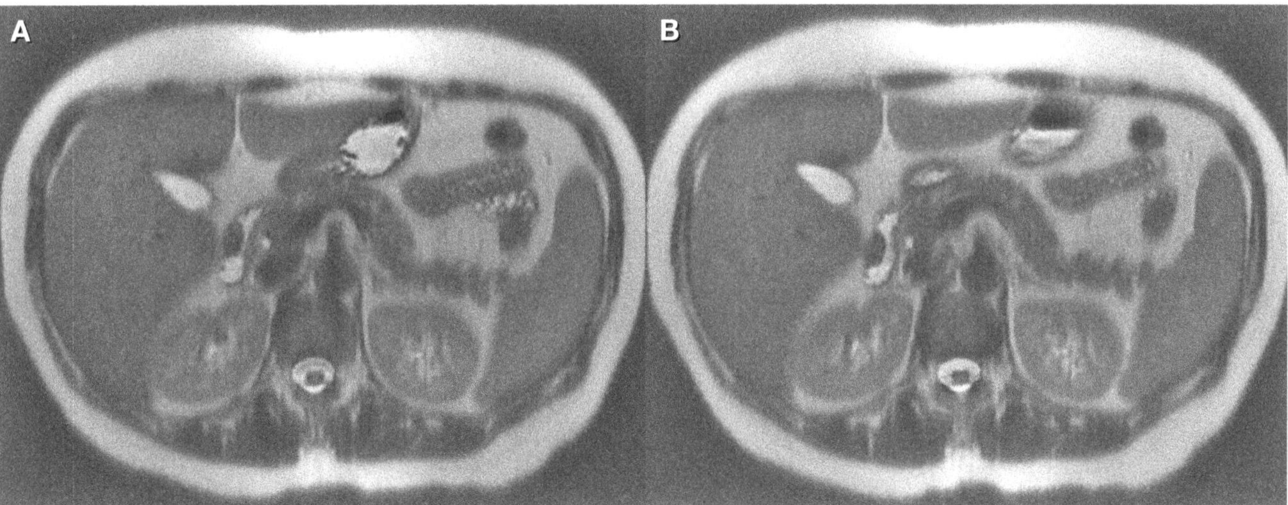

Figure 9.7.2

HISTORY: 44-year-old woman with a 2-year history of abdominal pain and bloating; CT identified a hepatic mass that was indeterminate but thought to most likely be a hemangioma, as well as a mass in the second portion of the duodenum

IMAGING FINDINGS: Axial arterial phase post-gadolinium 3D SPGR images (Figure 9.7.1) show an ovoid hyperenhancing mass in the lateral wall of the second portion of the duodenum. The mass appears relatively hypointense on axial SSFSE images (Figure 9.7.2).

DIAGNOSIS: Ectopic pancreatic tissue in the duodenum (pancreatic rest)

COMMENT: I remember being shown a case of a duodenal pancreatic rest on an upper GI scan as a first-year resident—a submucosal lesion with the classic central umbilication—and having no idea what it was. The GI staff radiologist was shocked at my ignorance (I hadn't been around long enough yet for them to stop being surprised when I missed cases), and of course, I subsequently never saw a real example at fluoroscopy or anywhere else until a couple of years ago, when this case was performed mostly to verify that the hepatic lesion seen on CT was a hemangioma (it was).

Ectopic pancreas is defined as pancreatic tissue lacking anatomic and vascular continuity with the rest of the gland. It is most often located in the stomach, duodenum, or jejunum. Although not a rare abnormality, with autopsy studies reporting an incidence of 0.6% to 13%, it is an uncommon finding at cross-sectional imaging and, particularly, MRI. Most lesions are small and asymptomatic and are discovered incidentally at endoscopy, surgery, or cross-sectional imaging. Lesions may become symptomatic when pancreatitis or a pancreatic tumor develops within the ectopic tissue.

Ectopic pancreas typically appears as an enhancing submucosal mass in the stomach or duodenum, for which the differential diagnosis includes GIST, neuroendocrine tumor, and leiomyoma. Since GISTs are much more common (especially in the stomach) and need to be resected, while ectopic pancreas and leiomyomas do not, it would be nice if there were a way to reliably distinguish these lesions. One CT paper claims 100% sensitivity and 82% specificity for diagnosing ectopic pancreas on the basis of the presence of 2 of the following 5 criteria: location in the prepyloric antrum or duodenum, endoluminal growth pattern, ill-defined border, prominent enhancement of the overlying mucosa, and a long diameter to short diameter ratio greater than 1.4. This example probably meets 4 of these criteria and therefore somewhat supports the investigators' argument, but their criteria are based on 14 ectopic pancreas lesions from a single center using a different imaging modality.

The appearance of central dimpling or umbilication in these lesions on upper GI tract barium studies or endoscopy has been considered a finding diagnostic of ectopic pancreas: The ectopic tissue is trying to form a duct. This sign is not apparent in this case, is not described in the limited CT and MR literature, and is not a universal finding. Endoscopic studies have documented this feature in only about one-third of pancreatic rests.

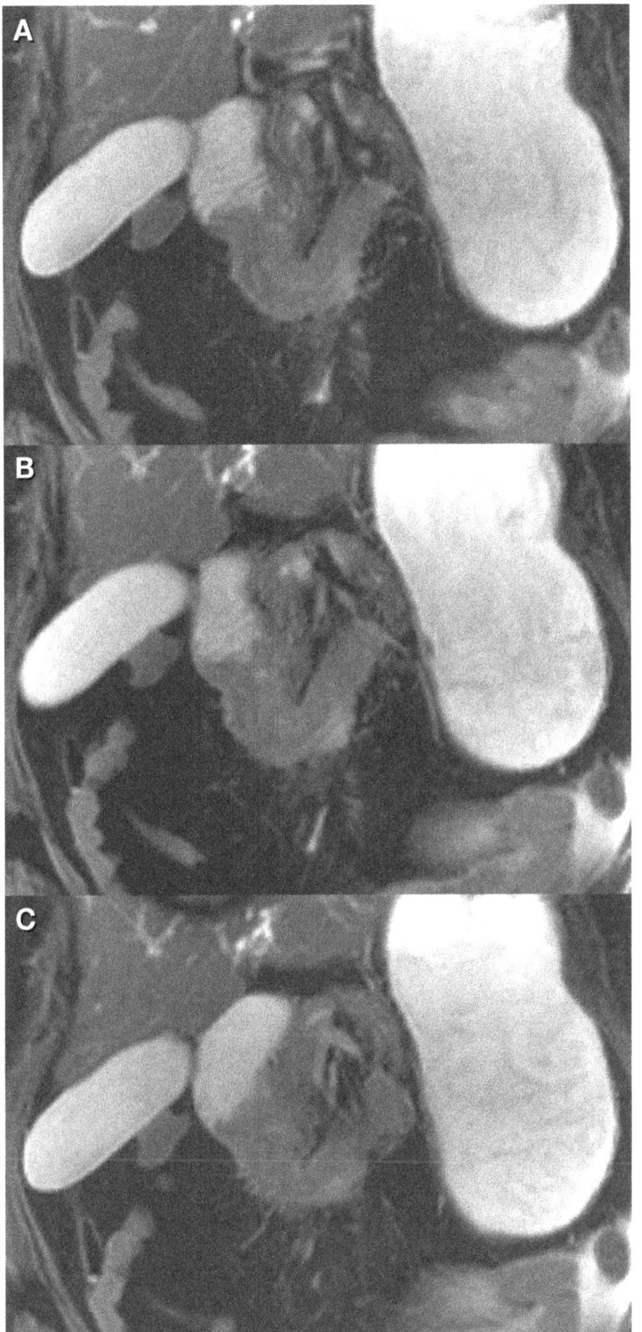

Figure 9.8.1

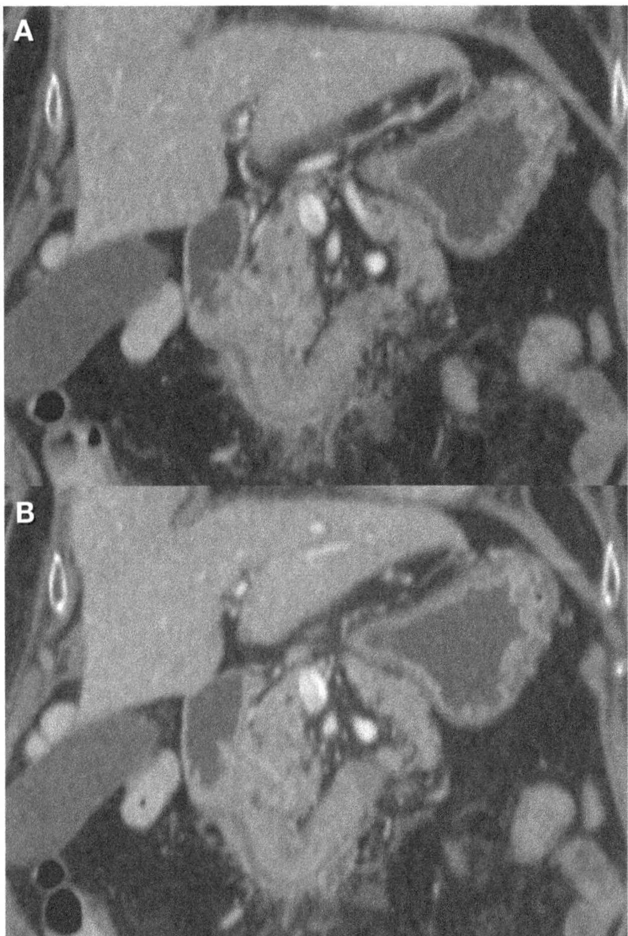

Figure 9.8.2

HISTORY: 79-year-old woman admitted to the hospital with obstructive uropathy and acute renal failure; cystoscopy showed a bladder mass obstructing the ureters. She also reports intermittent nausea and vomiting; a recent endoscopy noted duodenal stenosis

IMAGING FINDINGS: Coronal fat-suppressed 2D SSFP images (Figure 9.8.1) and coronal reformatted postcontrast CT images (Figure 9.8.2) demonstrate a fluid-filled, dilated stomach and proximal duodenum extending to an annular constrictive lesion in the third and fourth portions of the duodenum. Best seen on the CT images, subtle spiculation is apparent along the margins of the lesion and extending into the mesenteric fat.

DIAGNOSIS: Duodenal metastasis from bladder urothelial carcinoma

COMMENT: Without the clinical history of bladder carcinoma, a metastasis probably would not be on anyone's radar, and even with that history, it was not our first choice. We thought that the diagnosis was most likely a primary duodenal adenocarcinoma, which could have an identical appearance. The other, more common lesions in this differential are pancreatic carcinoma invading the duodenum and invasive ampullary carcinoma. Generally, both of these lesions will have prominent pancreatic and biliary ductal obstruction, but not always.

Two recent case reports of metastatic bladder urothelial carcinoma to the duodenum describe one causing massive upper GI tract bleeding and the other resulting in occult blood loss and a low hematocrit level. Bladder cancer accounts for more than 90% of urinary tract cancers, with 67,000 new cases in the United States annually and 13,000 deaths. At diagnosis, 75% of patients have superficial disease, 20% have a locally invasive tumor, and only 5% have distant metastases, most frequently to lymph nodes, liver, lungs, and bone. Intestinal metastases have been found in as many as 13% of patients in an autopsy series; however, they are rarely of clinical significance.

This case is unusual in that obstruction was the presenting symptom rather than bleeding, and no additional metastases could be identified.

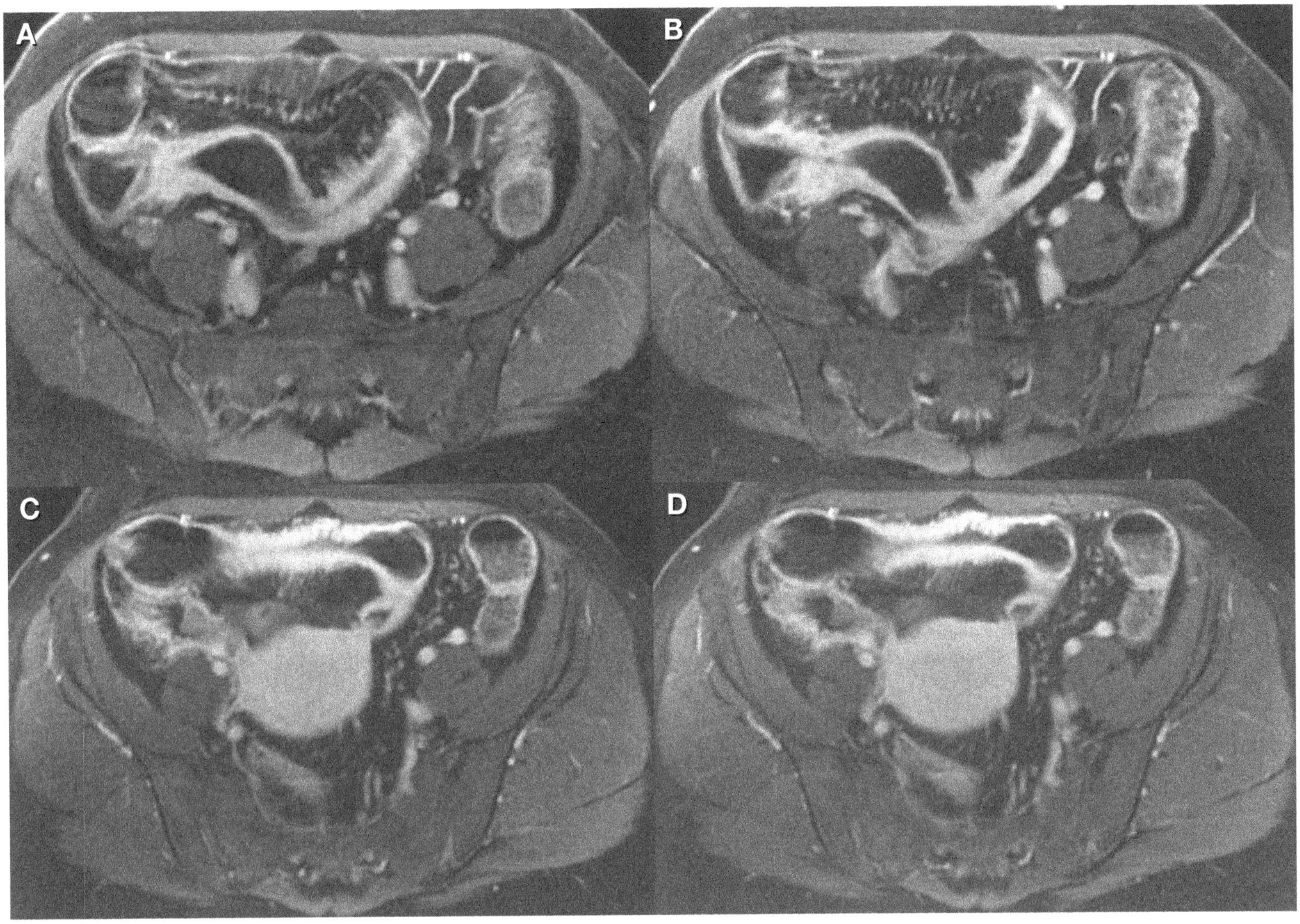

Figure 9.9.1

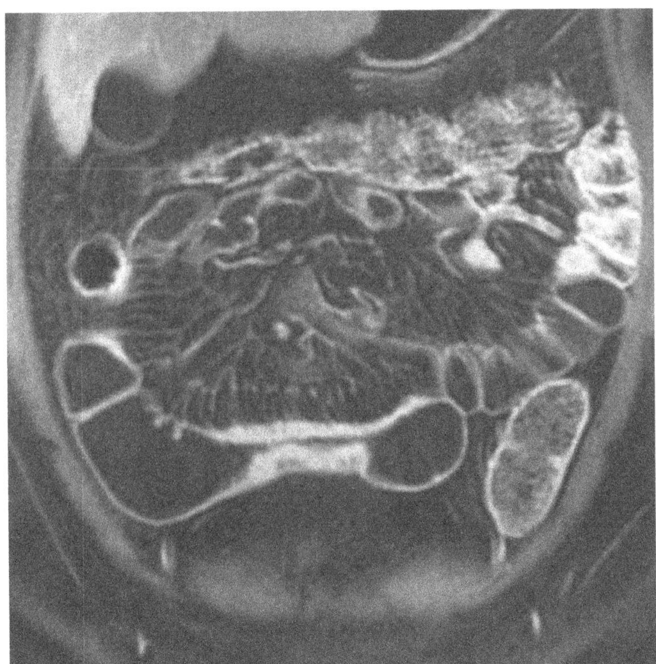

Figure 9.9.2

HISTORY: 35-year-old woman with chronic illness

IMAGING FINDINGS: Axial gadolinium-enhanced 3D SPGR images (Figure 9.9.1) demonstrate marked mural thickening and enhancement of the terminal ileum. At least 2 additional focal areas of involvement are seen in the distal ileum. The coronal 3D SPGR image (Figure 9.9.2) shows the more anterior lesion, with focal wall thickening and enhancement, prominence of the adjacent mesenteric vasculature, and pseudosacculations along the antimesenteric border.

DIAGNOSIS: Crohn disease with distal ileal involvement

COMMENT: MR enterography has become one of the most common examinations in our body MRI practice. Although this doesn't necessarily make all of us happy, it does make a lot of sense to switch from CT to MR enterography whenever possible in the IBD population, which for the most part consists of young patients who require multiple examinations throughout their lives.

It's not that difficult to obtain high-quality MR enterography images. Three key points to a successful examination are adequate distention of small bowel and, if possible, large bowel (a CT enteric agent containing sorbitol can be used); reduction of peristalsis (our protocol includes subcutaneous glucagon just before starting the examination, and an additional intravenous dose before gadolinium is administered); and time-efficient protocols—these patients are often uncomfortable and their cooperation can be described by an exponential decay curve. MR enterography protocols should emphasize fast T2-weighted sequences (SSFSE and SSFP) and dynamic gadolinium-enhanced 3D SPGR acquisitions in coronal and axial planes. The total imaging time need not exceed 20 minutes.

Crohn disease is a chronic inflammatory process involving the GI tract and usually follows a remitting and relapsing course. The etiology has remained uncertain despite extensive investigation, with current theories including an abnormal inflammatory response to unknown dietary antigens and an autoimmune process, with either or both involving a variable genetic component. The disease is most prevalent in the United States and Europe, with peak incidence between ages 15 and 25 years. For unknown reasons, the prevalence of IBD is increasing and has increased by 30% in the United States since 1991.

Any segment of the GI tract can be affected by Crohn disease, although small-bowel involvement is most common, occurring in more than 80% of cases, followed in frequency by colonic involvement. Crohn disease is characterized by erosions, ulcerations, and full-thickness mural inflammation. Bowel involvement is frequently segmental; *skip lesions* is the term used to describe diseased segments separated by regions of normal bowel. The earliest changes include aphthoid ulceration and lymphoid hyperplasia, progressing to mucosal ulceration and transmural ulceration, and eventually resulting in sinuses, fistulas, and abscesses. Chronic inflammation leads to fatty infiltration of the bowel wall, as well as fibrofatty proliferation in adjacent mesenteric fat. Chronic fibrotic changes can cause bowel strictures and consequent obstruction (fibrostenosis), which does not respond to medical therapy. This is in contrast to obstruction resulting from active mural inflammation, which improves when the intensity of the inflammatory response is diminished.

MRI findings in active Crohn disease include bowel wall thickening (usually defined as >3 mm), mural and mucosal hyperenhancement, irregularity and ulceration in bowel mucosa, prominent mesenteric vascularity (or edema) adjacent to an inflamed segment (comb sign), adjacent mesenteric adenopathy, sinus tract and fistula formation, and phlegmon or abscess adjacent to an inflamed segment. *Mural stratification* is a common descriptor used in IBD and refers to the appearance of hyperenhancing mucosal and muscularis propria layers separated by hypoenhancing edematous submucosa. The appearance on MR enterography in a patient with active disease is usually not subtle, and most studies have shown that the sensitivity of MR enterography for detecting Crohn disease ranges from 88% to 98%, with similar specificity. This case illustrates many of the classic findings on MRI: involvement of the distal and terminal ileum, marked mural thickening and hyperenhancement, skip lesions, and a prominent mesenteric comb sign.

The most common problem in our IBD enterography practice is poorly distended (or nondistended) bowel, which can give the appearance of mural thickening, as well as mural hyperenhancement. When the entire segment remains underdistended throughout the examination, you may be out of luck, but often, on 1 or 2 sequences you'll be able to appreciate a wave of peristalsis passing through the region and distending bowel to the point that its fundamental normality can be appreciated. (In fact, this idea also serves as the basis for a well-described accessory technique, in which the radiologist positions several multiphase SSFP slices over the loop in question, with a total acquisition time of 1 to 2 minutes, and looks for a normal wave of peristalsis to pass through the segment. If no normal peristalsis occurs, the segment is probably abnormal.) Another option for patients with poorly distended bowel is to get them up from the table and have them drink more oral contrast while waiting longer. Needless to say, this is not a popular option among patients, technologists, or nurses, and it won't work for patients with partial obstructions.

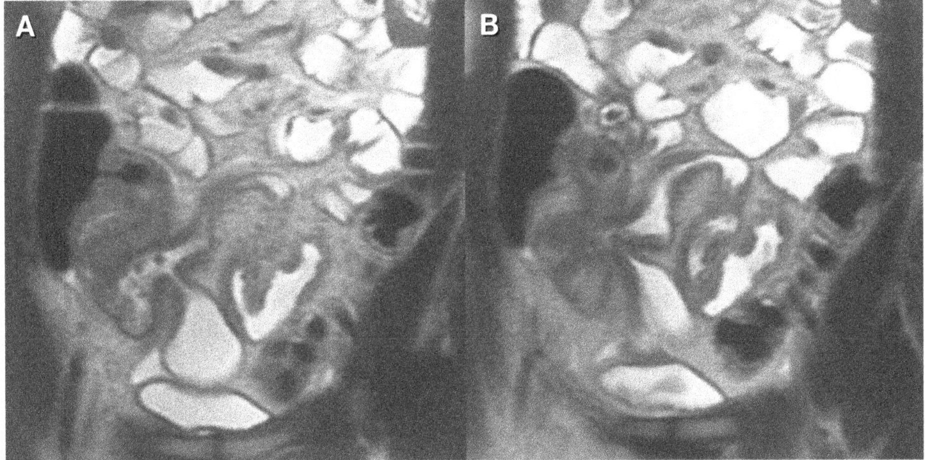

Figure 9.10.1

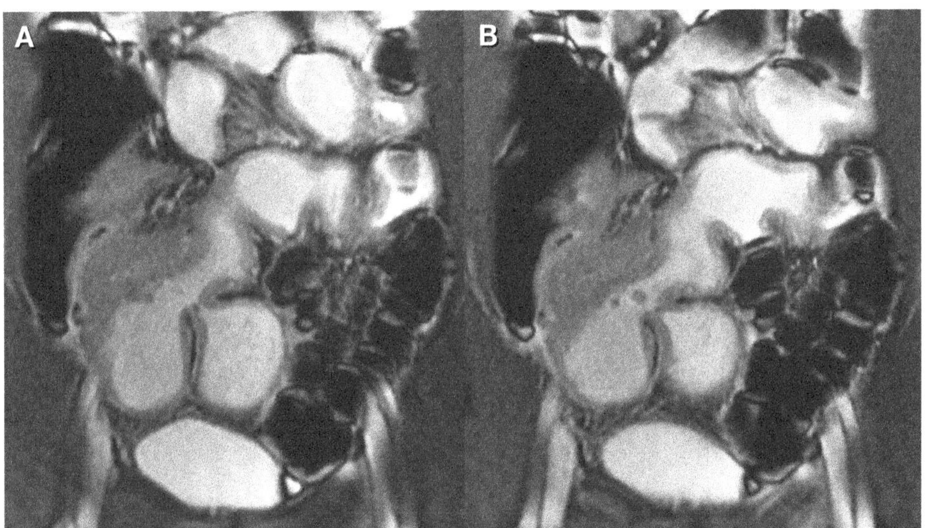

Figure 9.10.2

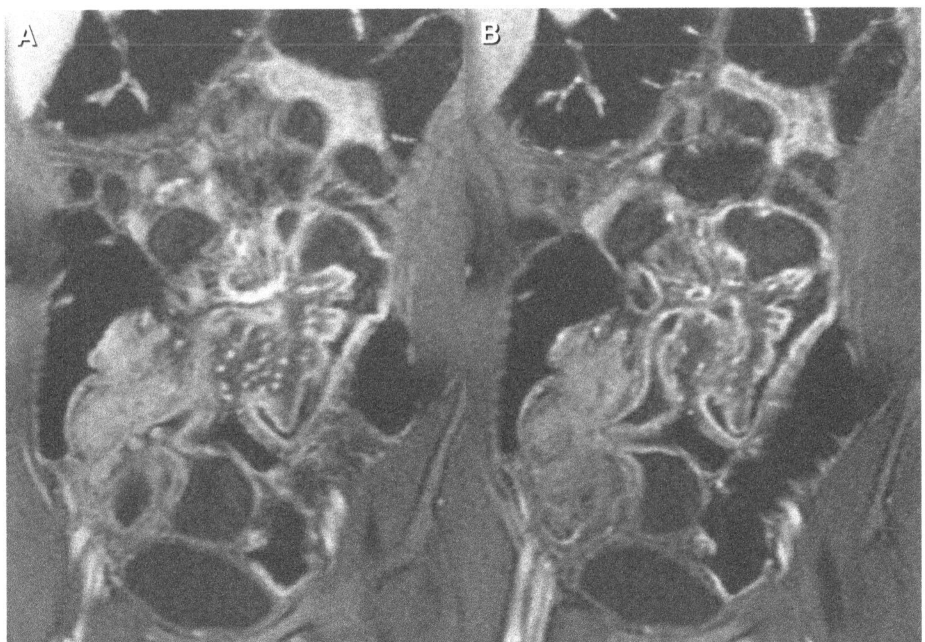

Figure 9.10.3

HISTORY: 24-year-old man with 5-year history of Crohn disease now with worsening right lower quadrant pain, difficulty eating, and diarrhea

IMAGING FINDINGS: Coronal SSFSE (Figure 9.10.1), fat-suppressed 2D SSFP (Figure 9.10.2), and postgadolinium 3D SPGR (Figure 9.10.3) images show marked thickening of the distal ileum, with matted loops of ileum in the right lower quadrant. Note the prominent enteroenteric fistula in the distal ileum.

DIAGNOSIS: Crohn disease with ileal involvement and enteroenteric fistula

COMMENT: Fistula formation is a hallmark of Crohn disease and occurs in up to one-third of patients at some point during the course of their disease. Most fistulas occur in the perianal region (see Case 9.26), but they can occur anywhere, with the enteroenteric fistula shown here a not-infrequent manifestation of severe disease. MR enterography is an excellent technique for detection of fistulas in Crohn disease, with most studies reporting sensitivity in the range of 85% to 100%.

Fistulas occur as a result of deep transmural ulcerations that cause inflammation of adjacent mesenteric tissue, leading to formation of blind-ending sinus tracts that may then extend to communicate with an adjacent bowel loop. Fistulas with a patent lumen containing fluid can be visualized fairly easily, provided you can recognize that they're not just another loop of bowel—which is sometimes easier said than done. Fistulas may show intense enhancement, which can be a helpful distinguishing feature when the adjacent bowel does not have a similar appearance. Fistulas occasionally generate a fibrotic or desmoplastic reaction in the adjacent mesentery, which can lead to a stellate appearance with distortion and tethering of adjacent bowel loops.

Sinus tracts or fistulas may lead to the development of intra-abdominal abscesses, which usually are straightforward to identify—again, provided you can recognize that they're distinct from adjacent bowel loops.

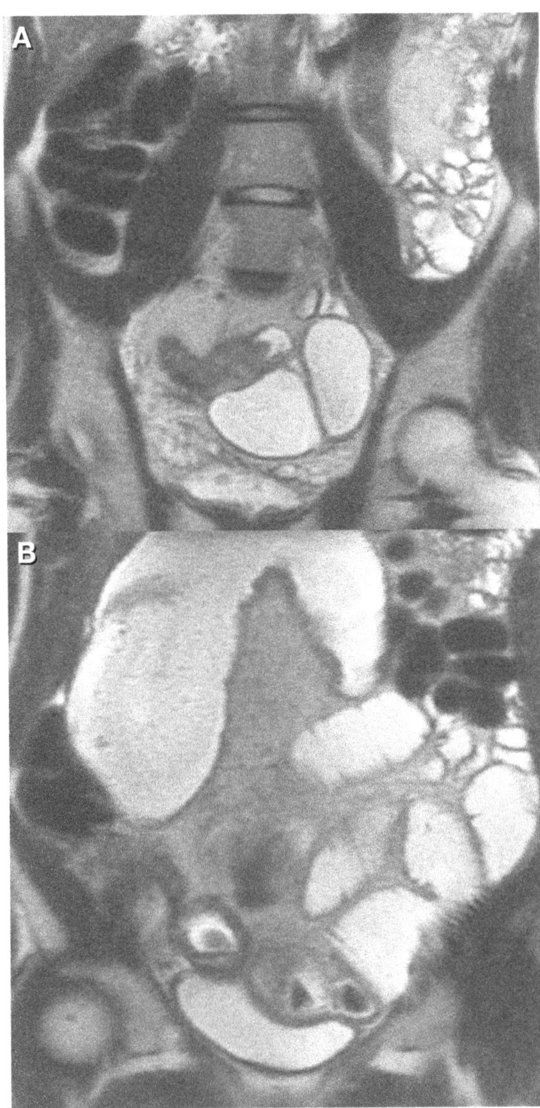

Figure 9.11.1

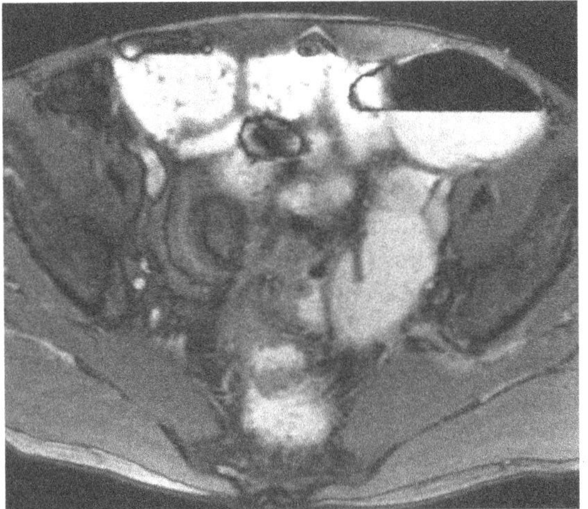

Figure 9.11.2

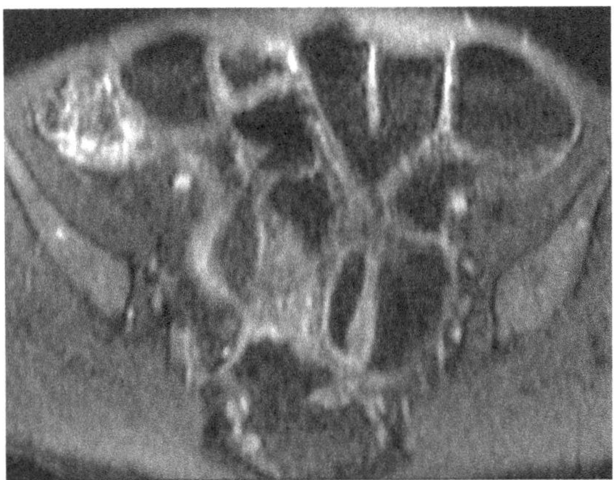

Figure 9.11.3

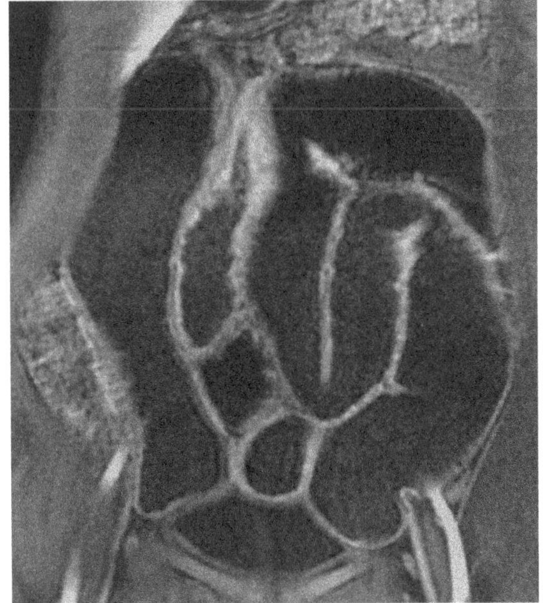

Figure 9.11.4

HISTORY: 33-year-old man with a 13-year history of Crohn disease and recent episodes of abdominal pain and cramping

IMAGING FINDINGS: Coronal SSFSE images (Figure 9.11.1) show thickening and narrowing of the terminal ileum. Fat-suppressed axial SSFP image (Figure 9.11.2) reveals no mural edema in this region, and an axial oblique reformatted 3D SPGR image (Figure 9.11.3) shows mild mural enhancement of the narrowed terminal ileum. Coronal post-gadolinium 3D SPGR image (Figure 9.11.4) shows substantial dilatation of proximal ileal loops, consistent with obstruction.

DIAGNOSIS: Crohn disease with obstructive fibrostenosis in the terminal ileum

COMMENT: *Fibrostenosis* has become one of the favorite buzzwords of the MR enterography literature and describes a fixed narrowing of bowel segment without any significant bowel wall thickening or inflammation. The stenosis, when severe enough, may lead to proximal obstruction. Identification of fibrostenosis is important in the clinical setting of obstruction, since it won't respond to anti-inflammatory therapy and needs to be resected surgically. The classic MRI appearance of a fibrostenotic segment is one with relatively minimal mural thickening, no hyperintensity on T2-weighted images (ie, no edema), and no appreciable enhancement after gadolinium administration. Physicians familiar with the appearance of fibrotic tissue in other anatomic locations will immediately recognize some problems with this definition. Fibrosis is sometimes bright on T2-weighted images and often shows late enhancement. In reality, it is rare to find a completely fibrotic segment with no residual inflammation; more often, it's a question of degree. This case is an illustration of this principle: The terminal ileum shows mild thickening and mild enhancement but not to the extent that we would consider it to demonstrate intense active inflammation. A useful finding in these situations (also present in this case but not shown) is a stable appearance of the segment in question over 2 or more examinations.

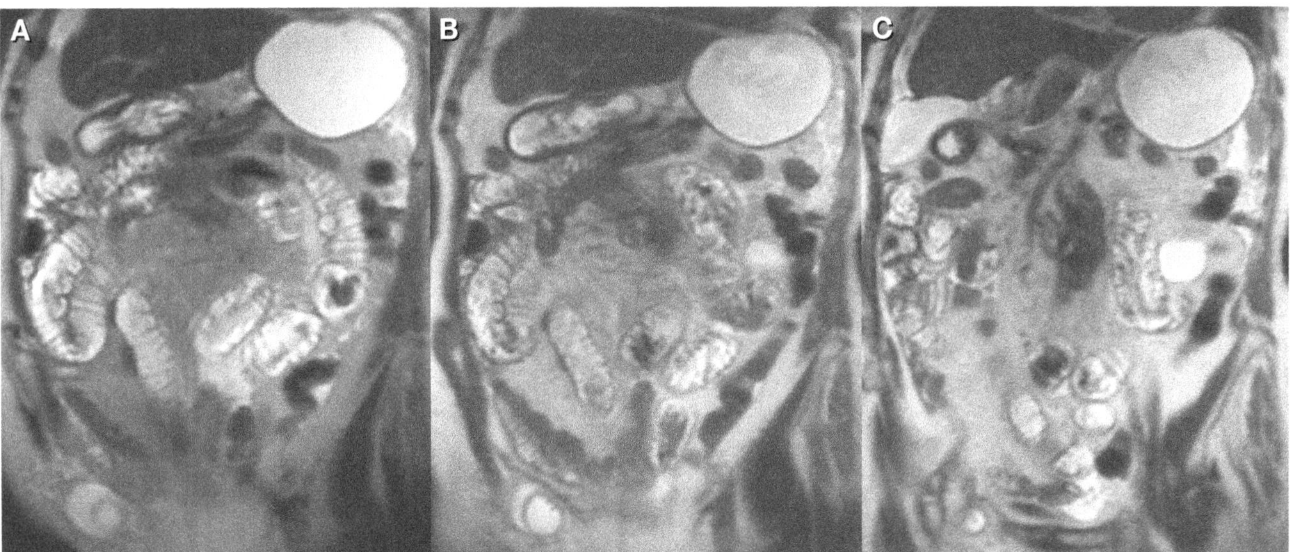

Figure 9.12.1

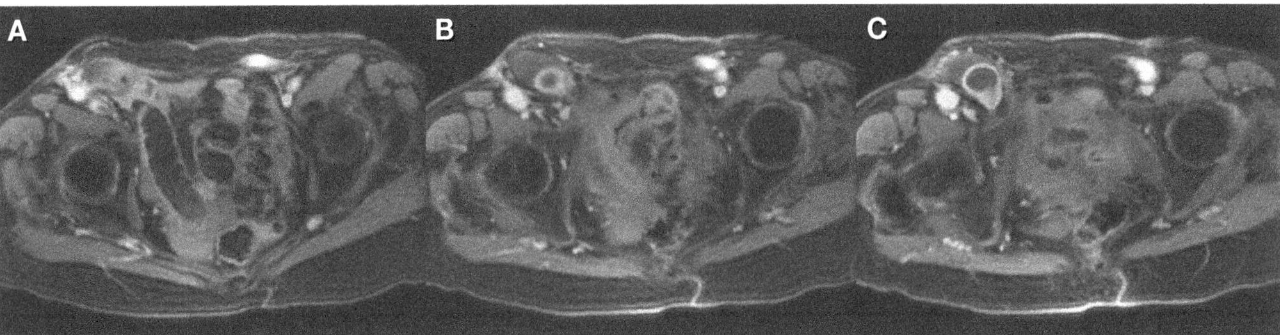

Figure 9.12.2

HISTORY: 89-year-old woman with abdominal pain and nausea and vomiting; abdominal MRA was requested to assess for mesenteric ischemia

IMAGING FINDINGS: Coronal SSFSE images (Figure 9.12.1) demonstrate protrusion of a loop of ileum into the right inguinal canal. Axial fat-suppressed 2D SPGR images (Figure 9.12.2) show moderate dilatation of ileum proximal to the hernia, thickening of the herniated loop, and a small amount of associated fluid within the hernia.

DIAGNOSIS: Incarcerated inguinal hernia

COMMENT: This case is yet another example of the importance of acquiring non-MRA sequences when performing thoracic or abdominal MRA. Mesenteric ischemia is not a bad guess at what's going on in an 89-year-old patient with severe vascular disease and abdominal pain, but it is not the only possibility. Even when the clinician has guessed right, you still want to assess the bowel for wall thickening or abnormal enhancement, the portal and mesenteric veins for signs of gas, and the peritoneum for free air. The inguinal hernia was visualized on the initial coronal SSFSE sequence and then additional postgadolinium 2D SPGR images were acquired through the hernia to show its location, as well as the proximal dilatation and wall thickening and enhancement of the herniated loop, suggestive of obstruction.

Abdominal hernias are common occurrences, with a lifetime risk of approximately 5% (when you exclude the near-ubiquitous hiatal hernia), and most (80%) are inguinal hernias. Inguinal hernias can be divided into direct and indirect types. Direct hernias extend directly through the inguinal canal, medial to the course of the inferior epigastric vessels; increase in incidence with age; are more common in men; and are less often associated with strangulation. Indirect inguinal hernias protrude into the inguinal canal through a fascial defect, generally arise lateral and superior to the course of the inferior epigastric vessels, and are more commonly associated with strangulation. Femoral hernias also occur in the same general area and can sometimes be mistaken for inguinal hernias. These are 10 times less common than inguinal hernias, occur more frequently in women, and are more frequently associated with strangulation than direct inguinal hernias. Femoral hernias exit inferior to the course of the inferior epigastric vessels just medial to the common femoral vein, often compressing the vein.

CASE 9.13

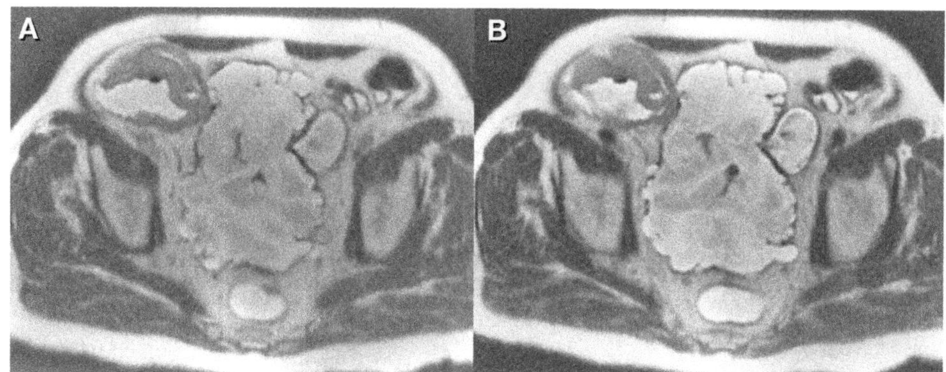

Figure 9.13.1

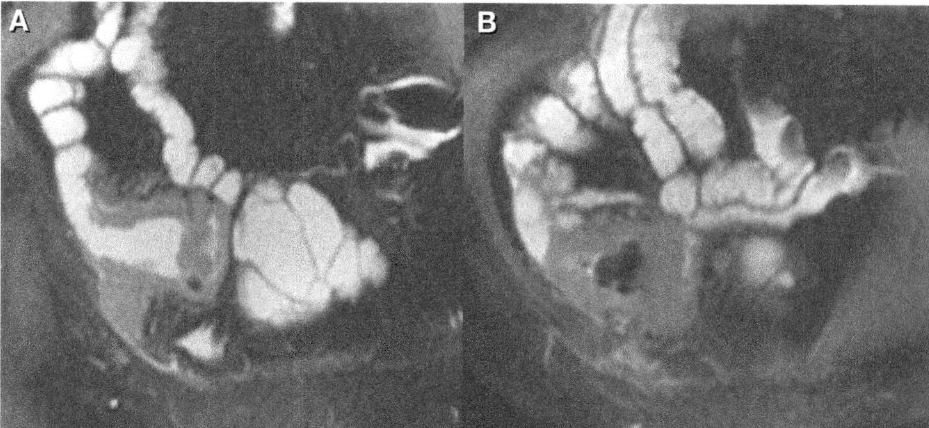

Figure 9.13.2

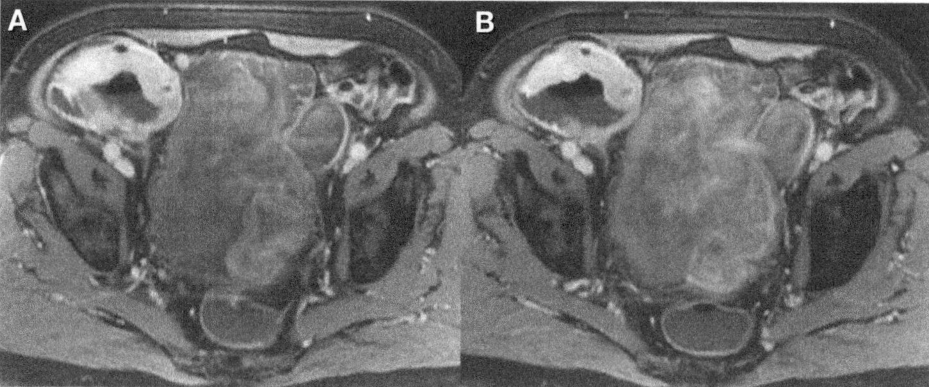

Figure 9.13.3

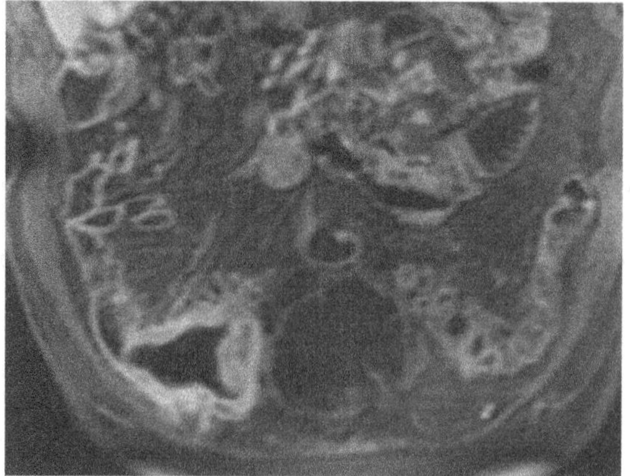

Figure 9.13.4

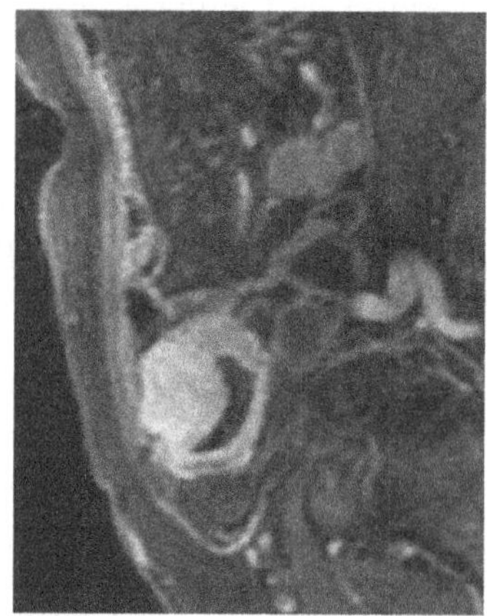

Figure 9.13.5

HISTORY: 86-year-old man with rectal bleeding; colonoscopy demonstrated a polyp in the ascending colon

IMAGING FINDINGS: Axial SSFSE images (Figure 9.13.1) and coronal fat-suppressed SSFP images (Figure 9.13.2) show focal mural thickening in the distal ileum. The underlying lumen is dilated, and no proximal obstruction is visible. Axial (Figure 9.13.3), coronal (Figure 9.13.4), and sagittal (Figure 9.13.5) postgadolinium 3D SPGR images demonstrate moderate homogeneous enhancement of the mass. Note the enlarged mesenteric nodes on the coronal and sagittal images. Incidentally noted is a dilated bladder with multiple diverticula, a consequence of chronic bladder outlet obstruction related to prostatic enlargement.

DIAGNOSIS: Ileal lymphoma

COMMENT: Small-bowel neoplasms are uncommon, representing 1% to 2% of all GI tract tumors. Lymphoma accounts for approximately 16% of these tumors. Secondary involvement of small bowel is more common than primary lymphoma, and histopathologically, the most common lesions are the non-Hodgkin B-cell type arising from mucosa-associated lymphoid tissue (ie, MALT lymphoma).

Small-bowel lymphoma can have various appearances on MRI, including an infiltrating form, a polypoid form, and multiple nodular filling defects, as well as diffuse fold thickening. Lymphomatous lesions may serve as a lead point for intussusception. Circumferentially infiltrating lymphoma, as seen in this case, causes mural thickening and effacement of folds. The lumen may be widened rather than narrowed, as is typical for adenocarcinoma, and this sign has been described as aneurysmal dilatation. Lymphoma generally does not evoke a desmoplastic reaction, and bowel obstruction is consequently uncommon even with relatively large masses.

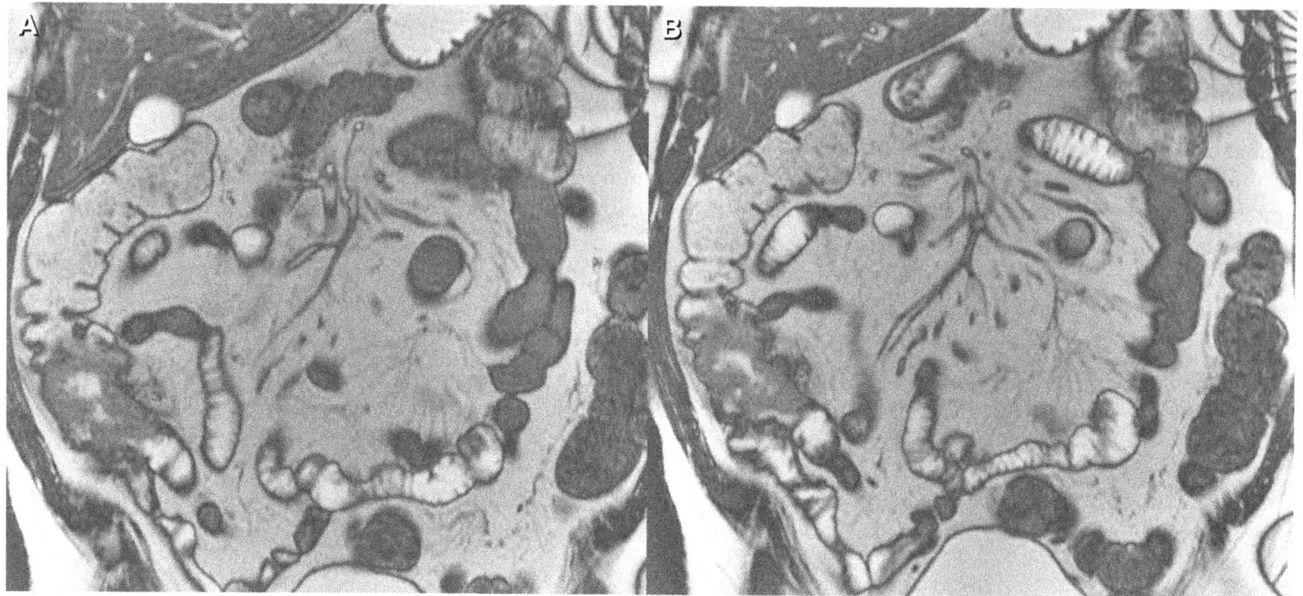

Figure 9.14.1

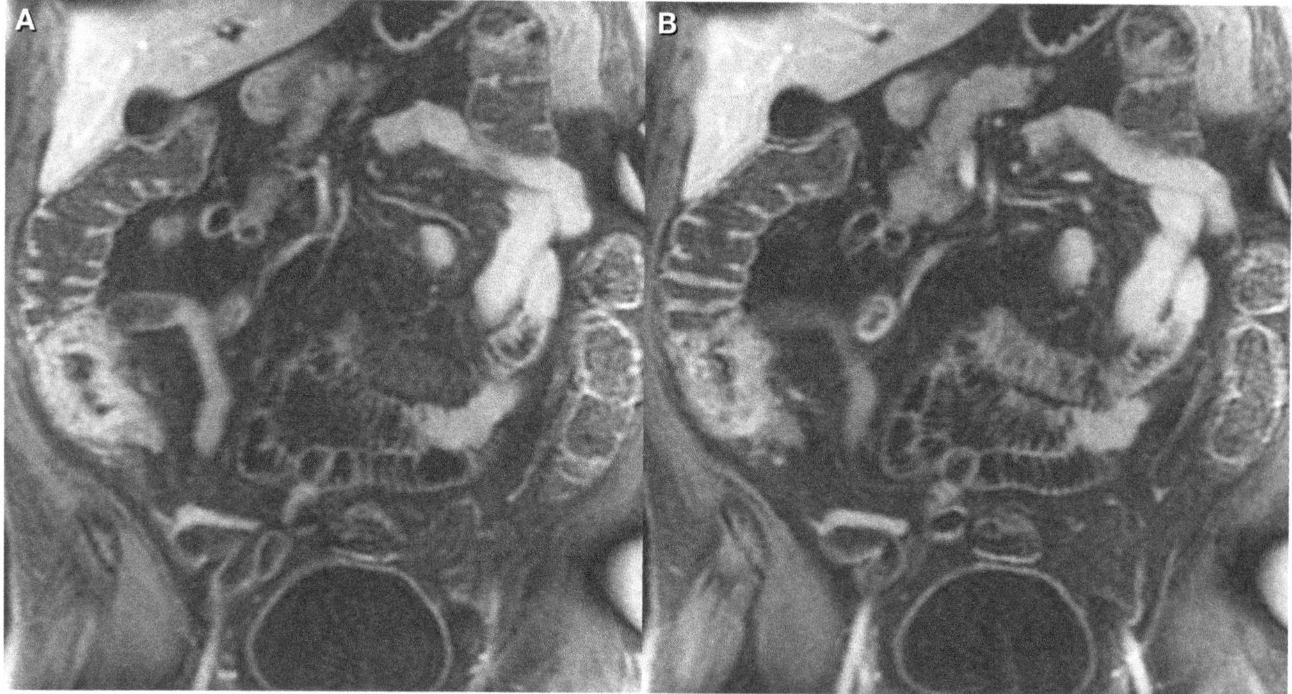

Figure 9.14.2

HISTORY: 60-year-old man with anemia and progressive fatigue

IMAGING FINDINGS: Coronal SSFP (Figure 9.14.1) and postgadolinium 3D SPGR (Figure 9.14.2) images show a focal nonobstructive mass in the cecum, with mural thickening and hyperenchancement.

DIAGNOSIS: Cecal adenocarcinoma

COMMENT: Colorectal carcinoma is the second leading cause of cancer death (after lung cancer) in the United States. Incidence rates have remained relatively stable over the past 30 years while the mortality rate has decreased, particularly in women. Most colorectal cancers arise from adenomatous polyps, which are common in middle-aged and elderly patients. Screening and autopsy studies describe an incidence of more than 30%, although less than 1% of these polyps become malignant.

The slow progression of asymptomatic adenomatous polyps to carcinoma over several years has led to the development of screening protocols, including colonoscopy and, more recently, CT colonography. Many authors also have investigated MR colonography, although the literature is very limited compared to CT colonography. Generally, MR colonography in small single-center studies is effective at detecting polyps greater than 1 cm in diameter, with sensitivities close to those of CT colonography. However, MR colonography is more expensive, has longer examination times, and requires both rectal and intravenous contrast agents (not fun for patients or for technologists who have to clean up after the occasional accident), and therefore has not seen widespread clinical application. So, unless you're in an academic center specializing in this kind of examination, most of the colon cancers seen at MRI are either incidental findings or known lesions visualized on 1 or 2 sequences while you're assessing the liver for metastases. The interesting exception to this rule is rectal carcinoma (Case 9.21 is devoted to this entity).

Presenting symptoms of colon cancer differ depending on the lesion location. Cancers in the ascending colon and cecum may become large without causing obstructive symptoms or alterations in bowel habits since stool is relatively liquid in this region, and ulceration and occult blood loss are more common characteristics of these lesions. Cancers in the descending colon are more likely to result in obstruction, and the annular, constricting "apple core" lesion is a more frequent presentation.

In this case, MR enterography was requested to look for a small-bowel lesion as a source of chronic blood loss; colonoscopy had been scheduled, but not yet performed, for evaluation of the colon. The appearance of the cecal adenocarcinoma is typical: Although there is nothing particularly distinctive about the lesion, it clearly looks like a neoplasm. Since adenocarcinoma is by far the most common colon tumor, it is the most likely diagnosis.

CASE 9.15

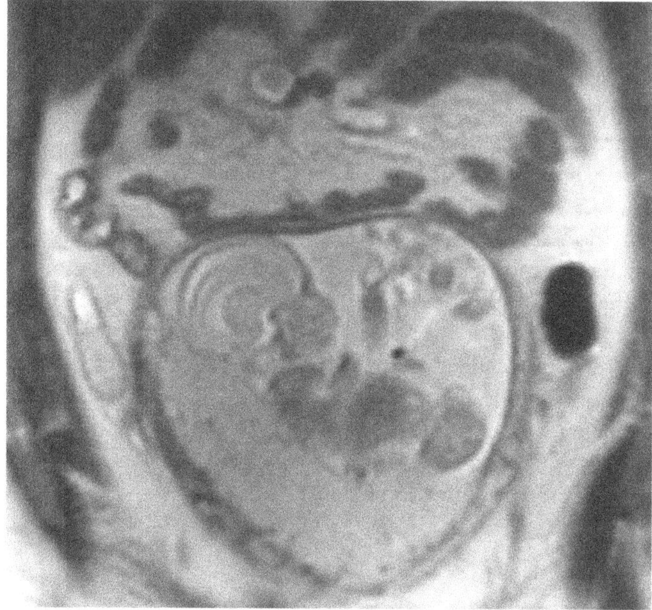

Figure 9.15.1

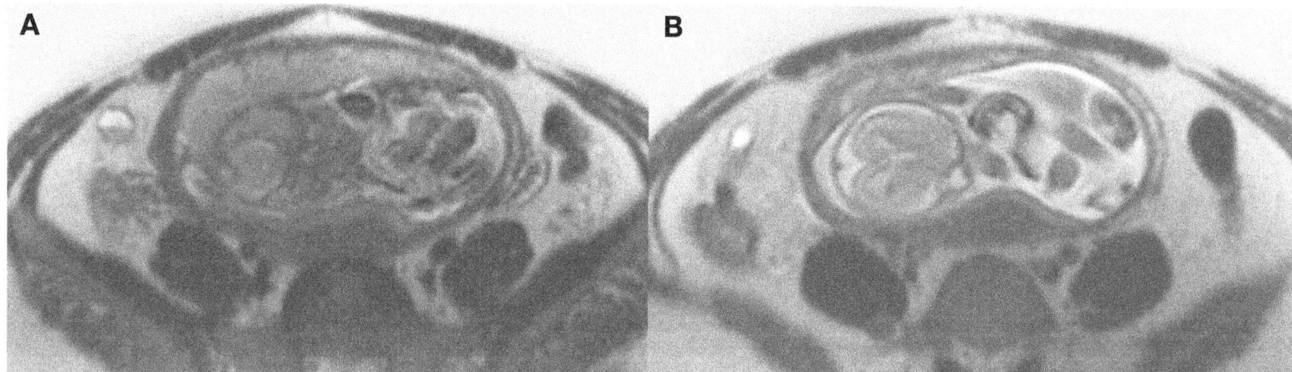

Figure 9.15.2

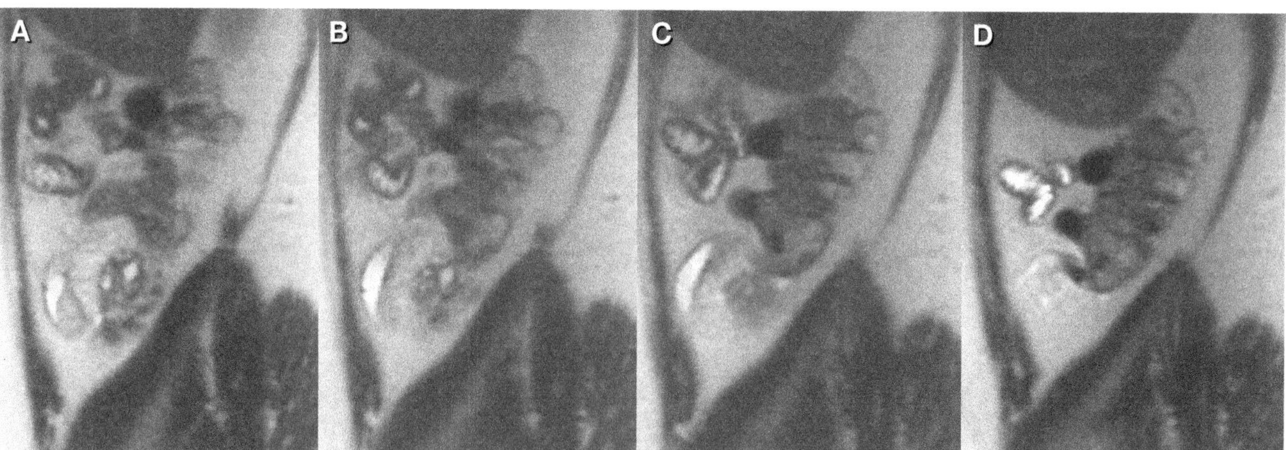

Figure 9.15.3

HISTORY: 23-year-old pregnant woman with worsening abdominal pain

IMAGING FINDINGS: Coronal (Figure 9.15.1), axial (Figure 9.15.2), and sagittal (Figure 9.15.3) SSFSE images show a dilated, fluid-filled appendix. A structure at the junction of the appendix and the cecum has low signal intensity and represents an obstructing appendicolith. Note also the mild edema and stranding in the periappendiceal fat.

DIAGNOSIS: Appendicitis

COMMENT: Acute appendicitis is the most common indication for abdominal surgery, performed in an estimated 7% to 12% of the general population at some point in their life. The peak incidence is in the second and third decades of life and men and women are affected equally. The mortality rate is relatively low (<1 per 100,000) but increases with delayed diagnosis and increasing risk of perforation. Luminal obstruction has long been considered the pathologic hallmark of appendicitis, but it can be identified in only 30% to 40% of cases. Mucosal ulceration is now thought to be the inciting event in the majority of patients. The classic clinical presentation of poorly localized periumbilical pain followed by nausea and vomiting and subsequent shift of pain to the right lower quadrant occurs in only 50% to 60% of cases. The confidence in a clinically based diagnosis is even lower in a pregnant patient, in whom signs and symptoms of appendicitis are more difficult to distinguish from physiologic and other pathologic causes.

MRI has become increasingly popular for assessing pregnant patients with suspected appendicitis, and some practices (mostly in Europe) are beginning to investigate its use in pediatric patients and young adults. A surprisingly large number of papers have been published on this topic, although the cumulative number of patients studied remains small in comparison to the CT and US literature. A recent meta-analysis assessing the performance of MRI in detection of appendicitis in adults reviewed 8 papers and 363 patients and found cumulative sensitivity and specificity of 97% and 95%. These are better results than a recent CT meta-analysis reported (91% and 90%) and are probably somewhat optimistic. Nevertheless, they suggest that even in the real world, where not every patient is an expert breath-holder whose appendix is surrounded by mesenteric fat, MRI can be an effective technique.

Most protocols for appendicitis (ours included) are designed with the pregnant patient in mind and consist mainly of thin-section SSFSE images in 2 or 3 planes, with at least 1 fat-suppressed acquisition. We also include fat-suppressed 2D SSFP images in 1 or more planes. Both of these are fast sequential acquisitions, which means that motion artifact from peristalsis is diminished and poor breath-holding is less problematic than almost any other pulse sequence. These fast acquisitions also help to minimize the total examination time—an important consideration in a pregnant patient with moderate or severe abdominal pain.

Several authors have used additional techniques, including conventional or breath-hold FSE or fast-recovery FSE sequences, SPGR in-phase/out-of-phase images, and post-gadolinium 3D SPGR images (in the nonpregnant population). One group, perhaps exerting undue influence given the relatively small number of patients studied, advocates use of oral superparamagnetic iron oxide contrast agents and a 2D time-of-flight acquisition, which may help distinguish the appendix from parametrial varices. These are not bad ideas, but remember that the progression of oral contrast to the cecum is variable and may be slowed in patients with appendicitis and a reactive ileus. When the oral contrast reaches the cecum, visualization of signal dropout in the appendix on time-of-flight or T2*-weighted images implies that the appendiceal orifice is not obstructed and effectively excludes the diagnosis of appendicitis (except in the cases where luminal obstruction is not the cause of the disease).

Three key elements comprise the appendicitis examination: finding the appendix, deciding whether it's normal or abnormal, and assessing for other potential causes of right lower quadrant or abdominal pain. We all know that the appendix originates from the cecum, usually 2 to 3 cm below the ileocecal valve, but there is considerable variability in the direction it will travel, a detail compounded in the pregnant patient, in whom the uterus displaces the cecum and appendix, especially in the third trimester.

We start the examination with overlapping axial and sagittal SSFSE or SSFP images, or both, and when the appendix is tentatively identified, we then prescribe oblique planes to optimize its visualization. Normally, the appendix has a diameter less than 6 mm, which makes it hard to detect, particularly when it's not surrounded by fat. However, most authors have been successful at identifying the normal appendix in 80% to 90% of patients. An abnormal appendix has a diameter greater than 6 or 7 mm, is distended with fluid, doesn't contain air in the lumen, and might have a thick wall (>3 mm). Localized periappendiceal inflammation is a useful sign when present and is easier to see on fat-suppressed images but can be difficult to identify in patients with ascites or generalized inflammation or edema. (See Figure 9.15.4 for a second example with more prominent wall thickening and periappendiceal edema.) You won't always see an obstructing appendicolith, as in this case, but it's worth looking for and can increase your confidence when present.

The differential diagnosis for appendicitis is broad. After documentation of a normal appendix, you should consider renal colic, cholecystitis, ovarian torsion or hemorrhagic cyst, and IBD. One entity that also presents with a distended appendix is a mucocele (see Case 9.16). Given the wide range of potential alternative diagnoses, it is a good idea to include at least 1 large field-of-view coronal acquisition that includes as much of the abdomen and pelvis as possible, to optimize your chances of spotting a nonappendiceal abnormality.

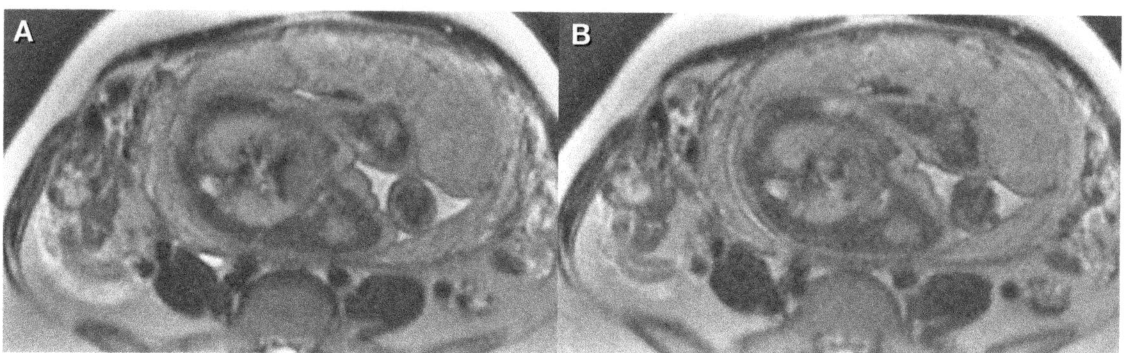

Figure 9.15.4

Axial SSFSE images of a 26-year-old pregnant woman with right lower quadrant pain show a thick-walled appendix with localized periappendiceal fluid and edema. Note that no significant luminal distention is seen in this case. Acute appendicitis was found at surgery.

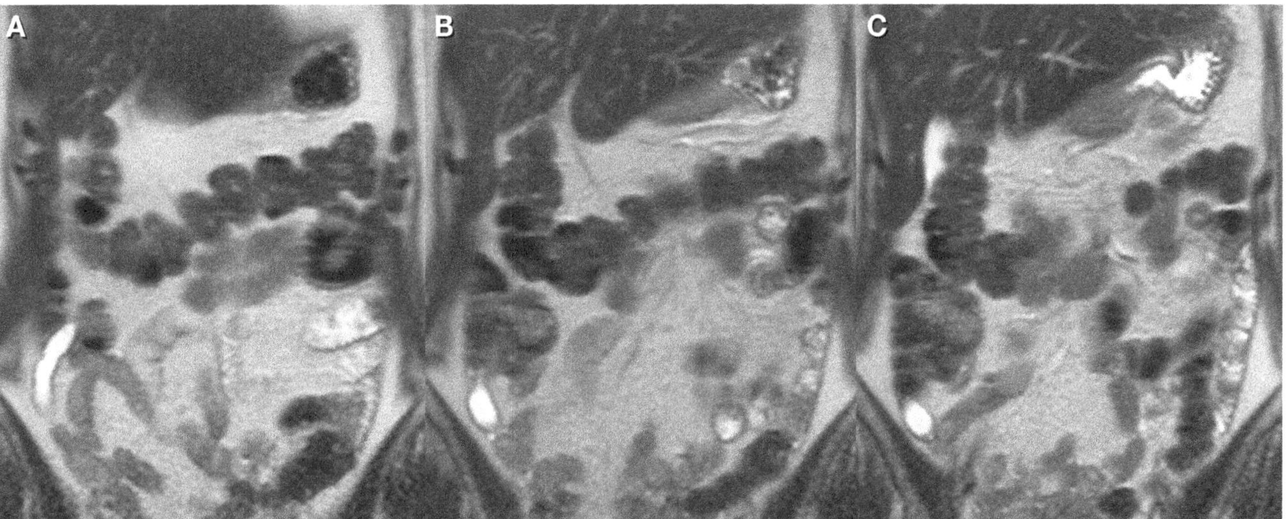

Figure 9.16.1

HISTORY: 54-year-old woman with a history of epigastric pain. MRA was requested to assess for mesenteric ischemia

IMAGING FINDINGS: Coronal SSFSE images (Figure 9.16.1) demonstrate a dilated, fluid-filled appendix without appreciable periappendiceal inflammation.

DIAGNOSIS: Appendiceal mucocele

COMMENT: *Appendiceal mucocele* is a generic term describing an appendix distended by mucus. A rare condition, appendiceal mucocele has a prevalence of 0.2% to 0.3% in appendectomy specimens. Mucoceles have been divided into 4 histologic subtypes: mucus retention cyst (the diagnosis in this case), mucosal hyperplasia, mucinous cystadenoma, and invasive mucinous cystadenocarcinoma. Most benign mucoceles are asymptomatic and are incidental findings at abdominal imaging or physical examination. Lesions may become symptomatic with superinfection, intussusception, or torsion.

It may not be possible to distinguish a mucocele from acute appendicitis in a patient presenting with right lower quadrant pain; however, the diagnosis usually can be made in an asymptomatic patient whose MRI is performed for a different indication. In general, the appendix is moderately to markedly distended, with minimal wall thickening and no appreciable periappendiceal inflammation. Marked distention of the lumen (>15 mm) should raise concern for malignancy.

Direct extension of an appendiceal mucinous cystadenocarcinoma into the peritoneal cavity with diffuse intraperitoneal accumulation of gelatinous material is known as *pseudomyxoma peritonei*. This term is somewhat ambiguous and has also been used to describe localized collections resulting from rupture of a benign mucocele.

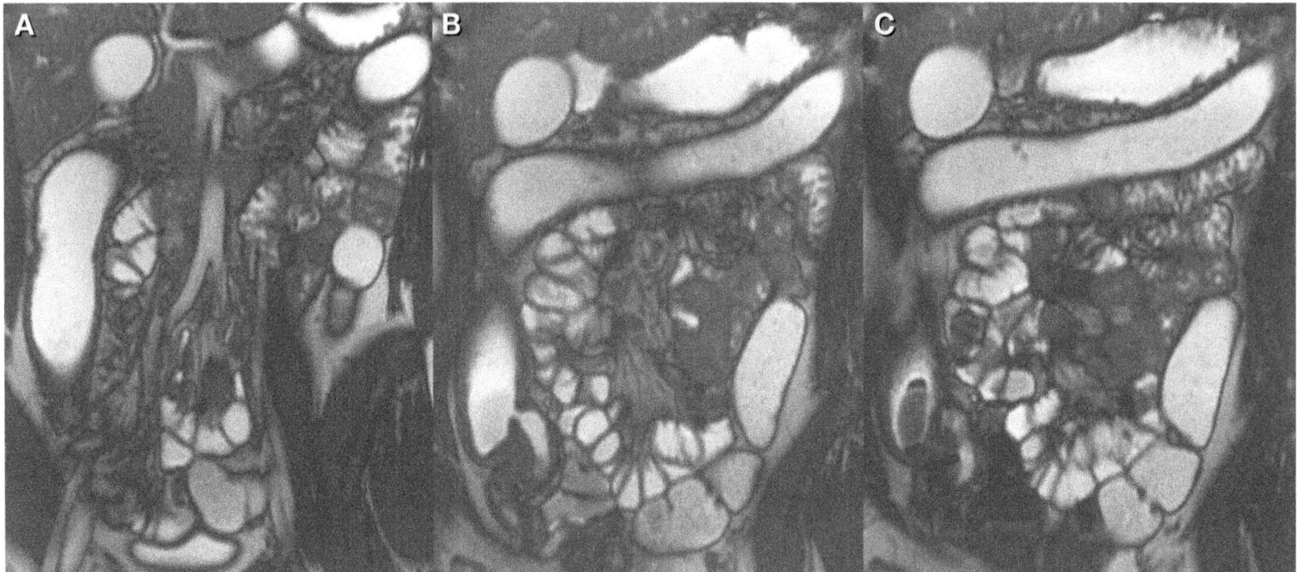

Figure 9.17.1

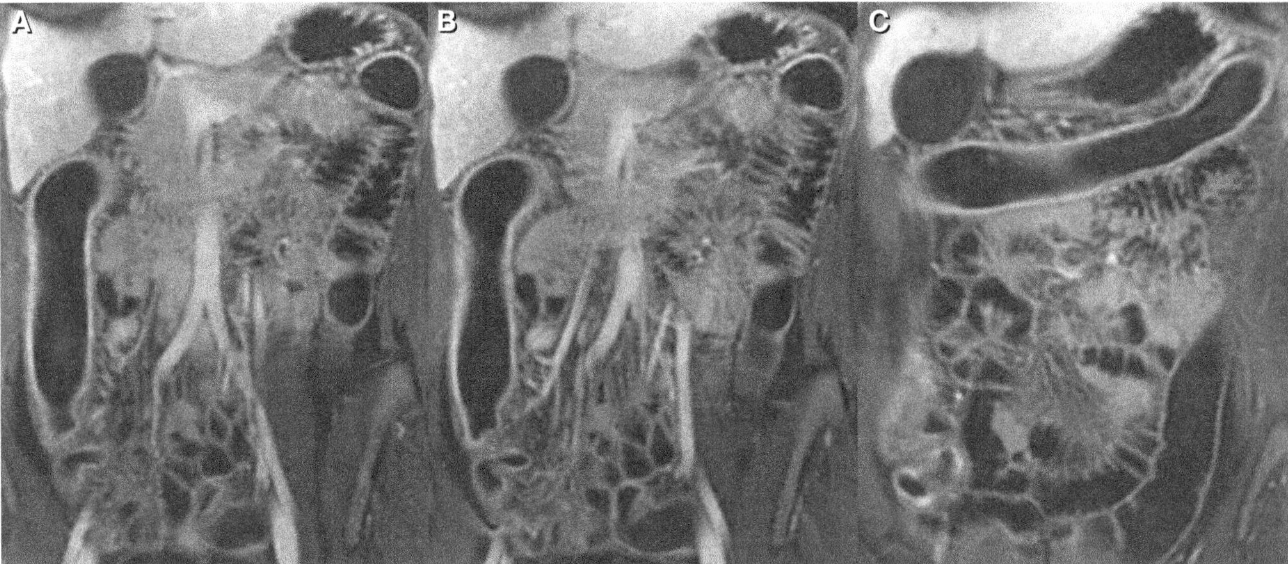

Figure 9.17.2

HISTORY: 35-year-old woman with a history of IBD and moderately active IBD symptoms

IMAGING FINDINGS: Coronal SSFP images (Figure 9.17.1) and coronal postgadolinium 3D SPGR images (Figure 9.17.2) show an ahaustral right and transverse colon with mild mural thickening and enhancement. Note the relatively normal appearance of the descending and sigmoid colon and the mild thickening and hyperenhancement of the terminal ileum.

DIAGNOSIS: Crohn colitis with ahaustral colon

COMMENT: An interesting (and curious) feature of the MR enterography literature on Crohn disease is that the colon is almost entirely ignored. Although it is true that the small bowel is more commonly affected than the colon, part of the reason for the discrepancy is that the various oral contrast recipes (the excruciating details of which account for an inordinate number of papers) do not reliably distend the colon, and therefore the colon is often difficult to evaluate. This case is included as a reminder to look at the colon when performing MR enterography in patients with Crohn disease. We have seen a few examples in our practice of rather obvious findings that were passed by in favor of describing subtle small-bowel abnormalities that may or may not have been present.

The classic teaching regarding Crohn colitis is that it predominantly affects the right colon. Involvement of the cecum and right colon is most common, with concomitant disease in the terminal ileum seen in a majority of cases. Rectal involvement is not rare, however, and may occur in as many as 30% to 50% of patients. Even so, right-sided colitis, particularly when skip lesions are present, should suggest Crohn disease rather than ulcerative colitis.

The clinical hallmark of Crohn colitis is diarrhea that is more intense and distressing than typically encountered in ulcerative colitis. By comparison, gross bleeding—a classic presentation of ulcerative colitis—is relatively rare in Crohn colitis.

The major pathologic abnormalities of Crohn colitis include penetrating ulcers or fissures, confluent linear ulcers, and mural thickening. The distinction between the superficial ulcerations of ulcerative colitis and the deep transmural ulcers of Crohn disease, which can be appreciated on double-contrast barium enema examinations, is generally not discernible on standard MR enterography examinations; however, mural thickening and hyperenhancement, loss of the normal haustral folds, and presence of sinus tracts or fistulas are common findings detectable on most examinations.

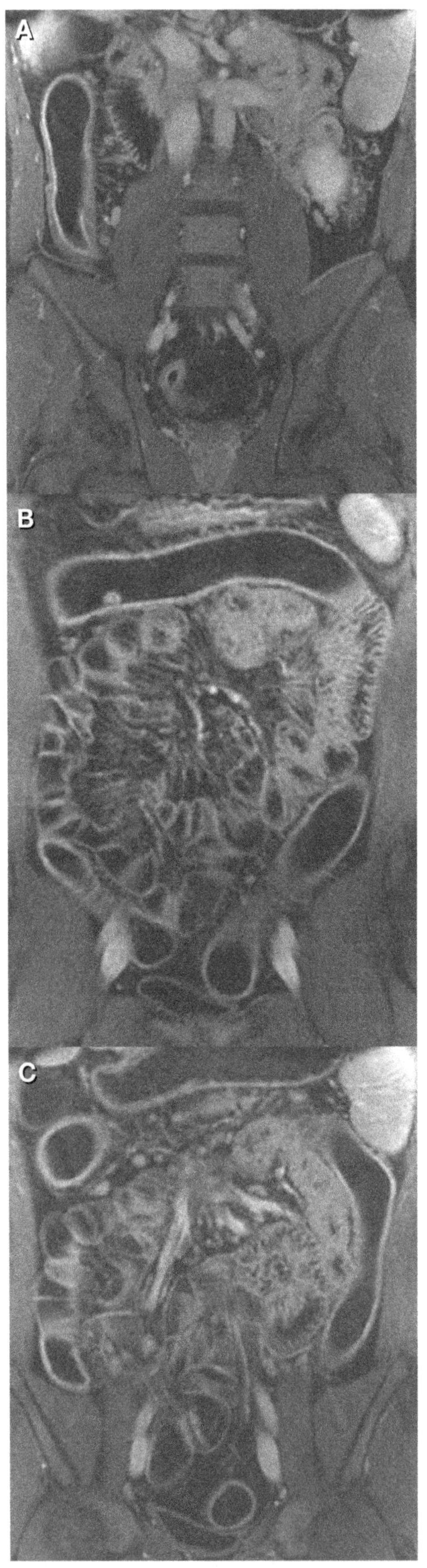

Figure 9.18.1

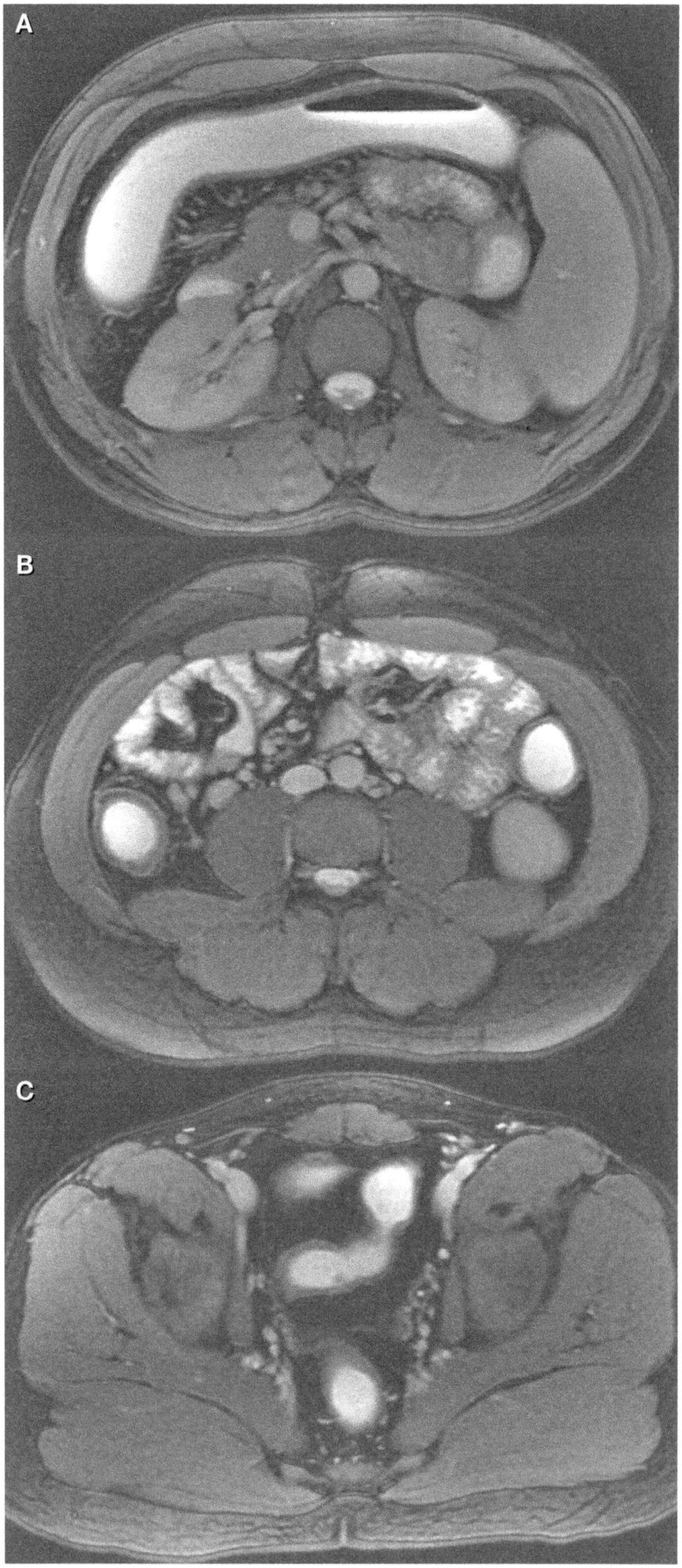

Figure 9.18.2

HISTORY: 20-year-old man with chronic GI symptoms, including bloody diarrhea

IMAGING FINDINGS: Coronal postgadolinium 3D SPGR images (Figure 9.18.1) demonstrate an ahaustral colon with mild, diffuse mural thickening and enhancement. Note the enhancing polyp in the transverse colon. Axial fat-suppressed 2D SSFP images (Figure 9.18.2) reveal similar findings, with the inferior image showing mild diffuse thickening of the rectosigmoid colon.

DIAGNOSIS: Ulcerative colitis with inflammatory polyp in the transverse colon

COMMENT: Ulcerative colitis, like Crohn disease, is primarily a disease of young adults, with a peak incidence between ages 20 and 40 years. The etiology remains obscure, with genetic, hypersensitivity, and autoimmune mechanisms among the favorite candidates. Ulcerative colitis is not a distinct histopathologic entity, and the inflammatory response in the colon can be seen in other diseases. However, in contradistinction to Crohn colitis, involvement is usually confined to the mucosa and submucosa. The distinction between mucosal or submucosal ulceration and transmural ulceration is generally too subtle to make on standard MR enterographic examinations, but the more common right-sided involvement of Crohn colitis (with rectal sparing when the case follows the classic teaching) vs the diffuse involvement of ulcerative colitis should be easily appreciated. Ulcerative colitis usually involves the rectum and extends proximally; about 40% to 50% of patients have disease limited to the rectosigmoid colon, 30% to 40% have disease beyond the sigmoid but not involving the entire colon, and 20% have diffuse colitis. Clinically, it typically presents with rectal bleeding, diarrhea, and crampy abdominal pain that waxes and wanes.

A number of extracolonic manifestations of ulcerative colitis can be appreciated occasionally on MR enterography examinations, including sacroiliitis and spondylitis. Most important, however, is the identification of sclerosing cholangitis (present in 1%-5% of IBD patients), which is associated with an increased risk of cholangiocarcinoma. Since most or all of the liver should be included in standard pre- and postgadolinium acquisitions of the MR enterography examination, it is important to look for such findings as segmental biliary dilatation and biliary wall thickening and enhancement to identify these patients. (The converse is also true; we have seen a few cases of MRI and MRCP examinations performed in patients with primary sclerosing cholangitis where obvious colonic thickening and enhancement were ignored in the report.)

Pseudopolyps are a well-known feature of ulcerative colitis and occur with extensive ulceration of the submucosal and mucosal linings. The pseudopolyps represent islands of residual mucosa or granulation tissue within large regions of denuded mucosa and submucosa. The polyp in the transverse colon in this case turned out to be inflammatory at biopsy, but the appearance of a single polyp, even within a clearly diseased segment of colon, is not sufficient to make a distinction between inflammatory and adenomatous polyps.

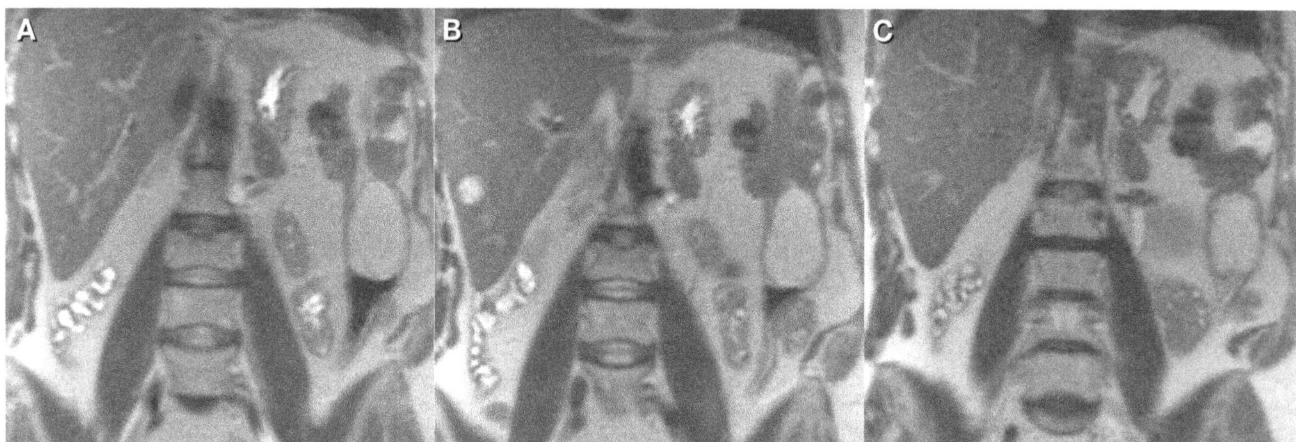

Figure 9.19.1

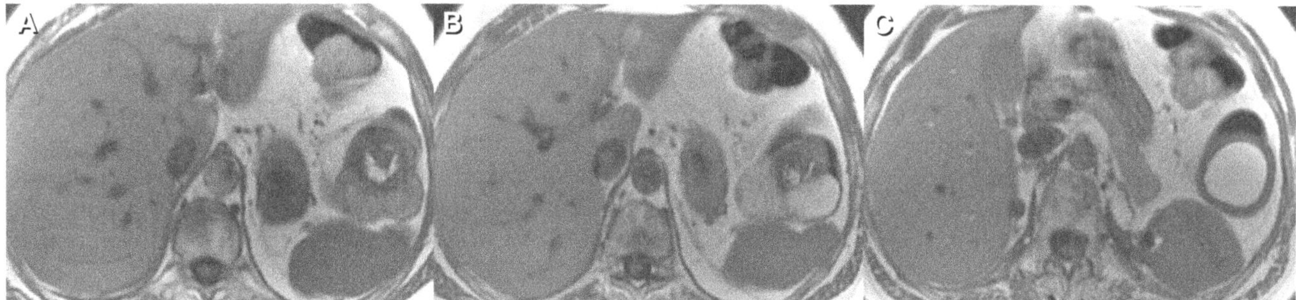

Figure 9.19.2

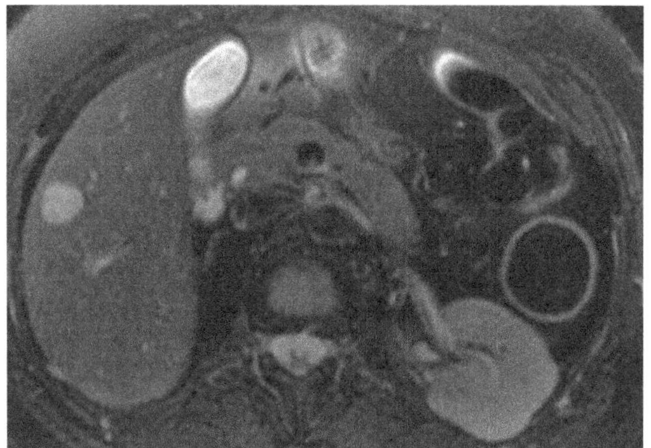

Figure 9.19.3

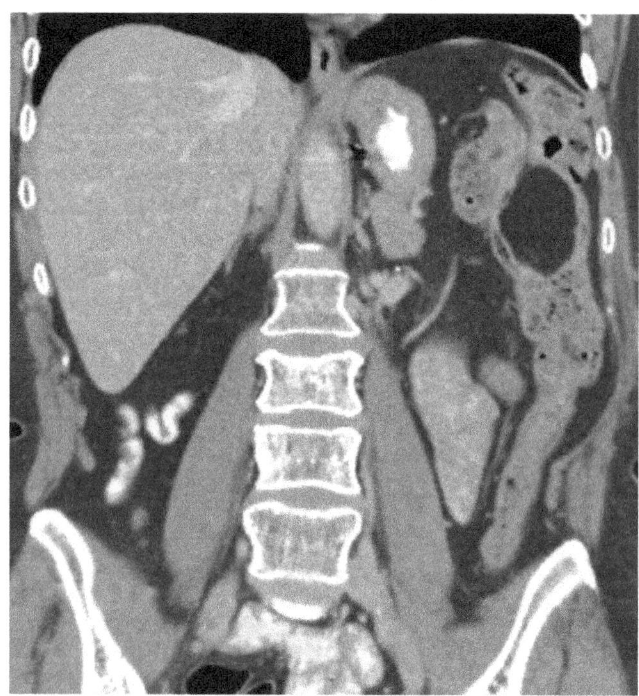

Figure 9.19.4

HISTORY: 54-year-old woman with intermittent abdominal cramps, bloating, and diarrhea

IMAGING FINDINGS: Coronal SSFSE images (Figure 9.19.1) demonstrate a large ovoid, T2-hyperintense lesion in the descending colon that serves as the lead point for an intussusception. Notice also a second, smaller lesion proximally in the descending colon. The lesions are hyperintense on axial T1-weighted images (Figure 9.19.2), with the top image showing the collapsed intussuscepting colon surrounded by mesenteric fat. A fat-suppressed T2-weighted image (Figure 9.19.3) shows signal dropout in the largest colonic lesion (and an incidental hepatic hemangioma). A coronal reformatted CT image (Figure 9.19.4) also shows fat density within the large lesion.

DIAGNOSIS: Giant colonic lipoma

COMMENT: Colonic lipomas are rare, benign mesenchymal tumors with an estimated incidence of 0.04% to 4.4%. The peak incidence is in the fifth and sixth decades of life, with a slight female preponderance. Lipomas are located in the cecum, ascending colon, and sigmoid colon, listed in decreasing order of frequency. Most colonic lipomas are small asymptomatic lesions detected incidentally at colonoscopy, surgery, or cross-sectional imaging, but lesions larger than 2 cm in diameter are more likely to cause symptoms. The most common presentations of patients with giant (obviously a relative term) colonic lipomas are abdominal pain, changes in bowel habits, intestinal obstruction, and bleeding.

Lipomas, even large ones, are notoriously easy to overlook, particularly when they are located in the intestine. On CT, the signal intensity is strikingly similar to intraluminal gas. Even with MRI, where you typically have multiple chances to avoid missing a lesion, the heterogeneous appearance of fecal material on all imaging sequences can be confounding. Generally, documentation of fat within a lesion is accomplished by showing signal loss from a non–fat-suppressed to a fat-suppressed T1- or T2-weighted sequence (or high signal intensity on a fat image and low signal intensity on the corresponding water image if Dixon pulse sequences are available).

The intussusception in this case is so prominent that it is somewhat difficult to appreciate; on the coronal SSFSE images, the colon at the splenic flexure is divided in 2 by the mesocolic fat of the intussuscipiens, which can also be seen on the axial T1 images.

CASE 9.20

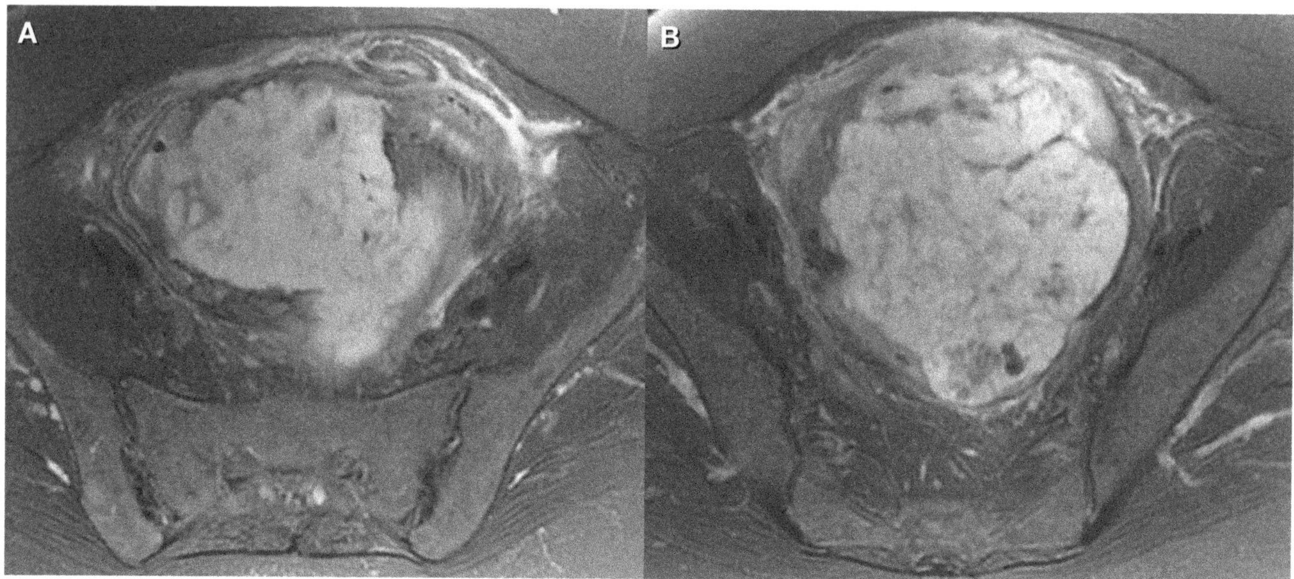

Figure 9.20.1

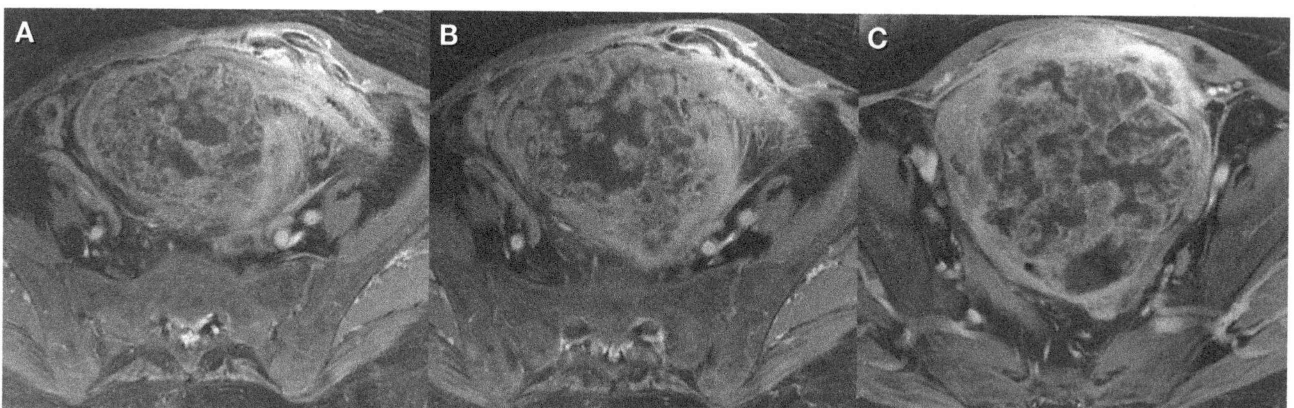

Figure 9.20.2

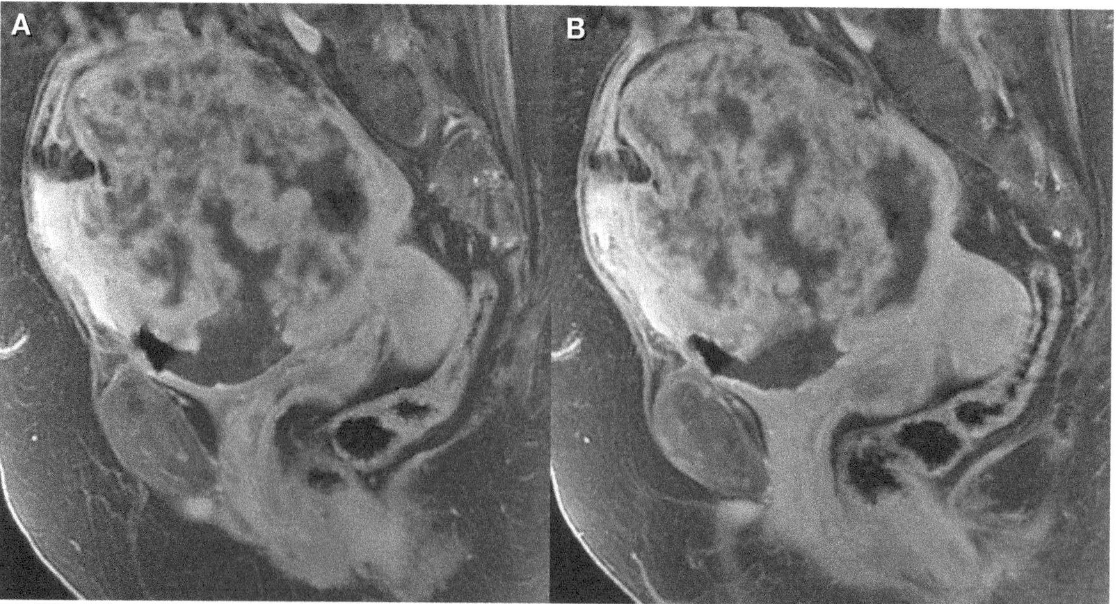

Figure 9.20.3

HISTORY: 70-year-old woman with 20-lb weight loss over the past 6 months and crampy lower abdominal pain

IMAGING FINDINGS: Axial fat-suppressed FSE T2-weighted images (Figure 9.20.1) and postgadolinium axial (Figure 9.20.2) and sagittal (Figure 9.20.3) 3D SPGR images demonstrate a large, heterogeneously enhancing mass in the pelvis, with markedly increased T2-signal intensity and multiple cystic regions on postcontrast images. The origin of the lesion from the sigmoid colon is difficult to discern, but it is probably best appreciated on the axial postgadolinium images. Note the invasion of the bladder dome, with a gas pocket in the anterior bladder.

DIAGNOSIS: Mucinous adenocarcinoma of the sigmoid colon invading the bladder

COMMENT: This appearance is unusual for colon cancer, but we have seen several cases of mucinous adenocarcinoma of the colon presenting as a large heterogeneous pelvic mass. Mucinous adenocarcinoma is generally defined as a lesion in which at least 50% of the tumor is composed of extracellular mucin. This subtype is thought to represent 6% to 20% of all colorectal carcinomas. Some controversy exists regarding whether the histologic subtype is a prognostic indicator, but in general, mucinous carcinoma is characterized by more extensive invasion at presentation and has a relatively poor prognosis. It has also been suggested that the location of mucinous tumors affects prognosis, with proximal lesions associated with a more favorable outcome.

The appearance of these lesions on MRI reflects the abundance of mucin and is characterized by high T2-signal intensity and low signal intensity on postgadolinium fat-suppressed T1-weighted images.

This case reflects a common dilemma with very large lesions: The site of origin is difficult to discern with certainty. The mass clearly involves the bladder dome and the sigmoid colon, but the ovaries were never definitely identified, and its appearance would also be consistent with an ovarian neoplasm. A good clinical history (something of a luxury in our practice), along with an optimal examination, including multiple imaging planes, probably gives you the best chance at correctly characterizing these lesions.

Since mucinous carcinomas tend to be more invasive at presentation, it's not unusual to see very large and aggressive recurrent lesions after resection. The images below are an example of recurrent mucinous adenocarcinoma that presented as a large, markedly T2 hyperintense lesion.

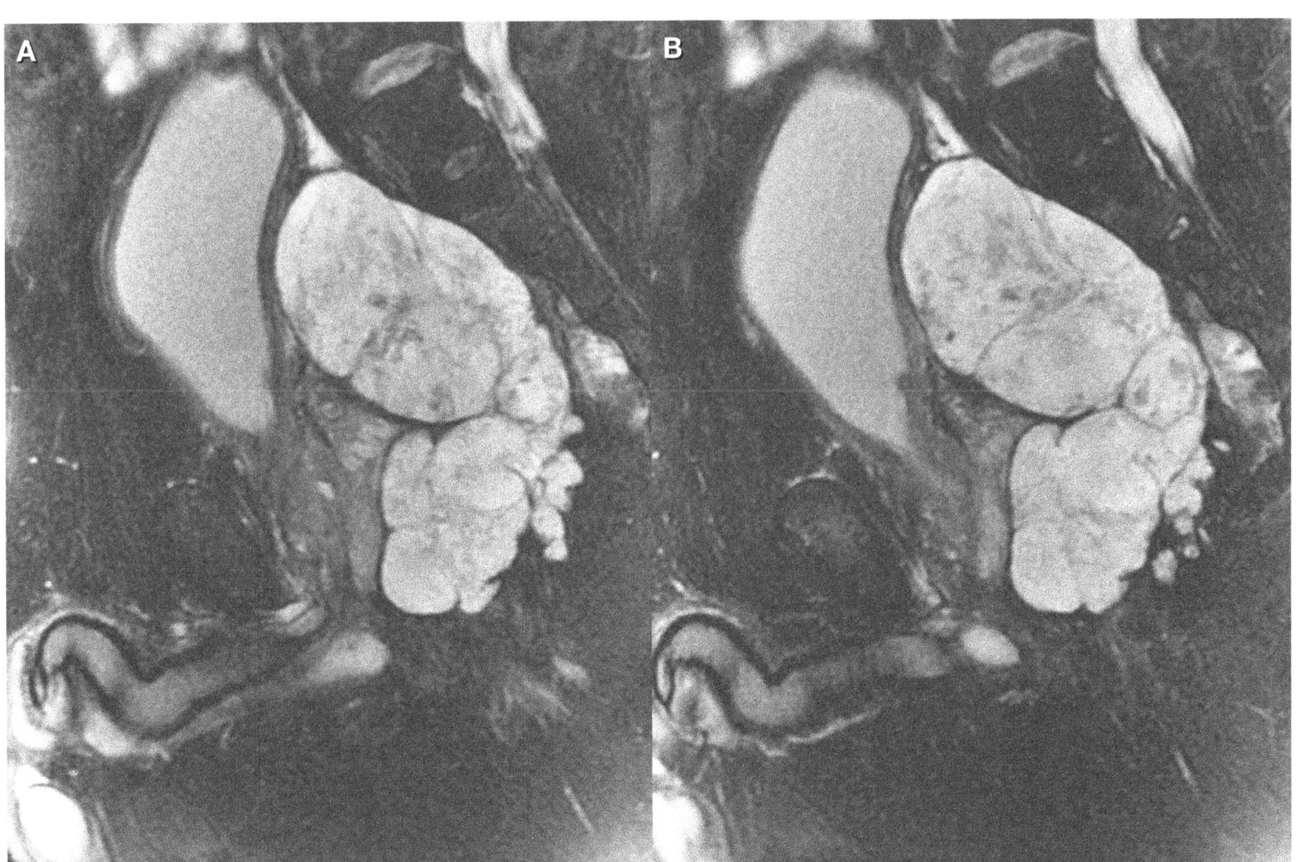

Figure 9.20.4

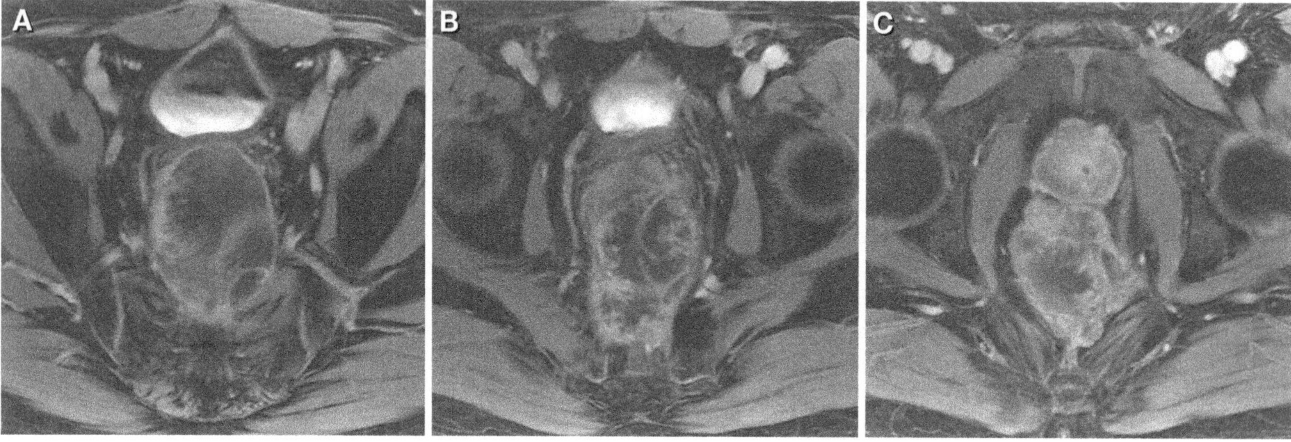

Figure 9.20.5

A 68-year-old man with a history of rectal carcinoma and proctocolectomy 2 years ago had a pelvic mass detected on recent CT, representing recurrent mucinous adenocarcinoma. Sagittal T2-weighted fat-suppressed FSE images (Figure 9.20.4) show a large lobulated lesion with high signal intensity. Axial postgadolinium 3D SPGR images (Figure 9.20.5) show predominantly low signal intensity with hyperenhancing margins.

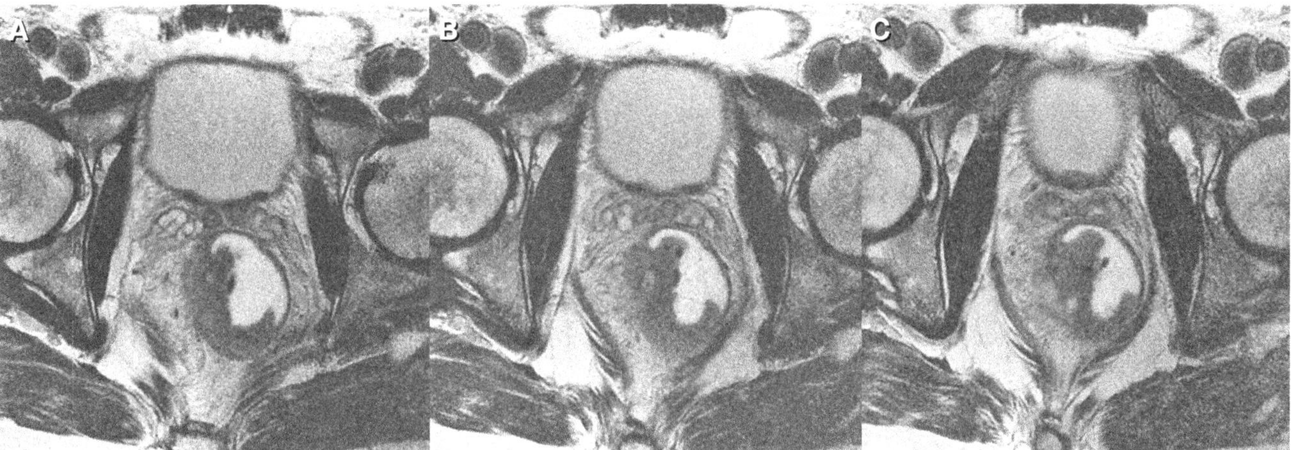

Figure 9.21.1

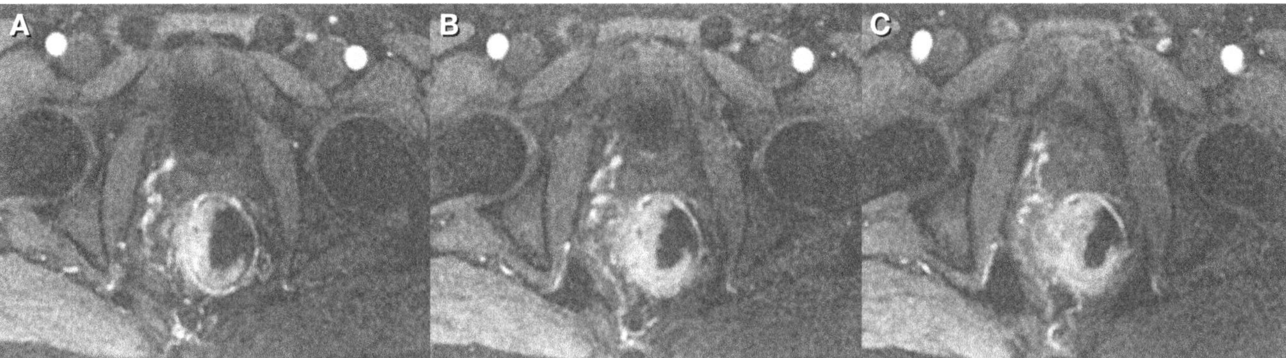

Figure 9.21.2

HISTORY: 50-year-old man with hematochezia; colonoscopy showed a rectal mass

IMAGING FINDINGS: Axial FSE T2-weighted images (Figure 9.21.1) obtained after endorectal administration of US gel show a crescentic mass involving the right and posterior walls of the rectum and extending into the lumen. Note the stranding in the mesorectal fat extending toward the margin of the mesorectal fascia and loss of delineation of the rectal wall. Axial arterial phase, postgadolinium 3D SPGR images (Figure 9.21.2) show early heterogeneous enhancement of the mass, as well as extramural extension with prominent perirectal veins. Note that the well-defined hyperenhancing rectal wall disappears in the region of the mass.

DIAGNOSIS: Rectal carcinoma

COMMENT: Rectal carcinoma is a common malignancy with a significant mortality rate. Locally advanced disease has a poor prognosis because of an increased frequency of metastasis and local recurrence, although improvements in surgical and oncologic management in the past 10 to 15 years have led to improved survival. Total mesorectal excision is the current surgery of choice for rectal cancer and is defined as resection of both the tumor and the surrounding mesorectal fat and local nodes, performed by dissecting along the surface of the mesorectal fascia. Total mesorectal excision as an isolated treatment is associated with recurrence rates of less than 10%; however, inadequate surgical excision with microscopic infiltration of the resection margins may result in local recurrence in as many as 83% of patients. This outcome has led to the concept of *circumferential resection margin*, defined as the surgical cut surface of the perirectal connective tissue. Tumor extension to or beyond the mesorectal fascia indicates a poor prognosis. MRI is highly accurate at predicting the circumferential resection margin. In many practices, treatment strategies are based on the MRI findings and offer concurrent chemotherapy and radiation therapy for tumor extending to within 5 mm of the mesorectal fascia, in hopes of downstaging the lesion before surgery.

The mesorectal fascia can be identified on non–fat-suppressed T2-weighted images as a thin, hypointense line defining the outer margin of the perirectal fat. In this case, it is best seen along the anterior left lateral margins of the rectum. In the low rectum, tumor extension to the margin of the levator muscle would also predict a poor outcome. In general, any soft-tissue thickening or stranding within the perirectal fat extending from the tumor to the mesorectal fascia counts as a positive margin, as seen in this case.

The specific techniques described in the literature for imaging rectal cancers differ, but nearly all authors emphasize the importance of high-resolution axial or axial oblique T2-weighted images without fat suppression. These images are most useful for identifying the mesorectal fascia and for defining the circumferential resection margin. Some authors advocate the use of endoluminal rectal contrast or endorectal coils in these examinations. Others contend that visualization of the primary tumor is not critically important since MRI has not proved particularly adept at distinguishing stage T2 tumors (involving the rectal wall) from stage T3 tumors (extending through the serosa), and the main point of the examination is identifying the circumferential resection margin. We favor the use of endorectal contrast (warmed US gel) because it is a little less invasive and slightly less uncomfortable than an endorectal coil, although luminal distention may not be optimal at the superior and inferior margins of the rectum. Endorectal coils are most helpful for visualizing low rectal lesions near the anal sphincter, where adequate luminal distention with gel is less likely to occur. Complete visualization of the primary tumor may not always be necessary, but it can be a useful landmark, and we have often been surprised at how even large lesions are essentially invisible in the undistended rectum.

Nearly every review article addressing the topic of MRI in rectal carcinoma notes that the use of gadolinium does not increase the accuracy of either tumor or circumferential resection margin staging. This is probably true, but what is often left unsaid is that nevertheless, nearly everyone uses gadolinium, for a couple of reasons. Postgadolinium images can be helpful in detecting pelvic bone and nodal metastases and are also reasonably accurate staging tools. The axial T2-weighted images, which everyone agrees are most important, should be obtained with submillimeter in-plane spatial resolution and a slice thickness of 3 to 4 mm. Because spatial resolution in MRI scales with acquisition time, these sequences can last 6 to 8 minutes. Although motion artifact is rarely encountered among the ideal patients of the MRI literature, it can be a substantial problem in the real world, and it's useful to have an alternative strategy (ie, postgadolinium 3D SPGR images) that can be performed quickly with minimal artifact.

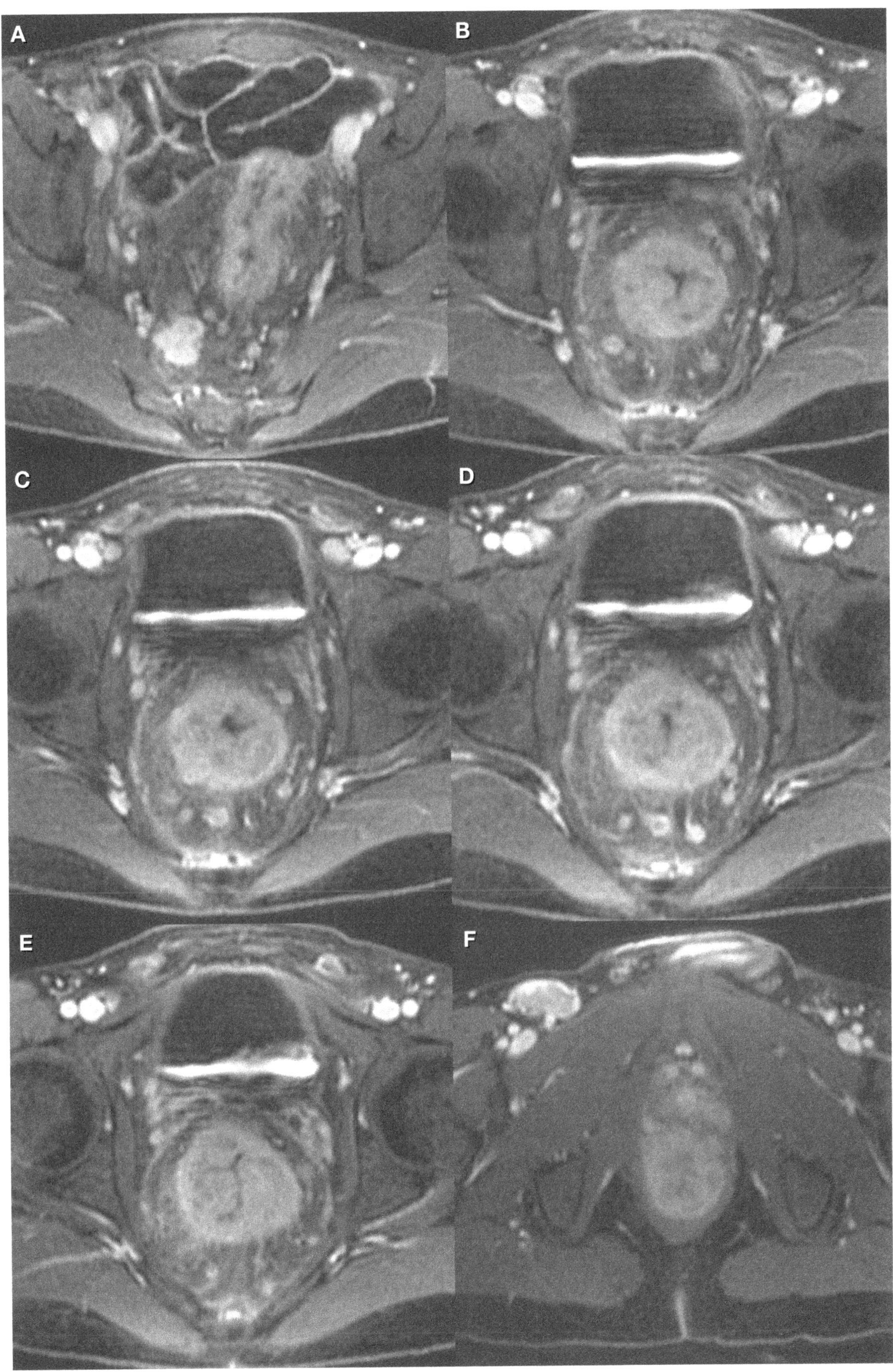

Figure 9.22.1

HISTORY: 23-year-old man with a history of Crohn disease and previous ileocecal resection, now with abdominal pelvic pain, bloody diarrhea, and a suspected perianal fistula

IMAGING FINDINGS: Axial postgadolinium 3D SPGR images (Figure 9.22.1) demonstrate moderate thickening of the sigmoid colon consistent with Crohn colitis and severe diffuse thickening and heterogeneous enhancement of the rectum. Note the prominent perirectal and right inguinal adenopathy, as well as perirectal fibrofatty proliferation that is likely secondary to chronic inflammation.

DIAGNOSIS: Rectal lymphoma

COMMENT: Primary colorectal lymphoma is a rare disease accounting for approximately 0.05% of all colonic neoplasms and 0.1% of primary rectal tumors. Colorectal lymphoma is almost always the non-Hodgkin type and is most frequent in men between the ages of 50 and 70 years. Symptoms of the disease are usually nonspecific (rectal bleeding and pain) and may mimic the presentation of rectal adenocarcinoma or, as in this case, an exacerbation of IBD.

Whether patients with IBD are at increased risk for lymphoma remains a subject of debate. The effect of chronic inflammation on carcinogenesis in IBD has long been recognized, and the risk of colorectal adenocarcinoma is estimated to be 1% annually. Some authors have suggested a similar link with lymphoma, but the few available population-based studies are unconvincing. A recent review from Mayo Clinic of 15 IBD patients with primary intestinal lymphoma found that the colon was the most common location (60%), and the most common presenting symptoms of pain and bloody diarrhea were difficult to distinguish from exacerbations of IBD. Overall 1- and 5-year survival rates were 67% and 40%, although a significant percentage of deaths were from causes other than lymphoma. Survival is correlated with the stage of disease at diagnosis, and treatment usually involves a combination of surgical resection and chemotherapy.

Rectal lymphoma on MRI usually presents as a homogeneous mural mass, with less obstruction than expected from a comparably sized adenocarcinoma. The mural thickening in this case is more than typically seen in uncomplicated Crohn disease or ulcerative colitis, and the presence of large nodes in the perirectal fat and right groin should suggest that something more than IBD may be occurring. This patient had been scanned 3 months previously, where a small perianal fistula had been identified. A substantial increase in rectal wall thickening, as well as the interval appearance of several large nodes, was noted in the report without any specific implication, but these findings were sufficient to prompt endoscopy and biopsy, which led to the diagnosis.

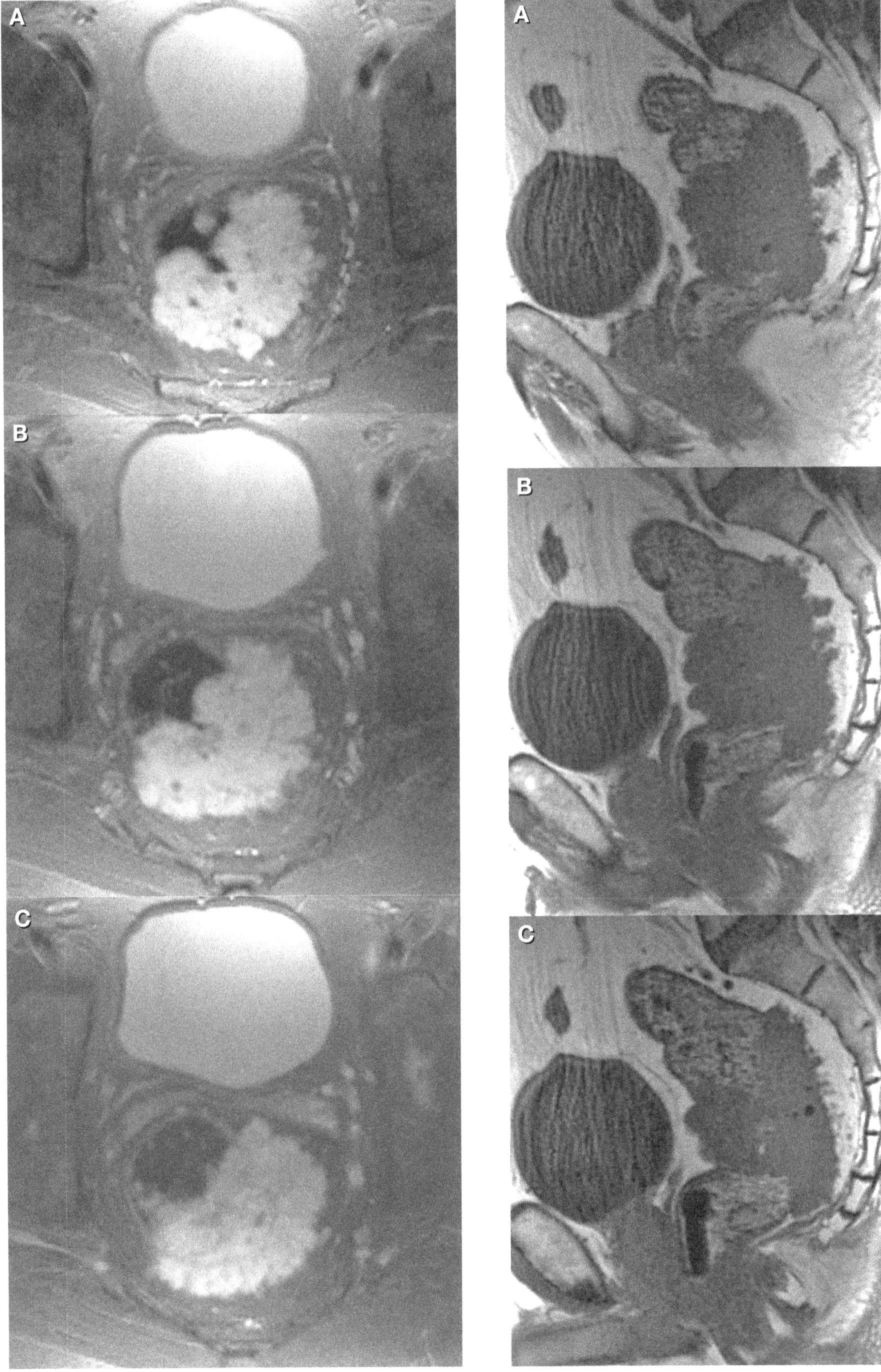

Figure 9.23.1

Figure 9.23.2

HISTORY: 66-year-old man with recent rectal bleeding underwent colonoscopy at an outside institution, where a biopsy was performed but yielded benign tissue. Sigmoidoscopy at Mayo Clinic suggested a vascular lesion, and pelvic MRI was requested for further evaluation

IMAGING FINDINGS: Axial fat-suppressed T2-weighted FSE images (Figure 9.23.1) reveal a markedly hyperintense, lobulated lesion surrounding, but not obstructing, the posterior and lateral margins of the rectum. Sagittal FSE T1-weighted images (Figure 9.23.2) again show the large nonobstructive lesion with fronds of tissue extending posteriorly.

DIAGNOSIS: Rectal hemangioma

COMMENT: Rectal hemangiomas are relatively rare lesions, with approximately 350 cases reported in the literature, but they are important to recognize because endoscopic biopsy is generally not a good idea and surgical strategies may differ from the standard approach to rectal adenocarcinoma. Not too long ago, MRI was performed only in cases where an unusual rectal lesion (ie, not an adenocarcinoma) was suspected at endoscopy, but now it is requested with increasing frequency for staging purposes (see Case 9.21). As this imaging algorithm becomes more popular, more uncommon rectal lesions will likely begin to appear at MRI. Rectal hemangiomas are particularly well suited for MRI since the appearance is diagnostic and the extent of the lesions can be demonstrated easily.

Rectal hemangiomas are most common in children and young adults, who typically present with recurrent, intermittent painless rectal bleeding. Additional symptoms may include melena, hematochezia, and anemia. Obstruction, intussusception, and perforation are rare complications of rectal hemangioma, but they have been reported. The symptoms are comparatively nonspecific, and this condition is frequently misdiagnosed as hemorrhoids. Most rectal hemangiomas are isolated findings; however, they sometimes are associated with systemic syndromes, such as Klippel-Trénaunay syndrome or Bean (blue rubber bleb nevus) syndrome.

Both capillary and cavernous types of rectal hemangioma have been described. Capillary hemangiomas consist of tightly packed capillaries lined with a single layer of endothelial cells and surrounded by a thin fibrous capsule. Cavernous hemangiomas are composed of large, dilated, blood-filled sinuses.

The typical appearance of a rectal hemangioma is a lobulated lesion with marked hyperintensity on fat-suppressed T2-weighted images and prominent enhancement after contrast agent administration. Multiple associated phleboliths can often be seen on CT but are more difficult to appreciate on MRI. These are soft lesions, and thus obstruction is relatively uncommon—it's not evident in this case—while an adenocarcinoma of this size would be more likely to have a typical apple-core appearance. Another feature of rectal hemangiomas not seen in this case but also typical is the presence of abnormal perirectal vessels arranged in a serpiginous or palisading pattern radiating from the rectum, with associated infiltration of the mesorectal fat (see the example below).

At colonoscopy, these lesions appear as multiple, bluish-purple submucosal masses representing the dilated blood vessels. Biopsy should be avoided because of the risk of uncontrollable bleeding. Surgical resection when possible is the treatment of choice.

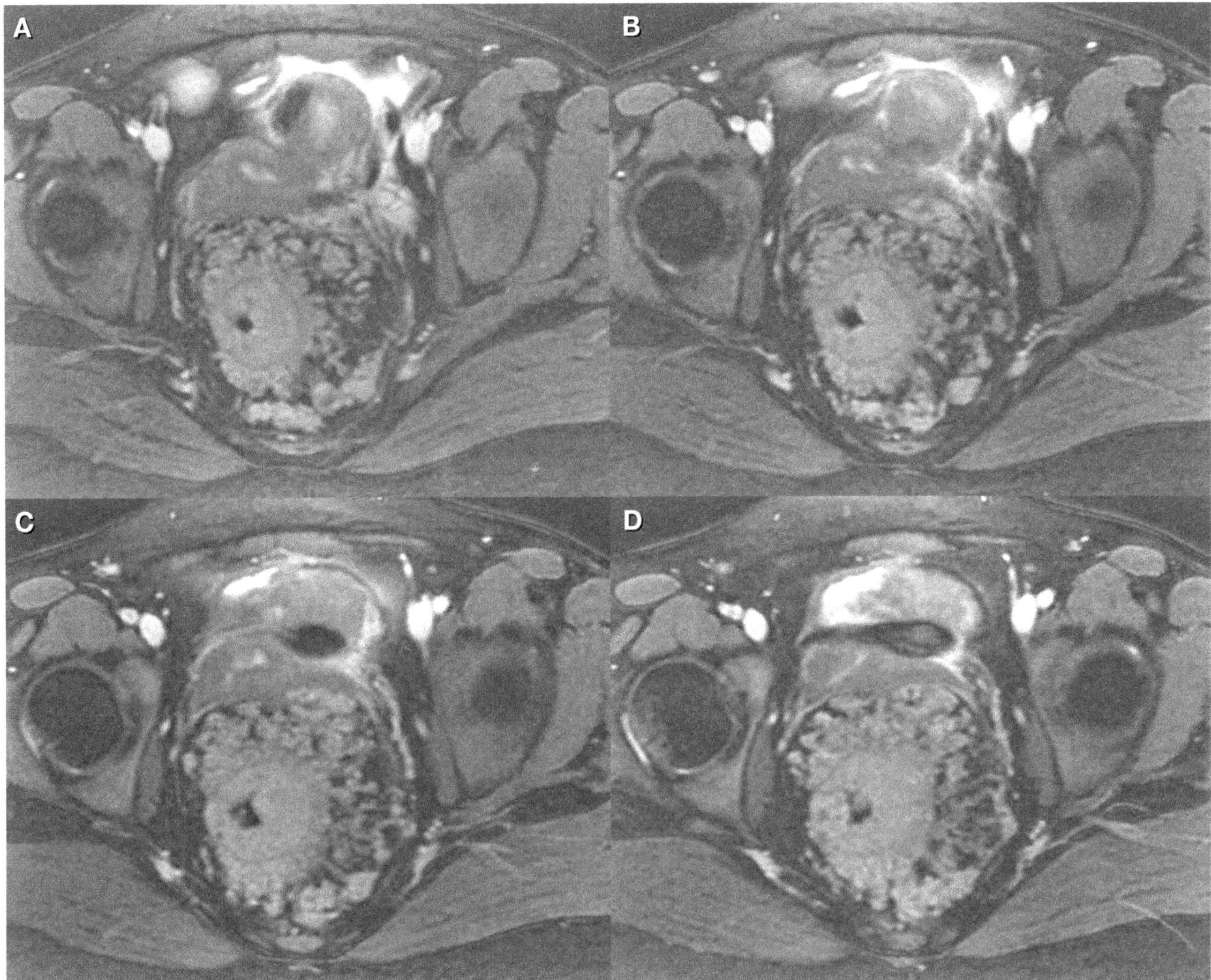

Figure 9.23.3

Axial fat-suppressed 2D SSFP images (Figure 9.23.3) in a 21-year-old patient with known rectal hemangioma and history of intermittent rectal bleeding. Notice the hyperintense rectal mass, as well as multiple dilated veins in the mesorectal fat radiating outward from the rectum.

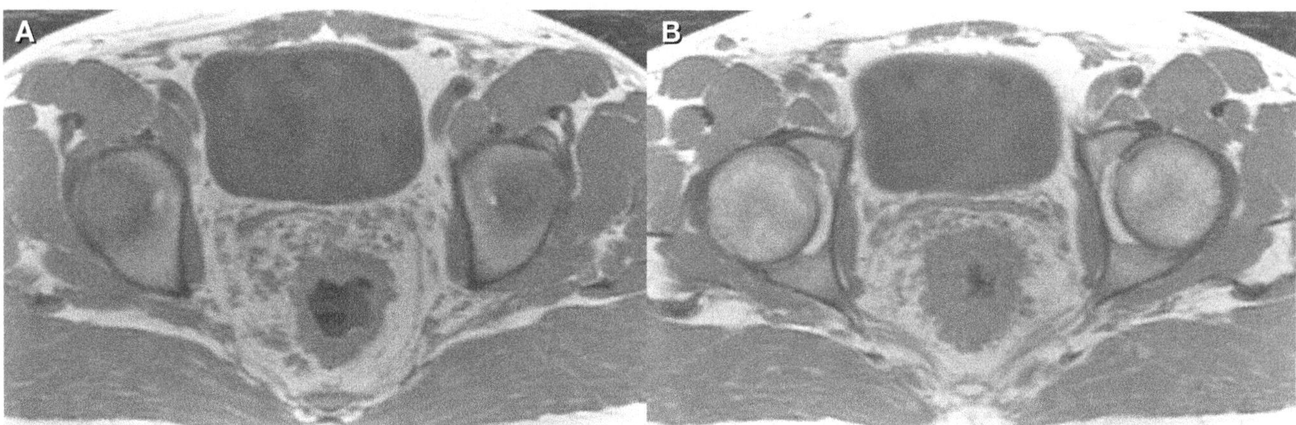

Figure 9.24.1

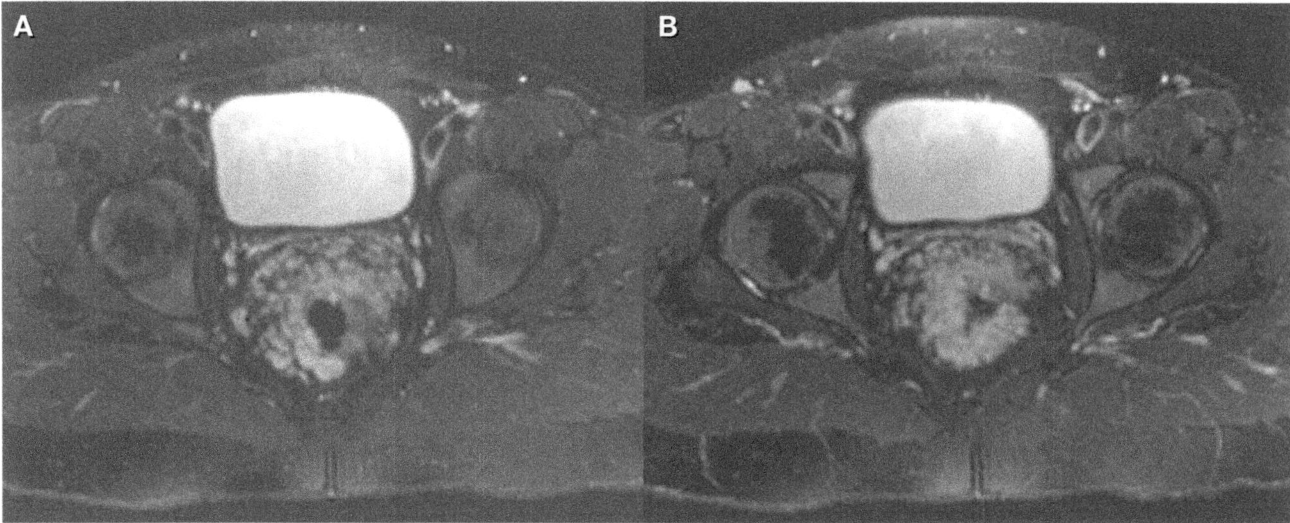

Figure 9.24.2

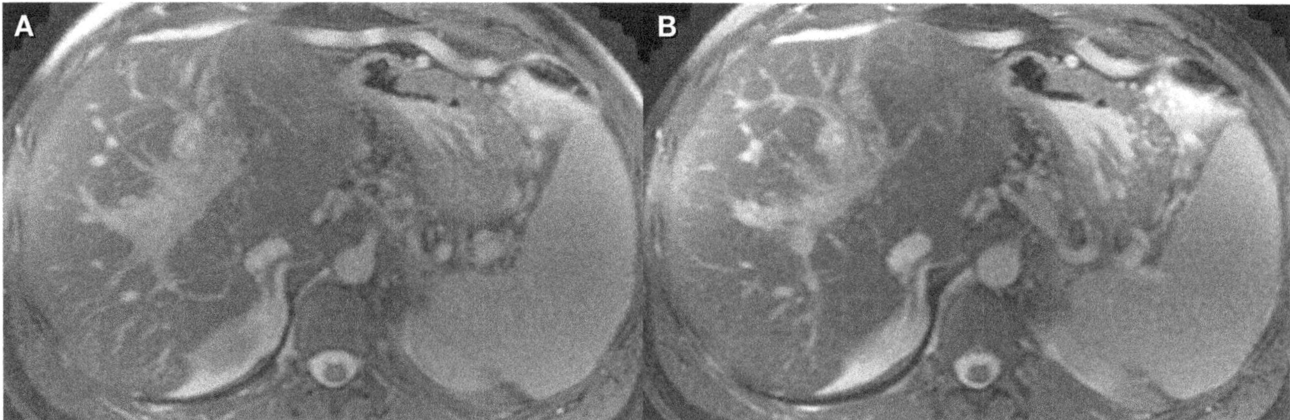

Figure 9.24.3

HISTORY: 45-year-old man with chronic portal and superior mesenteric vein thrombosis and new onset of rectal bleeding

IMAGING FINDINGS: Axial T1-weighted (Figure 9.24.1) and fat-suppressed T2-weighted (Figure 9.24.2) FSE images demonstrate nodular thickening of the rectal wall with surrounding serpiginous structures, all with high T2-signal intensity. Axial 2D fat-suppressed SSFP images (Figure 9.24.3) show cavernous transformation of the portal vein, as well as a large gastroepiploic collateral vein anteriorly.

DIAGNOSIS: Rectal varices in a patient with chronic portal and mesenteric vein thrombosis

COMMENT: You will notice that this case has a nearly identical appearance to the rectal hemangioma described in Case 9.23, a similarity that is not surprising since both entities involve multiple dilated venous channels in the rectal wall and surrounding mesorectal fat.

Rectal varices represent a portal systemic collateral pathway that develops in the clinical setting of portal hypertension or obstructed portal venous flow—in this instance, chronic portal vein thrombosis. The rectum has overlapping portal and systemic venous drainage through superior hemorrhoidal veins of the inferior mesenteric system and the middle and inferior hemorrhoidal veins of the iliac system.

Data regarding the prevalence of rectal varices in patients with portal hypertension are highly inconsistent, with reports ranging from 4% to 78% of cases. Many of the studies showing low prevalence were performed with endoscopy only and did not include endorectal sonography, so it's reasonable to conclude that the true prevalence is toward the middle to higher end of the spectrum. Rectal varices may be more common in patients with noncirrhotic portal hypertension, particularly extrahepatic portal venous obstruction, although these observations have not been widely confirmed.

Most authors agree that the incidence of clinically significant bleeding from rectal varices is relatively low in comparison to esophageal varices, occurring in 0.5% to 3.6%. Risk factors for bleeding include deep rectal varices (ie, within the rectal wall as opposed to perirectal varices), varices greater than 5 mm in diameter, and increased velocities within the varices.

As with rectal hemangiomas, these lesions frequently are mistaken for hemorrhoids. However, hemorrhoids are vascular cushions resulting from arteriolar venous communications in the hemorrhoidal plexus and have no direct communication with any portal venous system branches. Although hemorrhoids commonly cause rectal bleeding, they do not cause the massive blood loss that rarely can occur with bleeding rectal varices.

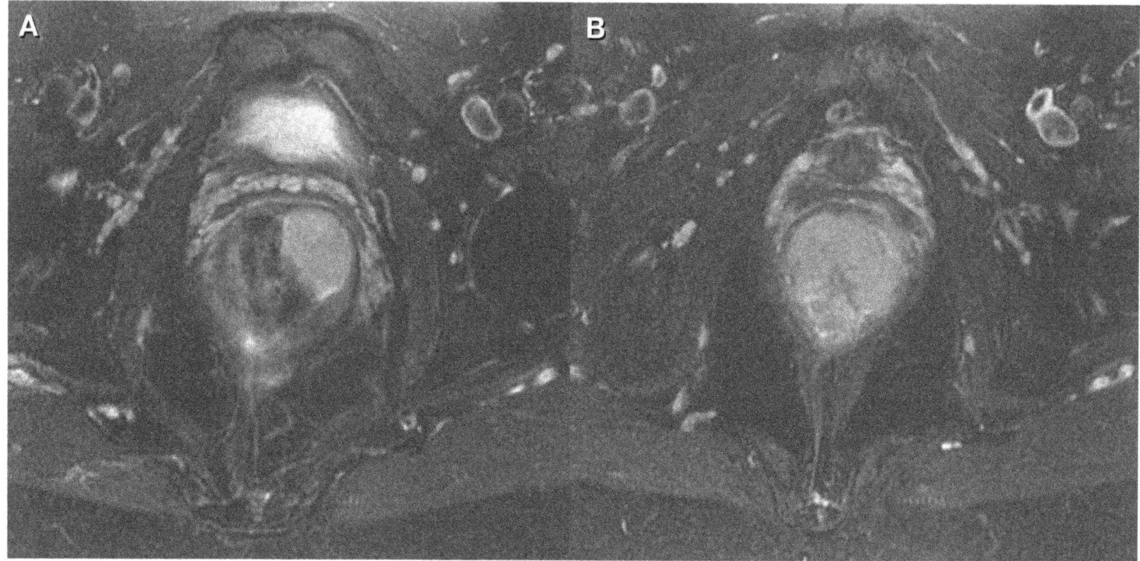

Figure 9.25.1

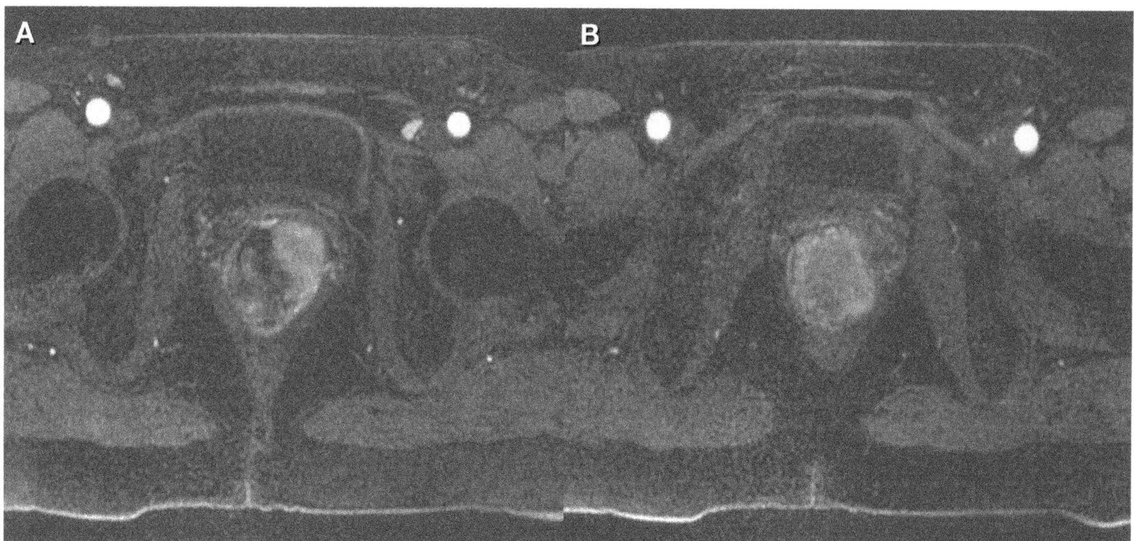

Figure 9.25.2

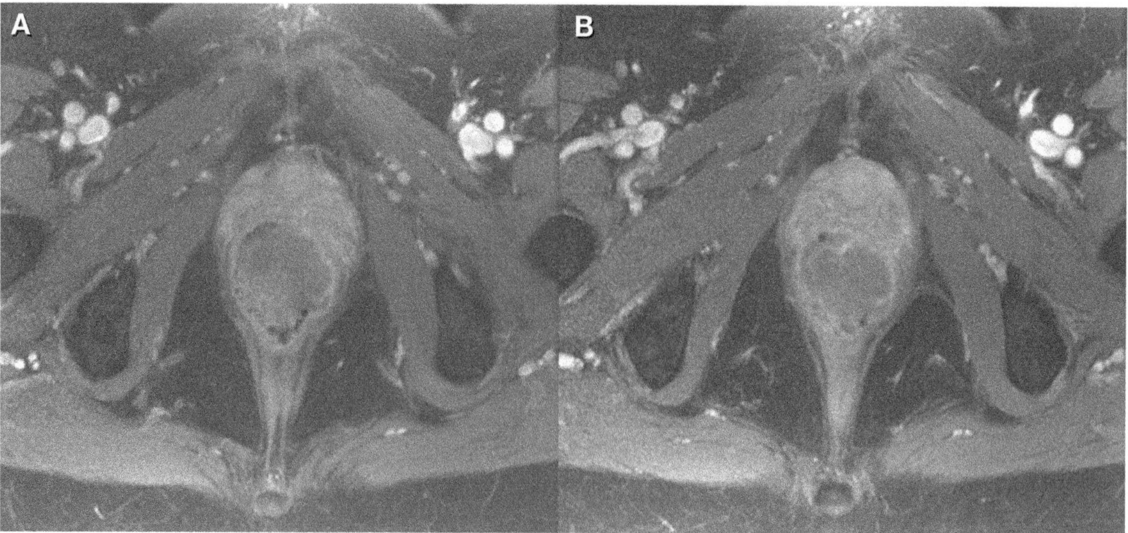

Figure 9.25.3

HISTORY: 68-year-old woman with gradual onset of occasional incontinence and bright red blood per rectum; colonoscopy showed a low rectal mass

IMAGING FINDINGS: Axial fat-suppressed FSE T2-weighted images (Figure 9.25.1) demonstrate a lobulated hyperintense mass in the low rectum and anus. Axial arterial phase (Figure 9.25.2) and equilibrium phase (Figure 9.25.3) 3D SPGR images show heterogeneous arterial phase enhancement with washout on equilibrium phase images.

DIAGNOSIS: Anorectal melanoma

COMMENT: Anorectal melanoma is a rare entity, accounting for 0.2% to 3.0% of all melanoma cases and 0.1% to 4.6% of all malignant tumors of the rectum and anus. Lesions can be melanotic or amelanotic and are usually not obstructive, with rectal bleeding the typical presenting symptom.

The largest series (N=8) described polypoid or fungating intraluminal masses with homogeneous or heterogeneous contrast enhancement. Adjacent lymphadenopathy was noted in all patients. The prognosis for these patients was poor, with 5-year survival rates ranging from 6% to 12%.

Whenever melanoma is discussed in the context of MRI, inevitably it is noted that melanomas may have increased signal intensity on T1-weighted images, a result of the paramagnetic properties of melanin. Melanin is in fact an interesting, somewhat amorphous material with an abundance of sterically protected unpaired electrons. We have seen a few cases of melanoma metastases in the liver that are clearly bright on precontrast T1-weighted images, but many aren't, and the diagnostic utility of this sign is ambiguous at best.

In this case, the lesion had no distinctive features that should lead you to the diagnosis of melanoma. The lesion was large and was not obstructive (although you can't really tell this from the images provided), which would be a little unusual for an adenocarcinoma. However, given the high prevalence of adenocarcinoma, it should still be at the top of the differential diagnosis. Other possibilities include GIST and metastasis.

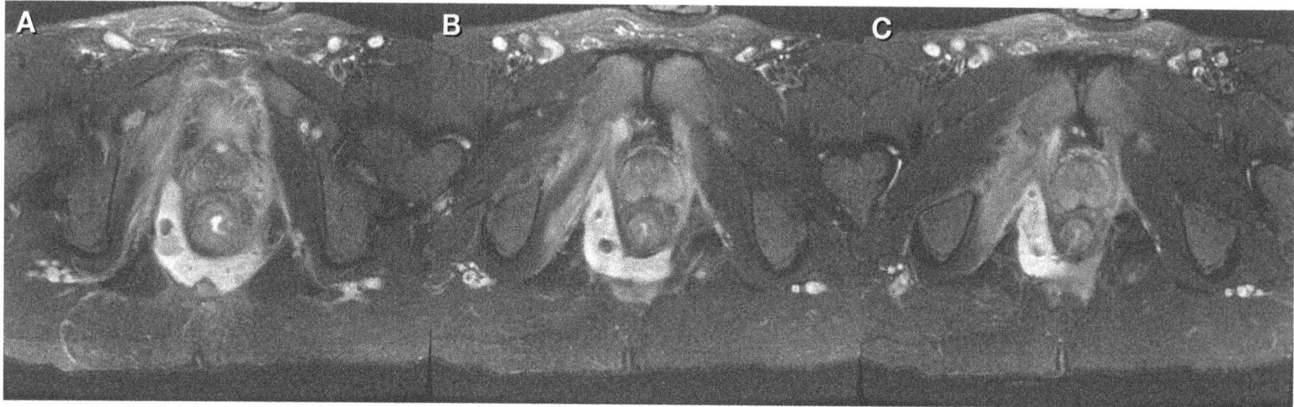

Figure 9.26.1

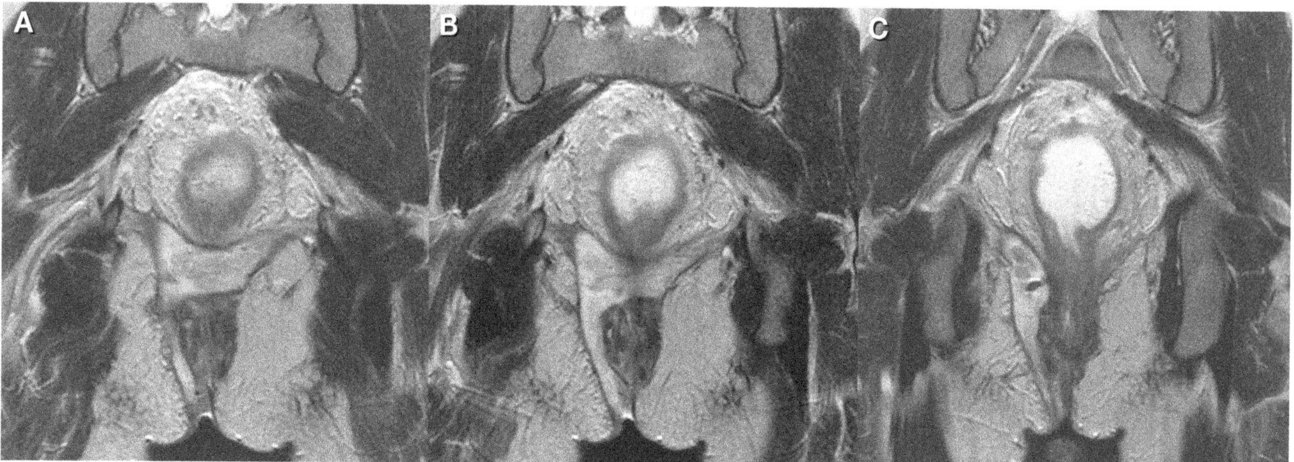

Figure 9.26.2

HISTORY: 23-year-old man with Crohn disease diagnosed at age 11 years, with large- and small-bowel involvement

IMAGING FINDINGS: Axial fat-suppressed FSE T2-weighted images (Figure 9.26.1) reveal a horseshoe-shaped fluid collection along the posterior and right lateral margin of the anus that contains foci of gas. Note the small, faintly visualized communication with the lumen of the anus on the most inferior image. Coronal FSE T2-weighted images (Figure 9.26.2) again show the large perianal fluid collection. Better seen on these images is a component extending inferiorly along the right gluteal fold.

DIAGNOSIS: Crohn disease with large transsphincteric perianal fistula and abscess

COMMENT: MRI is ideally suited for imaging perianal fistulas. The perianal region is one of the few, relatively motion-free segments of the GI tract, and therefore you can afford to spend some extra time to achieve the high spatial resolution necessary for documentation of small fistulous tracts. The excellent soft tissue contrast of MRI also provides an important advantage over CT. The literature on this topic is somewhat divided on whether an endoanal-endorectal coil is required for an optimal examination. To us, this technique is rarely necessary because these patients are fairly uncomfortable already, and the extra signal to noise ratio achieved with an endoanal coil often comes at the expense of distorted anatomy and increased motion artifact.

In our practice, nearly all perianal fistula examinations are performed in patients with Crohn disease. However, an additional group without inflammatory bowel disease (most often, middle-aged men) are also affected with perianal fistulas. In this population, cryptoglandular fistulas are thought to represent approximately 90% of such lesions, originating from infected anal glands located in the region of the dentate line dividing squamous epithelium of the anus and columnar epithelium of the rectum. Cryptoglandular fistulas are often treated surgically; in contrast, most fistulas resulting from Crohn disease are treated medically. Perianal fistulas are common in patients with Crohn disease. A perianal fistula will develop in about 35% to 40% of these patients, and as many as 35% of patients present with a perianal fistula as the initial symptom.

The anal canal consists of mucosal and submucosal layers surrounded by an internal smooth muscle sphincter, an intersphincteric space, and an outer striated muscle layer, the external sphincter, that is contiguous with the puborectalis muscle superiorly.

Fistulas are generally classified according to the Parks system, although a few additional, competing classifications are specific to MRI. Intersphincteric fistulas course from an internal opening in the anal canal through the internal sphincter and then travel in the intersphincteric space to reach the perineum. Transsphincteric fistulas cross both internal and external sphincters to travel in the ischioanal fossa to the perineum. Less common suprasphincteric fistulas travel over the top of the puborectalis muscle into the ischioanal fossa and perineum.

Axial oblique and coronal oblique images are usually the most important for identifying the fistula and determining its classification. Obtaining at least 1 axial acquisition oriented transverse to the anal plane from a sagittal localizer is useful for an undistorted view of the anatomy, although this is less true for fistulas originating from the lower rectum, a common occurrence in Crohn disease. Large fistulas are not diagnostic dilemmas, and the presence of fluid (and gas in this case) is seen as high signal intensity on T2-weighted images. In smaller fistulas, however, it can be tricky to distinguish between patent fistulas containing fluid and fistulas with intense inflammation—sometimes a consideration in deciding whether more aggressive treatment is necessary. In these cases, postgadolinium images are useful. Below is an example of a fistula with extensive inflammation and only minimal internal fluid.

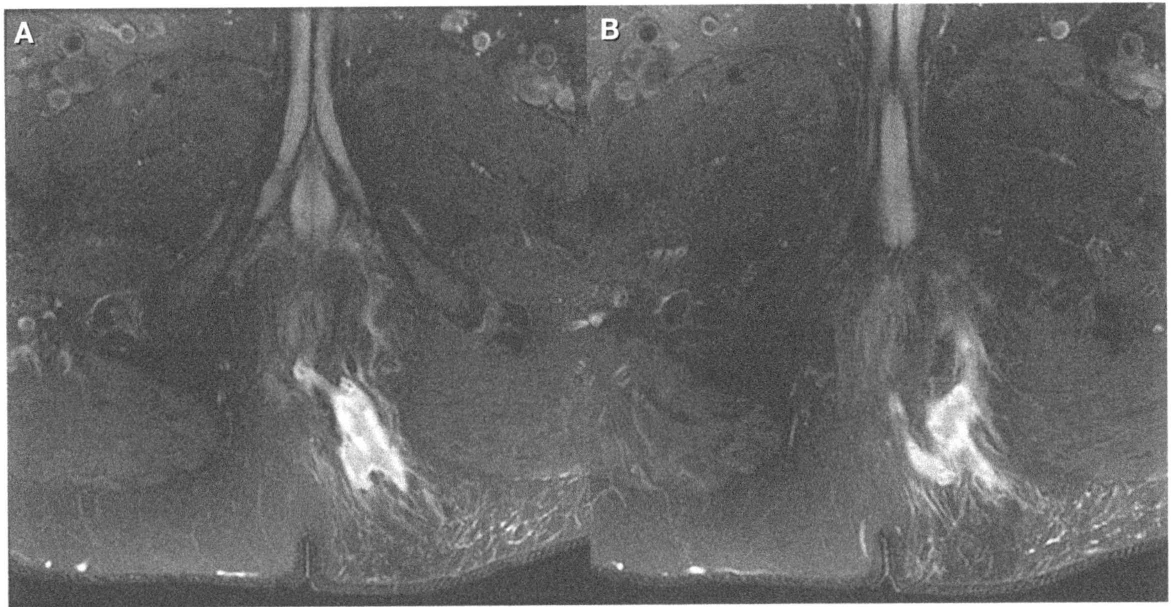

Figure 9.26.3

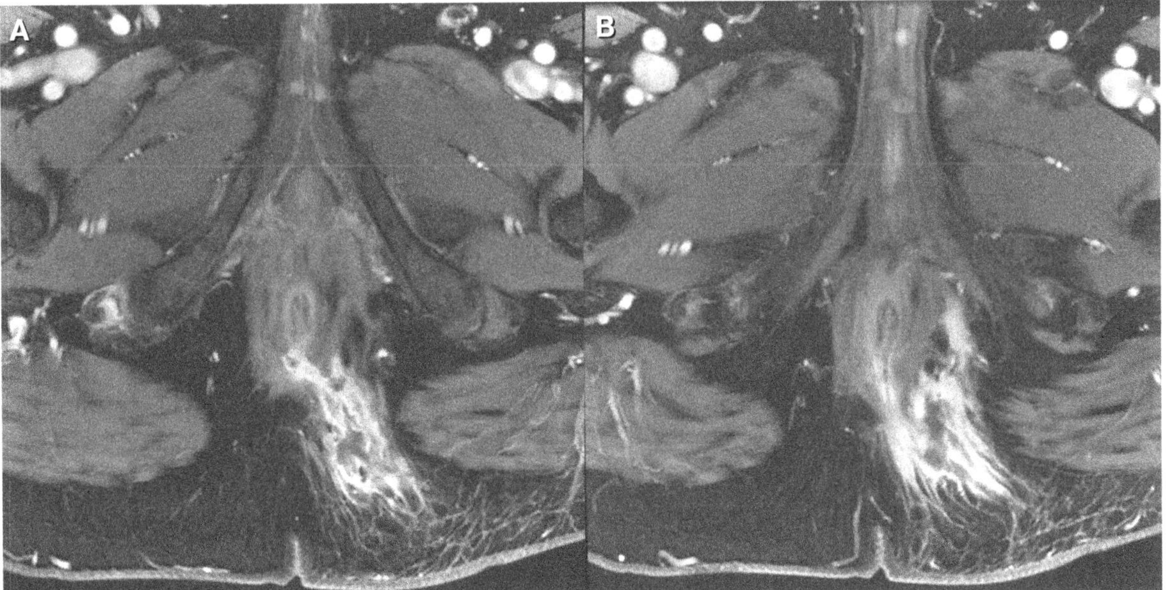

Figure 9.26.4

A 60-year-old man with history of Crohn disease now has perirectal pain and bleeding. Axial fat-suppressed FSE T2-weighted images (Figure 9.26.3) show a complex, branching transsphincteric fistula originating from the 6 o'clock position and extending posteriorly and laterally along the left gluteal fold. Axial postgadolinium fat-suppressed 2D SPGR images (Figure 9.26.4) demonstrate intense enhancement of the fistulous tract, which contains only a small amount of fluid.

CASE 9.27

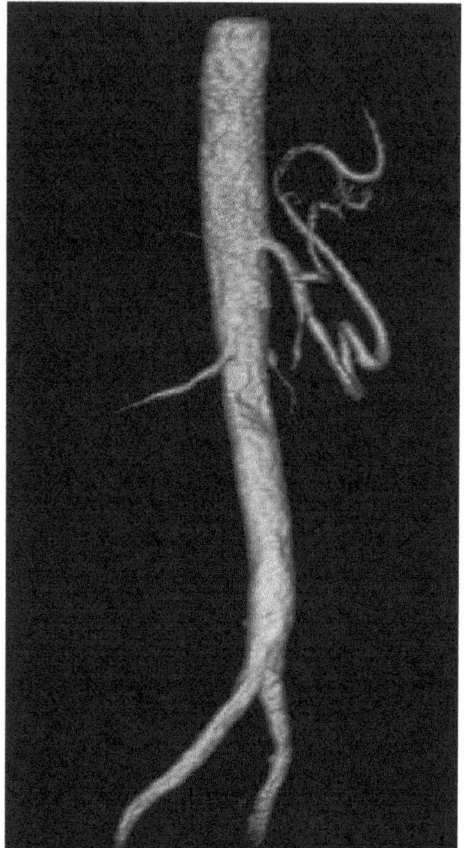

Figure 9.27.1

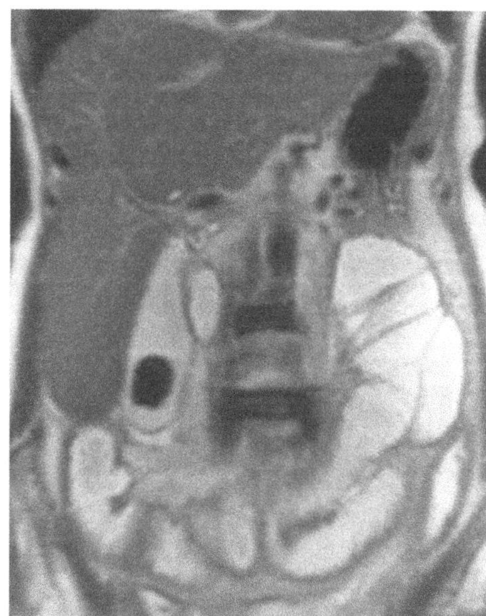

Figure 9.27.2

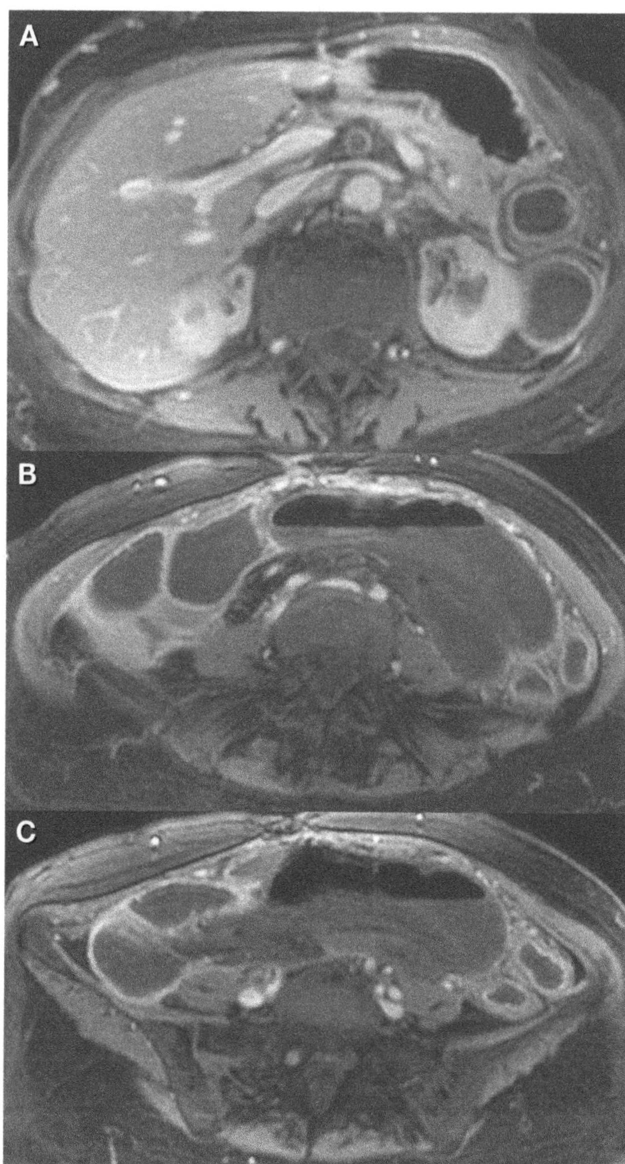

Figure 9.27.3

HISTORY: 59-year-old woman with abdominal pain and partial small-bowel obstruction visualized on plain radiographs

IMAGING FINDINGS: A volume-rendered image from 3D contrast-enhanced MRA (Figure 9.27.1) shows the presence of a single mesenteric vessel, the celiac artery. The SMA and the inferior mesenteric artery are not visualized. Coronal SSFSE (Figure 9.27.2) and axial postgadolinium fat-suppressed 2D SPGR images (Figure 9.27.3) demonstrate dilatation of multiple small bowel loops, with thickening and hyperenhancement of both large and small bowel. Note also the occlusive thrombus that distends the lumen of the proximal SMA on the most superior SPGR image.

DIAGNOSIS: Mesenteric ischemia

COMMENT: This case is an example of acute mesenteric ischemia. (See Case 16.6 for another example of mesenteric ischemia.) A large thrombus was seen within the SMA expanding the lumen and the patient's symptoms were relatively acute. Arterial embolism, usually in the SMA, is the underlying cause of mesenteric ischemia in 40% to 50% of cases, and mortality rates remain high.

Bowel findings, although nonspecific, are important to note. Mural thickening and hyperenhancement, often in conjunction with luminal distention, are common findings, but in the hyperacute setting (ie, those you are unlikely to see at MRI), mural hypoenhancement may be the more prominent feature.

In this case, mesenteric ischemia was suspected at initial examination and duplex sonography showed absence of flow in the SMA. An MRA was ordered to assess the other mesenteric vessels, as well as the aorta, in the patient, who was allergic to CT contrast. If you're not performing an examination specifically to assess for mesenteric ischemia, it is likely that you won't be doing an MRA, since it is not included in most enterography protocols. But standard MR enterography protocols should include coronal and axial postgadolinium 3D SPGR images, and these images should be sufficient in nearly all cases to document the patency (or lack thereof) of the mesenteric arteries.

Additional findings to support the diagnosis of ischemic bowel include pneumatosis and portal venous gas. The appearance is much more subtle on MRI than CT, but the diagnosis can often be made by the careful observer.

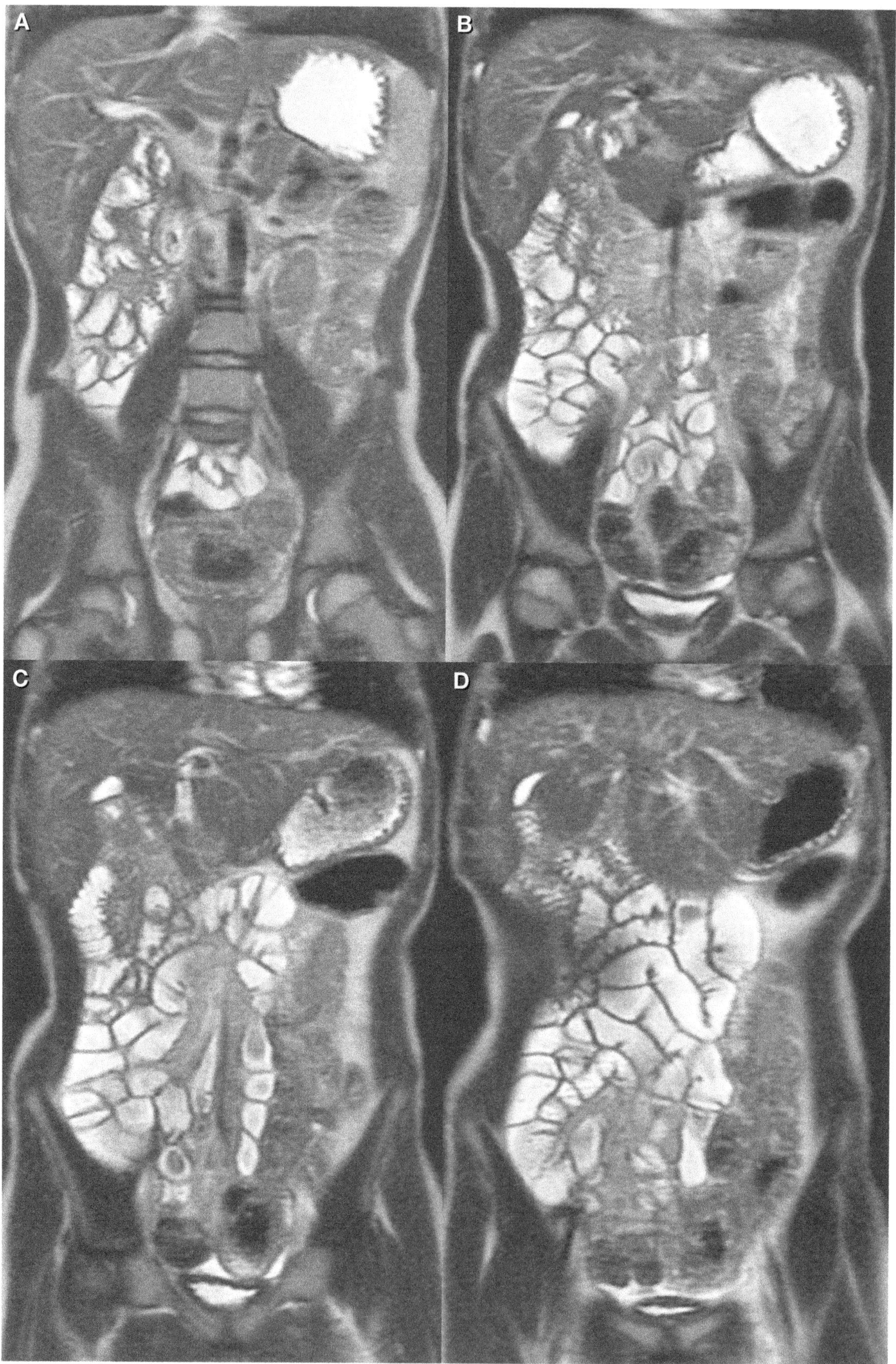

Figure 9.28.1

HISTORY: 11-year-old boy with suspected IBD

IMAGING FINDINGS: Coronal SSFSE images (Figure 9.28.1) demonstrate abnormal orientation of large and small bowel, with small bowel in the right abdomen and colon in the left abdomen.

DIAGNOSIS: Malrotation

COMMENT: Classic thinking regarding malrotation holds that most cases are detected within the first few months of life. However, in the new era of cross-sectional imaging for everyone, more and more adults with asymptomatic malrotations are noted and the true incidence is not entirely certain. Estimates in the literature range from 1 in 6,000 to 1 in 200 live births. Autopsy studies suggest that some form of malrotation exists in 0.5% to 1% of the population.

Errors in development can occur at any point in the complex process of GI tract development, leading to a wide spectrum of malrotations, some of which are likely to result in obstruction and volvulus. The abnormal location of bowel may not be problematic, but malrotated bowel is also not properly anchored. This characteristic can predispose to volvulus, and in addition, the mesentery may attempt to affix the malrotated colon to the posterior abdominal wall, resulting in fibrous peritoneal bands (Ladd bands) that can cause obstruction.

The classic presentation of malrotation is a newborn infant with bilious vomiting (ie, obstruction distal to the ampulla of Vater). Presentations beyond the neonatal period are usually less specific, and it's often not clear, as in this case, whether the patient's symptoms are actually related to malrotation and intermittent volvulus or whether the malrotation is simply an interesting, but incidental, finding.

This case shows a normally positioned stomach with small bowel located entirely in the right abdomen and colon entirely in the left abdomen. This variant of malrotation has been termed *nonrotation* and is thought to result from a relatively early embryologic arrest in bowel rotation.

MRI is not the test of choice in patients with suspected malrotation; a small bowel series is probably still preferred, but grossly malpositioned large and small bowel can be identified fairly easily and points of obstruction noted. In some forms of malrotation, the mesenteric root is abnormal, with the superior mesenteric vein positioned to the left of the SMA, in a reversal of the normal orientation. Although not specific for malrotation, this finding can be helpful as confirmatory evidence.

Treatment of symptomatic malrotation is surgical, generally an open or laparoscopic Ladd procedure, which includes lysis of all abnormal bands and adhesions, straightening of the duodenum so that it descends directly into the right lower quadrant, widening the small bowel mesentery, and performing an appendectomy. Treatment of asymptomatic patients is controversial. Many of them are expected to have no symptoms related to this diagnosis during their lives; however, the risk of a catastrophic event has led some surgeons to suggest that all malrotations should have surgical intervention.

ABBREVIATIONS

ADC	apparent diffusion coefficient
CT	computed tomography
FSE	fast-spin echo
GI	gastrointestinal
GIST	gastrointestinal stromal tumor
IBD	inflammatory bowel disease
IDH	intramural duodenal hematoma
MR	magnetic resonance
MRA	magnetic resonance angiography
MRCP	magnetic resonance cholangiopancreatography
MRI	magnetic resonance imaging
SMA	superior mesenteric artery
SPGR	spoiled gradient-recalled
SSFP	steady-state free precession
SSFSE	single-shot fast-spin echo
3D	3-dimensional
2D	2-dimensional
US	ultrasonography

10.

UTERUS

CASE 10.1

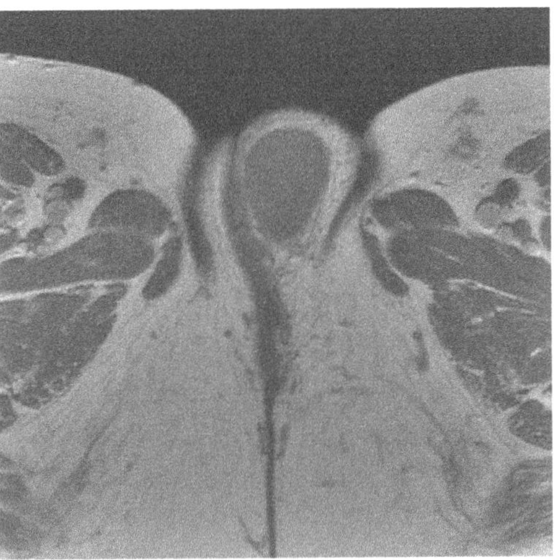

Figure 10.1.1

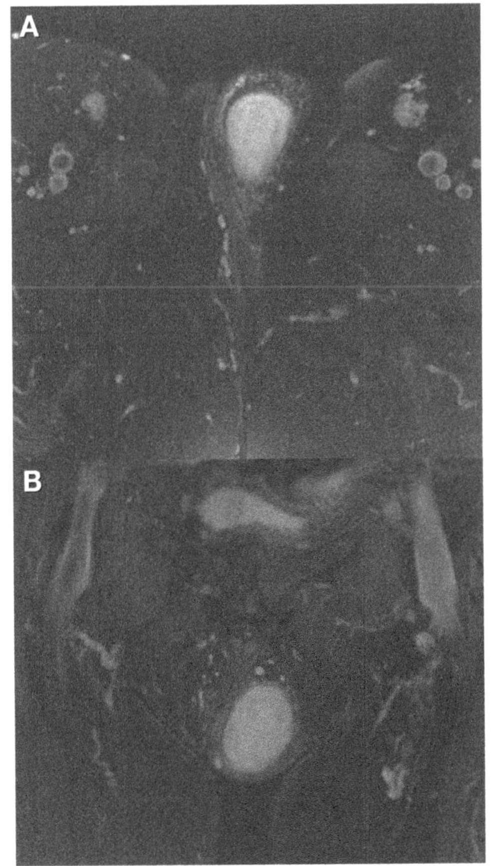

Figure 10.1.2

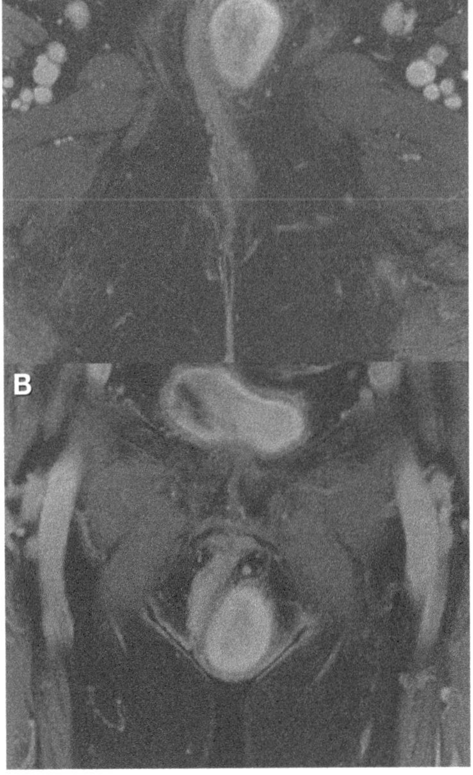

Figure 10.1.3

HISTORY: 69-year-old woman with chronic left labial swelling

IMAGING FINDINGS: Axial T1-weighted (Figure 10.1.1) and axial and coronal fat-suppressed T2-weighted (Figure 10.1.2) FSE images reveal a well-defined T2-hyperintense lesion in the left labia. Axial and coronal postgadolinium 2D SPGR images (Figure 10.1.3) show intense enhancement of the lesion.

DIAGNOSIS: Labial angiomyofibroblastoma

COMMENT: The differential diagnosis of a perineal or labial mass is broad and includes neurogenic tumors, angiomatous tumors, cysts, and abscesses. Angiomyofibroblastoma is an uncommon tumor first described by Fletcher in 1992 and is thought to occur predominantly in premenopausal women, usually in the vulva, labia, and vagina. Clinically, most tumors present as slowly growing, painless masses. Histopathologic features include a thin pseudocapsule, bundles of spindle cells with myofibroblastic differentiation, and thin-walled blood vessels. Imaging features have been reported in only a few cases, often with discrepant descriptions—we consider this case to be the most representative example, of course, and perhaps the most salient features are its well-circumscribed margins, high T2-signal intensity, and intense uniform enhancement after gadolinium administration.

Although these findings are nonspecific, they are useful in distinguishing angiomyofibroblastoma from a cyst or abscess. The pathology literature (or more accurately, the pathologist coauthors of the various case reports) emphasizes the importance of distinguishing the rare entity of angiomyofibroblastoma from the equally rare, aggressive angiomyxoma and cellular angiofibroma. These latter lesions are more invasive and require radical surgical treatment, as opposed to a simple excision for angiomyofibroblastoma.

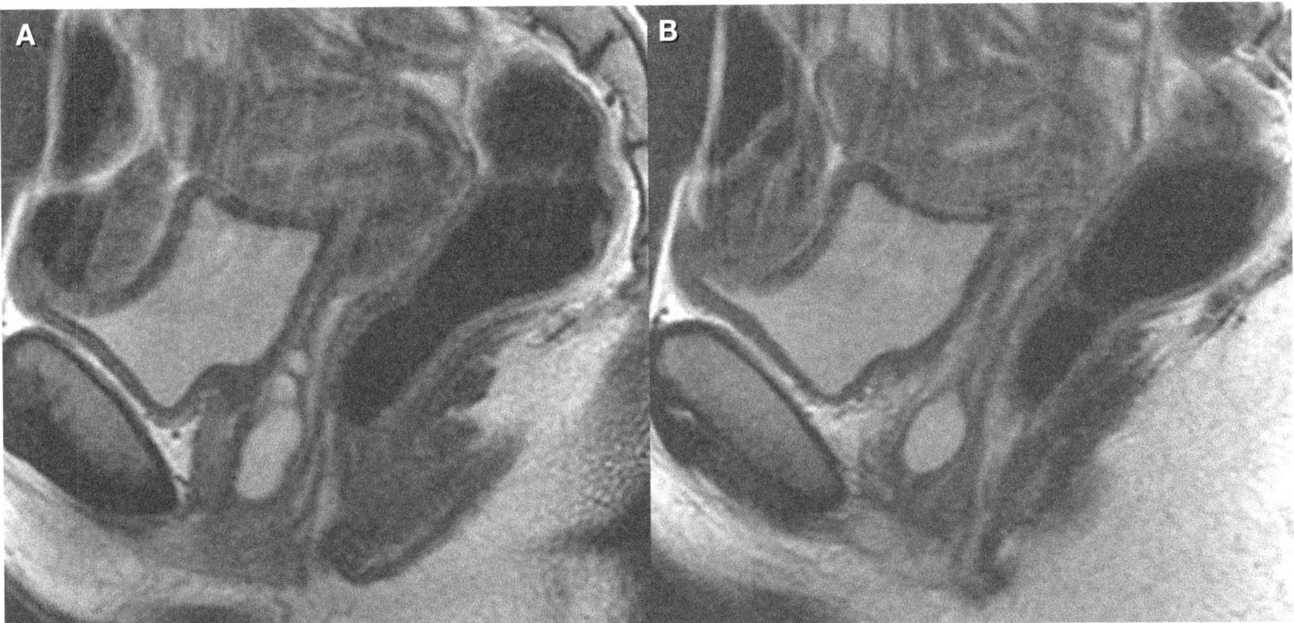

Figure 10.2.1

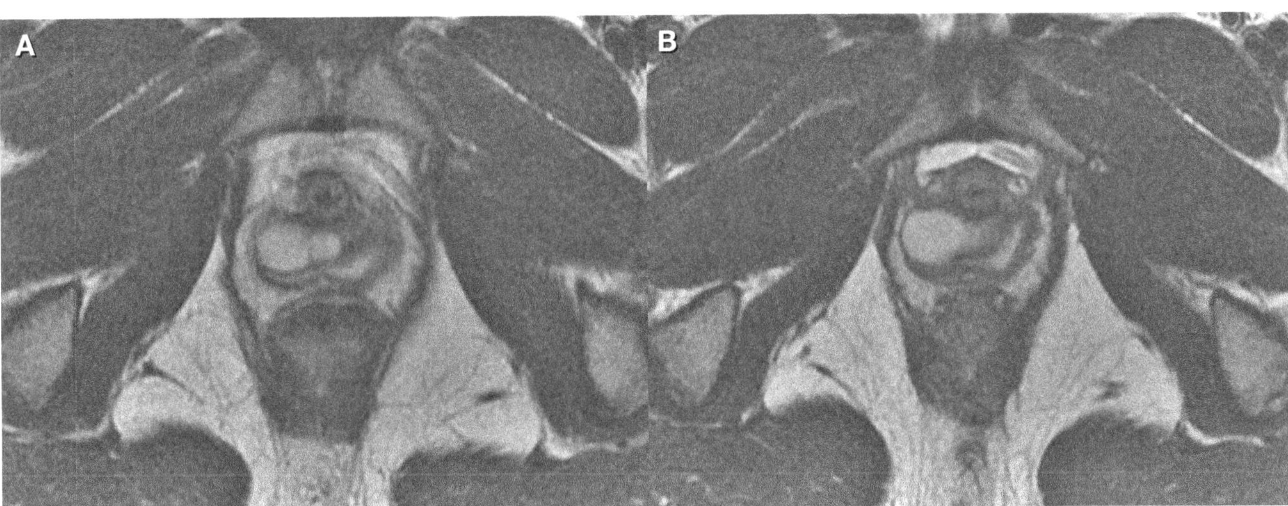

Figure 10.2.2

HISTORY: 15-year-old girl with imperforate hymen

IMAGING FINDINGS: Sagittal oblique (Figure 10.2.1) and axial (Figure 10.2.2) FSE T2-weighted images demonstrate cystic lesions along the anterior wall of the mid-distal vagina.

DIAGNOSIS: Gartner duct cysts

COMMENT: Gartner duct cysts represent remnants of the mesonephric or wolffian ducts that involute in the absence of a Y chromosome. These cysts arise from the anterolateral wall of the vagina above the level of the pubic symphysis and usually contain simple fluid. There is a small increased incidence of developmental anomalies of the genitourinary tract associated with the presence of Gartner duct cysts, and some authors have advocated large field-of-view coronal acquisitions to include the kidneys when a cyst is discovered on pelvic MRI. Logistically, this is often difficult to manage unless you simply include a large field-of-view 3-plane localizer in your routine female pelvis protocol.

Most vaginal cysts are asymptomatic and are incidental findings on physical examination or pelvic imaging. Symptomatic lesions may occur, with large cysts that cause mass effect or with infected cysts where the fluid may become more complex and rim enhancement may be seen.

Differential diagnosis includes other vaginal cysts. Bartholin gland cysts are thought to develop as a complication of infection of the vestibular glands of the vagina and occur in the posterolateral margins of the distal vagina near the introitus. Müllerian cysts are characterized by a mucin-secreting epithelial layer similar to the endocervix and can occur anywhere within the vagina. Because of the close proximity of the urethra and vagina, urethral cysts—including urethral diverticula and Skene gland cysts—are sometimes difficult to distinguish from vaginal cysts. Examples of these cysts are shown in Cases 8.1, 8.3, and 8.4.

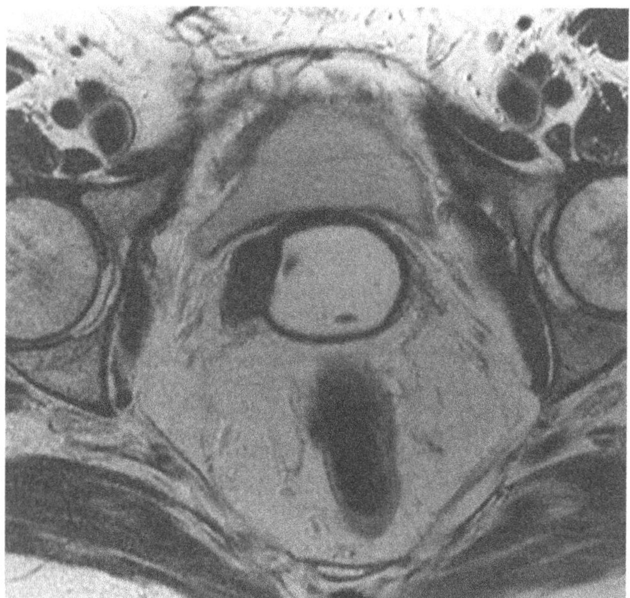

Figure 10.3.1

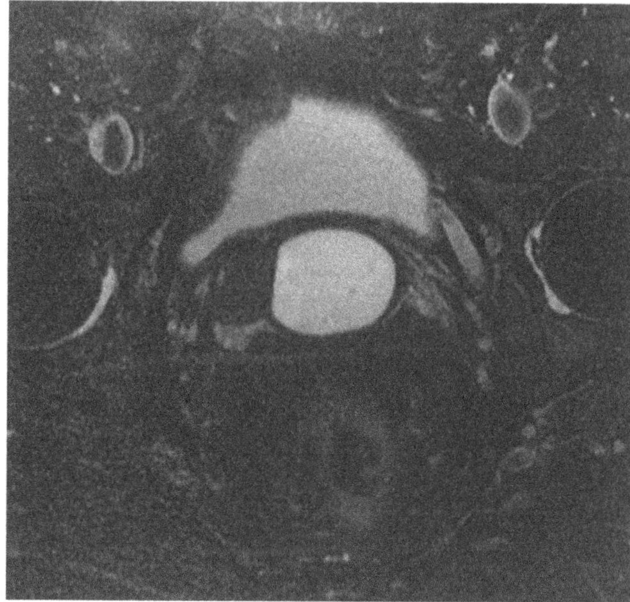

Figure 10.3.2

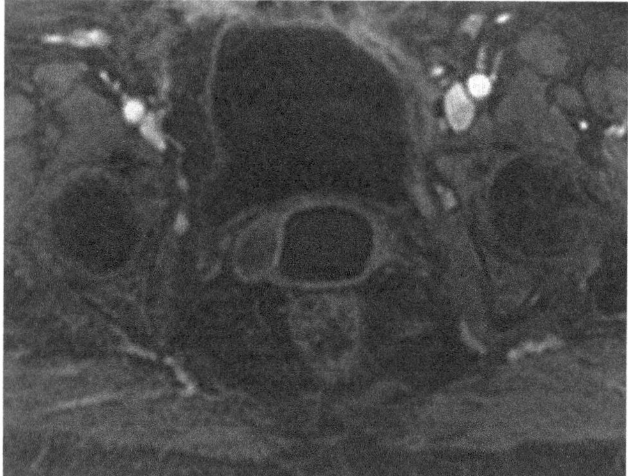

Figure 10.3.3

HISTORY: 69-year-old woman with a vaginal lesion noted on physical examination

IMAGING FINDINGS: Axial FSE T2-weighted images without (Figure 10.3.1) and with (Figure 10.3.2) fat suppression obtained following instillation of vaginal US gel demonstrate a uniformly hypointense lesion along the right lateral margin of the vagina. Axial postgadolinium 3D SPGR image (Figure 10.3.3) shows minimal central enhancement of the lesion and slight rim enhancement.

DIAGNOSIS: Vaginal leiomyoma

COMMENT: Uterine leiomyomas are common, occurring in 20% of women of reproductive age and found in 75% of hysterectomy specimens. Vaginal leiomyomas, by comparison, are unusual, although they are the most common mesenchymal neoplasms of the vagina. Many of these lesions are asymptomatic and are detected incidentally on physical examination, as in this case, although larger tumors may be associated with pain, dyspareunia, or even obstructive urinary symptoms.

Pathologically, vaginal leiomyomas resemble uterine fibroids, and tissue diagnosis is usually straightforward. Since the entity of vaginal leiomyoma is rare, there are no well-defined imaging criteria for making a definitive diagnosis, and the vast majority of lesions are resected. This case is a classic example of a fibrotic tumor with uniformly low signal intensity on T2-weighted images and minimal enhancement on relatively early postgadolinium images (delayed images might have shown significant enhancement). However, many leiomyomas are not typical and could have a more heterogeneous appearance with high T2-signal intensity, necrosis, and hyperenhancement. Leiomyoma was suggested as a diagnosis on the MRI report, but the lesion was resected anyway, providing pathologic proof for this case.

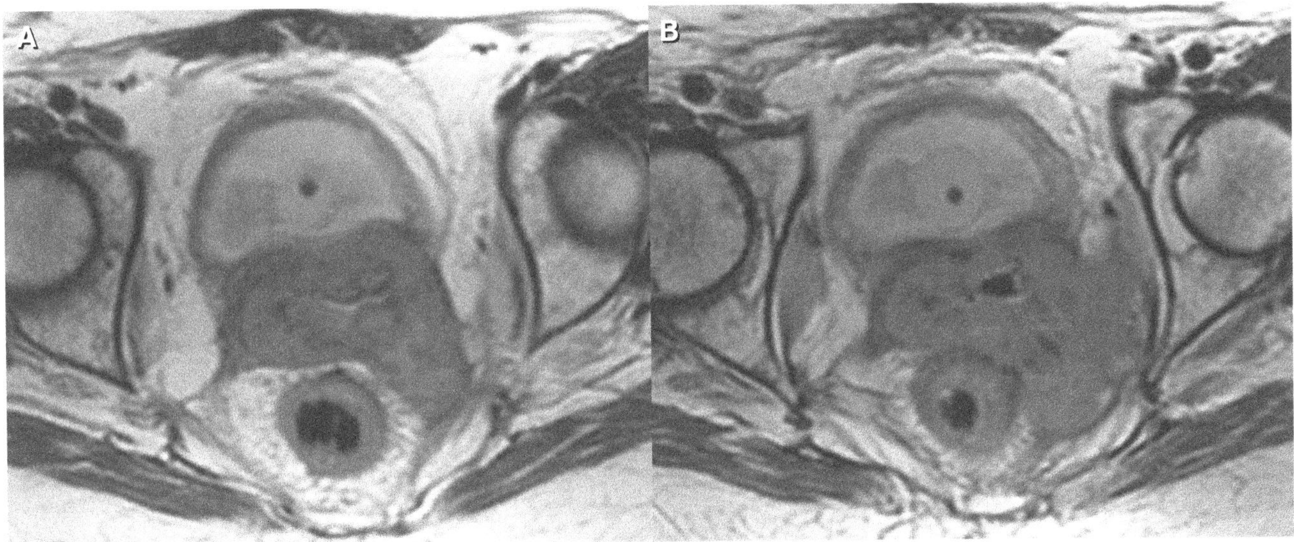

Figure 10.4.1

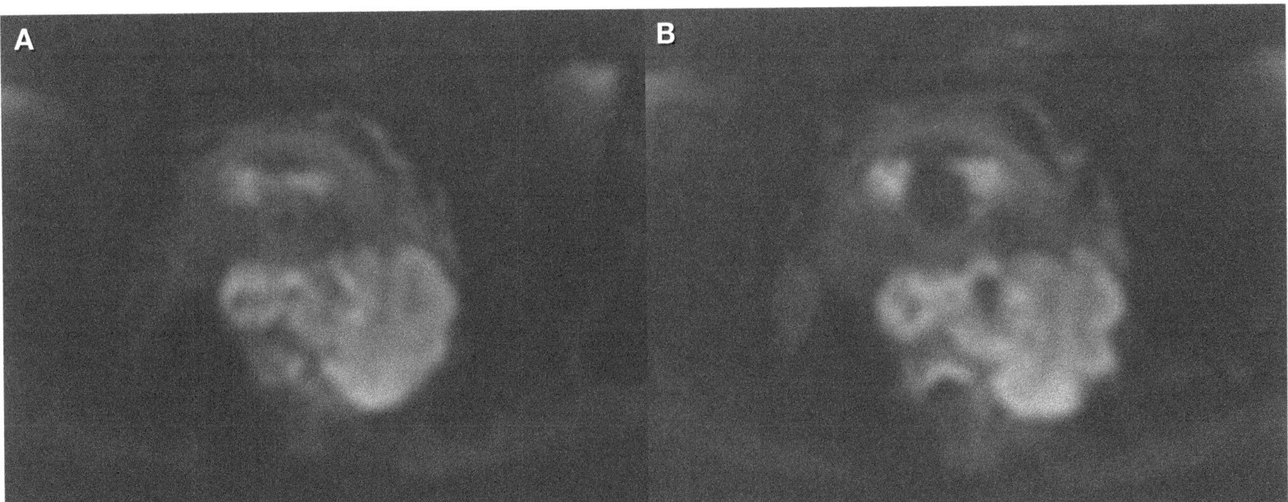

Figure 10.4.2

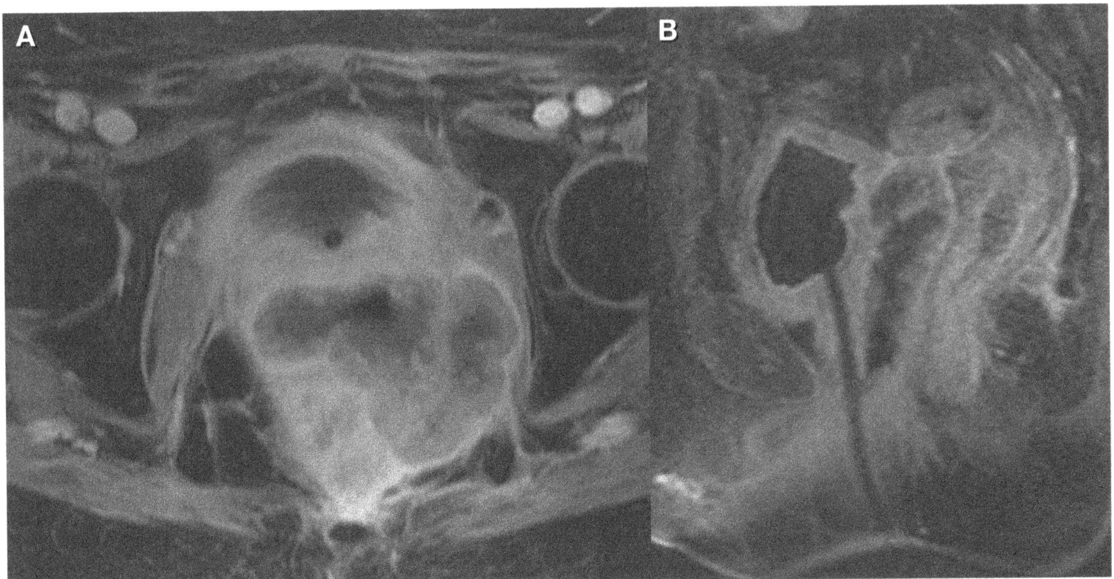

Figure 10.4.3

HISTORY: 69-year-old woman with vaginal bleeding

IMAGING FINDINGS: Axial FSE T2-weighted images (Figure 10.4.1) reveal a large infiltrative mass expanding the walls of the vagina and extending laterally into the left pelvic sidewall. Note that the tumor partially encases the rectum and extends into the posterior bladder wall. The lesion shows high signal intensity on axial DWI (b=800 s/mm^2) (Figure 10.4.2) and heterogeneous hypoenhancement on axial (Figure 10.4.3A) and sagittal (Figure 10.4.3B) postgadolinium 3D SPGR images.

DIAGNOSIS: Vaginal adenocarcinoma

COMMENT: *Primary vaginal carcinoma* is defined as arising solely from the vagina with no involvement of the cervix or vulva. SCC accounts for 85% of primary vaginal cancers and usually occurs in elderly women presenting with painless vaginal bleeding, pelvic pain, or a vaginal mass. Risk factors for development of vaginal SCC are similar to those for cervical cancer and include chronic human papillomavirus infection, immunosuppression, multiple sexual partners, and smoking. Vaginal SCC most often arises in the proximal third of the vagina, with a tendency to involve the posterior wall.

Vaginal adenocarcinoma accounts for 2% to 9% of all vaginal tumors and develops in approximately 2% of women exposed to diethylstilbestrol in utero. It frequently occurs in young women, with a peak incidence at age 20 years, and is thought to arise from regions of vaginal adenosis, endometriosis, wolffian rest remnants, and periurethral glands (since the vagina has a squamous epithelium). Vaginal adenocarcinoma occurs most frequently in the upper third and anterior wall of the vagina. Primary vaginal cancers are rare and account for only 1% to 2% of all gynecologic neoplasms. Metastatic involvement of the vagina is at least 4 to 5 times more frequent than primary vaginal neoplasms.

Vaginal carcinoma can appear as a focal mass or as focal or diffuse wall thickening. This case illustrates a large infiltrative lesion with diffuse vaginal wall thickening and left pelvic sidewall extension, as well as probable invasion of the bladder and rectum. MRI is most useful in this case for staging and surgical or radiation planning, rather than for arriving at a specific diagnosis. Diffusion-weighted acquisitions often beautifully delineate the margins of the tumor in vaginal, vulvar, and cervical carcinomas, which show high signal intensity against the dark background of normal tissue. Postgadolinium images can be helpful for characterizing the extent of disease and identifying metastatic disease.

Identification of a vaginal mass is not difficult in this case; the lesion is large and impossible to miss.

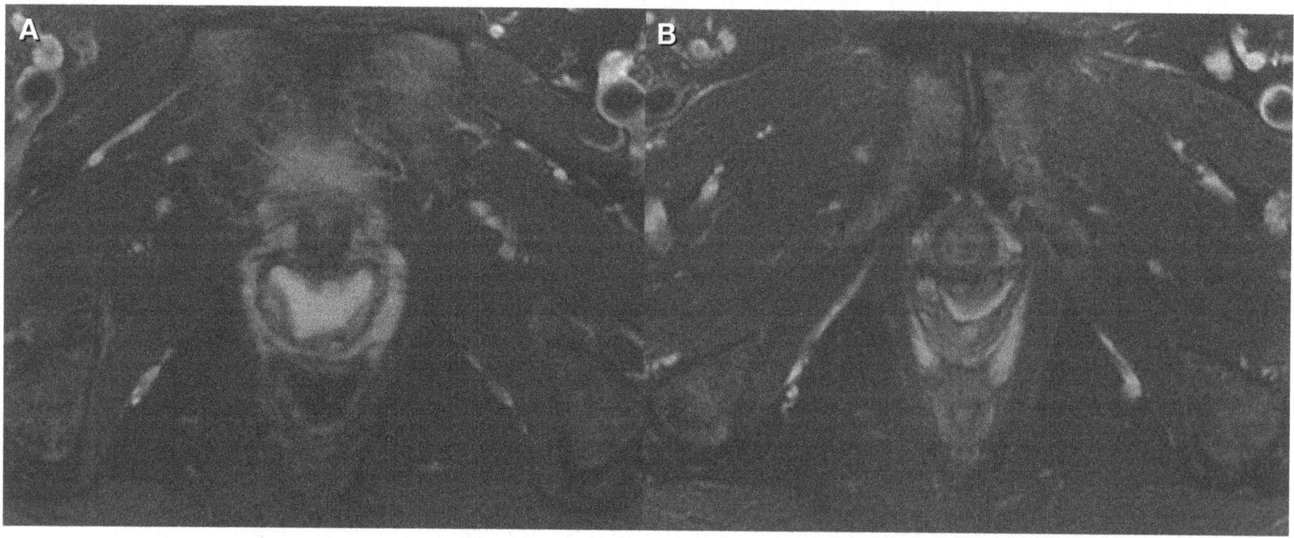

Figure 10.4.4

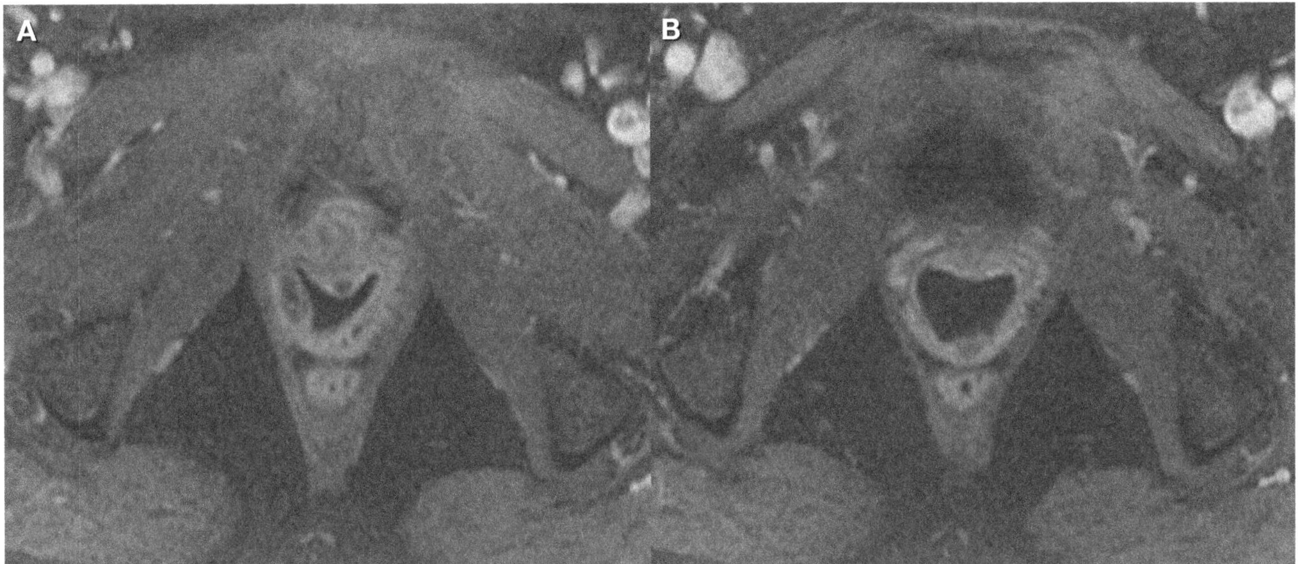

Figure 10.4.5

A much more subtle example of vaginal adenocarcinoma is shown in Figures 10.4.4 and 10.4.5 from a 43-year-old woman who had a vaginal lesion incidentally detected on physical examination. In this instance, vaginal US gel was helpful to distend the lumen and allow complete visualization of the vaginal walls, where the subtle T2-hyperintense and hypoenhancing nodule can be seen.

Axial FSE T2-weighted images (Figure 10.4.4) obtained after instillation of vaginal US gel demonstrate nodular thickening of the right lateral and posterior vaginal walls. These regions show focal hypoenhancement on axial postgadolinium 3D SPGR images (Figure 10.4.5).

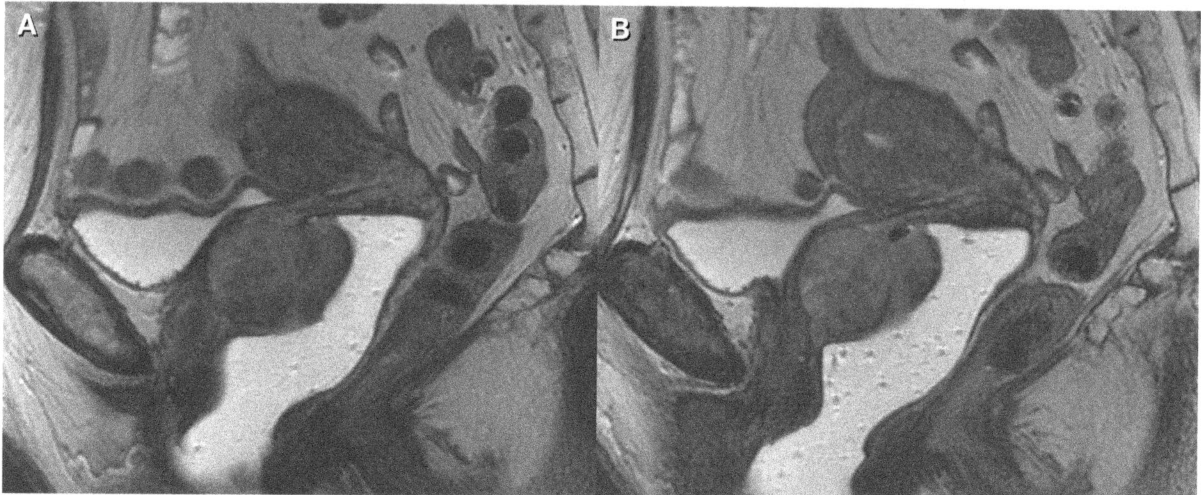

Figure 10.5.1

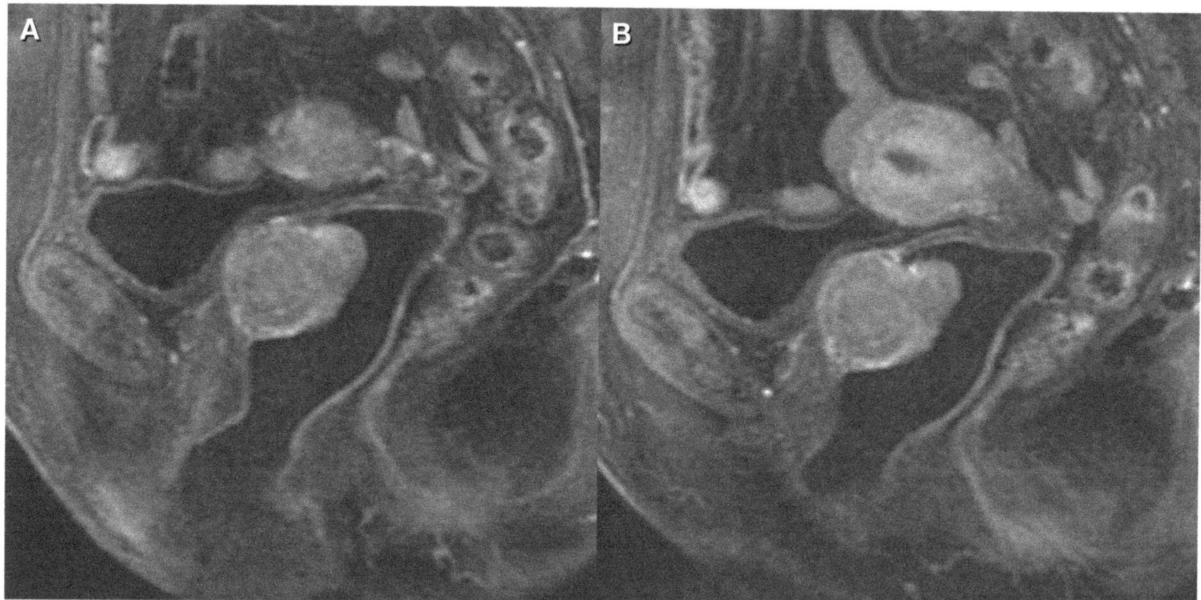

Figure 10.5.2

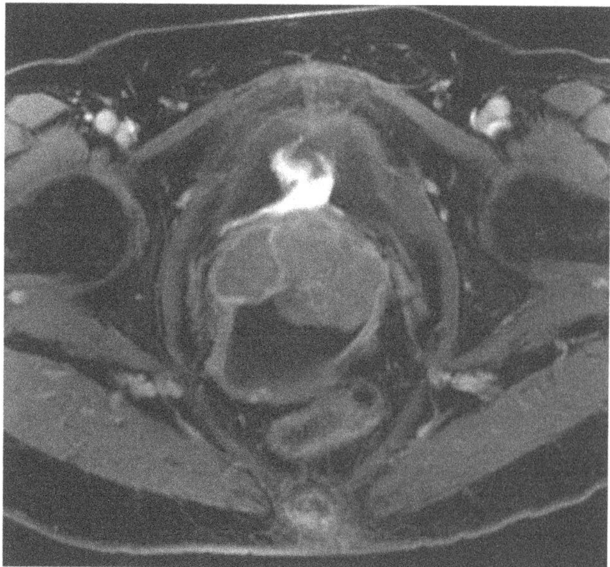

Figure 10.5.3

HISTORY: 81-year-old woman with abnormal Papanicoulaou smear

IMAGING FINDINGS: Sagittal FSE T2-weighted images (Figure 10.5.1) obtained after instillation of vaginal US gel demonstrate a large, mildly heterogeneous, well-defined lesion in the anterior proximal vagina. Sagittal arterial phase postgadolinium 3D SPGR images (Figure 10.5.2) reveal moderate diffuse enhancement of the lesion. Axial 3D SPGR image obtained 7 minutes after contrast injection (Figure 10.5.3) shows contrast washout with residual rim enhancement.

DIAGNOSIS: Vaginal melanoma

COMMENT: Vaginal melanoma is an unusual neoplasm, with fewer than 300 cases reported in the literature. Melanocytes derived from neural crest cells can be found in the basal portion of the vaginal epidermis in 3% of healthy women. Some of the melanocytes may be aberrantly located in the vaginal mucosa, and these are thought to represent potential sites of origin of vaginal melanoma. Vaginal melanoma accounts for 2% to 3% of all primary malignant tumors of the vagina and 0.4% to 0.8% of all malignant melanomas in women. These tumors typically present in the sixth and seventh decades and have a predilection for the anterior vaginal wall, most often in the lower third of the vagina. The most common presenting symptom is vaginal bleeding.

In general, vaginal melanoma is associated with a poor prognosis. A recent retrospective review revealed that the median survival in patients with localized disease was 19 months. Many radical surgical approaches have been described, but there is little evidence that they provide a significant survival benefit.

The imaging appearance of vaginal melanoma is that of a vaginal mass. After the presence of a mass has been confirmed, you can occasionally make an educated guess regarding the cause (leiomyoma) or even render a definitive diagnosis (Gartner duct cyst), but in general, a solid vaginal mass can be a primary carcinoma, metastasis, or some other rare lesion such as this case, and your main job after identifying it is to describe its location and look for local invasion or metastatic disease.

This case is a good example of fairly aggressive use of vaginal US gel. It probably wasn't necessary in this case since the mass was so large, but vaginal gel can be useful for sorting out anterior vs posterior location of smaller masses, as well as distinguishing cervical from vaginal involvement. Although endovaginal gel is often helpful, it usually degrades the quality of DWI, and so it's a good idea to acquire these images at the beginning of the examination before injecting the gel.

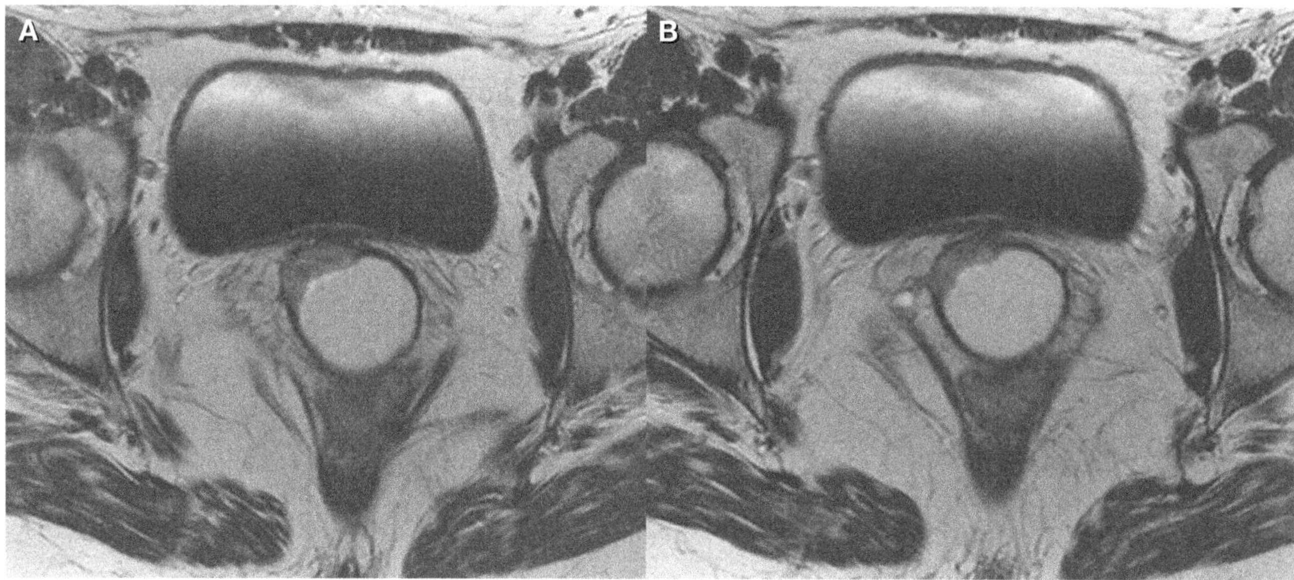

Figure 10.6.1

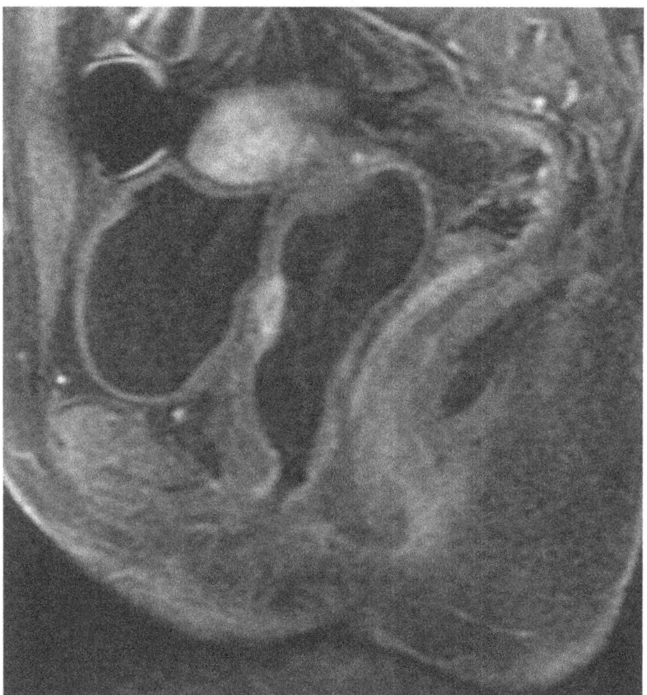

Figure 10.6.2

HISTORY: 40-year-old woman with metastatic breast cancer and an abnormal vaginal examination

IMAGING FINDINGS: Axial FSE T2-weighted images (Figure 10.6.1) reveal a crescentic, mildly hyperintense mass involving the right anterolateral vaginal wall. Sagittal arterial phase postgadolinium 3D SPGR image (Figure 10.6.2) shows intense enhancement of the lesion in the midanterior vagina.

DIAGNOSIS: Vaginal metastasis from breast carcinoma

COMMENT: Vaginal metastases are more common than primary vaginal neoplasms, a specific example of a more general truth. In fact, the vagina is the second most common site (after the ovary) of metastatic disease in the female genital tract. Most metastases are from primary cancers involving other areas of the genitourinary tract, and the 3 most common metastatic primary tumors are cervical, endometrial, and renal cell carcinomas. Only a few case reports have described breast cancer metastasizing to the vagina, although it is likely that these lesions are rarely imaged.

The appearance in this case is that of an infiltrative mass in the vaginal wall, with intense enhancement after gadolinium administration. This appearance is nonspecific; however, the value of MRI is in distinguishing this lesion from a potentially benign cause, such as a vaginal cyst, and in documenting the location, size, and local extent of the mass.

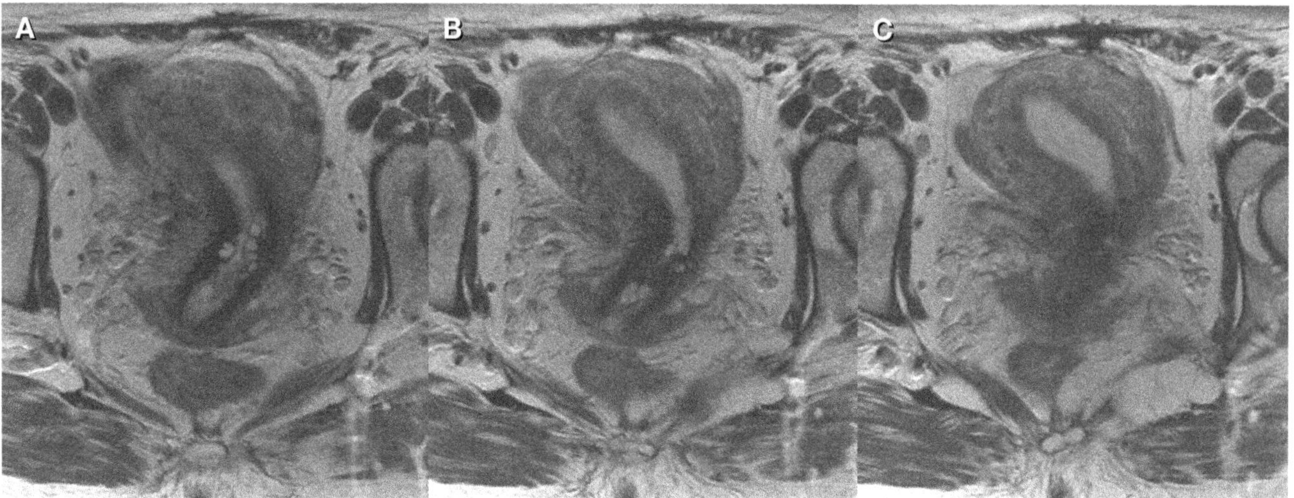

Figure 10.7.1

HISTORY: 45-year-old woman with abnormal uterine bleeding

IMAGING FINDINGS: Axial oblique FSE T2-weighted images (Figure 10.7.1) show a banana-shaped uterus with a single horn. Note also small nabothian cysts in the cervix.

DIAGNOSIS: Unicornuate uterus

COMMENT: Müllerian duct anomalies are not common, but their importance lies in the fact that some of them represent treatable causes of infertility. The female reproductive tract develops primarily from the paired müllerian ducts, which form the fallopian tubes, uterus, cervix, and upper two-thirds of the vagina. Normal development requires completion of organogenesis, fusion, and septal resorption. Failure of organogenesis leads to class I and class II anomalies (agenesis/hypoplasia and unicornuate uterus). Abnormalities of fusion result in bicornuate and didelphic configurations (class III and class VI). Incomplete or absent septal resorption results in a septate (class V) or arcuate (class VI) uterus.

The prevalence of müllerian duct anomalies has been estimated at 3.2% in women with normal reproductive outcomes, 5% to 10% in women with recurrent first-trimester miscarriages, and greater than 25% in women with late first- and early second-trimester miscarriages. Unicornuate uterus constitutes approximately 20% of all müllerian duct anomalies and is generally asymptomatic until menarche or pregnancy.

Unicornuate uterus is a class II uterine anomaly resulting from partial failure of organogenesis. There are 4 variants of unicornuate uterus. Isolated unicornuate uterus (shown herein) is the most common, with a reported frequency of 35%. When a rudimentary horn is also present, it is noncavitary in 33% of cases, cavitary noncommunicating in 22%, and cavitary communicating in 10%.

Abnormalities of the urinary tract are commonly associated with müllerian duct anomalies, with an overall incidence of 29%. The highest incidence occurs in patients with unicornuate uterus (40%). Renal agenesis is the most common abnormality and is nearly always ipsilateral to the rudimentary horn.

Patients with unicornuate uterus and a rudimentary horn have a higher incidence of dysmenorrhea, chronic pelvic pain, hematometra, and hematosalpinx, particularly when the rudimentary horn contains endometrium. Adenomyosis (in the rudimentary horn) and endometriosis (usually ipsilateral to the rudimentary horn) are also more frequent. Patients may present with infertility, multiple miscarriages or spontaneous abortions, preterm deliveries, intrauterine fetal demise, and ectopic pregnancies.

A pregnancy can develop in both communicating and noncommunicating rudimentary horns. Most rudimentary horn pregnancies occur in a noncommunicating horn (83%), and uterine rupture can result in as many as 90% of these cases in the second trimester. The diagnosis is therefore a critical one to make early in pregnancy and is treated with removal of the rudimentary horn and ipsilateral fallopian tube. This entity sometimes can be very difficult to distinguish from a pregnancy within 1 horn of a bicornuate uterus.

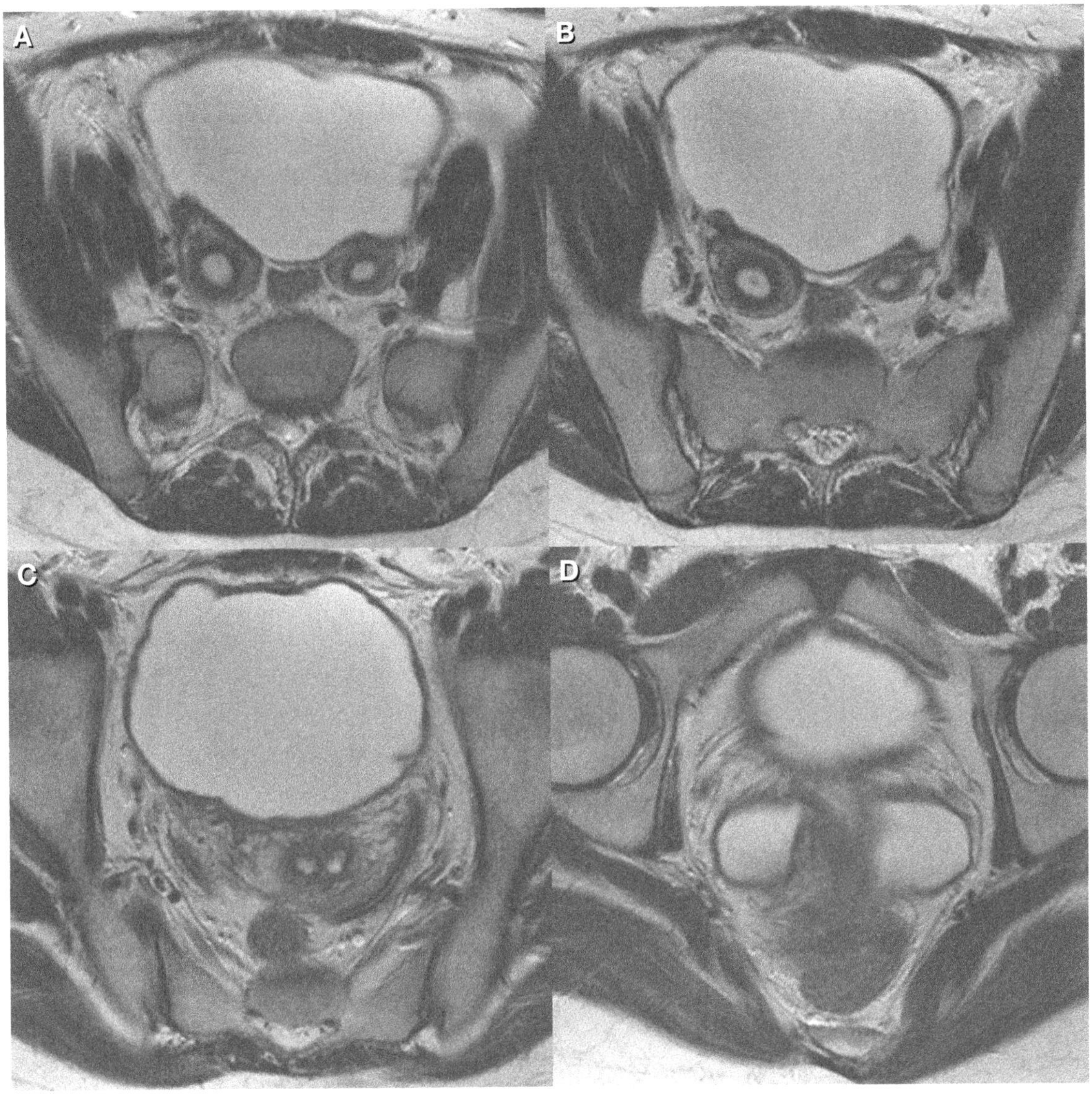

Figure 10.8.1

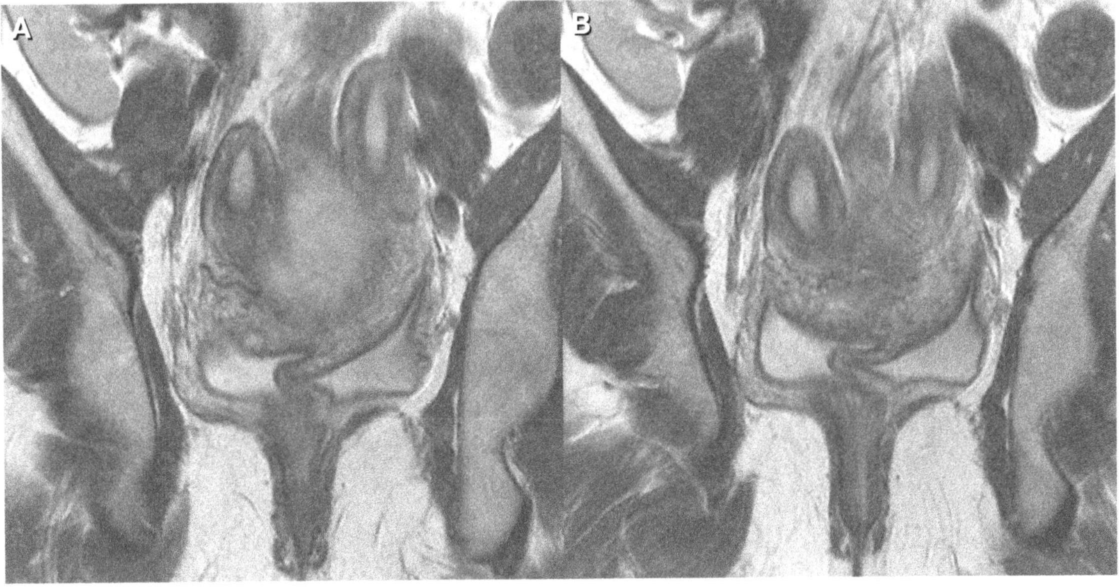

Figure 10.8.2

HISTORY: 20-year-old woman with a congenital uterine anomaly

IMAGING FINDINGS: Axial (Figure 10.8.1) and coronal (Figure 10.8.2) FSE T2-weighted images reveal 2 separate uterine horns and separate cervices. Note also 2 distinct vaginal canals, both distended with fluid.

DIAGNOSIS: Uterine didelphys with vaginal septum

COMMENT: Uterine didelphys represents a class III müllerian duct anomaly characterized by complete nonfusion of both müllerian ducts. The resulting uterus consists of widely separated uterine horns and a deep fundal cleft, 2 cervices, and nearly always a longitudinal or transverse vaginal septum or 2 vaginal cavities.

Uterine anomalies may be encountered as an incidental finding when performing pelvic MRI for another indication or may be found during an infertility work-up. Some patients present with symptoms directly related to the anomaly—for example, obstruction of 1 or both uterine or vaginal cavities, or a combination, in uterine didelphys.

Müllerian anomalies are associated with renal anomalies in 29% of patients and are also associated with infertility, as well as adverse pregnancy outcomes. Women with congenital uterine anomalies have a higher incidence of preterm delivery, premature rupture of membranes, breech presentation, cesarean section, and neonates who are small for their gestational age.

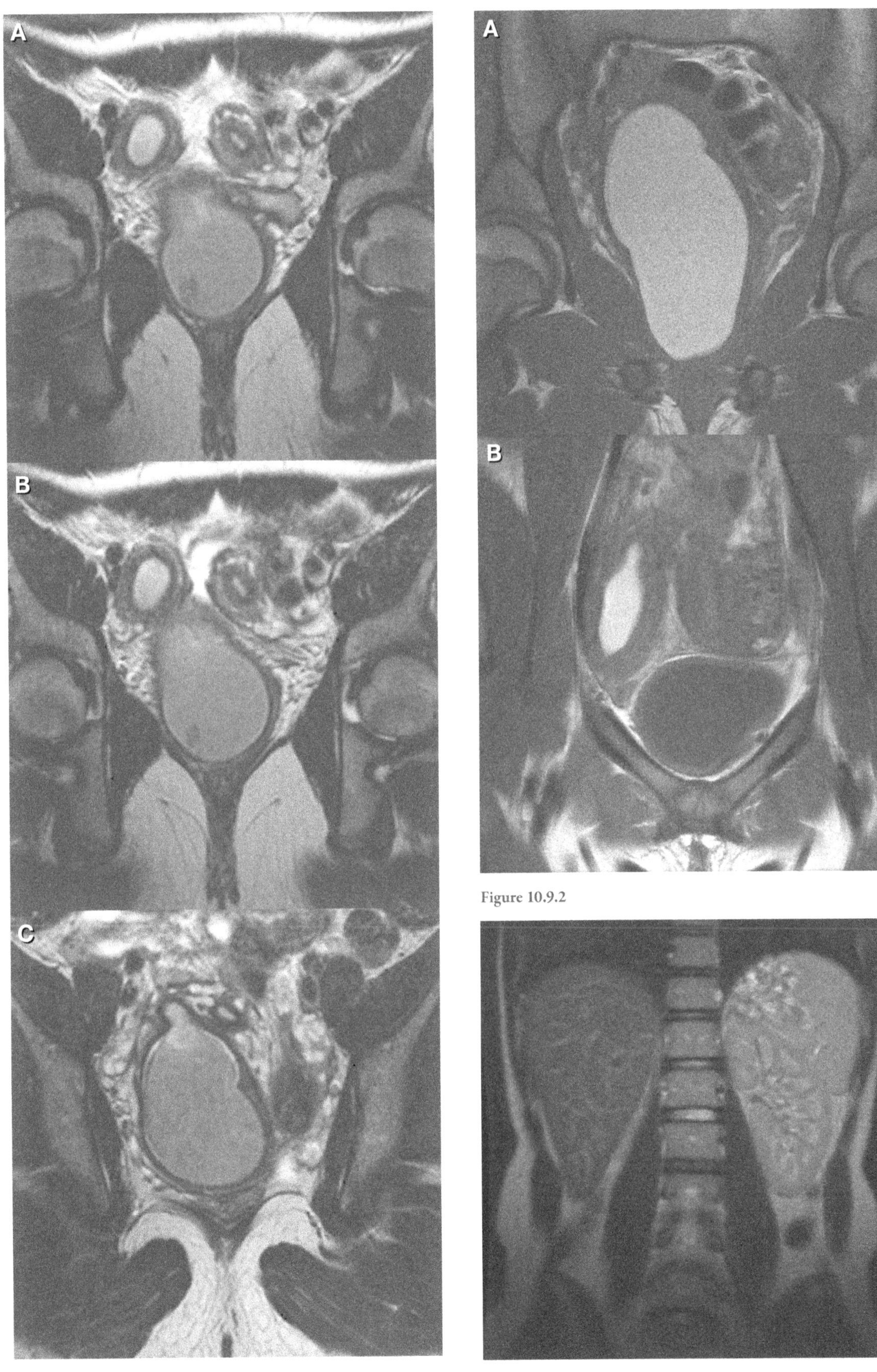

Figure 10.9.1

Figure 10.9.2

Figure 10.9.3

HISTORY: 15-year-old girl with abdominal pain, irregular periods, and suspected uterine anomaly

IMAGING FINDINGS: Coronal oblique FSE T2-weighted images (Figure 10.9.1) reveal 2 distinct uterine horns, with the right endometrial cavity distended with fluid. Note that 2 cervices are present on Figure 10.9.1C. There are 2 vaginal cavities: the right massively dilated and fluid-filled and the left collapsed and barely perceptible. Coronal oblique T1-weighted images (Figure 10.9.2) show hyperintense fluid within the right vaginal and uterine cavities. A coronal SSFSE image (Figure 10.9.3) of the abdomen demonstrates right-sided renal agenesis.

DIAGNOSIS: Uterine didelphys with vaginal septum, obstructed right hemivagina, and ipsilateral renal agenesis

COMMENT: Uterine didelphys is associated with a longitudinal vaginal septum in at least 75% of cases and a transverse vaginal septum in a smaller percentage. This patient had a combined longitudinal and transverse septum that resulted in obstruction of the right hemivagina and subsequent hematometrocolpos. This presentation of uterine didelphys is not unusual, and the constellation of didelphys, vaginal obstruction, and unilateral renal agenesis has been described in multiple case reports, although the entity has not acquired a distinct name to make it more popular in resident conferences.

As with other müllerian duct anomalies, uterine didelphys has an association with adverse reproductive outcomes, including a spontaneous abortion rate of 32%, preterm birth rate of 28%, and live birth rate of 56%. Although the Strassman metroplasty is a controversial procedure for women with didelphic uteri and reproductive loss, incision of the vaginal septum is indicated for an obstructed hemivagina and hematocolpos, dyspareunia, and pelvic pain.

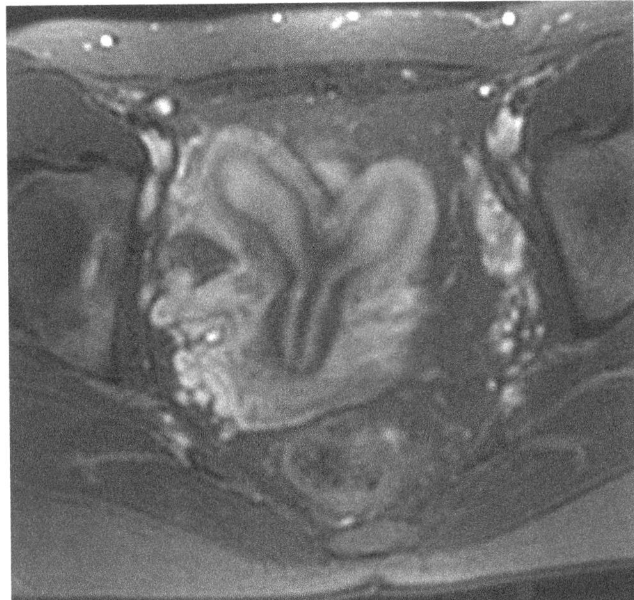

Figure 10.10.1

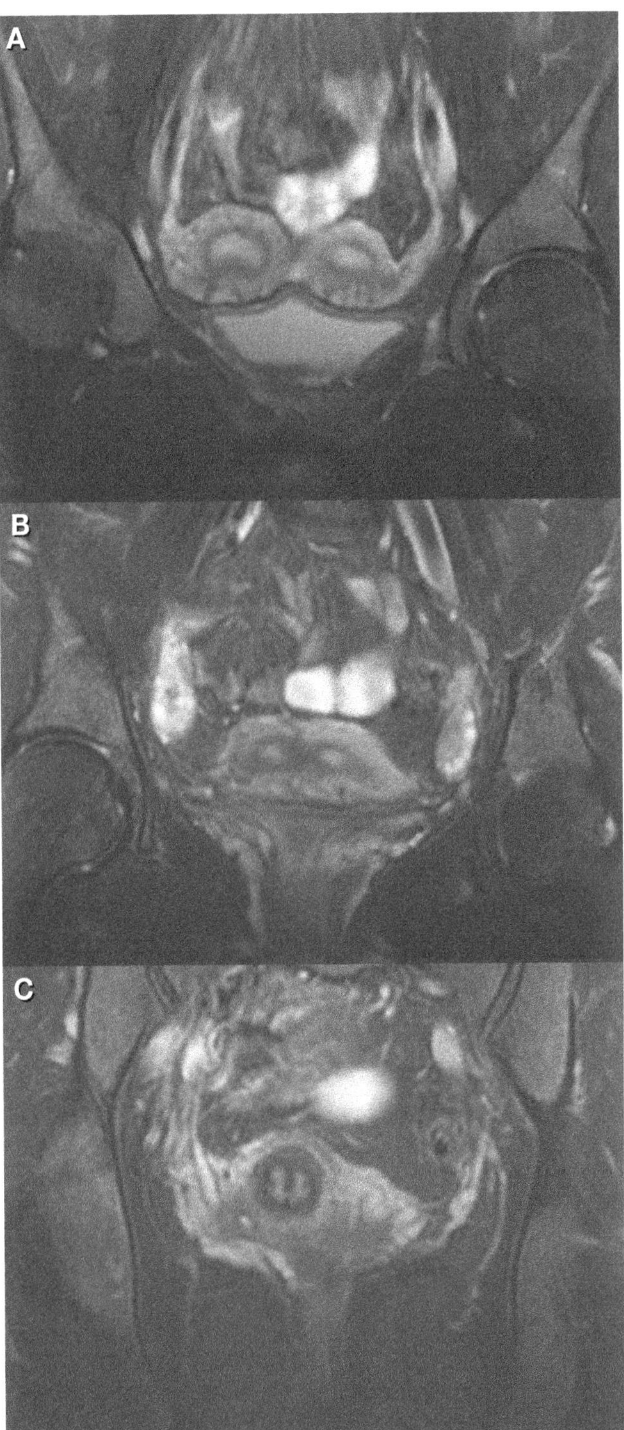

Figure 10.10.2

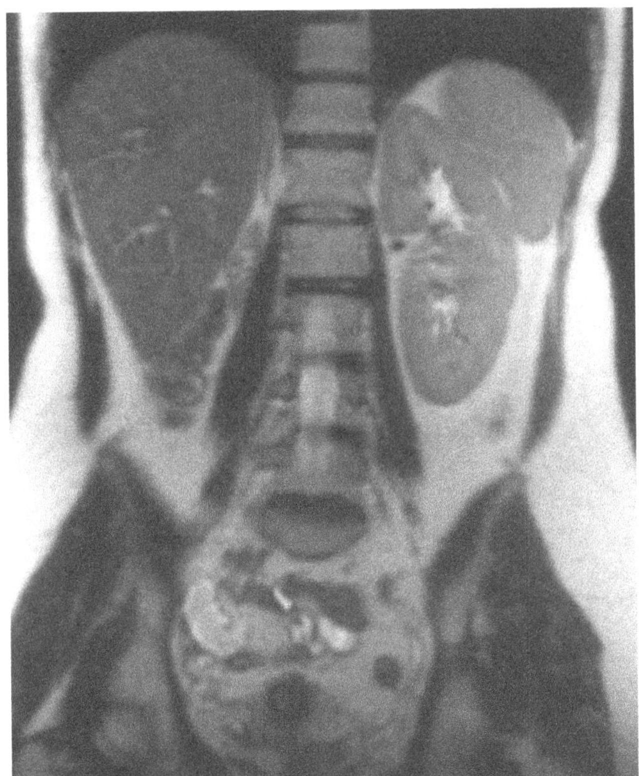

Figure 10.10.3

HISTORY: 30-year-old woman with a possible uterine anomaly on pelvic US

IMAGING FINDINGS: Axial (Figure 10.10.1) and coronal oblique (Figure 10.10.2) fat-suppressed FSE T2-weighted images reveal 2 uterine horns with a moderate uterine cleft and a septum extending throughout the endometrial cavity and cervix. A coronal large field-of-view SSFSE image (Figure 10.10.3) shows absence of the right kidney and compensatory hypertrophy of the left kidney.

DIAGNOSIS: Bicornuate uterus

COMMENT: Bicornuate uterus is a class IV müllerian duct anomaly representing incomplete fusion of the paired ducts and is characterized by distinct uterine horns with a fundal concavity or cleft greater than 1 cm in diameter. Partial fusion of the lower uterine segment and cervix occurs with a muscular or combined muscular and fibrous septum that may (bicollis) or may not (unicollis) extend to the external os. The vagina is usually normal.

Bicornuate uterus is associated with obstetrical complications in a fairly high percentage of patients, including a spontaneous abortion rate of 36% and preterm birth rate of 23%. The incidence of preterm delivery is much higher in patients with bicornuate bicollis than with unicollis uterus (66% vs 38%) and is probably related to diminished cavitary size, insufficient musculature, and impaired ability to distend.

A bicornuate uterus is generally considered a nonsurgical anomaly (in distinction with a septate uterus). However, metroplasty has been advocated for women with recurrent pregnancy loss, and cervical cerclage has been proposed as a remedy for the increased incidence of cervical incompetence associated with this disorder.

This case also illustrates the association of uterine and renal anomalies, occurring in 29% of patients with müllerian duct anomalies. Unilateral renal agenesis, as seen in this case, is the most commonly reported abnormality, accounting for 67% of cases, but ectopic kidney, horseshoe kidney, renal dysplasia, and duplicated collecting systems may also occur. For this reason, any pelvic MRI performed to investigate a potential uterine anomaly should include a large field-of-view acquisition through the abdomen to visualize the kidneys and document any abnormalities.

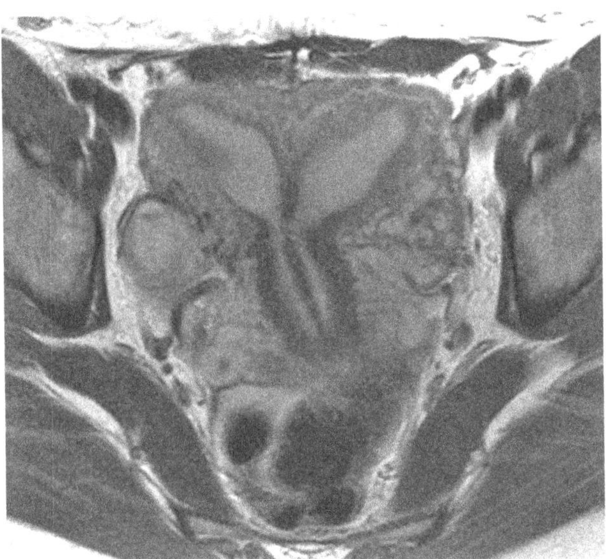

Figure 10.11.1

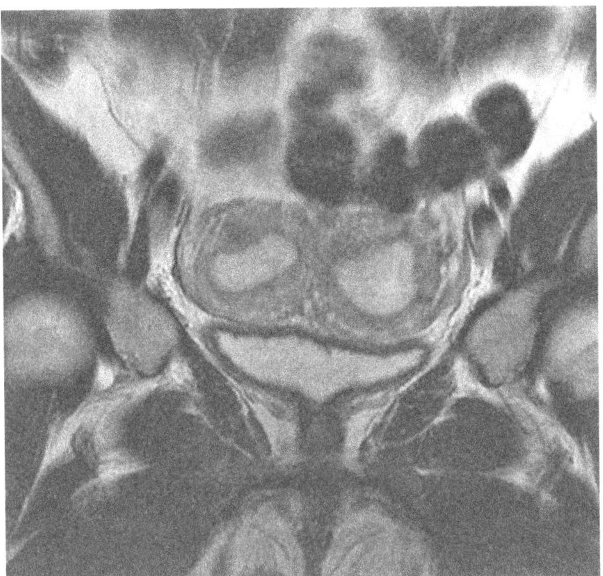

Figure 10.11.2

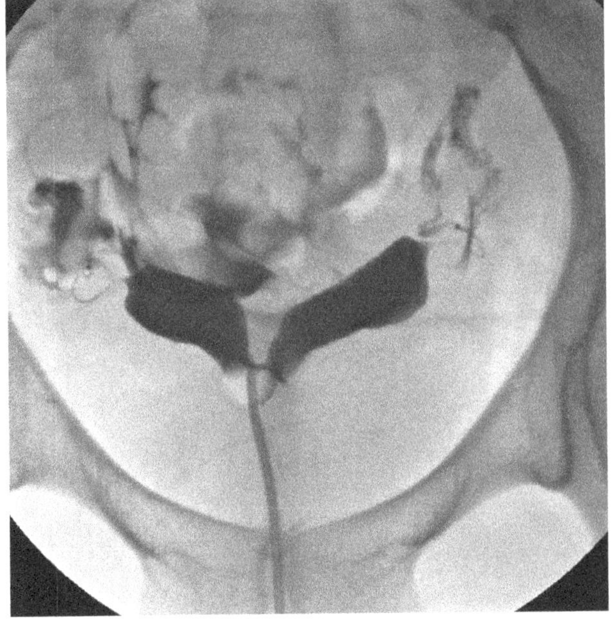

Figure 10.11.3

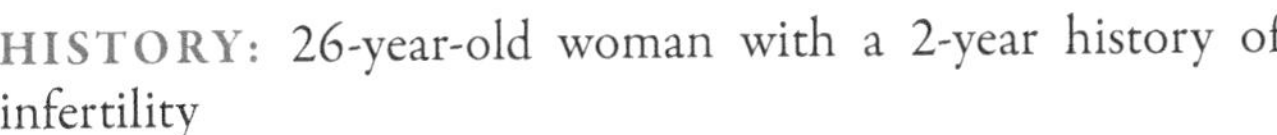

HISTORY: 26-year-old woman with a 2-year history of infertility

IMAGING FINDINGS: Axial oblique FSE T2-weighted image (Figure 10.11.1) reveals a minimally concave uterine fundal contour. There are 2 uterine horns, and the endometrial cavity and cervix are divided by a linear structure with dark T2-signal intensity. Coronal FSE T2-weighted image (Figure 10.11.2) through the uterine fundus again demonstrates that the 2 uterine horns are separated by myometrium. Image from hysterosalpingogram (Figure 10.11.3) shows contrast filling both uterine horns, with contrast spilling into the peritoneum.

DIAGNOSIS: Septate uterus

COMMENT: Uterine anomalies such as septate uterus are not always as straightforward as one might think after reading the standard MRI textbooks. In this case, for example, the 3 gynecologists who had seen the patient described her condition as didelphys, bicornuate, and septate and even once as unicornuate.

Magnetic resonance evaluation of uterine anomalies begins with assessment of the fundal contour. If the contour is convex or shows less than 1 cm of concavity (as in this case), then a septate or arcuate uterus is diagnosed (assuming that it is not normal). A concavity or fundal cleft of greater than 1 cm means that the diagnosis is either didelphic uterus or bicornuate uterus. Uterine didelphys is characterized by a deep fundal cleft, 2 separate uteri that may be joined at the body, 2 cervices, and a longitudinal or oblique vaginal septum. The fundal cleft of a bicornuate uterus is less prominent, the uterine horns are less widely separated, and a muscular or combined muscular-fibrous septum may (bicollis) or may not (unicollis) extend to the external os. The cervix is single or is divided by a septum, and a vaginal septum may be seen in some cases.

The septate uterus is characterized by a convex, flat, or minimally concave (<1 cm) fundal contour. The septum can be muscular or fibrous or a combination of the 2 and may be incomplete or extend to the external os. A single cervix should be present, which may be divided by a septum, and a vaginal septum is seen in approximately 25% of cases. (The uncommon occurrence of a septate uterus with 2 cervices is recognized by the American Society of Reproductive Medicine. Many clinicians automatically diagnose a didelphic uterus when they see 2 cervices, and from the radiologic perspective, it can be difficult to distinguish 2 cervices from a single cervix divided by a prominent septum.)

Septate uterus is the most common müllerian duct anomaly, accounting for approximately 55% of cases, and is associated with the poorest obstetrical outcomes, but it can be treated surgically. A fibrous septum can be repaired through hysteroscopy, whereas resection of a muscular septum generally requires a transabdominal approach.

Although sonography is generally the most common first examination in a patient with a suspected uterine anomaly, the results are sometimes ambiguous, particularly in large patients, patients with substantial amounts of bowel gas, those who cannot tolerate an endovaginal examination, or those with a retroflexed or retroverted uterus. In any case, visualization of the fundal contour is generally more operator dependent with sonography, and some authors advocate MRI as a first-line test for this indication. Hysterosalpingograms provide excellent visualization of the 1 or more uterine cavities (provided that they communicate with the cervix and vagina) and demonstrate patency of the fallopian tubes. However, as in this case, they often are not particularly helpful in diagnosing the particular variety of the anomaly, since the fundal contour is not visualized.

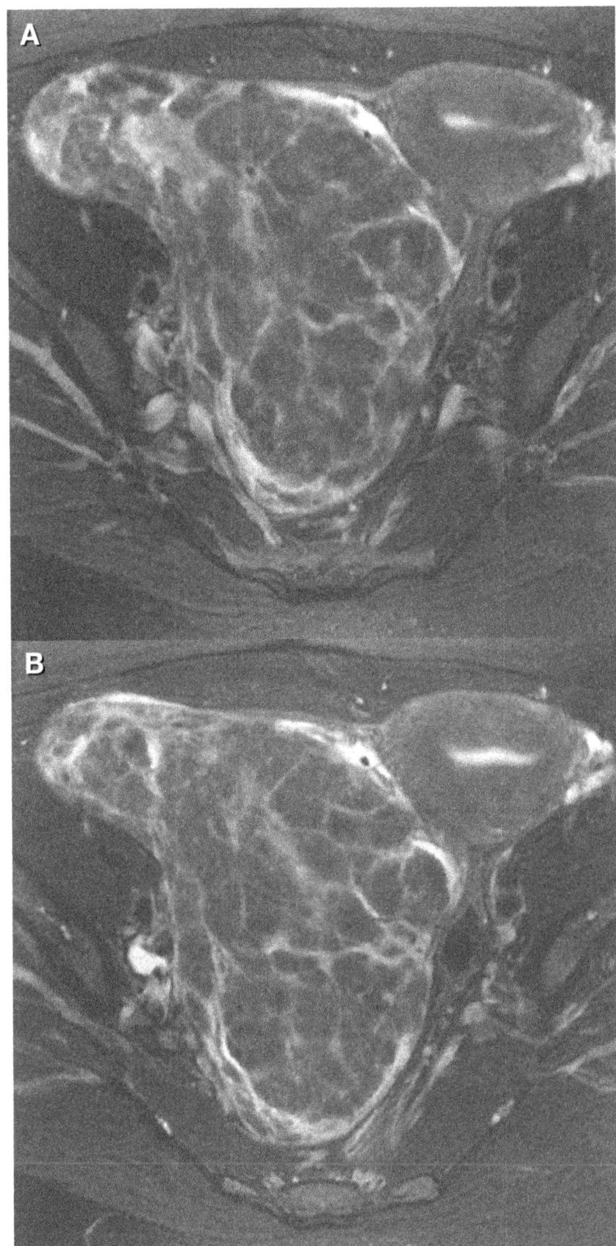

Figure 10.12.1

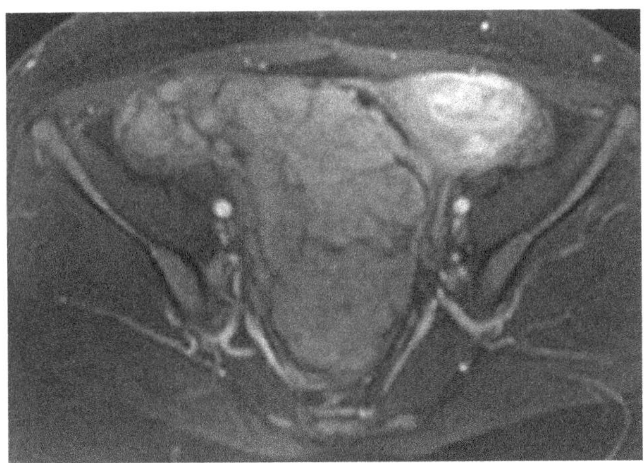

Figure 10.12.3

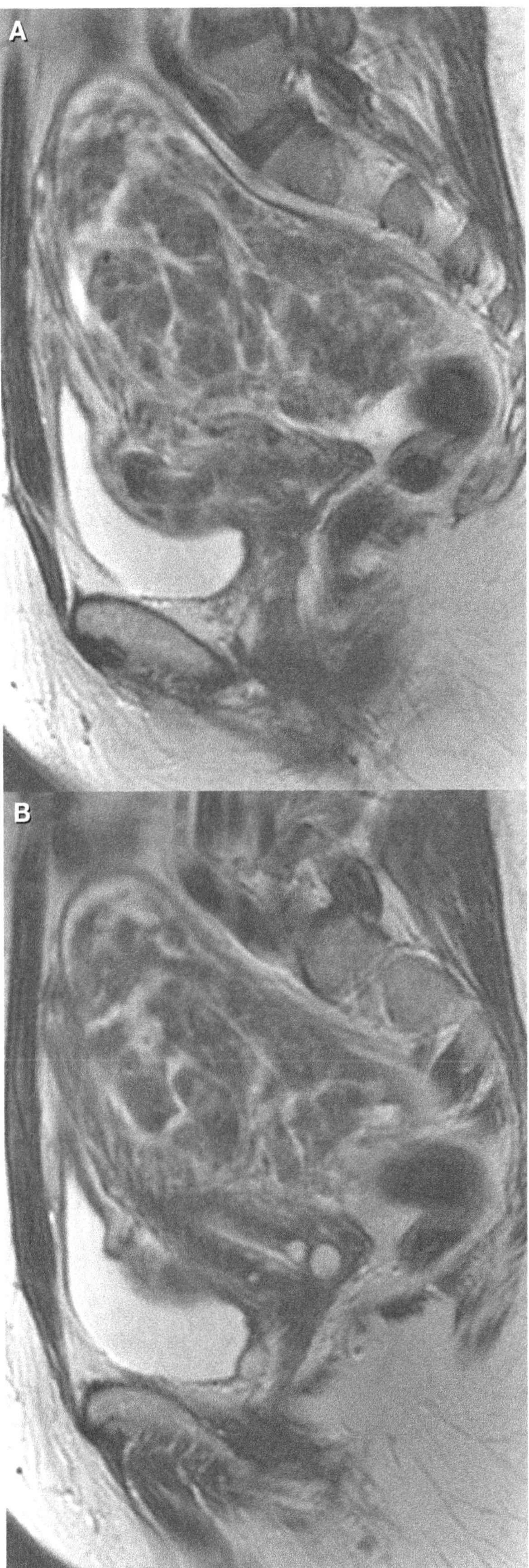

Figure 10.12.2

HISTORY: 49-year-old woman with a right-sided pelvic mass on physical examination

IMAGING FINDINGS: Axial fat-suppressed FSE T2-weighted images (Figure 10.12.1) and sagittal FSE T2-weighted images without fat suppression (Figure 10.12.2) demonstrate a large lobulated mass with low T2-signal intensity. An axial arterial phase postgadolinium 3D SPGR image (Figure 10.12.3) shows moderate diffuse enhancement of the lesion.

DIAGNOSIS: Exophytic subserosal uterine fibroid

COMMENT: Uterine fibroids (leiomyomas) are the most common gynecologic neoplasm and the most common cause of uterine enlargement (excluding pregnancy). They occur in 20% to 25% of women of reproductive age and have their highest prevalence in the fifth decade. Fibroids are benign, smooth muscle tumors that also contain variable amounts of connective tissue. Approximately 40% of fibroids have cells with a mutation that is thought to enhance the cellular response to corticosteroids and growth factors, and most cells also have a greater concentration of progesterone and estrogen receptors than normal myometrium, both of which probably contribute to enlargement of fibroids during pregnancy and in response to oral contraception.

Fibroids are symptomatic in approximately 50% of cases, with the presence and severity of symptoms depending to a large extent on the size and location of lesions. Submucosal fibroids (5%-10%) predispose to menorrhagia, infertility, miscarriages, dyspareunia, and pelvic pain. Intramural and subserosal fibroids are less likely to cause symptoms until they are large enough to exert significant mass effect.

This case demonstrates a fairly typical appearance of a large subserosal fibroid: a well-marginated lobulated lesion with predominantly low signal intensity on T2-weighted images. The vascular supply to fibroids is highly variable, but nondegenerated fibroids often show prominent early enhancement, as seen in Figure 10.12.3, although usually less than normal endometrium and myometrium. Verification of uterine origin is sometimes difficult, and in this case, it is best seen on the sagittal image, where a stalk attaches the fibroid to the superior fundus. In general, MRI is superior to sonography at confirming uterine or ovarian origin of a pelvic mass, but of course it isn't 100% successful. The differential diagnosis in these cases is usually a pedunculated fibroid vs a fibrous ovarian tumor.

A number of different forms of fibroid degeneration have been described. Hyaline degeneration often has a hypointense appearance on T2-weighted images, similar to that of normal fibroids, although concurrent calcification may introduce regions of signal loss corresponding to susceptibility artifact. Myxoid degeneration appears as high T2-signal intensity with low initial enhancement that increases on delayed acquisitions. Cystic degeneration also has high T2-signal intensity with minimal or no enhancement. Fibroids with hemorrhagic degeneration show increased precontrast T1-signal intensity with minimal enhancement. Degenerating fibroids may be the cause of worsening symptoms, but from the imaging standpoint, they are important mainly because the additional heterogeneity introduced can occasionally make the distinction between a leiomyoma and leiomyosarcoma difficult. Malignant degeneration of fibroids is rare, occurring in approximately 0.3% to 0.7% of cases. However, the incidence increases with age, and a 60-year-old woman has a 10-fold greater risk than a 40-year-old woman.

MRI is used with increasing frequency in screening patients with fibroids for potential nonsurgical therapy, including uterine artery embolization and focused US ablation. Several studies have shown that MRI often detects more lesions than sonography, particularly in patients with enlarged uteri, and that the additional information provided by MRI may sometimes lead to a change in treatment. For example, degenerated fibroids with little or no enhancement are not likely to respond to uterine artery embolization.

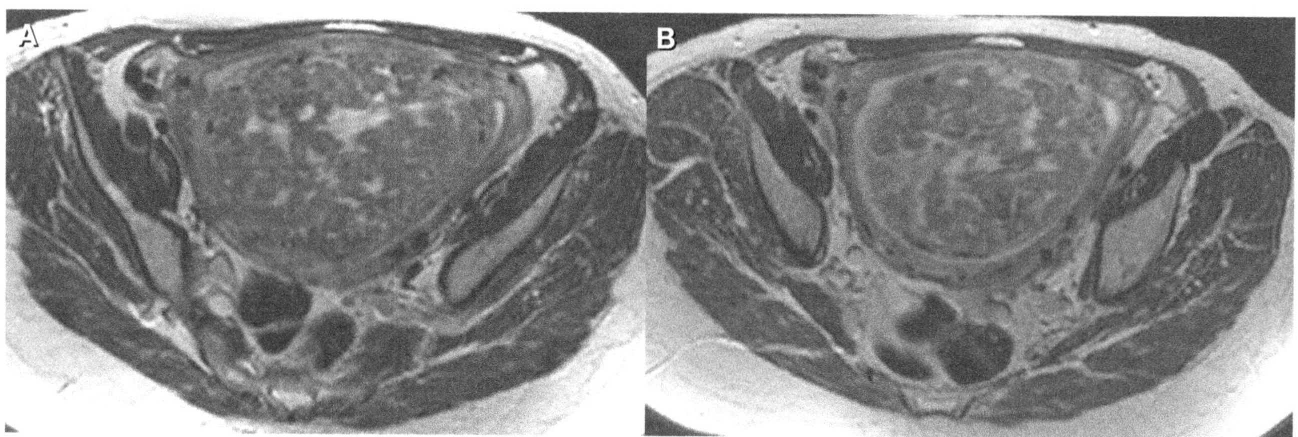

Figure 10.12.4

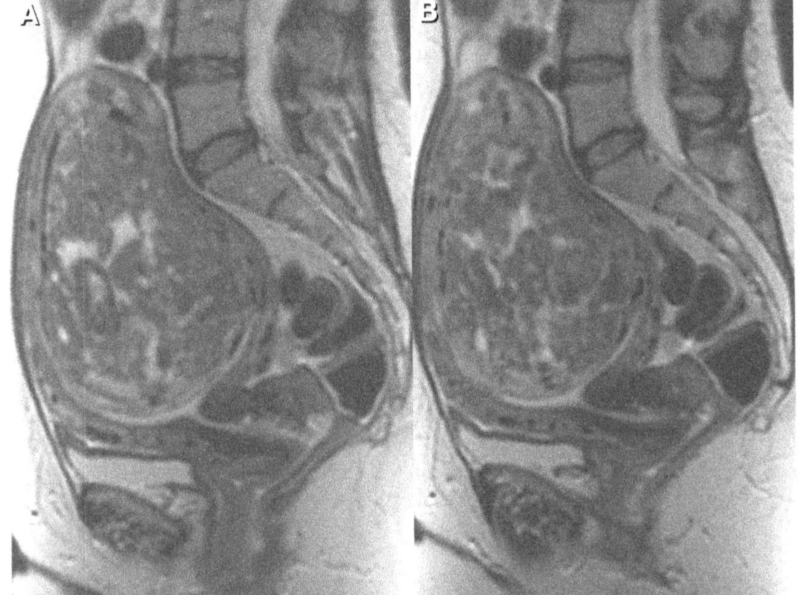

Figure 10.12.5

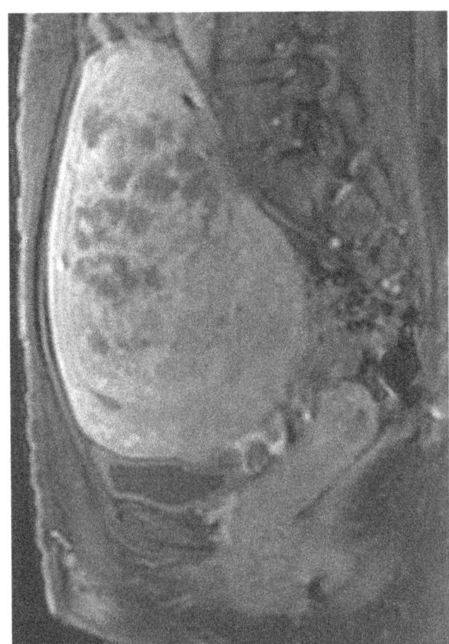
Figure 10.12.6

In a separate case of a 49-year-old woman with pelvic mass and menorrhagia, axial (Figure 10.12.4) and sagittal (Figure 10.12.5) FSE T2-weighted images show a large heterogeneous, lobulated uterine mass extending into the endometrial cavity. This mass has predominantly low T2-signal intensity, with small central foci of high signal intensity. A sagittal postgadolinium 2D SPGR image (Figure 10.12.6) shows moderate enhancement of the lesion interspersed with small cystic, nonenhancing regions.

The diagnosis was a large submucosal fibroid. This lesion has the classic appearance of a fibroid: predominantly low T2-signal intensity with interspersed regions of higher signal, likely representing foci of cystic degeneration (and showing no enhancement on postgadolinium images). The submucosal location is demonstrated by the splaying of the endometrial cavity seen on both sagittal and axial T2-weighted images.

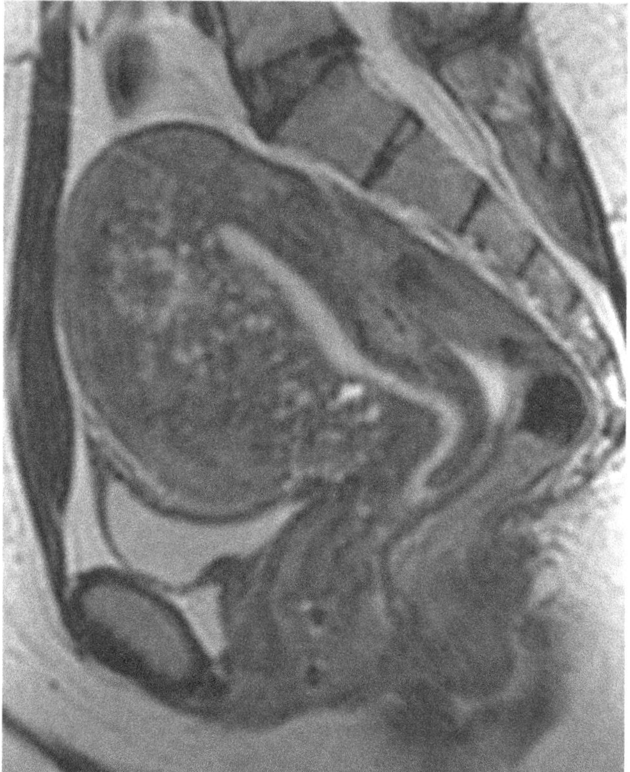

Figure 10.13.1

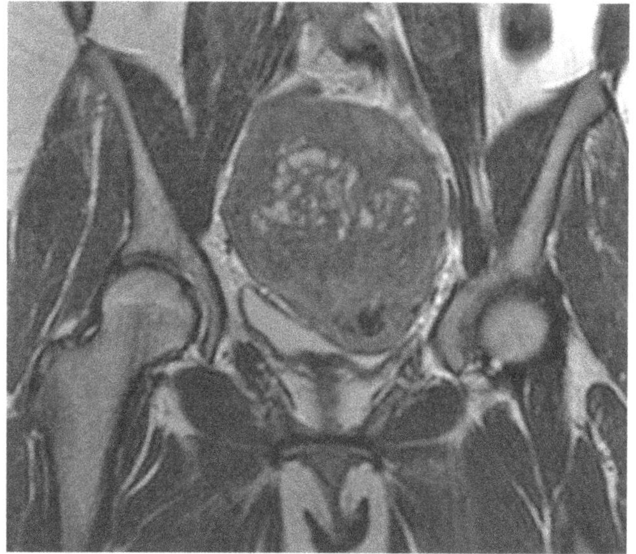

Figure 10.13.2

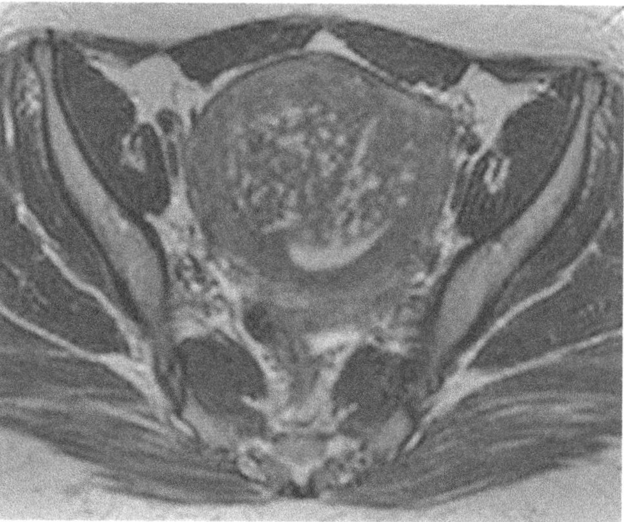

Figure 10.13.3

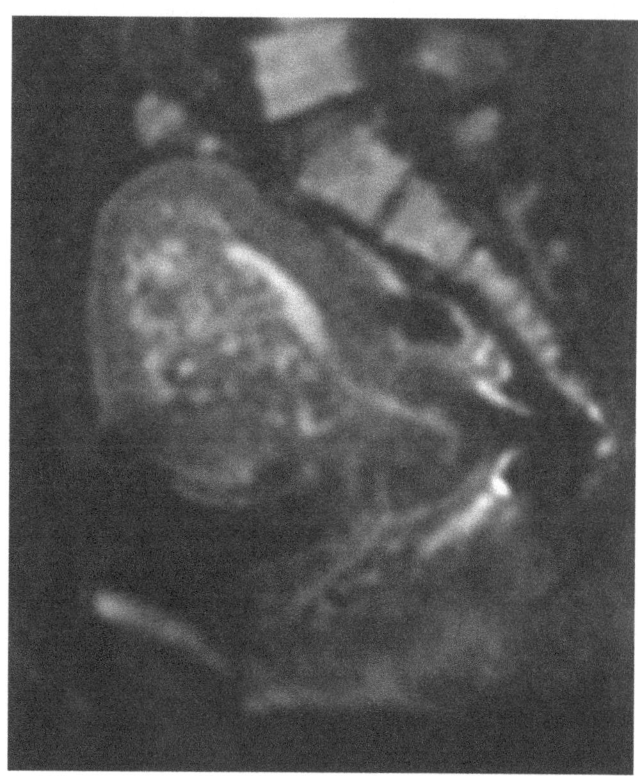

Figure 10.13.4

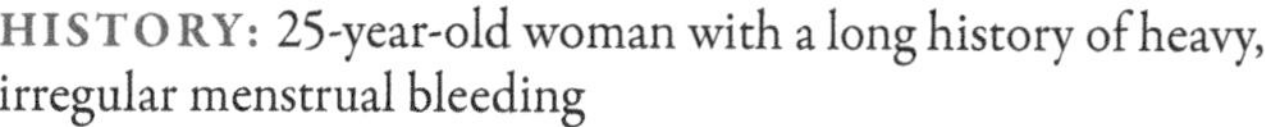

HISTORY: 25-year-old woman with a long history of heavy, irregular menstrual bleeding

IMAGING FINDINGS: Sagittal (Figure 10.13.1), coronal (Figure 10.13.2), and axial (Figure 10.13.3) oblique FSE T2-weighted images show expansion of the junctional zone in the inferior uterine body and fundus with multiple small, cystic lesions. Note also the small hypointense lesion inferiorly on the coronal image. Sagittal DWI (b=600 s/mm^2) (Figure 10.13.4) shows similar findings.

DIAGNOSIS: Adenomyosis and small leiomyoma

COMMENT: Adenomyosis is a nonneoplastic condition defined as the presence of endometrial glandular tissue within the myometrium. It typically affects premenopausal women, particularly those who are multiparous or who have had previous uterine surgery. Although many patients are completely asymptomatic, common presenting symptoms include dysmenorrhea, menorrhagia, and abnormal uterine bleeding.

There is some controversy in the pathology literature regarding the precise definition of how deeply the endometrial tissue must extend into the myometrium, and this in part has led to prevalence estimates for adenomyosis ranging from 5% to 70%. A hypertrophic reaction of the smooth muscle cells surrounding the ectopic glands is an important element of the histology and is responsible for the enlargement of the uterine junctional zone seen on MRI.

The junctional zone represents the interface between the endometrium and myometrium observed on MRI and corresponds to the innermost layer of myometrium. The myocytes of this layer actually have distinct morphologic characteristics and are arranged in concentric, rather than longitudinal, layers, and this arrangement is thought to explain its characteristic low signal intensity on T2-weighted images.

The normal junctional zone measures less than 8 mm in diameter, and a junctional zone thickness of greater than 12 mm indicates adenomyosis with an accuracy of 85%, sensitivity of 63%, and specificity of 96%. The presence of junctional zone microcysts, corresponding to ectopic endometrium surrounding small glands, is the most direct indication of adenomyosis, but these are seen in only about 50% of patients. The ectopic endometrium in adenomyosis does not typically exhibit the cyclical hormonal response seen in endometriosis. However, this cyclical pattern does occur in a relatively small percentage of patients, and therefore occasionally, hemorrhagic foci can be seen as punctate hyperintense foci on T1-weighted images.

Adenomyosis may involve the entire myometrium, resulting in a diffusely enlarged uterus, or it can present in a limited area. A more localized, masslike configuration can also occur, termed an *adenomyoma*, which can be difficult to distinguish from leiomyomas.

The differential diagnosis for adenomyosis includes normal variants (eg, the junctional zone can increase in diameter during the menstrual phase) and focal myometrial contractions, which generally should not persist during the entire examination. Adenomyomas are typically less well circumscribed than leiomyomas, and the presence of microcysts within a lesion can be diagnostic.

Adenomyosis is most commonly seen in premenopausal women; however, tamoxifen therapy for breast carcinoma is known to increase its incidence in the postmenopausal population. Adenomyosis has been linked with endometrial carcinoma and is seen in 20% of patients with endometrial cancer. The incidence of endometrial carcinoma in patients with adenomyosis is 1.4%—considerably higher than in the general population. The presence of adenomyosis may make the diagnosis of endometrial carcinoma less straightforward and occasionally can lead to difficulties in accurately staging myometrial extension.

Treatment of adenomyosis includes nonsteroidal anti-inflammatory medications and hormonal therapy. The definitive treatment is hysterectomy, reserved for severe cases that do not respond to medical therapy.

CASE 10.14

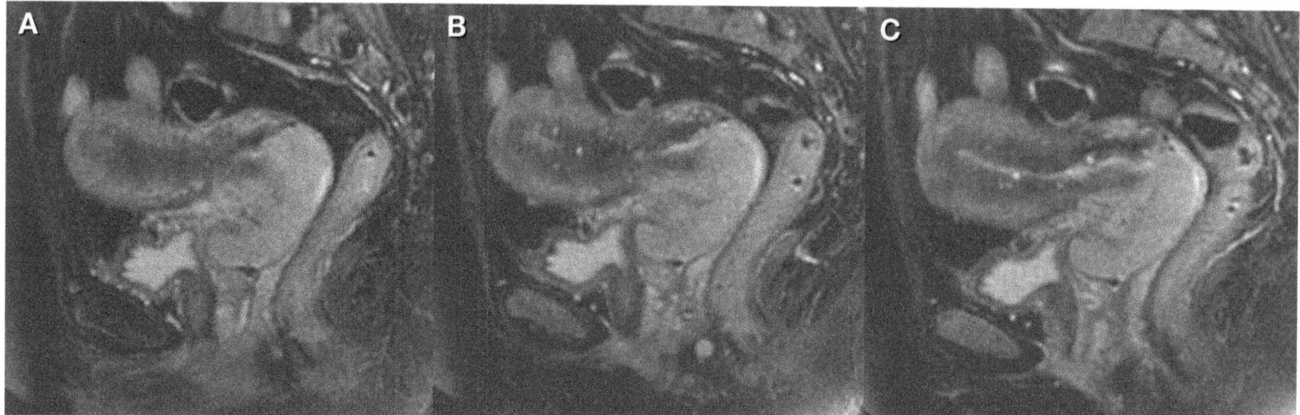

Figure 10.14.1

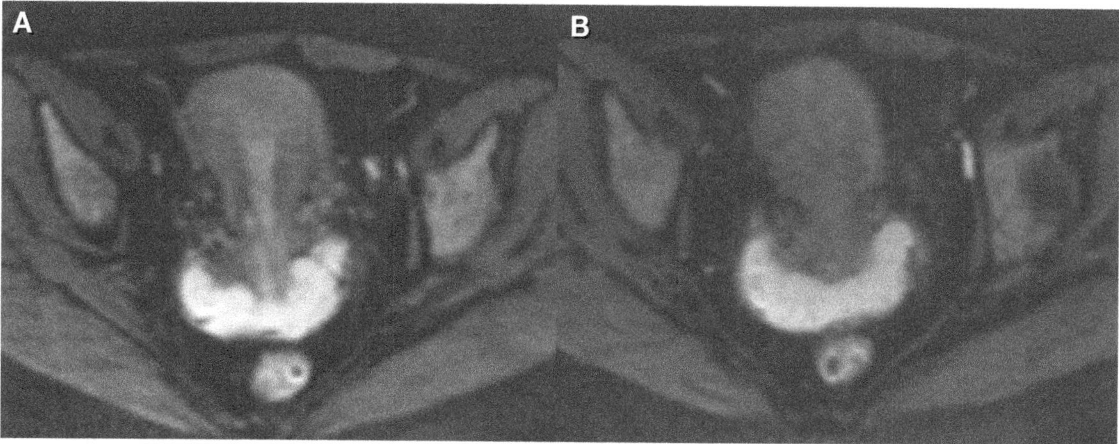

Figure 10.14.2

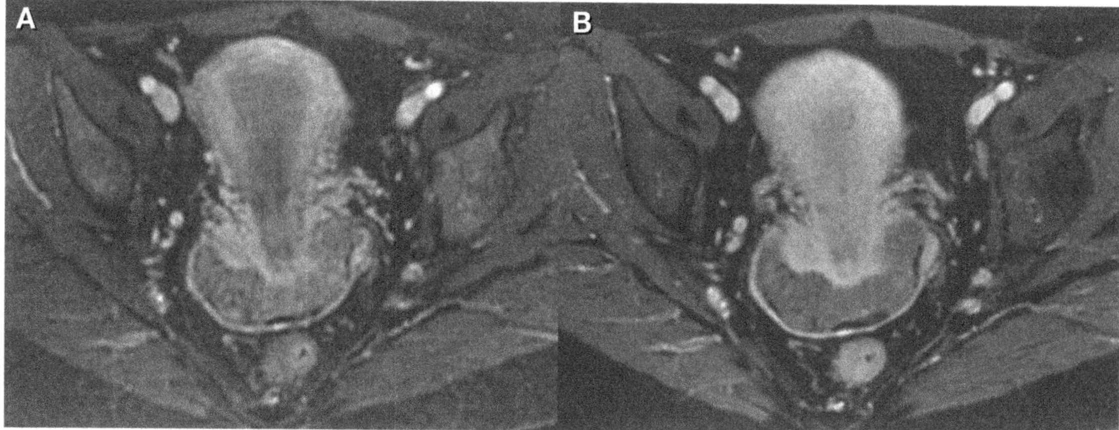

Figure 10.14.3

HISTORY: 53-year-old woman with abnormal uterine bleeding

IMAGING FINDINGS: Sagittal oblique fat-suppressed FSE T2-weighted images (Figure 10.14.1) reveal a hyperintense mass originating in the cervix and extending inferiorly into the upper vagina. Axial DWI (b=600 s/mm^2) (Figure 10.14.2) again shows the cervical mass, with marked hyperintensity. The lesion is hypointense relative to myometrium on postgadolinium axial arterial and equilibrium phase images (Figure 10.14.3). Note the thickening of the junctional zone, associated with small cystic lesions, on sagittal FSE images.

DIAGNOSIS: Cervical carcinoma and incidental adenomyosis

COMMENT: Cervical carcinoma is the third most common gynecologic malignancy, with more than 500,000 new cases diagnosed annually. Approximately 80% of new cases occur in developing countries with limited availability of screening procedures and, unfortunately, many women present with advanced, incurable disease. Cytologic screening with the Papanicolaou smear was introduced in the 1970s in British Columbia and has led to a pronounced decline in the frequency and mortality of cervical cancer in developed countries. Widespread application of vaccines against the human papillomavirus may lead to a further decline in cervical cancer incidence. Most cervical carcinomas (80%) are SCCs, with the remainder including adenocarcinoma, adenosquamous carcinoma, and undifferentiated carcinoma—all of which carry an unfavorable prognosis relative to squamous cell histology.

Cervical cancer is staged clinically according to the FIGO system, although the use of imaging is encouraged, and several studies have shown that both MRI and CT are more accurate than clinical staging.

- Stage 0 disease (carcinoma in situ) is treated with cervical conization.
- Stage I disease describes invasive carcinoma confined to the cervix.
- Stage II disease involves extrauterine extension to the upper two-thirds of the vagina (stage IIA) or the parametrium (stage IIB).
- Stage III includes extension to the pelvic sidewall or lower one-third of the vagina.
- Stage IV represents bladder or rectal invasion or distant metastases, or a combination.

Treatment of stage I-IIA lesions is generally surgical, and patients with advanced disease receive radiation and chemotherapy. Lymph node assessment is not part of the FIGO staging system (and is a limitation of MRI and CT), but nodal disease carries a worse prognosis and is present in approximately 1% to 8% of patients with stage IA disease and 16% to 18% of patients with stage IB disease (ie, clinically visible tumor).

Cervical carcinoma is generally slightly hypointense relative to normal endometrium on T2-weighted images and hyperintense to myometrium and cervical stroma. DWI can be useful in identifying the lesion, since the contrast between tumor and uterus, as seen in Figure 10.14.2, is often much greater than obtained with conventional T2-weighted images. Cervical carcinoma usually shows less enhancement than adjacent uterine tissue, and postgadolinium images can be useful in defining tumor extent.

One of the key discriminators between surgical and nonsurgical disease is the presence of parametrial extension. Many authors have emphasized the importance of obtaining transversely oriented T2-weighted images through the cervix and assessing for disruption of the low-signal-intensity cervical stroma by the tumor, an indication of parametrial extension. This sign is useful and can also be appreciated on postgadolinium images; however, its accuracy may be limited in cases such as this one, where the tumor is large and exophytic and extends into the vaginal vault but without vaginal invasion or obvious parametrial extension. This case probably would have benefited from the use of vaginal US gel, which would have helped to separate the cervical lesion from the vaginal wall and increase the level of confidence regarding the absence of vaginal invasion. This case was clinically staged as IB; however, enlarged iliac nodes were identified on MRI, and the patient received radiation therapy before hysterectomy with nodal dissection.

DWI, by virtue of its high contrast, is a useful technique for identifying all the pelvic nodes, which are so easy to miss on most other sequences. However, there is little evidence, despite numerous attempts, that measurement of nodal ADC values improves the specificity over standard size criteria for determination of tumor infiltration.

Functional imaging (parametric analysis of dynamic contrast-enhanced data and, to a lesser extent, analysis of ADC values from DWI) has been shown in a few small studies to be useful in evaluating treatment response (ie, distinguishing patients whose disease is resistant to chemoradiotherapy from the treatment responders). However, none of these techniques have seen widespread clinical application, and the actual clinical utility is uncertain.

Notice also the bonus diagnosis of adenomyosis in this case—mild, diffuse thickening of the dark transition zone (>12 mm) containing scattered small cystic lesions.

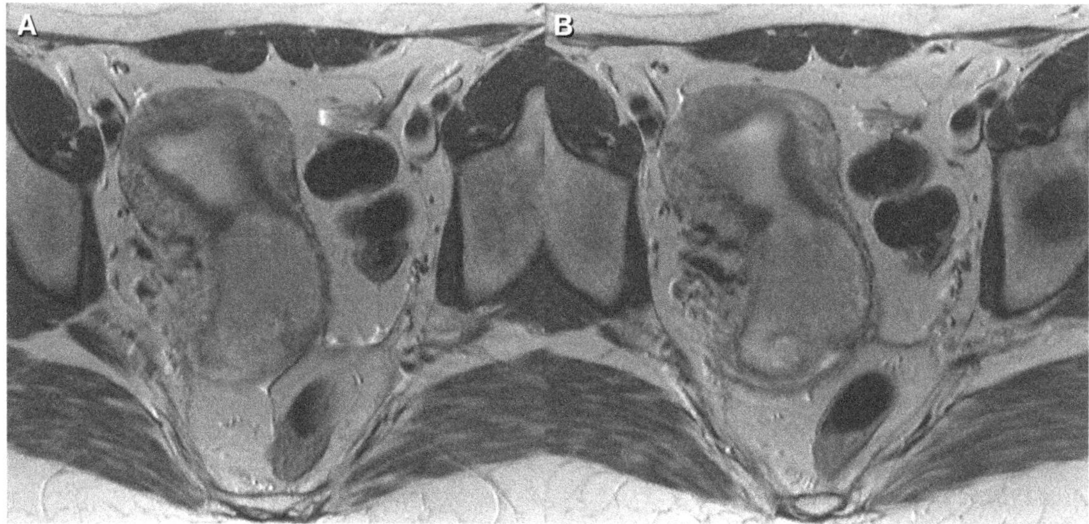

Figure 10.15.1

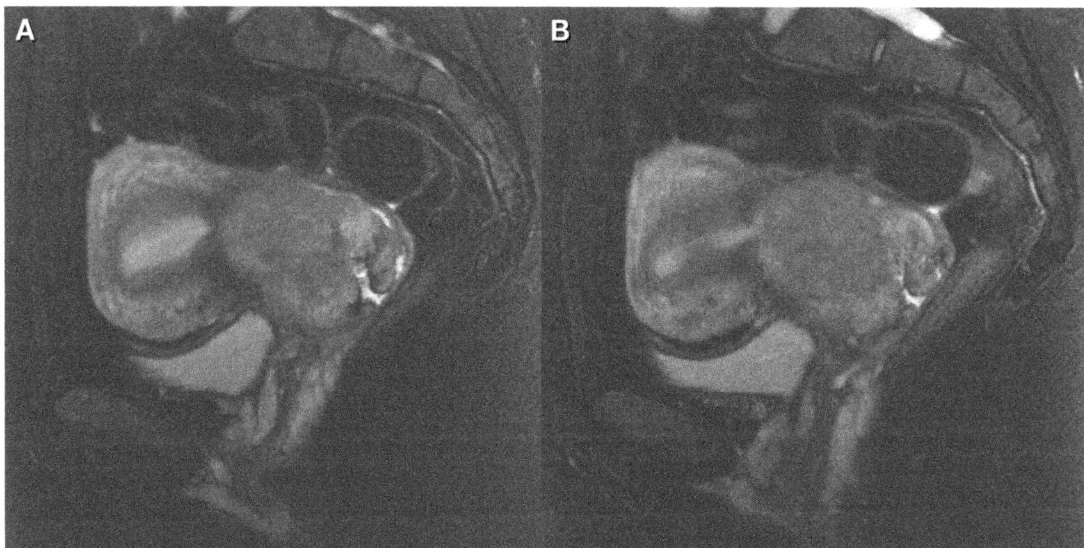

Figure 10.15.2

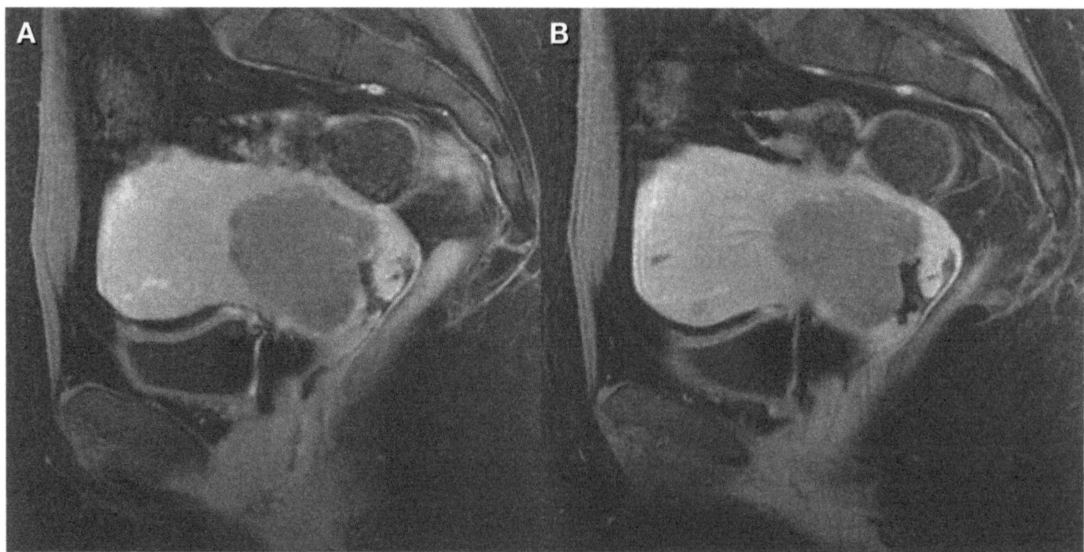

Figure 10.15.3

HISTORY: 34-year-old woman with abnormal uterine bleeding

IMAGING FINDINGS: Axial oblique FSE T2-weighted images (Figure 10.15.1) reveal a hyperintense mass originating in the cervix and extending into the lower uterine segment. Sagittal fat-suppressed FSE T2-weighted images (Figure 10.15.2) show similar findings, and postgadolinium sagittal 3D SPGR images (Figure 10.15.3) show a well-defined hypoenhancing lesion in the cervix, surrounded by a thin rim of normally enhancing tissue.

DIAGNOSIS: Cervical carcinoma (adenosquamous)

COMMENT: Approximately 20% of cervical carcinomas are of the non–squamous cell type, including adenocarcinoma, adenosquamous carcinoma, and undifferentiated carcinoma. Unlike SCC, with its incidence declining for the past few decades, the incidence of adenocarcinoma and adenosquamous carcinoma is increasing.

The influence of tumor histology on outcome for women with cervical cancer has been long debated in the literature. A recent large study involving 24,000 patients with cervical cancer and including more than 5,000 with adenocarcinoma/adenosquamous carcinoma found that women with adenocarcinoma/adenosquamous histology had reduced survival whether presenting with early stage or advanced disease.

The appearance of adenosquamous carcinoma (or adenocarcinoma) is not distinct on MRI. This case illustrates a typical cervical carcinoma—hypointense to endometrium on T2-weighted images (but hyperintense relative to myometrium) and well defined as a hypoenhancing lesion surrounded by stroma and myometrium on postgadolinium images. The intact low-signal-intensity cervical stroma, indicating a lack of parametrial extension (stage IA disease), is well seen on the axial T2-weighted images.

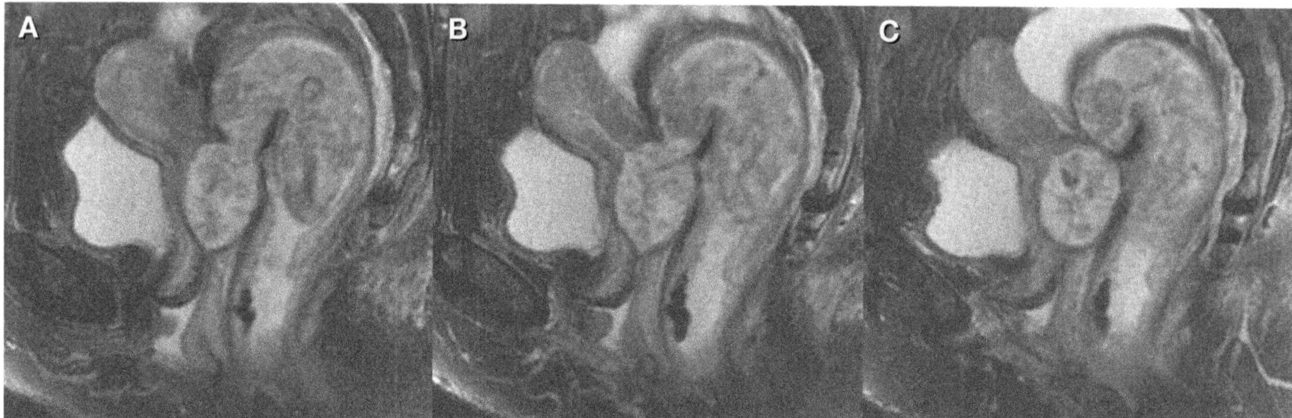

Figure 10.16.1

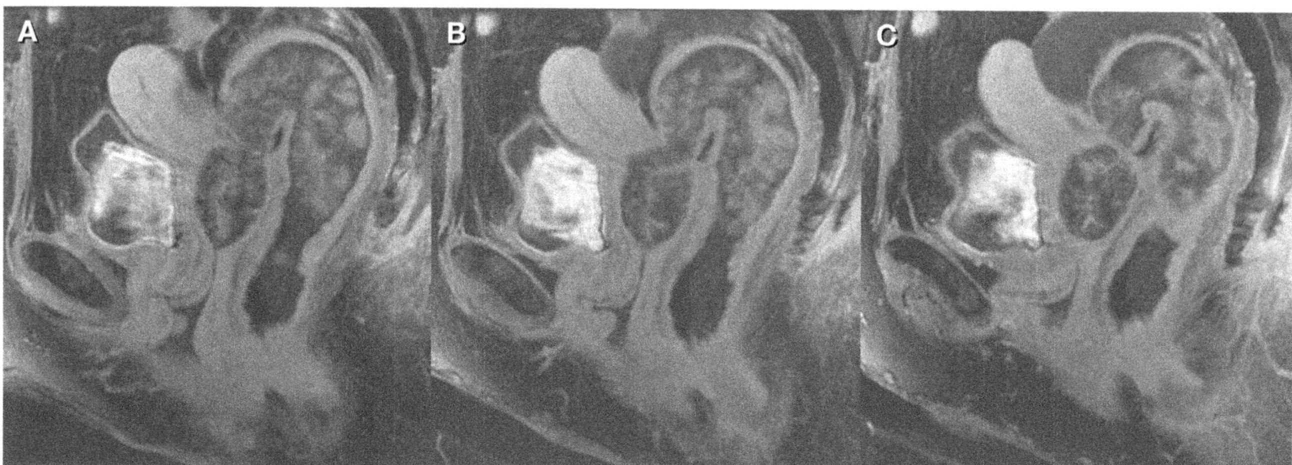

Figure 10.16.2

HISTORY: 68-year-old woman with a remote history of cervical cancer treated with cobalt therapy, now with rectal bleeding

IMAGING FINDINGS: Sagittal oblique fat-suppressed FSE T2-weighted (Figure 10.16.1) and postgadolinium 2D SPGR (Figure 10.16.2) images reveal a heterogeneous mass involving both the cervix and the rectosigmoid colon.

DIAGNOSIS: Rectal adenocarcinoma invading the cervix

COMMENT: As noted in Chapter 9, rectal and colon adenocarcinomas are sometimes aggressive and invasive, particularly the mucinous types, and this case illustrates a rectal lesion directly invading the cervix.

Cervical metastases are relatively uncommon, but most often they occur in the clinical setting of direct extension from colorectal or bladder carcinoma. Hematogenous or lymphatic metastases to the cervix are rare. It should be noted that cervical carcinoma also has a propensity for direct extension and invasion of the bladder or rectum, which is considered stage IVA disease. We have seen a few cases such as this one, where it is not entirely clear whether the primary lesion is cervical or rectal, although the distinction is to some extent a moot point since direct biopsy is relatively simple via either a vaginal or an endorectal approach.

This patient was treated by en bloc resection of the rectum, uterus, and upper vagina and has had no recurrence or metastasis in 5 years of follow-up.

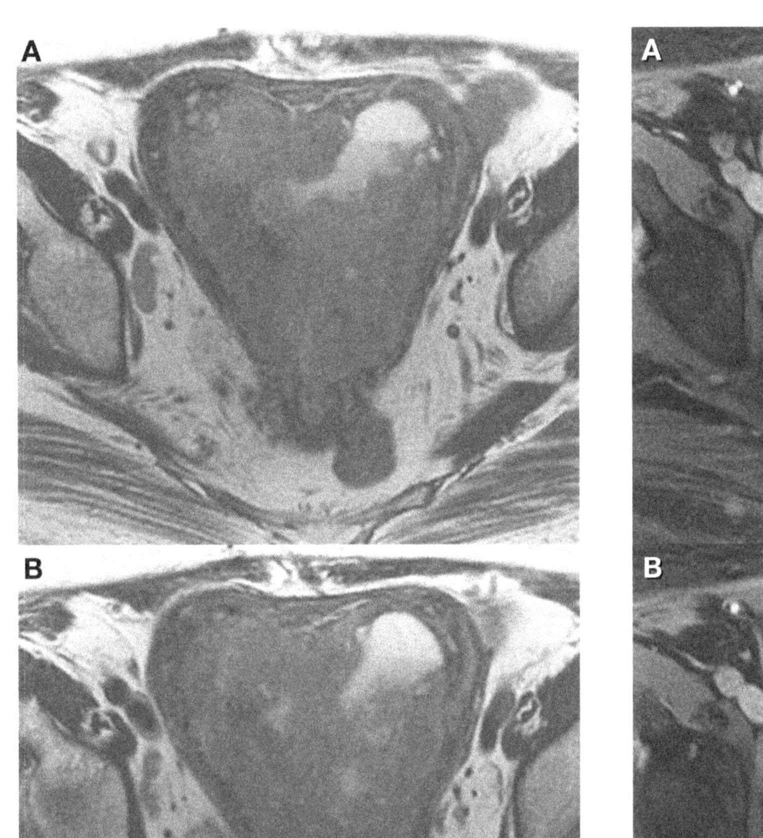

Figure 10.17.1

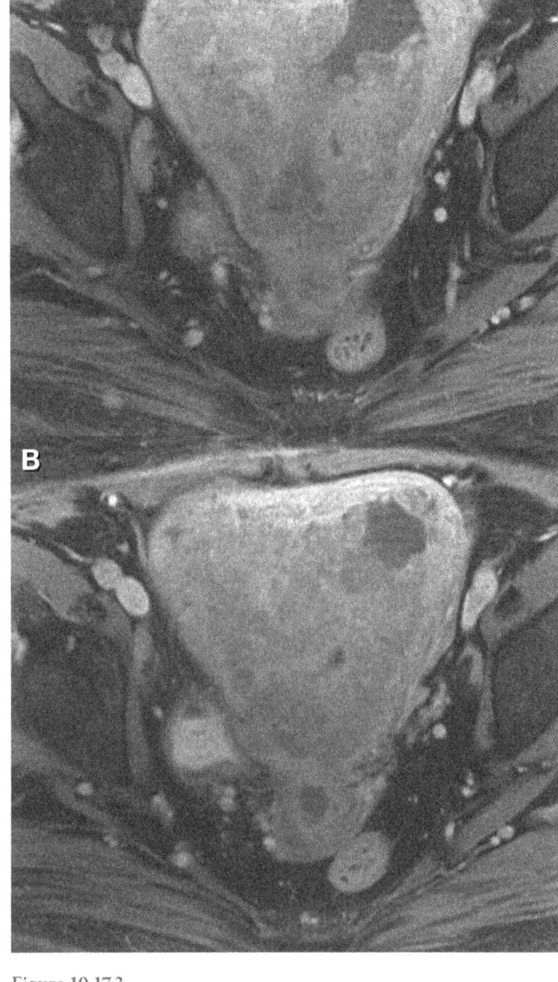

Figure 10.17.3

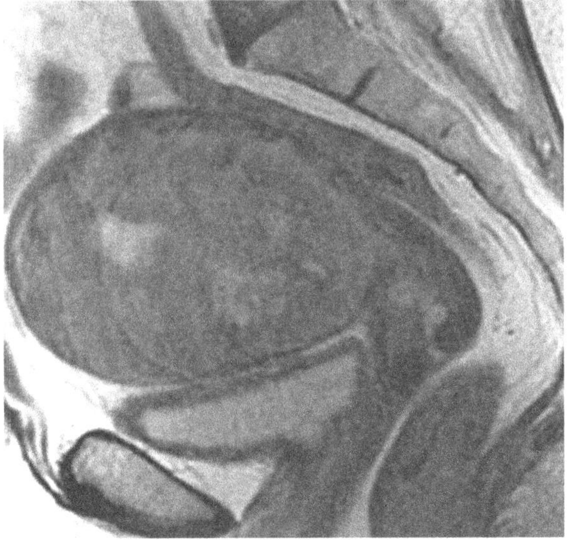

Figure 10.17.2

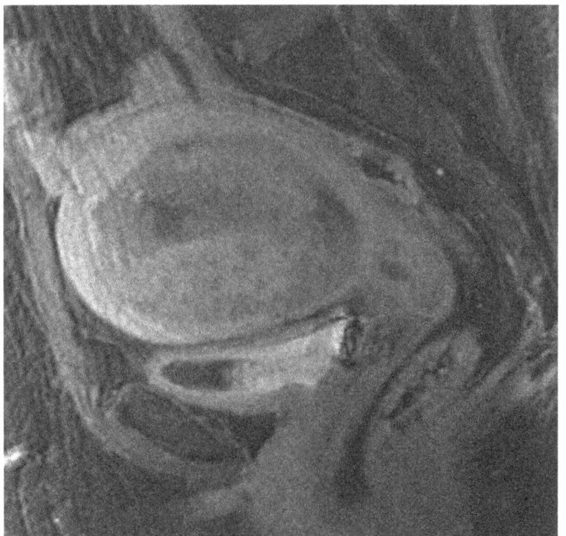

Figure 10.17.4

HISTORY: 64-year-old woman with a metastatic lesion in her right distal femur

IMAGING FINDINGS: Axial oblique (Figure 10.17.1) and sagittal oblique (Figure 10.17.2) FSE T2-weighted images and postgadolinium 2D SPGR images (Figures 10.17.3 and 10.17.4) reveal a large infiltrative mass expanding the endometrial cavity and invading the myometrium. Note also the mildly enlarged lymph node in the right pelvic sidewall.

DIAGNOSIS: Endometrial carcinoma (endometrioid)

COMMENT: Endometrial carcinoma is the most common cancer of the female genital tract, with an estimated lifetime risk of approximately 2.5%. The incidence is greatest in postmenopausal women, and associated risk factors include obesity, diabetes mellitus, nulliparity, and tamoxifen therapy. Most endometrial carcinomas (80%) are of the endometrioid type, and these carcinomas have been further subdivided into well-, moderately, and poorly differentiated grades. Additional tumor types include papillary serous, clear cell, small cell, mucinous, squamous cell, transitional cell, and undifferentiated carcinoma.

Most endometrial carcinomas are detected relatively early, presenting as vaginal bleeding in a postmenopausal woman; 75% to 80% of patients have stage I disease at diagnosis. The prognosis in this patient population is excellent, with 5-year survival rates of 85% to 90%. The primary treatment of endometrial carcinoma is surgical and may involve hysterectomy, bilateral salpingo-oophorectomy, and pelvic and para-aortic lymphadenectomy. Patients with higher-stage endometrial carcinoma also receive brachytherapy or external beam radiotherapy.

Staging of endometrial carcinoma is defined by the FIGO criteria and is based on surgery and pathology. Stage I disease is confined to the uterine body, with varying myometrial involvement; stage II has cervical extension; stage III has regional involvement of the pelvis, including uterine serosa, adnexa, peritoneum, vagina, or regional nodes; and stage IV includes bladder or bowel invasion, as well as distant metastases.

Although surgical staging remains the standard of care for endometrial carcinoma, MRI can be helpful in visualizing the primary lesion in cases where sonography is inadequate. MRI is also accurate in all aspects of staging except assessment of nodal involvement. (Use of superparamagnetic iron oxide, or SPIO, contrast agents was a promising technique for addressing that problem; however, those agents are no longer commercially available.)

Typically, endometrial carcinoma appears slightly hypointense to normal endometrium on T2-weighted images, although this is sometimes a relatively subtle distinction. Likewise, determining the extent of myometrial invasion on T2-weighted images alone can be challenging because the relative contrast between tumor and myometrium may be subtle and the normal dark junctional zone delineating endometrium and myometrium is not always visible in postmenopausal women. For this reason, postgadolinium imaging has long been included in most MRI protocols. As shown in Figures 10.17.3 and 10.17.4, endometrial carcinoma generally demonstrates less enhancement than myometrium, and often the tumor extent is better visualized on these images. (A second example of this is shown in Figure 10.17.5, in a patient with stage III disease [lymph node involvement]. This examination was performed using a dynamic postgadolinium protocol, and the images were acquired approximately 1 to 1.5 minutes after gadolinium injection. Notice the improved tumor-myometrial contrast obtained when multiple postgadolinium phases are obtained.)

This case shows a heterogeneous, bulky tumor with regions of necrosis expanding the endometrial cavity and invading the myometrium to nearly full thickness but without cervical or serosal extension. This appearance would represent stage IC disease; however, the patient unfortunately also had bone metastases at presentation.

Our standard protocol includes FSE T2-weighted images in 2 or 3 planes (oriented along the axes of the uterus) and postgadolinium images (3D SPGR) in at least 2 planes. There has been a long-standing prejudice against fat-suppressed T2-weighted images among some experts in female pelvic imaging, the reason for which has always eluded us. However, these images often show greater tumor-parenchymal contrast and have the additional benefit of less prominent phase ghosting artifact (the signal intensity of phase ghosts reflects the signal intensity of the ghost material, which is usually fat). Sometimes, serosal or parametrial extension is better seen without fat suppression, and so our protocol has at least 1 fat-suppressed and 1 non–fat-suppressed FSE T2-weighted acquisition. An antiperistaltic agent, such as glucagon, is a good idea to use when possible; if motion artifact is still problematic, it's worth remembering that respiratory-triggered acquisitions can be run in the pelvis just as easily as in the abdomen, although this does increase the acquisition time. Recently, we have also begun to use 3D FRFSE pulse sequences for these patients. The 3D acquisition means that thinner sections (1-2 mm) with correspondingly higher spatial resolution can be acquired with adequate signal to noise ratio, and this increased spatial resolution, along with the ability to obtain reformatted views in different planes, is occasionally helpful in tumor staging. DWI should be a part of any tumor identification or staging protocol in the female pelvis and should be acquired with a relatively high b value (800-1,000 s/mm^2). The contrast between tumor and endometrium-myometrium is almost always greater on DWI acquisitions than any other pulse sequence, and this technique is also excellent for identification (but not classification) of pelvic lymph nodes.

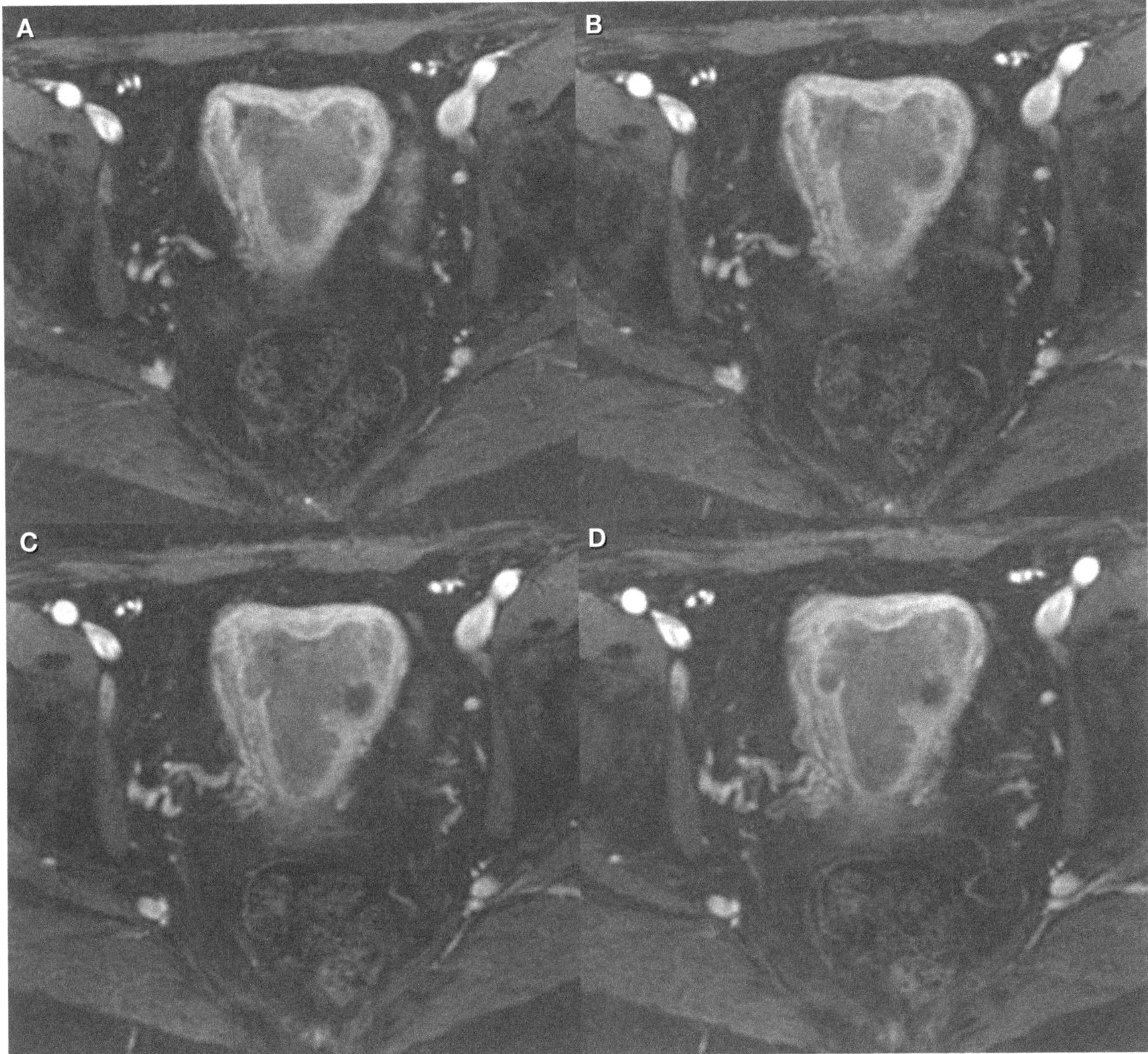

Figure 10.17.5

Axial 3D SPGR early venous phase postgadolinium images (Figure 10.17.5) demonstrate endometrial carcinoma in a 56-year-old woman. The tumor is hypointense relative to myometrium and involves nearly the entire thickness of myometrium on the left, but without serosal extension. Note the small right obturator node, which was positive for malignancy at surgery.

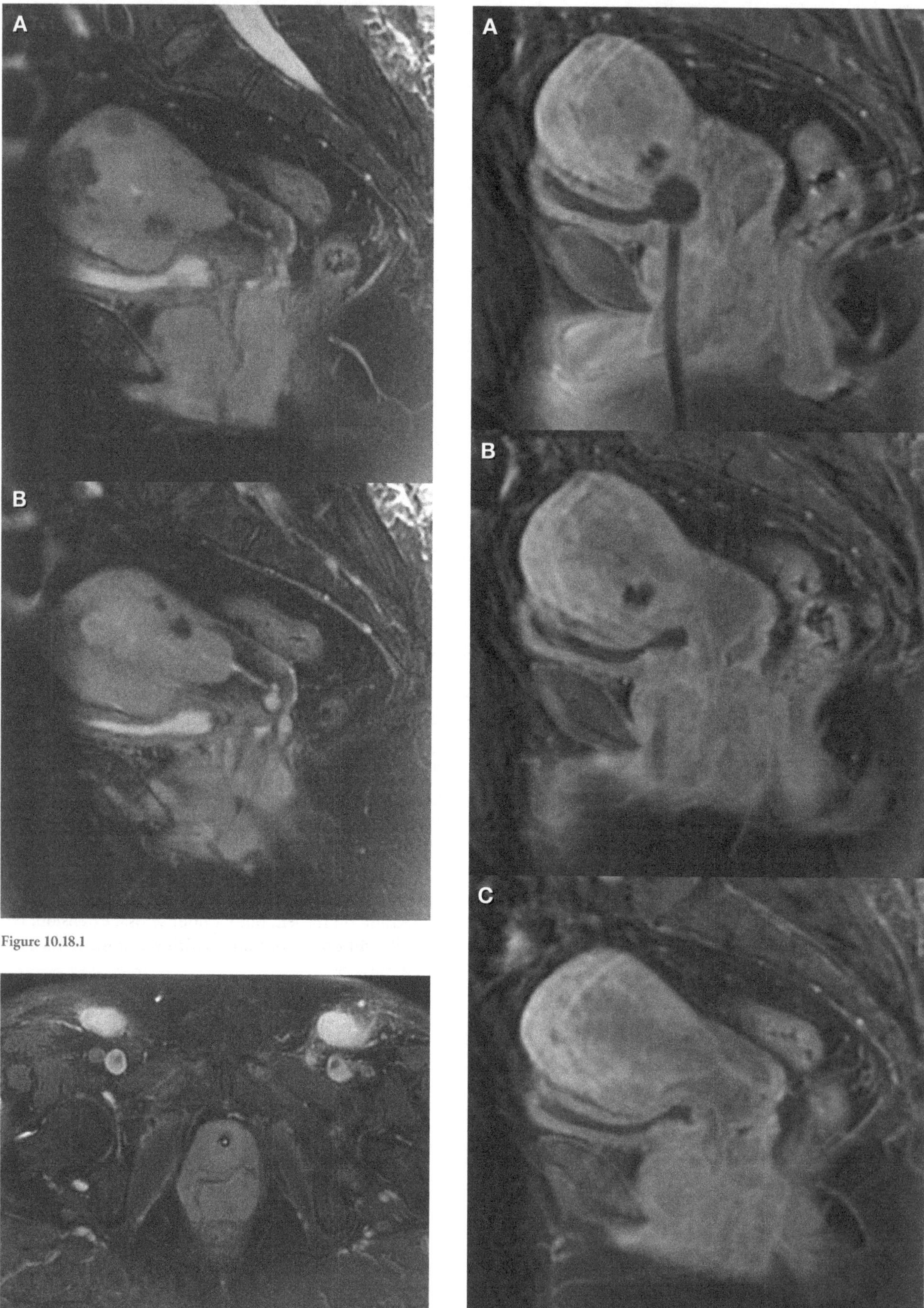

Figure 10.18.1

Figure 10.18.2

Figure 10.18.3

HISTORY: 72-year-old woman with vaginal bleeding

IMAGING FINDINGS: Sagittal fat-suppressed FSE T2-weighted images (Figure 10.18.1) demonstrate an ill-defined mass in the endometrial cavity that extends into the myometrium of the uterine fundus superiorly and protrudes into the lower uterine segment. There are multiple round, T2-hypointense fibroids within the uterine body and fundus. Notice the bulky, heterogeneously enhancing mass centered in the vagina and extending anteriorly to encase the urethra and bladder base and abutting the rectum posteriorly. Axial FSE T2-weighted image through the inferior pelvis (Figure 10.18.2) again shows an infiltrative mass involving the vagina and urethra, as well as large bilateral inguinal lymph nodes. Sagittal postgadolinium 2D SPGR images (Figure 10.18.3) again demonstrate the ill-defined uterine mass and the heterogeneously enhancing mass surrounding the vagina and urethra.

DIAGNOSIS: Endometrial carcinoma with vaginal and urethral involvement

COMMENT: This case is an example of stage IV disease with invasion of the bladder, urethra, and, possibly, the rectum, as well as inguinal nodal involvement. It also illustrates the value of using MRI to document the presence of advanced disease, suspected on clinical examination, and to thereby avoid surgery.

Notice the poor definition of the endometrial lesion on both FSE T2-weighted and postgadolinium 2D SPGR images. This case was performed several years ago, before DWI was routinely used in body MRI, and clearly would have benefited from DWI, which would have helped to define the uterine and extrauterine extent of the neoplasm. The postcontrast images were obtained a few minutes after hand injection of gadolinium and are adequate to demonstrate the extensive tumor involving the vagina and urethra; however, they probably would have been improved by using a power injector and a dynamic acquisition protocol.

Our dynamic protocol generally consists of 3 or more phases acquired at 30 seconds, 60 seconds, and 2 minutes after gadolinium injection, in an imaging plane tailored to the individual case. When the arterial phase images are more important (when imaging a hypervascular tumor, for example), a test bolus or fluoroscopic triggering can be used to optimize the timing of the arterial phase acquisition.

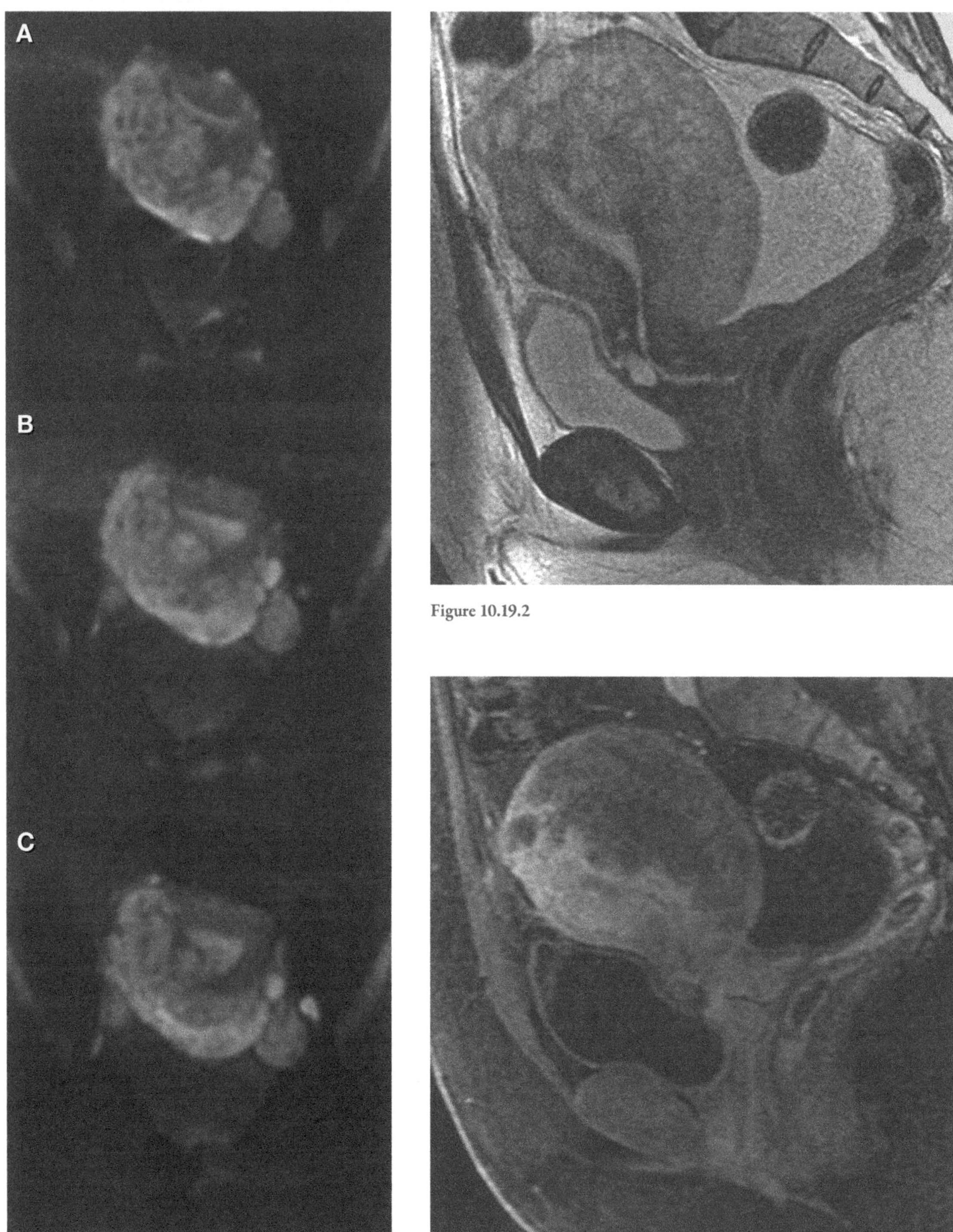

Figure 10.19.2

Figure 10.19.1

Figure 10.19.3

HISTORY: 38-year-old woman with a 2-week history of pelvic pain

IMAGING FINDINGS: Axial diffusion-weighted images (b=800 s/mm^2) (Figure 10.19.1) reveal an infiltrative mass centered in the posterior and right lateral myometrium with heterogeneous increased signal intensity. Sagittal oblique FSE image (Figure 10.19.2) again demonstrates the infiltrative mass along the posterior margin of the uterus. Sagittal postgadolinium 3D SPGR image (Figure 10.19.3) shows hypoenhancement of the mass relative to the myometrium.

DIAGNOSIS: Endometrial stromal sarcoma

COMMENT: Uterine sarcomas represent approximately 5% of uterine cancers and have an incidence of 17 per

1 million persons. Carcinosarcoma is the most common sarcoma (although recent evidence suggests that carcinosarcomas probably are best regarded as metaplastic carcinomas), followed in frequency by leiomyosarcoma and ESS. In general, the prognosis of uterine sarcoma is worse than endometrial carcinoma, and its clinical behavior tends to be more aggressive.

ESS is classified into low-grade ESS and undifferentiated endometrial sarcoma. Low-grade ESS is composed of cells reminiscent of endometrial stromal cells in proliferative phase that invade the myometrium and, often, the intramyometrial or parametrial vessels. Frequently, little cytologic atypia or pleomorphism is seen, and mitoses are scant. By comparison, undifferentiated endometrial sarcoma is a high-grade tumor lacking specific differentiation and any features of normal endometrial stroma.

Tumors are characterized histologically by hemorrhage and necrosis, frequent myometrial invasion, and marked nuclear pleomorphism and high mitotic activity. A high percentage of ESS cases have a chromosomal translocation resulting in the juxtaposition of 2 zinc finger genes. This translocation is also fairly common in endometrial stromal nodule (Case 10.21), implying that this lesion may progress to ESS. In contrast, it is less frequently observed in undifferentiated endometrial sarcoma, suggesting that this disease may not always result from malignant progression of ESS.

Low-grade ESS typically occurs in women aged 40 to 55 years, a slightly younger age-group than those presenting with other uterine sarcomas. The most common presenting symptoms include abnormal vaginal bleeding and pelvic or abdominal pain, although as many as 25% of women are asymptomatic at diagnosis.

ESS is difficult to differentiate from other uterine sarcomas at imaging, and the typical appearance is that of an infiltrative myometrial or endometrial mass with heterogeneous signal intensity on T2-weighted images, high signal intensity on DWI, and hypoenhancement after gadolinium administration. Uterine sarcomas tend to have a more heterogeneous appearance than endometrial carcinomas, but this distinction is often difficult to make with MRI.

DWI is in general a good idea when imaging any uterine mass—nearly all lesions have high signal intensity with high contrast against the background of normal myometrium and endometrium. Several early papers suggested that ADC measurements could reliably distinguish benign from malignant lesions. However, larger studies have not replicated those results, and there likely is considerable overlap between the ADC values of various lesions. The usual problem is distinguishing an atypical fibroid from a sarcoma, as illustrated in Case 10.20.

Among uterine sarcomas, ESS has a favorable prognosis. Patient outcome depends largely on the extent of the tumor at diagnosis. The 5-year survival for women with stage I and stage II tumors (confined to the uterus or within the pelvis) is 89% vs 50% for those with stage III and stage IV tumors (nodal or abdominal extension or distant metastases). Compared to ESS, undifferentiated endometrial sarcoma has a poor prognosis, and most women die within 2 years of diagnosis. Treatment of ESS is largely surgical, consisting of hysterectomy and bilateral salpingo-oophorectomy, which may be followed by radiation therapy or hormonal therapy, or both.

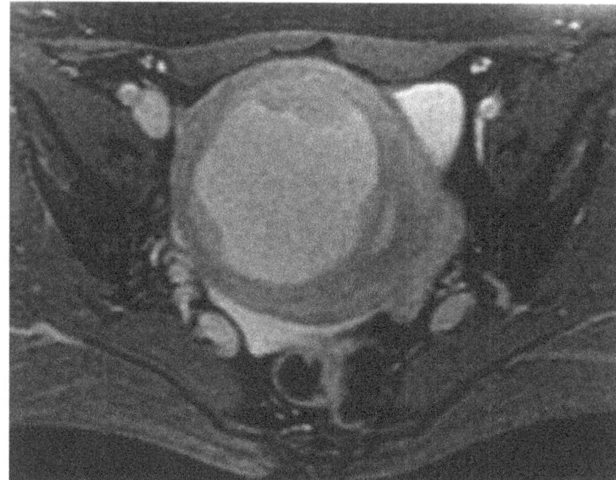

Figure 10.20.1

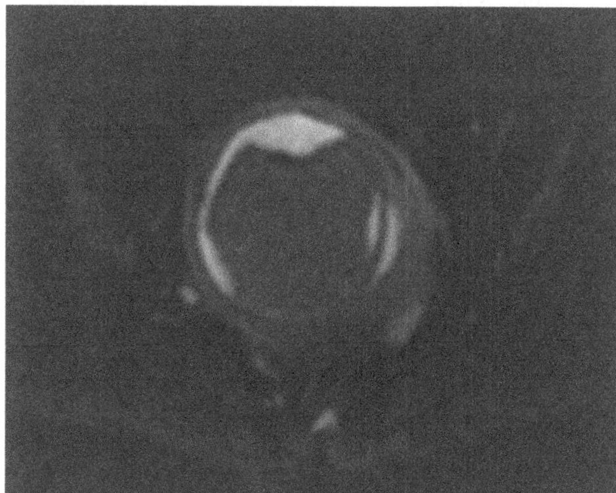

Figure 10.20.2

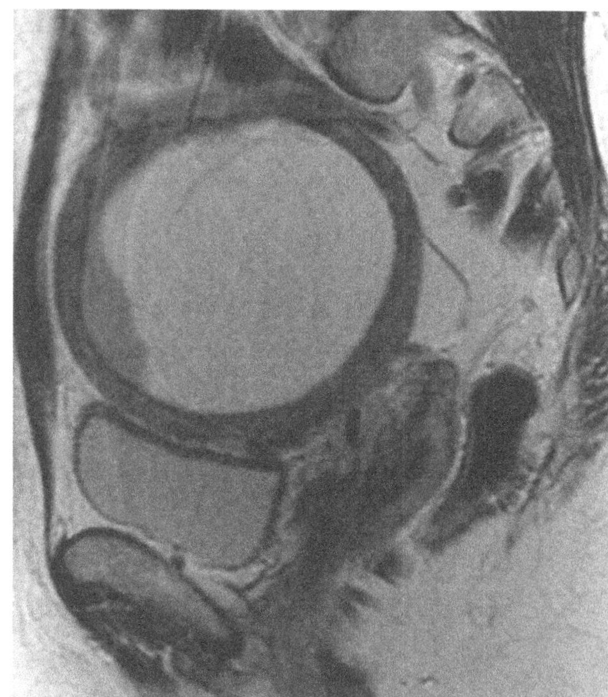

Figure 10.20.3

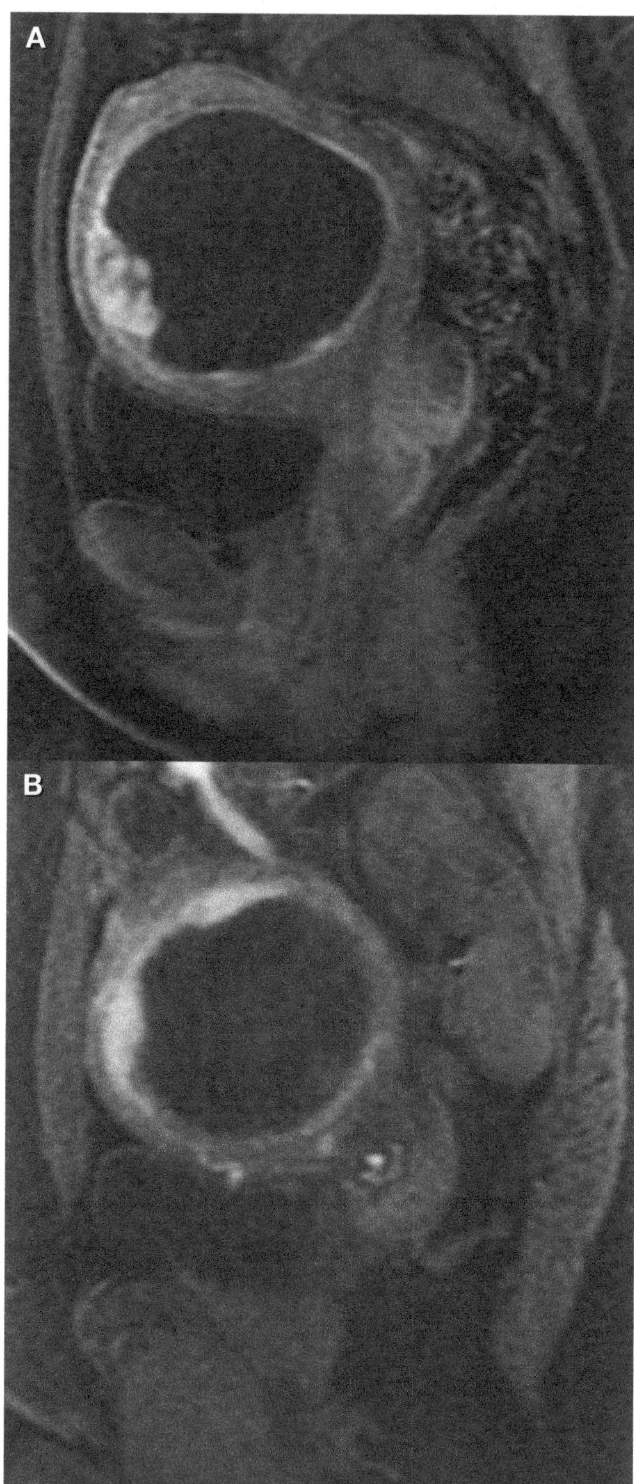

Figure 10.20.4

HISTORY: 43-year-old woman with a uterine mass

IMAGING FINDINGS: Axial fat-suppressed SSFP image (Figure 10.20.1) reveals a large, predominantly cystic mass in the uterine fundus that contains peripheral nodular soft tissue components. The soft tissue rim has high signal intensity on axial DWI (b=800 s/mm^2) (Figure 10.20.2). A sagittal T2-weighted FSE image (Figure 10.20.3) demonstrates similar findings. Arterial phase sagittal postgadolinium 3D SPGR images (Figure 10.20.4) show intense enhancement of the soft tissue component.

DIAGNOSIS: Endometrial stromal sarcoma

COMMENT: This patient was referred to MRI as a potential candidate for focused US ablation or uterine artery embolization of a known uterine fibroid. This case illustrates the difficulty in distinguishing well-defined sarcomas from degenerating leiomyomas. Of all women undergoing hysterectomy for a preoperative diagnosis of fibroids, approximately 0.5% are found to have a uterine sarcoma at surgery.

Cystic degeneration of leiomyomas is a well-known, albeit slightly uncommon, presentation; however, the presence of mural nodules with intense arterial phase enhancement is unusual, as is the very high signal intensity of the nodules on DWI. The presence of restricted diffusion (and low ADC value, although we didn't actually measure it) has been suggested as a diagnostic criterion for distinguishing uterine sarcomas from benign lesions. Nevertheless, the most likely diagnosis for a lesion with a similar appearance probably remains an atypical degenerating fibroid. We suggested the possibility of an unusual lesion, and the patient had a hysterectomy and received a subsequent diagnosis of ESS.

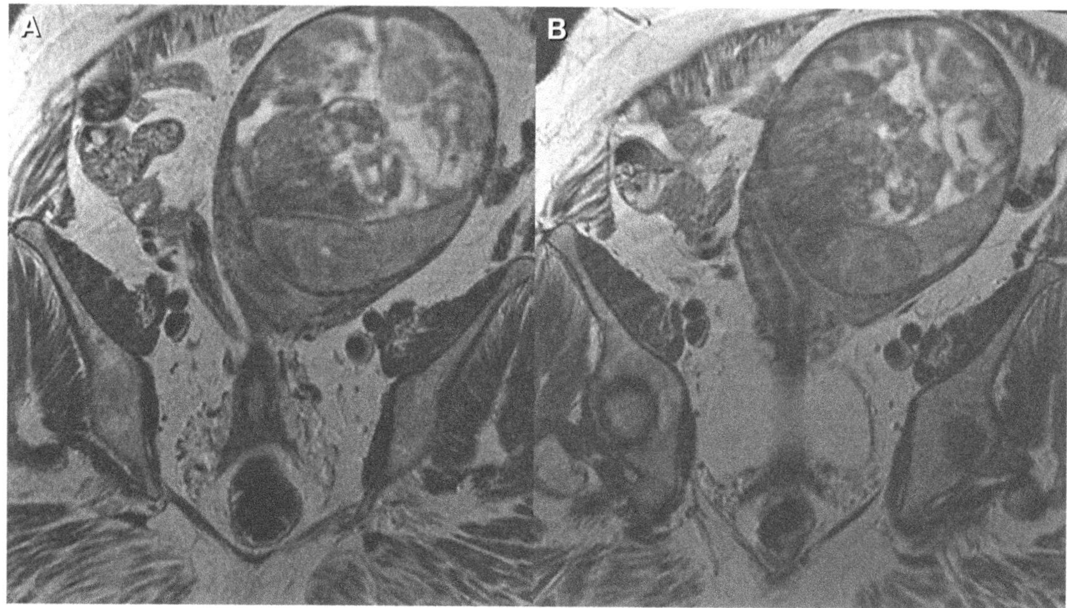

Figure 10.21.1

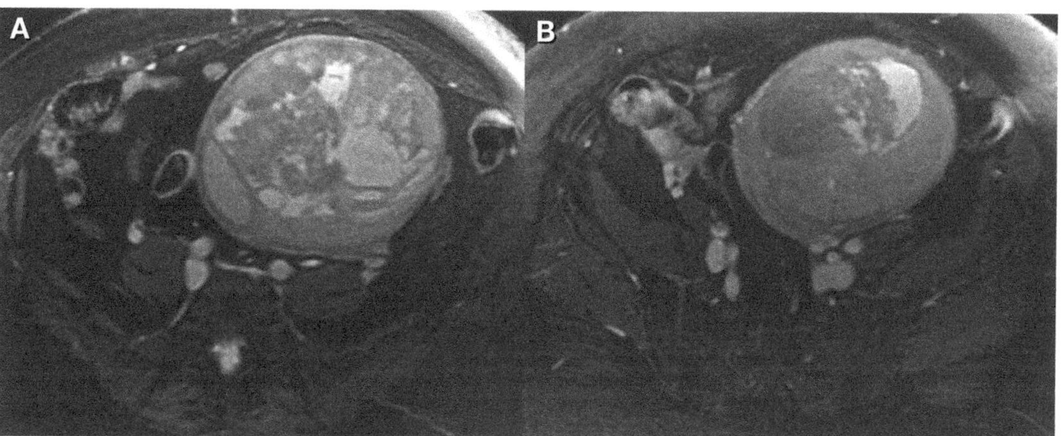

Figure 10.21.2

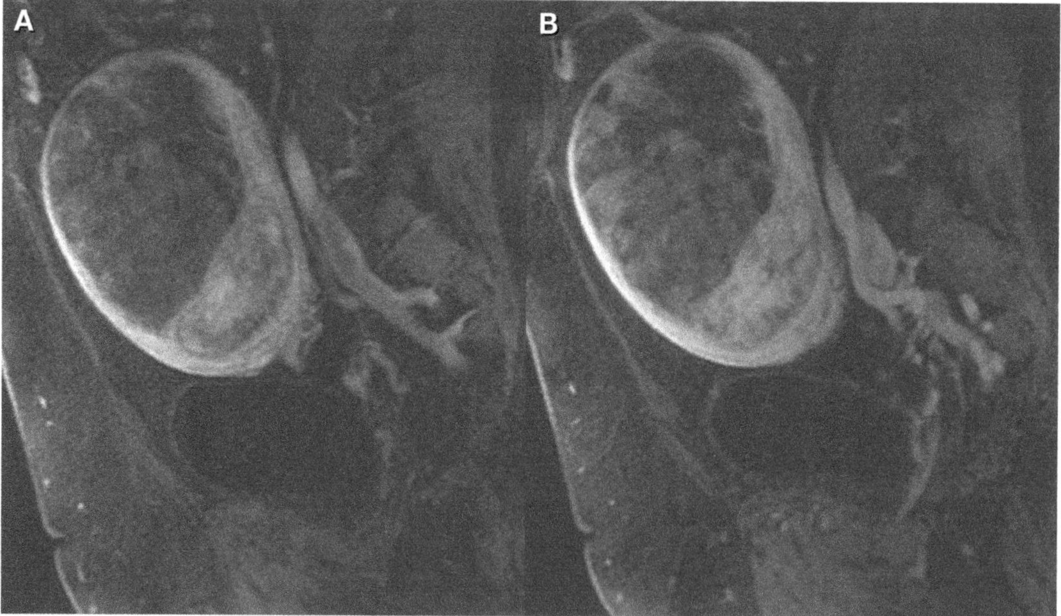

Figure 10.21.3

HISTORY: 48-year-old woman with an abdominal mass noted on physical examination

IMAGING FINDINGS: Coronal oblique FSE T2-weighted images (Figure 10.21.1), axial fat-suppressed SSFP images (Figure 10.21.2), and postgadolinium sagittal 3D SPGR images (Figure 10.21.3) demonstrate a large, complex mass arising from the uterine fundus. The mass has both cystic and solid components and shows heterogeneous enhancement after gadolinium administration.

DIAGNOSIS: Endometrial stromal nodule

COMMENT: ESN falls into the category of endometrial mesenchymal tumors, which also includes ESS and undifferentiated endometrial sarcoma and accounts for approximately 25% of these lesions. ESN is a benign tumor generally presenting as a well-defined lesion composed of cells that resemble proliferative phase stromal cells. It most commonly occurs in perimenopausal or postmenopausal women, who may be asymptomatic or present with vaginal bleeding or pelvic pain.

The molecular pathology of ESN includes a high incidence of a balanced chromosomal translocation resulting in a juxtaposition of 2 zinc finger genes, as noted in Case 10.19. This same translocation is seen in ESS and suggests the possibility that ESN can degenerate into ESS.

Distinction between ESN and ESS can be extremely difficult in a curettage specimen unless the margins can be fully evaluated. The distinction between ESN, ESS, and cellular leiomyomas is also problematic without examination of the entire tumor.

Since these lesions are generally well-defined masses, the differential diagnosis often involves complex or atypical fibroids and, in fact, that was the diagnosis suggested in this case. The complexity of the lesion is greater than typically seen in a fibroid and might indicate the possibility of a sarcoma, but in practice an unusual presentation of a degenerating fibroid is much more commonly encountered than an ESN.

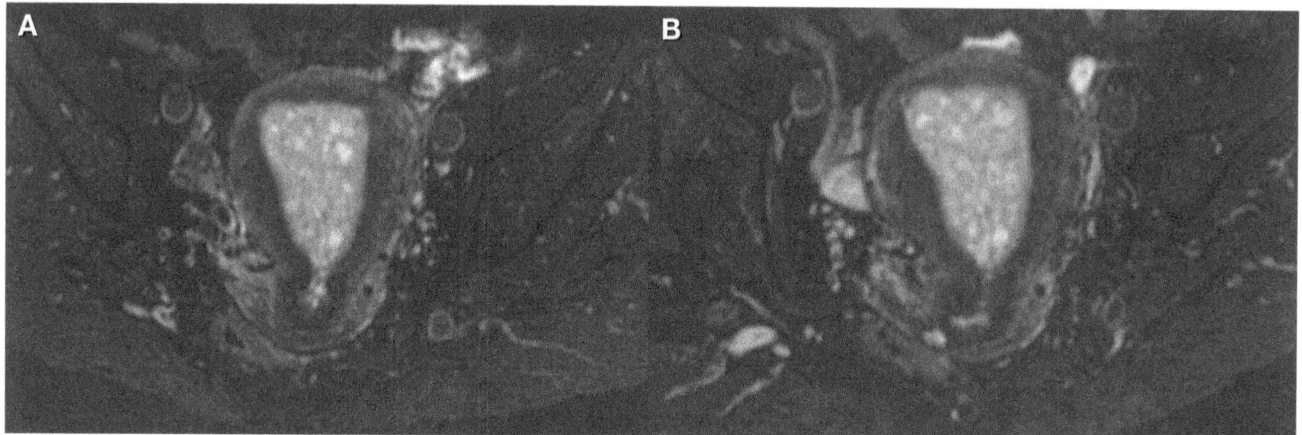

Figure 10.22.1

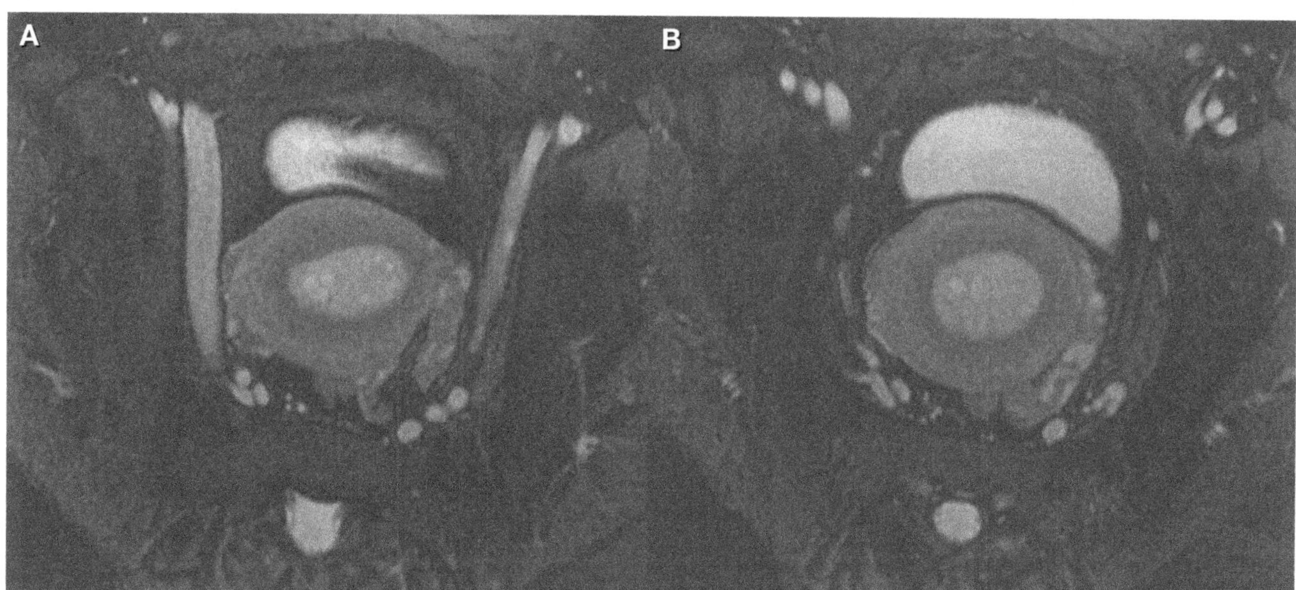

Figure 10.22.2

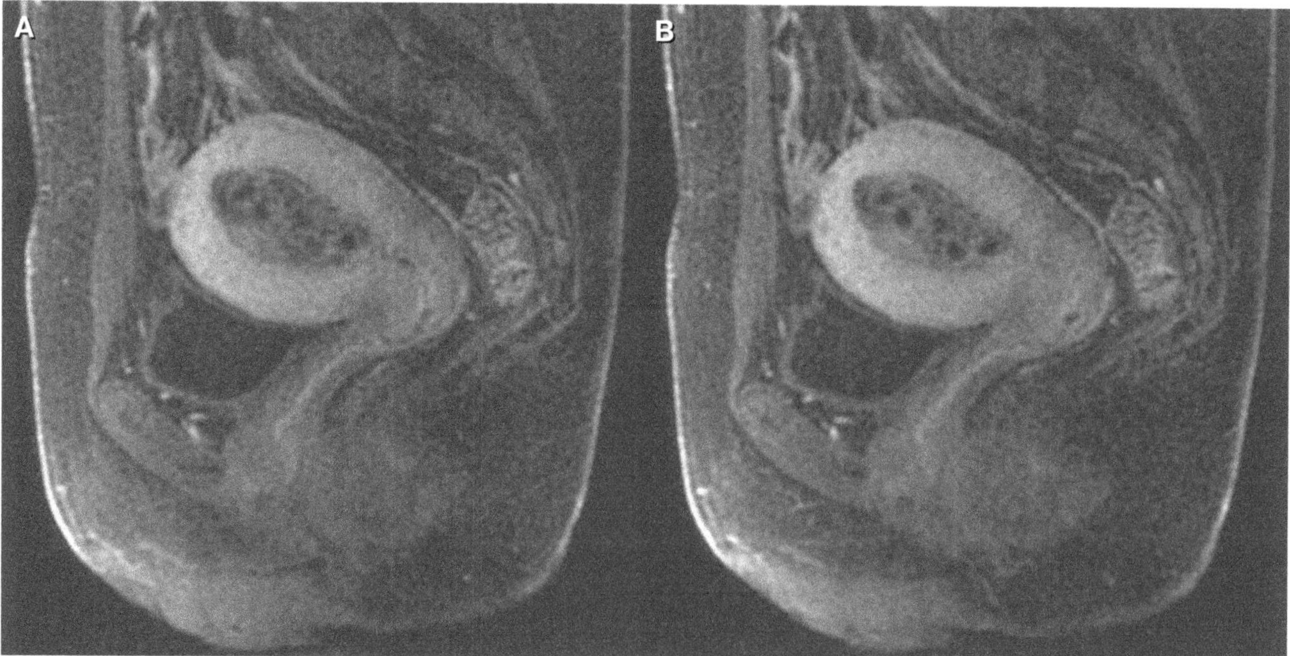

Figure 10.22.3

HISTORY: 58-year-old postmenopausal woman with abnormal uterine bleeding

IMAGING FINDINGS: Axial oblique fat-suppressed 3D FRFSE T2-weighted images (Figure 10.22.1) reveal diffuse irregular thickening of the endometrial cavity with multiple small cystic lesions. Similar complex cystic expansion of the endometrium is also seen on coronal oblique fat-suppressed SSFP images (Figure 10.22.2). Postgadolinium sagittal 3D SPGR images (Figure 10.22.3) show heterogeneous enhancement of the endometrial lesions.

DIAGNOSIS: Müllerian adenosarcoma

COMMENT: Uterine sarcomas represent 1% to 3% of gynecologic cancers, of which müllerian adenosarcoma is one of the more uncommon examples, accounting for 8% of the total. Adenosarcomas arise most often within the endometrium (83% of cases) but also can originate from the cervix or myometrium and rarely from the fallopian tubes or ovaries.

Müllerian adenosarcoma is a mixed epithelial-mesenchymal tumor, a pathologic category that includes adenofibroma and carcinosarcoma. Adenosarcoma is in the middle of the spectrum and contains benign glandular epithelial elements and malignant mesenchymal elements. Adenofibromas have benign epithelial and benign mesenchymal elements; carcinosarcomas contain malignant epithelial and mesenchymal stroma.

Adenosarcoma typically affects postmenopausal women who present with uterine bleeding, and an association with tamoxifen therapy has been suggested. One-third of adenosarcoma patients are premenopausal, however. The clinical scenario described most frequently in case reports is a polypoid mass expanding the endometrial cavity and protruding through the cervical os on physical examination. This case contains imaging features similar to many of the lesions reported in the literature, including a multicystic appearance with high T2-signal intensity. Larger lesions may become more heterogeneous, and extension into the cervix or the myometrium may be seen. The multicystic nature of the lesion was best appreciated on a high-resolution 3D FRFSE acquisition, which allowed a section thickness of 2 mm.

Adenosarcomas are frequently misdiagnosed initially at pathology as adenofibromas or polyps because of the heterogeneous nature of the lesions and the low-grade histology of the sarcomatous stroma. The prognosis is intermediate between adenofibroma (excellent) and carcinosarcoma (poor), with recurrence after hysterectomy occurring in 20% to 30% of patients. Recurrences and metastases are often composed solely of sarcomatous elements, usually of higher grade than the initial lesion.

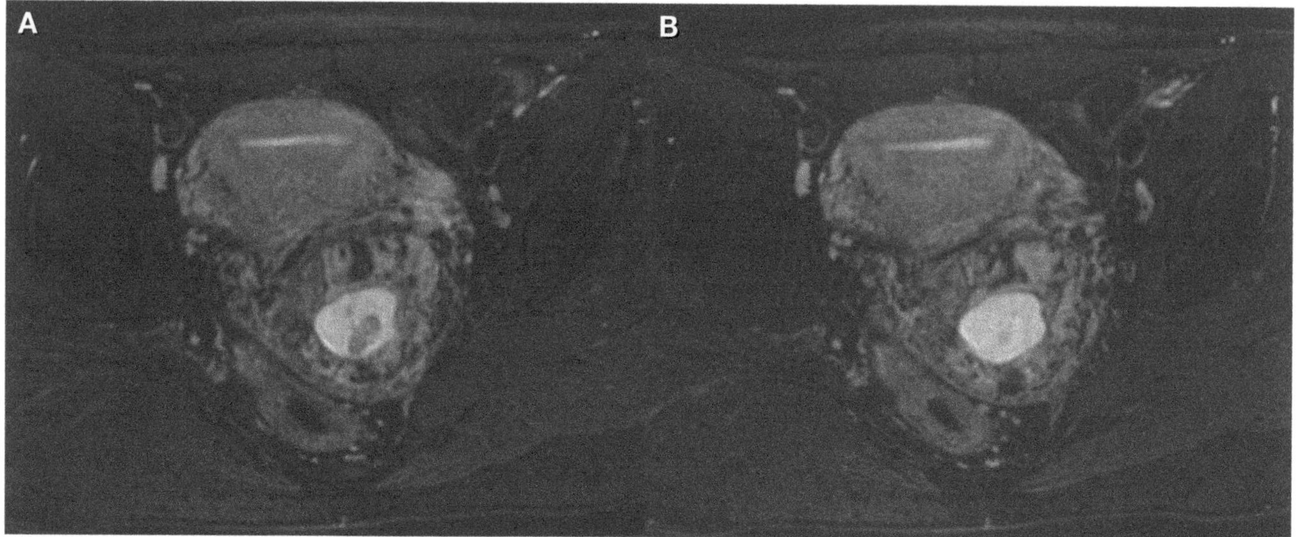

Figure 10.23.1

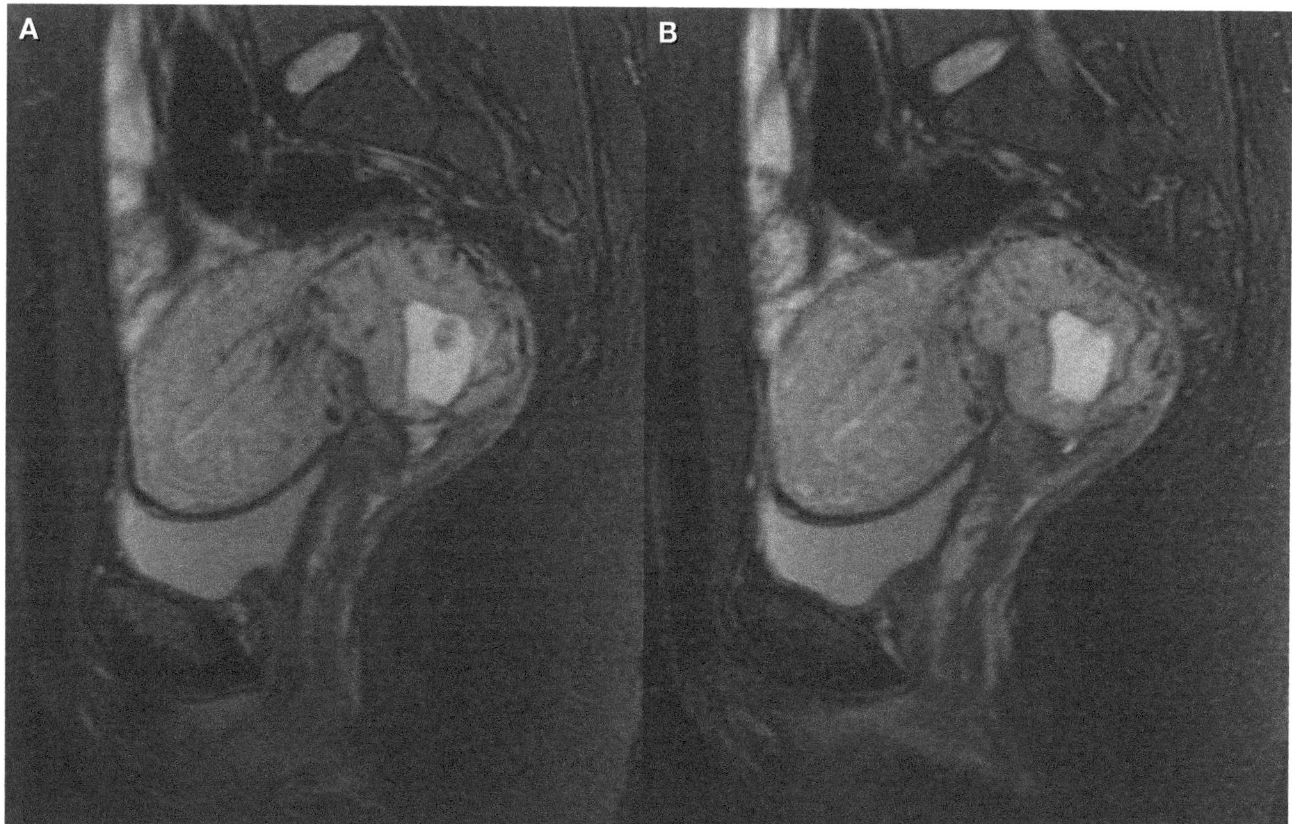

Figure 10.23.2

HISTORY: 24-year-old pregnant woman with recent uterine bleeding

IMAGING FINDINGS: Axial oblique 3D FRFSE (Figure 10.23.1) and sagittal oblique 2D FSE (Figure 10.23.2) images show a complex mass along the margin of the cervix with a central cystic region containing a small soft tissue structure.

DIAGNOSIS: Cervical ectopic pregnancy

COMMENT: Ectopic pregnancy is a leading cause of maternal mortality in the first trimester and accounts for more than 70% of all deaths. The vast majority (95%) of ectopic pregnancies occur in the fallopian tubes. Nontubal ectopic pregnancies, although uncommon, have much higher morbidity and mortality rates. The incidence of nontubal ectopic pregnancy is rising, and this is thought to result from increasing rates of uterine surgery (primarily cesarean sections) with associated damage to the endometrium and cervix, as well as the increasing use of assisted reproductive technologies.

Cervical ectopic pregnancies account for less than 1% of all ectopic pregnancies, with an estimated incidence ranging from 1 in 1,000 to 1 in 95,000 pregnancies, and are defined as pregnancy implanted into the cervical mucosa below the level of the internal os. Although the traditional treatment of cervical ectopic pregnancy was once surgical, the associated morbidity and mortality were high and conservative management is now preferred, most commonly through systemic or local injection of methotrexate.

Conservative techniques are most successful when the cervical ectopic pregnancy is detected early; most case series have reported successful outcomes in more than 95% of cases. Advanced pregnancies, however, often require multiple treatments and have a higher incidence of complications—most commonly, hemorrhage.

MRI is obviously not a first-line examination for suspected ectopic pregnancy, but it is occasionally useful for confirming the diagnosis in cases where sonography is indeterminate—that was the indication in this case, and the MRI showed a well-vascularized gestational sac arising from the region of the cervix and containing a fetal pole. This patient was treated with systemic methotrexate, as well as direct injection of potassium chloride into the gestational sac, with a successful result.

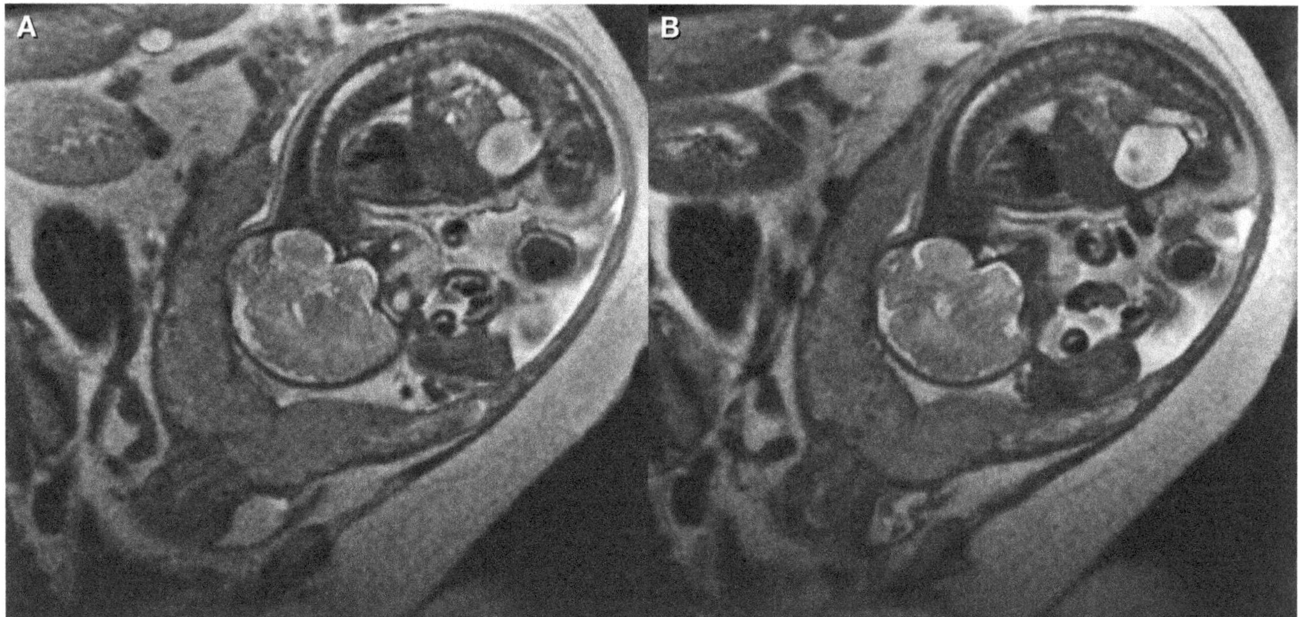

Figure 10.24.1

HISTORY: 36-year-old woman with abnormal obstetric US

IMAGING FINDINGS: Coronal oblique SSFSE images (Figure 10.24.1) demonstrate the placenta completely covering the cervical os.

DIAGNOSIS: Placenta previa

COMMENT: MRI is not generally required to make the diagnosis of placenta previa, but it can be helpful in complicated cases and in patients for whom sonography is less than optimal. The placenta is named after the Greek term *plakuos* (flat cake) and serves as a barrier between maternal and fetal tissue while simultaneously providing a pathway for transmission of nourishment from mother to fetus and removal of waste in the opposite direction. The normal placenta appears as a fairly homogeneous structure of intermediate T2-signal intensity on SSFSE and SSFP images or conventional T2-weighted FSE images.

Placenta previa refers to abnormal implantation of the placenta in the lower uterine segment overlying or near the internal cervical os and is one of the most common causes of bleeding during pregnancy. Normally, the inferior placental border should be at least 2 cm from the margin of the internal os; if it isn't, a placenta previa is diagnosed. The diagnosis should not be made before 15-weeks gestational age, since approximately 25% of pregnancies at this stage have a placenta previa, whereas expansion of the lower uterine segment reduces this percentage to 1% by the end of the third trimester. Placenta previa is subdivided according to the position of the placenta relative to the internal os as low lying, marginal, and complete.

Placenta previa occurs with higher frequency in multiparous women, women with prior cesarean sections, smokers, and cocaine users. Placenta previa is associated with a higher incidence (10%) of placenta accreta, increta, and percreta, which describe an abnormal invasion of the myometrium by the chorionic villi of the placenta. Superficial invasion of the basalis layer is termed *placenta accreta* (75% of cases); deeper invasion of the myometrium, *placenta increta*; and complete extension to the uterine serosa, *placenta percreta*. Undiagnosed placenta accreta is associated with increased maternal morbidity and mortality due to intrapartum hemorrhage, uterine rupture, abscess formation, and bladder or rectal invasion. The incidence of placenta accreta has increased more than 10-fold in the past 30 years, to approximately 1 in 2,500 deliveries, and is thought to be related to the increased prevalence of uterine surgery that leaves decidual defects, thereby allowing placental ingrowth. The combination of placenta previa and prior instrumentation leads to development of placenta accreta in 50% to 67% of patients.

Several studies have compared the relative abilities of US and MRI to diagnose placenta accreta, increta, and percreta, with most concluding that MRI is somewhat more sensitive. These results have led to more frequent use of MRI as a problem-solving technique for patients at high risk or those with inconclusive US examinations. MRI signs described in the literature include abnormal thinning of the myometrium underlying the placenta, T2 dark bands within the placenta, and direct visualization of placental invasion of the myometrium. Some authors have advocated the use of conventional FSE pulse sequences with respiratory triggering, noting the soft tissue contrast is improved relative to SSFSE and SSFP acquisitions and that motion artifact is somewhat less problematic for this application.

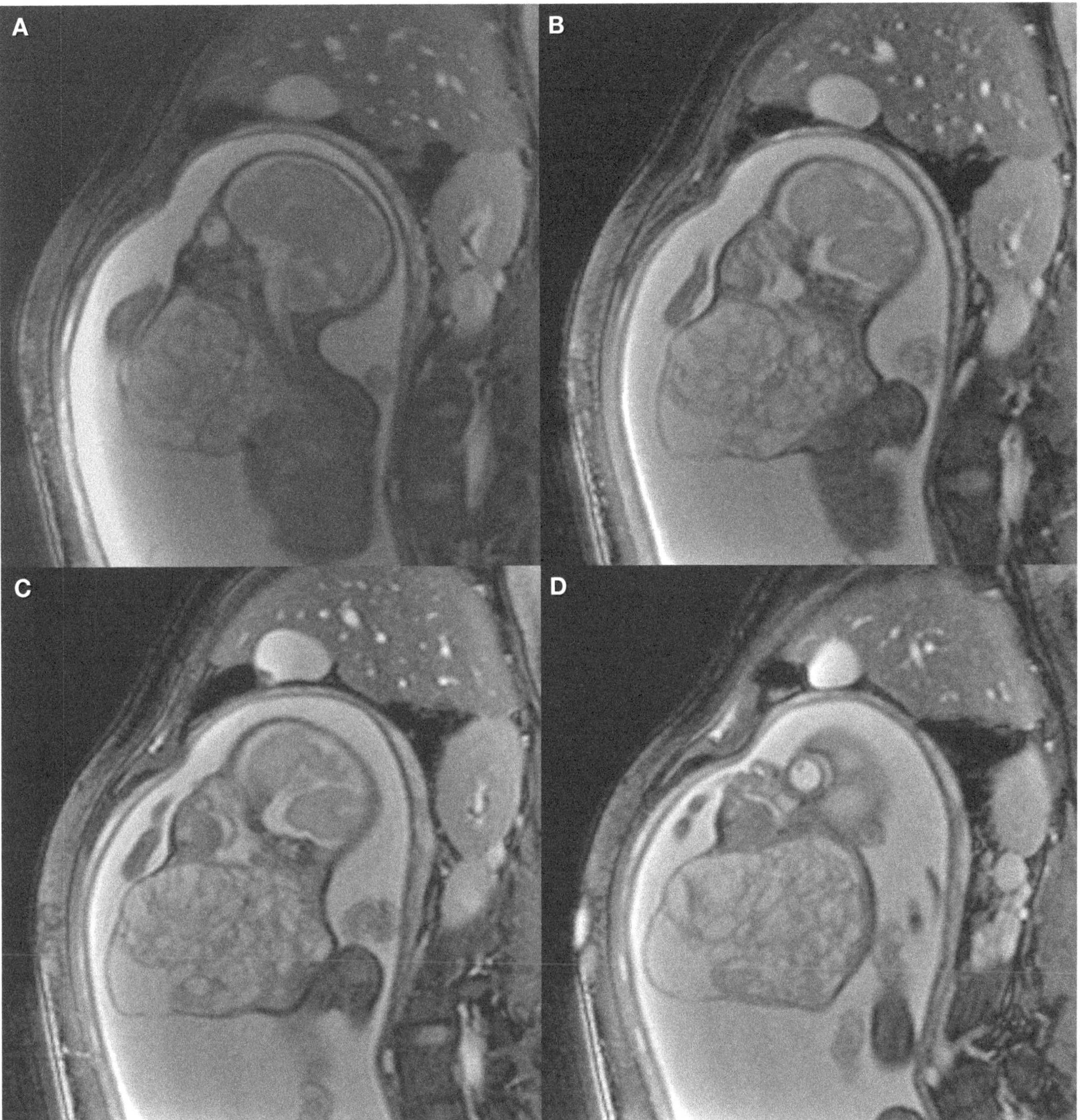

Figure 10.25.1

HISTORY: 35-year-old pregnant woman with abnormal obstetric US

IMAGING FINDINGS: Sagittal oblique fat-suppressed 2D SSFP images (Figure 10.25.1) demonstrate a large complex, multiloculated, and predominantly cystic mass in the anterior fetal neck, with some solid components. Note also polyhydramnios.

DIAGNOSIS: Fetal cervical teratoma

COMMENT: This is a companion case to the fetal intracranial teratoma case (Case 10.26) and illustrates a more common extracranial fetal teratoma. The sacrococcygeal region is the most common location for teratomas, accounting for 70% to 80% of lesions, with the head and neck the next most frequent sites of origin. Tumors can arise from the thyrocervical region, palate, or nasopharynx and are usually seen as large masses containing both cystic and solid components. Calcifications are essentially diagnostic of teratomas, but they can be seen in only one-half of all lesions (based on fetal US) and are even more difficult to visualize with MRI. Polyhydramnios is a common associated finding and is generally the result of direct esophageal compression and consequent compromise of fetal swallowing.

The major differential diagnosis for cervical teratoma is cystic hygroma. The imaging features of these 2 conditions overlap considerably; however, cervical teratomas are more anterior in location and cystic hygromas should have few, if any, solid components. The large neck mass often compromises the airway, as well as the esophagus, and is a major reason for the substantial antenatal mortality associated with cervical teratomas.

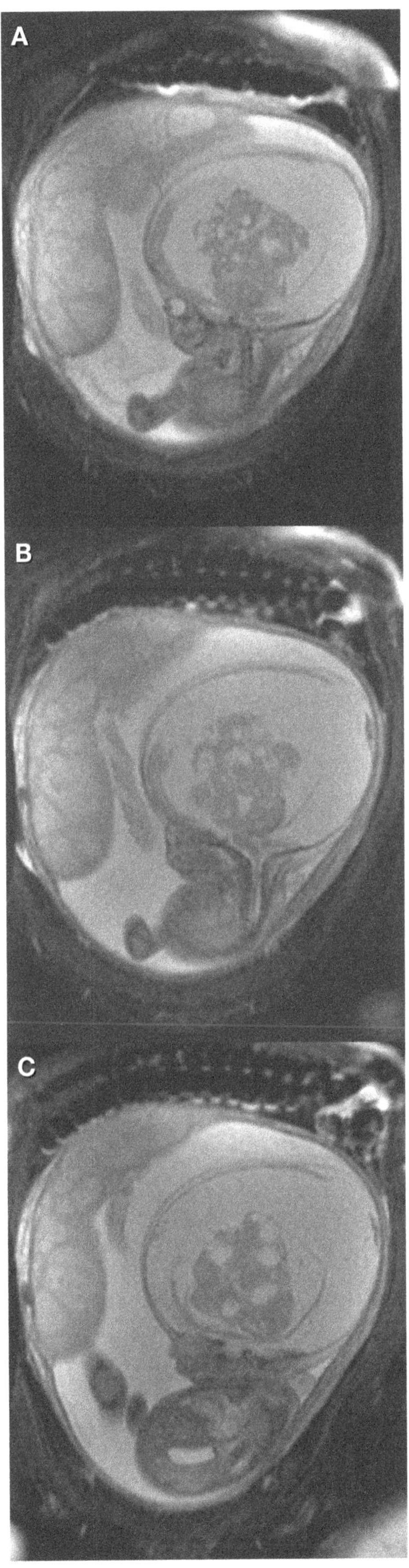

Figure 10.26.1

HISTORY: 32-year-old woman with abnormal obstetric US

IMAGING FINDINGS: Coronal oblique fat-suppressed 2D SSFP images (Figure 10.26.1) show a complex cystic and solid supratentorial mass replacing most of the fetal brain. Note also macrocephaly and polyhydramnios.

DIAGNOSIS: Fetal intracranial teratoma

COMMENT: Fetal and congenital tumors represent less than 3% of all tumors diagnosed before age 15 years. The reported incidence of congenital tumors ranges from 1.7 to 13.5 per 100,000 live births and is likely greater in stillborn and aborted fetuses. If the definition of *congenital tumors* excludes hamartomas, hemangiomas, and lymphangiomas (usually, but not always, the case among expert reviewers), the most common lesions are extracranial teratomas, neuroblastomas, and soft tissue tumors.

Congenital intracranial tumors constitute 0.5% to 1.9% of all childhood brain neoplasms, and teratomas represent about one-half of this total. Teratomas are thought to arise from unincorporated pluripotential germ cells left in various midline locations during their migration from the yolk sac to the genital ridge that fail to involute and continue to undergo mitosis. Teratomas are composed of all 3 germ cell layers—ectoderm, mesoderm, and endoderm. Ectodermal and mesodermal components are more common in fetal teratomas than endodermal components. Teratomas are classified histologically as either mature or immature. Immature elements, not surprisingly, are common in fetal teratomas.

Macrocephaly is the most common finding of fetal intracranial teratoma on prenatal US, either as a direct result of tumor growth or secondary to hydrocephalus. Polyhydramnios is also a frequent finding and is caused by depressed swallowing. The tumor itself appears as a complex solid and cystic lesion. The presence of calcification (probably more easily detected on US than MRI) strongly suggests the diagnosis of teratoma. The differential diagnosis for a fetal intracranial mass also includes astrocytoma, ependymoma, craniopharyngioma, choroid plexus cyst, and hemorrhage.

The prognosis of fetal intracranial teratoma is poor, with a reported mortality rate of approximately 90%. The tumor frequently replaces much of the normal brain tissue and prevents normal neural development.

The subject of fetal MRI has stimulated many papers and has become the major interest of a few academic radiologists; however, it remains a niche application in our practice. The images are sometimes spectacular, but in general, MRI rarely provides more information than conventional obstetric US, and the associated expense and inconvenience are usually not justified. We use it in our practice as an occasional problem-solving or confirmatory technique. In this case, the examination was requested to assess whether there was enough normal brain tissue for viability. A diminutive brainstem and cerebellum can be seen on the center image, but no normal supratentorial structures are identifiable.

Since motion artifact is a potential problem when imaging most fetuses (and sometimes their mothers), most of these examinations are performed using a combination of SSFSE and SSFP techniques. Both of these pulse sequences acquire images rapidly and sequentially, generally with acquisition times of 1 second or less per image and with soft tissue contrast that is usually adequate for visualization of most fetal abnormalities.

ABBREVIATIONS

ADC	apparent diffusion coefficient
CT	computed tomography
DWI	diffusion-weighted imaging
ESN	endometrial stromal nodule
ESS	endometrial stromal sarcoma
FIGO	International Federation of Obstetrics and Gynecology
FRFSE	fast-recovery fast-spin echo
FSE	fast-spin echo
MRI	magnetic resonance imaging
SCC	squamous cell carcinoma
SPGR	spoiled gradient-recalled echo
SSFP	steady-state free precession
SSFSE	single-shot fast-spin echo
3D	3-dimensional
2D	2-dimensional
US	ultrasonography

11.

OVARIES

CASE 11.1

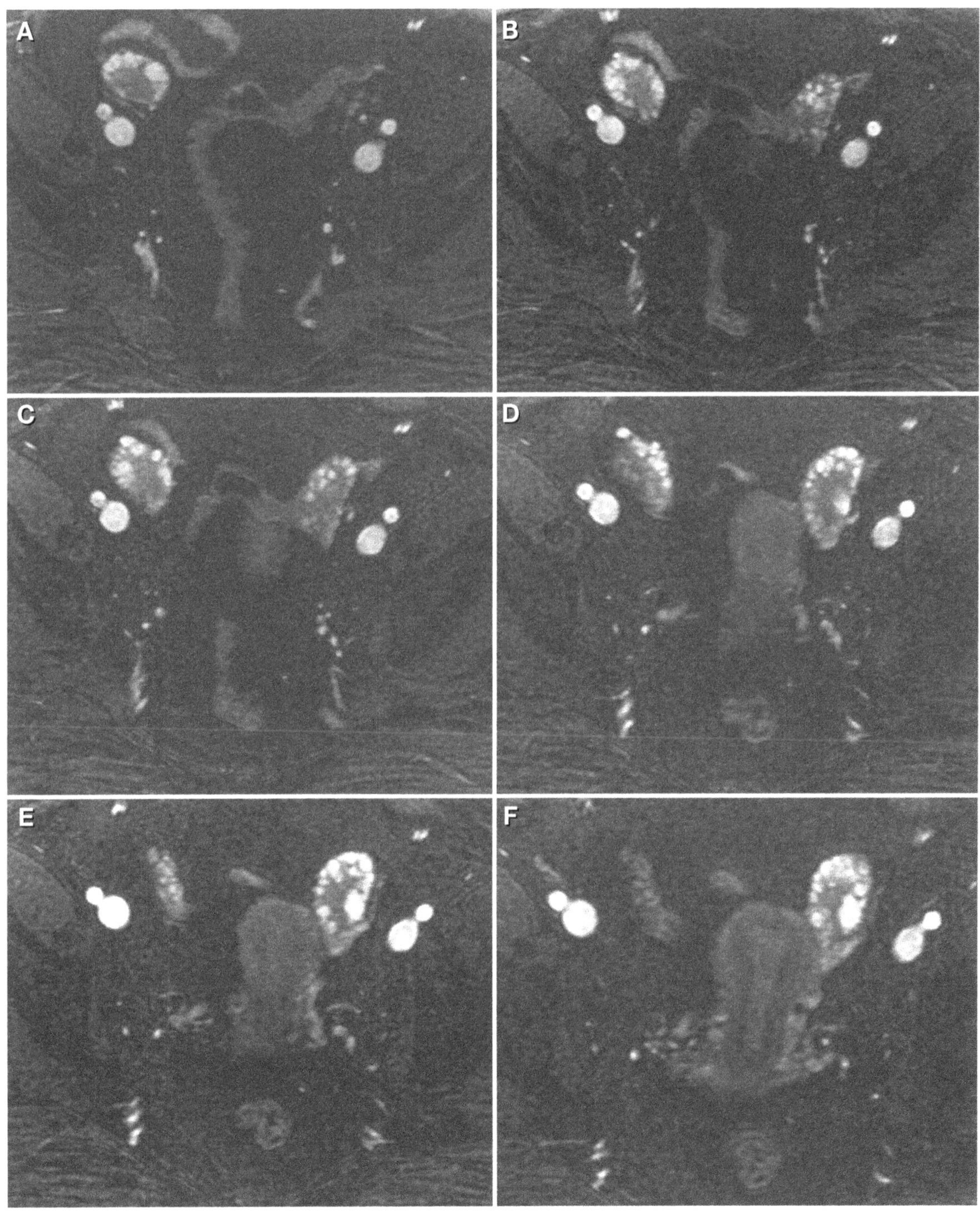

Figure 11.1.1

HISTORY: 28-year-old woman with secondary amenorrhea and hirsutism

IMAGING FINDINGS: Axial fat-suppressed 2D SSFP images (Figure 11.1.1) demonstrate multiple follicles arranged in the periphery of the ovaries bilaterally.

DIAGNOSIS: Polycystic ovary syndrome

COMMENT: PCOS is the most common endocrine disorder in women of reproductive age, affecting between 6% and 15%, depending on the criteria used for diagnosis. It typically presents with anovulatory or oligo-ovulatory menstrual cycles leading to oligomenorrhea, polycystic ovaries, and clinical and biochemical hyperandrogenism. PCOS is also associated with increased risk of obesity, insulin resistance, diabetes mellitus, metabolic syndrome, and infertility.

The Rotterdam criteria for diagnosis of PCOS include oligo-ovulation or anovulation, clinical and biochemical signs of hyperandrogenism, and polycystic ovaries. Polycystic ovaries are defined on pelvic US as the presence of at least 12 follicles measuring 2 to 9 mm in diameter or an increased ovarian volume of more than 10 mL. The addition of imaging criteria in the Rotterdam criteria compared with the previous guidelines from the National Institutes of Health was and continues to be somewhat controversial because several studies have demonstrated that US features of PCOS can be found in 20% to 60% of normal women.

Nevertheless, US is widely used in the diagnostic algorithm for suspected PCOS, always with the caveat that accompanying clinical evidence of the syndrome must be present. Since US is sometimes limited for visualizing the ovaries, particularly in large patients, MRI has been proposed as a potential alternative, and several papers have demonstrated that greater numbers of follicles are seen in patients with PCOS and that ovarian volumes are correspondingly larger—results similar to those of the more numerous US studies.

The classic appearance of PCOS on either US or MRI is enlarged ovaries containing multiple peripheral follicles. This is not universally true, however, and enlarged ovaries may be the predominant finding or the multiple cysts may be interspersed throughout the ovaries. Visualization of small ovarian follicles is a task well suited to SSFSE and SSFP pulse sequences, which emphasize fluid-containing structures, and 3D FSE or SSFP acquisitions may be helpful for those who are counting follicles.

Treatment of PCOS includes combined estrogen-progestin contraceptives, antiandrogen therapies, and insulin sensitizers, as well as weight loss.

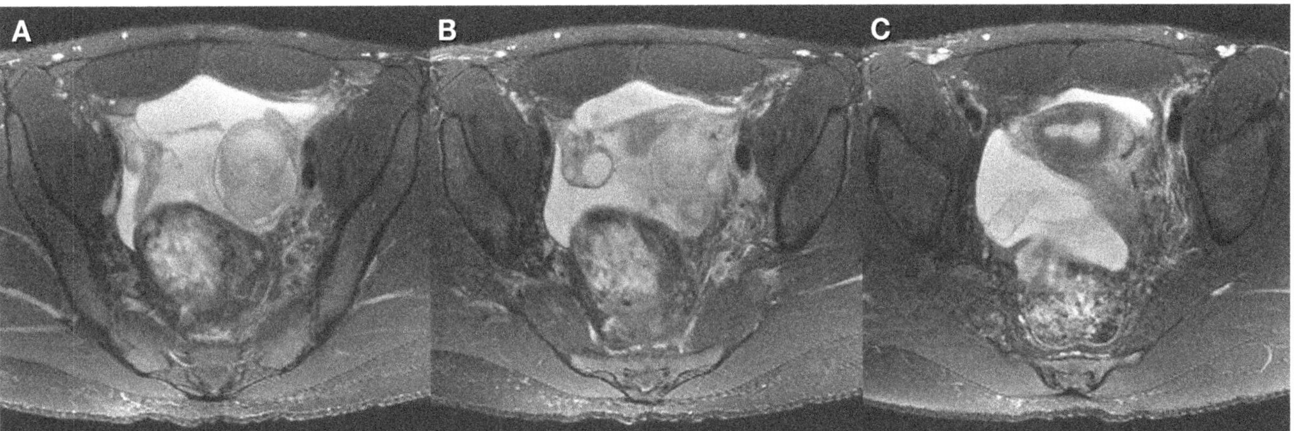

Figure 11.2.1

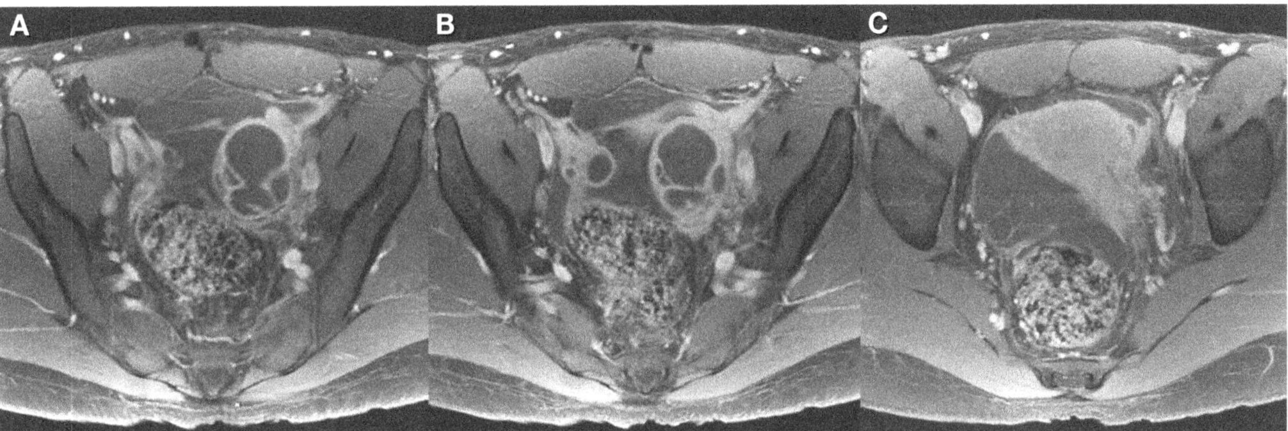

Figure 11.2.2

HISTORY: 31-year-old woman with a history of Crohn colitis and rectovaginal fistula, now presenting with new, left lower quadrant pain

IMAGING FINDINGS: Axial fat-suppressed FSE T2-weighted images (Figure 11.2.1) demonstrate a complex high-signal-intensity lesion in the left adnexa. Notice also pelvic ascites and a tubular cystic structure traversing the ascites within the posterior right pelvis. Axial postgadolinium 2D SPGR images (Figure 11.2.2) reveal similar findings. The left adnexal lesion is predominantly cystic, with a thick enhancing rim and septations.

DIAGNOSIS: Tubo-ovarian abscess

COMMENT: Tubo-ovarian abscess is almost always the result of pelvic inflammatory disease, an ascending infection in the female genital tract usually originating in the vagina or cervix. The most common causative organisms are *Neisseria gonorrhoeae* and *Chlamydia trachomatis*. Progressive infection and inflammation may eventually result in tissue destruction and formation of an inflammatory mass encompassing both the fallopian tube and ovary.

Patients typically present with abdominal or pelvic pain, fever, vaginal discharge, or urinary symptoms; however, not all patients are severely symptomatic, and as many as 20% have a normal white blood cell count and are afebrile.

On MRI, tubo-ovarian abscesses have an appearance similar to abscesses in other locations: a thick-walled, rim-enhancing complex fluid collection, often associated with adjacent inflammatory changes and free fluid. In this case, the distal portion of the ipsilateral fallopian tube was involved in the abscess at surgery but is not clearly visible at MRI, although the right-sided hydrosalpinx is apparent. Gas may occasionally be visualized within tubo-ovarian abscesses and is usually more easily appreciated at CT, but it can be seen as signal void on gradient echo images.

The diagnosis is usually apparent on the basis of MRI findings and clinical symptoms; however, it is not always possible to distinguish this entity from an ovarian neoplasm in patients without fever or an elevated white blood cell count. In these patients, the finding of a dilated, thickened fallopian tube is helpful because this is more commonly encountered in pelvic inflammatory disease and tubo-ovarian abscess.

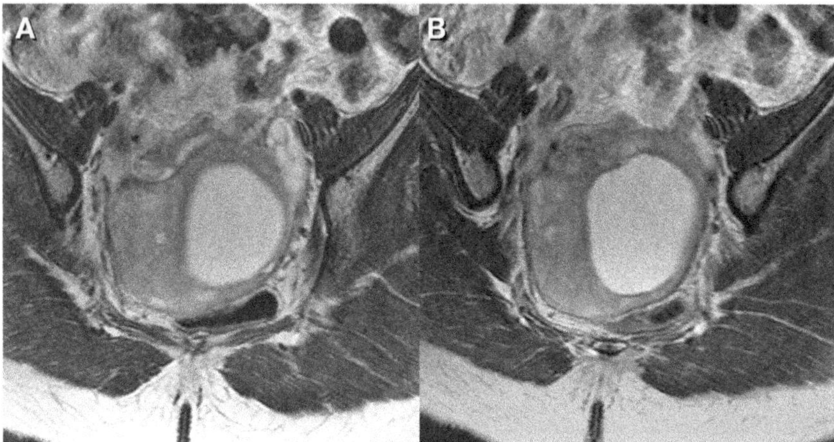

Figure 11.3.1

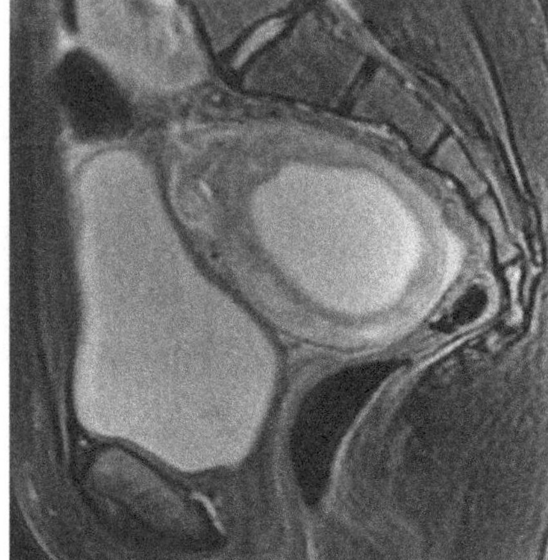

Figure 11.3.2

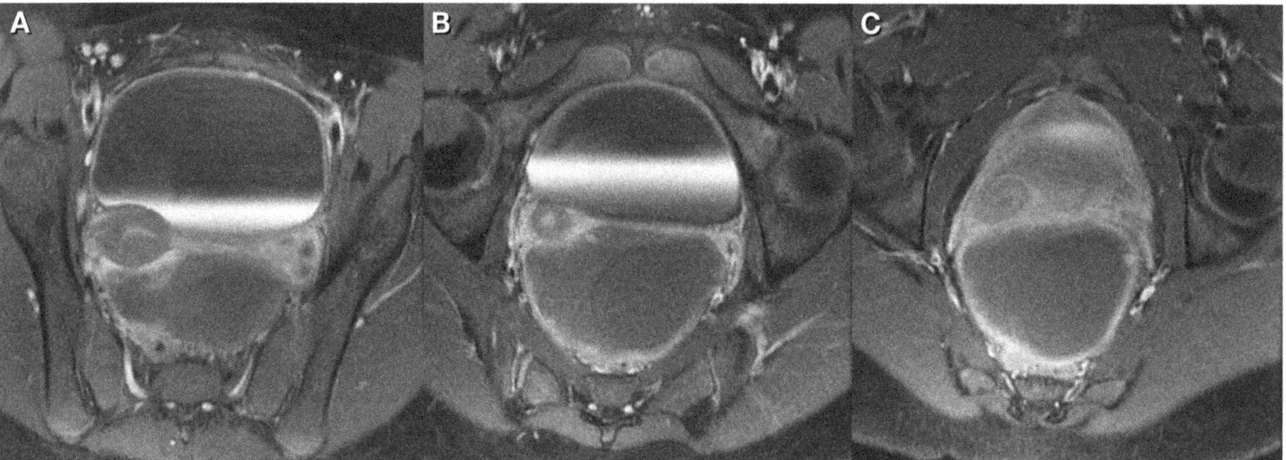

Figure 11.3.3

HISTORY: 11-year-old girl with a 3-month history of increasing intermittent right lower quadrant pain

IMAGING FINDINGS: Coronal oblique FSE T2-weighted images (Figure 11.3.1) demonstrate a markedly enlarged right ovary that contains a prominent cyst (the normal left ovary can be seen along the left superior margin of the right ovary, with multiple small follicles). Sagittal fat-suppressed FSE T2-weighted image (Figure 11.3.2) reveals similar findings. Axial postgadolinium 2D SPGR images (Figure 11.3.3) show faint rim enhancement of the right ovary and no internal enhancement.

DIAGNOSIS: Right ovarian cyst with adnexal torsion

COMMENT: *Adnexal torsion* is probably the preferred term for this entity rather than *ovarian torsion*, since the fallopian tube is frequently involved and rarely undergoes torsion without involvement of the associated ovary. Adnexal torsion is a rare gynecologic emergency that occurs when the ovary and its vascular pedicle twist along the long axis of the ovary. Torsion initially compromises low-pressure venous flow, resulting in congestion and edema of the ovary. This eventually leads to arterial obstruction and subsequent hemorrhagic infarction and necrosis of the ovary.

Torsion occurs most frequently in girls and premenopausal women and is associated with an adnexal lesion in as many as 80% of cases, with corpus luteal cysts and dermoids the most commonly associated masses. Predisposing factors include pregnancy, ovarian hyperstimulation for in vitro fertilization, long ovarian ligaments, and polycystic ovaries.

The classic clinical presentation is colicky lower quadrant pain radiating to the ipsilateral flank or groin with adnexal tenderness and a palpable mass. As is often the case, the classic presentation is rare, and the differential diagnosis for a young woman presenting with lower abdominal or pelvic pain is long, particularly when the symptoms are subacute or intermittent, as in this case. This problem is illustrated by a recent study documenting that only 58% of 135 women with adnexal torsion received a correct diagnosis at their initial presentation.

US is generally considered the initial imaging modality of choice for a potential diagnosis of adnexal torsion. However, many patients have ambiguous examinations, and it's also true that the clinical presentation of some patients directs their work-up toward the appendicitis algorithm and abdominal-pelvic CT. Regardless of the initial imaging strategy, MRI is reasonable as both a follow-up examination in patients with ambiguous US or CT findings or an initial test for a patient with suspected torsion.

This case illustrates many of the typical findings of adnexal torsion. The ovary is markedly enlarged, which is one of the most consistent findings in the literature. Some authors have described increased T2-signal intensity of ovarian stroma secondary to edema or hemorrhage. This distinction can be subtle, but displaced or absent follicles in the same region can be a helpful clue. Subacute hemorrhage is best demonstrated as high signal intensity on fat-suppressed T1-weighted FSE or SPGR images and, more specifically, a high-signal-intensity rim along the outer margin of the affected ovary, indicating a subacute hematoma rather than an endometrioma or other hemorrhagic mass. Minimal or no enhancement following gadolinium administration is a fairly specific sign, but remember that the presence of ovarian enhancement does not exclude torsion and can be seen in cases of intermittent torsion or in early torsion where only venous outflow is compromised. In fact, these are important cases to identify, since the enhancing ovary is generally viable and can be saved with prompt surgery. Direct visualization of the twisted vascular pedicle is emphasized by many authors, and this is certainly the most direct confirmation of the diagnosis when confidently identified; however, it is seen in less than one-third of patients on CT and MRI.

In this case, the edematous vascular pedicle can probably be seen along the superior right margin of the ovary on the coronal FSE images and superiorly on the sagittal FSE image; however, this is a much easier diagnosis to make in retrospect. Acquisition of overlapping thin-section 2D SSFP images in 1 or more planes (a technique not available when this case was performed) should help in visualizing the twisted vascular pedicle.

Adnexal torsion may also be associated with mural thickening and dilatation of the associated fallopian tube, pelvic ascites, and deviation of the uterus (a highly nonspecific sign). Treatment of adnexal torsion is surgical, with preservation of viable ovarian tissue whenever possible.

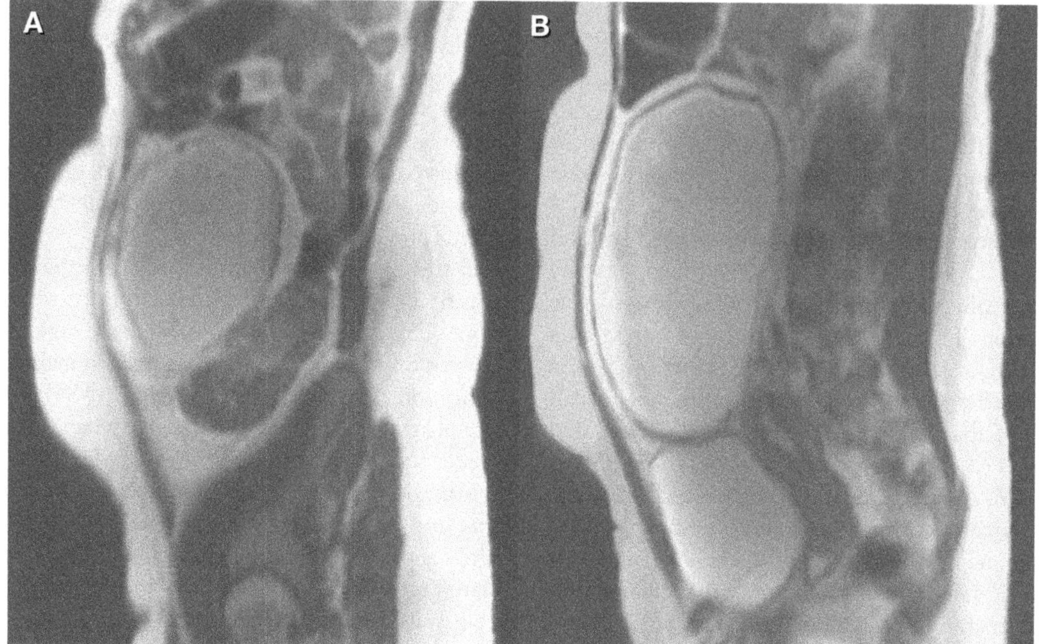

Figure 11.4.1

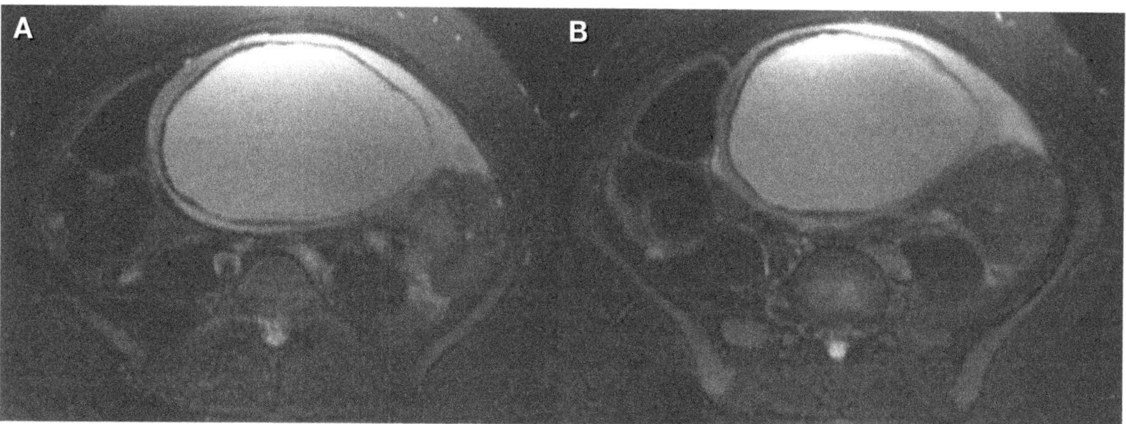

Figure 11.4.2

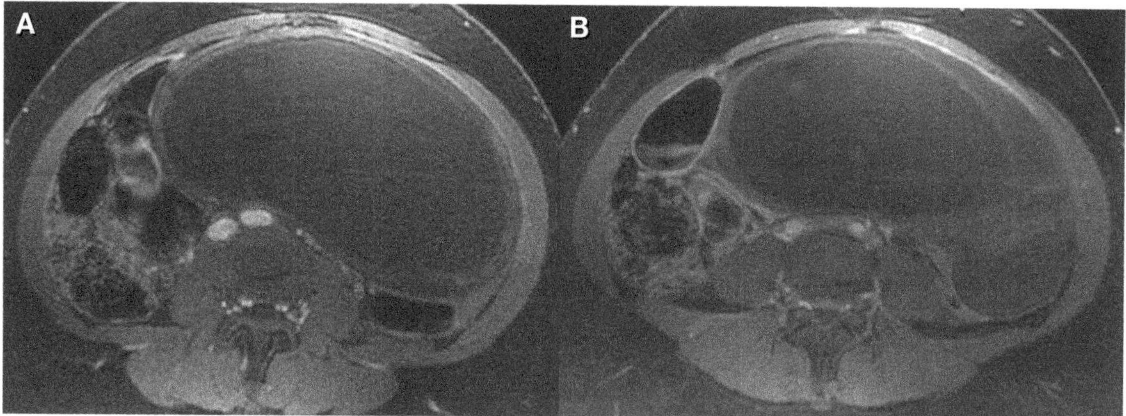

Figure 11.4.3

HISTORY: 21-year-old woman with sudden onset of severe abdominal pain

IMAGING FINDINGS: Sagittal images from a 3-plane SSFSE localizer (Figure 11.4.1) demonstrate an enlarged low-signal-intensity ovary with a large adjacent tubular cystic structure. Axial fat-suppressed FSE T2-weighted images (Figure 11.4.2) again reveal a large hypointense left ovary containing a few small follicles, as well as an adjacent large cystic structure medially with a thickened edematous wall and a small amount of associated free fluid. Axial postgadolinium 2D SPGR images (Figure 11.4.3) show no enhancement of either the left ovary or the adjacent cystic lesion.

DIAGNOSIS: Torsion of the left ovary and fallopian tube

COMMENT: This companion case of adnexal torsion demonstrates impressive involvement of the fallopian tube, with marked hydrosalpinx, substantial mural thickening, and a small fluid-debris level best seen on the sagittal scout images. The ovary is also enlarged and shows diffuse low T2-signal intensity, consistent with infarction. As in Case 11.3, the postgadolinium images confirm the diagnosis, demonstrating virtually no enhancement of the dilated fallopian tube and left ovary. The torsive vascular pedicle is probably represented by the amorphous, mildly hyperintense structure in the ovarian hilum on the superior, most axial FSE image, but even in retrospect it is difficult to identify with certainty.

This case provides another illustration of the value of fast imaging in patients with severe pain. Although the axial FSE and postgadolinium SPGR images are diagnostic, only a few images in each of these acquisitions were relatively free from motion artifact, and a few series were repeated as a result of severe artifact. On the other hand, the 3-plane SSFSE localizer is actually diagnostic and relatively artifact-free. Often, the best plan for the very uncomfortable patient is to begin with SSFSE or SSFP acquisitions in 1 or 2 planes and proceed as rapidly as possible to postcontrast acquisitions if necessary. It's worth remembering that a completed diagnostic examination with pedestrian image quality is always better than a failed attempt to obtain high-quality images from a problematic patient.

CASE 11.5

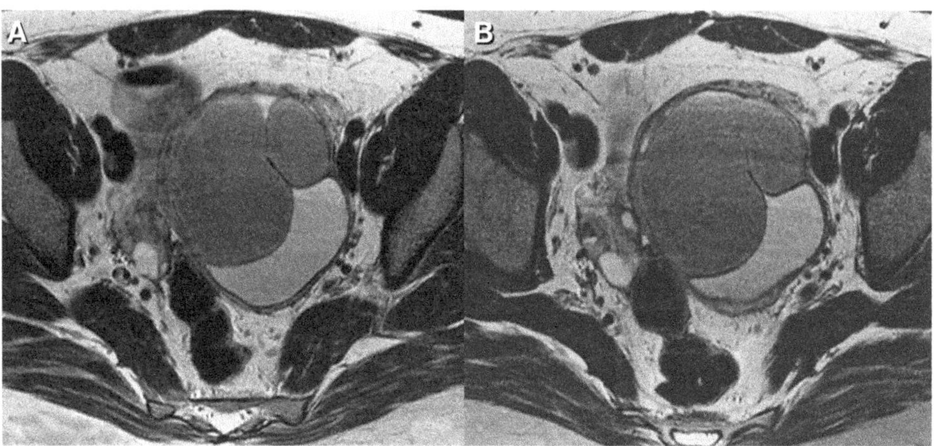

Figure 11.5.1

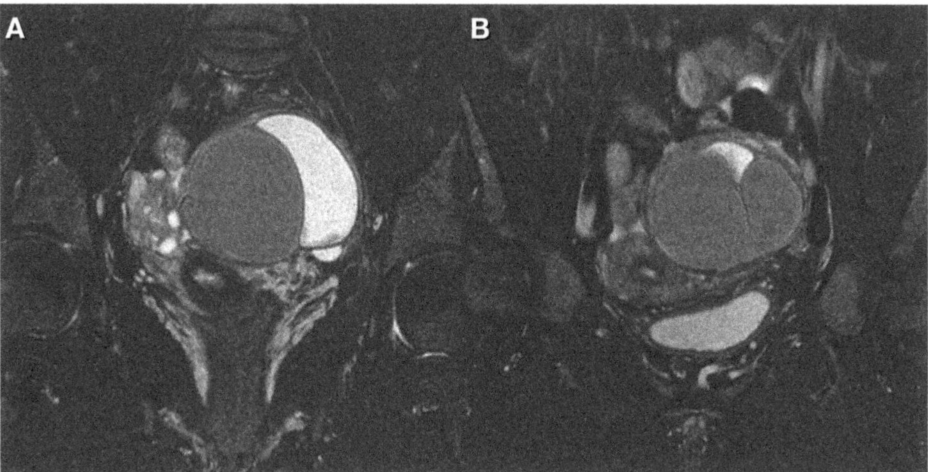

Figure 11.5.2

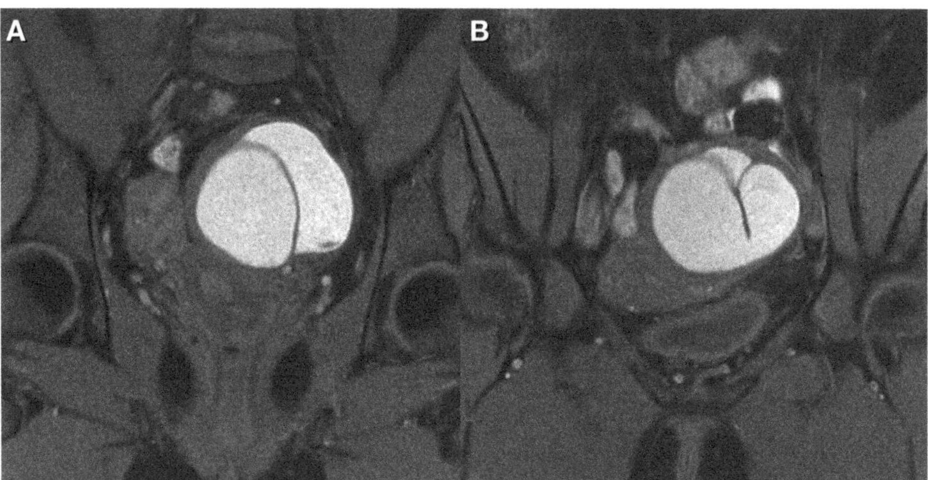

Figure 11.5.3

HISTORY: 27-year-old woman with left lower quadrant pain and a history of endometriosis

IMAGING FINDINGS: Axial FSE T2-weighted images (Figure 11.5.1) demonstrate a large, lobulated left adnexal lesion with regions of high and low signal intensity. Coronal fat-suppressed FSE T2-weighted images (Figure 11.5.2) reveal similar findings. Coronal fat-suppressed FSE T1-weighted images (Figure 11.5.3) show marked hyperintensity throughout the lesion, as well as prominent septations.

DIAGNOSIS: Endometrioma

COMMENT: Endometriosis, characterized by growth of endometrial tissue outside of the uterus, is a common disorder affecting 6% to 10% of women of reproductive age and as many as 5% of postmenopausal women. Pelvic pain and infertility are typical presenting symptoms; however, many women have minimal or no symptoms.

The most common sites of involvement in endometriosis are the ovary, uterine ligaments, rectovaginal septum, cul-de-sac, and peritoneum. Although the diagnostic criteria for endometriosis require pathologic demonstration of extrauterine endometrial glands and stroma, MRI has proven fairly successful in detecting implants, with reported sensitivities in the range of 90%.

MRI findings of endometriosis are often distinctive, and this is particularly true in the ovaries, where endometriomas are frequently larger and more easily visible in comparison to more subtle extraovarian disease. Endometriomas are cysts with a fibrous wall lined by functional endometrial tissue and filled with blood products of various ages. The most characteristic and sensitive finding is homogeneous very high signal intensity on fat-suppressed FSE or SPGR T1-weighted images, a result of the paramagnetic blood breakdown product methemoglobin. Although it is true that other ovarian lesions may be hemorrhagic, the signal intensity on T1-weighted images tends to be less bright and the lesions are often more complex and nonuniform. T2-weighted images often demonstrate low signal intensity within endometriomas, but this is a less frequent and less sensitive finding. The unfortunate term *shading* has been applied to this appearance, borrowed from the US literature without regard for the actual meaning of the word. Low T2-signal intensity is likely a reflection of the T2* effect of blood by-products, best described as *low signal intensity*. Fluid-fluid levels may occasionally be seen on T1- or T2-weighted images, representing layers of blood products of different ages. Endometriomas are frequently multiple, thought to occur as a result of repeated cyst rupture from repetitive cycles of hemorrhage.

An associated neoplasm develops in approximately 1% of women with endometriosis, which most frequently is endometrioid or clear cell ovarian carcinoma. These tumors generally appear at a younger age than typical ovarian epithelial carcinomas and are associated with a better prognosis. The appearance of an enhancing nodule within an endometrioma should raise suspicion for this uncommon complication.

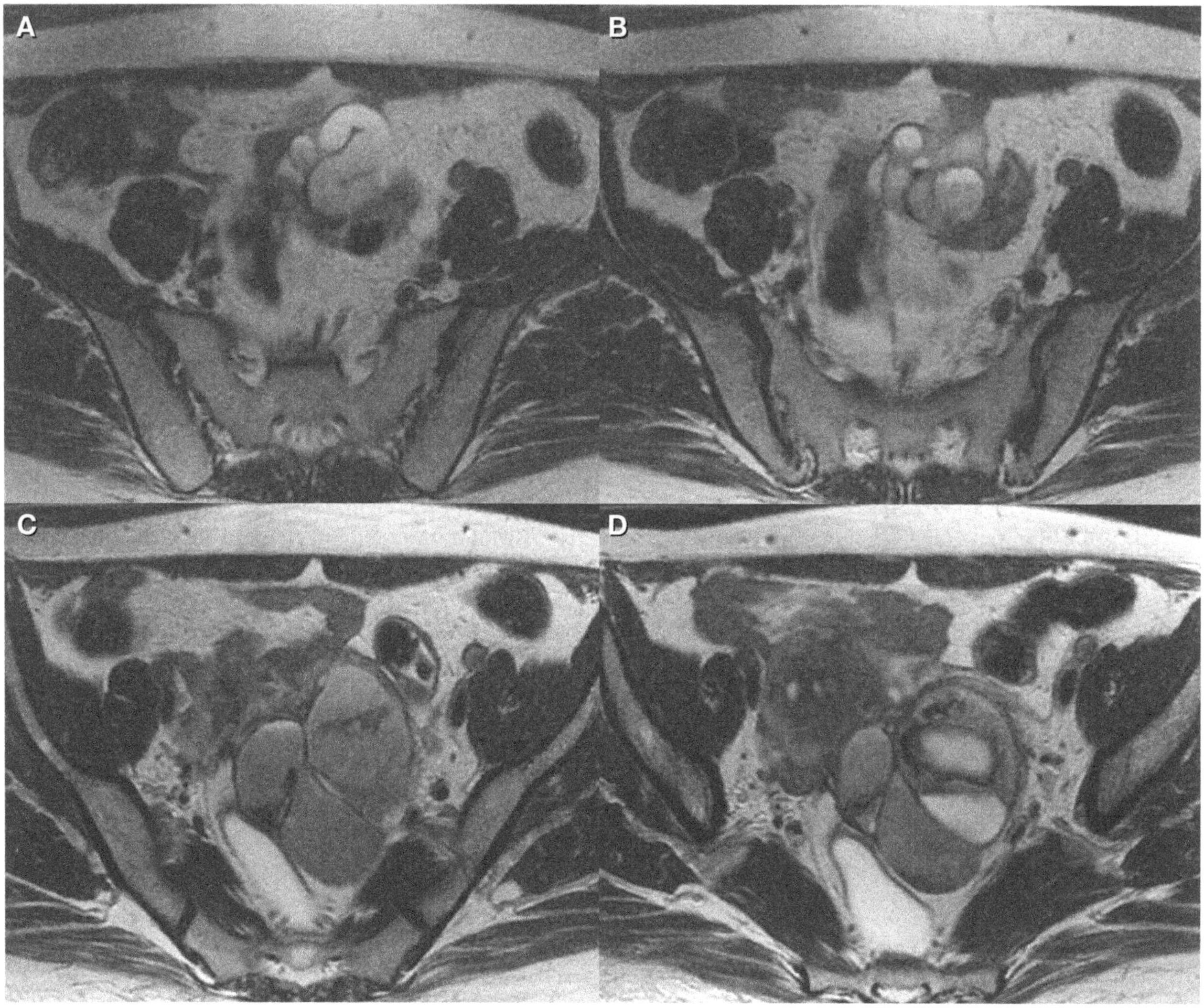

Figure 11.6.1

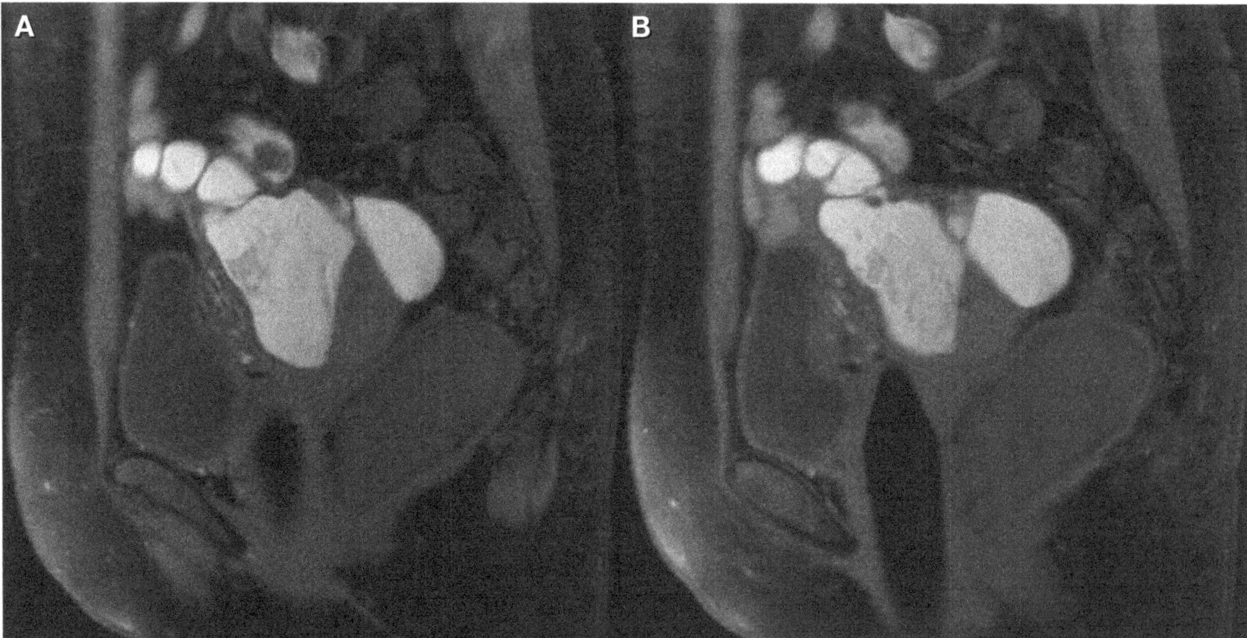

Figure 11.6.2

HISTORY: 50-year-old woman with intermittent rectal bleeding

IMAGING FINDINGS: Axial FSE T2-weighted images (Figure 11.6.1) demonstrate a dilated serpiginous cystic structure in the upper pelvis that connects to larger complex fluid collections inferiorly. Sagittal fat-suppressed FSE T1-weighted images (Figure 11.6.2) show high signal intensity within the tubular structure.

DIAGNOSIS: Endometriosis with chronic salpingitis and hematosalpinx

COMMENT: This patient had a history of endometriosis diagnosed at a previous laparoscopy, and the intermittent rectal bleeding also is suggestive of this diagnosis. At surgery, endometrial implants were seen involving the left fallopian tube and also along the posterior margin of the bladder, probably represented by the very small foci of high T1-signal intensity on the fat-suppressed T1-weighted FSE images (Figure 11.6.2).

Hydrosalpinx usually results from obstruction of the fimbriated end of the fallopian tube and resultant internal accumulation of fluid, blood, or pus, although implants from endometriosis or pelvic adhesions can affect the tube throughout its extrauterine course. Serosal and subserosal implants are the most common site of tubal endometriosis, and recurrent hemorrhage may lead to tubal adhesions and hydrosalpinx. Pelvic adhesions involving the fallopian tubes are seen in 26% of women with endometriosis, while direct endometrial implants involving the fallopian tubes are less common, occurring in 6%. Hyperintense tubal fluid on T1-weighted images usually represents hematosalpinx and is suggestive of endometriosis, although less commonly it can be seen in association with ectopic pregnancy, torsion, infection, or neoplasm.

MRI is often a useful technique for distinguishing hydrosalpinx from a cystic ovarian lesion: A dilated fallopian tube usually folds on itself to form a C- or S-shaped structure, often with incomplete septations corresponding to tubal plicae. Finding an ovary distinct from the dilated tube is of course helpful in correctly identifying hydrosalpinx, and the acquisition of images in multiple planes generally allows visualization of an extended tubular structure in 1 or more orientations.

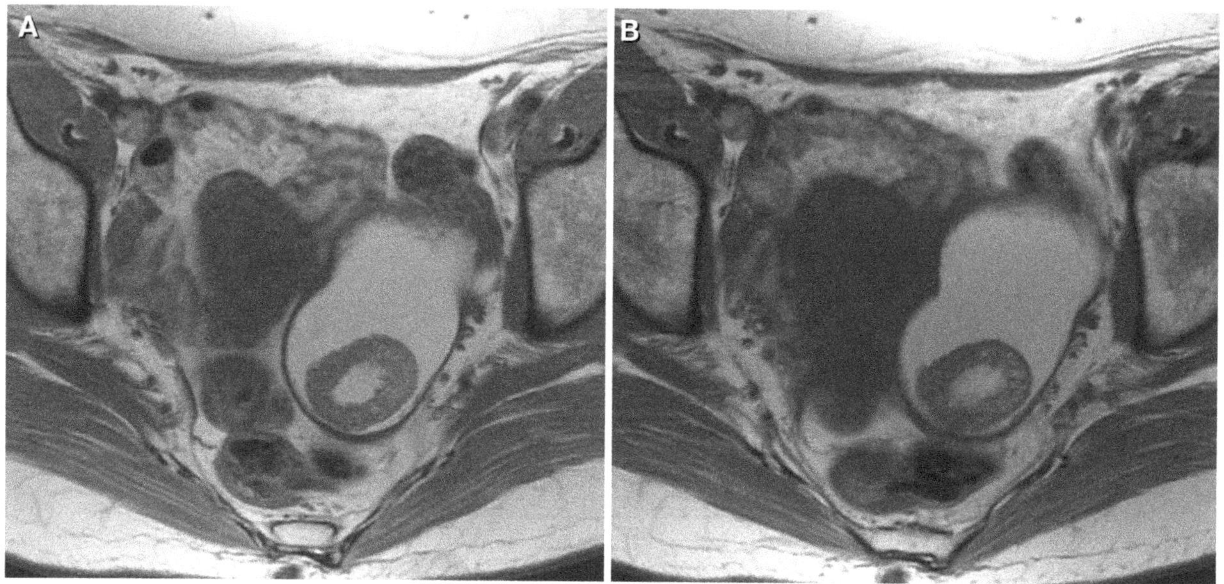

Figure 11.7.1

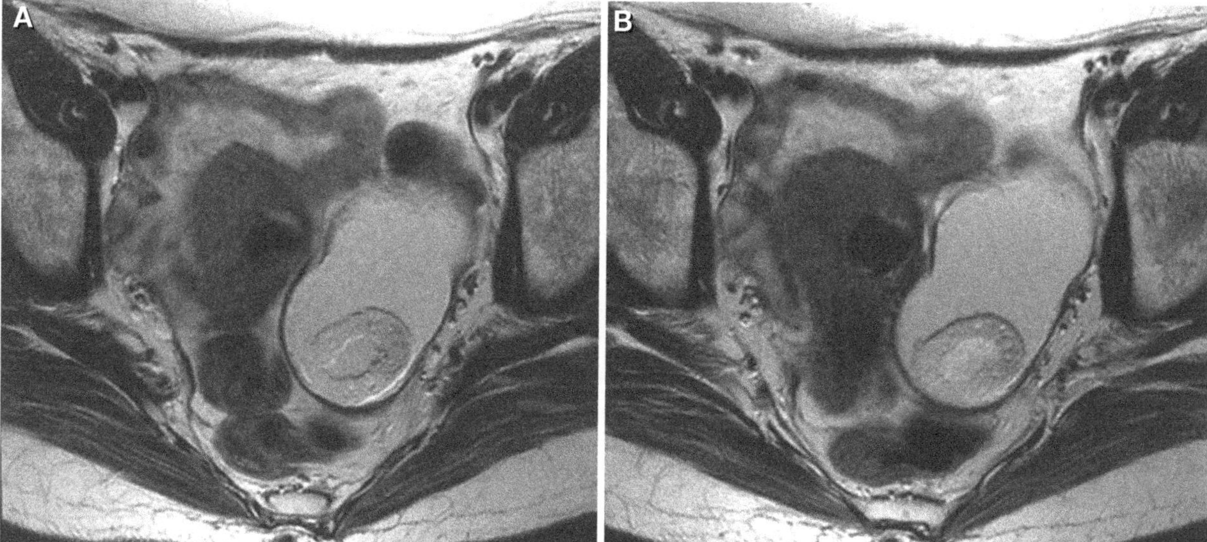

Figure 11.7.2

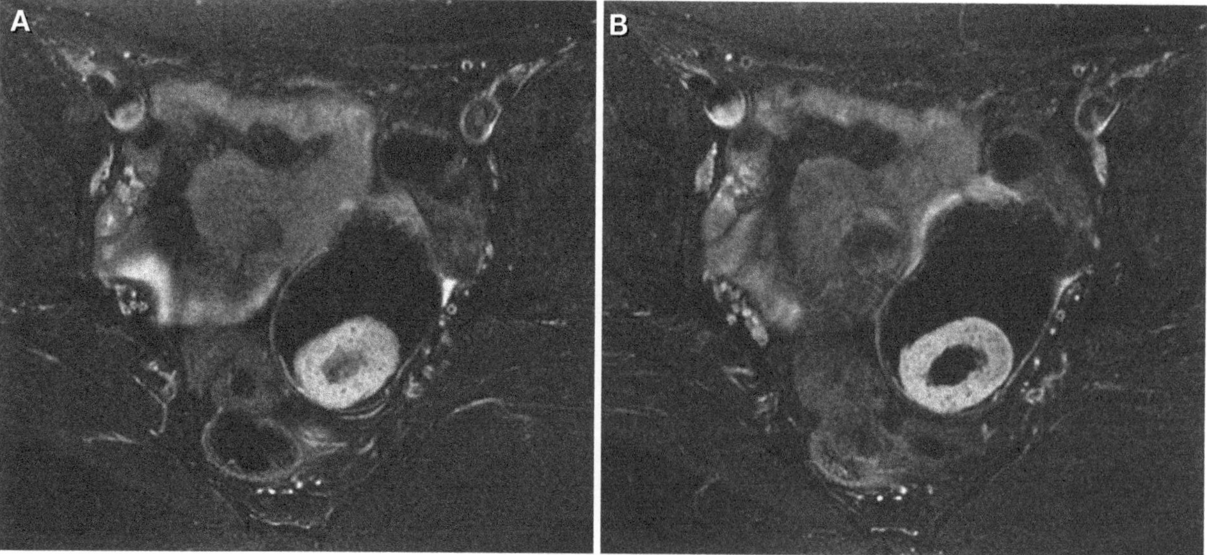

Figure 11.7.3

HISTORY: 50-year-old perimenopausal woman with intermittent mild abdominopelvic pain

IMAGING FINDINGS: Axial FSE T1-weighted images (Figure 11.7.1) demonstrate a large left adnexal mass with predominantly high signal intensity containing a donut-shaped internal nodule with lower signal intensity along the posterior margin of the lesion. Axial FSE T2-weighted images (Figure 11.7.2) reveal similar findings—a predominantly cystic appearance with a focal internal nodule. Axial fat-suppressed FSE T2-weighted images (Figure 11.7.3) show complete loss of signal in the majority of the lesion, as well as in the center of the internal nodule.

DIAGNOSIS: Mature cystic teratoma (dermoid cyst)

COMMENT: Dermoid cysts are the most common ovarian germ cell neoplasms, the most common benign ovarian tumor in women younger than 45 years, and, in some series, the most commonly resected ovarian neoplasm, accounting for 20% to 30% of all ovarian tumors. Mature teratomas are cystic lesions composed of well-differentiated cells arising from at least 2 of the 3 germ cell layers (ectoderm, mesoderm, and endoderm). The term *dermoid* derives from the predominance of dermal elements within most of these tumors, including hair, sebum, and keratin.

Most dermoids are asymptomatic lesions detected in young women in their second and third decades; however, pelvic pain or other nonspecific symptoms may occur in some patients. The estimated incidence is 8.9 per 100,000 women.

Dermoids are usually unilocular lesions filled with liquid sebaceous material and lined with squamous epithelium. The Rokitansky nodule or dermal plug, a raised protuberance projecting into the cyst cavity and well seen in this case, is often the location for bones or teeth when these are present. Ectodermal elements are present in virtually all lesions; mesodermal tissue (ie, fat, bone, muscle, and cartilage) is found in more than 90% of cases.

Confident diagnosis of a dermoid rests on identification of lipid or fat within the mass. Since this is something MRI is particularly good at showing, these lesions are rarely missed or misidentified. There are a few potential pitfalls, however, because other lesions (endometriomas, for instance) can have a similar appearance on T1-weighted images. Therefore, it is important to obtain both fat-suppressed and non–fat-suppressed T1- or T2-weighted images. Which of these are acquired doesn't matter and you can do both if you're particularly motivated or obsessive, but a female pelvis protocol that doesn't fulfill this basic requirement will cause trouble sooner or later. A few papers have described dermoids containing only a small amount of lipid within the wall of the lesion or only within the Rokitansky nodule. In these cases, IP-OP images may be more sensitive than fat-suppressed and non–fat-suppressed images for demonstrating signal loss. A convenient way of acquiring all these data within a single breath-hold is a Dixon 3D SPGR acquisition, which is illustrated in Case 11.8.

The demonstration of fat or lipid within an ovarian lesion is generally considered convincing evidence of a benign lesion. However, it is worth remembering that 1) immature teratomas may contain lipid and frequently demonstrate clinically malignant behavior and 2) mature cystic teratomas have a small, but real, incidence (probably <1%) of malignant degeneration, most frequently to squamous cell carcinoma. Malignant degeneration usually occurs in patients in their sixth and seventh decades. Immature teratomas represent less than 1% of all ovarian teratomas and contain immature tissue from the 3 germ cell layers. These lesions are generally more complex, occur in a younger age-group, and contain more prominent solid components, often with internal necrosis or hemorrhage. Scattered small foci of fat are more characteristic of immature teratomas than the prominent uniform lipid of dermoid cysts.

Germ cell tumors are the second most common ovarian neoplasms after epithelial tumors, mostly because of the high prevalence of dermoids, and represent 15% to 20% of all ovarian tumors. This group also includes immature teratomas, dysgerminomas, endodermal sinus tumor, embryonal carcinoma, and choriocarcinoma—all very uncommon neoplasms and all malignant.

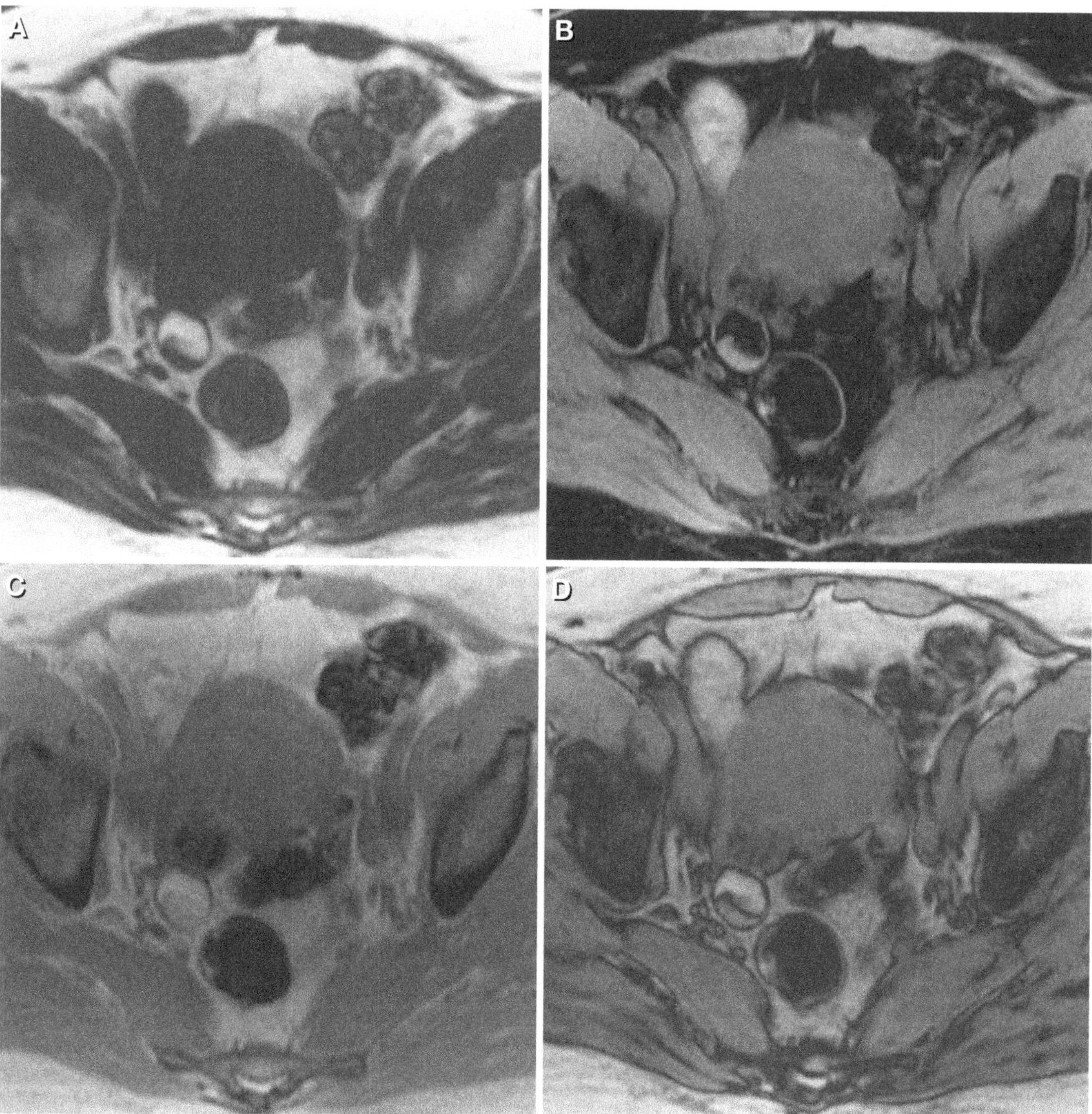

Figure 11.8.1

HISTORY: 50-year-old perimenopausal woman with intermittent mild abdominopelvic pain

IMAGING FINDINGS: Fat, water, IP, and OP images from a 3D SPGR Dixon acquisition (Figure 11.8.1) reveal a posterior right adnexal lesion with a fluid-fluid level. The anterior nondependent layer is lipid, which appears bright on the fat image and dark on the water image. Notice also the chemical shift artifact appearing at the fat-fluid interface on the OP image.

DIAGNOSIS: Mature cystic teratoma (dermoid cyst)

COMMENT: This case is another example of a mature cystic teratoma, diagnosed in a single breath-hold with a 3D Dixon SPGR acquisition, which allows reconstruction of fat, water, and IP-OP images. This technique has the obvious advantage of being much faster than 2 separate FSE acquisitions with and without chemical fat suppression and can be applied in a general female pelvis protocol as a substitute for a standard FSE T1-weighted sequence. The fat images are useful for detecting marrow lesions in patients with malignant disease and possible metastases; the water images generally display more uniform fat suppression than standard 3D SPGR acquisitions and are sensitive for detection of hemorrhagic material (in endometriomas, for example).

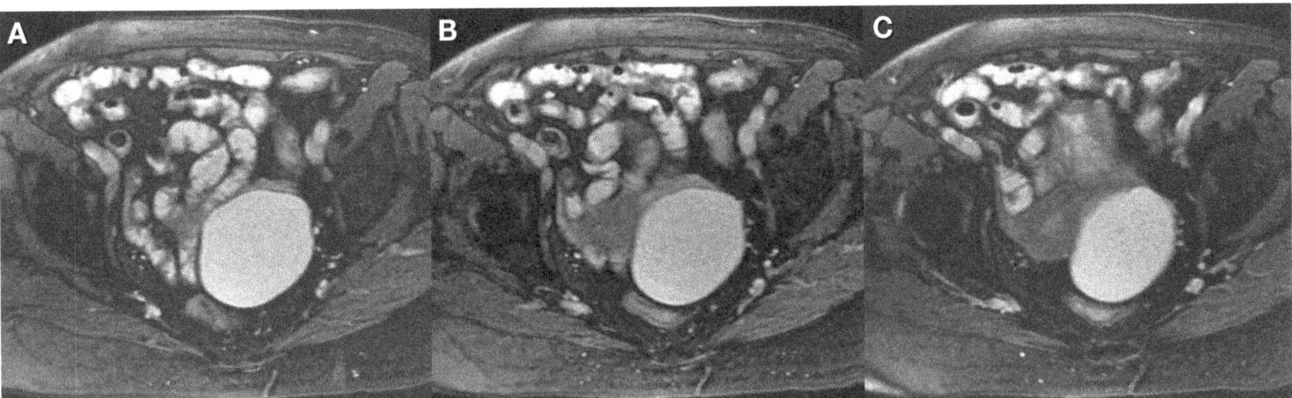

Figure 11.9.1

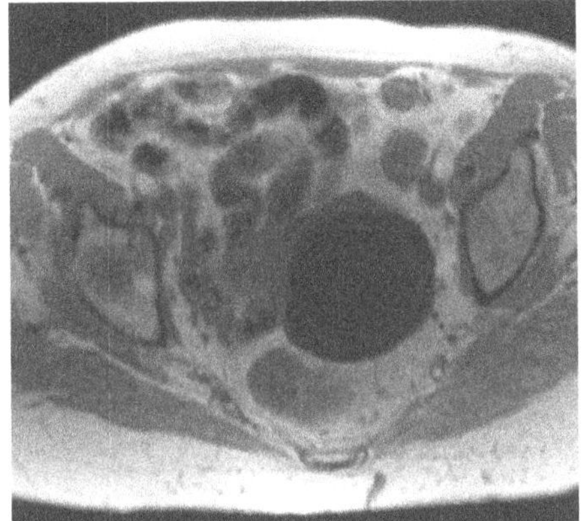

Figure 11.9.2

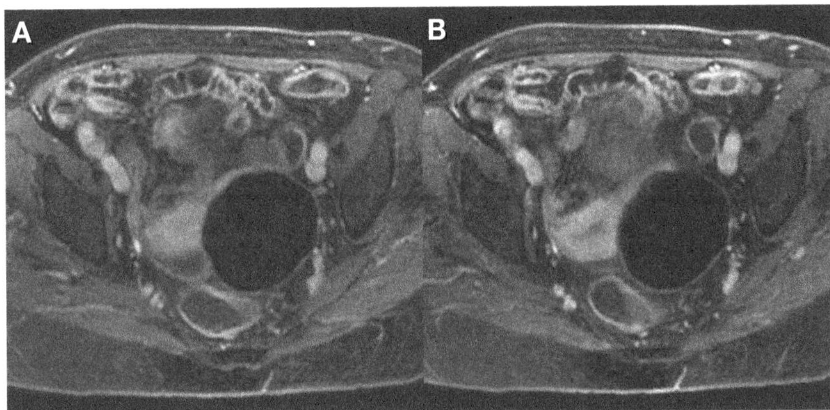

Figure 11.9.3

HISTORY: 75-year-old woman with a 6-month history of anorexia and weight loss

IMAGING FINDINGS: Axial fat-suppressed 2D SSFP images (Figure 11.9.1) demonstrate a cystic lesion in the left adnexa with a thin wall and no internal features. Axial IP T1-weighted 2D SPGR image (Figure 11.9.2) shows uniform low signal intensity within the lesion. Axial postgadolinium 3D SPGR images (Figure 11.9.3) reveal minimal rim enhancement and no internal enhancement.

DIAGNOSIS: Serous cystadenoma

COMMENT: Serous cystadenomas are common lesions, accounting for 25% of benign ovarian neoplasms and occurring more frequently in postmenopausal women, with peak incidence in the fourth and fifth decades. Bilateral lesions are not unusual and are seen in 12% to 24% of patients with serous cystadenoma. At the time they are detected, serous cystadenomas are often fairly large (average diameter, 10 cm). This neoplasm has generated a string of sensationalized case reports describing massive tumors, often accompanied by intraoperative photographs, analogous in many ways to stories featuring winners of the giant pumpkin contest at a regional fair found occasionally in the local news.

Approximately 60% of serous ovarian epithelial neoplasms are benign, with 15% borderline and 25% frankly malignant. The imaging appearance of benign serous cystadenomas is typified by this case: a large cystic mass with no internal complexity that is distinguishable from a functional cyst by its failure to resolve on follow-up imaging. As the complexity of the serous cystadenoma increases, particularly in the form of solid mural nodules, the likelihood of malignancy also increases. The presence of a thick irregular wall, prominent enhancing internal septations, ascites, and adenopathy is also a clue that the ovarian lesion may not be benign.

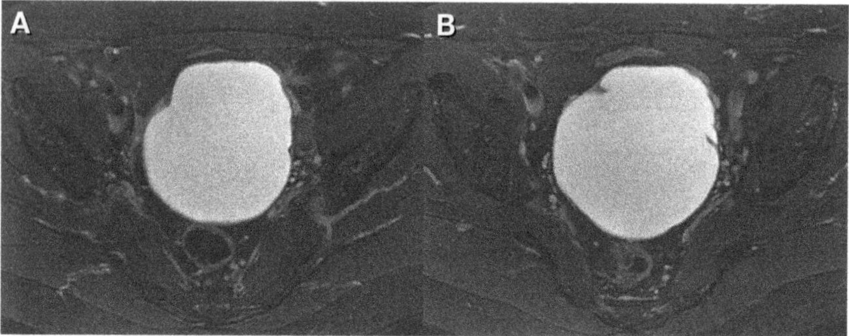

Figure 11.10.1

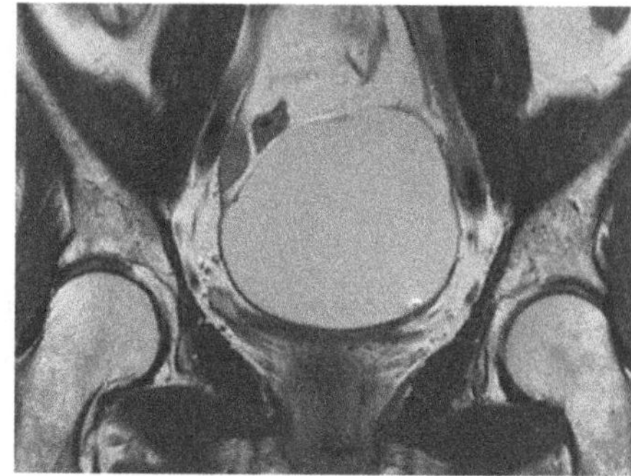

Figure 11.10.2

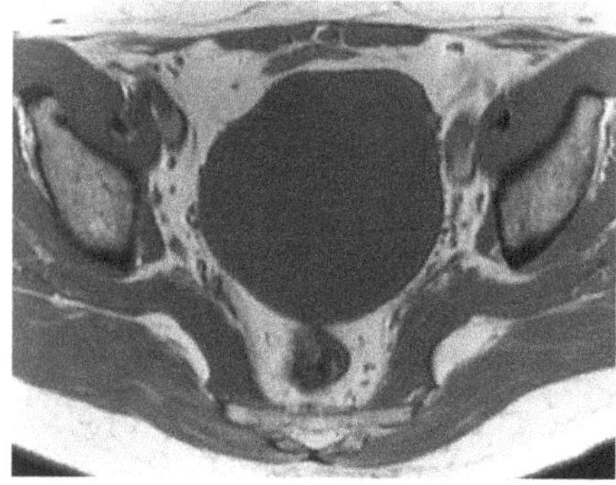

Figure 11.10.3

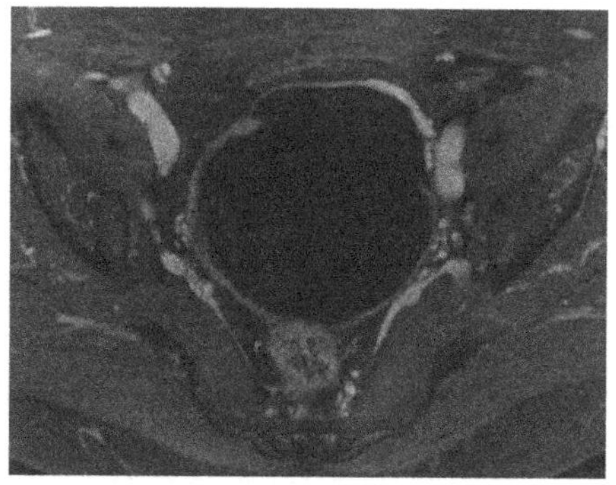

Figure 11.10.4

HISTORY: 57-year-old asymptomatic woman with a pelvic mass palpated during routine physical examination

IMAGING FINDINGS: Axial fat-suppressed FSE T2-weighted images (Figure 11.10.1) reveal a large cystic lesion in the pelvis, with a partial septation anteriorly. Coronal FSE T2-weighted image (Figure 11.10.2) shows similar findings. An axial FSE T1-weighted image (Figure 11.10.3) demonstrates diffuse low signal intensity throughout the mass, and an axial postgadolinium 3D SPGR image (Figure 11.10.4) reveals minimal enhancement of the lesion wall with no central enhancement.

DIAGNOSIS: Mucinous cystadenoma

COMMENT: This is an atypical presentation of mucinous cystadenoma in that mucinous cystadenomas are more frequently multilocular lesions than serous cystadenomas, which tend to be unilocular. Since our only other example of mucinous cystadenoma is also unilocular, we include this example of a benign cystic epithelial tumor that happens to be mucinous rather than serous.

Mucinous cystadenomas typically present in premenopausal women, with peak incidence in the fourth and fifth decades. Although serous cystadenomas are more common than mucinous cystadenomas, accounting for 25% vs approximately 20% of all ovarian tumors, a slightly greater percentage of mucinous tumors (75%-85%) are benign in comparison with serous tumors. Bilateral lesions are relatively uncommon, occurring in only 2% to 3% of patients with mucinous cystadenoma.

The MRI appearance of a mucinous cystadenoma is sometimes distinctive (ie, a multiseptate cystic lesion); however, as in this example, these features are not always apparent. The presence of mucin sometimes alters the signal characteristics of the cystic components of the lesion so that there is lower signal intensity on T2-weighted images and higher signal intensity on T1-weighted images, in comparison to simple fluid, and occasionally variable signal intensity is seen within different locules of the same mass. As is true of most tumors, the presence of solid nodules or papillary projections with significant enhancement is suggestive of a borderline or malignant lesion, and the likelihood of this increases with the proportion of solid tissue.

Ruptured mucinous cystadenomas were once thought to be responsible for a large percentage of pseudomyxoma peritonei. However, the current view is that this complication results almost exclusively from mucinous appendiceal neoplasms.

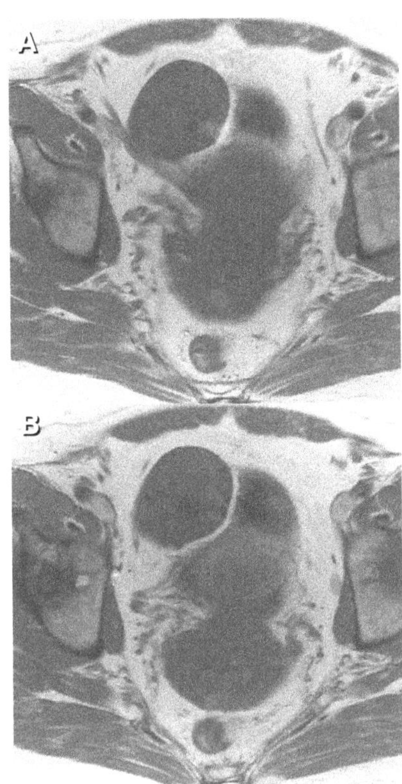

Figure 11.11.1

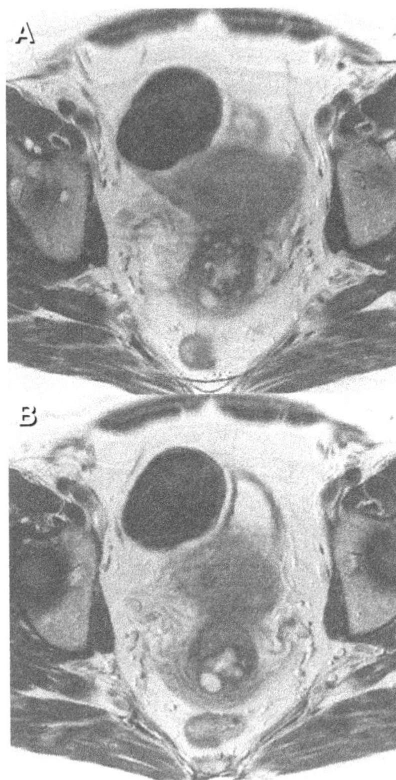

Figure 11.11.2

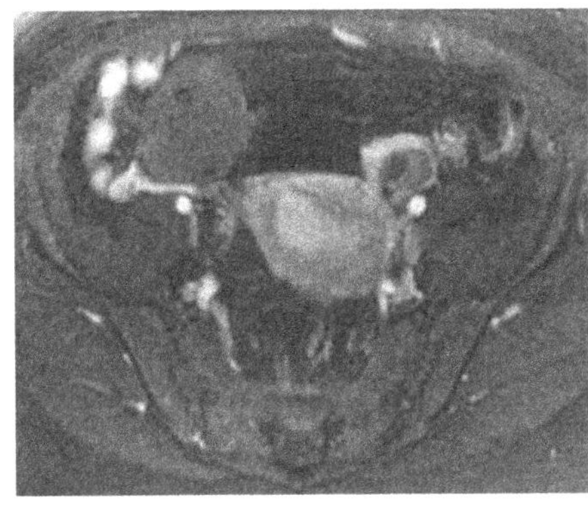

Figure 11.11.3

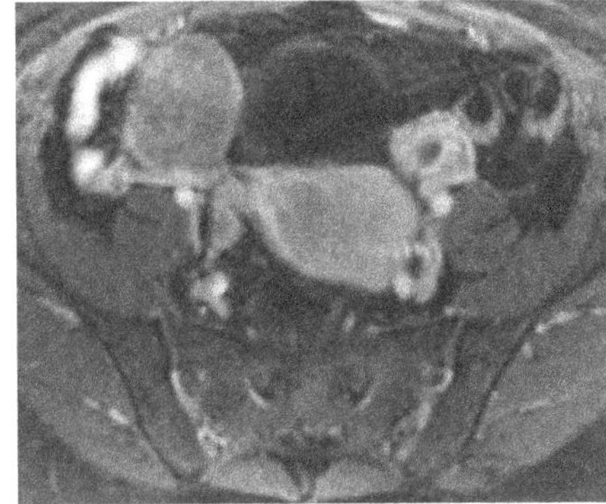

Figure 11.11.4

HISTORY: 50-year-old woman with an ovarian mass incidentally detected on screening CT colonography

IMAGING FINDINGS: Axial FSE T1-weighted (Figure 11.11.1) and T2-weighted (Figure 11.11.2) images demonstrate a low-signal-intensity ovoid mass in the right adnexa anterior to the uterus. Axial arterial phase postgadolinium 3D SPGR image (Figure 11.11.3) reveals minimal early enhancement of the lesion. The mass shows mild diffuse enhancement on a 5-minute delayed axial postgadolinium 3D SPGR image (Figure 11.11.4).

DIAGNOSIS: Fibroma

COMMENT: Fibromas are relatively rare benign tumors, accounting for approximately 4% of all ovarian neoplasms. They are, however, the most common sex cord stromal tumor, as well as the most common solid benign ovarian tumor, and are composed of intersecting bundles of spindle cells embedded in a collagenous stroma. Fibrothecomas are similar lesions, also categorized as benign sex cord stromal tumors, and contain spindle cells with lipid-rich cytoplasm that resemble theca interna cells. They also may have interspersed lutein cells, which can produce estrogen and may occasionally lead to symptoms related to excessive estrogen production, such as irregular bleeding, amenorrhea, and endometrial hyperplasia.

Fibromas can occur in all stages of life but are most common in middle age and appear with similar frequency in pre- and postmenopausal women. Fibrothecomas, by comparison, are much more common in postmenopausal women. Most lesions are asymptomatic and are detected incidentally either during physical examination or on pelvic imaging, but larger lesions can cause abdominal fullness or pain. Fibromas are also associated with Meigs syndrome, which describes the presence of ascites and pleural effusions in association with an ovarian fibroma, as well as Gorlin-Golz syndrome (nevoid basal cell carcinoma syndrome).

This case illustrates the classic appearance of fibromas on MRI: uniform low signal intensity on both T1- and T2-weighted images, with mild enhancement following gadolinium administration. Low T2-signal intensity is of course the defining feature since essentially all ovarian masses, excluding dermoids and endometriomas, have low signal intensity on T1-weighted images. Some of the early papers describing the MRI properties of fibromas were careful to relate the signal intensity of the lesion to an internal reference, usually skeletal muscle, but in reality, this is almost always unnecessary since the distinction is usually obvious to anyone who has looked at a few normal ovaries. Larger lesions tend to be more likely to exhibit atypical features, which may include regions of increased T2-signal intensity, representing both edema and cystic changes.

One of the main differential diagnoses for ovarian fibromas is a pedunculated uterine fibroid. The pedunculated fibroid is a particular problem for sonographers and, in some respects, is a friend of MR specialists since they are probably responsible for a sizable percentage of pelvic MRI referrals. Even so, distinguishing a fibroid from an ovarian mass is not always trivial, since nondegenerated fibroids often exhibit similar low signal intensity on T2-weighted images. This is particularly true when you follow a standard protocol without regard to the location of the mass. A better strategy is to tailor the examination to the lesion and orient the acquisition planes accordingly. Postgadolinium high-spatial-resolution 3D SPGR images are often helpful in delineating the presence or absence of a rim of normal myometrial tissue continuous with the uterus.

Fibromas are benign tumors with an excellent prognosis. Most symptomatic lesions are resected, and a sizable percentage of patients with asymptomatic lesions also have surgery, since the imaging appearance may not be absolutely diagnostic. Case 11.12 illustrates an atypical fibroma that might easily be mistaken for a more serious lesion.

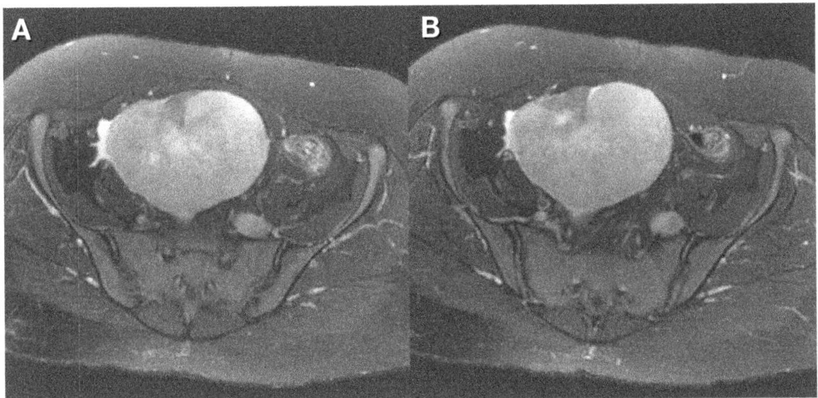

Figure 11.12.1

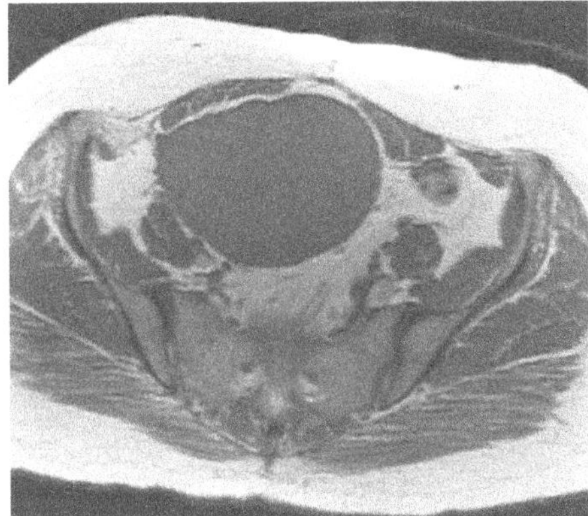

Figure 11.12.2

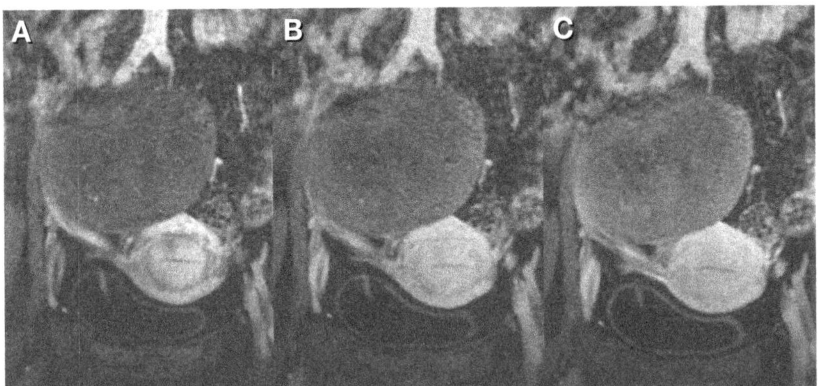

Figure 11.12.3

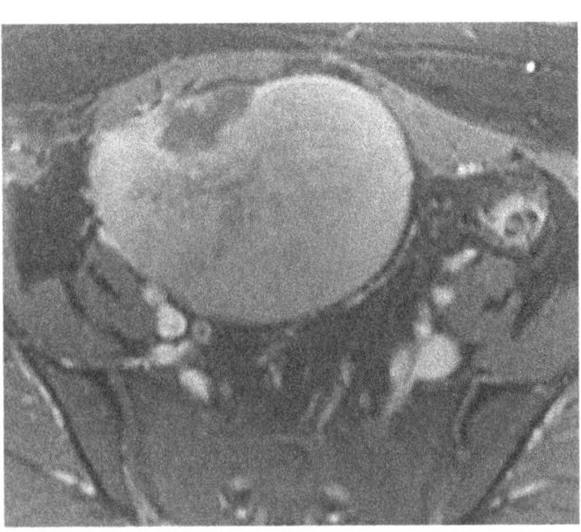

Figure 11.12.4

HISTORY: 46-year-old woman with pelvic pain and dysuria; pelvic US demonstrated an adnexal mass

IMAGING FINDINGS: Axial fat-suppressed FSE T2-weighted images (Figure 11.12.1) demonstrate a large right adnexal lesion with moderately high signal intensity except for a small anterior component. Axial FSE T1-weighted image (Figure 11.12.2) reveals diffusely low signal intensity throughout the mass. Coronal arterial, venous, and 3-minute delayed postgadolinium 3D SPGR images (Figure 11.12.3) show mild enhancement of the lesion, with increasing enhancement on the delayed image. The mass shows intense late enhancement on an axial 8-minute delayed 2D SPGR image (Figure 11.12.4), with the exception of the small anterior region with corresponding low T2-signal intensity.

DIAGNOSIS: Fibroma

COMMENT: This is a companion case to the prior classic fibroma (Case 11.11) and illustrates a lesion with mild heterogeneity and moderately increased T2-signal intensity. The presence of high signal intensity (although more commonly interspersed within a background of low signal intensity) is seen more frequently in larger lesions, as is hemorrhagic and cystic degeneration. The finding of gradual enhancement following contrast administration is not well described in the literature, but in our experience it is a frequent characteristic of fibromas, provided that you wait long enough after contrast administration to see it. Notice how much less impressive the enhancement is on the 3-minute delayed image compared with the 8-minute delayed image.

CASE 11.13

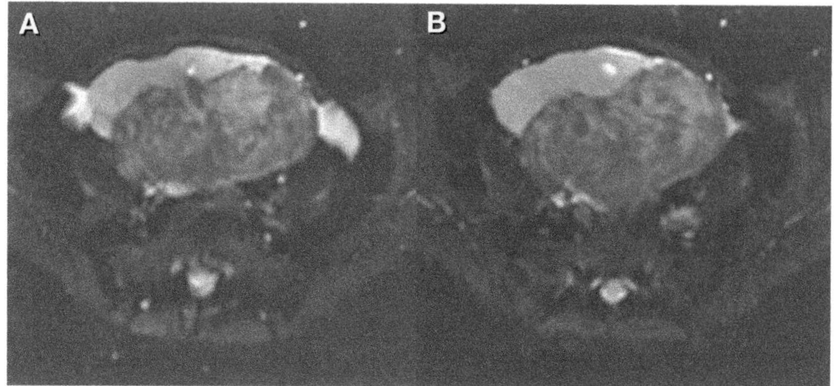

Figure 11.13.1

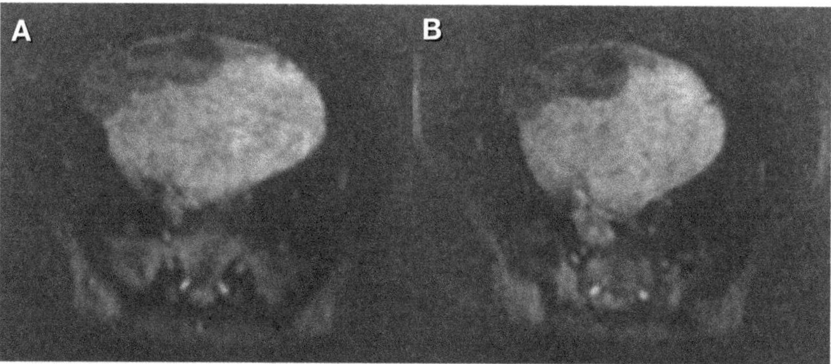

Figure 11.13.2

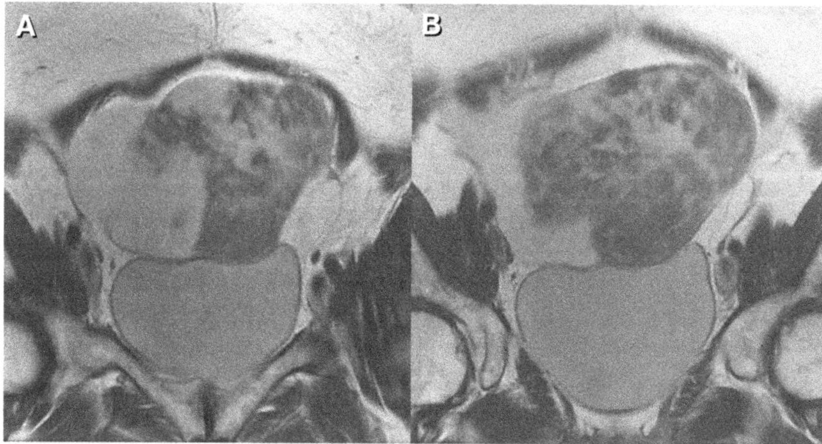

Figure 11.13.3

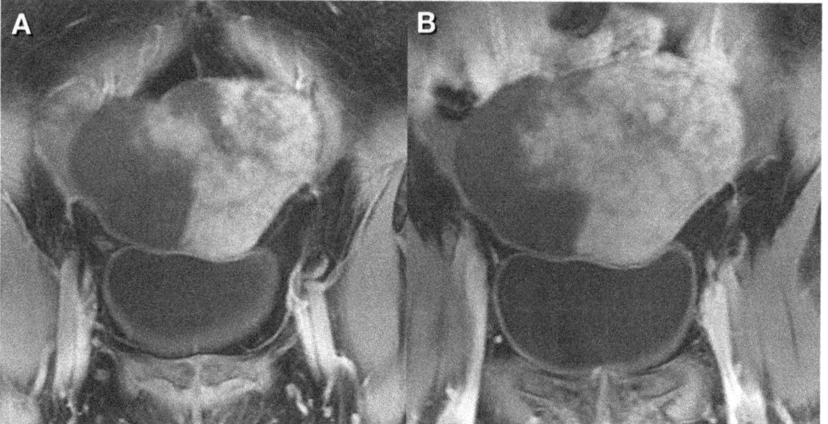

Figure 11.13.4

HISTORY: 54-year-old postmenopausal woman with vague pelvic pain

IMAGING FINDINGS: Axial T2-weighted images from a DWI acquisition (b=0 s/mm^2) (Figure 11.13.1) demonstrate a complex central pelvic mass containing an anterior cystic component, as well as a lobulated posterior solid component with mixed, but predominantly low, signal intensity. Corresponding axial diffusion-weighted images (b=800 s/mm^2) from the same acquisition (Figure 11.13.2) show moderately high signal intensity within the solid component of the mass. Coronal FSE T2-weighted images (Figure 11.13.3) again reveal a cystic and solid mass with both high- and low-signal-intensity components within the solid portion of the lesion. Coronal postgadolinium 2D SPGR images (Figure 11.13.4) demonstrate heterogeneous enhancement of the solid portion of the mass.

DIAGNOSIS: Serous cystadenofibroma

COMMENT: Ovarian cystadenofibromas are rare ovarian tumors that account for approximately 1% to 2% of all ovarian neoplasms. They are derived from both epithelial and stromal components but are classified as epithelial tumors, even though the fibrous stroma is the dominant component. (When the stroma occupies an area greater than the cystic portion, the suffix *fibroma* is added.) These lesions are further subclassified on the basis of epithelial types as serous, endometrioid, mucinous, clear cell, or mixed. The degree of epithelial proliferation also determines whether the tumor is characterized as benign, borderline, or malignant (eg, cystadenocarcinoma fibroma).

Most women are middle-aged at diagnosis, but a wide age range has been reported, and both pre- and postmenopausal women can be affected. Presenting symptoms are vague, generally consisting of abdominal pain, vaginal bleeding, or a palpable mass, and many patients are asymptomatic. Elevated CA 125 levels were reported in 25% of patients in 1 series.

An early paper described a characteristic low signal intensity of the solid component of cystadenofibromas on T2-weighted images, and this finding was recently replicated in the largest reported MRI series of 47 cystadenofibromas. In that study, a solid component was identified in 85% of lesions and low signal intensity in 75% on T2-weighted images, defined as signal intensity similar to or lower than skeletal muscle. In contrast, 2 other recent papers (with smaller numbers) have described discrepant results: The larger of the 2 series found purely cystic lesions with no visible solid components in 50% of cases, and the other paper reported the presence of solid nodules with low T2-signal intensity in only 43% of cases.

Even though there is no firm consensus in the literature regarding how frequently a solid component with low T2-signal intensity is seen in cystadenofibromas, this does seem to be the most reliable and characteristic imaging feature and is demonstrated in this case. This sign is probably most useful in distinguishing cystadenofibromas from ovarian epithelial carcinoma but is not unique to cystadenofibromas, since it is also a characteristic feature of ovarian fibromas, Brenner tumors, and ovarian metastases from gastrointestinal tract tumors.

This case also illustrates the utility of images obtained from DWI acquisitions with a b value of 0 s/mm^2. Our residents sometimes forget that these are actually T2-weighted images that often exhibit superior fat suppression and less motion artifact than corresponding FSE images. The occasional advantage of DWI of b equals 0 s/mm^2 is in part related to the fact that it's very tempting to acquire images in the pelvis without respiratory gating, since the 3 planes of high-spatial-resolution FSE images included in most female pelvis protocols represent a time-intensive proposition. Most DWI acquisitions are single-shot pulse sequences with short acquisition times (and theoretically infinite TRs). These characteristics help to reduce respiratory motion artifact, as well as artifact from peristalsis, which is often only partially eliminated on FSE acquisitions by subcutaneous injection of glucagon or a similar agent.

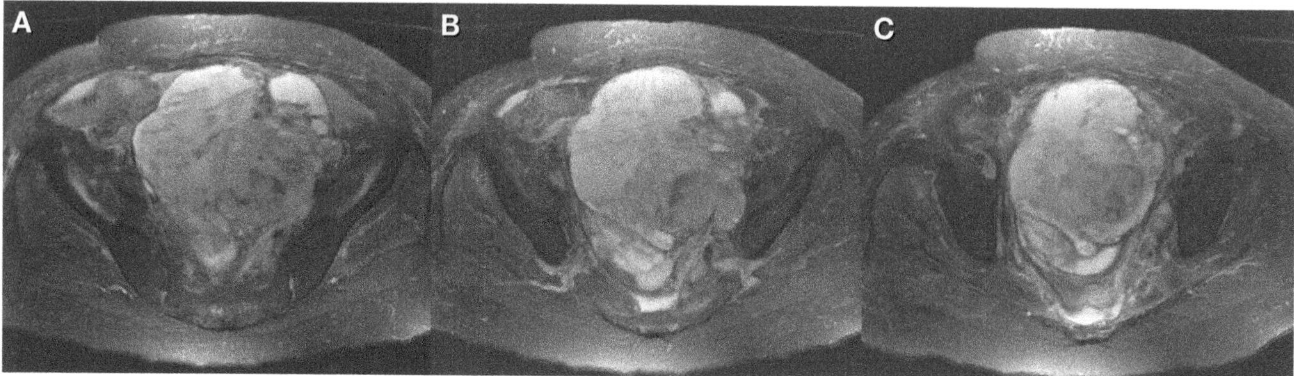

Figure 11.14.1

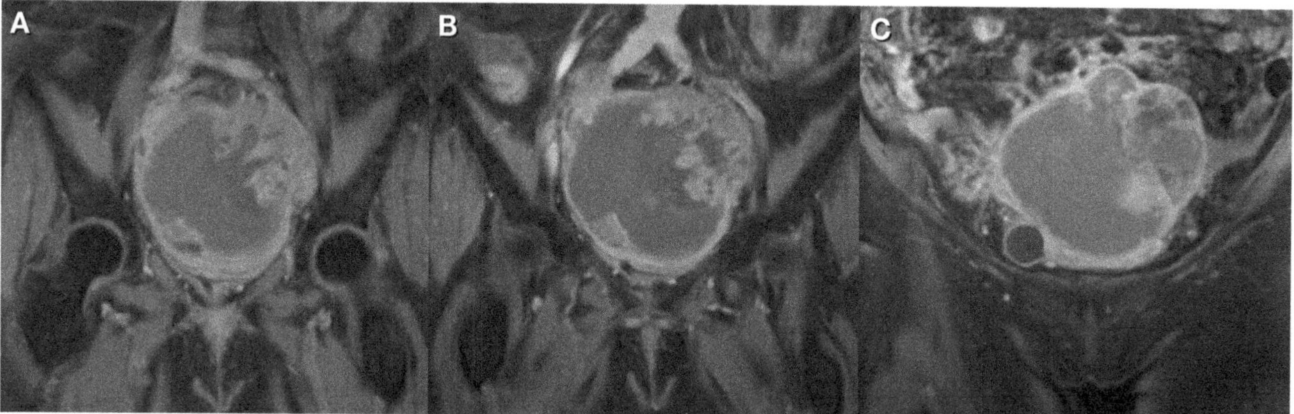

Figure 11.14.2

HISTORY: 82-year-old woman with a distended, mildly painful abdomen and palpable pelvic mass

IMAGING FINDINGS: Axial fat-suppressed FSE T2-weighted images (Figure 11.14.1) demonstrate a large complex mass in the central pelvis containing both cystic and solid elements. Coronal postgadolinium 2D SPGR images (Figure 11.14.2) again reveal a large, predominantly cystic lesion containing prominent mildly enhancing papillary projections. Note the Foley catheter balloon in the collapsed bladder on the most anterior image.

DIAGNOSIS: Papillary serous ovarian cystadenocarcinoma

COMMENT: Ovarian cancer is the leading cause of death from gynecologic cancers, with approximately 15,000 deaths and 22,000 new cases annually in the United States. Ovarian tumors are classified as epithelial, germ cell, sex cord-stromal, or metastatic on the basis of the cell of origin, with epithelial tumors accounting for more than 90% of malignant lesions. Epithelial carcinomas are subdivided into serous, mucinous, clear cell, endometrioid, or transitional (Brenner) tumors on the basis of cell type and are further characterized as benign, borderline, or malignant. Serous cystadenocarcinoma is the most common malignant epithelial tumor, accounting for more than two-thirds of cases, although it is worth remembering that the cystadenocarcinoma's benign counterpart, serous cystadenoma, is also a common lesion and that approximately 60% of serous tumors are benign, 15% are borderline, and 25% are malignant.

To further add to an already confusing picture, serous carcinoma is divided into high-grade and low-grade varieties, which according to the current pathology literature are fundamentally different tumor types and different diseases. Low-grade serous carcinomas are uncommon, accounting for less than 5% of all cases, and are indolent, slow-growing neoplasms most likely resulting from progression of serous borderline tumors beyond microinvasion.

High-grade serous carcinomas represent the most common ovarian malignancy, and recent investigations based on examination of pathologic specimens of women with *BRCA* mutations who had prophylactic oophorectomies suggest that these tumors, rather than arising exclusively from the ovarian surface epithelium, may evolve instead from tubal intraepithelial carcinoma of the distal fallopian tube. Most high-grade serous carcinomas are aggressive, rapidly growing tumors, with 1 study estimating an average doubling time of less than 3 months. This characteristic probably explains the high percentage of women who present with advanced disease and also illustrates one of the difficulties in implementing a cost-effective screening program for women at high risk for ovarian cancer.

Benign adnexal lesions are fairly common (complex ovarian cysts were found in 3% of postmenopausal women in 1 study) and ovarian malignancy is relatively rare. Therefore, it's important to be able to characterize benign disease with a high accuracy, and this is one of the major advantages of MRI. Several benign lesions, including simple cysts or cystadenomas, endometriomas, fibromas, and dermoids, can be characterized with a high degree of confidence. On the other hand, MRI is too expensive to serve as a general screening examination, and so most referrals result from an indeterminate lesion first identified on pelvic US or CT. The second advantage of MRI with respect to US and CT has to do with staging ovarian cancer, and this is discussed in greater detail in Case 11.15.

An effective MRI examination for characterization of an indeterminate adnexal lesion requires several elements, including high-spatial-resolution T2-weighted images in at least 2 planes, fat-suppressed T1-weighted images to identify subacute blood products in endometriomas, and at least 1 set of T1- or T2-weighted images with and without fat suppression to document the presence of fat in dermoid cysts. We use subcutaneous glucagon for all of these examinations, to help reduce motion artifact from peristalsis.

Additional artifact reduction techniques include the use of anterior (covering the subcutaneous fat) and superior saturation bands to minimize artifact from both respiratory motion and peristalsis, and swapping the phase and frequency encoding directions on axial oblique acquisitions (ie, the phase encode direction is right-to-left rather than anterior-to-posterior), which helps to move phase ghosting artifacts away from the ovaries. Respiratory triggering is also an effective technique for minimizing respiratory artifact and should always be considered in cases of refractory motion artifact; however, it can be quite time intensive, particularly when acquiring high-resolution FSE T2-weighted images in 3 planes. DWI is most useful in detecting peritoneal implants, as noted in Case 11.15.

Although many authors have tried to apply apparent diffusion coefficient cutoff values in complex cystic and solid ovarian masses to distinguish benign from malignant lesions, the results have not been particularly impressive. Dynamic contrast-enhanced acquisitions are important to delineate enhancing solid components of ovarian masses. This technique has also stimulated interest among enthusiasts of enhancement curve analysis. The general idea is that malignant lesions show more rapid and intense enhancement than borderline or benign lesions, and additional confidence regarding the diagnosis of a complex ovarian mass can be obtained by either analyzing the general shape of the enhancement curve or establishing cutoff values of associated parameters. Several papers have demonstrated promising results in small series of patients, but the specifics of the acquisition (such as the temporal resolution), as well as the optimal parameters to measure, are all uncertain. It also can be difficult in complex lesions containing multiple papillary projections to identify the most suspicious-appearing portion of the mass for more detailed analysis.

In our practice, most epithelial ovarian carcinomas referred to MRI are unfortunately not diagnostic dilemmas. As in this case, they are large complex lesions containing cystic and solid components, with prominent enhancing papillary projections, mural nodules, and thick septations—all features suggestive of malignancy.

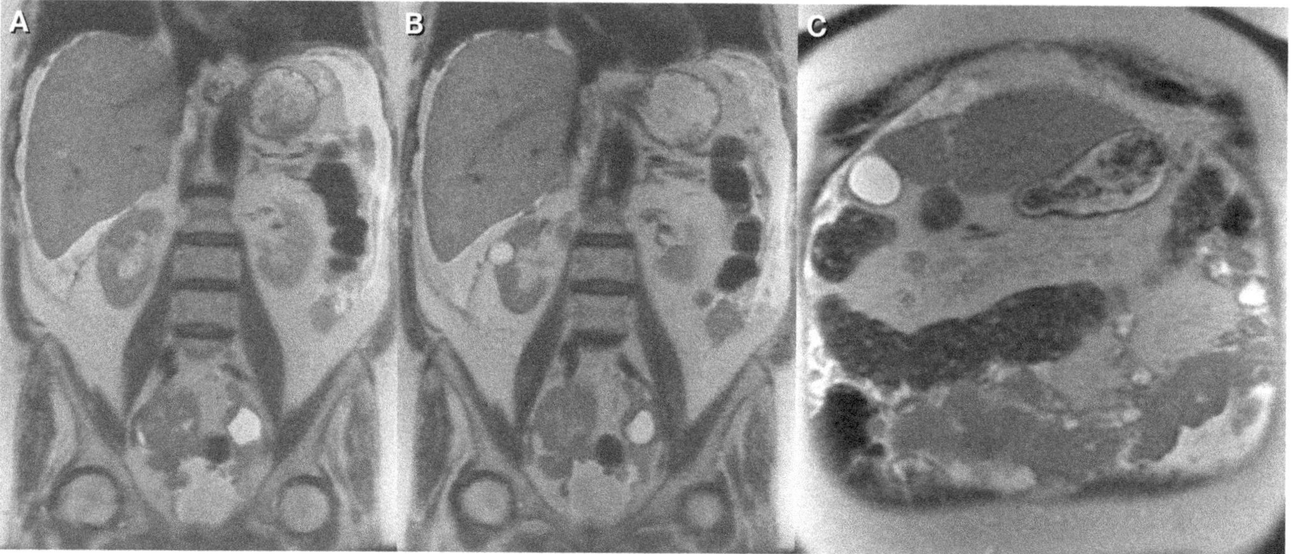

Figure 11.15.1

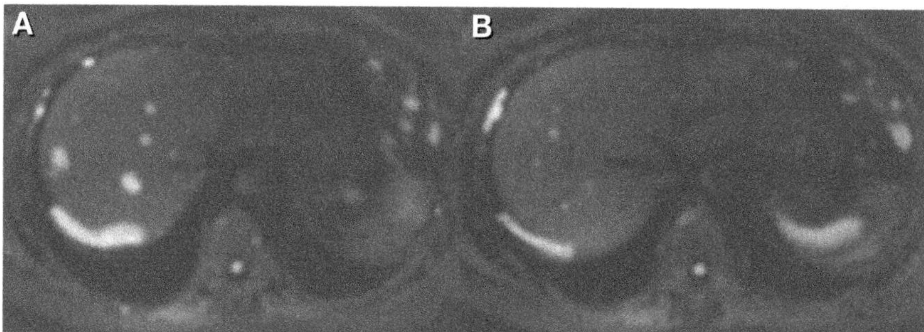

Figure 11.15.2

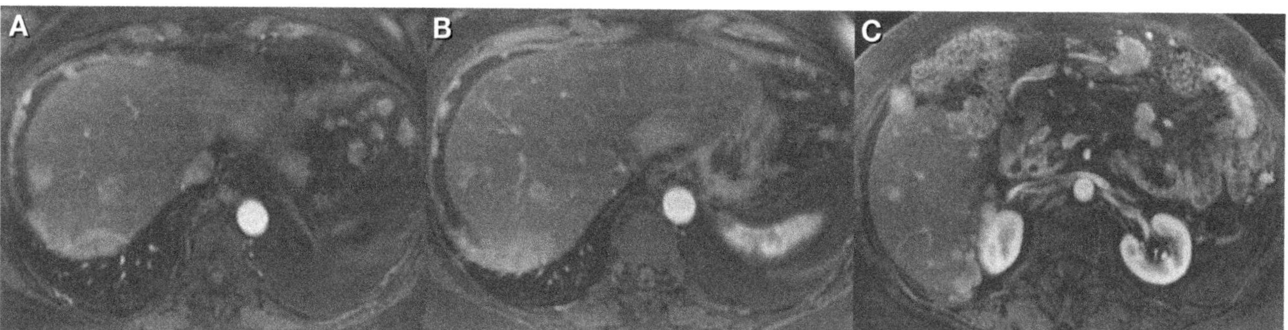

Figure 11.15.3

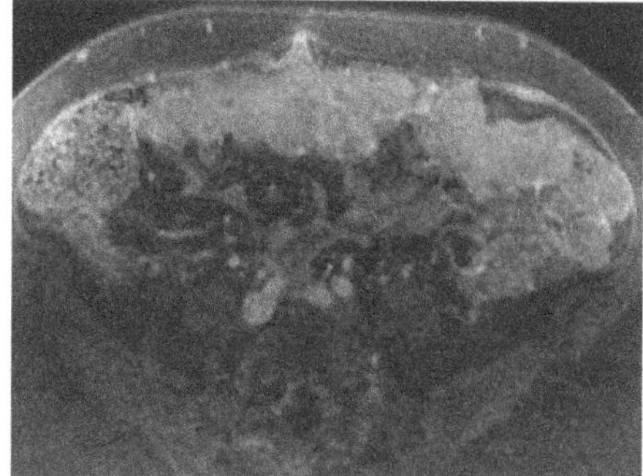

Figure 11.15.4

HISTORY: 70-year-old woman with a history of ovarian carcinoma

IMAGING FINDINGS: Coronal SSFSE images (Figure 11.15.1) demonstrate a large, predominantly solid right adnexal mass, with a simple-appearing cystic lesion in the left ovary. Note the abdominal pelvic ascites and small solid nodules between the diaphragm and liver, as well as confluent omental masses below the transverse colon on the most anterior image. Axial diffusion-weighted images (b=600 s/mm^2) (Figure 11.15.2) reveal multiple discrete and confluent implants along the diaphragm and liver, with several additional nodules in the left upper abdomen, as well as multiple hepatic lesions. Axial arterial phase postgadolinium 3D SPGR images (Figure 11.15.3) demonstrate enhancement of the diaphragmatic and hepatic capsular implants and additional hyperenhancing lesions in the liver. A more inferior venous phase 3D SPGR image (Figure 11.15.4) shows diffuse masslike thickening and enhancement of the omentum.

DIAGNOSIS: Metastatic ovarian serous cystadenocarcinoma with peritoneal, omental, and hepatic metastases

COMMENT: Ovarian cancer is the fifth most common cause of cancer death in women in the Western world and is the most lethal gynecologic cancer. Although survival statistics have been gradually improving, 75% of patients present with advanced disease (stage III or IV), and in these women the 5-year survival rates are relatively poor, ranging from 25% to 37%. These statistics predominantly reflect the course of epithelial ovarian cancers, which account for more than 90% of all ovarian cancers.

Since advanced disease is relatively common at diagnosis, it is important not only to characterize the adnexal mass, but also to assess for extraovarian spread when imaging these patients with MRI. The International Federation of Obstetrics and Gynecology staging system does not include imaging, instead relying primarily on surgical findings, but MRI can be helpful in identifying possible sites of unsuspected disease and in documenting disease in patients who are not able to have staging laparotomy or laparoscopy.

Stage I describes tumors primarily confined to 1 or both ovaries, with stage IC representing capsular rupture, tumor on the ovarian surface, or malignant cells in ascites or peritoneal washings. Stage II is characterized by local extension of tumor to the uterus or fallopian tubes (IIA) or to additional pelvic structures (IIB), with stage IIC representing extraovarian pelvic extension with malignant cells in ascites or peritoneal fluid. Stage III describes peritoneal metastasis outside of the pelvis (microscopic lesions [IIIA], macroscopic lesions [IIIB], and lesions >2 cm or regional nodal involvement [IIIC]). Stage IV represents distant metastases beyond the peritoneal cavity.

The distribution of peritoneal implants is thought to reflect, at least in part, the circulation of peritoneal fluid, with the pouch of Douglas, right paracolic gutter, omentum, and perihepatic space representing frequent sites of metastatic deposits.

MRI is probably more sensitive than CT for detection of small peritoneal implants, and this has to do with the high conspicuity of small lesions on diffusion-weighted and postgadolinium 2D or 3D SPGR images. DWI should be performed with a b value high enough to eliminate the signal from simple ascites (typically, 600-800 s/mm^2), leaving high-signal-intensity implants conspicuous against a dark background, as illustrated in this case. DWI is probably most successful in the upper abdomen and pelvis, where peristalsis is less problematic for imaging. In the midabdomen, motion artifact occasionally results in reduced image quality, even after glucagon administration, because of the relatively long acquisition times required. Postgadolinium 3D SPGR acquisitions with fat suppression are much faster and also provide relatively high contrast to noise ratios between enhancing peritoneal implants and dark pelvic fluid and fat. The relative contrast is somewhat less than what is seen with DWI, but these acquisitions are less artifact-prone and can be obtained relatively quickly in patients who are reasonably good breath-holders. Even though acquisition times are much shorter, peristalsis can still degrade image quality, and so use of antiperistalsis agents is usually a good idea.

Dense omental disease (omental caking), as seen in this case, is usually an easy diagnosis on either MRI or CT. We have seen a few cases where what was in retrospect fairly obvious disease was missed on an abdominal examination ordered to look for or to follow subcapsular hepatic implants. This can happen because 1) the omentum is best seen on sequences that we tend not to pay much attention to, such as the localizer and coronal SSFSE images, and 2) we may not think specifically about the omentum while performing and reading an abdominal examination. For that reason, it's worthwhile to include at least 1 large field-of-view coronal series and 1 axial series extending more inferiorly than usual (SSFSE, SSFP, and 3D SPGR are all good candidates) in patients with ovarian cancer.

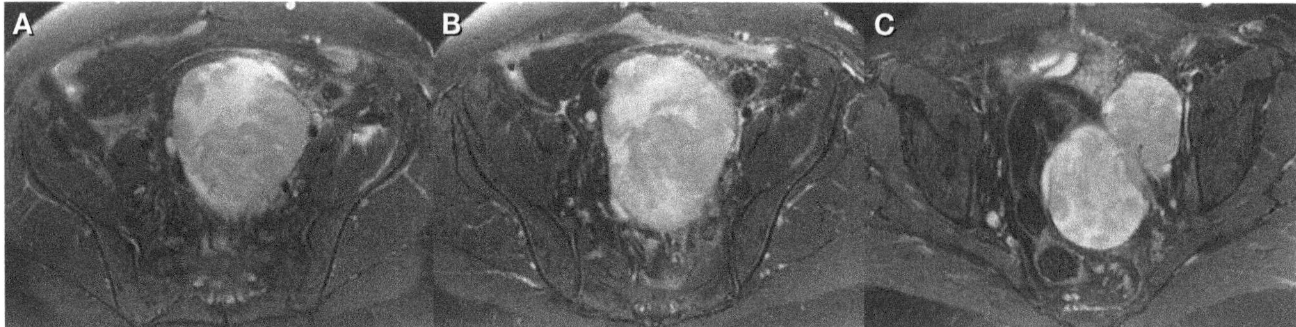

Figure 11.16.1

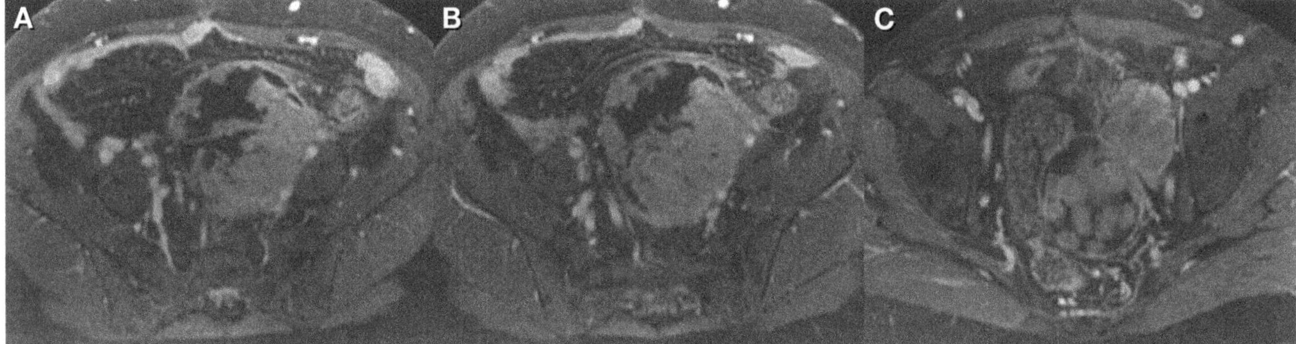

Figure 11.16.2

HISTORY: 57-year-old woman with a pelvic mass

IMAGING FINDINGS: Axial fat-suppressed FSE T2-weighted images (Figure 11.16.1) demonstrate a large heterogeneous mass in the central and right pelvis with regions of high and intermediate signal intensity. Axial postgadolinium 3D SPGR images (Figure 11.16.2) reveal heterogeneous enhancement of the lesion with anterior and inferior cystic or necrotic regions.

DIAGNOSIS: Clear cell ovarian carcinoma

COMMENT: Epithelial ovarian carcinomas constitute 90% to 95% of all cases of ovarian cancer. The epithelial tumors are a heterogeneous group of neoplasms and include serous, mucinous, endometrioid, clear cell, transitional, and squamous cell tumors. Clear cell carcinoma is now recognized as the second most common histologic subtype of the epithelial tumors (and, by extrapolation, the second most common type overall), accounting for 5% to 25% of all ovarian cancers.

Clear cell carcinoma is 1 of the 2 ovarian neoplasms associated with endometriosis (endometrioid carcinoma is the other). This association is fairly common: Several authors now believe that most clear cell carcinomas arise from endometriomas. However, 1 recent study identified endometriosis in only 45% of patients with newly diagnosed clear cell ovarian carcinoma.

Women with clear cell carcinoma present at a younger age than those with serous epithelial carcinoma (the most common ovarian cancer), with a mean age at presentation of 55 years, and also have frequent thromboembolic events (40% of patients in 1 study, and roughly double the rate of serous ovarian tumors). The prognosis of patients with clear cell carcinoma is somewhat ambiguous. A higher percentage of women present with early stage disease (stages I and II) relative to serous ovarian carcinoma, and their survival rates are higher. However, patients presenting with late-stage disease (stages III and IV) frequently have disease resistant to standard chemotherapies and therefore have poor outcomes.

There is little evidence in the literature to suggest that MRI is able to distinguish among the various types of epithelial ovarian cancers with any degree of accuracy; however, it is usually able to distinguish benign from malignant lesions and is generally better in staging disease than CT. This case demonstrates a large heterogeneous pelvic mass with predominantly solid components but also has anterior and inferior cystic or necrotic regions—a typical appearance for an epithelial ovarian malignancy. The large mass containing prominent solid components with at least moderate signal intensity on T2-weighted images leaves little doubt that this is a malignant lesion, and although the ovaries cannot be identified, they certainly represent the most likely site of origin, especially since the patient has had a hysterectomy.

Postgadolinium 3D SPGR images, as well as diffusion-weighted images, are helpful for detecting peritoneal disease, which is illustrated in Case 11.15, and several small studies have suggested that data from dynamic contrast-enhanced images (ie, analysis of enhancement curves and tissue perfusion) may help to distinguish complex benign lesions from malignant tumors and to assess the response of tumors to chemotherapy.

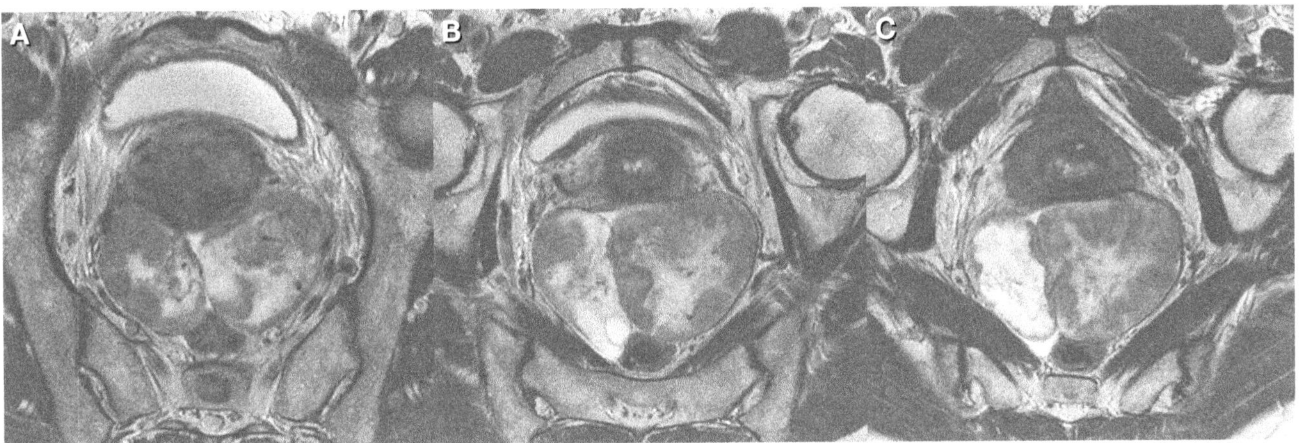

Figure 11.17.1

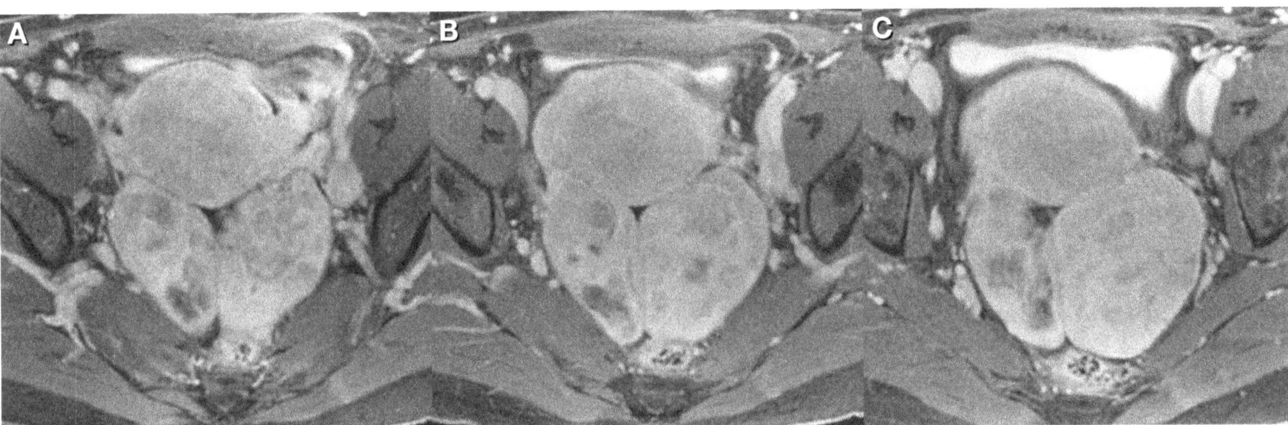

Figure 11.17.2

HISTORY: 51-year-old woman with a 1-month history of increasing lower abdominal pain

IMAGING FINDINGS: Axial oblique FSE T2-weighted images (Figure 11.17.1) reveal enlarged ovaries bilaterally that contain elements of high and low signal intensity, as well as a small cystic component in the inferior right ovary. Axial oblique postgadolinium 2D SPGR images (Figure 11.17.2) demonstrate heterogeneous enhancement of the enlarged ovaries.

DIAGNOSIS: Bilateral Krukenberg metastases from mucinous carcinoma of the appendix

COMMENT: Although the term *Krukenberg tumor* is known by virtually every radiology resident, the precise definition has always been somewhat ambiguous and the term is often used (incorrectly) to refer to any ovarian metastasis.

The first description of Krukenberg tumor in the literature actually predates Friedrich Krukenberg's 1896 paper: James Paget discussed a distinct form of ovarian cancer associated with breast cancer or gastric cancer in 1854, and there are probably several even earlier descriptions. Krukenberg, a student of the pathologist Felix Marchand (who deserves credit for not relegating his student to second author status), described 5 cases of a unique ovarian tumor that he designated a fibrosarcoma and emphasized its occurrence in young patients, the frequent presence of ascites, and bilaterality. The metastatic nature of the tumor was recognized shortly thereafter by several authors, and Wagner in 1902 related the morphologic characteristics of the primary gastric cancer to the appearance of the ovarian lesions and was the first to use the eponym *Krukenberg tumor* in his paper.

The designation of Krukenberg tumor should be reserved for lesions with an appreciable component (>10%) of mucin-producing signet-ring cells and no evidence in support of the diagnosis of a primary ovarian tumor containing signet ring cells, such as clear cell carcinoma. These are relatively uncommon lesions, representing 2% of all ovarian cancers, and account for 30% to 40% of all ovarian metastases. Pathologic distinction between a Krukenberg tumor and a primary mucinous epithelial neoplasm is not trivial, and the validity of many older series describing mucinous ovarian neoplasms is questionable because they likely contain a sizable percentage of metastatic lesions. The majority (76%) of Krukenberg tumors originate in the stomach, and not surprisingly the incidence of Krukenberg tumors reflects the prevalence of gastric carcinoma, which is more common in Japan and less frequent in North America. Colorectal carcinoma accounts for 11% of lesions, with breast, biliary, and appendiceal tumor each responsible for approximately 3%. Signet-ring carcinomas are associated with ovarian metastases more frequently than other carcinomas by a ratio of 4:1, for reasons that are not entirely clear. A fairly high percentage of young women presenting with gastric carcinoma (55% in 1 series) have ovarian involvement.

Most women presenting with Krukenberg tumors are 40 to 50 years old and a majority of them are premenopausal. Symptoms are highly variable; however, those related to the ovarian tumors are usually predominant, since only 25% to 30% of these patients present with a known primary lesion. Abdominal pelvic pain and a palpable mass are fairly common; ascites is present in approximately 50%; and since Krukenberg tumors can cause stromal luteinization and hormone production, uterine bleeding is occasionally seen.

The appearance of Krukenberg tumors on MRI is not distinctive. Bilaterality is probably the most common and most distinctive feature, but undifferentiated and serous primary ovarian carcinomas are also frequently bilateral. Endometrioid and mucinous features in bilateral ovarian tumors, by comparison, are much more likely to represent metastatic rather than primary ovarian neoplasms. Krukenberg tumors are typically well-defined lesions with a heterogeneous internal appearance on T2-weighted images and hypointense solid elements reflecting the presence of dense stromal proliferation, as well as cystic hyperintense mucinous components. Low signal intensity on T2-weighted images is also seen in fibromas and fibrothecomas; however, these are more frequently unilateral and tend to have a more pronounced and uniform hypointense component. Postgadolinium images similarly demonstrate heterogeneous enhancement, often with internal cystic components. One paper has described rim enhancement of intratumoral cysts as a relatively specific, if not sensitive, sign for Krukenberg tumors, although this finding has not been widely replicated and is not apparent in this case.

The prognosis of patients with Krukenberg tumors is generally poor, with median survival of 7 to 14 months.

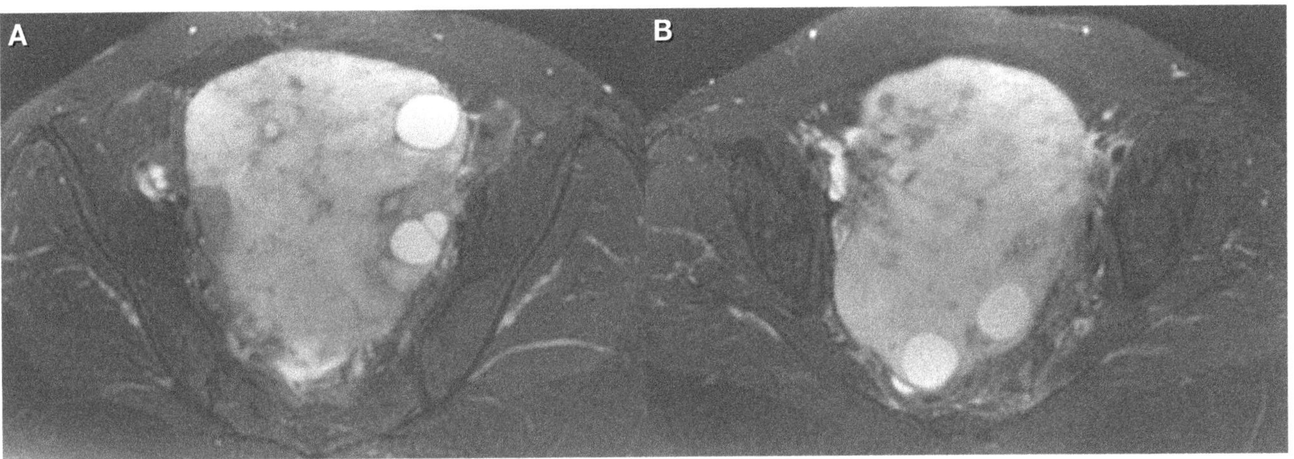

Figure 11.18.1

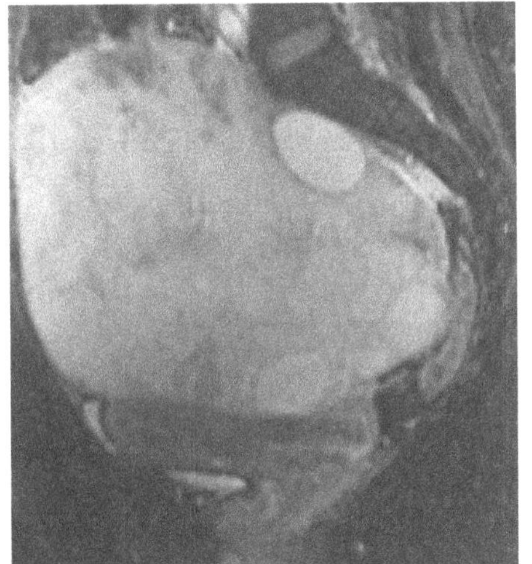

Figure 11.18.2

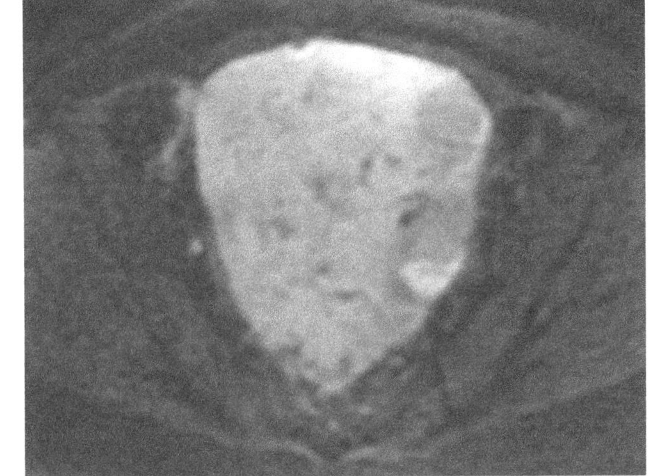

Figure 11.18.3

Figure 11.18.4

HISTORY: 46-year-old woman with history of appendiceal goblet cell carcinoid, resected 3 years previously, who underwent MRI to assess for hepatic metastases

IMAGING FINDINGS: Axial fat-suppressed FSE T2-weighted images (Figure 11.18.1) and sagittal fat-suppressed 2D SSFP image (Figure 11.18.2) reveal a large, mildly heterogeneous mass in the central pelvis superior to the uterus with diffusely high signal intensity and a few scattered cystic components. Axial diffusion-weighted image (b=800 s/mm^2) (Figure 11.18.3) again demonstrates high signal intensity throughout the mass. Axial postgadolinium 3D SPGR images (Figure 11.18.4) show diffuse enhancement of the solid component of the lesion, as well as rim enhancement of the cystic portions.

DIAGNOSIS: Metastatic adenocarcinoma of the appendix with neuroendocrine features

COMMENT: This case is a second example of ovarian metastasis that can also be considered a Krukenberg tumor. The lesion involved only the right ovary at surgery, which is somewhat atypical for Krukenberg tumors. Primary appendiceal cancers are rare, representing 0.5% of all gastrointestinal cancers, which translates into an incidence of approximately 0.12 cases per 1 million people per year in the United States. However, appendiceal tumors do have a propensity to metastasize to the ovaries. One recent study of 48 women with primary appendiceal cancer found a 38% incidence of ovarian metastasis, which was bilateral in 83% of cases. The authors also noted that most of these women presented with symptoms related to their ovarian tumor, the appendix was evaluated intraoperatively in less than half of these cases, and appendectomy or right hemicolectomy was performed in only 16%. Although the deficiencies of gynecologic surgeons always make for entertaining reading, it's only fair to note that these same failings may well apply to radiologic evaluation of ovarian masses—always remember to look for a potential primary tumor in patients with bilateral lesions.

This case provides a better illustration of the rim-enhancing cystic components on postgadolinium images described by 1 group as characteristic of Krukenberg tumors, although a unilateral mass with fairly homogeneous high signal intensity on T2-weighted images is a less classic appearance.

This case also illustrates a dilemma faced by our clinicians when ordering MRIs: The choice between an abdomen and an abdominal-pelvic examination is the difference between 1 or 2 slots on the schedule, which has implications for both the cost of the examination and how soon it can be scheduled. Almost invariably, when an abdominal-pelvic examination is ordered for follow-up imaging of a resected neoplasm, we never see anything in the pelvis, and when only the abdomen is requested, we'll either miss findings in the pelvis entirely or notice them after the patient has left, preventing complete characterization. This case is the rare exception to that rule. The large pelvic metastasis was found on an appropriately ordered abdominal-pelvic examination. However, on retrospective review of the coronal SSFSE images from the abdominal examination performed the year before, a smaller lesion was visible in the pelvis, emphasizing the importance of 1) looking at all images in the examination and 2) paying attention to all the anatomy included.

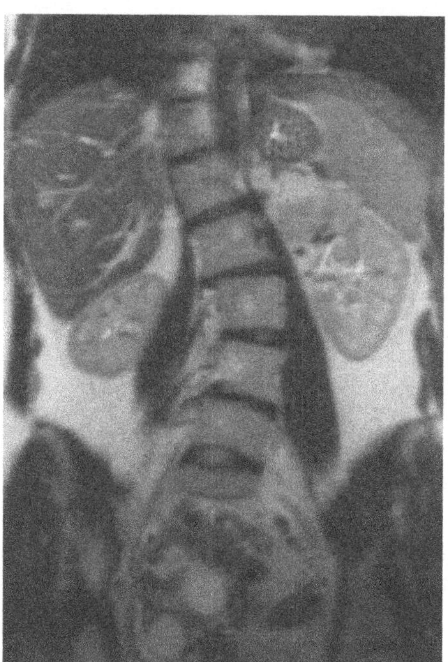

Figure 11.18.5

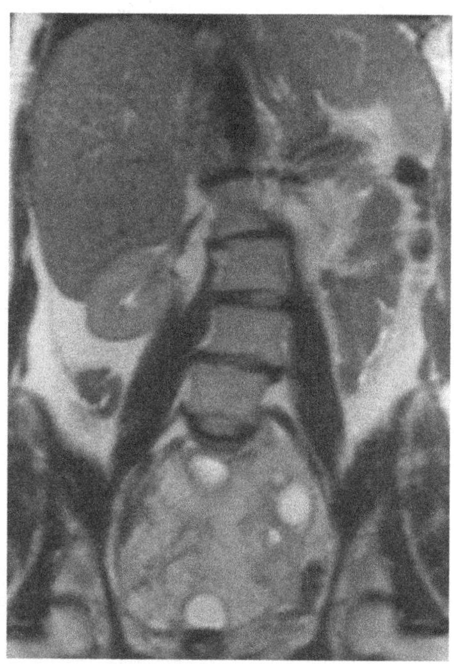

Figure 11.18.6

Coronal SSFSE image from the previous year's abdominal MRI (Figure 11.18.5) and corresponding SSFSE image from the current abdominal-pelvic examination (Figure 11.18.6) of this patient are shown. Notice the loss of signal in the pelvis on the prior examination, resulting from selection of the abdominal portion of the phased array coil. Nevertheless, a right ovarian mass can be visualized.

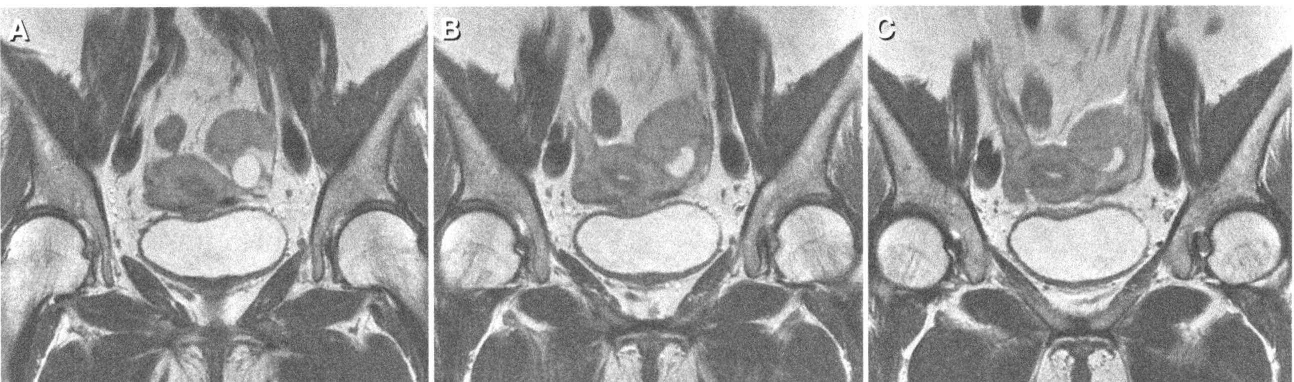

Figure 11.19.1

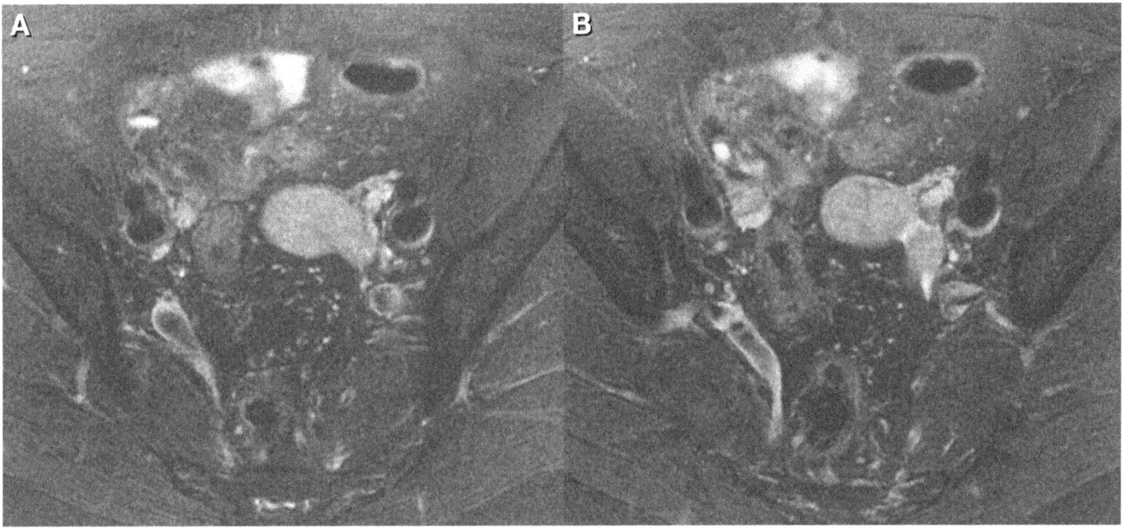

Figure 11.19.2

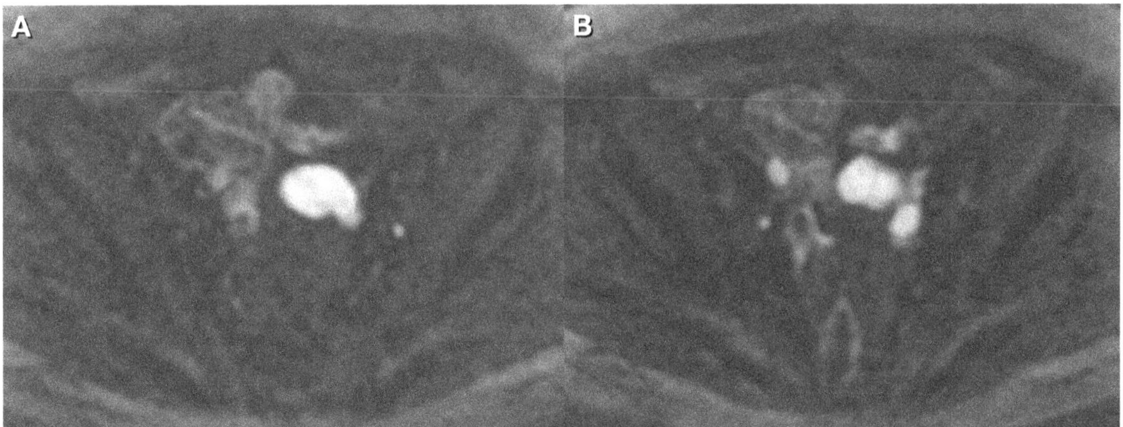

Figure 11.19.3

HISTORY: 53-year-old postmenopausal woman with recently diagnosed breast cancer and 6-month history of bloody vaginal discharge

IMAGING FINDINGS: Coronal FSE T2-weighted images (Figure 11.19.1) demonstrate an ovoid soft tissue mass expanding the ampulla and isthmus of the left fallopian tube, with a small associated cystic lesion adjacent to the isthmus. Axial fat-suppressed FSE T2-weighted images (Figure 11.19.2) reveal similar findings, and axial diffusion-weighted images (b=800 s/mm^2) (Figure 11.19.3) show high signal intensity within the mass.

DIAGNOSIS: Primary fallopian tube serous carcinoma

COMMENT: PFTC is generally considered the least common gynecologic malignancy, accounting for 0.3% to 1% of all tumors; however, recent evidence suggests that it may be much more common and, in fact, may be responsible for most ovarian epithelial carcinomas. This hypothesis is based on pathologic examination of salpingo-oophorectomy specimens from patients with a genetic predisposition to ovarian carcinoma who underwent prophylactic surgery. A high prevalence of fallopian tube in situ or invasive carcinoma was found, rather than the expected ovarian lesions. Other authors have showed that nearly 60% of conventionally classified ovarian carcinomas are associated with tubal intraepithelial carcinoma. PFTC most often arises in the ampulla, and the most common histologic subtype is serous adenocarcinoma, followed by endometrioid and transitional cell carcinoma.

The clinical presentation of PFTC is generally nonspecific. Typically, the patients are postmenopausal and in their sixth and seventh decades, and they may have abdominal pain, vaginal bleeding, or an adnexal mass. Two named clinical signs occasionally show up on written board examinations or as questions in case conferences reserved for the overconfident resident: 1) the Latzko triad, consisting of intermittent serosanguineous vaginal discharge, colicky pelvic pain relieved by vaginal discharge, and an adnexal mass and 2) hydrops tubae profluens, an intermittent vaginal discharge that is spontaneous or caused by pressure, followed by shrinkage of the adnexal mass. Both signs are uncommonly detected (in 5%-10% of patients) and are related to secretion of fluid into the fallopian tube by the carcinoma, which eventually is discharged either into the uterus or peritoneum. CA 125 is a nonspecific marker of malignancy, and elevated levels of CA 125 are found in approximately 80% of patients with PFTC.

Most clinical series of PFTC report that the vast majority of patients receive an incorrect diagnosis before surgery, generally of ovarian carcinoma, tubo-ovarian abscess, or hydrosalpinx or pyosalpinx; the very limited MRI literature suggests that a prospective diagnosis can be made in many patients. The appearance on MRI depends to some extent on the amount of fluid in the fallopian tube, as well as the location of the mass. In the presence of hydrosalpinx, PFTC typically appears as an ovoid or tubular cystic lesion containing an eccentric solid mural nodule or nodules, whereas a solid ovoid or sausage-shaped tubal mass is the predominant feature when hydrosalpinx is absent, as in this case. The solid components generally show mild enhancement following gadolinium administration, typically less than uterine myometrium. Notice also the very high lesion to background contrast on diffusion-weighted images obtained with a b value high enough to eliminate the signal from any adjacent fluid, which would have been more important had this tumor been associated with a prominent hydrosalpinx.

Obviously, the correct diagnosis depends on recognition of the tubal location of the lesion, and this may not always be possible for advanced, complex lesions. However, it is probably true that the multiplanar capabilities of MRI, along with its superior soft tissue contrast, offer the best chance for a correct diagnosis and accurate local staging compared with CT and US.

Prognosis of PFTC is variable but is generally considered better than ovarian epithelial carcinoma, probably because more lesions are diagnosed at an earlier stage. T1 lesions are confined to the fallopian tubes, T2 lesions have pelvic extension, and T3 disease includes metastatic disease beyond the pelvis. Dissemination of PFTC is similar to ovarian carcinoma, occurring principally through transperitoneal shedding of tumor cells that can then implant throughout the peritoneal cavity. Direct invasion of adjacent structures is also fairly common, with hematogenous metastases occurring late in the disease course. Five-year survival rates ranging from 22% to 57% have been reported.

ABBREVIATIONS

CA 125	cancer antigen 125
CT	computed tomography
DWI	diffusion-weighted imaging
FSE	fast-spin echo
IP	in-phase
IP/OP	in-phase and out-of-phase
MR	magnetic resonance
MRI	magnetic resonance imaging
OP	out-of-phase
PCOS	polycystic ovary syndrome
PFTC	primary fallopian tube carcinoma
SPGR	spoiled gradient-recalled echo
SSFP	steady-state free precession
SSFSE	single-shot fast-spin echo
3D	3-dimensional
2D	2-dimensional
TR	repetition time
US	ultrasonography

12.

MALE PELVIS

CASE 12.1

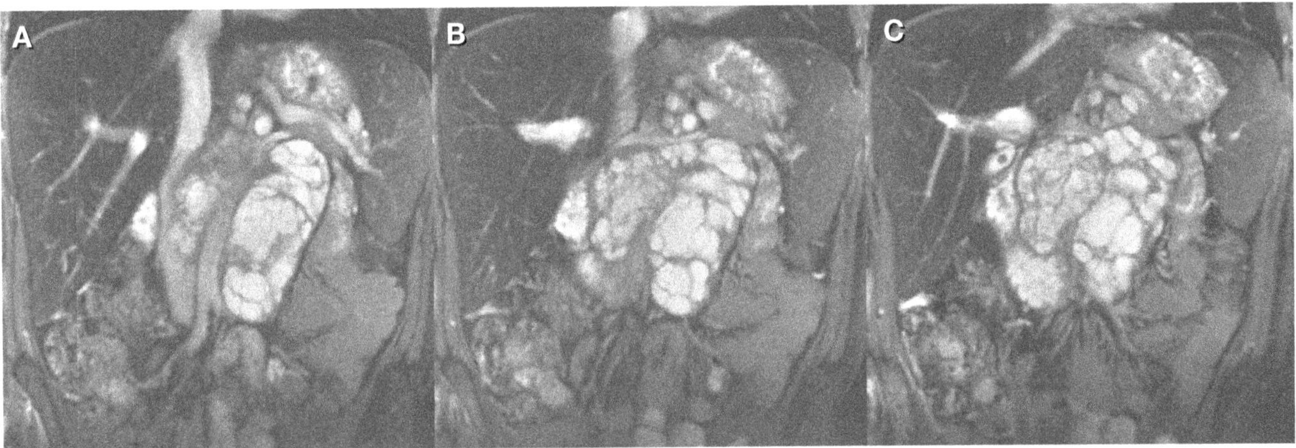

Figure 12.1.1

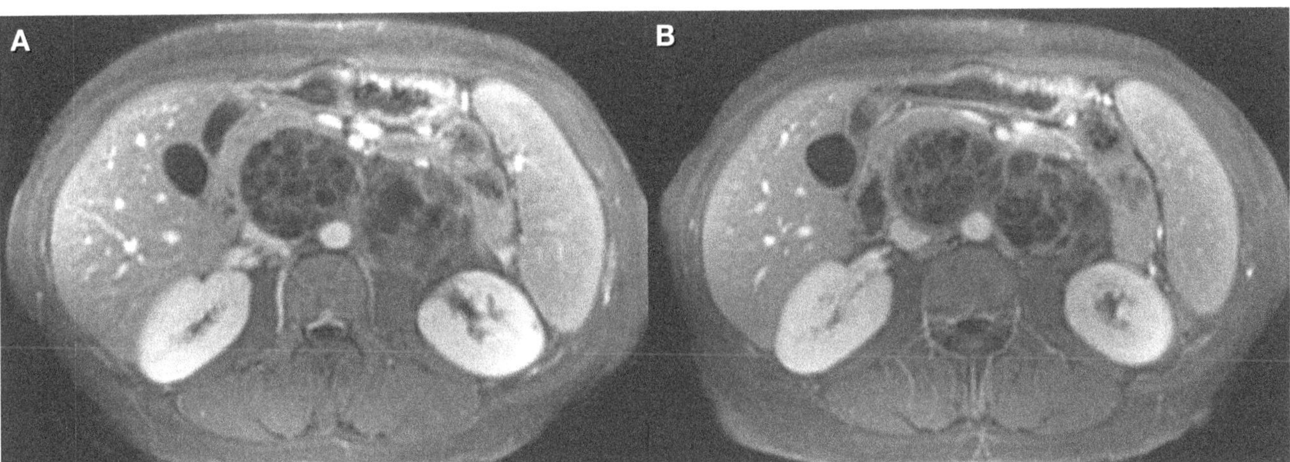

Figure 12.1.2

HISTORY: 36-year-old man with a history of previous orchiectomy for testicular carcinoma

IMAGING FINDINGS: Coronal fat-suppressed 2D SSFP images (Figure 12.1.1) reveal large, septated, predominantly cystic retroperitoneal masses in the periaortic and aortocaval regions of the midabdomen. Axial postgadolinium 3D SPGR images (Figure 12.1.2) demonstrate multiple prominent septations with mild enhancement.

DIAGNOSIS: Metastatic testicular carcinoma (mixed germ cell tumor)

COMMENT: Testicular cancer accounts for approximately 1% of all cancers in men; however, it is the most common solid tumor in young men between the ages of 15 and 35 years. Germ cell tumors constitute 95% of all testicular cancers, and they are divided evenly between seminomas and nonseminomatous germ cell tumors. Advances in treatment (largely involving chemotherapy) have dramatically improved survival among patients with testicular cancer and metastatic disease, with overall survival rates greater than 90% for all stages.

Of the nonseminomatous testicular carcinomas, mixed germ cell tumors containing more than 1 germ cell component are much more common than any of the pure histologic forms and constitute 32% to 60% of all germ cell tumors. Essentially all combinations of the different cell types can occur; however, embryonal carcinoma is the most common component, in combination with teratoma, seminoma, and yolk sac tumors.

Testicular carcinomas tend to spread initially via the lymphatic system rather than hematogenously. This accounts for the classic appearance of massive retroperitoneal adenopathy at the level of the renal hila in patients with metastatic disease, since the testicular lymphatics follow the course of the testicular veins, which normally drain into the left renal vein and inferior vena cava. The observation that patients with testicular carcinoma often have nodal masses with strikingly low attenuation was reported fairly early in the CT literature, and the MRI correlate of this can be seen in this case, in which the lesions are almost entirely cystic and show little enhancement. This appearance at least partially reflects another interesting feature of germ cell tumors, namely that their metastases can have different histologic characteristics from the primary tumor, reflecting their totipotential nature.

It is not uncommon for germ cell tumor metastases to evolve into mature teratomas, in which cystic components feature prominently, and this transformation can also occur in response to chemotherapy. Several authors have examined the histologic features of retroperitoneal nodes resected after treatment and have found that roughly 40% of the nodes became necrotic, 40% evolved into mature teratomas, and 20% contained residual tumor (all these components were found in this patient at surgery). There is no convincing evidence that either MRI or CT is particularly effective for distinguishing between necrotic nodes, teratomas, and viable tumor, and so most treatment protocols call for resection of retroperitoneal masses after chemotherapy, which is not always a trivial operation. (Even if you could make this distinction, teratomas would still need to be removed, since they have the potential to differentiate into a more aggressive tumor.)

The differential diagnosis for cystic nodal masses in the retroperitoneum is fairly short, and testicular carcinoma should definitely be at the top of the list for a young male patient. Other more esoteric possibilities include tuberculosis, treated lymphoma, and squamous cell carcinoma.

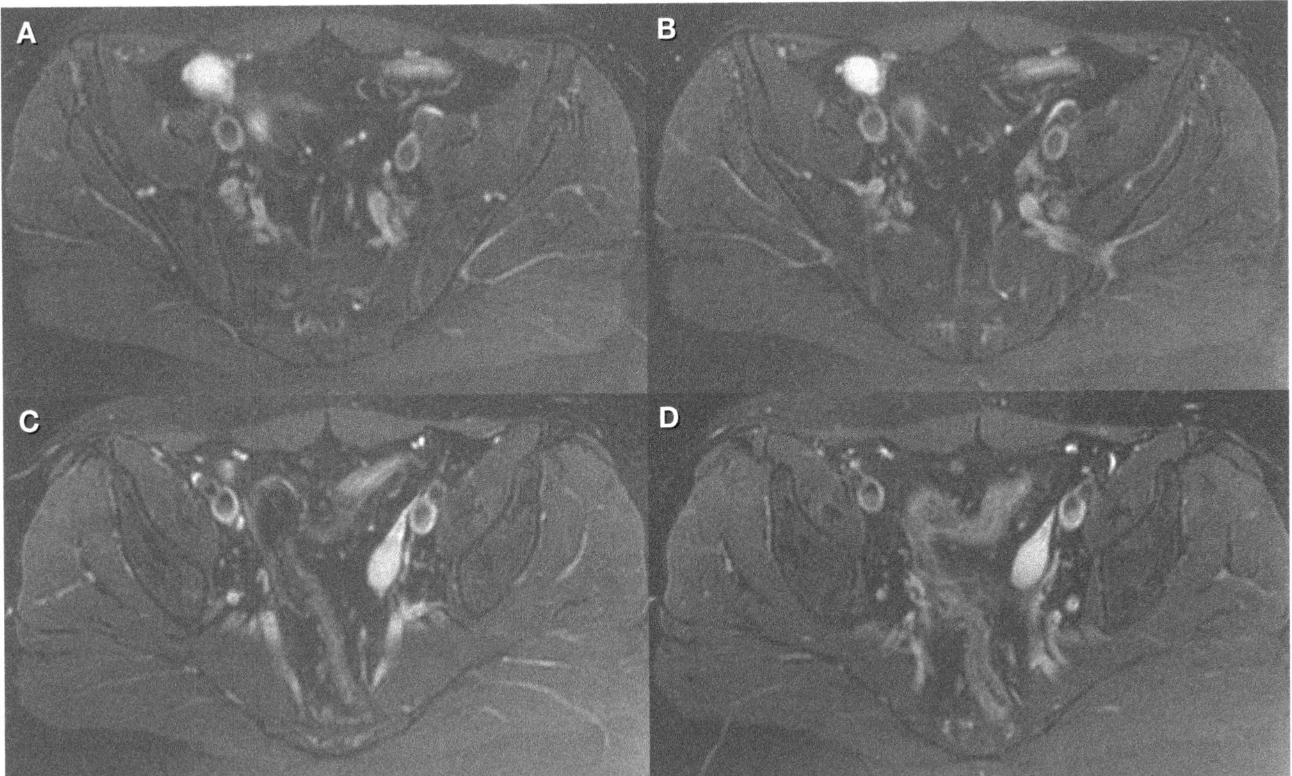

Figure 12.2.1

HISTORY: 32-year-old man with infertility and azospermia

IMAGING FINDINGS: Axial fat-suppressed FSE T2-weighted images (Figure 12.2.1) reveal 2 ovoid hyperintense structures in the anterior right pelvis and lateral left pelvis.

DIAGNOSIS: Bilateral undescended testicles

COMMENT: Cryptorchidism is the most common genitourinary anomaly in male infants, occurring in 1% to 3% of term infants and in up to 30% of premature infants. Boys with cryptorchidism are at increased risk for infertility and testicular cancer, with the incidence of both complications increasing the longer the testicle remains undescended; therefore, orchiopexy is generally recommended at 12 months of age.

An undescended testis may be found adjacent to the kidney or anywhere else along the path of testicular descent into the scrotum; occasionally, it appears in ectopic locations. With careful physical examination, an undescended testis may be found at or distal to the internal inguinal ring in 70% of cases. Regardless of whether the undescended testis is palpable or not, all boys with cryptorchidism require surgery to retrieve a viable testicle to the scrotum and to remove nonviable testicular tissue. The surgical literature reports sensitivities and specificities of nearly 100% for laparoscopic localization of a testis or confirmation of its absence, and so the utility of imaging in these cases is far from clear. US is frequently requested by pediatricians before surgery, in spite of a meta-analysis reporting net sensitivity of 45% and specificity of 78% for correctly identifying a nonpalpable testis. MRI fares a little better, with most articles reporting sensitivities and specificities ranging from 80% to 95% (a discrepant article did report a much lower sensitivity of 43%, although interestingly there were no radiologist coauthors).

At first glance, it may seem somewhat surprising that MRI is not almost perfect in detecting the undescended testicle (and it is true that the techniques used by most authors could have been improved), but keep in mind the general problem of imaging the infant, particularly one who is sedated and not anesthetized. The small size of the patient (and the very small size of the object of interest) means that high spatial resolution is required, generally with a higher number of signal averages to maintain an adequate SNR, thereby increasing the opportunity for motion artifact. There are currently no governmental or societal guidelines recommending imaging as a part of the diagnosis and treatment algorithm for cryptorchidism. (We generally don't put much stock in the recommendations of such committees, whose members often approach their work through the strong bias of their academic orientations—except, of course, when we agree with them.)

That being said, a more reasonable argument for imaging could probably be made for the rare adult patient (such as in this case) with cryptorchidism, where the territory to be explored laparoscopically is much larger and the probability of additional complications (eg, a testicular mass or other related or unrelated pathology) is much higher. Also, MRI of the cooperative adult patient is a much easier proposition, and the odds of successful detection of an undescended testicle are probably higher. In this case, the diagnosis is obvious on a simple fat-suppressed FSE T2-weighted acquisition, where the testicles appear as bright ovoid structures. If these initial attempts are unsuccessful, additional techniques to consider include DWI (the undescended testicle will show high signal intensity against a dark background) or 3D FSE or SSFP acquisitions with high spatial resolution.

CASE 12.3

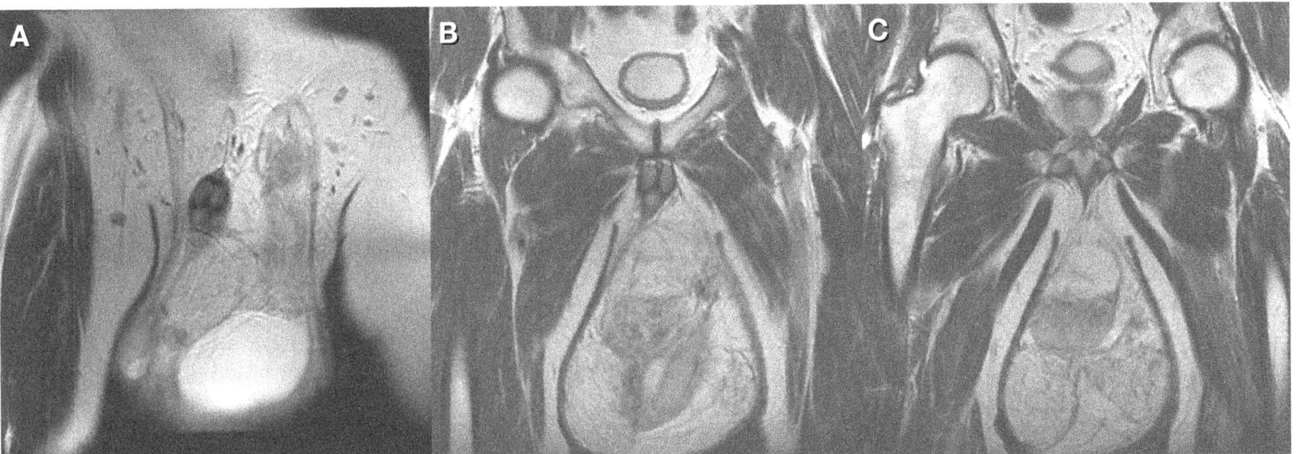

Figure 12.3.1

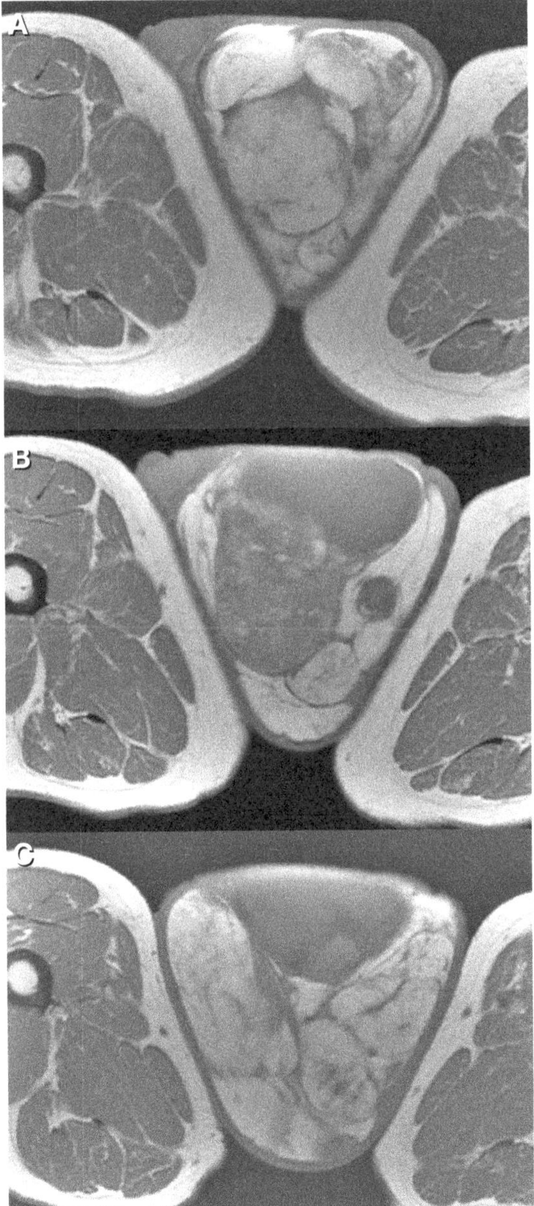

Figure 12.3.2

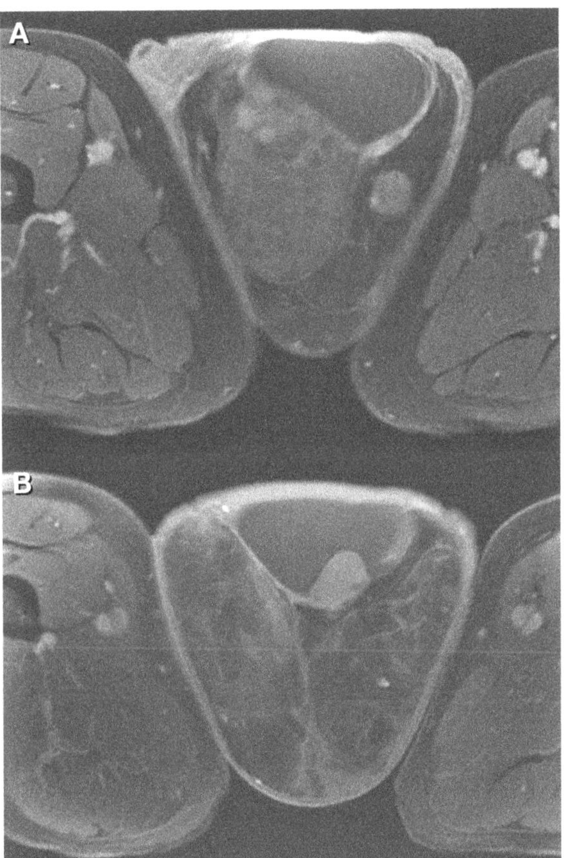

Figure 12.3.3

HISTORY: 73-year-old man with a gradually enlarging scrotal mass

IMAGING FINDINGS: Coronal T2-weighted FSE images (Figure 12.3.1) demonstrate a complex predominantly fatty scrotal mass with prominent septations as well as a nodular nonfatty central component and a small hydrocele. Note that the lesion extends superiorly into the inguinal canal. Axial FSE T1-weighted images (Figure 12.3.2) reveal similar findings. Axial postgadolinium 2D SPGR images (Figure 12.3.3) demonstrate mild enhancement of the scrotal lesion with a few small enhancing nodules.

DIAGNOSIS: Spermatic cord liposarcoma (dedifferentiated)

COMMENT: Spermatic cord liposarcomas are rare lesions, with approximately 200 cases described in the literature. Most patients are middle-aged or elderly, although liposarcomas have been reported to occur in male patients as young as 16 years. Liposarcomas are the most common soft tissue sarcoma and can occur anywhere in the body; however, the spermatic cord is a rare location and is thought to account for approximately 0.1% of all lesions.

Spermatic cord liposarcomas typically grow below the external inguinal ring and therefore more frequently present as a scrotal rather than an inguinal mass, although several have been discovered during surgery for what was intended to be an inguinal hernia repair.

Liposarcomas are classified into 5 categories: well differentiated, dedifferentiated, myxoid, pleomorphic, and mixed. Well-differentiated tumors are low-grade neoplasms with no metastatic potential. Dedifferentiated lesions do have metastatic potential, the likelihood of which depends on the amount and histologic grade of the dedifferentiated components.

The treatment of choice is radical orchiectomy with high ligation of the spermatic cord. The prognosis is excellent for well-differentiated tumors and poor for the less common high-grade lesions with high metastatic potential, but all lesions have a propensity for local recurrence, with reported rates ranging from 25% to 70%.

Diagnosis may be relatively simple, as in this case, or extremely difficult, as in the setting of a nearly homogeneous fatty lesion that is indistinguishable from a simple lipoma, which is one of the most common scrotal-inguinal masses. A fat-containing lesion (ie, a true mass rather than herniated fat) involving the inguinal canal or scrotum is either a lipoma or a liposarcoma with a few rare exceptions. In this case, the presence of numerous thick septations and enhancing soft tissue nodules makes the diagnosis of liposarcoma much more likely than lipoma. When imaging any potentially fatty lesion, it is important to include a combination of T1- or T2-weighted images with and without fat suppression to document the presence of macroscopic fat.

Spermatic cord liposarcomas, while rare, nevertheless comprise 10% to 20% of all malignant extratesticular scrotal tumors. Other lesions that occur in this region and could be considered in the differential diagnosis (but which do not contain fat) include lymphoma, malignant fibrous histiocytoma, and mesothelioma.

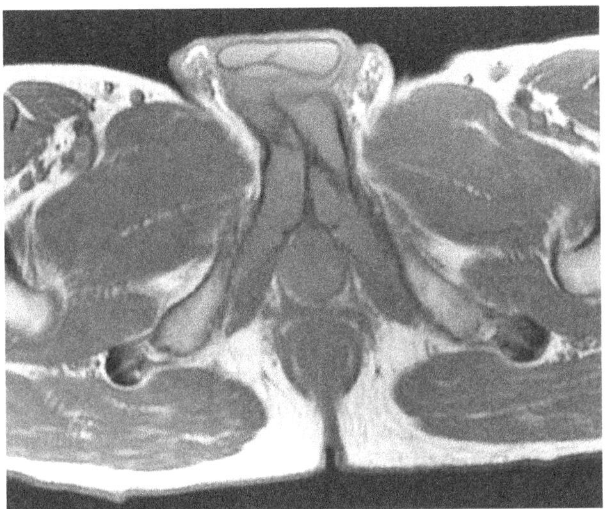

Figure 12.4.1

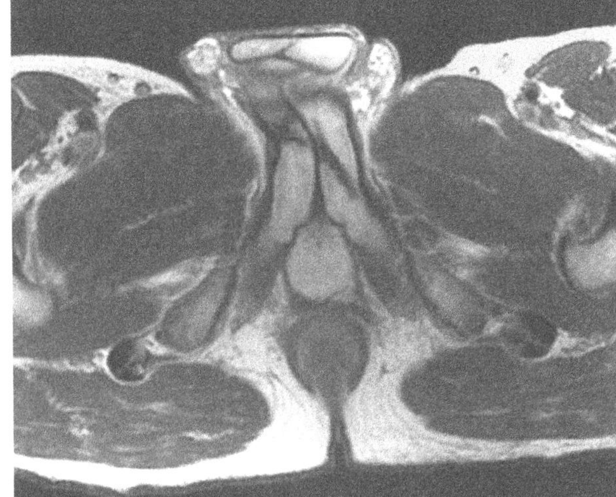

Figure 12.4.2

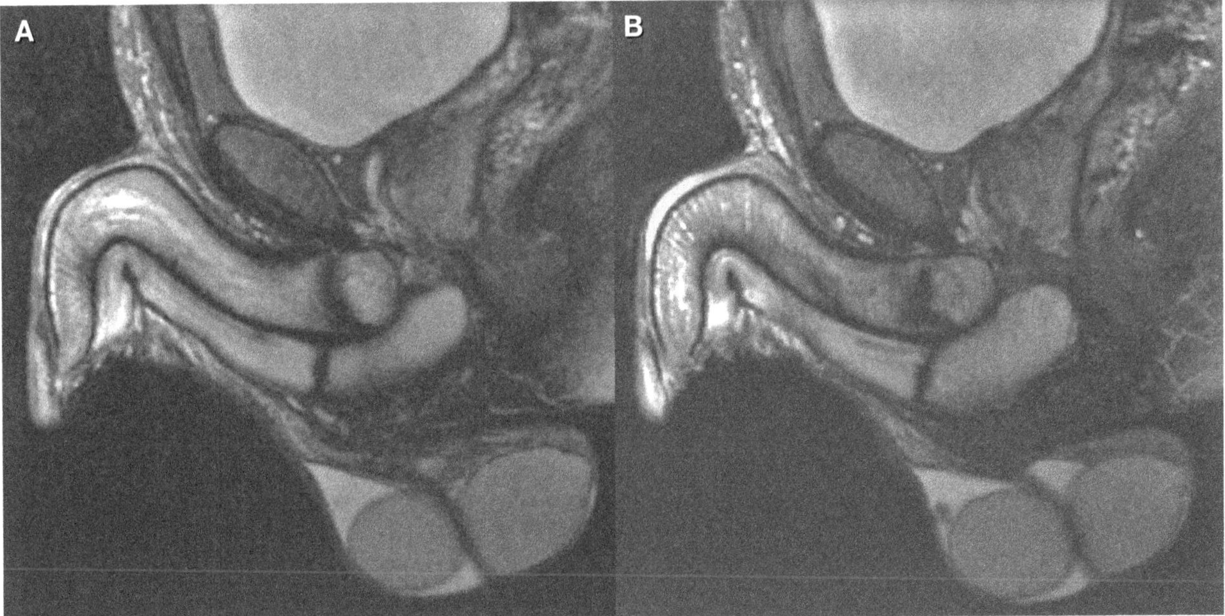

Figure 12.4.3

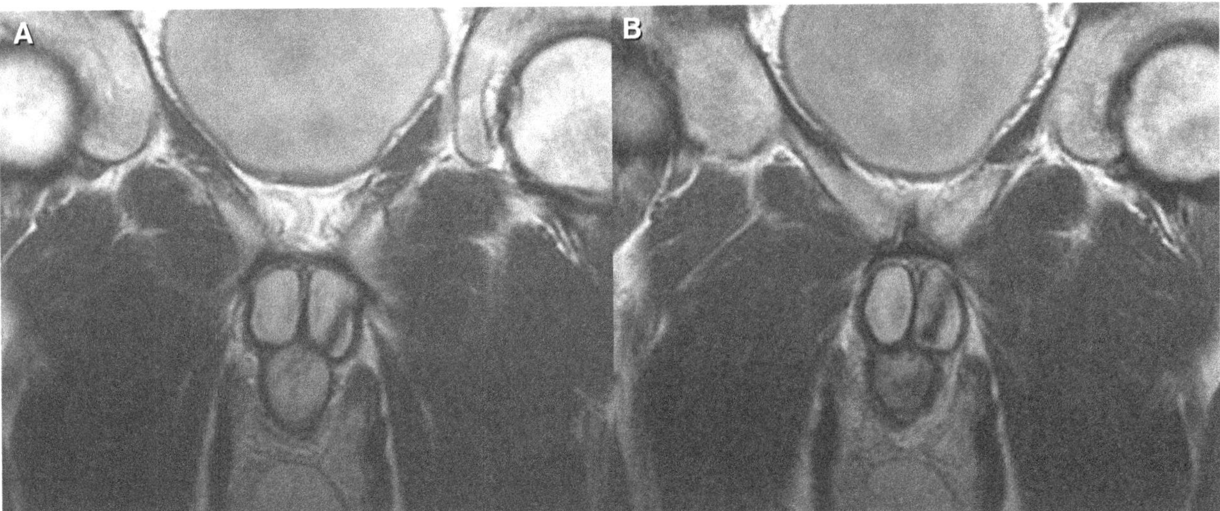

Figure 12.4.4

HISTORY: 41-year-old man with previous pelvic trauma, now with erectile dysfunction

IMAGING FINDINGS: Axial FSE T1-weighted (Figure 12.4.1) and T2-weighted (Figure 12.4.2) images demonstrate a hypointense linear defect crossing the corpora cavernosa of the proximal penis. Sagittal (Figure 12.4.3) and coronal (Figure 12.4.4) FSE T2-weighted images show similar findings and also demonstrate involvement of the corpus spongiosum.

DIAGNOSIS: Penile straddle injury

COMMENT: MRI is used infrequently for patients who have penile injuries, with the occasional exception of penile fracture, a rare traumatic injury that usually results in unilateral rupture of the tunica albuginea and occurs most frequently during sexual intercourse. Identification of focal disruption of the low-signal-intensity tunica albuginea with MRI can confirm the diagnosis in difficult cases and may aid in surgical planning.

In this case, the injury occurred several years earlier; however, disruption of the tunica albuginea was not confirmed and the patient was managed conservatively. The finding of a low-signal-intensity linear band crossing the corpora cavernosa and spongiosum at the site of the patient's prior straddle injury indicates fibrosis, and this is likely responsible for his erectile dysfunction.

The most common cause of penile fibrosis is Peyronie disease, which typically manifests with erectile dysfunction, penile curvature, and a palpable plaque in the tunica albuginea or corpora cavernosum (or both). These plaques also appear as low-signal-intensity foci on both T1- and T2-weighted images, although occasionally postgadolinium enhancement, which is thought to indicate active inflammation, may be seen. The signal abnormalities in this case have a linear nature that corresponds to the site of prior injury and are much more consistent with posttraumatic scarring than with Peyronie disease, in which the plaques tend to be distributed more randomly.

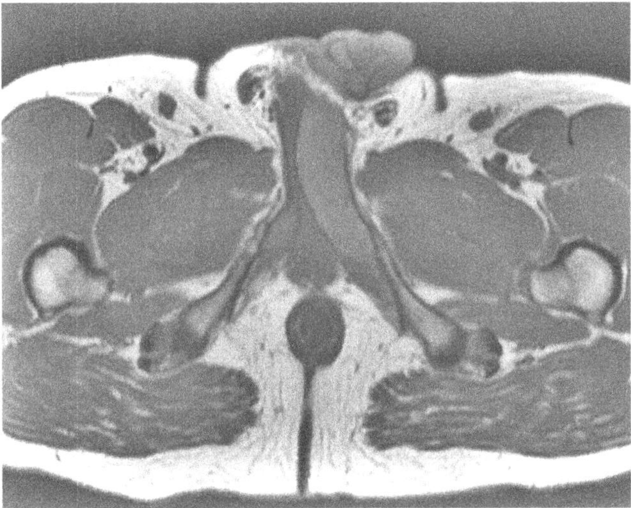

Figure 12.5.1

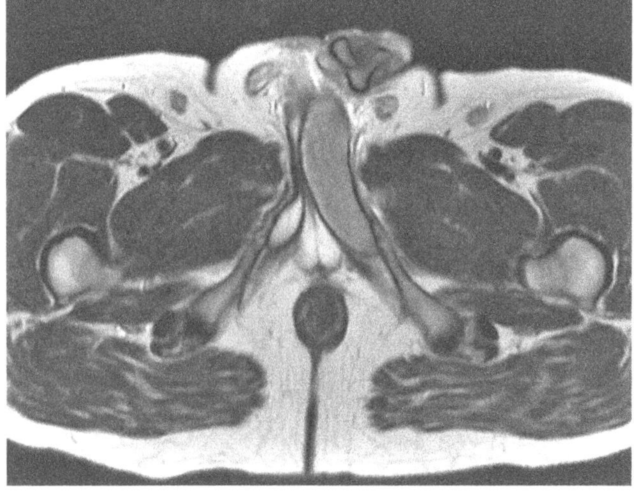

Figure 12.5.2

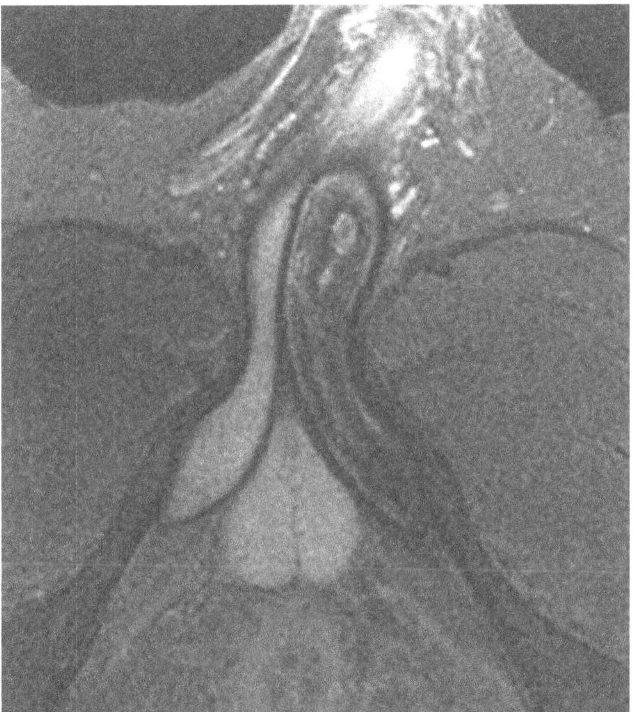

Figure 12.5.3

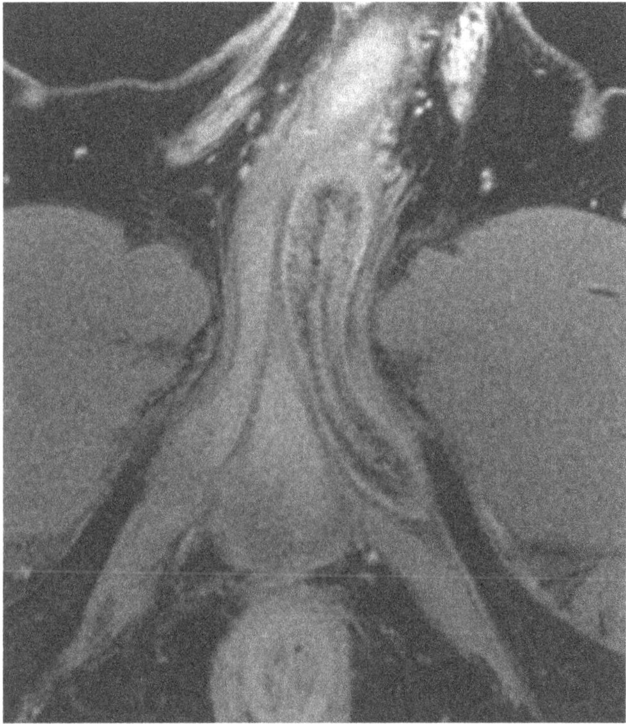

Figure 12.5.4

HISTORY: 49-year-old man with mild pain and a palpable abnormality at the base of the penis

IMAGING FINDINGS: Axial T1-weighted (Figure 12.5.1) and T2-weighted (Figure 12.5.2) FSE images demonstrate homogeneous focal expansion of the left corpora cavernosum at the base of the penis with increased T1-signal intensity and decreased T2-signal intensity in relation to the normal cavernosal signal. Axial fat-suppressed T2-weighted FSE image (Figure 12.5.3) and axial postgadolinium 2D SPGR image (Figure 12.5.4) from an examination performed 3 months later demonstrate interval evolution of the lesion, which now has a prominent rim of low signal intensity.

DIAGNOSIS: Corpora cavernosum hematoma

COMMENT: The cause of this patient's lesion remains a mystery. He was initially thought to have a clotting disorder, but further investigation revealed no abnormality, and he could not recall a history of trauma that could explain development of a hematoma. Either a spontaneous hematoma or a cavernosal infarct or thrombosis could account for the imaging appearance, and 2 urologists postulated 1 or the other explanation. A third urologist at another medical facility decided that the lesion was actually a mass, possibly a hemangioma, an explanation not supported by any imaging findings that we were aware of, and this led to surgical evacuation of what was described on the pathology report as an old hematoma.

This diagnosis is consistent with the imaging appearance of the lesion, which initially shows mildly increased T1-signal intensity and decreased T2-signal intensity, consistent with subacute blood products. The follow-up examination demonstrates the development of a rim of low-signal-intensity hemosiderin. The absence of enhancement is, of course, reassuring that there is not an underlying mass, which should be a concern whenever a hematoma occurs spontaneously in a patient who does not have a bleeding disorder or who is not receiving anticoagulation therapy.

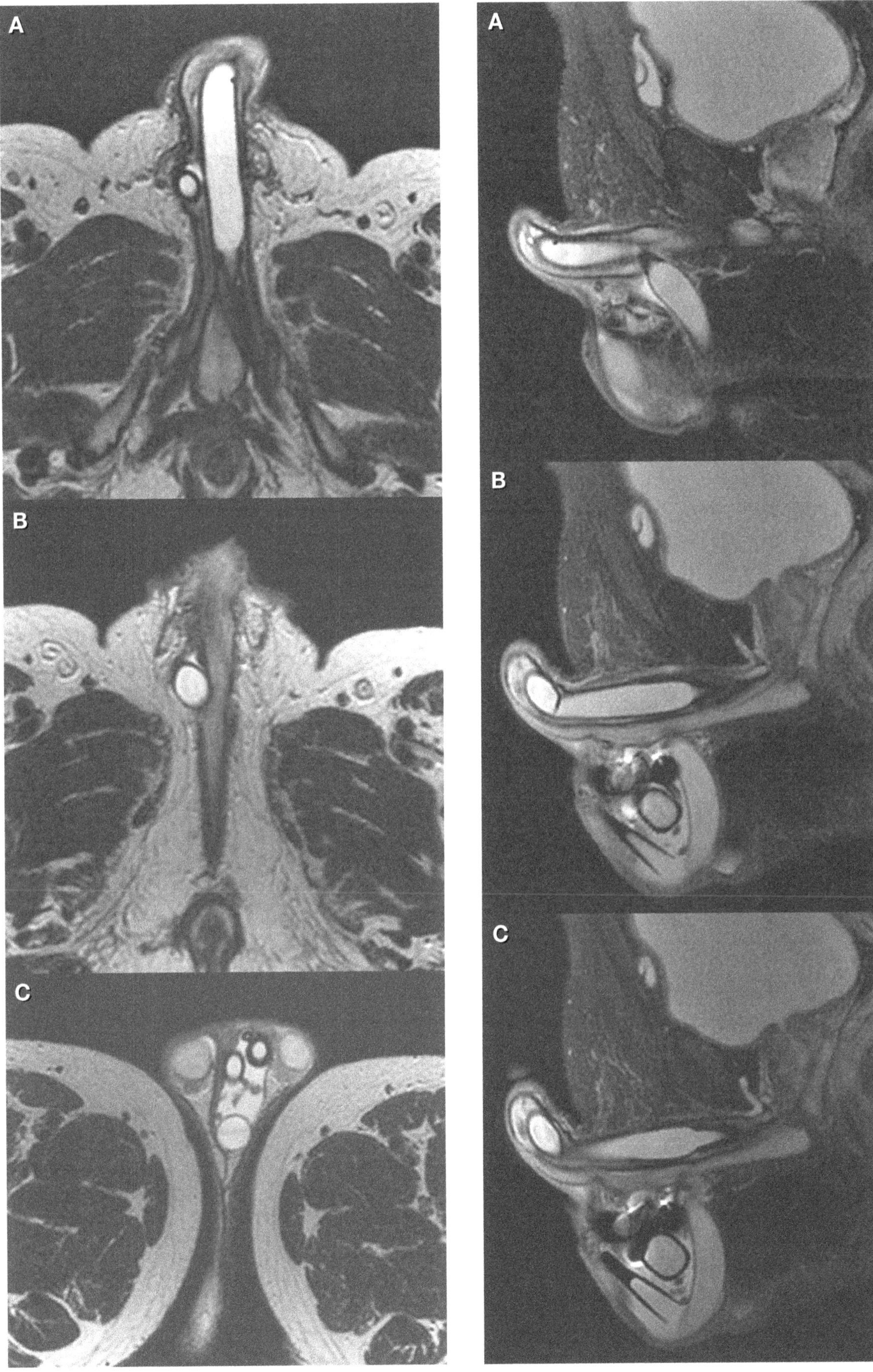

Figure 12.6.1

Figure 12.6.2

HISTORY: 56-year-old man with a malfunctioning penile prosthesis

IMAGING FINDINGS: Axial FSE T2-weighted images (Figure 12.6.1) and sagittal fat-suppressed FSE T2-weighted images (Figure 12.6.2) demonstrate marked displacement of the right-sided penile prosthesis cylinder, the majority of which is contained within the scrotum. Note that the reservoir is incompletely visualized in the pelvis anterior to the bladder.

DIAGNOSIS: Penile prosthesis displacement

COMMENT: Assessment of the dysfunctional penile prosthesis is an uncommon examination in our practice, but it does arise a few times every year. The protocol consists of FSE T2-weighted imaging with or without fat suppression in axial, coronal, and sagittal oblique planes oriented along the axes of the penis (fat suppression is not particularly important for the interpretation of the examination but can reduce phase ghosting artifact when this is problematic). The examination is done with the prosthesis inflated and deflated. (The patient usually takes care of the inflation and deflation. We did have a patient who didn't know how to do this, which probably explained why his prosthesis wasn't working.)

The 3D FSE or FRFSE techniques that have become widely available are also potentially useful. In the ideal case, you could perform 1 acquisition with high spatial resolution (ie, section thickness of 1-2 mm), allowing reconstruction of the other planes without actually acquiring them. Also helpful are 3D SSFP acquisitions, particularly in the setting of motion artifact or a difficult patient, since the acquisition times are quite short. Penile positioning is an important element of the examination because the straighter the penis (and this may not always be possible), the easier it is to visualize the anatomy and follow the prosthetic elements on successive images. We generally position the penis along the anterior abdominal wall between 2 rolled towels, with the surface coil lying on top.

Surgical implantation of a penile prosthesis is a treatment option for patients with organic erectile dysfunction not responsive to medical therapy. Although most devices are successfully implanted with high patient satisfaction, problems are occasionally encountered, and patient complaints may include discomfort, inadequate inflation, visible deformity, and painful intercourse. If the history and physical examination are adequate to determine that the prosthesis needs to be removed, then of course MRI is not necessary, but often imaging is helpful to determine whether a significant abnormality is present and, if so, whether it can be corrected without removing the prosthesis. The standard prosthesis consists of 2 cylinders implanted in the corpora cavernosa and attached to a fluid-filled reservoir. The cylinders should be reasonably symmetrical and contained entirely within the corpora. Inflated cylinders should not show any focal constrictions or buckling, which might suggest corporal fibrosis.

The literature on this subject is extremely limited, with fewer than 100 reported cases; however, MRI does seem to be fairly accurate at detecting obvious defects in the prosthesis, including migration or herniation, focal angulation or buckling of the cylinder, cylinder aneurysm, loss of fluid in the reservoir, and periprosthetic fluid collections. The defect in this case could probably have been detected with a good physical examination, since the right-sided cylinder had almost entirely herniated into the scrotum. The finding is also easily appreciated on MRI and indicates a problem requiring surgical correction.

CASE 12.7

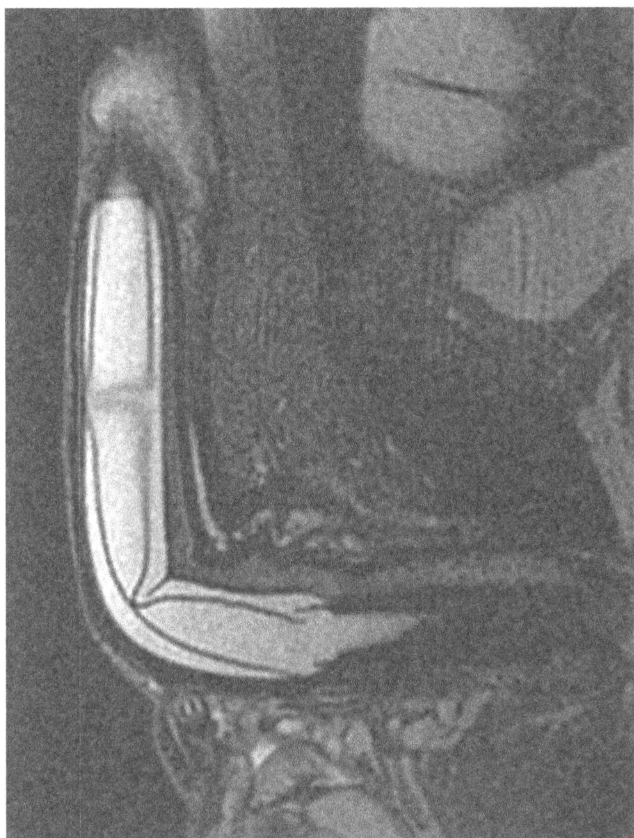

Figure 12.7.1

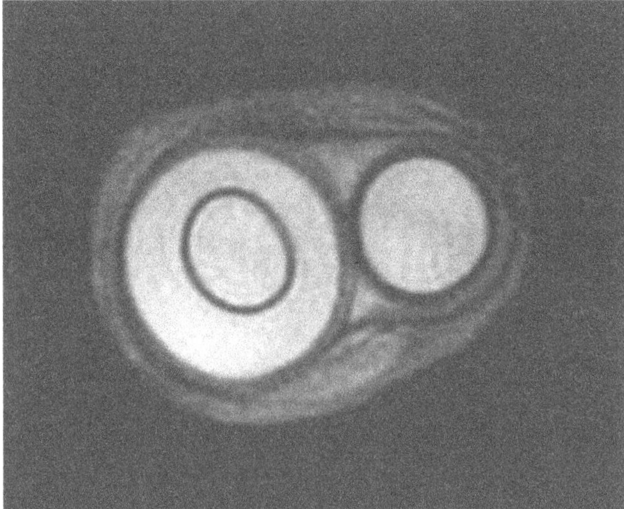

Figure 12.7.3

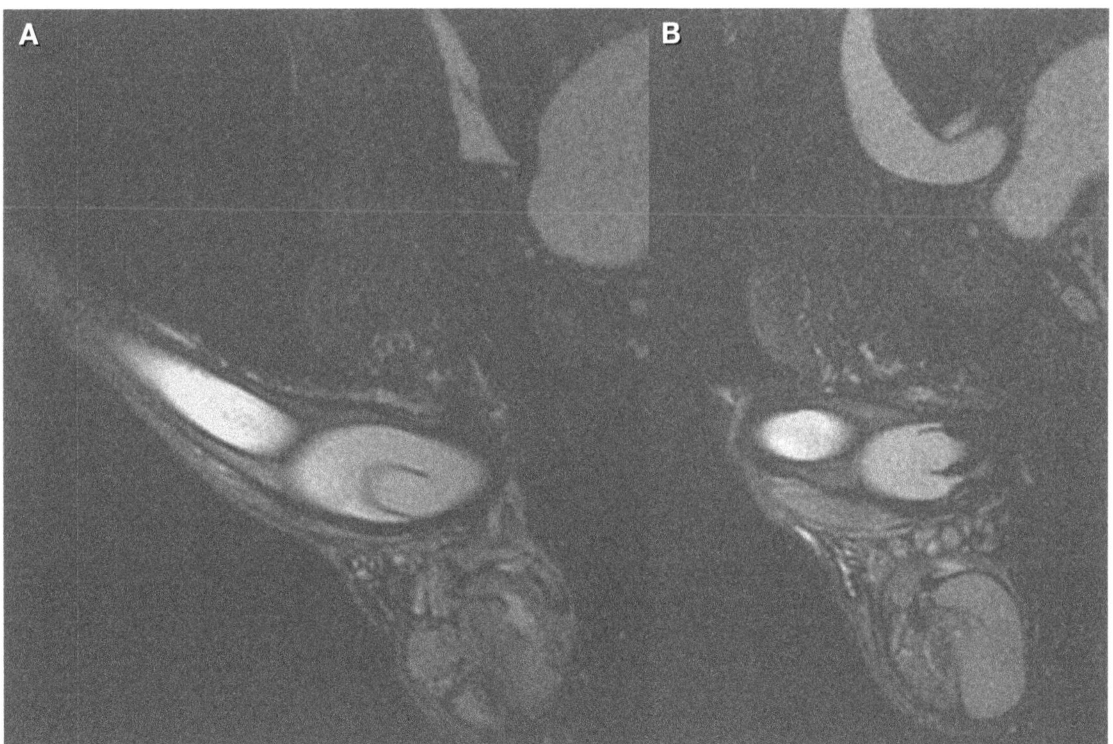

Figure 12.7.2

HISTORY: 74-year-old man with a penile prosthesis and a new enlargement and discomfort of the right penile shaft

IMAGING FINDINGS: Sagittal fat-suppressed FSE T2-weighted image (Figure 12.7.1) through the right corporus cavernosum demonstrates fluid surrounding the cylinder of the penile prosthesis. Note also the focal angulation at the base of the cylinder with discontinuity of the prosthesis components. Sagittal oblique postinflation FSE T2-weighted images (Figure 12.7.2) through the base of the penis reveal complete separation between the base of the cylinder and the more distal portion. Axial oblique postinflation FSE T2-weighted image (Figure 12.7.3) demonstrates fluid surrounding the right cylinder. Note that the right cylinder is smaller than the left.

DIAGNOSIS: Penile prosthesis rupture

COMMENT: This case is another example of a penile prosthesis problem, which appears fairly obvious on MRI but was in fact ambiguous to the clinician. In this case, physical examination was indeterminate. The patient had presented to the emergency department a few weeks previously with a focal bulge, but the urologist could not visualize any focal abnormality or asymmetry, and the prosthesis could be inflated.

The appearance on MRI is analogous to that of a ruptured breast implant, with fluid outside the cylinder where it isn't supposed to be, and a cylinder diameter that is smaller than the diameter of the intact cylinder on the other side. Periprosthetic fluid could also occur in the setting of prosthetic infection or a postoperative hematoma, but visualization of the ruptured cylinder is diagnostic. One could argue that the postinflation views were unnecessary since the defect was already apparent on the deflated images, but this would imply that someone had carefully checked the images before continuing, which doesn't always happen. The possibility of doing additional harm by inflating the prosthesis is a minor consideration, since that procedure had already been performed several times by the patient and the urologist.

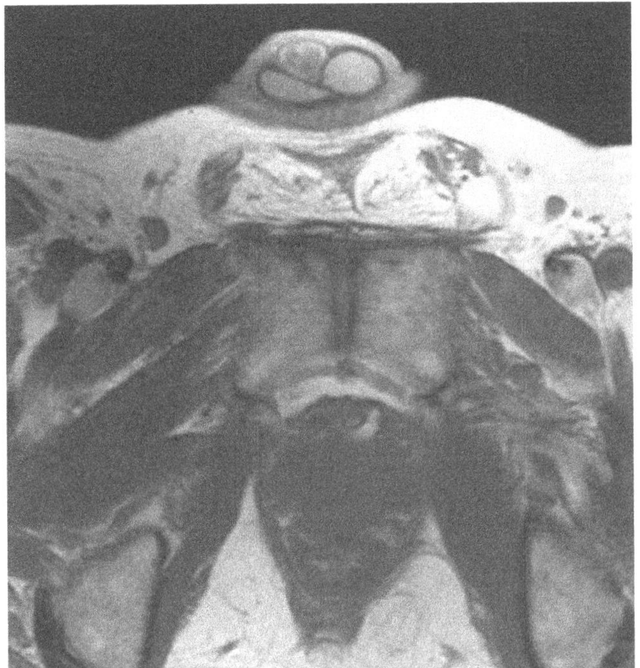

Figure 12.8.1

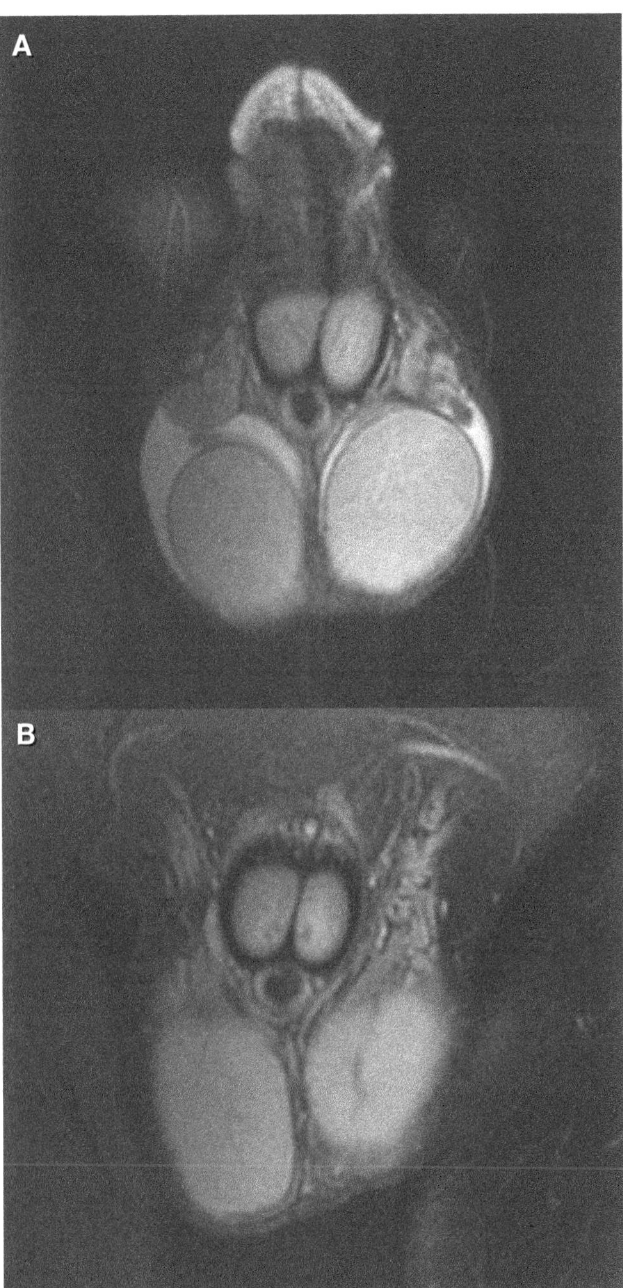

Figure 12.8.2

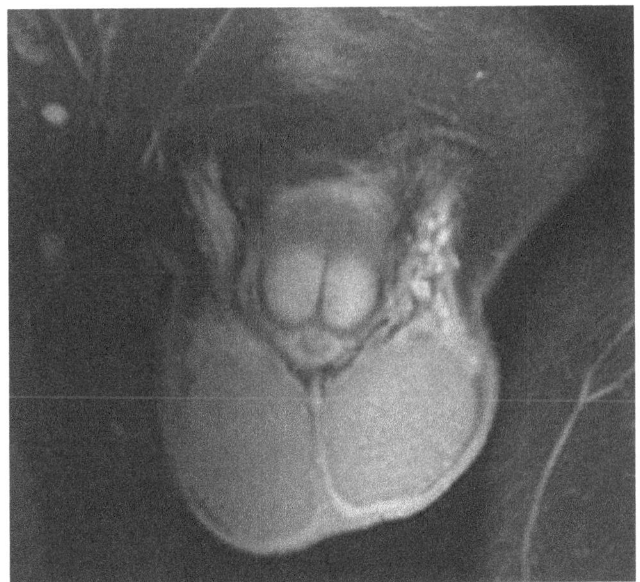

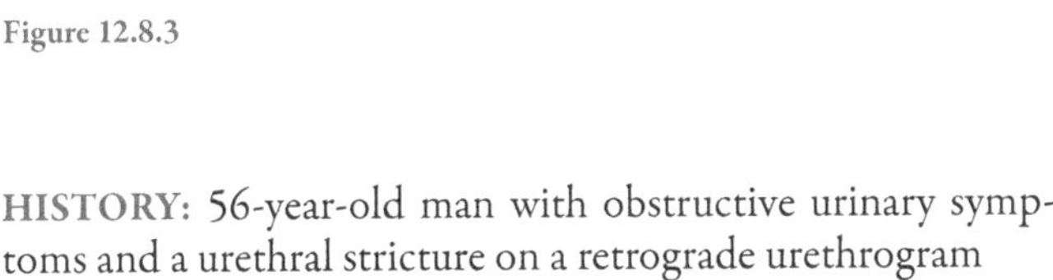

Figure 12.8.3

HISTORY: 56-year-old man with obstructive urinary symptoms and a urethral stricture on a retrograde urethrogram

IMAGING FINDINGS: Axial FSE T1-weighted image (Figure 12.8.1) reveals a hypointense lesion centrally in the mid–penile urethra. The lesion is markedly hypointense on coronal oblique fat-suppressed T2-weighted FSE images (Figure 12.8.2). Coronal oblique postgadolinium 2D SPGR image (Figure 12.8.3) shows mild enhancement of the lesion.

DIAGNOSIS: Urethral amyloid

COMMENT: Amyloidosis is usually a systemic disorder, and systemic or localized involvement has been described in nearly every organ in the body (hence, amyloidosis appears in many chapters of this book). Amyloidosis is characterized by the deposition of amyloid proteins into the extracellular matrix of the involved organ. These proteins are arranged in a β pleated sheet configuration and form insoluble amyloid fibrils, which stain pink with Congo red dye and show characteristic apple-green birefringence when viewed with polarized light at light microscopy.

Amyloidosis is classified as primary (AL) or secondary (AA) on the basis of the involved protein precursors. Primary amyloidosis deposits contain immunoglobulin light chain proteins; secondary amyloidosis deposits contain serum protein A, an acute-phase reactant that may be produced in response to underlying chronic inflammatory diseases or multiple myeloma.

Unfortunately, 80% to 90% of amyloidosis is the systemic variety, which is generally progressive and rapidly fatal, with death resulting from cardiac or renal failure. Systemic amyloidosis is usually diagnosed by demonstrating the presence of amyloid protein in subcutaneous fat, bone marrow, urine, or blood serum, whereas localized amyloidosis is demonstrated by excluding systemic involvement. In general, localized amyloidosis occurs much less frequently, but it is the more common variety in the urinary tract.

The appearance of urethral amyloidosis on MRI has been described in only a handful of case reports, and so there are no reliable diagnostic criteria; however, the periurethral lesion in this case could be considered a typical example, with indistinct margins, low signal intensity on T2-weighted images, and gradual enhancement after contrast administration. Patients may present with obstructive urinary symptoms, as in this case, and typically proceed to endoscopy and biopsy. Localized urethral amyloidosis is considered to be benign, and treatment is based on symptomatic relief.

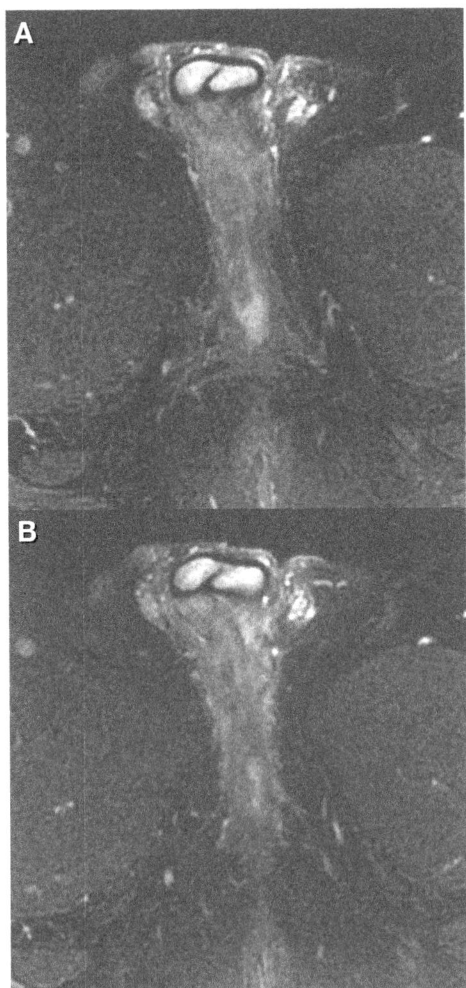

Figure 12.9.1

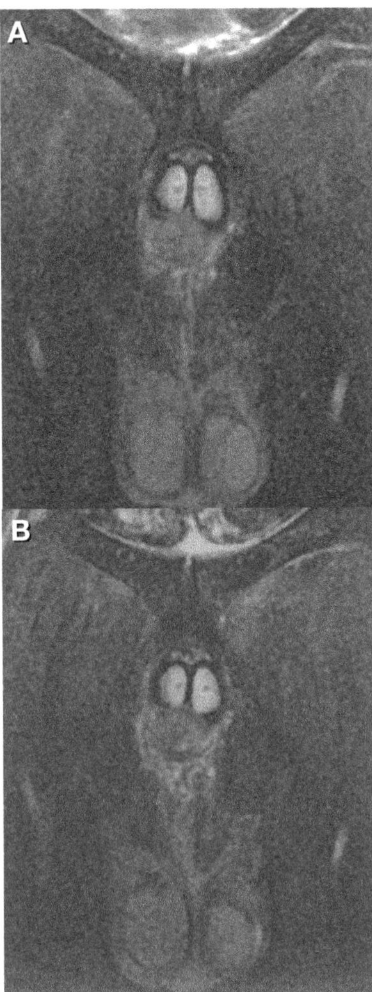

Figure 12.9.2

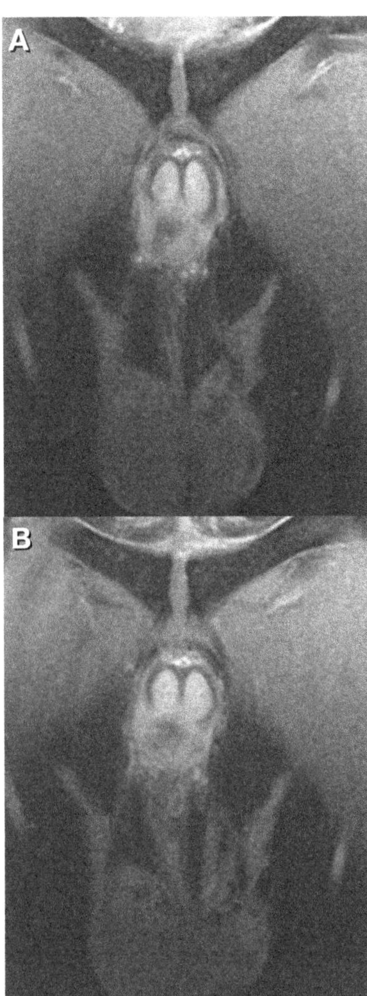

Figure 12.9.3

HISTORY: 34-year-old man with dysuria and urinary frequency

IMAGING FINDINGS: Axial (Figure 12.9.1) and coronal (Figure 12.9.2) fat-suppressed FSE T2-weighted images reveal a hypointense infiltrative mass surrounding the bulbous and penile urethra. Coronal postgadolinium 2D SPGR images (Figure 12.9.3) show heterogeneous enhancement of the lesion and irregular margins. Notice on both T2-weighted and postgadolinium coronal images disruption of the normal low-signal-intensity rim of the tunica albuginea with extension into the corpora cavernosa.

DIAGNOSIS: Urethral squamous cell carcinoma

COMMENT: Tumors of the male urethra are rare (<1% of all urologic neoplasms) and usually occur in middle-aged or older men. Presenting symptoms include a palpable mass, irritation, and obstructive voiding. Chronic urethritis with associated urethral strictures, chronic toxic exposures, and venereal or viral disease are all known risk factors for development of urethral carcinoma.

Male urethral tumors are categorized according to location and histologic type. The bulbomembranous urethra is most frequently involved (60%), followed by the penile urethra (30%) and the prostatic urethra (10%). Squamous cell carcinoma is the most common histologic type (68%-80%), followed by transitional cell carcinoma (15%-18%) and adenocarcinoma (5%). The prostatic urethra is involved by transitional cell carcinoma in 90% of cases and by squamous cell carcinoma in 10%. The bulbomembranous urethra is involved by squamous cell carcinoma in 80%, by transitional cell carcinoma in 10%, and by adenocarcinoma in 10%. In the penile urethra, squamous cell carcinoma is also the predominant lesion (90%), with transitional cell carcinoma in 10%.

Urethral carcinoma has a tendency to invade adjacent structures (the corpora cavernosa in this case) and to metastasize to pelvic lymph nodes. Hematogenous metastases are uncommon except in advanced disease. Stage I tumors are confined to the subepithelial connective tissue; stage II lesions have invaded the corpus spongiosum, prostate, or periurethral muscle; stage III includes masses invading the corpus cavernosum and bladder neck or extending beyond the prostate capsule; and stage IV tumors have invaded adjacent organs. Tumors of the penile urethra tend to present earlier, are more easily resected, and in general carry a better prognosis than lesions involving the posterior urethra, which present at more advanced stages, often with local invasion and pelvic lymph node involvement. Five-year survival rates are 65% to 70% for low-stage tumors and 33% for high-stage lesions.

MRI is a useful technique for identifying and staging disease. Since the corpus spongiosum normally demonstrates high signal intensity on T2-weighted images, lesions surrounding and expanding the urethra tend to appear hypointense against the high background signal. (This is an exception to the rule that tumors are hyperintense on T2-weighted images, with prostate cancer the most important example.) The tunica albuginea, the fibrous sheath enveloping the erectile bodies, is a useful anatomical marker for tumor extension. This normally appears as a dark band surrounding the corpora cavernosa and spongiosum on both T1- and T2-weighted images; therefore, tumor spreading across the tunica albuginea is relatively easy to visualize, as in this case.

In any examination involving the penis, the most important keys to success are proper positioning (usually with the penis lying as straight as possible along the anterior abdominal wall, supported anteriorly and on either side by towels), selection of a small surface coil, and image acquisition with a small FOV and high spatial resolution. This is a good application for high-field (3-T) imaging, since the SNR is increased at no additional cost (assuming that you don't count the extra million dollars or so you spent on the magnet, or the interesting new artifacts), and judicious use of 3D FSE/FRFSE acquisitions can provide visualization of the tumor with excellent contrast and spatial resolution. Dynamic gadolinium-enhanced images are almost always worth obtaining since the acquisition times are short and the images are usually free of motion artifact, with the optimal acquisition plane depending on the size and location of the tumor. Remember to include larger FOV acquisitions of the pelvis to document adenopathy, local extension, and bone metastases. As always, MRI is not at its best in distinguishing benign from malignant lymph nodes, pending the reintroduction of superparamagnetic iron oxide contrast agents.

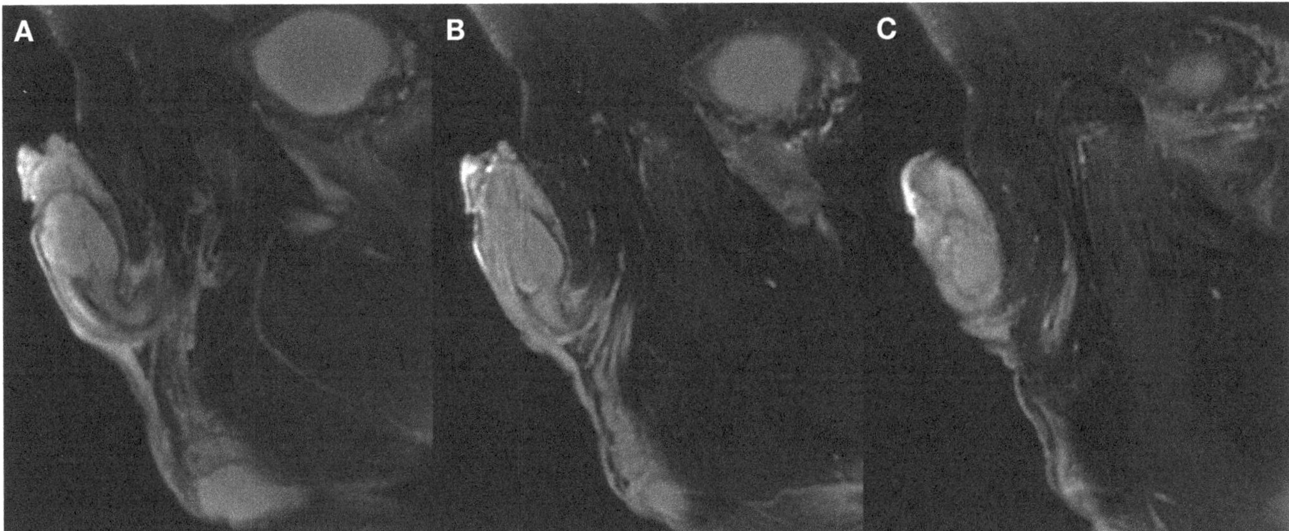

Figure 12.10.1

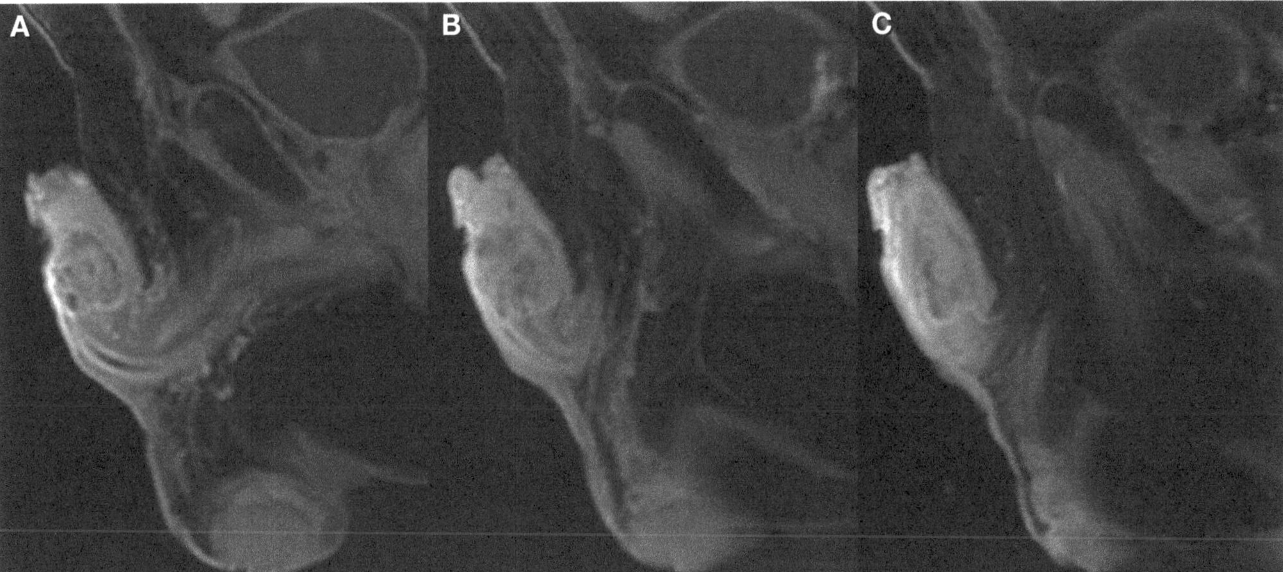

Figure 12.10.2

HISTORY: 53-year-old man with a penile mass

IMAGING FINDINGS: Sagittal fat-suppressed FSE T2-weighted images (Figure 12.10.1) demonstrate a lobulated ill-defined mass in the tip of the penis involving both the corpora cavernosa and the corpus spongiosum. Sagittal post-gadolinium 2D SPGR images (Figure 12.10.2) reveal heterogeneous enhancement of the lesion without clear visualization of the tunica albuginea.

DIAGNOSIS: Penile carcinoma (squamous cell carcinoma)

COMMENT: Penile carcinoma is a rare disease in the developed world, accounting for approximately 0.4% of all malignancies in men in the United States. The incidence is much higher in parts of Asia, Africa, and South America, where it constitutes 10% to 20% of cancers in men. Penile carcinoma is most common in older men, with peak incidence in the sixth and seventh decades. Risk factors include the presence of a foreskin (risk is 3 times higher in uncircumcised men than in circumcised men), chronic inflammatory conditions, smoking, and infection with human papillomavirus.

Squamous cell carcinoma is the dominant histologic type, representing 95% of all neoplasms. The remaining 5% include sarcoma, melanoma, basal cell carcinoma, and lymphoma. Verrucous carcinoma, a unique variant of squamous cell carcinoma, is a locally aggressive lesion that rarely metastasizes, and an example is included in this chapter (Case 12.11). Penile carcinoma may occur anywhere throughout the organ, but the glans is the most common location (48%), followed by the prepuce (21%). Papillary and flat growth patterns have been described.

The presence of lymph node metastases is the most important prognostic factor in penile carcinoma. In an older study, the 5-year survival decreased from 95% for patients without nodal disease to 81% for patients with 1 to 3 positive inguinal lymph nodes, 50% for patients with 4 or more positive inguinal lymph nodes, and 0% for patients with positive pelvic lymph nodes. The presence of nodal disease is related to the local stage, occurring in 20% with T1 disease (invasion of subepithelial connective tissue) and in 45% to 65% with T2, T3, or T4 lesions (T2 indicates corporal invasion; T3, invasion of the urethra or prostate; and T4, local invasion of adjacent structures).

MRI is helpful in surgical planning: Small, distal, superficial lesions are readily treated with conservative surgery, while more invasive and proximal lesions require a more radical approach. In the largest study of patients with penile carcinoma (55 patients), there was good correlation between radiologic and histologic staging, and MRI accurately predicted corpora cavernosa invasion with 100% accuracy. Interestingly, the authors attributed much of their success to the use of an intracavernosal prostaglandin E_1 injection to achieve artificial erection, a practice that has very few advocates in the United States. MRI protocols should rely primarily on small-FOV, high-spatial-resolution T2-weighted and postgadolinium 3D SPGR acquisitions in 2 or 3 planes, preferably obtained with a 3-T system in conjunction with a small phased-array surface coil, which depicts penile carcinoma as hypointense and hypoenhancing relative to adjacent corpora. The tunica albuginea can be seen on both sequences as a dark rim surrounding the corpora cavernosa and the corpus spongiosum, and violation of this rim by the tumor is highly correlated with histologic evidence of invasion.

This case is an older one that is not particularly photogenic. You can see why prostaglandin injection might have been helpful; however, the images are adequate to depict the large heterogeneous mass obliterating the corpora and violating the tunica albuginea.

MRI is currently much less useful for staging nodal disease. Size criteria are well known to be only mildly accurate. In fact, approximately 60% of patients with newly diagnosed penile carcinoma have palpable inguinal adenopathy, of which less than half are positive for metastatic disease. A few small articles have suggested that PET-CT may be very accurate for nodal staging in penile carcinoma, and, of course, MRI might fare much better should the ultrasmall superparamagnetic iron oxide lymph node contrast agents become commercially available.

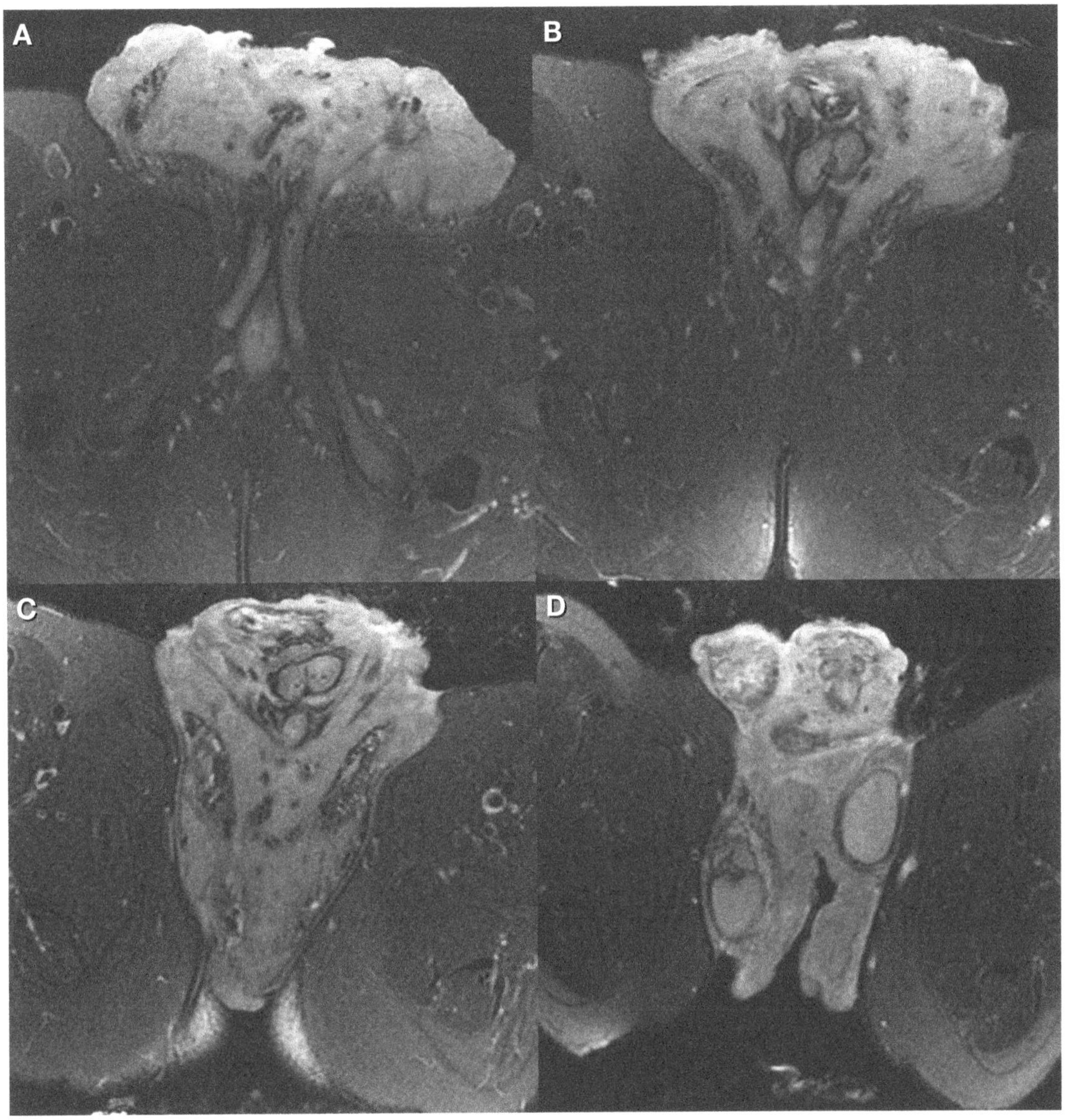

Figure 12.11.1

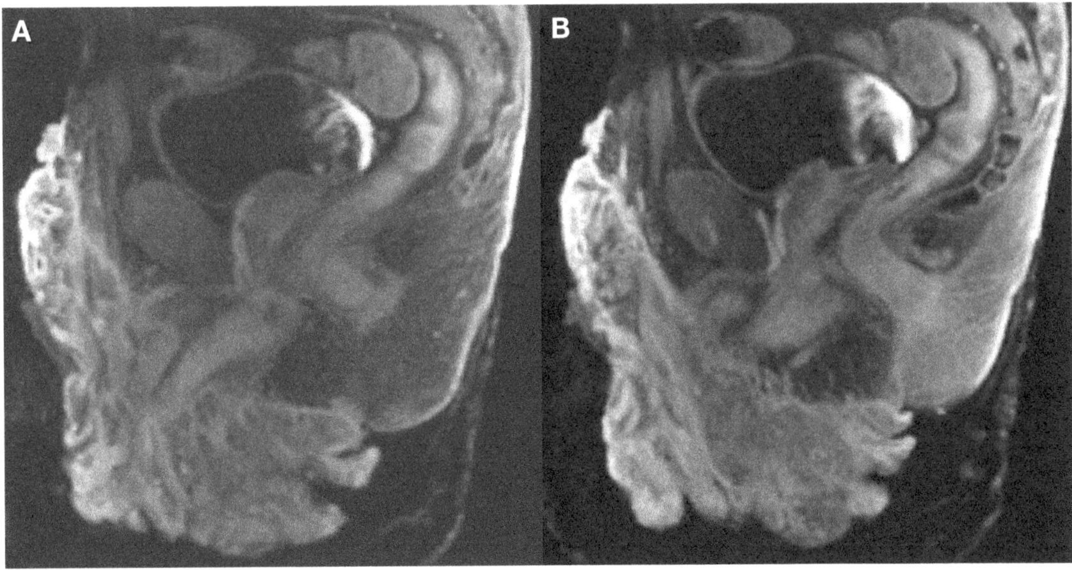

Figure 12.11.2

HISTORY: 58-year-old man with a history of a fungating penile mass that has grown slowly over 2 to 3 years

IMAGING FINDINGS: Axial fat-suppressed FSE T2-weighted images (Figure 12.11.1) and sagittal postgadolinium 3D SPGR images (Figure 12.11.2) reveal a large mass involving the penis, scrotum, and perineum with multiple frondlike projections demonstrating mild heterogeneous enhancement.

DIAGNOSIS: Verrucous carcinoma

COMMENT: Verrucous carcinoma is a rare form of squamous cell carcinoma initially reported in 1948 by Ackerman, who described a mass in the oral cavity. Similar lesions involving the penis had been discussed in an earlier article in 1925 by Buschke and Löwenstein, who noted an appearance intermediate between condyloma acuminatum (genital wart associated with human papillomavirus) and squamous cell carcinoma. Subsequently, the terms *Buschke-Löwenstein tumor, giant condyloma acuminata,* and *verrucous carcinoma* have been used somewhat interchangeably, generating much confusion in the literature.

These lesions typically manifest as a large mass originating from the penis, vulva, or perineum with a broad base and an ulcerated, cauliflower, or cobblestone surface. Histologically, verrucous carcinoma is characterized by minimal cytologic atypia, absent koilocytosis (nuclear enlargement, increased staining of the nucleus, perinuclear halo, and other features resulting from human papillomavirus infection), a "pushing" margin (rather than an invasive one characteristic of most squamous carcinomas), and a broad base separating the neoplasm from the underlying stroma. The appearance is similar to that of a condyloma acuminata but pathologically distinguishable in most cases.

Verrucous carcinoma typically exhibits slow growth and local invasion, with a low incidence of metastatic disease. Treatment guidelines are not clearly defined, but most authors have advocated wide surgical excision with or without adjuvant chemotherapy. Recurrence rates are high (60%-70%), and the associated mortality is 20% to 30%.

To our knowledge, there are no reports in the literature describing the MRI appearance of verrucous carcinoma. These lesions are rare but, as in this case, not subtle; MRI likely adds little value in confirming the diagnosis. In this case, imaging was helpful to delineate the depth of the tumor and the extent of local invasion and to assess for regional adenopathy or metastatic disease.

CASE 12.12

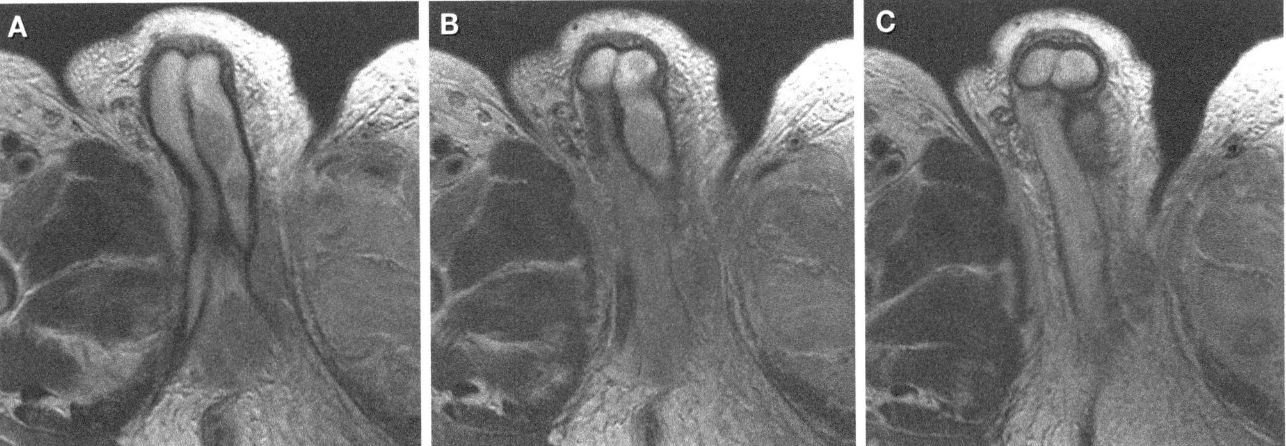

Figure 12.12.1

HISTORY: 54-year-old man with a history of a prior cystectomy for bladder urothelial cell carcinoma

IMAGING FINDINGS: Axial FSE T2-weighted images (Figure 12.12.1) reveal multiple hypointense masses in both corpora cavernosa (more prominent in the left than in the right) and in the base of the corpus spongiosum.

DIAGNOSIS: Penile metastases from urothelial cell carcinoma

COMMENT: Metastatic penile tumors are relatively rare and are usually indicative of terminal disease. The largest series (110 cases) was reported in the Japanese literature and demonstrated that urogenital tract cancers were by far the most common primary disease (69%), followed by gastrointestinal tract cancers (19%). Of the urogenital cancers, bladder was the most frequent source (29% of all metastases) followed by prostate (23%).

Common presenting symptoms include a painless or painful penile mass, priapism, pain at erection, and dysuria.

Penile metastases typically appear as multiple masses in the corpora cavernosa and corpus spongiosum, as in this case, generally with low signal intensity on T1- and T2-weighted images relative to the adjacent penile tissue. Postgadolinium images generally show hypoenhancing lesions against the strong background enhancement of the corpora.

The differential diagnosis for penile metastases is relatively short, particularly if, as in this case, the patient has a history of metastatic urogenital tract carcinoma. However, the differential diagnosis may also include infectious causes in the proper clinical context.

Radiotherapy and chemotherapy are the usual treatments for penile metastases. In general, though, the prognosis is poor, mostly because these lesions usually appear in patients who have widespread metastatic disease from their primary tumor.

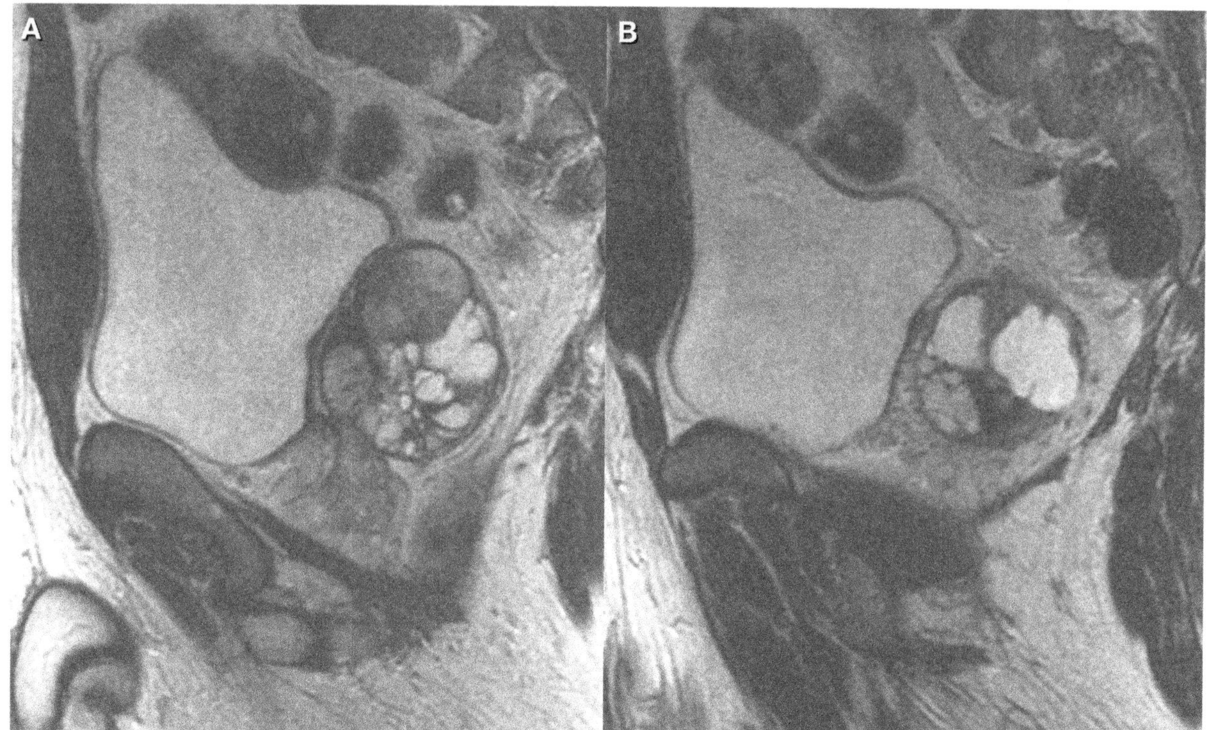

Figure 12.13.1

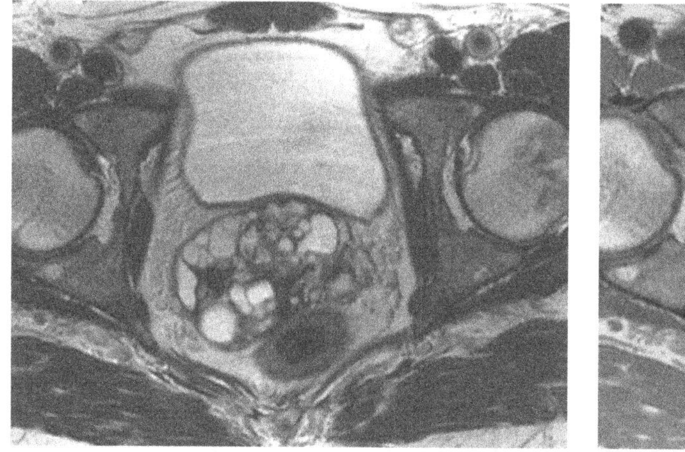

Figure 12.13.2

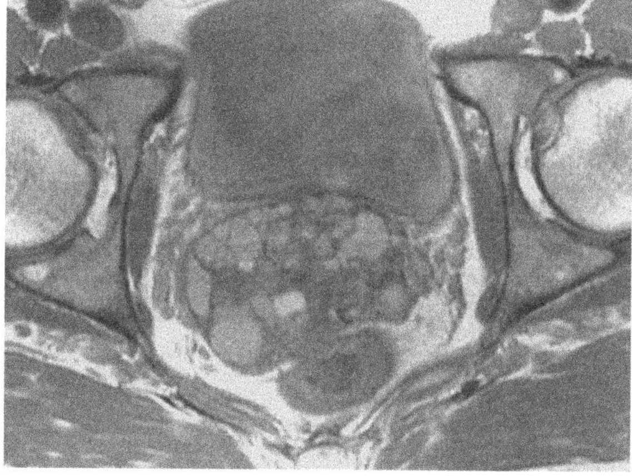

Figure 12.13.3

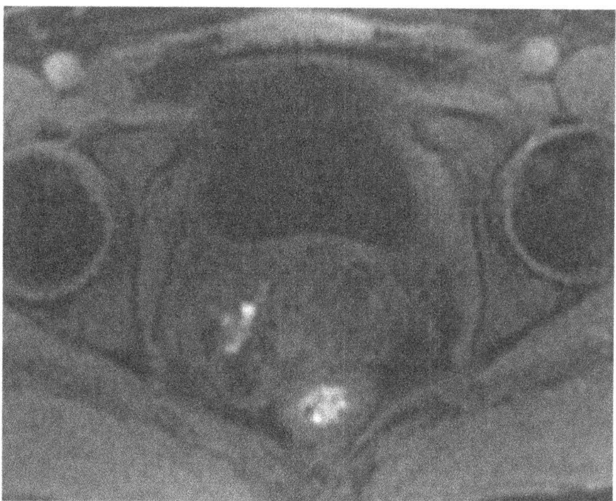

Figure 12.13.4

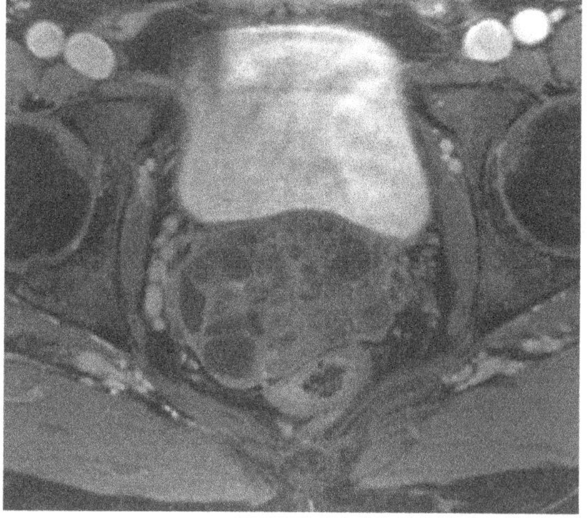

Figure 12.13.5

HISTORY: 46-year-old asymptomatic man with a palpable mass above the prostate on digital rectal examination

IMAGING FINDINGS: Sagittal (Figure 12.13.1) and axial (Figure 12.13.2) FSE T2-weighted images reveal a complex multicystic lesion involving the right side of the seminal vesicle. Axial T1-weighted FSE image (Figure 12.13.3) demonstrates that many of the small components have increased signal intensity. Precontrast 3D SPGR image (Figure 12.13.4) shows diffuse low signal intensity throughout the lesion with the exception of a few small bright foci centrally. Postgadolinium 3D SPGR image (Figure 12.13.5) demonstrates mild enhancement of the septations.

DIAGNOSIS: Seminal vesicle teratoma

COMMENT: Seminal vesicle lesions are uncommon once secondary invasion by prostate, bladder, and rectal cancer is excluded. Cysts are probably seen most frequently and are often associated with other genitourinary tract anomalies, including ipsilateral renal agenesis or dysgenesis. Cystic dilatation of the seminal vesicles may occur with obstruction, and dilatation of the proximal portion of the ejaculatory duct may appear as a seminal vesicle cyst. More complex masses have been reported infrequently in the literature; the only other description of a seminal vesicle teratoma comes from our institution and, coincidentally, uses this case but with slightly different images.

Teratomas arise from pluripotential germ cells that fail to involute and continue to undergo mitosis. By definition, teratomas are composed of all 3 germ cell layers (ectoderm, mesoderm, and endoderm). The usual key to the diagnosis is demonstration of fat within the lesion (along with nonfatty components that let you know it's not a lipoma)—this arises most frequently with ovarian dermoids.

In the past, pelvic imaging experts insisted that confirmation of fat within a dermoid could be accomplished only by obtaining T1-weighted FSE images with and without chemical fat suppression. In reality, though, any pulse sequence will do, including T2-weighted FSE, T1-weighted 2D or 3D SPGR, or even SSFP sequences. What will occasionally get you into trouble is a fat-suppressed T2-weighted acquisition in combination with non–fat-suppressed T1-weighted images, or vice versa, where it is theoretically possible that blood products of the correct age may mimic the signal changes of fat.

A Dixon sequence (FSE or SPGR), which reconstructs both fat and water images, is now the most elegant technique for confirming the presence of fat. Demonstration of fat within the teratoma does not achieve elegance in this case, although a comparison of the FSE T1-weighted and precontrast fat-suppressed 3D SPGR images, which show signal dropout of high-signal-intensity regions with fat suppression, should be reasonably convincing.

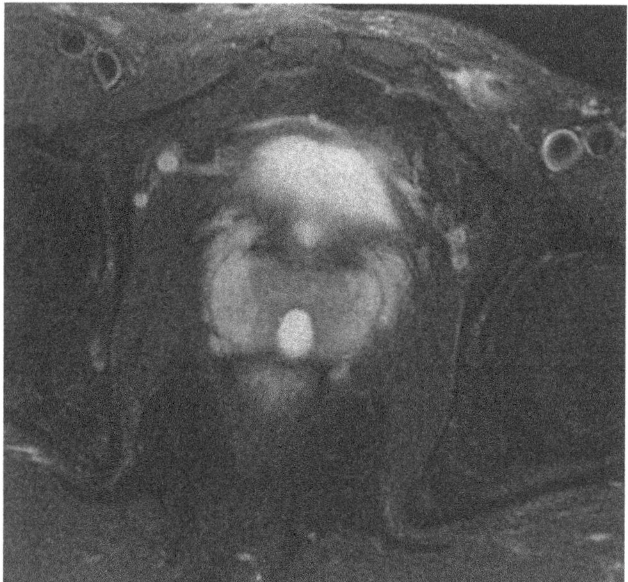

Figure 12.14.1

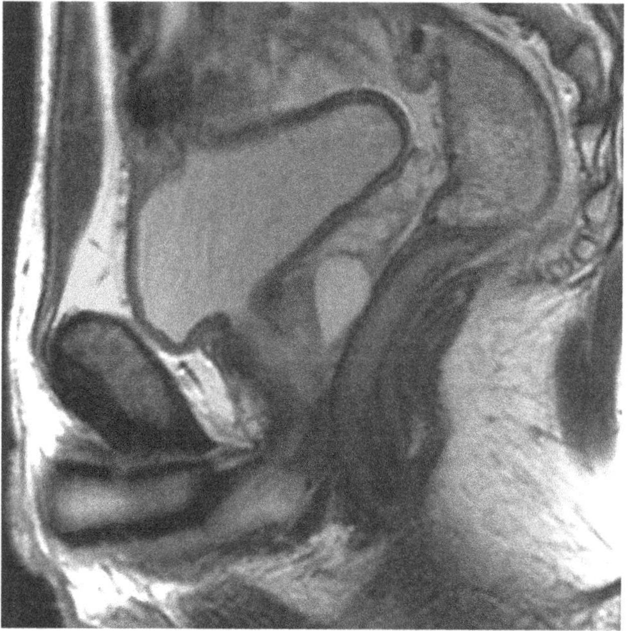

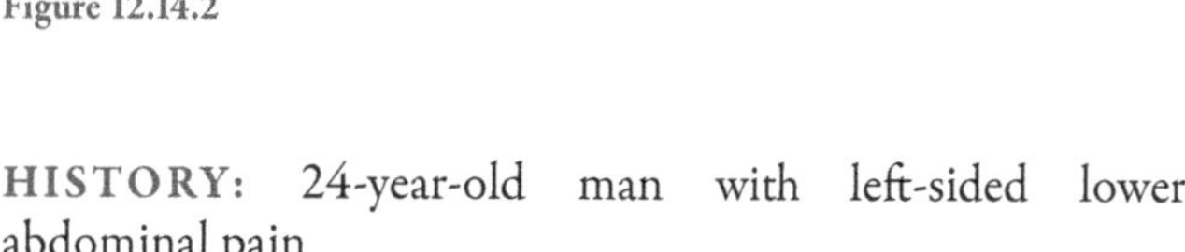

Figure 12.14.2

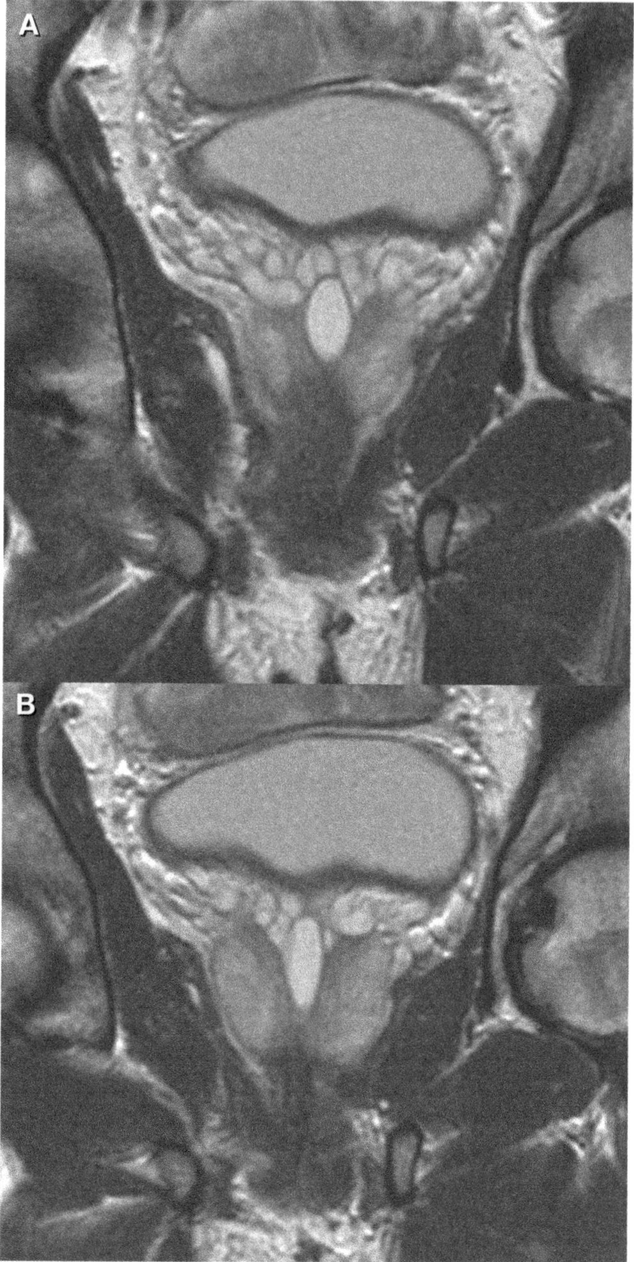

Figure 12.14.3

HISTORY: 24-year-old man with left-sided lower abdominal pain

IMAGING FINDINGS: Axial (Figure 12.14.1), sagittal (Figure 12.14.2), and coronal (Figure 12.14.3) FSE T2-weighted images demonstrate a small midline cystic lesion in the posterior portion of the prostate base.

DIAGNOSIS: Prostatic utricle cyst

COMMENT: Cystic lesions of the prostate constitute a surprisingly large differential diagnosis, and some lesions can be indistinguishable from one another on virtually any imaging modality, including MRI. This of course begs the question of whether there's really any point in trying to make the distinction (an idea infrequently voiced but often thought by residents, who live in fear of appearing indifferent to their mentor's lifework and thereby acquiring a reputation for laziness and sarcasm). Nevertheless, there are a few implications for treatment and prognosis depending on the diagnosis, and questions occasionally arise on board examinations, and so we forge ahead.

Cystic lesions can be classified in several ways. One of the most useful is to distinguish midline lesions from lateral lesions. Truly midline lesions include prostatic utricle cysts, müllerian duct cysts, and defects related to TURP; ejaculatory duct and vas deferens cysts are near-midline lesions, which are generally included in this category. Müllerian duct cysts and utricle cysts are separate entities that can have an identical appearance. Müllerian duct cysts arise from remnants of the müllerian duct, which regresses in male embryologic development and gives rise to the prostatic utricle and the appendix testis. (Wolffian ducts develop into the epididymis, vas deferens, seminal vesicles, and ejaculatory ducts.) Müllerian duct cysts may arise from the region of the verumontanum (a structure located posteriorly at the angle of the prostatic urethra, which contains the utricle, the orifices of the ejaculatory ducts, and the orifices of the prostatic glandular ductules) but often extend cephalad to the prostate gland. Müllerian duct cysts may also extend slightly lateral to midline, corresponding to the location of the cephalic portion of the ducts. Therefore, a larger central cyst extending well above the superior margin of the prostate and slightly lateral to midline is more likely a müllerian duct cyst than a prostatic utricle cyst.

Utricle cysts originate from the prostatic utricle, a blind pouch on the verumontanum just superior to the ejaculatory duct orifices. They always have a midline location and are usually smaller than müllerian duct cysts, measuring on average about 1 cm in length and tapering toward the verumontanum. Utricle cysts are usually detected in the first 2 decades of life and are associated with a variety of genitourinary anomalies, including hypospadias, cryptorchidism, and unilateral renal agenesis. Müllerian duct cysts are most often diagnosed in men in their third or fourth decades and have no association with genitourinary anomalies. Endoscopic visualization of a utricle origin is the gold standard for distinguishing utricle cysts from müllerian duct cysts. Müllerian duct cysts do not contain spermatozoa upon aspiration, and utricle cysts rarely do, in contrast to vas deferens and ejaculatory duct cysts. Both utricle and müllerian duct cysts are associated with an increased risk of prostate carcinoma, which can be endometrial, clear cell, or squamous cell carcinoma. These lesions are often clinically silent and are detected incidentally, but patients can present with obstructive and irritative urinary tract symptoms, hematuria, and pelvic pain. Urine may pool in utricle cysts and result in the classic clinical sign of postvoid dribbling. When large enough, utricle cysts and müllerian duct cysts may obstruct the ejaculatory ducts and result in infertility.

Ejaculatory duct cysts result from congenital or acquired obstruction of the ejaculatory duct and appear as cystic lesions along the expected course of the ejaculatory ducts, slightly lateral to midline in the base of the prostate and closer to midline near the verumontanum. Ejaculatory duct cysts contain spermatozoa upon aspiration and may be associated with cystic dilatation of the ipsilateral seminal vesicle. Stone formation within these cysts is relatively common.

Prostatic cysts not associated with a characteristic midline or near-midline location include cystic degeneration of BPH, typically seen within the hyperplastic transitional zone, and retention cysts resulting from obstruction of prostatic glandular ductules and consequent acinar dilatation. Retention cysts can occur within any zone of the prostate, and both entities are most often seen in older patients, who usually have no associated symptoms.

Prostatic abscesses also have a cystic appearance but are usually easily distinguished on the basis of signs and symptoms of prostatitis, including fever, chills, urinary frequency and urgency, pain, dysuria, and hematuria. *Escherichia coli* is the most common causative organism, and abscesses are more frequent in diabetic patients. Abscesses in the prostate, as in most other organs, typically have thick walls with prominent rim enhancement following contrast administration.

Examples of more unusual diffuse cystic processes are also included in this chapter. Remember that prostate carcinoma can rarely have a cystic presentation, and so a cystic prostate lesion, particularly with nodular or enhancing components, should never be automatically dismissed as a benign entity.

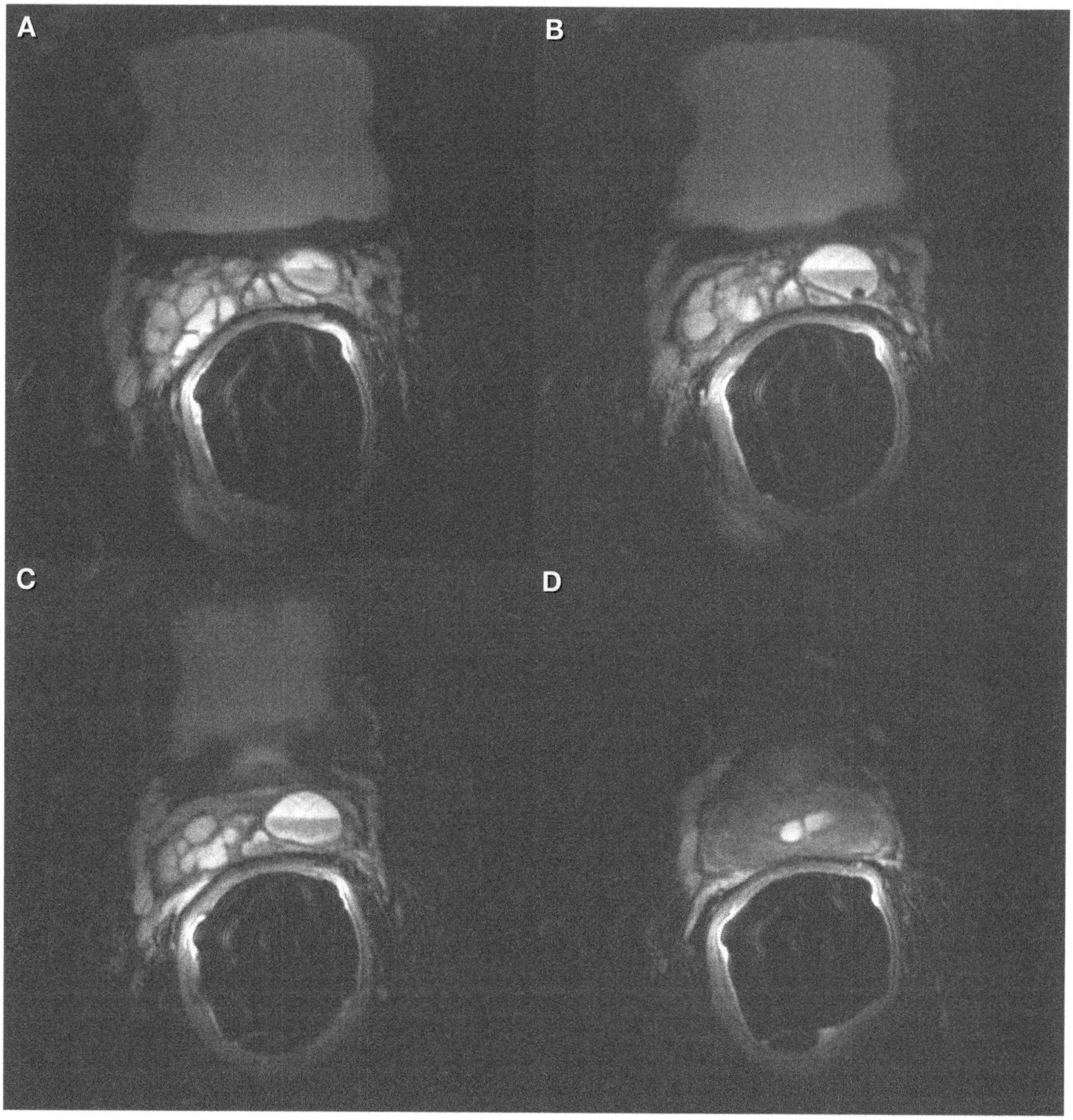

Figure 12.15.1

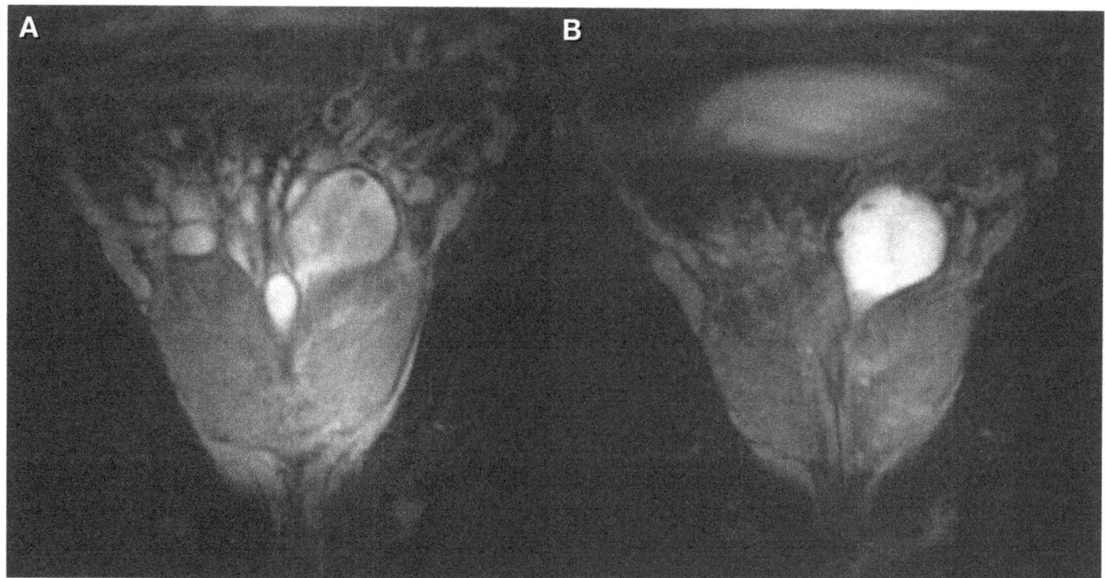

Figure 12.15.2

HISTORY: 42-year-old man with painless hematospermia

IMAGING FINDINGS: Axial fat-suppressed T2-weighted FRFSE images (Figure 12.15.1) obtained with an endorectal coil demonstrate a cystic lesion containing a fluid-fluid level as well as a hypointense calculus originating in the left seminal vesicle and extending inferiorly into the prostate. Note that on the most inferior image there is a second smaller midline cyst. Coronal fat-suppressed T2-weighted FRFSE images (Figure 12.15.2) also reveal a large ovoid cystic lesion involving the left seminal vesicle and prostate and a smaller midline prostatic cyst.

DIAGNOSIS: Ejaculatory duct cyst and prostatic utricle cyst

COMMENT: While hematospermia is an alarming sign to most patients, it is rarely associated with significant urologic disease. Some form of imaging is usually performed, though, to exclude a malignant lesion and reassure the patient. This case illustrates another variety of prostatic cyst, a near-midline ejaculatory duct cyst, in conjunction with an additional small utricle cyst.

The ejaculatory ducts arise from the wolffian ducts and travel from the seminal vesicles to the verumontanum, with an orientation that is slightly lateral to midline at the base of the prostate and becomes midline as the ducts reach the verumontanum. Ejaculatory duct cysts result from an obstruction of the duct, which may be congenital or acquired (one could argue that this case resulted from obstruction caused by the small utricle cyst), are usually larger than utricle cysts and often extend above the prostate, and will yield spermatozoa if aspirated. Hemorrhagic debris and calculi are fairly common findings in ejaculatory duct cysts.

Patients who have ejaculatory duct cysts may be completely asymptomatic or have dysuria, perineal pain, hematospermia, and ejaculatory pain. Ejaculatory duct obstruction can be associated with infertility, low ejaculate volume, and azoospermia.

Diagnosis with MRI is usually straightforward. T2-weighted FSE or FRFSE acquisitions through the prostate and seminal vesicles in 2 or 3 planes are usually sufficient to visualize the near-midline cystic prostatic lesion and to make a reasonable guess at its etiology. The use of an endorectal coil is probably not necessary for this diagnosis, particularly if you use a 3-T magnet. Three-dimensional T2-weighted FRFSE or FSE pulse sequences can display the cyst and adjacent prostate parenchyma with high spatial resolution and excellent contrast, and a 3D SSFP acquisition is a fast and simple technique for making the diagnosis.

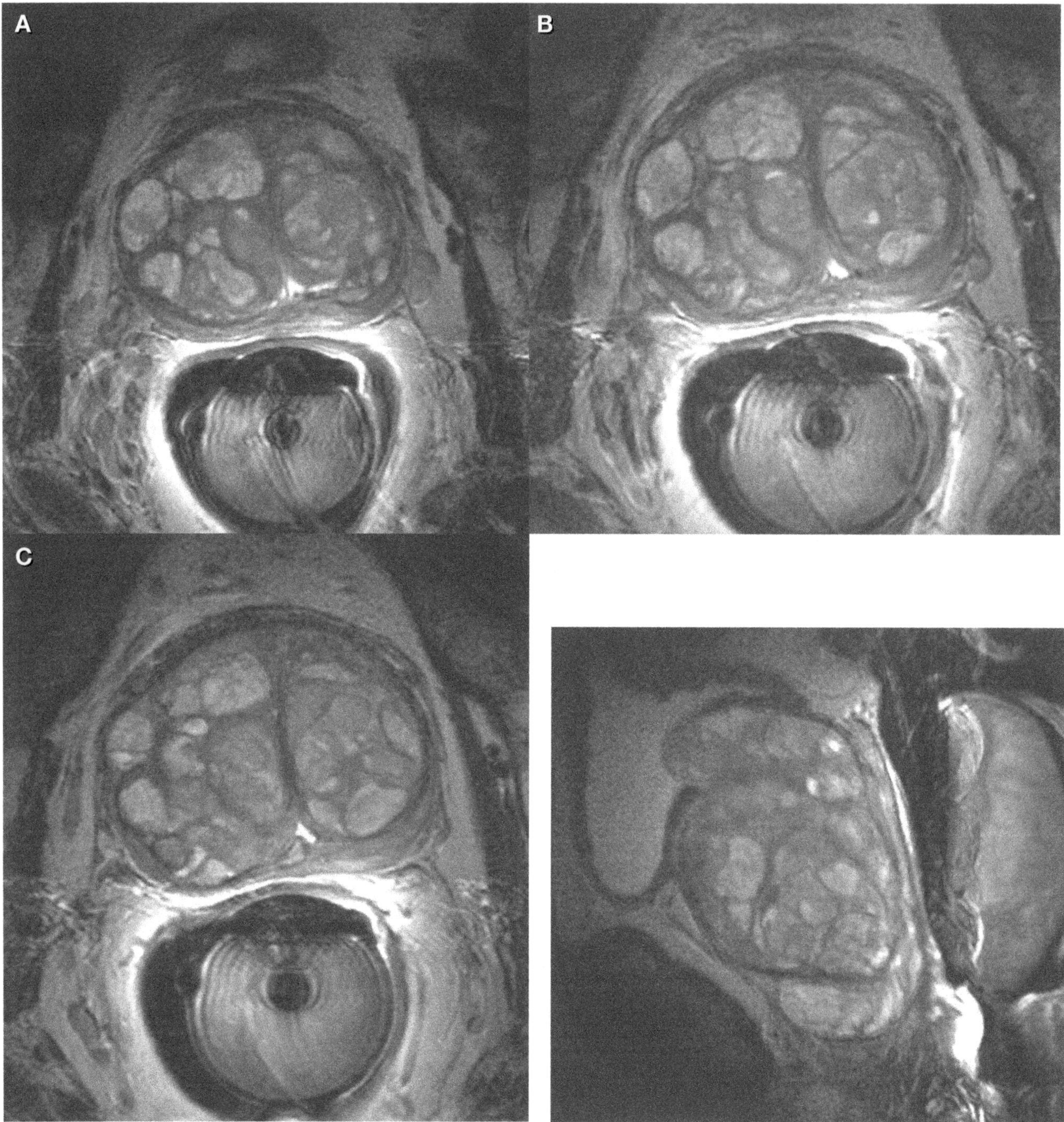

Figure 12.16.1

Figure 12.16.2

HISTORY: 61-year-old man with an elevated PSA on routine physical examination

IMAGING FINDINGS: Axial (Figure 12.16.1) and sagittal (Figure 12.16.2) T2-weighted FRFSE images obtained with an endorectal coil demonstrate marked enlargement of the central gland of the prostate, which contains numerous heterogeneous nodules of variable signal intensity. The peripheral zone is compressed and difficult to visualize on the axial images, but it can be seen as a thin lip of tissue projecting along the posterior margin of the prostate on the sagittal image.

DIAGNOSIS: Benign prostatic hyperplasia

COMMENT: BPH is considered the most common benign neoplasm in men in the United States. It is associated with progressive lower urinary tract symptoms, including nocturia, incomplete bladder emptying, urinary hesitancy or frequency, and acute urinary retention. The estimated prevalence of BPH increases from approximately 50% at 60 years of age to 90% in men older than 85 years.

Histologically, BPH arises predominantly in the transition zone of the prostate (this is the tissue surrounding the prostatic urethra and normally accounting for 5% of the prostate volume) and consists of nodules composed of a mixture of glandular and stromal elements of variable percentages. Glandular elements may undergo cystic dilation, and cystic foci are not uncommon in patients with BPH.

The etiology of BPH is likely multifactorial and has not been completely elucidated. Metabolic factors, including insulin resistance, obesity, and elevated low-density lipoprotein cholesterol have all been associated with BPH. An inflammatory component is also suspected, since histologic studies of BPH have frequently documented inflammatory changes in pathologic specimens, and there is likely a correlation between the intensity of inflammation and the severity of clinical symptoms.

This case is a fairly typical example of BPH. The central gland is enlarged and has a multinodular appearance, with a variable signal intensity of individual nodules on T2-weighted images. Notice also that since the transition zone includes the periurethral tissue at the base of the bladder, focal enlargement of this region with nodular indentation of the bladder base is a classic pattern of BPH and can resemble a bladder mass on axial images—sagittal images are very helpful when this is a consideration.

When BPH is discussed in the context of prostate MRI, it is usually as a confounding factor in the diagnosis of prostate cancer. Although a majority of prostate carcinomas originate in the peripheral zone, 25% occur within the transition zone and 5% occur within the central zone, and distinguishing foci of central gland carcinoma from nodules of BPH can be extremely challenging. Findings that support a diagnosis of transition zone carcinoma include a dominant low T2-signal intensity nodule disrupting the low-signal-intensity margin of the central gland (often, but not always, seen with BPH). A few papers have assessed the ability of DWI and DCE imaging to distinguish BPH from carcinoma in the transition zone. In general, there is significant overlap in the measured ADC values and parametric kinetic parameters, although criteria based on a combination of the 2 have shown some promise in this regard.

Treatment of BPH is shifting away from invasive surgical techniques, including TURP and prostatectomy, to medical therapy involving α blockers and 5 α-reductase inhibitors. Both types of drugs are generally effective and have relatively few side effects.

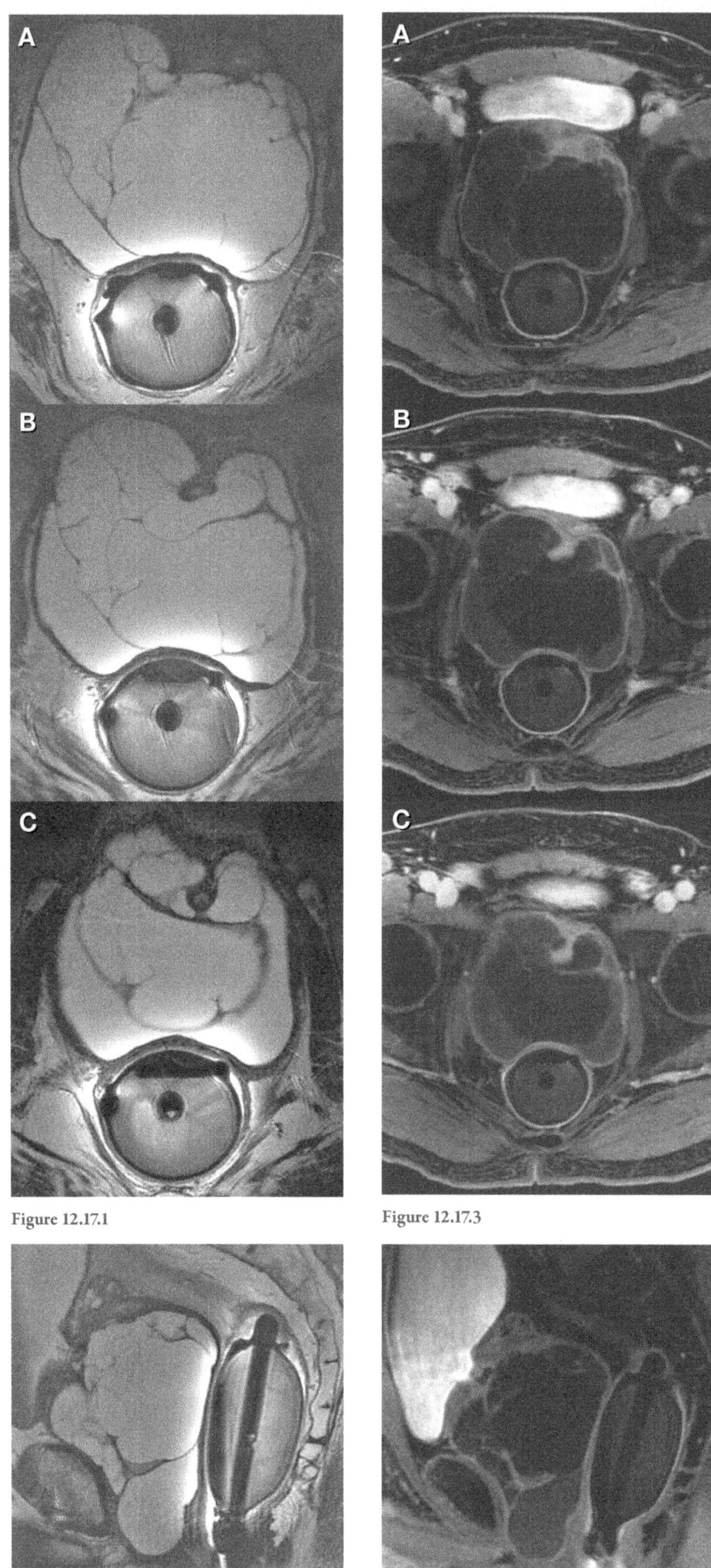

Figure 12.17.1

Figure 12.17.3

Figure 12.17.2

Figure 12.17.4

HISTORY: 62-year-old man with difficulty voiding and occasional dysuria and urinary frequency; a cystic prostatic lesion has been followed for more than 30 years at another medical institution

IMAGING FINDINGS: Axial (Figure 12.17.1) and sagittal (Figure 12.17.2) FRFSE T2-weighted images and axial (Figure 12.17.3) and sagittal (Figure 12.17.4) postgadolinium 3D SPGR images reveal that the prostate has been largely replaced by a complex cystic lesion containing multiple septations of varying thickness that show mild enhancement on postgadolinium images.

DIAGNOSIS: Inflammatory cystic degeneration of the prostate

COMMENT: This unusual case has few if any counterparts in the literature. The patient eventually underwent TURP primarily to relieve his obstructive symptoms, and pathology indicated benign prostatic tissue with scattered inflammatory cells and calcifications. The consensus among the many urologists who saw the patient was that this appearance probably represented an unusual end-stage prostatitis with glandular obstruction and eventual cystic degeneration. The term *cavitary prostatitis* has been used to describe a form of chronic prostatitis in which prolonged infection and fibrosis lead to glandular ductal constriction and acinar dilatation, eventually resulting in a "Swiss cheese" appearance of the prostate with multiple small cysts scattered throughout the gland. This case likely is an extreme example of this phenomenon.

The absence of any significant residual prostatic tissue except for a thin periurethral rim and the lack of nodular enhancing soft tissue components is somewhat reassuring for a chronic benign process, and this is particularly true in light of the 30-year history of the lesion. However, it is important to recognize that prostate carcinoma occasionally manifests in a cystic form (Case 12.20) and that other rare cystic neoplasms of the prostate (cystadenoma and cystadenocarcinoma) should be considered in the differential diagnosis.

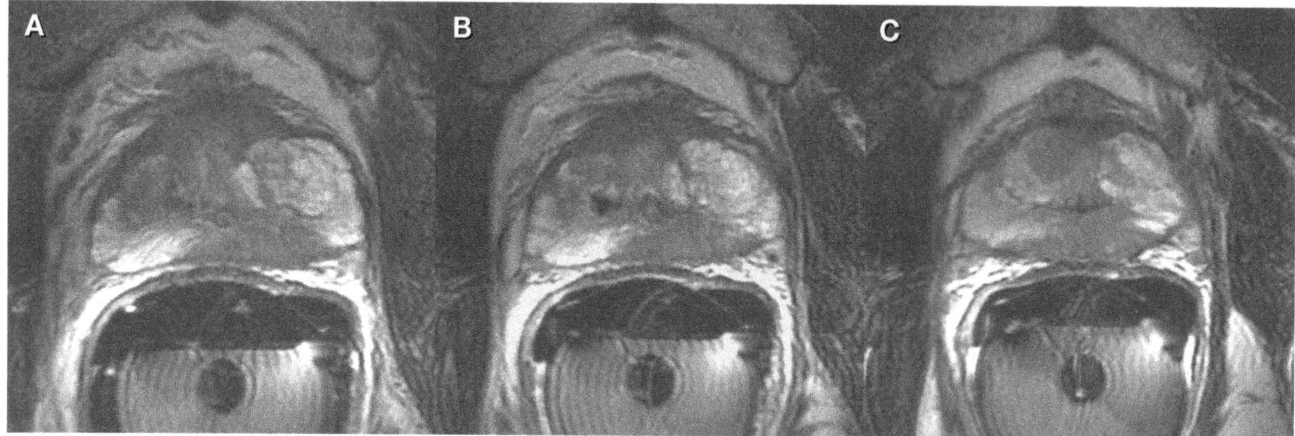

Figure 12.18.1

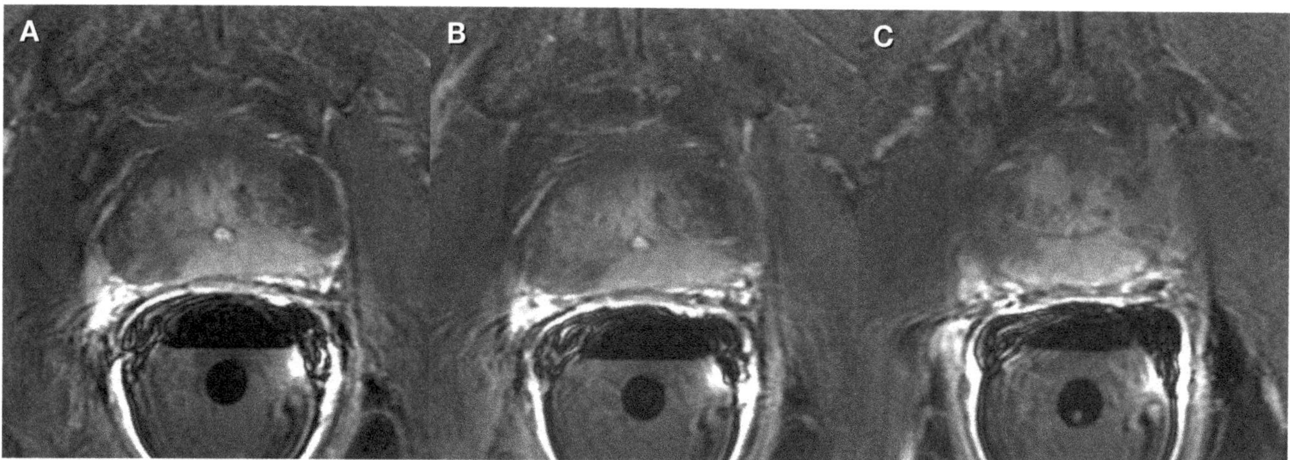

Figure 12.18.2

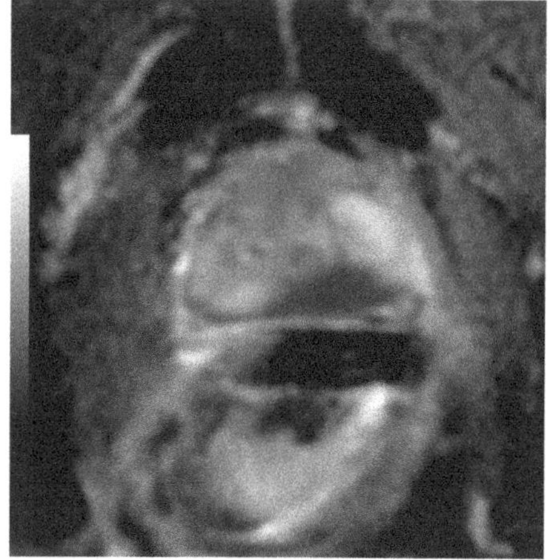

Figure 12.18.3

HISTORY: 62-year-old man with a recent diagnosis of prostate cancer; the Gleason score is 7 (3+4) on the left and 6 on the right

IMAGING FINDINGS: Axial FRFSE T2-weighted images (Figure 12.18.1) obtained with an endorectal coil demonstrate a triangular region of low signal intensity within the peripheral zone of the prostate centrally. There is more heterogeneous decreased signal intensity in the anterior right peripheral zone and in the central zone. Axial arterial phase postgadolinium 3D SPGR images (Figure 12.18.2) demonstrate early enhancement in the peripheral zone corresponding to the

T2-signal abnormality. The axial ADC map (Figure 12.18.3) from diffusion-weighted acquisition (b=1,000 s/mm^2) reveals restricted diffusion (decreased ADC) corresponding to the abnormal T2-signal intensity and enhancement.

DIAGNOSIS: Prostate adenocarcinoma

COMMENT: Prostate carcinoma is the most common cancer in men, accounting for 25% of all malignancies, and is the second leading cause of death after lung cancer. Prostate cancer will develop in 16% of men during their lifetime. The prevalence of prostate cancer increases with age, and it is estimated that as many as 70% of men older than 80 years have histologic evidence of prostate cancer. Survival rates have dramatically improved in recent decades. Although this improvement is related at least in part to the lead time bias of early diagnosis, there has been real progress, and the 5-year survival is essentially 100% when the disease is local or regional but drops to 34% with distant metastases. The most important prognostic factors are the Gleason score and the clinical stage at diagnosis.

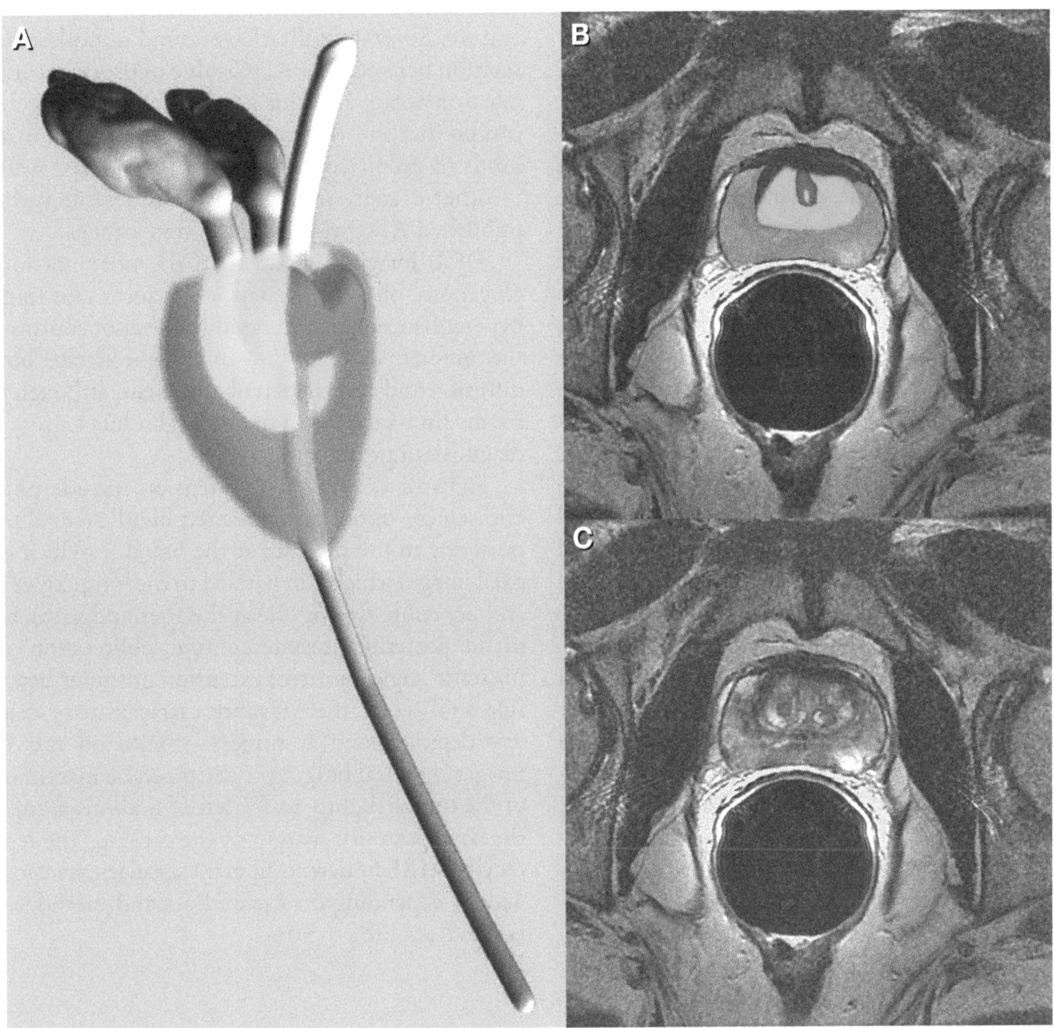

Figure 12.18.4 (A, Used with permission of Benjamin H. Lee.)

The anatomy of the prostate deserves brief consideration (Figure 12.18.4). The prostate is divided into the *transition zone* (red), which surrounds the urethra and contains 5% of the glandular tissue; the *central zone* (green), which posteriorly envelops the transition zone and contains 20% of the prostate volume; and the outer *peripheral zone* (tan), which contains 70% to 80% of the prostate volume and increases in size from base to apex. There is also the anterior fibromuscular stroma (brown), which is less often referenced on MRI reports. Most prostate carcinoma is adenocarcinoma originating within the prostate gland, with 70% arising in the peripheral zone, 25% in the transition zone, and 5% in the central zone.

While the significant decline in mortality from prostate cancer is encouraging, much remains that is strange and mysterious in its diagnosis and treatment, particularly with regard to the role of MRI. Screening for prostate cancer is based primarily on digital rectal examination (which nearly everyone agrees is unpleasant and has poor sensitivity and specificity) and on serum levels of PSA. The widespread use of PSA screening is controversial, since 70% to 80% of patients with elevated PSA levels (>4 ng/mL) do not have prostate cancer, and approximately 27% of patients with biopsy-proven cancers present with PSA values in the normal range.

Be that as it may, when there is a clinical suspicion of prostate cancer based on a palpable abnormality or elevated PSA, the next step is generally an ultrasound-guided prostate biopsy. *Ultrasound-guided* is a relative term. Since at least 40% of prostate cancers are not visualized on US, ultrasound guidance is primarily used to provide anatomical landmarks for a systematic biopsy in a sextant or octant pattern. The concept of saturation biopsy, performed with minimal imaging guidance, is unique to the prostate and, not surprisingly, carries a fairly high false-negative rate (10%-38%).

When prostate cancer is found at biopsy, histologic evaluation is performed with the Gleason grading system. Tumors are assigned a primary grade on the basis of the predominant pattern of differentiation and a secondary grade on the basis of the second most common pattern. The sum of the 2 numbers is the Gleason score. For example, a tumor classified as Gleason 4+3 has a Gleason score of 7. Cancers with Gleason scores less than 6 are considered well differentiated and are associated with a good prognosis. Cancers with Gleason scores of 8 to 10 have the worst prognosis and the highest risk of recurrence. Cancers with a Gleason score of 7 have a variable prognosis and an intermediate risk of recurrence. Tumor staging also has important implications for treatment and prognosis. Stage 1 lesions are nonpalpable, incidentally detected lesions confined to the prostate; stage 2 lesions are palpable but remain confined within the prostate capsule; and stage 3 tumors extend beyond the prostate. Patients with stage 1 or 2 cancers are candidates for local therapy, including radical prostatectomy and radiotherapy; stage 3 lesions require systemic combination therapy.

The traditional role of MRI in prostate cancer has been local staging for patients who have known lesions. Cancer in the peripheral zone (as in this case) generally appears as a hypointense lesion on T2-weighted images relative to the normal high signal intensity of the peripheral zone. It should be noted that this is not a particularly specific sign, since hemorrhage, prostatitis, scarring, and prior radiotherapy can all lead to a similar appearance. The reported sensitivity and specificity of T2-weighted imaging alone (long the standard practice) vary widely, with sensitivities of 77% to 91% and specificities of 27% to 61% reported for studies performed with an endorectal coil.

In several small studies, the addition of DWI and DCE imaging has led to increased sensitivity and specificity. As with most other tumors, diffusion is reduced or restricted in prostate cancer, and this is manifested as high signal intensity on diffusion-weighted images or reduced signal intensity on ADC parametric images. Relatively high b values (b=800-1,000 s/mm^2) are generally used in prostate imaging, although as with DWI for most other organs, there is not a strong justification for this choice in the literature. Several studies have found a modest negative correlation between the ADC value of prostate cancers and the Gleason score, and this has led some to suggest that DWI can predict the aggressiveness of the lesion; however, these kinds of predictions have not always fared well for masses in other organs, and there is considerable variation in the published ADC values for prostate cancer.

DCE imaging is based on the phenomenon of neoangiogenesis, often associated with cancer and leading to early hyperenhancement and rapid washout of contrast agent from the tumor. In this case, the cancer demonstrates both restricted diffusion and early hyperenhancement, although this is by no means always the case, nor is it an absolute requirement for the diagnosis of prostate cancer.

Signs of extracapsular extension include obliteration or encasement of the neurovascular bundle (small punctate foci posterior to the prostate at the 5 and 7 o'clock positions on axial images which run parallel to the long axis of the prostate and penetrate the capsule at the apex and base), focal bulging of the posterior prostate contour, obliteration of the rectoprostatic angle, or direct extension of tumor beyond the capsule. In this case, there is subtle extracapsular extension, which was demonstrated at surgery—notice on the T2-weighted images the focal bulging of the prostatic margin in the region of the tumor slightly to the left of midline, along with loss of the dark posterior margin of the capsule. The reported accuracy of MRI in detecting extracapsular extension has varied widely, depending on the authors and methods, but mostly ranges from 60% to 90%.

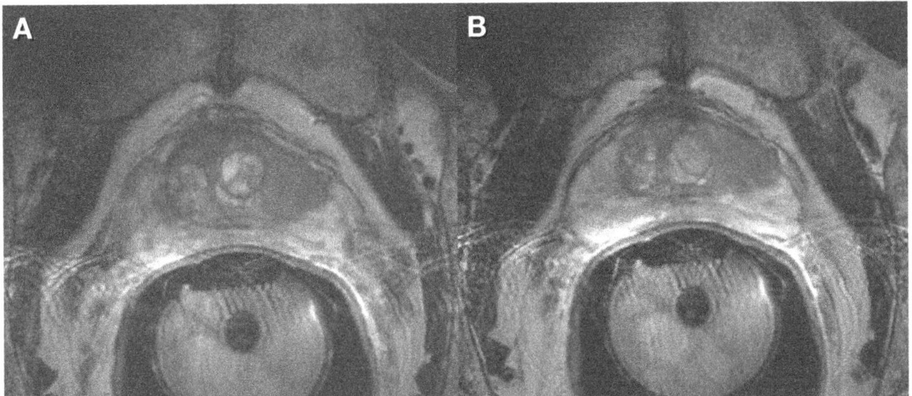

Figure 12.19.1

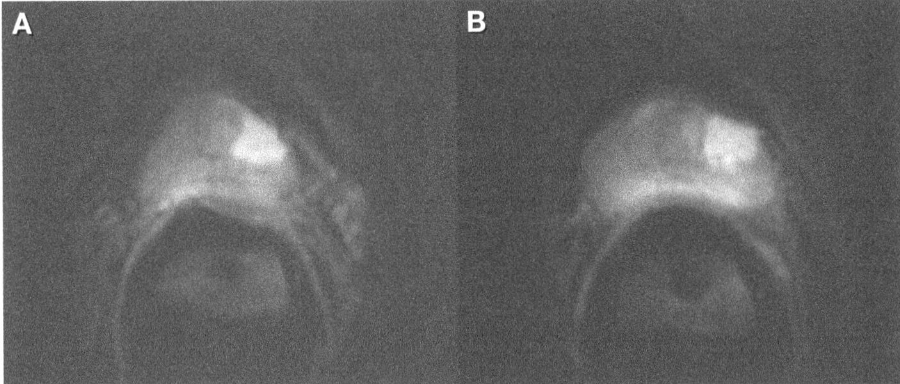

Figure 12.19.2

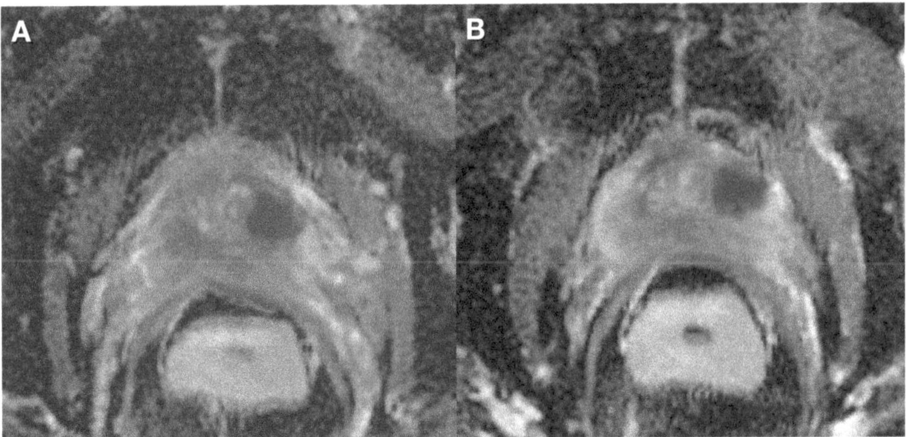

Figure 12.19.3

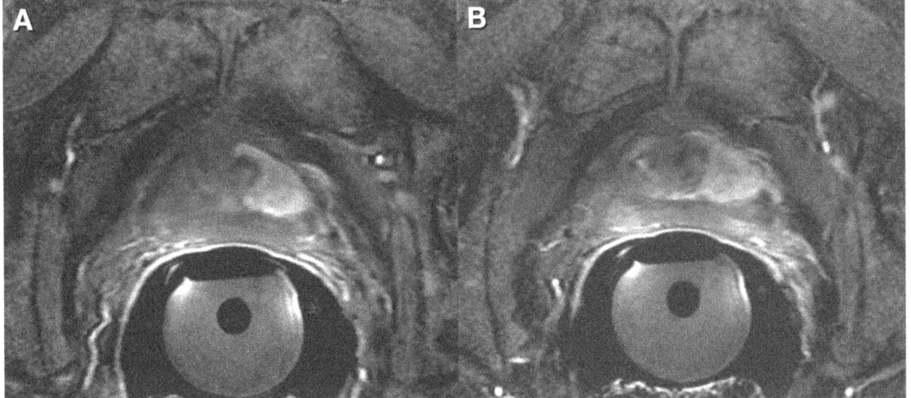

Figure 12.19.4

HISTORY: 62-year-old man with a history of prostate carcinoma (Gleason score 3+3) on ultrasound-guided biopsy

IMAGING FINDINGS: Axial T2-weighted FRFSE images (Figure 12.19.1) obtained with an endorectal coil demonstrate a hypointense lesion in the left anterior peripheral zone with probable involvement of the central gland. The lesion shows high signal intensity on axial diffusion-weighted images (b=1,000 s/mm^2) (Figure 12.19.2) and low ADC values relative to normal prostate on ADC parametric images (Figure 12.19.3). Axial arterial phase postgadolinium 3D SPGR images (Figure 12.19.4) reveal intense enhancement of the lesion above the level of normal prostate, including the central gland.

DIAGNOSIS: Prostate carcinoma

COMMENT: This case is another fairly classic example of prostate cancer, showing low T2-signal intensity, restricted diffusion, and early hyperenhancement on DCE images. In this case, involvement of the central gland is not a serious impediment to detection since the predominant peripheral zone component is readily visualized and the entire lesion is well delineated on the diffusion and postgadolinium images.

Detection of central gland cancer is not always so easy, however, and this can be a significant problem since approximately 30% of prostate cancers occur in this region. The major confounding factor is BPH, which is nearly ubiquitous in older men and leads to a heterogeneous appearance of the transition zone. While DCE imaging and DWI may be helpful in detecting central gland lesions, as in this case, there is often considerable overlap in the appearance of the stromal elements of BPH and prostate cancer, and some lesions are difficult to detect. Distinguishing cancer from BPH on T2-weighted images is even more problematic, although a dominant low-signal-intensity lesion in the central gland that breaches the low-signal-intensity rim often seen surrounding BPH should certainly raise suspicion.

As noted in Case 12.18, the role of MRI in prostate cancer may be undergoing a transformation. Until very recently, MRI was used primarily to stage known lesions for extracapsular extension, invasion of the seminal vesicles, and metastatic disease in the pelvis—it's clearly better than CT or US for these tasks, although not highly accurate, and does not perform well at all in predicting nodal involvement.

As the technology for MR-guided prostate biopsy becomes more widely available, it seems logical to use the best imaging modality to guide biopsies. Small studies have demonstrated an increased yield with MR-guided biopsies in patients with a strong clinical suspicion of prostate cancer and a negative first biopsy. Compared with ultrasound-guided biopsies, MR-guided biopsies have also shown better agreement in Gleason score with prostatectomy specimens. The logical ultimate step would seem to be a protocol in which a patient with a palpable mass or elevated PSA value then proceeds to MRI, with directed biopsy of any visible lesions or no biopsy if there are no suspicious findings.

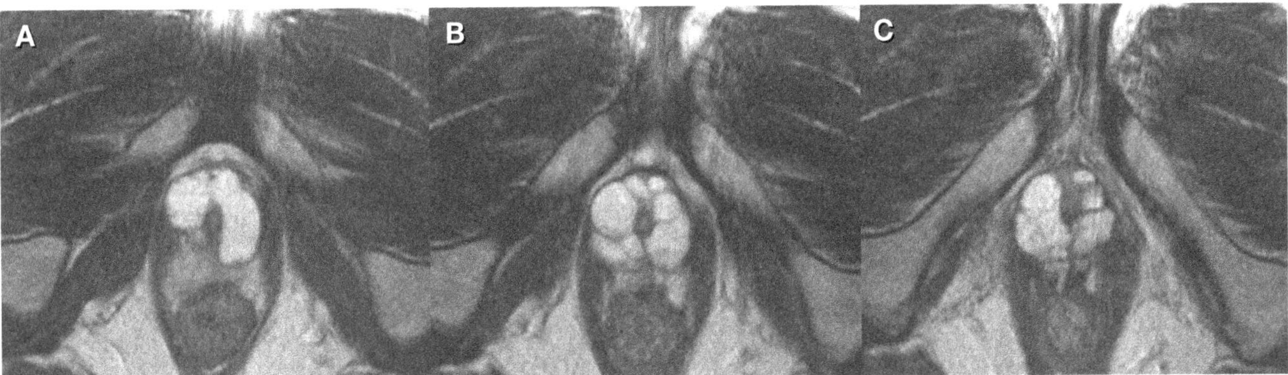

Figure 12.20.1

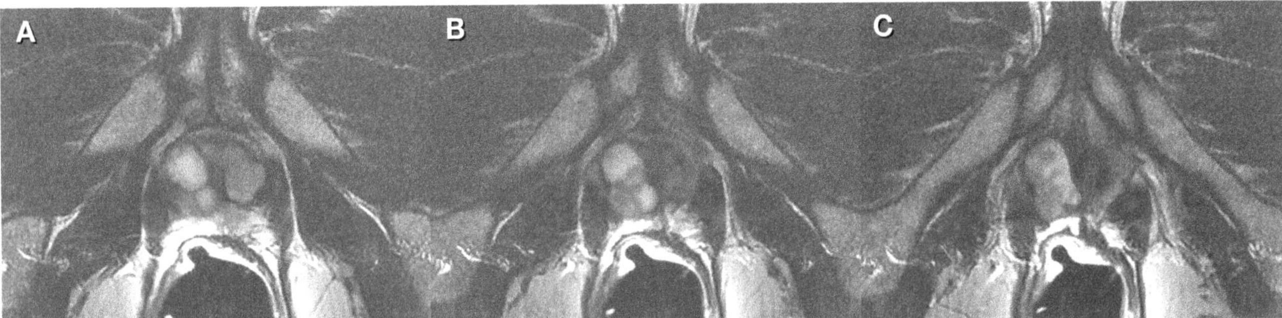

Figure 12.20.2

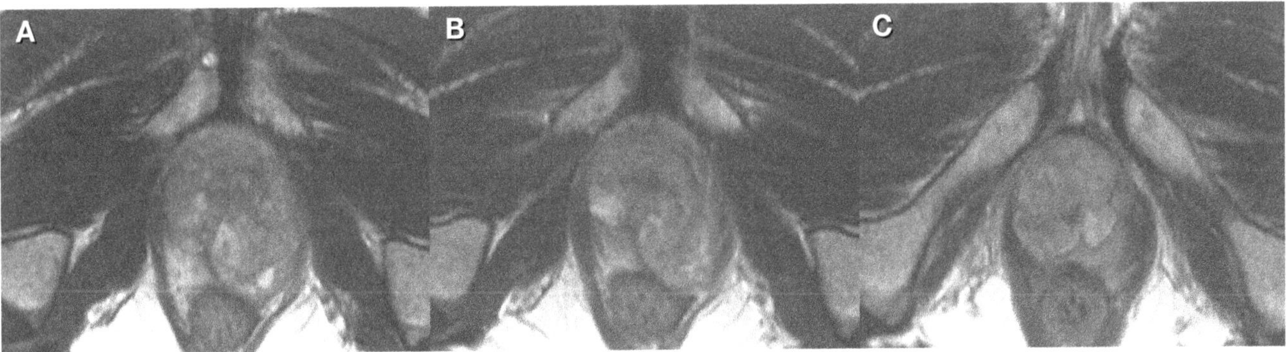

Figure 12.20.3

HISTORY: 46-year-old man with hematuria

IMAGING FINDINGS: Axial T2-weighted FRFSE images (Figure 12.20.1) demonstrate a multilobulated cystic lesion with several thin septations in the prostate apex. Axial FRFSE images from an examination performed 1 year later (Figure 12.20.2) demonstrate decreasing size of the cystic lesions but with new soft tissue nodularity. Axial FRFSE images from an examination performed 2 years later (Figure 12.20.3) reveal marked enlargement of the mass, with the cystic components replaced by heterogeneous soft tissue.

DIAGNOSIS: Cystic prostate carcinoma

COMMENT: This case is an unusual cystic manifestation of prostate adenocarcinoma, originating from what was probably a benign cystic lesion. The initial images show a cystic lesion in the apex of the prostate without any visible soft tissue components. On biopsy, the lesion contained benign prostatic tissue with mixed inflammatory cells. At the follow-up examination 1 year later, multiple new soft tissue nodules were, unfortunately, considered debris within the cystic lesion (gadolinium was administered and, in retrospect, there was minimal enhancement of some of the nodular components). In the 2-year follow-up images, the prostate adenocarcinoma is obvious, with a large heterogeneous soft tissue component replacing the cystic lesion.

The lessons from this case are that not all cystic lesions in the prostate are benign and that any lesion should be inspected carefully for suspicious elements.

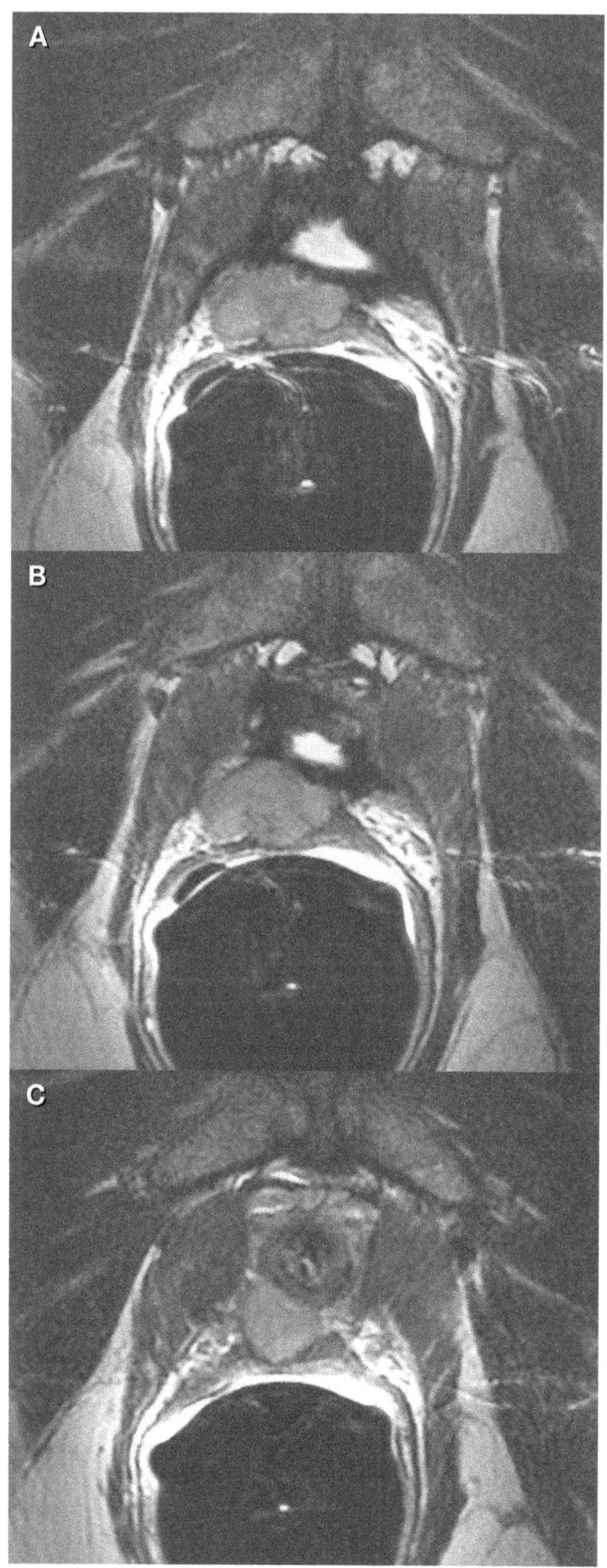

Figure 12.21.1

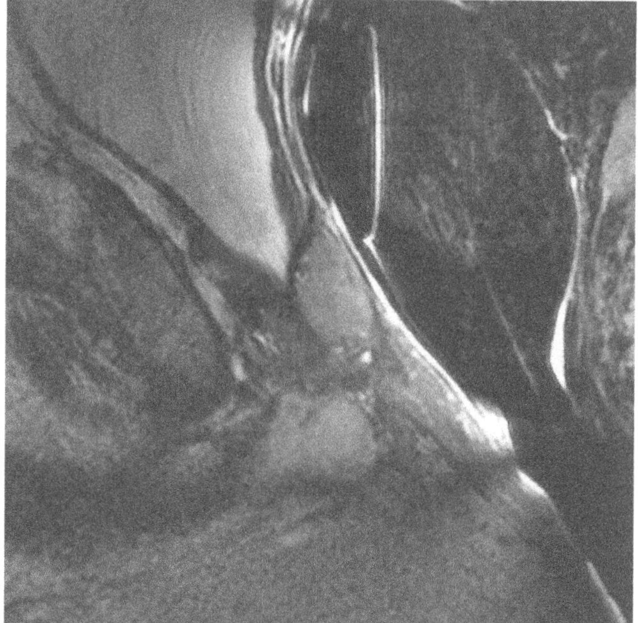

Figure 12.21.2

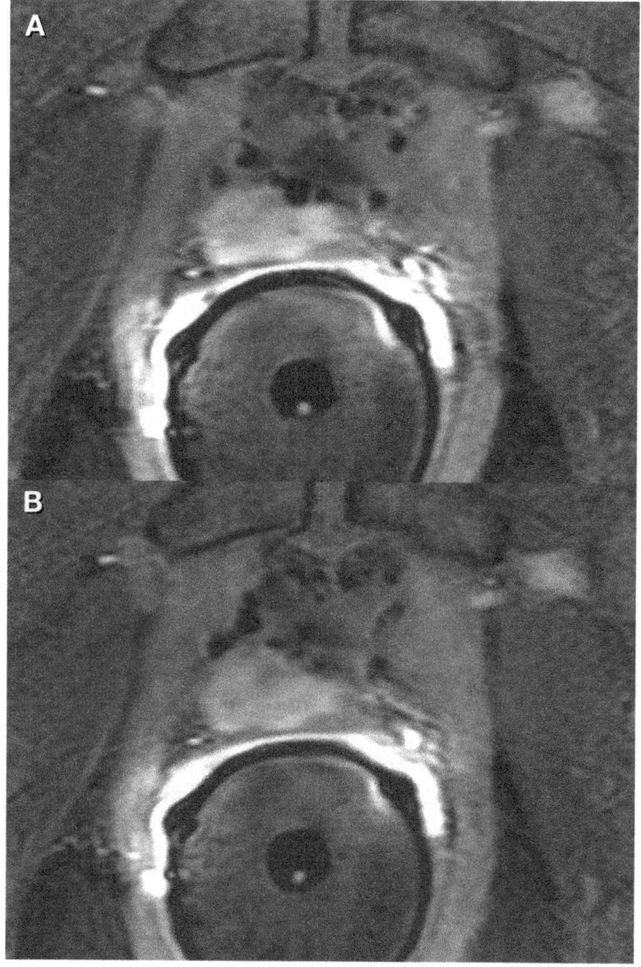

Figure 12.21.3

HISTORY: 53-year-old man who underwent robotic prostatectomy 4 years ago with a small positive margin in the right apex; PSA was initially zero postoperatively, but it has been slowly increasing in the past year

IMAGING FINDINGS: Axial (Figure 12.21.1) and sagittal (Figure 12.21.2) T2-weighted FRFSE images obtained with an endorectal coil demonstrate a lobulated mass with mildly increased signal intensity along the right posterior margin of the bladder outlet extending inferiorly into the prostatectomy bed. Axial arterial phase postgadolinium 3D SPGR images (Figure 12.21.3) reveal intense focal enhancement of the lesion. Notice the mildly prominent susceptibility artifact on the 3D SPGR images from surgical clips in the prostatectomy bed.

DIAGNOSIS: Prostate cancer recurrence

COMMENT: Unfortunately, recurrence of prostate cancer after prostatectomy or radiotherapy is fairly common, with rates ranging from 12% to 67%, depending on patient risk factors. Patients are monitored with PSA levels after local therapy, and abnormally sustained or increasing PSA levels typically indicate either local recurrence or metastatic disease. MRI is an excellent technique for detecting local recurrence and relies primarily on visualizing an early enhancing lesion in the prostatectomy bed. Occasionally, there is a small amount of residual prostate tissue that can be seen as symmetric periurethral enhancement, but in general there should be no enhancing soft tissue in the prostatectomy bed, and anything that does enhance should be regarded with suspicion unless it's clearly a blood vessel or some other recognizably benign structure. Similarly, the postradiation prostate should consist of fibrotic tissue without significant enhancement, and any early enhancing foci should raise concern for recurrent disease.

The patient in this case has a fairly large lesion that is clearly seen even on T2-weighted images. This is somewhat unusual in our practice, where patients generally undergo scanning fairly soon after a positive PSA level has been documented, and often the small recurrent lesions are seen only on DCE images.

Occasionally, surgical clips, adjacent metal, or radiation seeds generate significant susceptibility artifact on dynamic postgadolinium 3D SPGR images. This is most problematic for 3-T systems, and if we see a patient with severe artifact on the precontrast 3D SPGR acquisition, we try to move him to a 1.5-T magnet and, if necessary, take additional steps to minimize artifact, including use of a higher receiver bandwidth and shorter TE. This is logistically difficult, however, particularly for an examination requiring an endorectal coil. The addition of DCE imaging has led to much greater success at detecting local recurrence; recent papers have reported sensitivities of 84% to 88% and specificities of 89% to 100%.

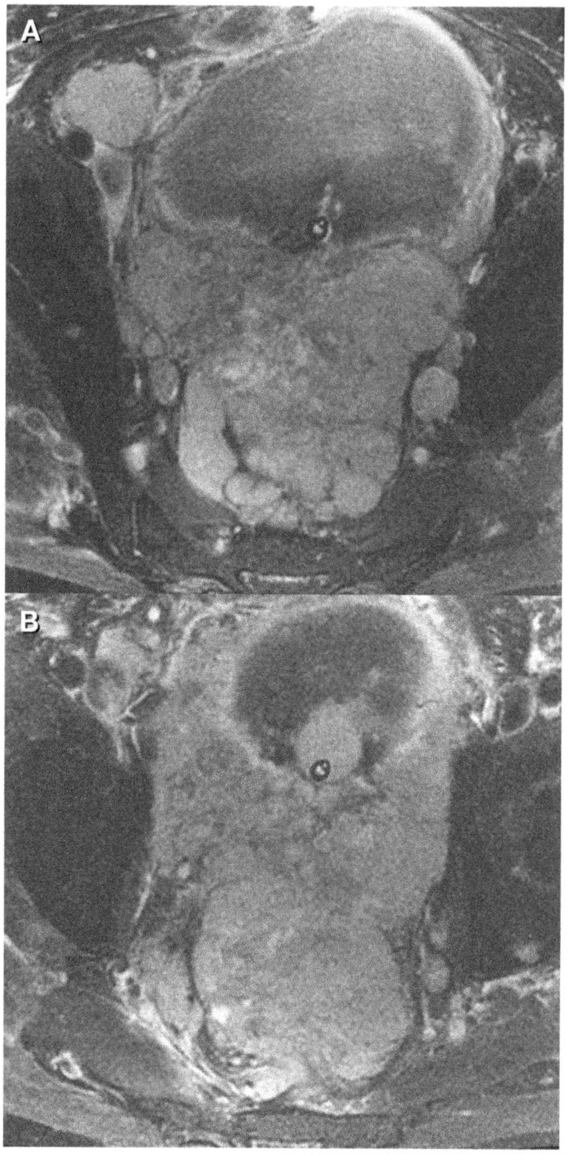

Figure 12.22.1

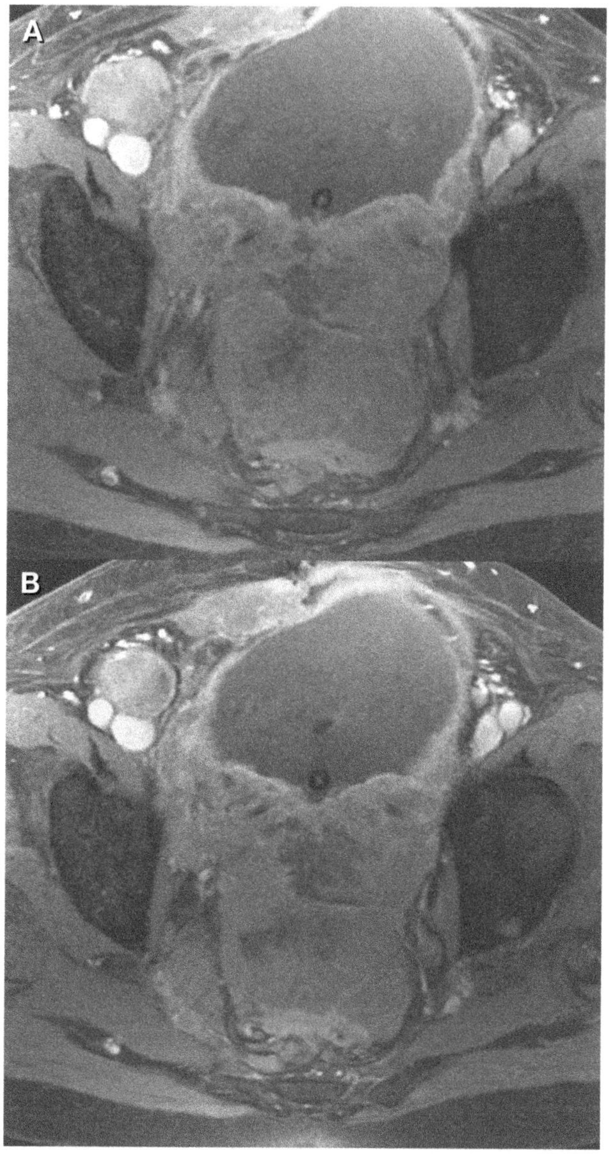

Figure 12.22.3

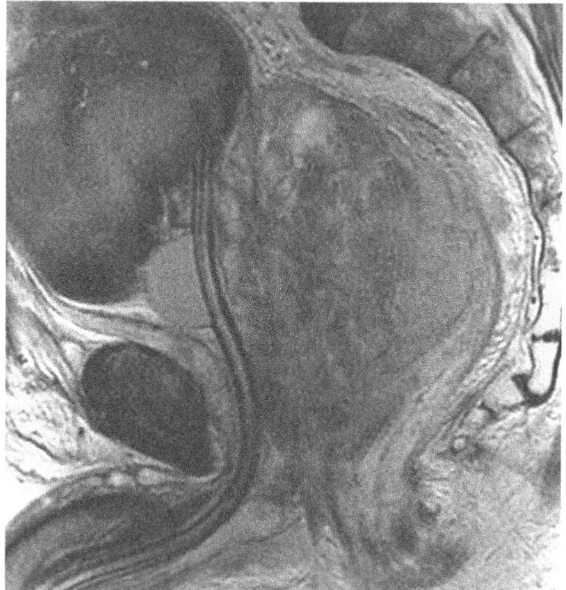

Figure 12.22.2

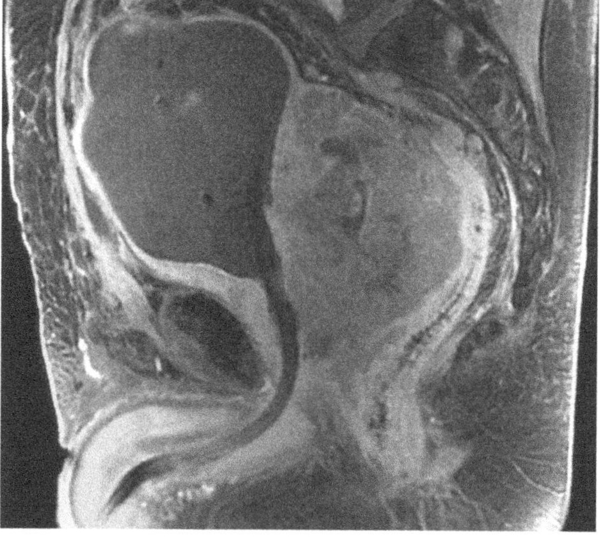

Figure 12.22.4

HISTORY: 70-year-old man with a history of prostate cancer diagnosed 12 years ago and treated with radical prostatectomy; a recurrence diagnosed 2 years later was treated with radiotherapy, and he now presents with nausea and signs of bladder outlet obstruction

IMAGING FINDINGS: Axial fat-suppressed (Figure 12.22.1) and sagittal (Figure 12.22.2) FSE T2-weighted images reveal a large mass in the prostatectomy bed. The mass invades the posterior wall of the bladder anteriorly and partially encases the rectum posteriorly. There is also extensive adenopathy in the pelvis. Axial (Figure 12.22.3) and sagittal (Figure 12.22.4) postgadolinium 2D SPGR images demonstrate similar findings. Note a small enhancing lesion in the posterior left acetabulum with high signal intensity on the corresponding T2-weighted axial image.

DIAGNOSIS: Recurrent and metastatic prostate carcinoma

COMMENT: In many respects, this case illustrates a worst-case scenario for prostate cancer. The patient initially had localized disease, which then recurred in the prostatectomy bed, for which he received radiotherapy. His PSA levels continued to rise slowly without definite evidence of metastatic disease. He eventually was placed on hormonal therapy, which led to a decline in PSA levels for approximately 1.5 years, after which they rose again. Ultimately, he presented with signs and symptoms of bladder outlet obstruction, and MRI demonstrated a massive recurrent lesion in the prostatectomy bed as well as extensive pelvic adenopathy and a small bone metastasis. CT of the chest and abdomen demonstrated widespread metastatic disease.

Therapy for locally advanced prostate cancer may involve surgery, radiotherapy, systemic chemotherapy, and hormonal therapy. Hormonal therapy is frequently used in patients with metastatic disease; however, the cancer tends to escape hormonal control after 13 to 21 months.

This case presents no diagnostic dilemma, although it is difficult to appreciate that the patient has had a prostatectomy. For small locally recurrent lesions, sensitivity is improved by using an endorectal coil and obtaining small FOV DCE images through the prostate bed, as illustrated in Case 12.21. (It's important for whoever inserts the coil to exercise restraint when resistance is encountered, both to avoid patient injury in the case of advanced disease and to preserve image quality. An examination performed without an endorectal coil is always preferable to one degraded by motion artifact or canceled by a patient in too much pain to continue.) Remember to obtain at least 1 or 2 large FOV acquisitions through the entire pelvis (in our protocol these include precontrast and postcontrast Dixon 3D SPGR images and diffusion-weighted images), so that enlarged lymph nodes and bone metastases can be detected.

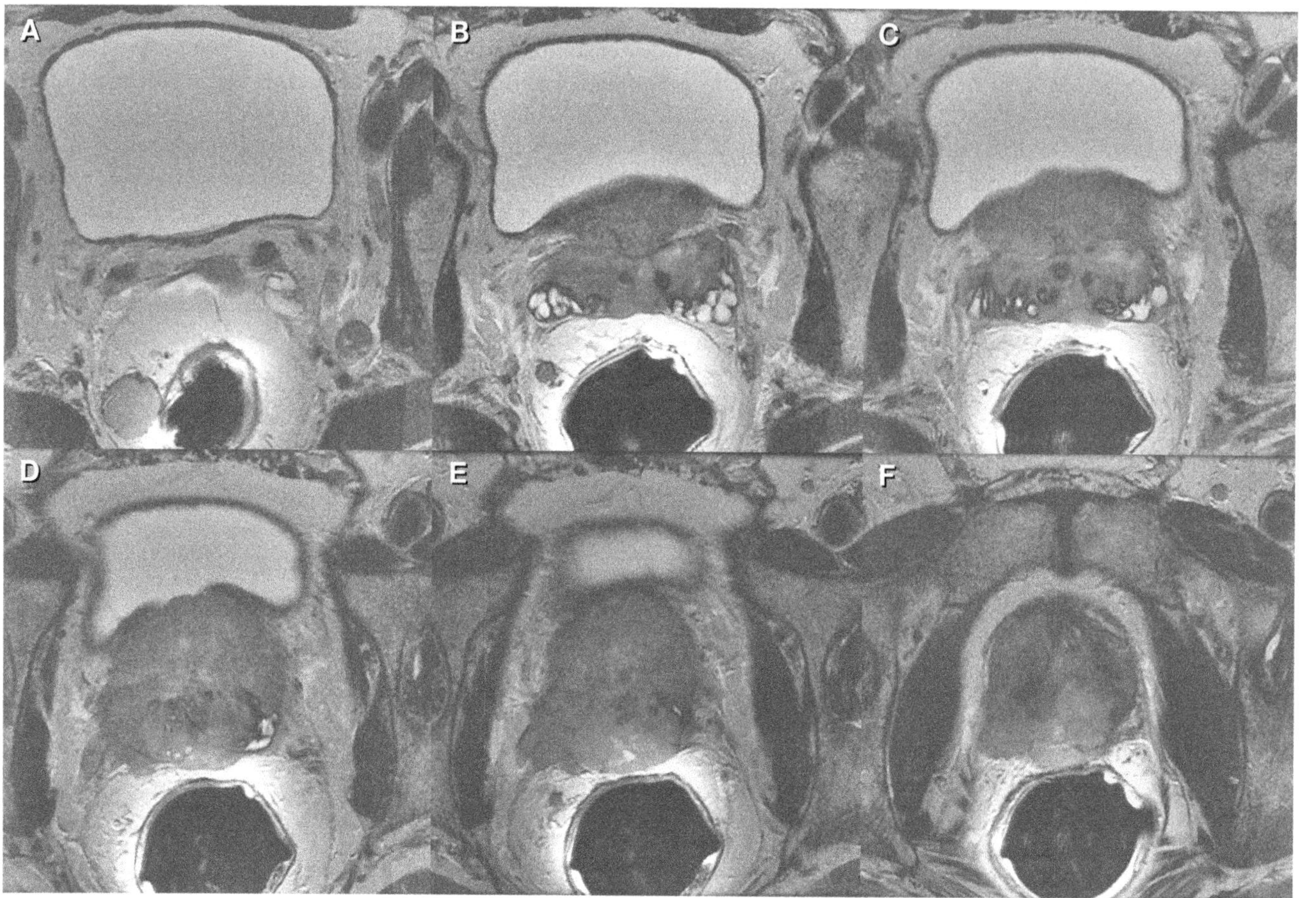

Figure 12.23.1

HISTORY: 45-year-old man with hematuria and difficulty voiding

IMAGING FINDINGS: Axial T2-weighted FRFSE images (Figure 12.23.1) obtained using an endorectal coil demonstrate a large infiltrative mass in the peripheral zone of the prostate. The mass invades the seminal vesicles and extends into the central zone in the apex. Note the loss of the well-defined posterior capsular margin indicating extracapsular extension, involvement of the right and probably the left neurovascular bundles, continuity of the mass with the anterior wall of the rectum, and the large perirectal lymph node on the first image.

DIAGNOSIS: Small cell prostate carcinoma

COMMENT: SCPCa, also described as neuroendocrine SCPCa, is a rare form of prostate cancer that generally follows an aggressive and rapidly fatal course. It is thought to account for approximately 2% of all prostate carcinomas and most commonly occurs in association with adenocarcinomatous elements, sometimes appearing in recurrent tumors following androgen deprivation therapy. In roughly one-third of cases, the histology is pure SCPCa. Small cell carcinomas are rare outside the lung, but 10% occur in the prostate, making it one of the most common extrapulmonary sites.

The clinical presentation may be indistinguishable from prostate adenocarcinoma but is often characterized by rapidly progressive symptoms, a large prostatic mass, and a high frequency of locally advanced or metastatic disease. Bone metastases are less frequent than conventional adenocarcinoma, and they tend to be lytic, with a higher frequency of lung and liver metastases. Another unique feature of SCPCa is the development of paraneoplastic syndromes in approximately 10% of patients, and elevations in corticotropin, calcitonin, parathyroid hormone, and other neuroendocrine markers can be seen. PSA levels may be elevated, particularly in patients with mixed tumors; however, because the neuroendocrine component does not secrete PSA, the value of PSA as a marker of disease burden or therapeutic response is limited.

Treatment has generally been modeled after therapy for small cell lung cancer, with chemotherapy having a leading role along with surgery or radiotherapy (or both) for local control. Nevertheless, prognosis is poor for most patients (median survival, 9-10 months; 5-year survival, <1%).

Few reports in the literature describe the imaging appearance of SCPCa, with most emphasizing the aggressive primary lesions and frequent metastases. This case illustrates a large lesion involving essentially the entire peripheral zone with invasion of the seminal vesicles, extension into the central zone, and possible involvement of the anterior rectal wall. We don't see anything unique in this presentation to lead to a consideration of SCPCa rather than a high-grade adenocarcinoma. This patient had extensive pelvic adenopathy at diagnosis but no bone or visceral metastases. He had a complete response to chemotherapy and no recurrence after 3 years of follow-up.

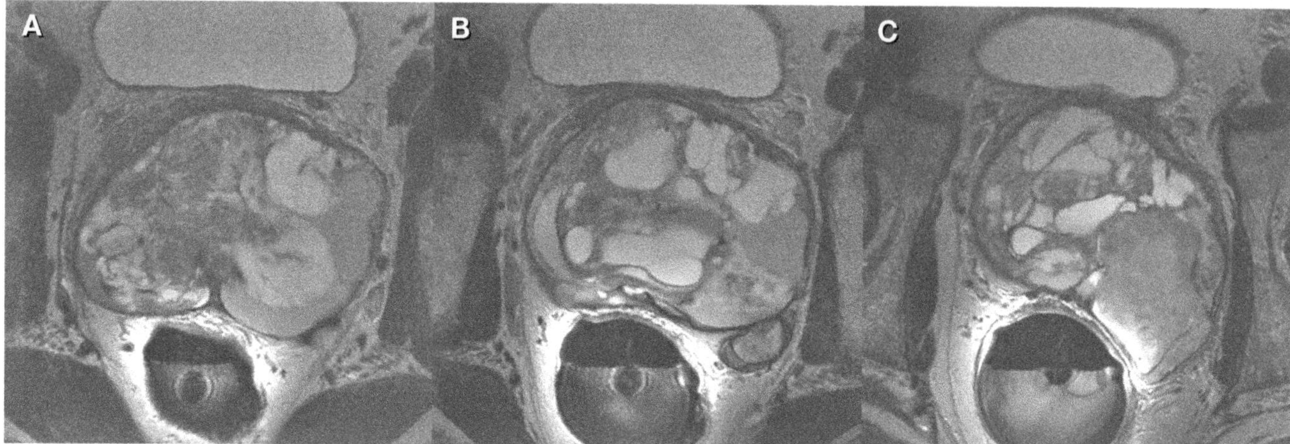

Figure 12.24.1

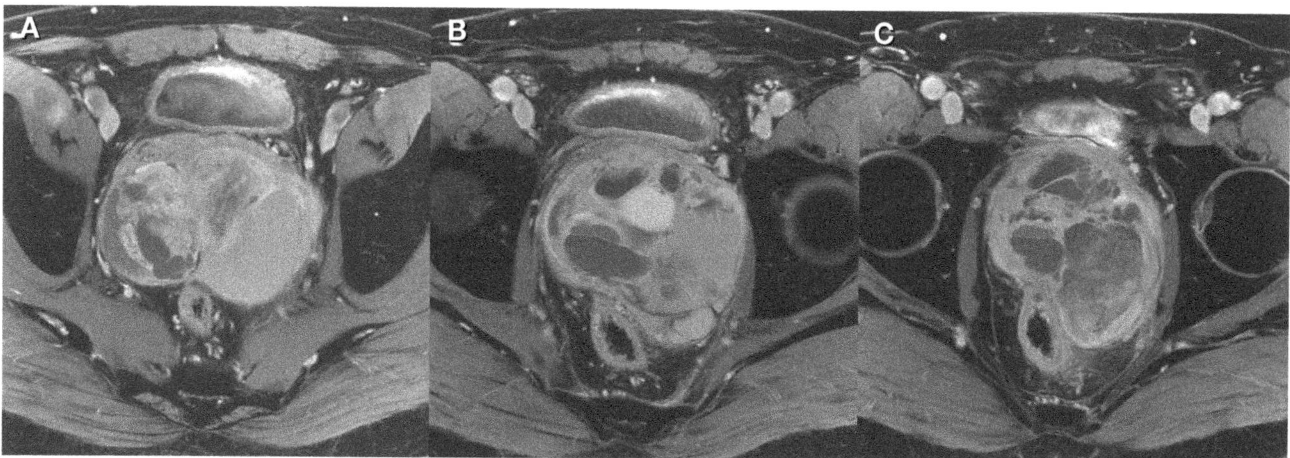

Figure 12.24.2

HISTORY: 50-year-old man with an elevated PSA level and an enlarged prostate on physical examination

IMAGING FINDINGS: Axial FSE T2-weighted images (Figure 12.24.1) obtained with an endorectal coil reveal a heterogeneous mass containing cystic and solid components replacing the prostate. Postgadolinium axial 2D SPGR images (Figure 12.24.2) also demonstrate a large mass with heterogeneous enhancement and multiple cystic or necrotic regions. (Notice also that the endorectal coil has been removed for patient comfort.)

DIAGNOSIS: Malignant phyllodes tumor of the prostate

COMMENT: Phyllodes tumor of the prostate is a rare neoplasm consisting of hyperplastic and neoplastic glandular-stromal proliferation, first reported by Cox and Dawson in 1960 and subsequently described by many different names, including cystic adenoma of the prostate, cystadenoleiomyofibroma, cystic epithelial stromal tumor, phyllodes type of atypical hyperplasia, and cystosarcoma phyllodes. Phyllodes tumor of the prostate is analogous to the more widely known breast lesion and can display significant variation in histologic appearance and clinical behavior.

Approximately 60 cases have been reported in the literature; most of the patients presented with symptoms of recurrent urinary obstruction. Reports of the imaging appearance on CT or MRI are quite limited, but they emphasize heterogeneous lesions with mixed cystic and solid components. This case demonstrates a large, bizarre lesion with multiple cystic and solid components involving the entire gland and showing heterogeneous enhancement following gadolinium administration. The appearance would be very unusual for a prostate adenocarcinoma (although cystic varieties do occur, as in Case 12.20) and might be more likely to be confused with extensive BPH, which frequently undergoes cystic degeneration. The differential diagnosis would also include leiomyosarcoma and rhabdomyosarcoma, which can be excluded histologically by the absence of immunostaining for muscle markers (desmin and smooth muscle actin).

The consensus in the literature is that most phyllodes tumors follow a benign course, but malignant behavior has been reported and is seen in this case. Pathologic features suggesting malignancy include infiltrating margins, increased numbers of mitoses, and atypia of stromal cells. The tumor in this case had focal high-grade sarcomatous stromal overgrowth but no evidence of local invasion or metastatic disease. Since the imaging findings of malignant phyllodes tumor have not been described, we can postulate without fear of contradiction that worrisome findings on MRI include the large solid nodule in the left gland with heterogeneous enhancement; the bulging, irregular left capsular margin; and the overall large size and heterogeneity of the lesion.

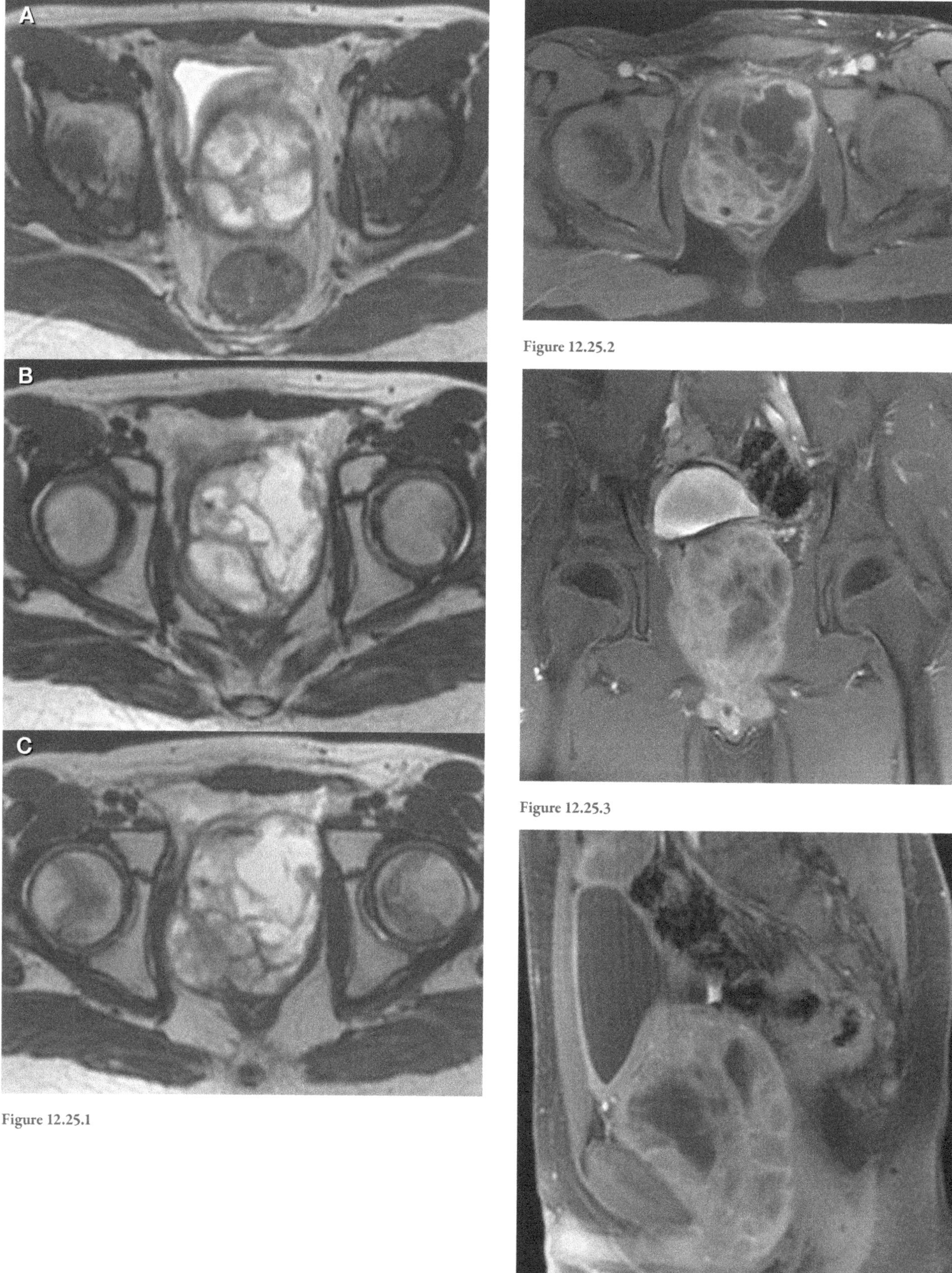

Figure 12.25.1

Figure 12.25.2

Figure 12.25.3

Figure 12.25.4

HISTORY: 7-year-old boy with urinary retention and a pelvic mass

IMAGING FINDINGS: Axial T2-weighted 3D FSE images (Figure 12.25.1) reveal a heterogeneous high-signal-intensity mass replacing the prostate. Axial (Figure 12.25.2), coronal (Figure 12.25.3), and sagittal (Figure 12.25.4) postgadolinium 2D SPGR images demonstrate a large prostate mass with heterogeneous enhancement and regions of necrosis.

DIAGNOSIS: Prostate rhabdomyosarcoma

COMMENT: Rhabdomyosarcoma is the most common tumor of the lower genitourinary tract in children and comprises 5% to 10% of the malignant tumors of childhood, with approximately 250 new cases diagnosed annually in the United States. Genitourinary rhabdomyosarcomas may involve the penis, testicles, perineum, vagina, and uterus, but they most commonly affect the bladder and prostate. Distinguishing between bladder and prostate origin can be difficult, since the tumors are often large and infiltrating, and many authors include them in a single category.

Most rhabdomyosarcomas appear sporadically, but a few occur in association with neurofibromatosis, fetal alcohol syndrome, and basal cell nevus syndrome. The median age at presentation is 7 years, and most patients present with bladder outlet obstruction, pain, dysuria, and urinary tract infection.

Rhabdomyosarcoma shares histologic features with fetal muscle cells (rhabdomyoblasts) of various maturational stages, and diagnostic criteria include demonstration of actin and myosin filaments and immunohistochemical markers for myoglobin, desmin, actin, and the *MYOD1* gene. Rhabdomyosarcomas are classified into embryonal, botryoid, alveolar, and pleomorphic subtypes; the embryonal subtype is the most common in bladder and prostate tumors.

The typical MRI appearance of rhabdomyosarcoma includes heterogeneous increased T2-signal intensity and heterogeneous enhancement following gadolinium administration, often with focal regions of hemorrhage and necrosis. Many lesions involve both the bladder and the prostate, but in this case, it is fairly clear that the prostate represents the epicenter of the lesion and the bladder is displaced rather than invaded.

There isn't much of a differential diagnosis for a large, aggressive, heterogeneous prostate mass in a child. When the bladder is more extensively involved, rhabdomyosarcoma can be difficult to distinguish from an inflammatory myofibroblastic tumor (an example is Case 8.12 in Chapter 8), and other bladder lesions, including polyps, hemangiomas, and focal cystitis, can occasionally present diagnostic dilemmas.

Treatment typically involves chemotherapy or radiotherapy (or both) followed by surgical resection. Outcomes for children with bladder or prostate rhabdomyosarcoma have improved considerably in the past few decades, with as many as 70% to 80% of patients experiencing long-term survival without recurrence.

ABBREVIATIONS

ADC	apparent diffusion coefficient
BPH	benign prostatic hyperplasia
CT	computed tomography
DCE	dynamic contrast-enhanced
DWI	diffusion-weighted imaging
FOV	field of view
FRFSE	fast-recovery fast-spin echo
FSE	fast-spin echo
MR	magnetic resonance
MRI	magnetic resonance imaging
PET	positron emission tomography
PSA	prostate-specific antigen
SCPCa	small cell prostate carcinoma
SNR	signal to noise ratio
SPGR	spoiled gradient recalled
SSFP	steady-state free precession
TE	echo time
3D	3-dimensional
TURP	transurethral resection of the prostate
2D	2-dimensional
US	ultrasonography

13.

THORAX AND HEART

CASE 13.1

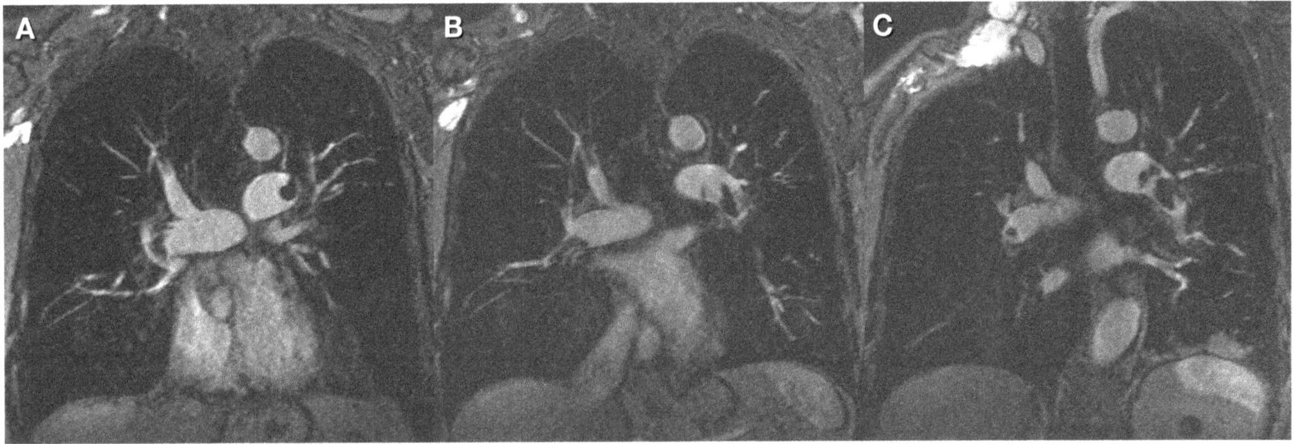

Figure 13.1.1

HISTORY: 80-year-old man with a left lower lobe adenocarcinoma, for which he is receiving radiotherapy, presents with cough and shortness of breath; MRI was requested to evaluate for pulmonary embolus

IMAGING FINDINGS: Coronal oblique images from 3D contrast-enhanced pulmonary MRA (Figure 13.1.1) reveal filling defects in the left main pulmonary artery and both lobar arteries.

DIAGNOSIS: Pulmonary emboli

COMMENT: MRA as an alternative technique for diagnosis of pulmonary embolus has lost some of its relevance in the age of nephrogenic systemic fibrosis, although interestingly in this case MRI was requested on the basis of mild renal insufficiency. CTA has evolved to the extent that the latest generation of equipment can scan the chest in 1 second or less, often with fairly low overall radiation doses. Although CT pulmonary embolus studies can still be of truly abysmal quality (we can personally attest to this), the point is that the gap between CTA and MRA for this indication seems to be widening rather than narrowing.

Nearly everyone who gives talks about MRA has examples like this case with beautiful, high-resolution, artifact-free images showing pulmonary emboli. The real problem is that these patients can be some of the worst candidates for MRA: By definition, they are dyspneic and often cannot hold their breath for more than a few seconds, if at all. Breathing artifacts are more problematic with MRA than with CTA since the MRA acquisition is truly volumetric, and each second contributes data that are used in the reconstruction of every image. In addition, MRA acquisition times are generally much longer and are therefore more susceptible to motion artifacts.

The MRI literature, as is often the case, supports a wide range of opinions on the subject. Many single-center studies, for example, achieved sensitivities greater than 90% for detection of pulmonary emboli, often with an astonishingly small proportion of examinations degraded by artifact. In contrast, the largest multicenter trial, the PIOPED III study with 371 patients in 7 hospitals, had disappointing results. Examinations were technically inadequate for 25% of patients, with an overall sensitivity of 57% for detection of pulmonary emboli; the sensitivity increased to 78% when the inadequate examinations were excluded. Unfortunately, there were no uniform standards for MRA performance and no imaging parameters were published, so it is difficult to know whether the poor results accurately reflect the state of the art or were at least partially a consequence of poor technique.

Our approach in these increasingly rare cases is to sacrifice spatial resolution for acquisition time in the typical dyspneic patient. We aim for acquisition times of 10 seconds or less, typically in an axial plane with a section thickness of 3 to 4 mm, and usually cut off the apical and basilar sections of the lungs since most of the vessels there are too small to evaluate. This is also probably a good indication for using a blood-pool contrast agent: If the breath-hold is inadequate the first time, the acquisition can be repeated until the results are acceptable.

We are occasionally asked to diagnose pulmonary embolism without the use of a contrast agent, typically for a pregnant patient. This is even more challenging, but usually central emboli (lobar and segmental) can be identified with a combination of overlapping 2D SSFP images in 1 or 2 planes and occasionally a navigator-gated 3D SSFP sequence. In our practice, the diagnosis of pulmonary embolism arises most often as an incidental finding (or a missed incidental finding) on an examination (usually cardiac) performed for a completely different purpose.

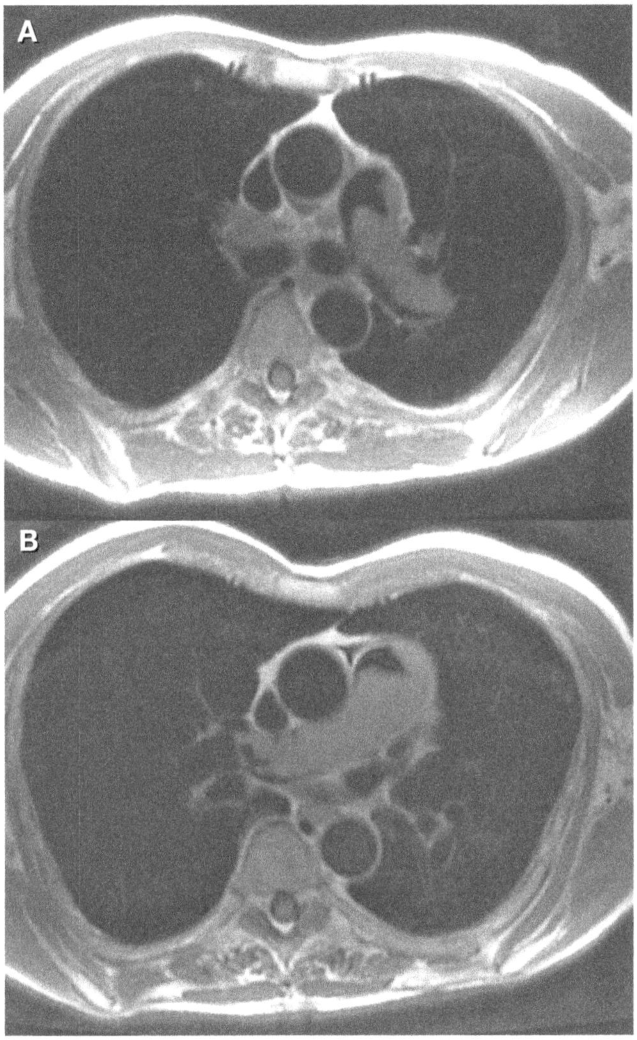

Figure 13.2.1

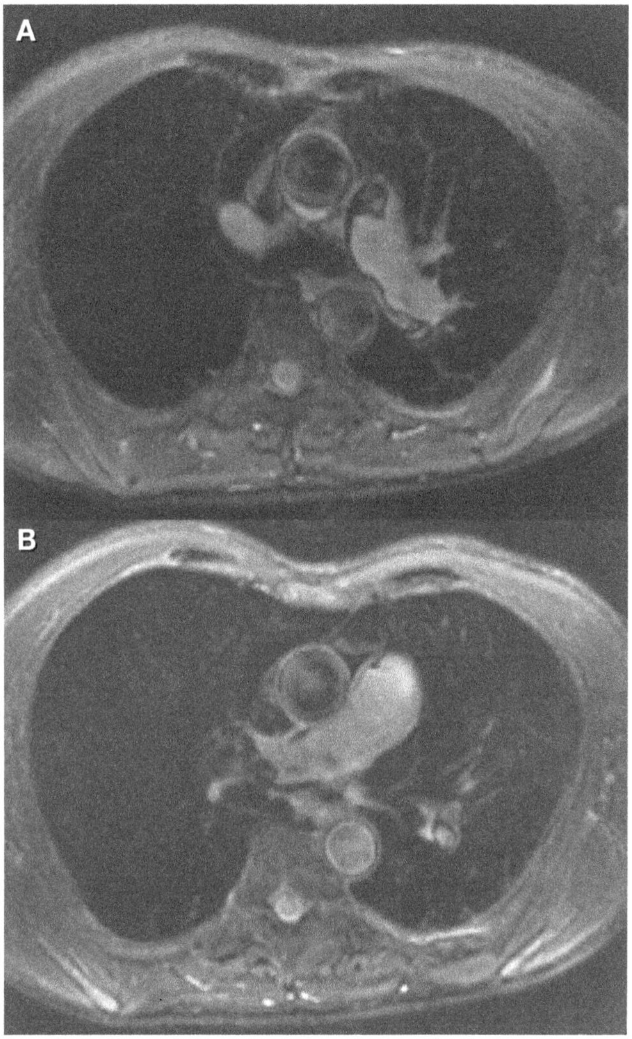

Figure 13.2.2

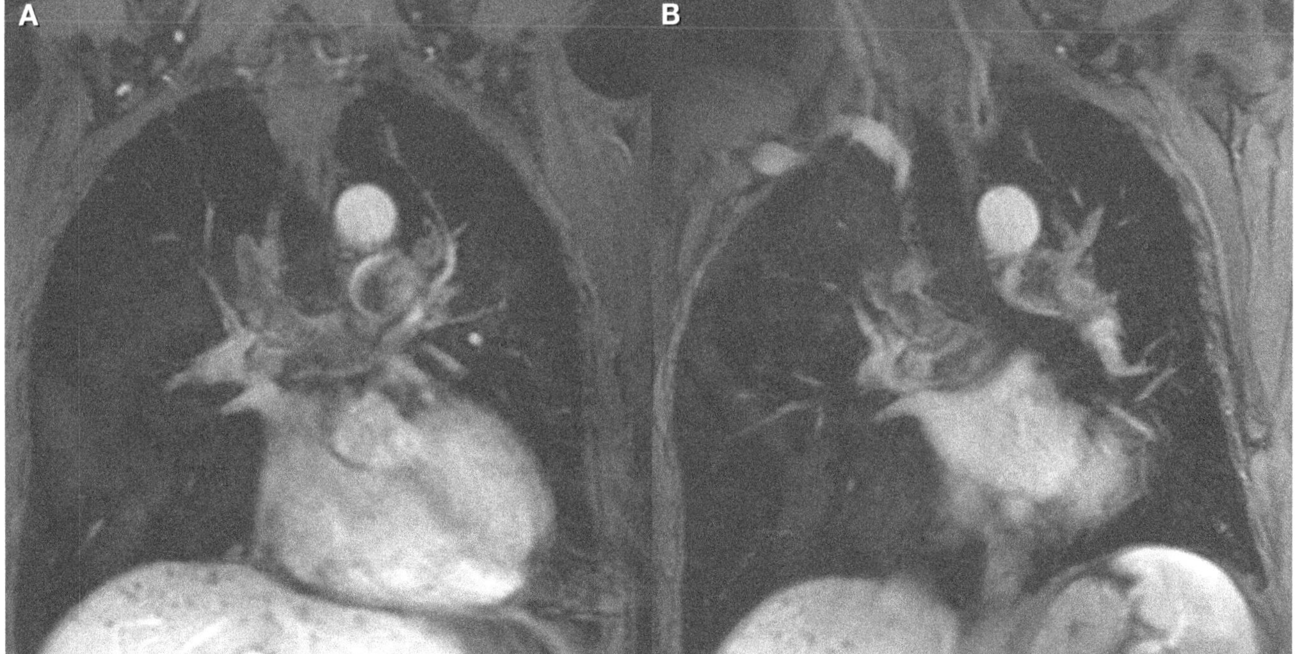

Figure 13.2.3

HISTORY: 74-year-old man with shortness of breath and fatigue; CT showed large central pulmonary emboli

IMAGING FINDINGS: Axial double inversion recovery (Figure 13.2.1) and triple inversion recovery (Figure 13.2.2) proton density-weighted and T2-weighted ECG-gated FSE images reveal a nearly occlusive soft tissue mass with increased T2-signal intensity in the main pulmonary artery and extending into the right and left main pulmonary arteries. Coronal postgadolinium 3D SPGR images (Figure 13.2.3) demonstrate regions of linear enhancement within the mass.

DIAGNOSIS: Pulmonary artery sarcoma

COMMENT: Pulmonary artery sarcomas are rare tumors that carry a generally dismal prognosis. The first case was reported in 1923 by Mandelstamm as an autopsy study; since then, descriptions of 250 to 300 cases have been published. The diagnosis is still often made at autopsy or occasionally as a surprising result during pulmonary thromboendarterectomy. Patient symptoms often mimic those of pulmonary embolism, and these lesions are frequently misdiagnosed as emboli, with the diagnosis suspected when there is no response to anticoagulation therapy. We have seen 3 cases with MRI, and all were initially treated as saddle emboli after initial misdiagnosis on CTA.

Clues to help distinguish tumor from thrombus may be found in the higher signal intensity on double and triple inversion recovery T1- and T2-weighted images or diffusion-weighted images and in enhancement within the mass following gadolinium administration. MRI, with its superior soft tissue characterization, is probably better than CT for making this distinction, but most of the time you can (retrospectively) find worrisome features on the initial CT. Most lesions arise from the main pulmonary artery, with approximately one-third involving the pulmonic valve. Extension of the mass through the vessel wall is diagnostic of a neoplasm and generally occurs when there is already a large intraluminal component. Pulmonary artery sarcomas may invade the pericardium or other adjacent mediastinal structures, and the presence of pulmonary, mediastinal, or other distant metastases should be documented. The presenting symptoms are often paradoxically less severe than would be expected for a simple pulmonary embolus. In this case, for example, the patient was only mildly dyspneic and could hold his breath for nearly 20 seconds in spite of nearly complete occlusion of the main pulmonary arteries. This likely reflects the relatively slow growth of the tumor compared to the sudden onset of most emboli.

Histologically, pulmonary artery sarcomas include undifferentiated sarcoma, leiomyosarcoma, fibrosarcoma, rhabdomyosarcoma, angiosarcoma, and many others; however, the histologic features do not seem to affect the prognosis, which is poor. In a literature review including 60 patients, median survival was 36 months among patients undergoing attempted curative resection, 24 months among patients receiving multimodality treatment, and less than 1 year among patients receiving single-modality treatment or undergoing incomplete resection.

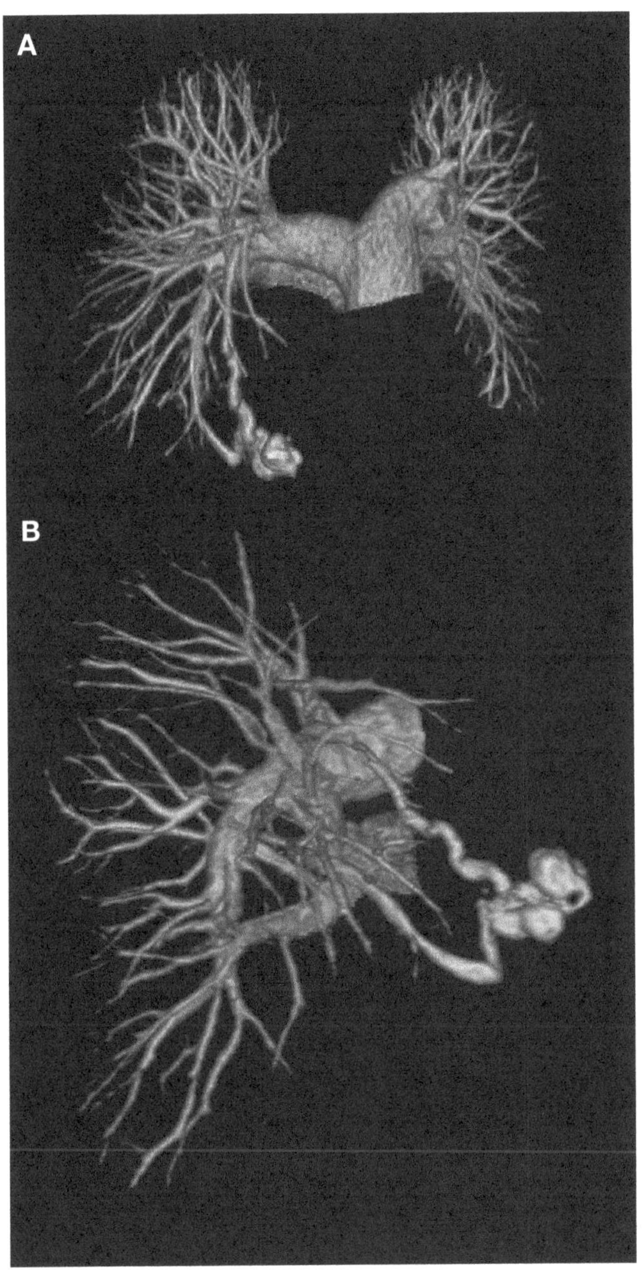

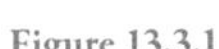
Figure 13.3.1

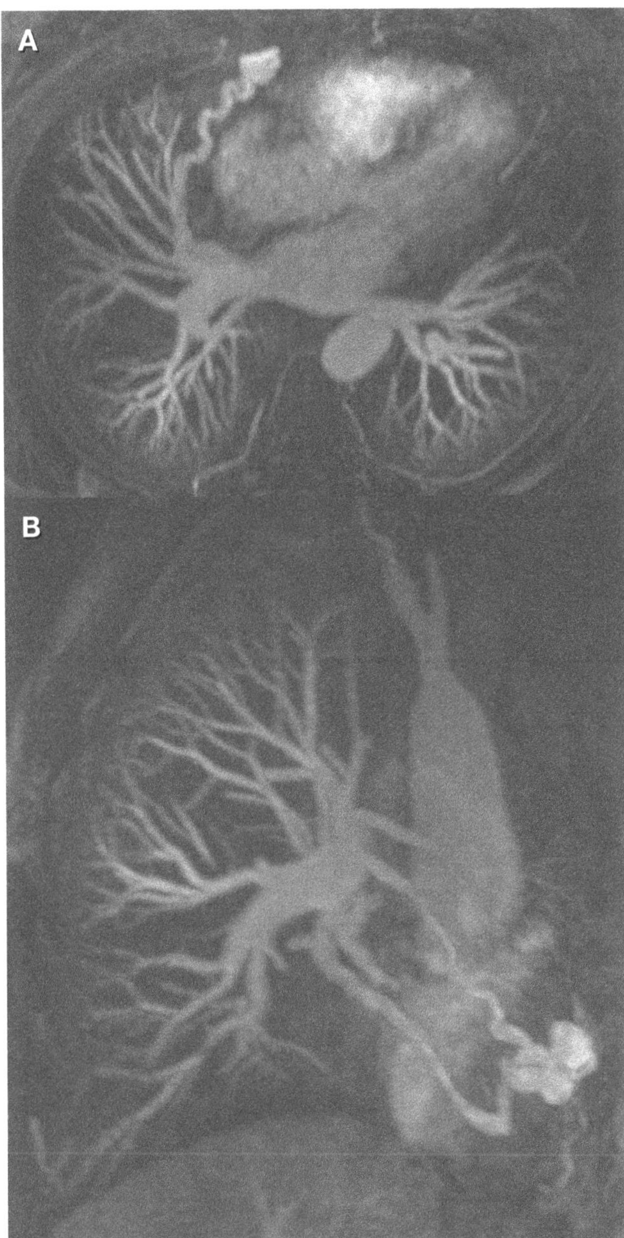

Figure 13.3.2

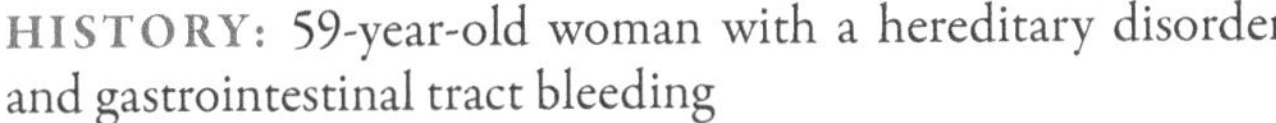
HISTORY: 59-year-old woman with a hereditary disorder and gastrointestinal tract bleeding

IMAGING FINDINGS: VR images (Figure 13.3.1) and subvolume maximum intensity projection images (Figure 13.3.2) from gadolinium-enhanced 3D MRA demonstrate a lobulated vascular structure in the anterior medial right lung with a prominent feeding artery and draining vein.

DIAGNOSIS: Pulmonary arteriovenous malformation in a patient with HHT

COMMENT: Pulmonary AVMs are strongly associated with HHT—a study of more than 200 consecutive pulmonary AVMs established a diagnosis of HHT in 94% of patients. The percentage of HHT patients with pulmonary AVMs varies depending on the surveillance technique used. In a CT-based study, 37% of patients were affected, while an investigation that used echocardiography with agitated saline (microbubble) contrast found that 59% of patients had evidence of a pulmonary shunt.

The original descriptions of familial epistaxis were made by Sutton in 1864 and Babington in 1865; however, their public relations skills were apparently no match for Osler, Parkes-Weber, and Rendu, who are generally given credit. (Osler's ego was strong enough that he stipulated in his will that his brain should be sent to the Wistar Institute in Philadelphia, where postmortem studies of prominent men were performed to search for distinguishing anatomical features of genius.) In recent years, *HHT* has become the more common term for this disorder. HHT is an autosomal dominant disorder with an incidence of 1 in 5,000 to 1 in 8,000 and is characterized by the presence of multiple AVMs that lack intervening capillaries, resulting in direct communication between arteries and veins.

Small AVMs are called telangiectasias and are commonly found on the lips, tongue, face, and fingers and the nasal, buccal, and gastrointestinal tract mucosa. Epistaxis is the most common presenting symptom of HHT patients and generally occurs in childhood. Approximately 25% of HHT patients have episodes of gastrointestinal tract bleeding, with the responsible telangiectasias almost always located in the upper gastrointestinal tract. Gastrointestinal tract bleeding usually occurs in adults and may become increasingly severe with increasing age.

AVMs occur most frequently in the liver, lung, and brain. Cerebral AVMs occur in 10% of patients, and most are present at birth; in contrast, hepatic and pulmonary AVMs may appear and grow throughout a person's life. Hepatic abnormalities are found in 74% of patients on CT, but most patients are asymptomatic. Focal nodular hyperplasia, telangiectasias, and AVMs occur with increased frequency; therefore, diagnosis of a non-HHT–related lesion can be problematic, especially since biopsy in these patients is not encouraged.

Pulmonary AVMs can cause high-output cardiac failure, pulmonary hypertension, and desaturation of arterial blood. The right-to-left shunts in the lung provide a pathway for bland or septic venous emboli to reach the arterial circulation and cause stroke or cerebral abscesses. One study reported significant neurologic events in 30% to 40% of HHT patients who had pulmonary AVMs with feeding artery diameters of 3 mm or greater. Other studies have not found a significant correlation between neurologic events and AVM size.

Screening for pulmonary AVMs is important for HHT patients and is generally performed with either contrast echocardiography or CT. MRI is an attractive alternative to both of these tests since it avoids the radiation of CT while providing visualization of the feeding arteries useful for planning interventional procedures. Gadolinium probably isn't necessary to identify the larger lesions, but 3D contrast-enhanced MRA is the easiest (and fastest) way to perform the examination. In this case, we used a coronal acquisition with 2D parallel imaging that allowed complete coverage of the lungs with reasonably high spatial resolution (<2 mm^3 voxel size) in a breath-hold of 22 seconds—a good choice for a healthy patient with a normal breath-hold capacity but not the protocol you want to use for an examination to exclude a pulmonary embolus.

CASE 13.4

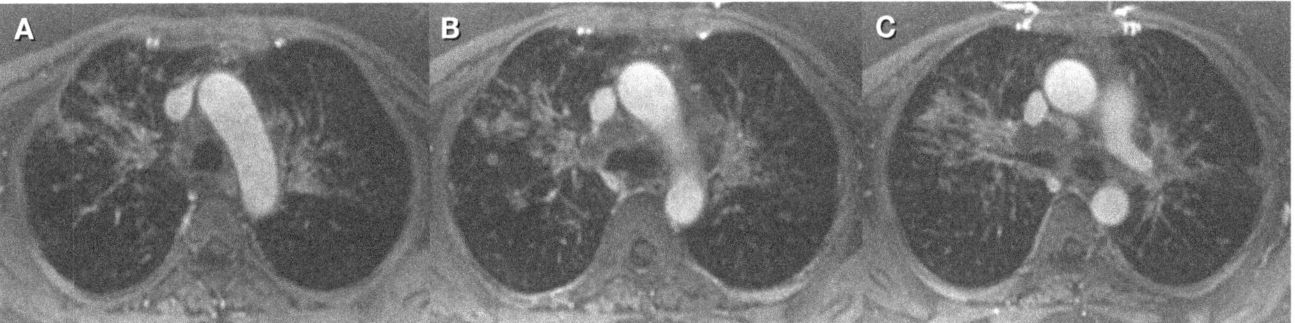

Figure 13.4.1

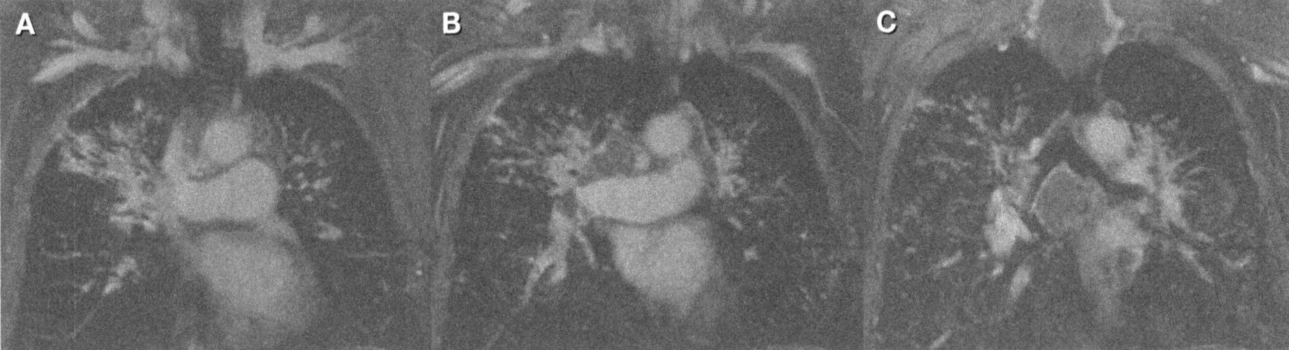

Figure 13.4.2

HISTORY: 60-year-old woman with chronic pulmonary disease and upper extremity swelling

IMAGING FINDINGS: Axial (Figure 13.4.1) and coronal (Figure 13.4.2) postgadolinium 3D SPGR images show extensive perihilar infiltrates, hilar and mediastinal adenopathy, and mild enlargement of the central pulmonary arteries.

DIAGNOSIS: Sarcoidosis

COMMENT: We hope that no one has ever recommended MRI as the test of choice for detection of pulmonary sarcoid (in this case, MRI was performed to exclude superior vena cava syndrome). This example, however, does show that you can see pulmonary findings on MRI if you're willing to look for them. (This reluctance seems to be particularly acute among cardiologists reading cardiac MRI, whose vision often extends only as far as the pericardium. To be fair, though, the number of missed cardiac findings on chest CT is nothing to be proud of either.)

Sarcoidosis is a multisystem disease of unknown etiology that can affect virtually any organ, but most commonly involves the lungs, liver, skin, and eyes. The estimated prevalence is 10 in 100,000 to 40 in 100,000 in the United States and Europe, with a higher incidence among women, African Americans, and Scandinavians.

An interesting feature of sarcoidosis is that many patients are asymptomatic. Treatment is generally limited to symptomatic patients, and in most series only about 50% require long-term therapy. Pulmonary involvement has been classified by chest radiography and CT according to the modified Scadding criteria: stage 0, no findings; stage I, hilar and mediastinal adenopathy; stage II, adenopathy and pulmonary infiltrates; stage III, pulmonary infiltrates alone; and stage IV, pulmonary fibrosis. In a study of patients with stage II or III disease, 20% had spontaneous improvement without therapy within 6 months, but in 40%, the disease worsened and the patients required corticosteroid therapy.

The classic findings of nodular perihilar infiltrates following a bronchovascular distribution appear more reliably on CT; however, they are easily seen in this case, and mediastinal adenopathy is readily appreciated on MRI.

When a patient is known to have sarcoidosis, body MRI is probably most often requested to evaluate for cardiac involvement. Cardiac sarcoid is found in 20% to 30% of patients in autopsy series and is likely associated with a worse prognosis; however, only 5% of patients with sarcoidosis have clinical manifestations of cardiac disease. Arrhythmias are the most common and dangerous manifestations of cardiac involvement and include bundle branch block, complete heart block, and ventricular tachyarrhythmias. MRI is generally considered the most sensitive test for detection of cardiac sarcoid. Classic findings include MDE in a nonischemic pattern, often in an epicardial or mid-myocardial distribution and sometimes associated with myocardial edema manifested as increased signal intensity on T2-weighted images.

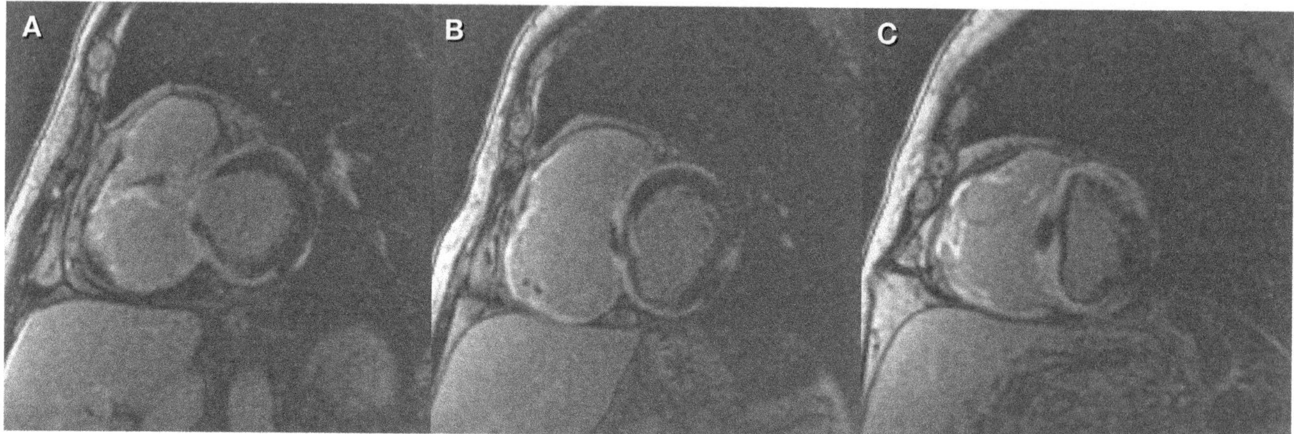

Figure 13.4.3

Figure 13.4.3 is an example of a positive cardiac examination in a 73-year-old man with exertional dyspnea and shortness of breath. Short-axis postgadolinium MDE images demonstrate extensive enhancement of the right ventricular free wall and inferior wall as well as epicardial enhancement of the left ventricular myocardium. Right ventricular endomyocardial biopsy was consistent with sarcoid.

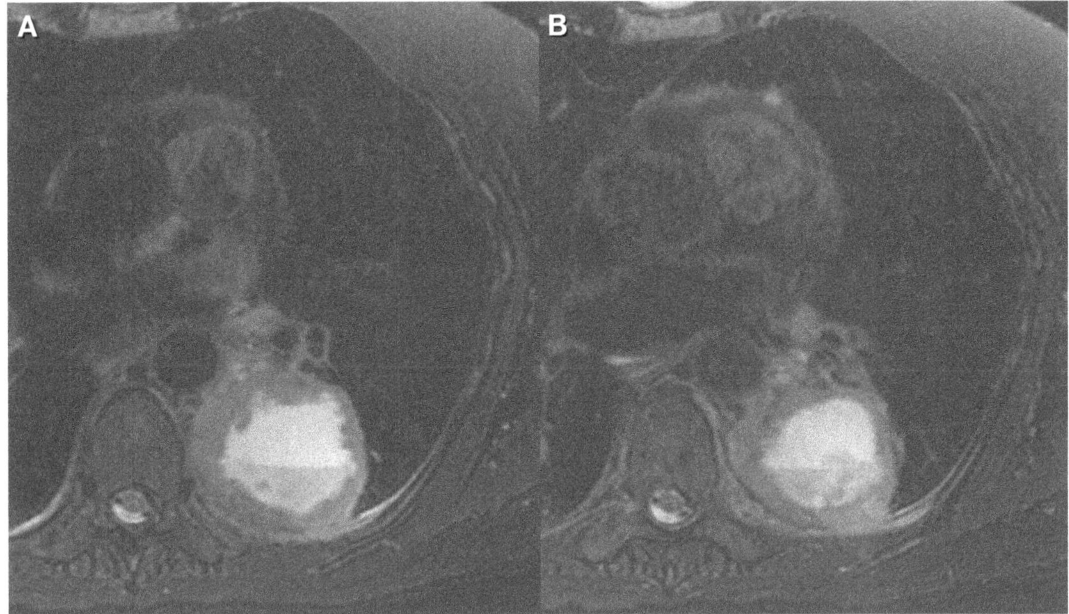

Figure 13.5.1

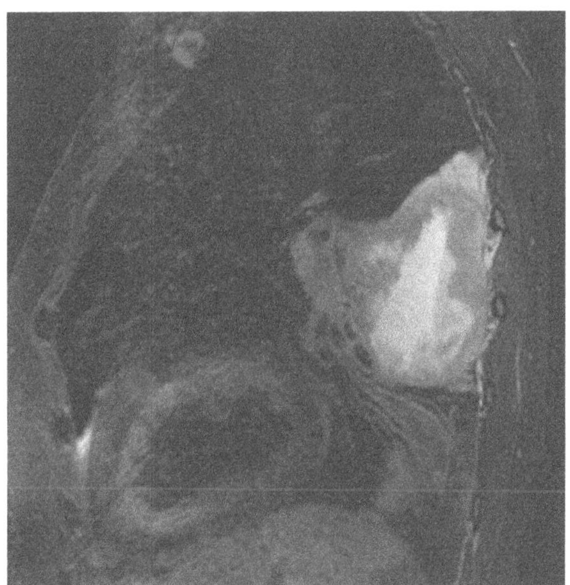

Figure 13.5.2

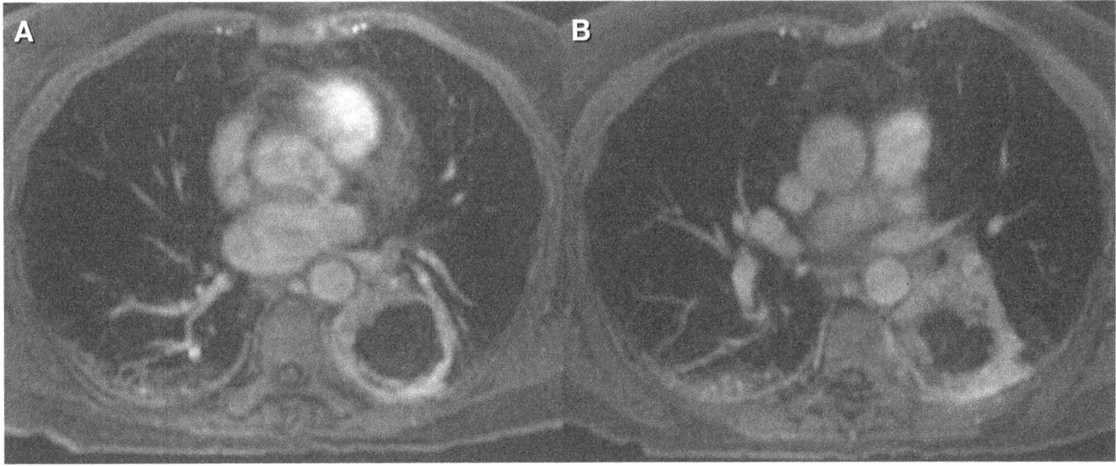

Figure 13.5.3

HISTORY: 72-year-old woman with a nonproductive cough and a mass on chest radiograph

IMAGING FINDINGS: Axial (Figure 13.5.1) and sagittal (Figure 13.5.2) fat-suppressed FSE T2-weighted images reveal a large centrally necrotic mass in the posterior left lower lobe. Notice the subtle tail of soft tissue extending across the pleura with minimal extension into the chest wall. Axial postgadolinium 3D SPGR images (Figure 13.5.3) demonstrate similar findings.

DIAGNOSIS: Squamous cell lung carcinoma with pleural and subtle chest wall invasion

COMMENT: Lung cancer is an uncommon indication for MRI, and in our practice, MRI is performed most frequently to assess for extrathoracic extension in patients with Pancoast tumors (superior pulmonary sulcus tumors). Occasionally, MRI is requested to confirm a metastatic lesion involving the thoracic skeleton or chest wall or to evaluate whether direct invasion of the chest wall has occurred (the indication in this case). CT and PET-CT are much more useful in detecting and staging lung cancer in most patients, but occasionally the superior soft tissue contrast of MRI is useful in problematic cases.

Lung cancer is the leading cause of cancer-related death in the United States, with 220,000 new diagnoses and 157,000 deaths per year. Lung cancer is classified as small cell cancer (treated with chemotherapy or radiotherapy or both) or non-small cell cancer (potentially resectable), and squamous cell carcinoma, a type of non-small cell lung cancer, accounts for approximately 20% of all tumors. Squamous cell carcinoma is highly associated with smoking, and chronic injury to the bronchial epithelium is thought to lead to squamous metaplasia and eventually frank malignancy. Two-thirds of squamous cell carcinoma lesions are central, with the remaining one-third peripheral. Although tumor growth is generally slower in comparison to other lesions, patients often have advanced disease at presentation, with invasion of hilar and mediastinal structures. Cavitation occurs in 10% to 15% of squamous cell carcinoma lesions, occurring more frequently in larger tumors and typically with a thick, irregular wall.

In lung cancer staging, MRI can be used to distinguish potentially surgical disease (mostly stages I and II) from nonsurgical disease (mostly stages III and IV). Stage III tumors, also described as locally advanced disease, have 2 subtypes, with stage IIIA characterized by nodal disease involving the ipsilateral mediastinum or subcarinal region (N2) and stage IIIB (unresectable) characterized by contralateral or supraclavicular nodal disease. Stage III disease can also include tumor invasion of the chest wall, diaphragm, mediastinal pleura, or parietal pericardium (T3). Since PET is much more accurate for distinguishing nodal involvement, MRI is usually used to characterize mediastinal or chest wall invasion.

FSE T2-weighted images obtained with respiratory triggering and moderately high spatial resolution and postgadolinium 3D SPGR images are most useful in this regard, although T1-weighted images can be helpful if a prominent layer of subpleural fat is present, since dark tumor extending across the bright fat is easily detected. Diffusion-weighted images are occasionally useful, but their value can be limited by susceptibility artifact from adjacent lung. Remember that you're allowed to obtain images from more than 1 plane and that sagittal or coronal acquisitions (or something in between) frequently provide the most valuable information.

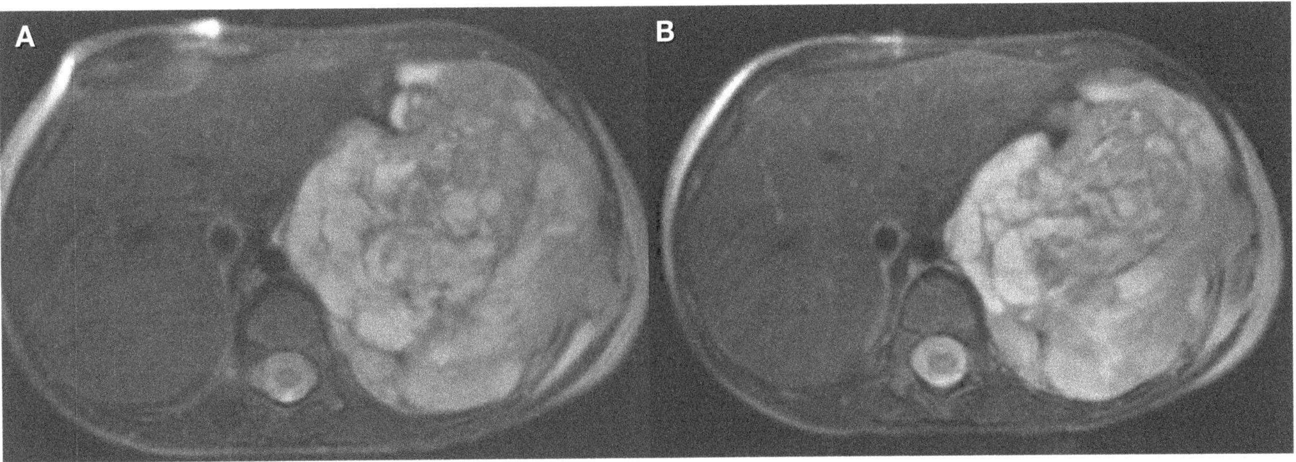

Figure 13.6.1

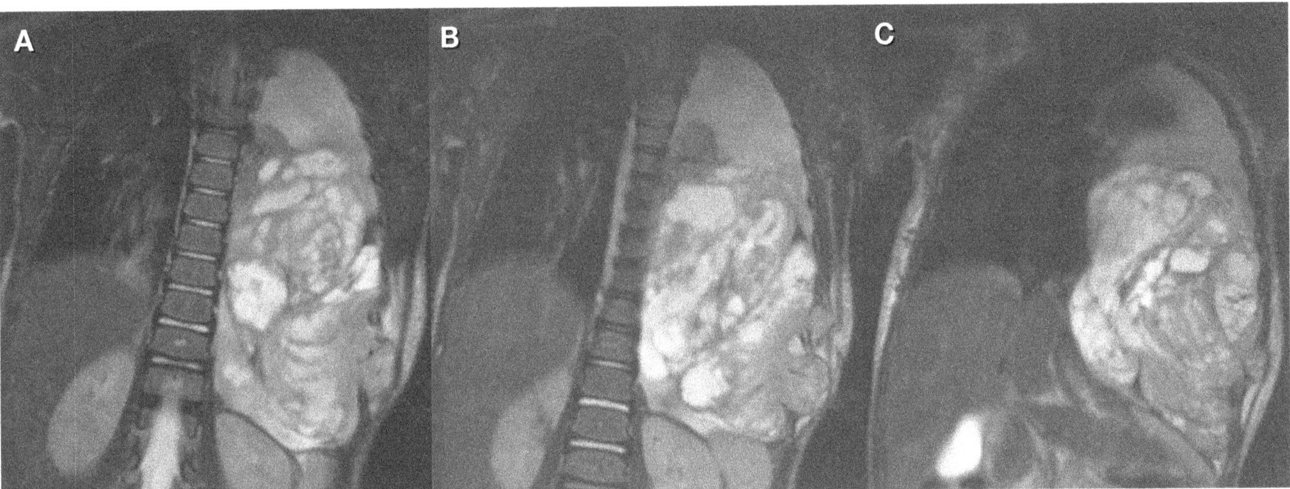

Figure 13.6.2

HISTORY: 3-year-old girl with a chest wall mass that her mother noticed

IMAGING FINDINGS: Axial (Figure 13.6.1) and coronal (Figure 13.6.2) FSE T2-weighted images demonstrate a large heterogeneous mass that has multiple regions of high signal intensity and occupies much of the left hemothorax. Note involvement of the lateral chest wall and a lower rib best seen on the coronal images.

DIAGNOSIS: Ewing sarcoma

COMMENT: Askin et al in 1979 described a rare malignant small cell tumor arising in the soft tissues of the chest wall in children and young adults. The tumors were initially known as Askin tumors and were subsequently classified as PNETs. More recently, PNETs have been recognized as belonging to the same family of tumors as Ewing sarcoma, which is characterized by the presence of small round cells with neural differentiation, probably arising from embryonal neural crest cells. Ewing sarcoma and PNET share the same genetic abnormality, a translocation of the long arms of chromosomes 11 and 22. The terms *Askin tumor*, *PNET*, and *Ewing sarcoma* are used interchangeably in the medical literature.

Chest wall lesions develop either as a solitary mass or as multiple masses with eccentric growth. They can originate from the ribs, sternum, scapula, or clavicles, or they may have an extraskeletal origin. Large tumors, as in this case, may grow into the thoracic cavity and displace or invade the lung.

On MRI, Ewing sarcoma has the appearance of an aggressive neoplasm, with heterogeneous regions of increased signal intensity on T2-weighted images and heterogeneous enhancement following gadolinium administration, with interspersed regions of necrosis and hemorrhage. The differential diagnosis includes other aggressive or invasive tumors, such as osteosarcoma or other sarcomas, neuroblastoma, and non-Hodgkin lymphoma. Standard treatment of these lesions includes neoadjuvant chemotherapy, surgical excision, and postoperative chemotherapy and radiotherapy. The long-term prognosis is relatively poor, with a reported 6-year survival of 14%.

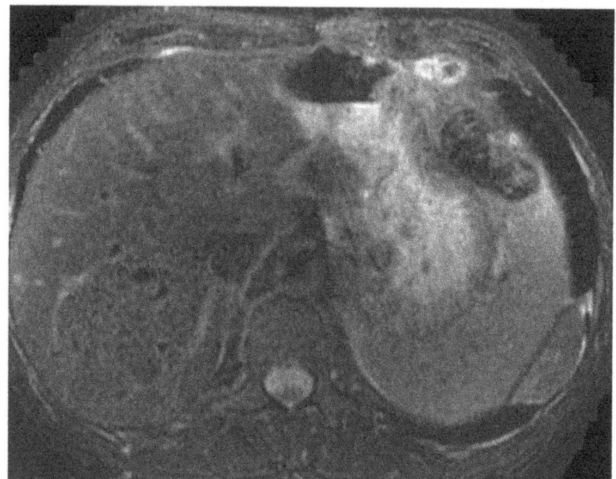

Figure 13.7.1

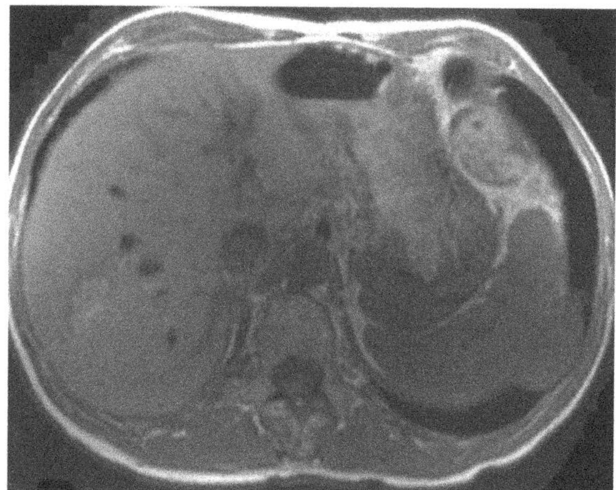

Figure 13.7.2

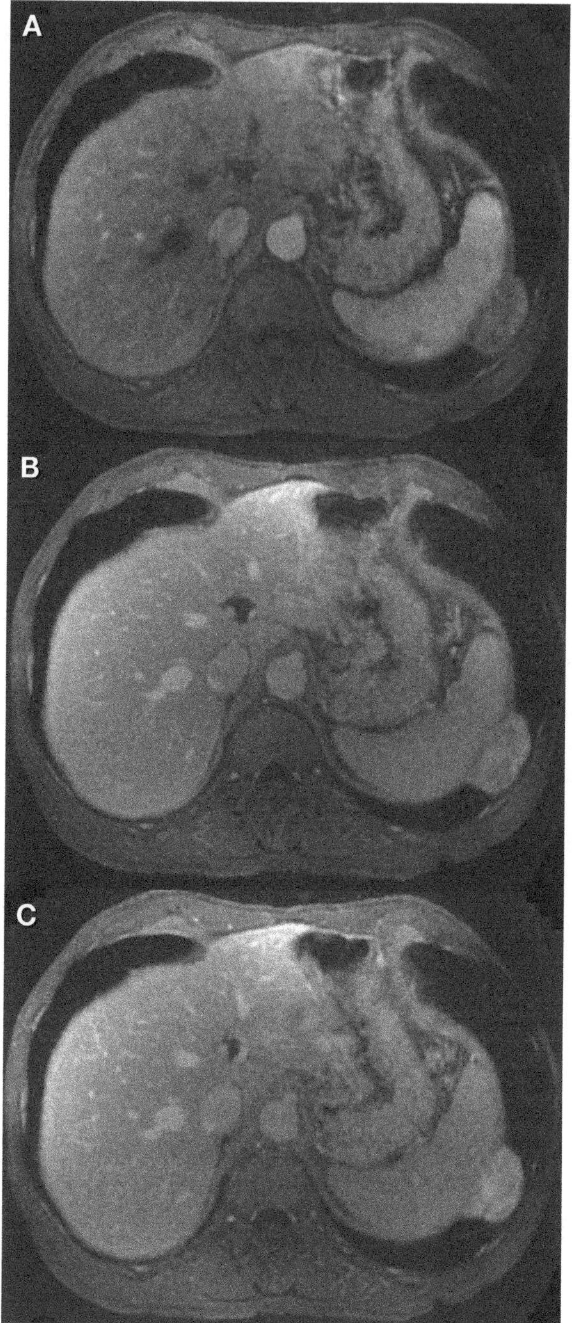

Figure 13.7.3

HISTORY: 75-year-old man with a pleural mass on chest radiograph

IMAGING FINDINGS: An elliptical lesion in the left costophrenic angle shows mildly heterogeneous low signal intensity on axial fat-suppressed FRFSE T2-weighted image (Figure 13.7.1) and intermediate signal intensity on axial T1-weighted FSE image (Figure 13.7.2). Arterial (Figure 13.7.3A), venous (Figure 13.7.3B), and 6-minute delayed phase (Figure 13.7.3C) 3D SPGR postgadolinium images demonstrate hypoenhancement relative to the liver and spleen in the arterial phase, with gradual accumulation of gadolinium. The mass is markedly hyperintense on the 6-minute delayed image. Note the small hemangioma in the hepatic dome.

DIAGNOSIS: Solitary fibrous tumor of the pleura

COMMENT: Previously, solitary fibrous tumor of the pleura was also referred to as benign fibrous tumor of the pleura;

however, several examples of malignant tumors have been reported, and it is now believed that as many as 20% of these neoplasms are malignant. This description is therefore no longer applicable, and resection of all lesions has become the standard treatment.

Solitary fibrous tumors are rare neoplasms of mesenchymal origin that account for less than 2% of all soft tissue tumors. The pleura is by far the most common location, but solitary fibrous tumors have also been described in the mediastinum, lung, pericardium, thyroid, kidneys, breast, epiglottis, and salivary glands. Men and women are equally affected, and patients typically present between the ages of 40 and 60 years. Most patients are asymptomatic at diagnosis, but symptoms associated with solitary fibrous tumor of the pleura include chest pain, cough, and dyspnea. Hypertrophic pulmonary osteoarthropathy and hypoglycemia have also been reported.

The histologic appearance of solitary fibrous tumor of the pleura consists of predominantly fibrotic components containing spindle cells and connective tissue arranged in alternating hypocellular and hypercellular areas. Less commonly, tumor cells are arranged adjacent to irregular branching vessels in a pattern reminiscent of hemangiopericytomas. Tumor cells are reactive for CD34 and CD39 and are usually negative for cytokeratins and desmin.

The classic appearance of solitary fibrous tumor of the pleura on MRI (this case is a good example) is a reflection of the fibrotic component: fairly homogeneous on all imaging sequences, low signal intensity on T2-weighted images, and gradual accumulation of contrast after gadolinium administration, often with striking enhancement on delayed images obtained 5 to 10 minutes after the initial gadolinium injection. This appearance is similar to that of other fibrotic lesions, such as ovarian fibromas, cardiac fibromas (see Case 13.25), and uterine leiomyomas, but, of course, not every lesion follows this pattern. To some extent, increasing heterogeneity, increased T2-signal intensity, and increasing size have been associated with malignant degeneration, and 1 recent report has suggested that restricted diffusion with a low ADC value at DWI may also suggest malignancy. No large series have been published to indicate whether any of these features can be used to reliably distinguish between benign and malignant solitary fibrous tumor of the pleura; therefore, all lesions are resected.

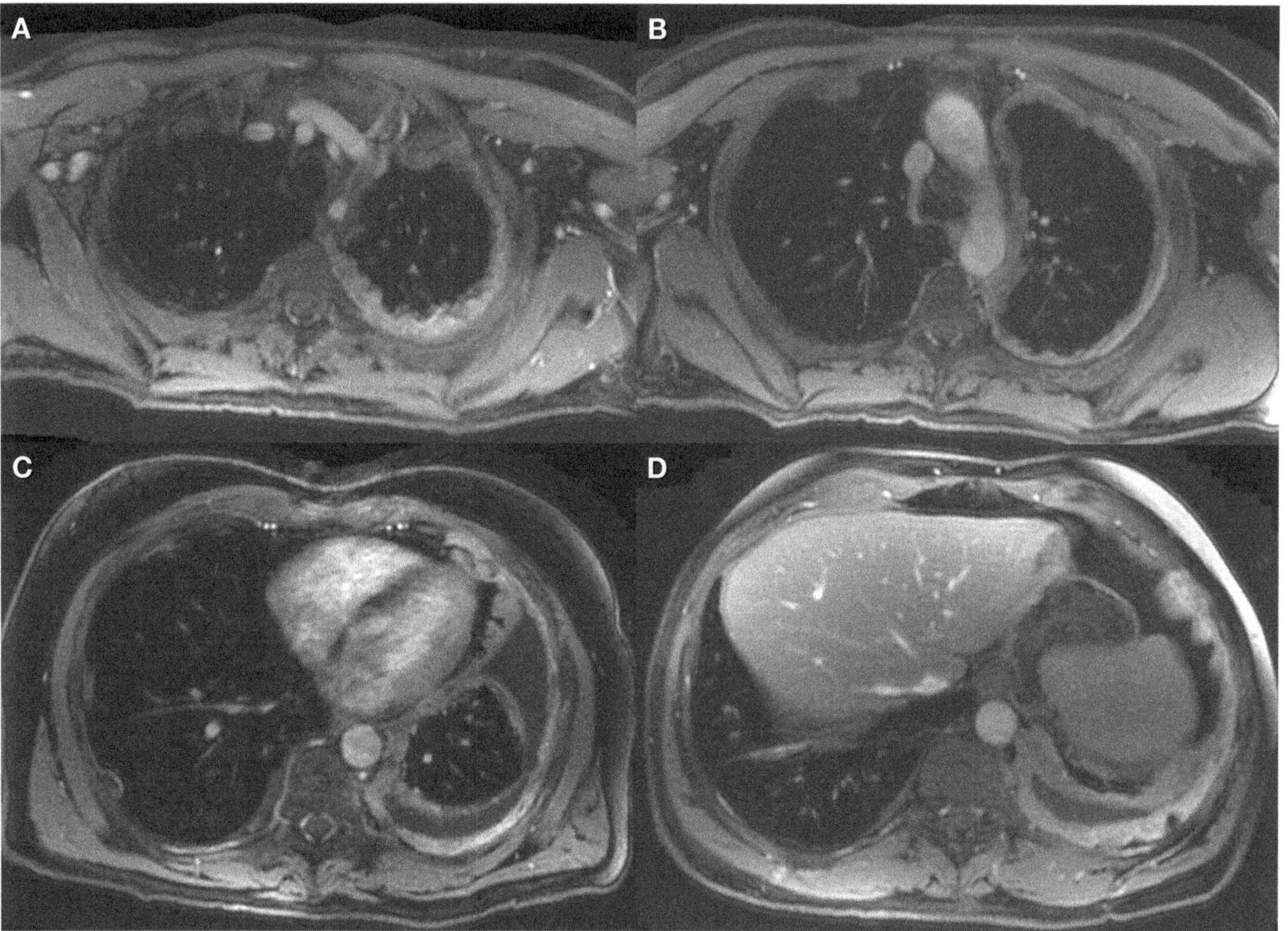

Figure 13.8.1

HISTORY: 62-year-old man with shortness of breath and an abnormal chest CT

IMAGING FINDINGS: Axial 3D SPGR postgadolinium images (Figure 13.8.1) demonstrate diffuse thickening and enhancement of the left pleura, with a few minimally enhancing, focal right-sided pleural plaques.

DIAGNOSIS: Malignant pleural mesothelioma

COMMENT: Malignant pleural mesothelioma is a rare neoplasm that originates from the mesothelial cells lining the visceral and parietal pleura. The incidence of malignant pleural mesothelioma in the United States is 15 cases per million; there is a strong correlation with asbestos exposure. Malignant pleural mesothelioma is divided into 3 histologic subtypes: epithelial (55%-65%), sarcomatoid (10%-15%), and mixed (20%-35%). Patients with epithelial malignant pleural mesothelioma have the best prognosis, and among those with limited disease who undergo extrapleural pneumonectomy (removal of the pleura, lung, hemidiaphragm, and part of the pericardium), survival is longer (5-year survival, 39%) than among all patients (median survival, 8-18 months after diagnosis).

As is true for most cancers, several staging systems have been proposed. The most common, from the International Mesothelioma Interest Group, divides tumor stage into involvement of the pleura (T1), invasion of the ipsilateral lung or diaphragm (or both) (T2), locally advanced but potentially resectable tumors invading the chest wall or mediastinal fat (T3), and locally advanced unresectable tumors (T4). Nodal staging is similar to lung cancer staging, with N1 and N2 indicating ipsilateral mediastinal and hilar lymph nodes and N3 indicating contralateral or supraclavicular (or both) lymph nodes. Stage I indicates T1N0 disease, stage II indicates T2N0 disease, and stage III indicates any combination containing T3, N1, and N2. Patients with stage I, II, or III disease are potential surgical candidates; stage IV patients (with N3 or T4 disease, or distant metastases) are not.

CT is usually the initial imaging technique for diagnosis and staging of malignant pleural mesothelioma. MRI has been advocated when ambiguous chest wall or mediastinal invasion might affect surgical staging. PET-CT is superior to either CT or MRI for nodal staging. One paper suggested that

PET-CT might also be more accurate for assessing chest wall, mediastinal, and diaphragmatic invasion, although this is a somewhat unexpected result given the low spatial resolution of this technique.

Mesothelioma typically appears as a unilateral rind of pleural thickening, often in a nodular configuration, with moderate diffuse enhancement after gadolinium administration. Invasion of the chest wall and mediastinum can usually be appreciated on T2-weighted, SSFP, or postgadolinium 3D SPGR images. Obtaining these images in at least 2 planes is useful, and 3D SPGR acquisitions are preferable to 2D because of the higher spatial resolution and because of their tendency to exhibit less cardiac pulsation artifact (likely on the basis of shorter TR and TE). Diffusion-weighted images show high signal intensity within the pleural tumor, and 1 paper has suggested that ADC measurement may allow epithelial subtypes (with higher ADC values) to be distinguished from non-epithelial tumors.

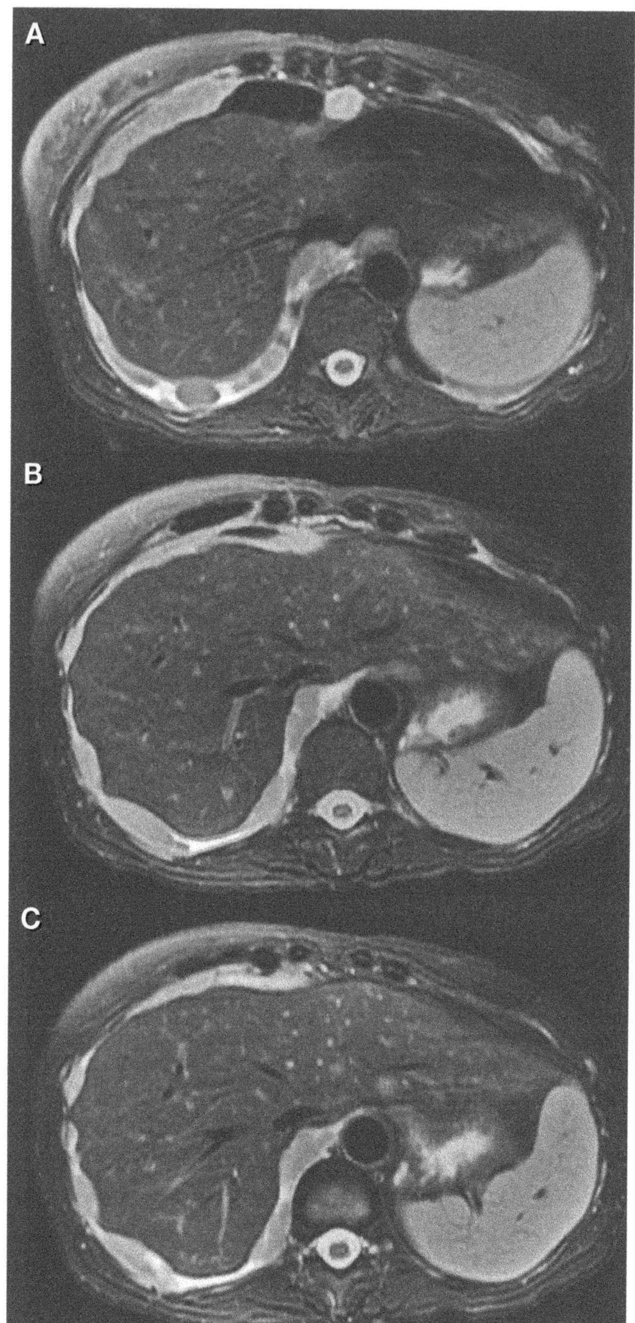

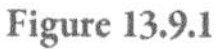

Figure 13.9.1

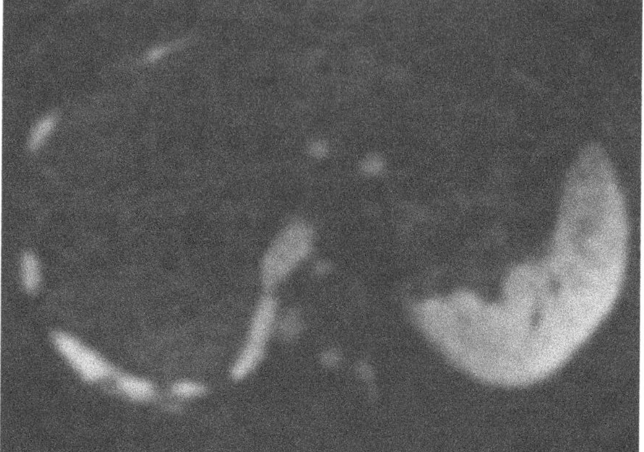

Figure 13.9.2

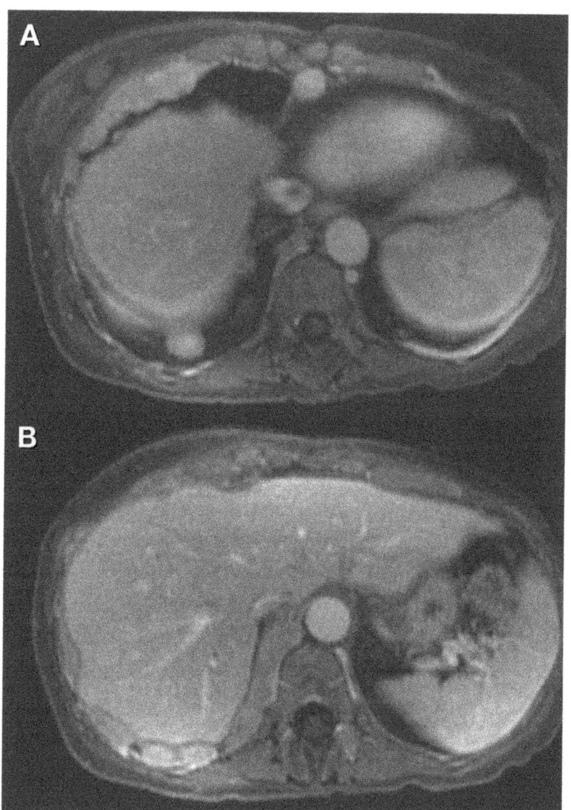

Figure 13.9.3

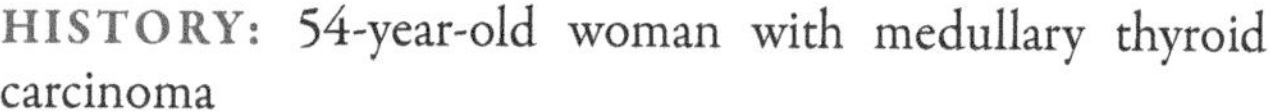

HISTORY: 54-year-old woman with medullary thyroid carcinoma

IMAGING FINDINGS: Axial fat-suppressed FSE T2-weighted images (Figure 13.9.1) demonstrate nodular soft tissue thickening of the pleura at the right lung base. Diffusion-weighted image (b=600 s/mm^2) (Figure 13.9.2) reveals high-signal-intensity pleural lesions and focal lesions in the left hepatic lobe and thoracic spine, which are more conspicuous than in the T2-weighted images. Axial postgadolinium 3D SPGR images (Figure 13.9.3) also show enhancement of the nodular pleural lesions. Faint hypoenhancing lesions are seen in the left hepatic lobe.

DIAGNOSIS: Pleural metastases

COMMENT: Although the utility of MRI is limited in the assessment of lungs, MRI is competitive with CT (if not superior) for evaluating pleural disease. In general, this is not a particularly useful distinction since an examination is rarely performed solely to image the pleura, but there are a few occasions when pleural imaging with MRI can be a useful problem-solving technique (eg, to evaluate chest wall invasion). This case is not one of those times—it was an abdominal examination performed to assess the hepatic metastases, and the pleural disease happened to be included in the field of view.

Pleural metastasis is the most common cause of malignant pleural thickening, with lung cancer, breast cancer, and lymphoma accounting for the majority of cases. Large pleural metastases can be detected on virtually any pulse sequence; our favorites include fat-suppressed respiratory-triggered FSE T2-weighted images, diffusion-weighted images, and postgadolinium 3D SPGR images. Remember that there is no rule against nonaxial acquisitions—sagittal and coronal planes are often very useful for visualizing the entire pleural space in a more time-efficient manner. In the presence of pleural effusion, diffusion-weighted images should be obtained with a moderately high b value (b=600-800 s/mm^2) to suppress the signal from pleural fluid.

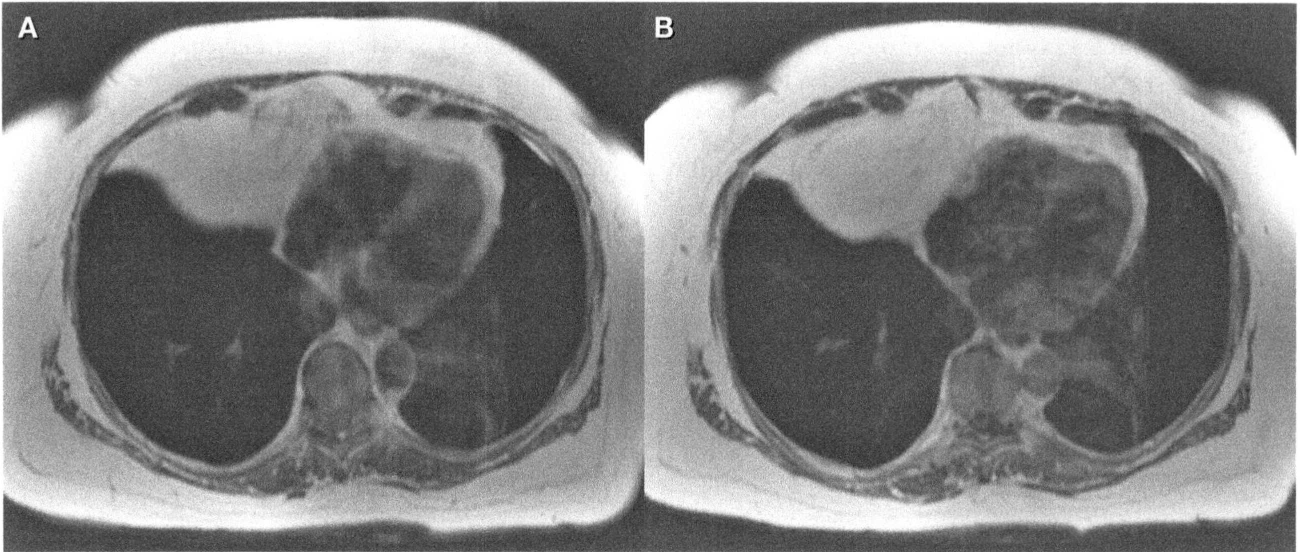

Figure 13.10.1

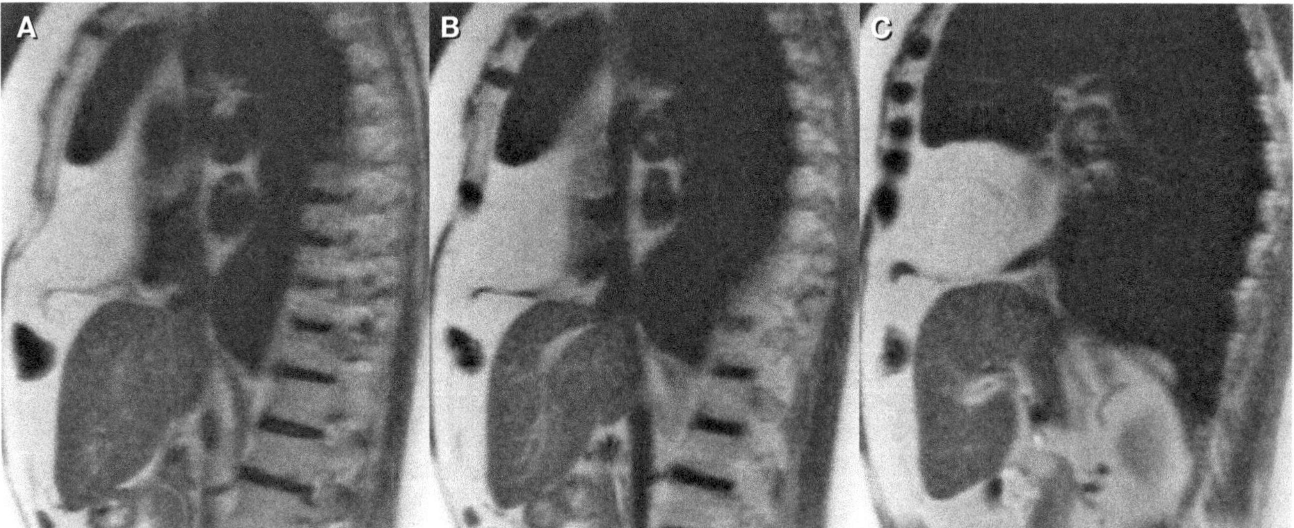

Figure 13.10.2

HISTORY: 66-year-old woman with a mediastinal mass incidentally seen on chest radiograph; thoracic CT revealed a fatty mass along the right anterior heart border

IMAGING FINDINGS: Axial T1-weighted FSE images (Figure 13.10.1) and sagittal T2-weighted SSFSE images (Figure 13.10.2) reveal herniation of fat through an anterior diaphragmatic defect into the mediastinum anterior to the right side of the heart.

DIAGNOSIS: Morgagni hernia

COMMENT: Giovanni Battista Morgagni included a description of a congenital anterior diaphragmatic hernia in his 1761 treatise, *On the Seats and Causes of Disease Investigated by Anatomy*. By comparison, the Bochdalek hernia is a relatively recent discovery, first described by Victor Bochdalek in 1848.

Both entities are caused by regions of relative weakness in the diaphragm—in this case, the foramen of Morgagni, which is located anteriorly and slightly to the right of midline in 90% of cases. Large hernias in neonates with cyanosis or respiratory distress are serious abnormalities and require urgent surgical repair. Small (or large) hernias in adults are often incidental findings, as in this case, and patients may be asymptomatic. When present, symptoms may involve obstruction of herniated bowel or mass effect on adjacent structures from large hernias.

The main differential diagnosis in this case is an anterior mediastinal lipoma or liposarcoma, which was the indication for the MRI. A prominent epicardial fat pad is also a consideration, although in this case the size of the lesion and its focal nature would be unusual for this entity. Of course, the hernia could have been demonstrated just as easily on the CT from an outside hospital if sagittal reformatted views had been reconstructed. Liposarcomas, particularly low-grade lesions, may have very little nonfatty soft tissue to distinguish them from focal fatty proliferation or from a simple lipoma; however, the presence of a Morgagni hernia makes this consideration improbable.

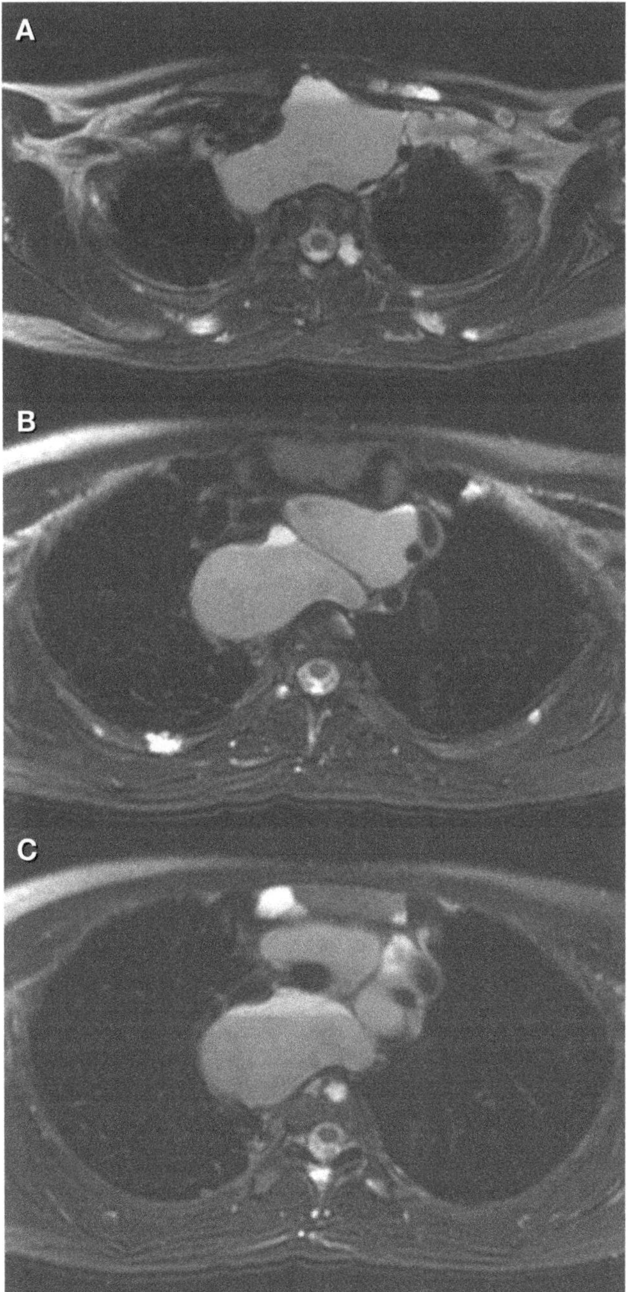

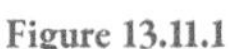
Figure 13.11.1

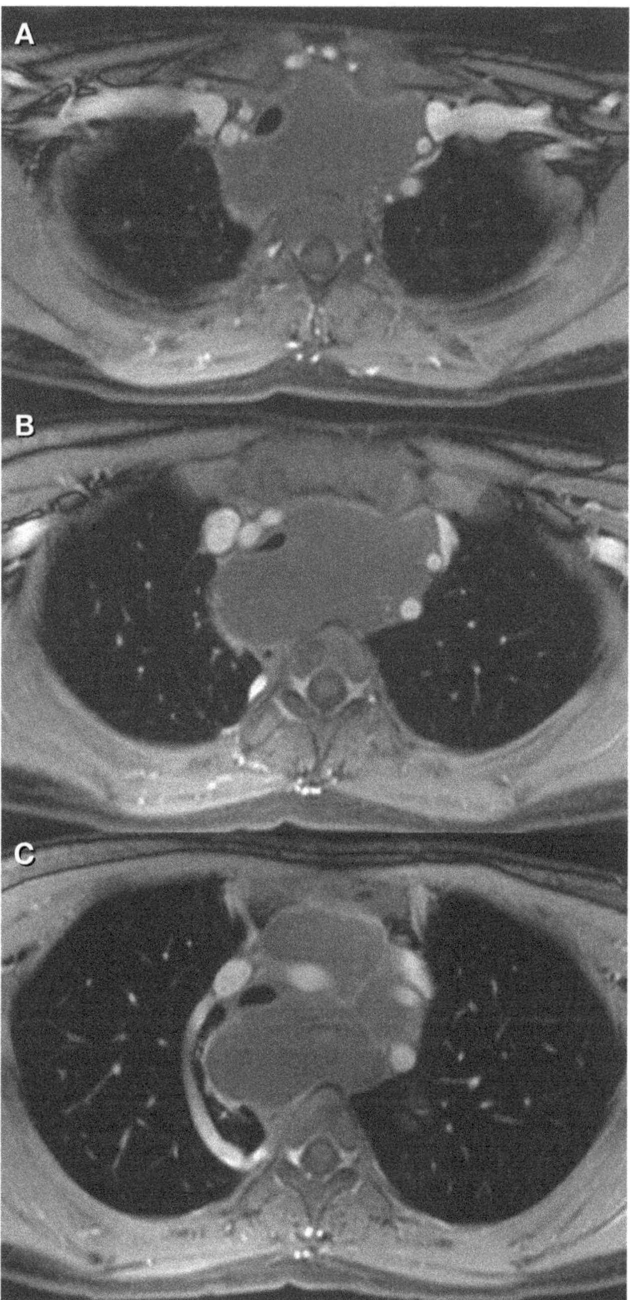

Figure 13.11.2

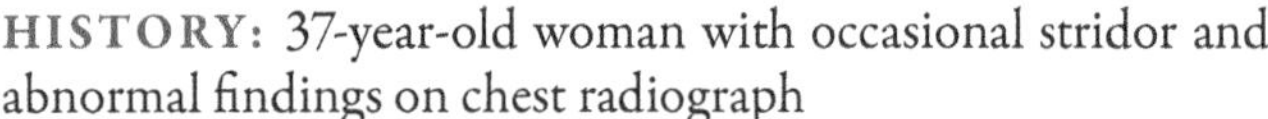
HISTORY: 37-year-old woman with occasional stridor and abnormal findings on chest radiograph

IMAGING FINDINGS: Axial fat-suppressed T2-weighted FSE images (Figure 13.11.1) reveal a thoracic inlet cystic lesion that deviates and compresses the trachea and contains several fluid-fluid levels. Axial postgadolinium 3D SPGR images (Figure 13.11.2) demonstrate minimal enhancement of the rim of the lesion and thin septations. Note also partial encasement of the mediastinal great vessels.

DIAGNOSIS: Thoracic lymphangioma

COMMENT: Lymphangiomas are benign lesions that account for 0.7% to 4.5% of all mediastinal tumors in adults. Lymphangiomas involve the neck and axillary region in 80% of cases, the thorax in 10%, and other locations in the remainder. Lesions in infants most commonly involve the neck and mediastinum; when detected in adults, however, lesions are more often confined to the mediastinum. Adults with mediastinal lymphangiomas are often asymptomatic, and the lesions are detected incidentally on chest radiography or CT; however, they may cause symptoms related to mass effect and compression of mediastinal structures, as in this case.

There is some controversy in the pathology literature regarding the etiology of lymphangiomas, with theories including developmental, hamartomatous, or neoplastic origin. Lymphangiomas are classified as simple (capillary), cavernous, or cystic (hygroma) depending on the size of the lymphatic channels, with cystic lesions occurring most frequently.

Cystic lymphangiomas appear as cystic lesions, often with thin septations. They have characteristically high signal intensity on T2-weighted images, often with fluid components of slightly different intensity (reflecting the presence of protein or blood products) and leading to the fairly common finding of fluid-fluid levels. Enhancement after contrast administration is minimal but may be more prominent in capillary lesions. Lymphangiomas may present as well-circumscribed masses, but often they insinuate between various mediastinal structures and involve multiple mediastinal compartments. Therefore, complete surgical resection is sometimes difficult, and postoperative recurrence is not uncommon.

The differential diagnosis includes other cystic mediastinal lesions, such as teratoma, thymic cyst, bronchogenic cyst, esophageal duplication cyst, and necrotic tumors or lymph nodes.

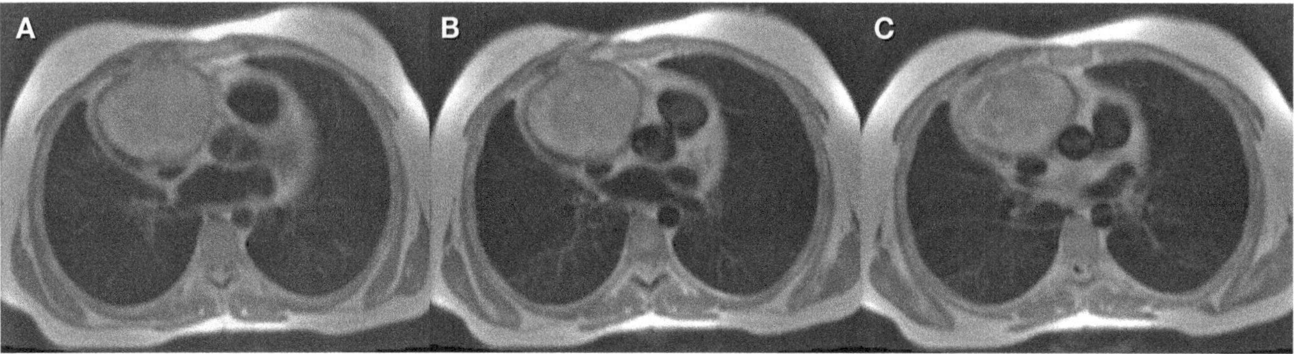

Figure 13.12.1

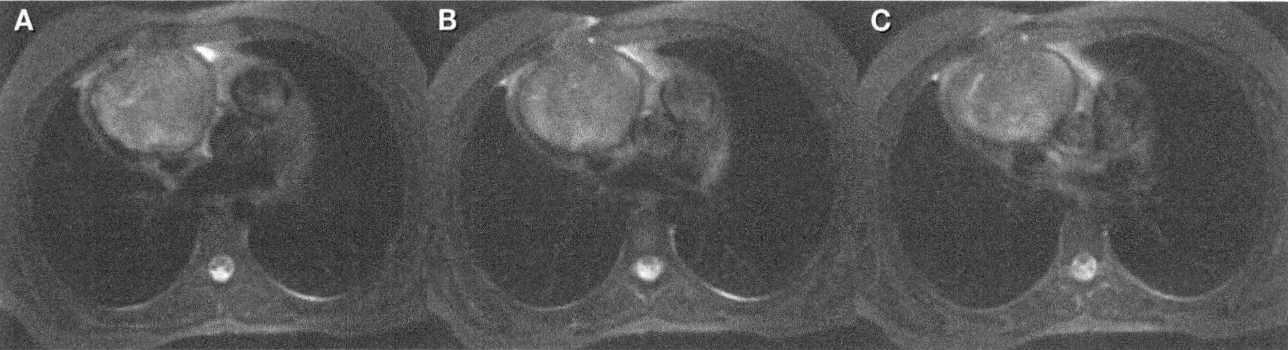

Figure 13.12.2

HISTORY: 52-year-old woman with chest discomfort; chest CT revealed an indeterminate mediastinal lesion

IMAGING FINDINGS: Axial proton density-weighted double inversion recovery FSE images (Figure 13.12.1) demonstrate a large mildly heterogeneous lesion with moderately increased signal intensity relative to adjacent skeletal muscle and a well-defined low-signal-intensity capsule. Axial T2-weighted triple inversion recovery FSE images (Figure 13.12.2) also show mild heterogeneity with regions of mild hyperintensity.

DIAGNOSIS: Thymoma

COMMENT: Thymic epithelial tumors, which include thymoma and thymic carcinoma, are the most common neoplasms of the anterior mediastinum. Thymoma is the most common variety and accounts for 20% of all mediastinal tumors. The 2004 World Health Organization histologic classification identifies 5 types of thymomas (types A, AB, B1, B2, and B3) and thymic carcinoma; this system broadly reflects the clinical and prognostic features of the tumors. The Masaoka staging system is also frequently used: stage I, completely encapsulated lesions; stage II, invasion into mediastinal fat or pleura; stage III, invasion into adjacent organs; and stage IV, metastatic disease. There is little evidence that MRI is particularly helpful for distinguishing the particular tumor subtype; however, uniform encapsulated lesions are likely to correspond to low-stage tumors, whereas heterogeneous, infiltrative lesions without capsules are likely to have a higher stage and carry a worse prognosis.

Thymomas usually occur in middle-aged adults (average age at diagnosis, 50 years). Patients with encapsulated thymomas are typically asymptomatic but may present with chest pain, cough, dyspnea, dysphagia, or hoarseness; patients with invasive lesions are generally symptomatic. Thymomas are well known for their association with paraneoplastic syndromes, of which myasthenia gravis is the most common manifestation. Approximately 10% to 20% of patients with myasthenia gravis have thymoma, and 35% to 40% of patients with thymoma have myasthenia gravis. Other paraneoplastic syndromes associated with thymoma include pure red cell aplasia, acquired hypogammaglobulinemia, and nonthymic cancers.

On MRI, thymoma appears as a solid anterior mediastinal mass with heterogeneity and aggressive features that correlate with invasiveness and malignancy. In this case, we obtained ECG-gated double and triple inversion recovery acquisitions rather than conventional respiratory-triggered FSE images. The main advantages of these techniques include the black-blood effect, which improves the distinction between mass and vessel, and the reduction of cardiac and vascular pulsation artifacts. Limitations include multiple breath-holds of 10 to 15 seconds per slice and relatively low signal to noise ratios since the number of signal averages is constrained by the need for breath-holding. MRI is probably slightly superior to CT in delineating invasion of mediastinal structures, such as the pericardium and heart, but there are no demonstrated advantages of MRI in the differential diagnosis of anterior mediastinal masses, which include lymphoma, mature teratoma, malignant germ cell tumor, thymic cyst, and thymic hyperplasia.

Complete resection is the mainstay of treatment for thymomas, and resection with negative margins is probably the most important prognostic factor. Adjuvant radiotherapy is helpful in patients with higher-stage disease or incomplete resections.

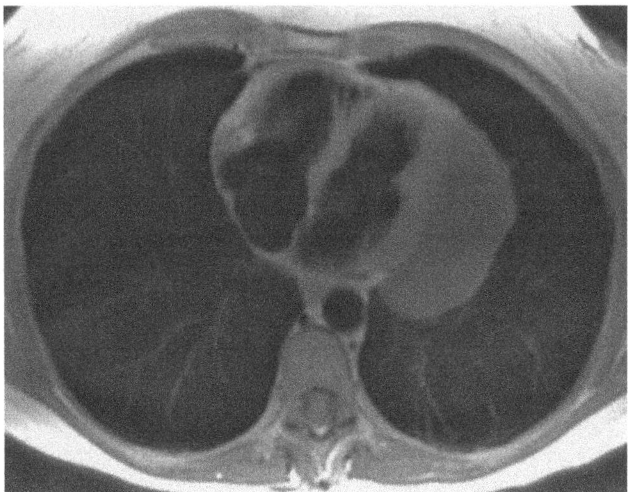

Figure 13.13.1

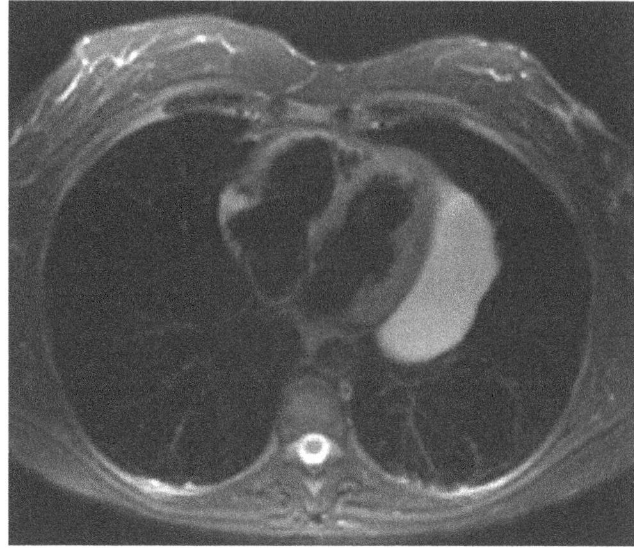

Figure 13.13.2

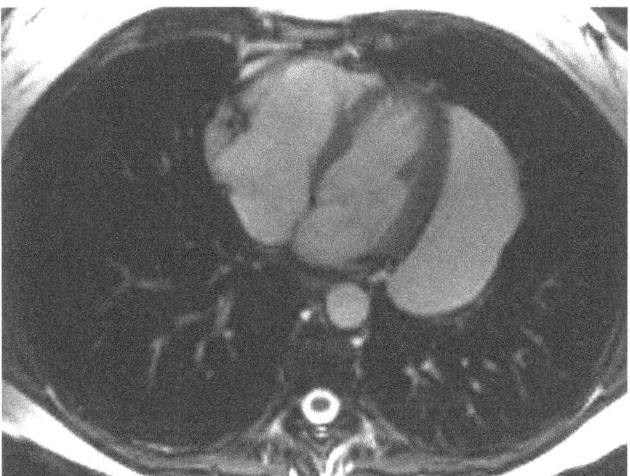

Figure 13.13.3

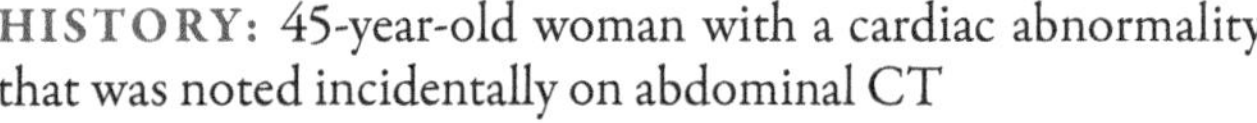

HISTORY: 45-year-old woman with a cardiac abnormality that was noted incidentally on abdominal CT

IMAGING FINDINGS: Axial double (Figure 13.13.1) and triple (Figure 13.13.2) inversion recovery FSE images and axial SSFP image (Figure 13.13.3) demonstrate an ovoid cystic lesion containing simple fluid along the left heart border.

DIAGNOSIS: Pericardial cyst

COMMENT: Pericardial cysts are benign lesions that comprise 7% of all mediastinal tumors and have an estimated prevalence of 1 in 100,000. The most common location is the right cardiophrenic angle (50%-70%) followed by the left cardiophrenic angle (28%-38%), but pericardial cysts may occur at any location adjacent to the pericardium.

Pericardial cysts are thought to form during embryogenesis when a portion of the pericardium is pinched off and becomes isolated from the rest of the pericardial cavity. They are lined by a single layer of mesothelial cells, and most contain simple fluid. The classic teaching that pericardial cysts never exert mass effect on the heart (unlike a loculated pericardial effusion, which often does) is generally true for small cysts but not necessarily so for larger cysts.

Most patients are asymptomatic, and the lesion is detected as an incidental finding on chest radiography, CT, or echocardiography; however, a small percentage of patients have chest pain or dyspnea; rarely, cysts are aspirated or resected to relieve severe symptoms.

The major goal of MRI in these cases is to document the lesion and to strongly emphasize its benign nature in the report. A well-circumscribed cystic lesion in a typical location should have no real differential diagnosis; however, it is important to verify that the lesion is truly cystic. We have seen 1 or 2 cases of homogeneous solid masses that were labeled pericardial cysts on outside examinations performed without contrast. If there is any doubt, gadolinium should be administered to verify the absence of internal enhancement.

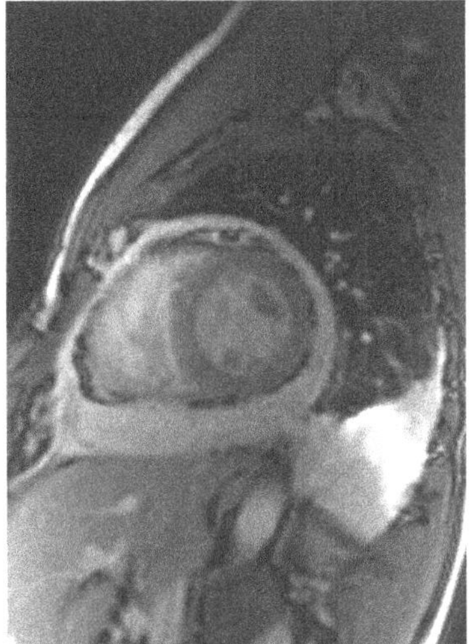

Figure 13.14.1

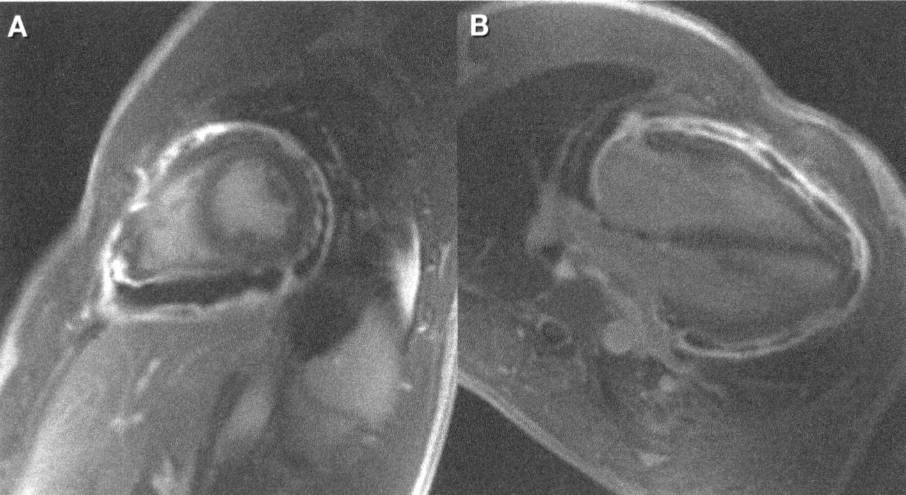

Figure 13.14.2

HISTORY: 25-year-old man with multiple episodes of pleuritic chest pain

IMAGING FINDINGS: Short-axis SSFP image (Figure 13.14.1) reveals a small, predominantly inferior pericardial effusion, a small left pleural effusion, and left base atelectasis. Short-axis and horizontal long-axis LGE inversion recovery T1-weighted images (Figure 13.14.2) demonstrate diffuse thickening and intense enhancement of the pericardium, with the nonenhancing pericardial fluid separating the fibrous and visceral pericardial layers.

DIAGNOSIS: Pericarditis

COMMENT: Once every year or 2, a patient comes through our emergency department with complaints of abdominal and lower extremity swelling, has a negative duplex US for lower extremity deep vein thrombosis, and then gets an abdominopelvic CT to exclude a mass compressing the inferior vena cava, where on the first 1 or 2 images you can see extensive calcification of the pericardium. The resident usually notices this finding and remarks on it in the report, but whether the term *constrictive pericarditis* is actually mentioned is more variable, and occasionally these patients have been discharged without being evaluated by a cardiologist.

Generally, you can't look at a single MRI image and make the diagnosis of pericardial constriction, as you can with circumferential pericardial calcification on CT. However, MRI does allow a more comprehensive assessment, with easier visualization of small pericardial effusions, higher sensitivity for detecting pericardial enhancement, and the ability to perform free-breathing functional imaging to assess for ventricular interdependence.

Pericarditis describes inflammation of the pericardium, the thin sac enclosing the heart whose functional utility is thought by many to be similar to that of the appendix. The classic symptom of acute pericarditis is pleuritic chest pain, although the presentation can sometimes simulate ischemic injury. In severe cases, cardiac biomarkers may be mildly elevated, most often with myopericarditis, and of course pericarditis can occur in association with acute myocardial infarction. The most common cause of pericarditis is thought to be viral infection. A few of the many additional causes are myocardial infarction (Dressler syndrome); bacterial, fungal, or tuberculous infection; autoimmune diseases; uremia; malignancy; and radiation injury.

Pericarditis has a broad range of appearances on MRI. Usually the pericardium is thickened (normal, <3 mm), often with a pericardial effusion of variable size that may be simple or complex. Pericardial thickening is best appreciated on ECG-gated double inversion recovery FSE images or LGE images. The pericardium anterior to the right ventricular free wall is usually the easiest to identify since it's almost always surrounded by fat and stands out as a dark structure with fat on either side on double inversion recovery images. In contrast, the pericardium adjacent to the left ventricle and atria usually adheres to the surface of these structures and is difficult to visualize unless an effusion is present or there is significant enhancement. Pericardial effusions have signal characteristics of fluid and are easily identified on cine SSFP images, although sometimes the effusion is nearly identical in signal intensity to the adjacent epicardial fat.

Enhancement of the pericardium on LGE images is a sensitive and fairly specific finding of pericardial inflammation, although it likely can also reflect fibrotic changes in patients with chronic pericarditis.

Constrictive pericarditis describes the situation in which the pericardium is rigid and reduces diastolic filling and ventricular preload. Right and left ventricular pressures are coupled (ventricular interdependence), and this is manifested as an abnormal septal motion, or septal bounce, which has a pronounced respiratory variation—more prominent on inspiration and less prominent on expiration. Additional signs of constrictive pericarditis include severely dilated atria, tubular ventricles, and significant dilatation of the inferior vena cava and hepatic veins. Constrictive pericarditis has classically been considered a surgical disease; however, pericardiectomy has a high associated morbidity and mortality, and therefore many patients now receive a trial of corticosteroids or nonsteroidal anti-inflammatory drugs. If diffuse calcification is present, medical therapy is likely to be unsuccessful, and in this regard CT would be favored as a diagnostic tool. However, the most common cause of calcific pericarditis is tuberculosis, with a decreasing prevalence, and MRI is better able to detect and characterize noncalcific pericardial disease. Pericardial calcification on MRI typically appears as low signal intensity on all imaging sequences, without significant enhancement after gadolinium administration.

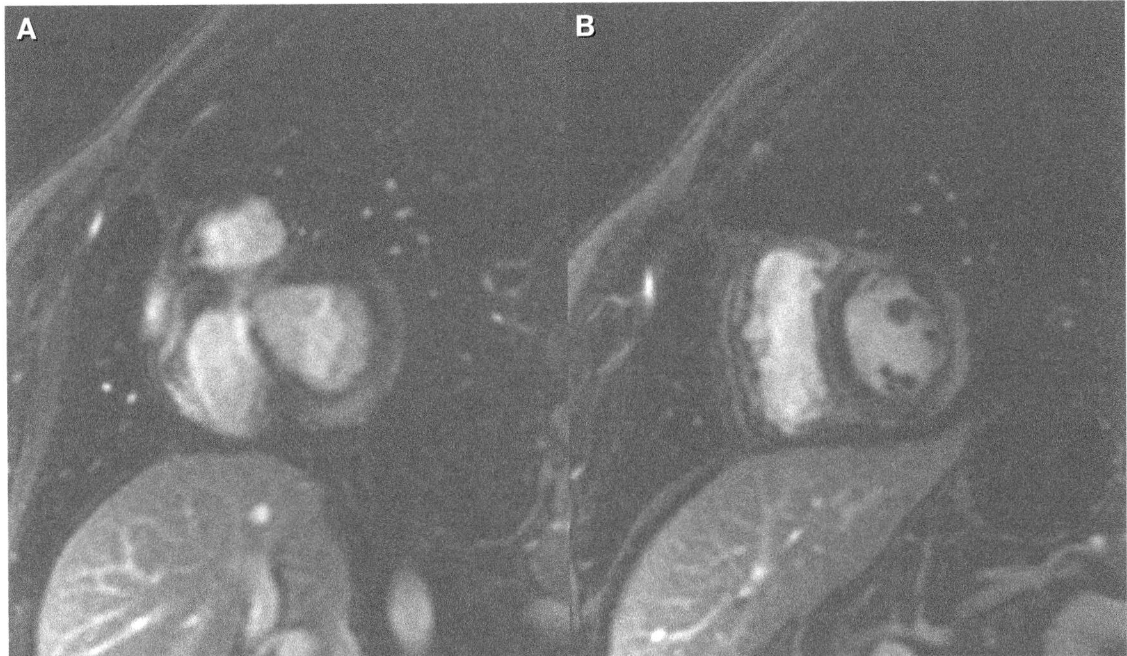

Figure 13.15.1

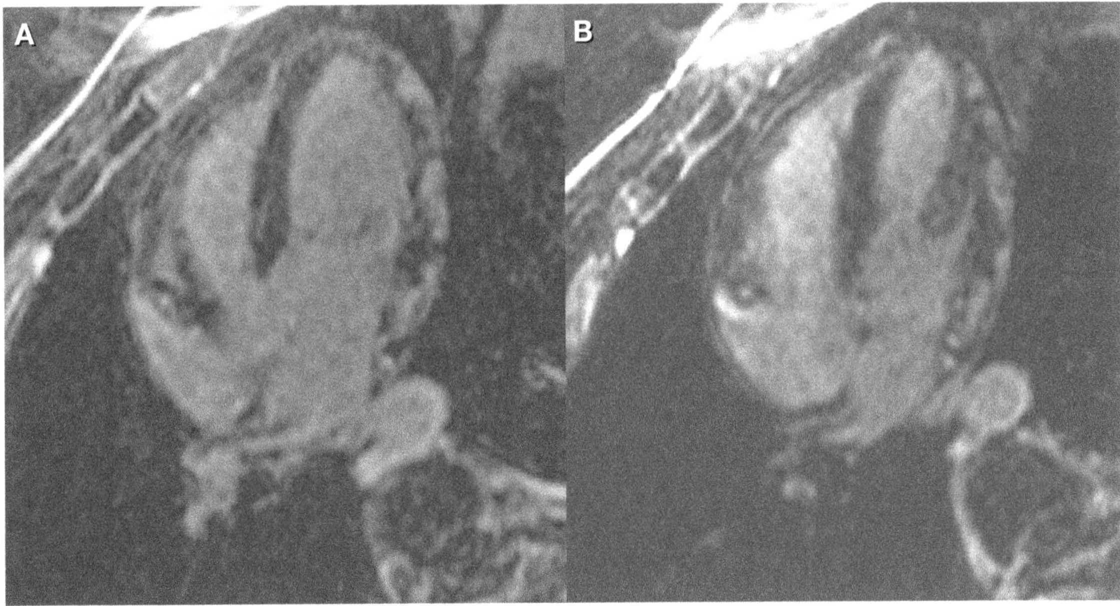

Figure 13.15.2

HISTORY: 34-year-old man with chest pressure and elevated troponin levels

IMAGING FINDINGS: Short-axis MDE images obtained 2 minutes after gadolinium injection (Figure 13.15.1) and horizontal long-axis MDE images obtained 10 minutes after gadolinium injection (Figure 13.15.2) demonstrate early heterogeneous enhancement of the lateral and inferior left ventricular myocardium and late patchy enhancement predominantly involving the lateral wall in an epicardial, nonischemic distribution.

DIAGNOSIS: Myocarditis

COMMENT: *Myocarditis* is defined as inflammation of the myocardium and constitutes a wide spectrum of clinical disease ranging from minimal symptoms to cardiac failure and sudden death. Myocarditis can occur in patients of any age; however, young adults are most frequently affected, and autopsy findings from young adults with sudden cardiac death suggest that myocarditis is the cause in 12% to 22%. Infectious, autoimmune, and toxic factors have been implicated in the development of myocarditis, with viral infection considered the most common cause.

The classic manifestation of myocarditis is similar to that of acute coronary syndrome—patients may have chest pain or pressure, fatigue, shortness of breath, and palpitations along with elevated myocardial enzyme levels and ECG changes. This invariably leads to an ischemic workup (as it should), and after myocardial ischemia or infarction has been excluded, then myocarditis becomes the presumptive diagnosis.

Myocarditis usually has a fairly benign course, and most patients recover full cardiac function within a few weeks. In some patients, however, arrhythmias or heart block develops, leading to sudden cardiac death; in some, persistent left ventricular dysfunction eventually results in dilated cardiomyopathy and heart failure; and in others, development of extensive fibrosis can cause restrictive cardiomyopathy.

Until recently, myocarditis was largely a diagnosis of exclusion. Once the ischemic workup was negative, myocarditis became the presumptive diagnosis. Myocardial biopsy was rarely performed because of its relatively low yield, invasiveness, and small but significant complication rate.

Cardiac MRI offers a noninvasive alternative path to diagnosis with a higher sensitivity than biopsy. Three findings have been described in patients with acute myocarditis: 1) myocardial edema, visible on T2-weighted double or triple inversion recovery images; 2) early myocardial enhancement, seen 1 to 2 minutes after gadolinium injection; and 3) LGE, seen on standard inversion recovery T1-weighted SPGR images 10 to 20 minutes after contrast administration. (Cine SSFP images are also important for demonstrating the degree of ventricular dysfunction, but they are not specific for the diagnosis of myocarditis.)

The Lake Louise Criteria (the work of an expert consensus panel) specify that when 2 of the 3 findings above are present, myocarditis can be diagnosed with a sensitivity of 67% and a specificity of 91%. The general criteria are sound; however, they lose some credibility in the details, which specify the use of edema and early enhancement ratios generated by comparing the signal intensity of myocardium to an internal reference of skeletal muscle. This is an unreliable measurement at best, and it may fail completely in patients with inflammatory diseases who might also have skeletal muscle inflammation. (An additional failing is the specification of a conventional ECG-gated spin echo T1-weighted acquisition for early enhancement measurements. This is one of the most artifact-prone techniques available in cardiac MRI, and many of the published positive examples may simply reflect the presence of increased phase ghosting artifacts overlying the myocardium in patients who are sicker than normal controls.)

Nevertheless, all these findings are legitimate signs of myocarditis, and we recommend that all postgadolinium T1-weighted acquisitions be performed with a standard breath-held or respiratory-triggered inversion recovery MDE technique. LGE is probably the most reproducible and consistent finding, although myocardial edema and early enhancement are helpful in distinguishing acute from chronic disease. LGE in myocarditis has a nonischemic distribution; the enhancement is typically subepicardial rather than subendocardial, as is seen in ischemic lesions. Transmural enhancement can occur in either ischemia or myocarditis, and if that's the only pattern visible, then distinguishing between the two is very difficult based on imaging findings alone; however, there are often regions where the enhancement becomes predominantly subepicardial or endocardial.

The meaning and prognostic implications of LGE in myocarditis are somewhat controversial. Some authors assert that LGE is synonymous with irreversible injury, while others have found a significant reduction in LGE at follow-up MRI performed in patients with resolving disease.

CASE 13.16

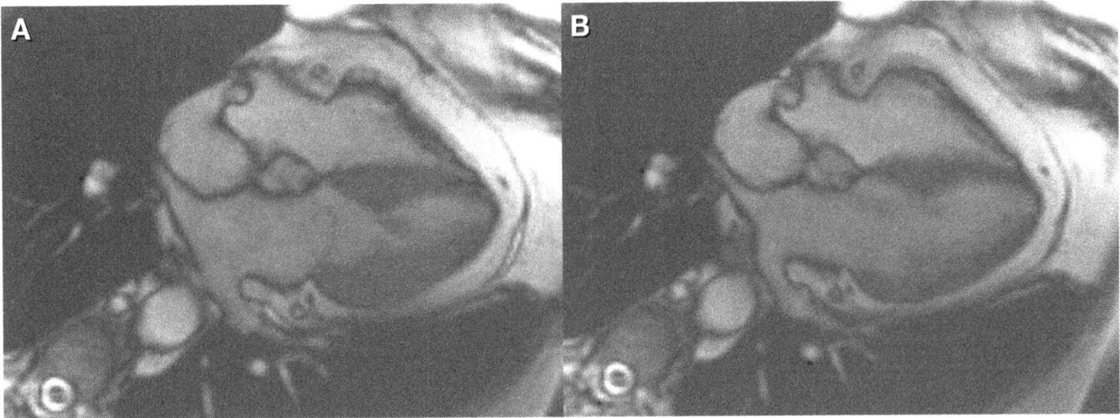

Figure 13.16.1

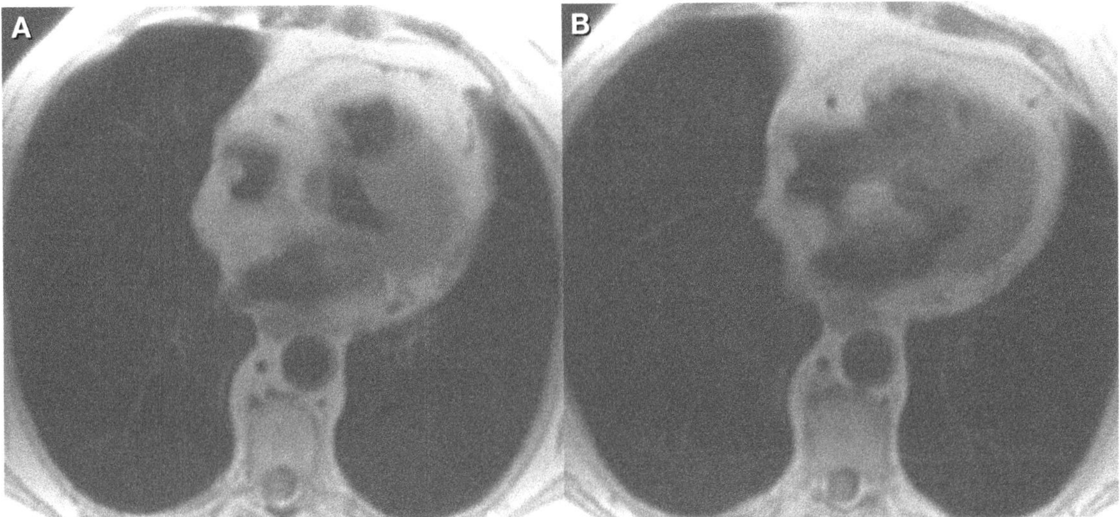

Figure 13.16.2

HISTORY: 72-year-old woman with known coronary artery disease; echocardiography noted a possible left atrial mass, and MRI was suggested for further assessment

IMAGING FINDINGS: Horizontal long-axis images from a cine SSFP acquisition (Figure 13.16.1) demonstrate dumbbell-shaped widening of the interatrial septum with uniform high signal intensity. Axial double inversion recovery FSE proton density-weighted images (Figure 13.16.2) show fatty replacement of the interatrial septum. Also note prominent epicardial fat, fatty replacement of the right ventricular free wall, and fatty replacement of the crista terminalis along the posterior wall of the right atrium.

DIAGNOSIS: Lipomatous hypertrophy of the interatrial septum

COMMENT: LHIAS is another in a long list of entities (see also the discussion of ventricular noncompaction in Case 13.22) whose incidence increases as the frequency and quality of imaging improve. LHIAS is fatty infiltration of the interatrial septum, classically sparing the fossa ovalis, which accounts for its dumbbell-shaped configuration. LHIAS was first described in 1964, and estimates of its prevalence range from 1% to 8%. Histologically, the lesion is composed of adipocytes infiltrating the interatrial septum along with interspersed myocytes and myocardial fibers. LHIAS is distinguished from a true intracardiac lipoma by its lack of a capsule and its heterogeneous mixture of both mature adipocytes and fetal fat cells or brown fat.

LHIAS is thought to be more prevalent in obese patients and possibly more common in women. This case illustrates the usual constellation of LHIAS, prominent epicardial fat (ie, the layer of fat between the pericardium and the myocardium), and fatty infiltration of the right ventricular free wall. The presence of fat in the right ventricular free wall used to be considered strong evidence of ARVD; however, this finding has been observed in 15% to 20% of normal patients, and an overreliance on this sign has probably had a prominent role in the decidedly mixed performance of MRI in the diagnosis of ARVD.

The clinical importance of LHIAS is somewhat controversial. Most cases—this case is a typical example—are detected incidentally on an examination performed for another indication. Occasionally, this entity is mistaken on echocardiography for a genuine atrial mass, such as a myxoma; MRI or CT should easily allow the correct diagnosis. Another interesting feature of LHIAS is the occasional significantly increased FDG uptake on PET scans, which is usually attributed to the presence of brown fat and is a potential mimic of a malignant lesion.

Generally, LHIAS is a benign and incidental finding, but it has been associated with atrial arrhythmias, altered P-wave configurations, chronic pulmonary disease, obstruction of the superior vena cava or inferior vena cava, and sudden death. The mechanism of atrial arrhythmias is presumably fatty infiltration interfering with the conducting pathways through the interatrial septum.

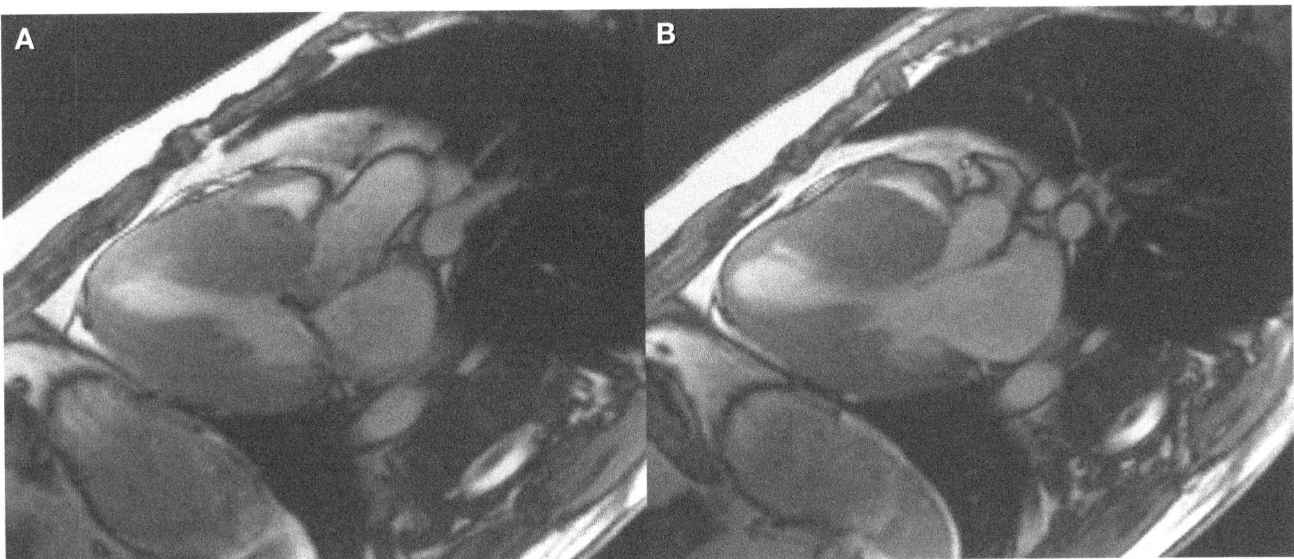

Figure 13.17.1

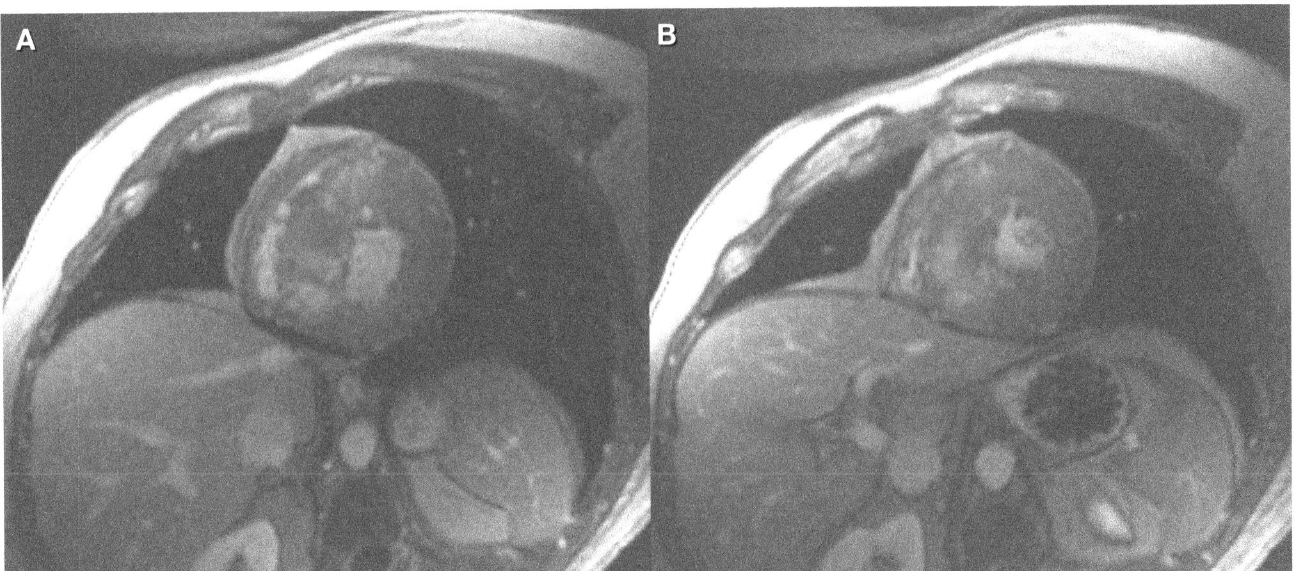

Figure 13.17.2

HISTORY: 38-year-old man with progressive chest pressure and dyspnea

IMAGING FINDINGS: Systolic (Figure 13.17.1A) and early diastolic (Figure 13.17.1B) frames from a 3-chamber cine SSFP acquisition demonstrate thickening of the basal anteroseptal wall. Note in systole the dark jet of mitral insufficiency directed posteriorly. Short-axis MDE images (Figure 13.17.2) show patchy enhancement of the thickened septal wall in a nonischemic pattern.

DIAGNOSIS: Hypertrophic cardiomyopathy

COMMENT: *HCM* is defined as left ventricular hypertrophy in the absence of left ventricular dilatation or any other underlying condition that could be responsible for significant hypertrophy. HCM is one of the most common genetic disorders, with autosomal dominant inheritance and a prevalence estimated at 0.1% to 0.2% (or 1 in 500) in the general population.

The genetic underpinnings of HCM are diverse, and hundreds of different mutations have been identified in affected patients, but most involve sarcomeric protein alterations that reduce contractility at the myocyte level. This in turn leads to hypertrophy (as a compensatory mechanism to reduce afterload) and myocardial fibrosis.

The histologic appearance of HCM is striking, with patchy regions of severely hypertrophied myocytes, connective tissue, and fibrosis in a whorled pattern (the descriptive term *myocardial disarray* is often used). Myocardial fibrosis is a prominent feature of HCM and is thought to be important in the development of arrhythmias and abnormal myocardial compliance. The coronary vasculature is also abnormal in these regions; frequent thrombosis and obliteration of smaller vessels likely predispose patients to ischemia and may contribute to the development of fibrosis.

Many distinct patterns of left ventricular hypertrophy have been reported, and the right ventricle may be variably affected as well; however, the asymmetrical septal hypertrophy in this case is most common. Basal septal hypertrophy obstructs the LVOT in approximately 70% of patients either at rest or with physiologic provocation. The pressure gradient across the LVOT during systole draws the anterior mitral valve leaflet forward (known as systolic anterior motion of the mitral valve), which exacerbates the LVOT obstruction and also leads to a posteriorly directed jet of mitral regurgitation, as seen in this case.

Although HCM is thought to be the most common cause of sudden death in young adults, the life expectancy of patients with HCM is similar to that of normal cohorts. Symptoms in HCM patients are highly variable and may be related to LVOT obstruction (dyspnea on exertion or exertional syncope), mitral regurgitation, or atrial fibrillation. Atrial fibrillation occurs in up to 30% of older patients and is generally associated with advanced disease and clinical deterioration. Development of atrial fibrillation is likely related to the fundamental diastolic dysfunction, increased filling pressures, and significant mitral regurgitation.

MRI is well suited for screening of family members of known HCM patients or for assessing the severity of disease. MRI is the most accurate technique for measuring myocardial thickness (patients with an end-diastolic thickness of >30 mm have a high risk of significant arrhythmias and often have prophylactic placement of an AICD), ventricular mass, and ventricular function. The severity of LVOT obstruction and the degree of mitral regurgitation can be quantified with cine phase contrast velocity encoding techniques; however, this procedure is usually more straightforward with echocardiography, which in our practice is invariably performed for these patients.

MDE is commonly seen in HCM patients. Some authors have reported that MDE occurs in as many as 80% of patients, but in our experience the incidence is closer to 50%. The typical appearance is within the hypertrophied ventricular septum near the insertion points of the right ventricle in a nonischemic distribution (ie, not subendocardial), but MDE can appear in segments of normal thickness. Several authors have noted a correlation between adverse cardiac events and the amount of myocardial fibrosis quantified by MRI. Eventually, large amounts of scarring may become an additional indication for AICD placement.

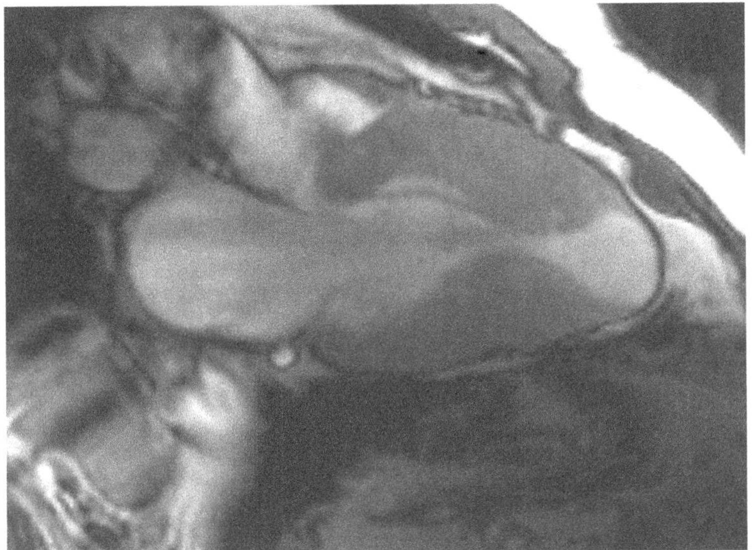

Figure 13.18.1

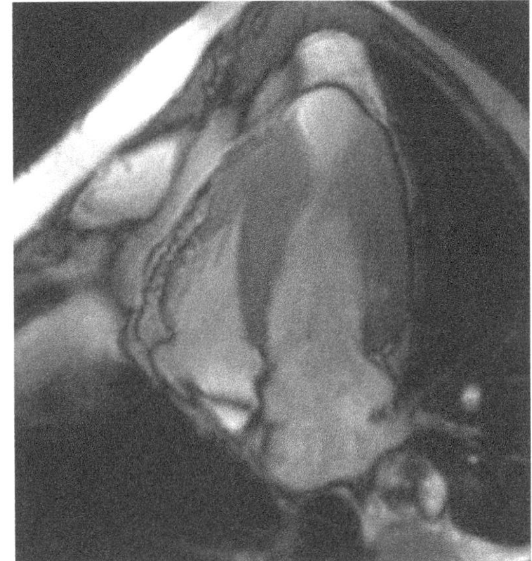

Figure 13.18.2

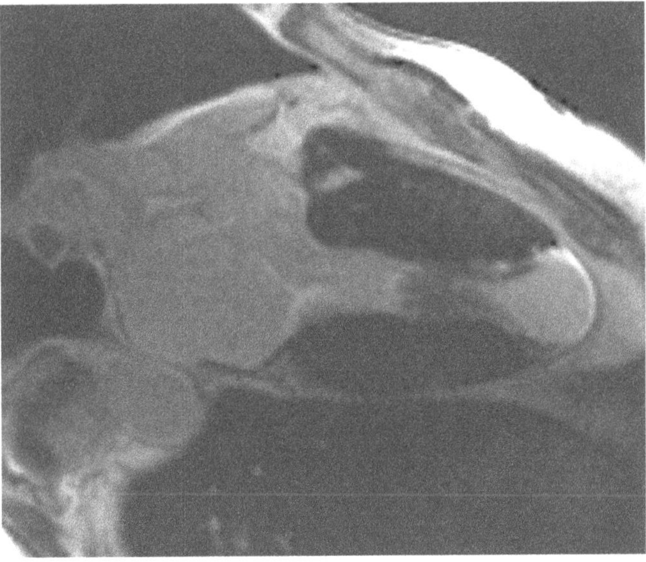

Figure 13.18.3

HISTORY: 76-year-old man with progressive exertional dyspnea

IMAGING FINDINGS: Two-chamber (Figure 13.18.1) and 4-chamber (Figure 13.18.2) systolic frames from cine SSFP acquisitions demonstrate hypertrophy of the mid myocardium sparing the base of the left ventricle and severe thinning of the apex. Two-chamber postgadolinium MDE image (Figure 13.18.3) reveals transmural enhancement of the thinned apex.

DIAGNOSIS: Midventricular variant HCM with apical aneurysm

COMMENT: HCM occurs in many distinct morphological subtypes; the basal septal variant shown in Case 13.17 is most common. Involvement of the midventricle is less well characterized, but this variant is thought to place patients at risk of apical aneurysms, as seen in this case.

Assessment of the left ventricular and right ventricular apices is notoriously difficult with transthoracic echocardiography, and apical hypertrophy (a variant first described in Japan and characterized by giant inverted T waves on

ECG) is frequently overlooked if the only examination performed is echocardiography. Similarly, apical aneurysms may not be appreciated, and certainly documentation of diffuse infarction or fibrosis with delayed enhancement imaging is not possible.

In a study of 1,300 patients with HCM, 2% had apical aneurysms, and echocardiography identified only 57% of the lesions. The patients who had apical aneurysms had a much higher rate (43%) of adverse cardiac events in an average of 4 years of follow-up.

The definition of *ventricular aneurysm* is, to some extent, in the eye of the beholder. A variable degree of focal dilatation is usually expected in the setting of an apical infarct or scar, although there are no widely accepted numerical criteria, and this requirement is often relaxed in the presence of focal dyskinesis (ie, the aneurysm dilates during systole).

Many theories have been advanced to explain the development of apical aneurysms, including a distinct genetic defect and the development of increased apical stress and subsequent ischemia due to mid cavitary obstruction.

CASE 13.19

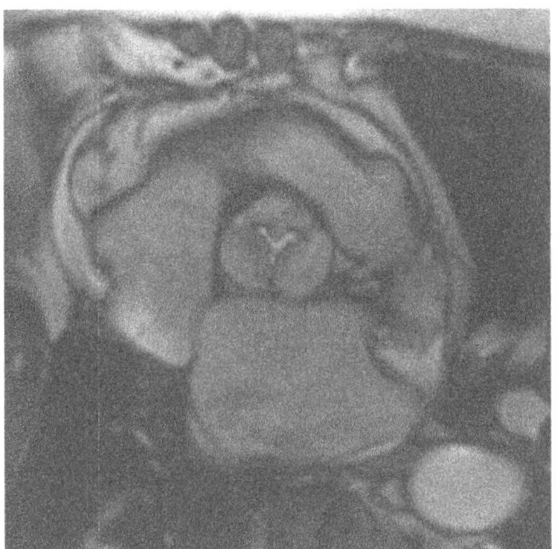

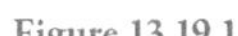

Figure 13.19.1

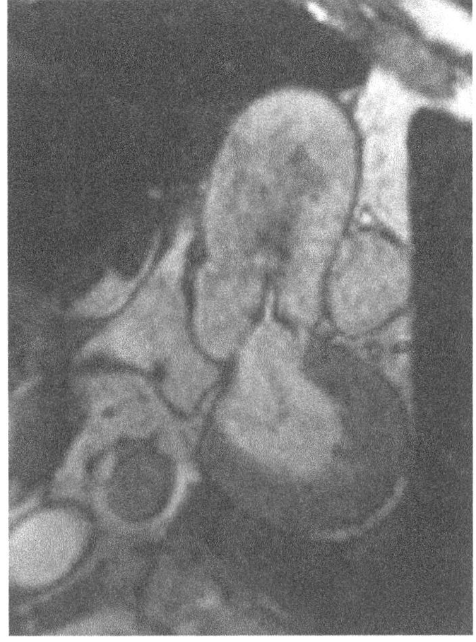

Figure 13.19.2

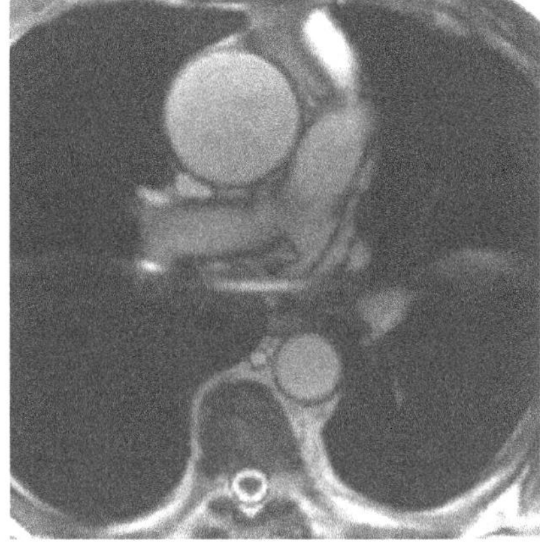

Figure 13.19.3

HISTORY: 74-year-old woman with hypertension; a dilated aorta was noted on chest CT

IMAGING FINDINGS: SSFP images obtained at end systole through the aortic valve in transverse (Figure 13.19.1) and coronal oblique (Figure 13.19.2) orientations demonstrate a tricuspid aortic valve with minimal excursion of the valve leaflets. Axial SSFP image at the level of the right main pulmonary artery (Figure 13.19.3) reveals dilatation of the ascending aorta.

DIAGNOSIS: Aortic stenosis

COMMENT: Evaluation of aortic valve disease with MRI has generated a large number of papers since the late 1990s, although it remains uncertain whether this indication will ever progress beyond the realm of academic curiosity: Echocardiography is in many respects an ideal technique for valve assessment and is faster, cheaper, and more inclusive than MRI. Nevertheless, it is true that transthoracic echocardiography is occasionally unsuccessful or successive examinations provide discrepant results, and in these cases MRI may be a useful alternative. MRI also allows a comprehensive assessment of left ventricular and valvular function and an accurate measurement of the aortic diameter. In theory, this application embodies the concept of the "one-stop cardiac shop" first advanced by Elias Zerhouni in the 1980s. This notion remains a powerful marketing tool for cardiac MRI but is still rarely applied in the real world.

The most common causes of aortic stenosis (in descending order) are idiopathic degeneration of a normal valve, degeneration of a bicuspid valve (typically occurring with earlier onset), and rheumatic heart disease. Classic symptoms include dyspnea on exertion, exertional syncope, and angina accompanied by a holosystolic murmur. Symptoms usually appear late in the course of the disease, and patients often experience a rapid decline (75% mortality within 3 years) if the valve is not replaced. Aortic stenosis causes obstruction of the LVOT, elevated left ventricular pressures, diminished cardiac output, and compensatory left ventricular hypertrophy.

Visualization of aortic stenosis with MRI is usually straightforward: 3-chamber and coronal oblique cine SSFP images are obtained through the LVOT, and these orthogonal views are used to prescribe transverse acquisitions through the aortic valve. These 3 sets of cine images allow visualization of the limited excursion of the valve leaflets, congenital abnormalities such as a bicuspid valve, and systolic jets of high-velocity flow in the ascending aorta, seen as dark flow voids. Additional short-axis SSFP images through the left ventricle are useful to assess ventricular function and document left ventricular hypertrophy, and of course the maximal diameter of the ascending aorta should be measured.

The severity of the aortic valve lesion can be assessed in several ways. One of the easiest is planimetry, in which the maximal opening area of the valve is manually traced on SSFP or cine phase contrast images. This measurement has been shown to correlate fairly well with echocardiographic estimation of effective orifice area (the easy-to-remember cutoff value for severe stenosis is <1.0 cm^2). One of the somewhat legitimate complaints about this method is that the corresponding echocardiographic technique is based on velocity measurements and is therefore more physiologic. The same analysis can be performed with MRI by acquiring cine phase contrast measurements in the LVOT and at the site of peak velocity just above the valve. On the basis of the principle of conservation of flow, the areas under the 2 time-velocity curves should be equivalent. Since the area of the LVOT can be directly measured from the magnitude images, the equation can be solved for the effective valve area. Several studies have shown that the MRI measurements agree reasonably well with those obtained with echocardiography. Cine phase contrast images can also be used to measure the peak velocities across the valve, and these in turn can be used to estimate the peak valvular pressure gradient with the modified Bernoulli equation ($\Delta P=4v_{max}^2$, where P is the pressure in millimeters of mercury and v is the velocity in meters per second).

Attention to detail is very important in obtaining accurate cine phase contrast velocity and flow measurements. The VENC gradient should be set to a value slightly higher than the expected peak velocity, slices should be positioned perpendicular to the direction of flow, and temporal and spatial resolution need to be adequate to assure accurate depiction of the vessel border and complete visualization of rapid flow components (with the unfortunate caveat that improving either temporal or spatial resolution results in a longer acquisition time).

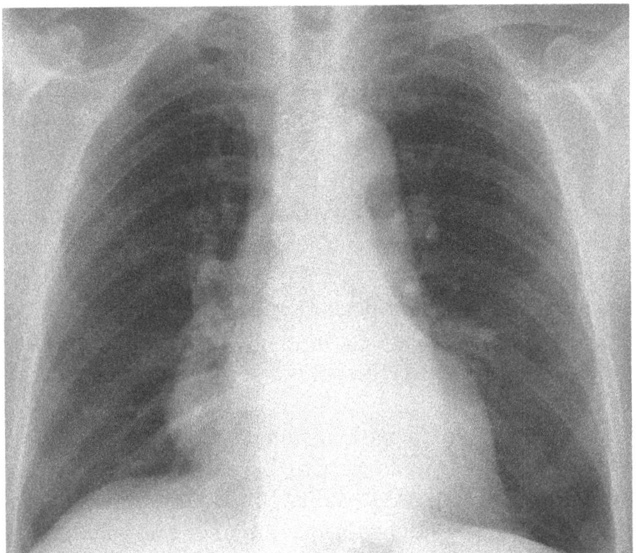

Figure 13.20.1

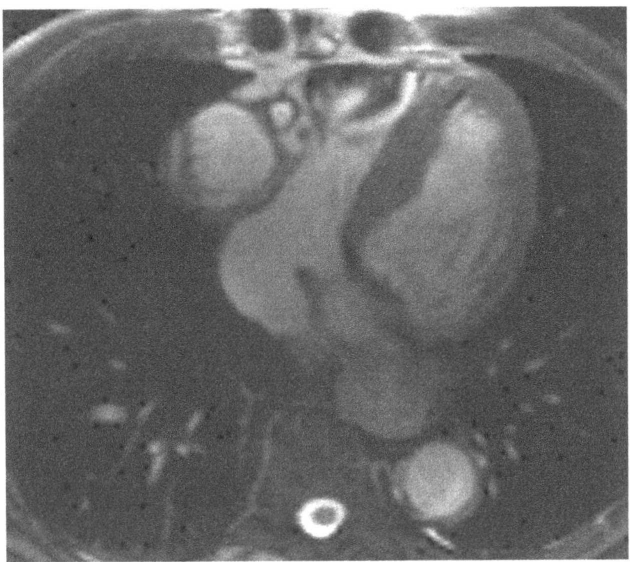

Figure 13.20.2

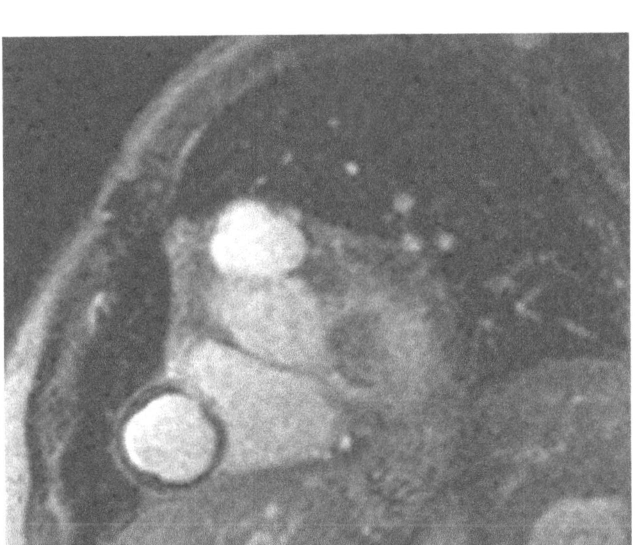

Figure 13.20.3

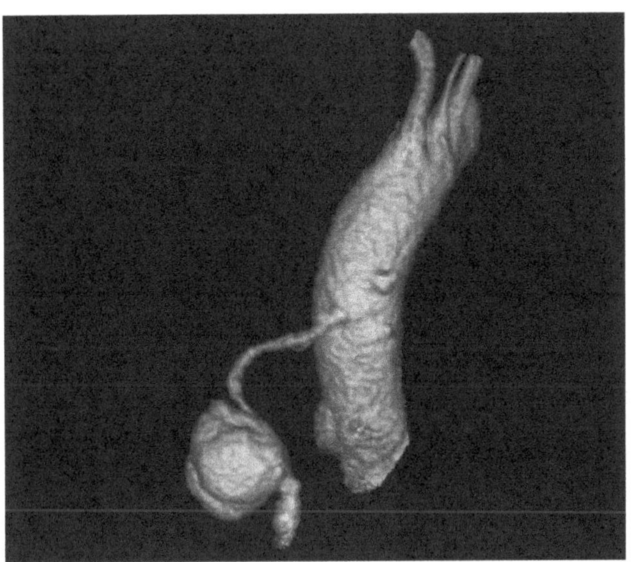

Figure 13.20.4

HISTORY: 79-year-old man with a history of CABG surgery 15 years ago now has gradually increasing chest pain and shortness of breath; chest radiography demonstrated a mass along the right heart border, and echocardiography identified a corresponding lesion, likely a vascular structure, adjacent to the right atrium

IMAGING FINDINGS: Posteroanterior chest radiograph (Figure 13.20.1) demonstrates a lobulated mass projecting along the right heart border. Axial 2D SSFP image (Figure 13.20.2) shows an ovoid lesion indenting the lateral border of the right atrium with signal intensity similar to the blood pool. Coronal oblique MDE postgadolinium image (Figure 13.20.3) demonstrates central enhancement of the lesion equivalent to the blood pool with a nonenhancing rim. VR image from 3D ECG-gated gadolinium MRA (Figure 13.20.4) connects the lesion to a CABG extending from the proximal ascending aorta.

DIAGNOSIS: CABG aneurysm

COMMENT: CABG aneurysms are uncommon. A Mayo Clinic retrospective analysis of 28,603 patients who underwent CABG surgery found only 16 patients with aneurysms, although this is almost certainly an underestimation of the true prevalence, since many patients are likely asymptomatic. Aneurysmal dilatation of a CABG was first reported in 1975 by Riahi and colleagues, and subsequently, 75 to 100 cases have been described in the literature. True aneurysms, which usually develop in the middle of the vein graft and are likely caused by atherosclerosis, are distinguished from pseudoaneurysms, which more commonly occur at the proximal or distal anastomosis.

The favorite CABG technique uses the left internal mammary artery as a graft. The artery is dissected from its retrosternal location and is typically anastomosed to the left anterior descending artery or to 1 of its branches. This arterial graft requires only 1 distal anastomosis, generally lasts longer than venous grafts, and has a lower restenosis rate. Unfortunately, patients have only 1 left internal mammary artery, although sometimes the right internal mammary artery is also used, and so the next alternative is to dissect a segment of the saphenous vein to form a conduit from the ascending aorta to a distal native coronary artery. Veins are not designed to withstand the high intraluminal pressure of an artery, and some grafts respond poorly, most often by rapidly developing stenosis and eventually thrombosis, but occasionally by aneurysm formation.

CABG aneurysms are subject to the same complications of aneurysms as in any other location: rupture with catastrophic bleeding, thrombosis, and distal embolization, all of which can lead to ischemia and myocardial infarction. Fistulization into the right atrium and right ventricle has also been described. When CABG aneurysms are detected, they are repaired on an emergent or elective basis, depending on the patient's symptoms.

CABG aneurysms are occasionally detected incidentally as a mediastinal mass on chest radiograph or noncontrast CT, although the increasing popularity of coronary CTA has led to more frequent noninvasive surveillance of coronary artery grafts and concomitant detection of the various associated complications. Coronary MRA is generally recognized as being a distant second-place alternative to coronary CTA, but it can be effective at determining whether grafts are patent or thrombosed, and it certainly can be used to detect large aneurysms.

In this case, we recognized immediately that the lesion was an aneurysm and then tried both noncontrast (ECG and navigator-gated 3D SSFP) and contrast-enhanced (ECG-gated 3D SPGR) MRA techniques. The gadolinium MRA generated the best images for this particular patient, mainly because he was a good breath-holder, but he had uneven respirations, which led to significant artifact on the 3D SSFP images.

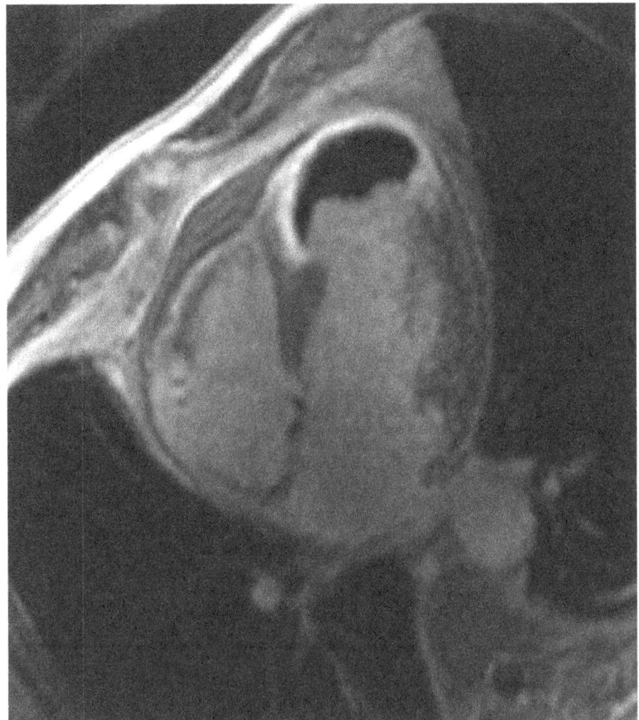

Figure 13.21.1

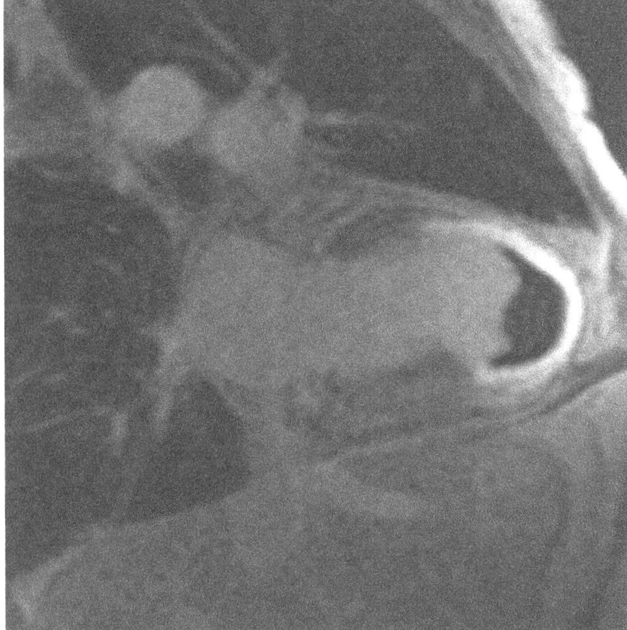

Figure 13.21.2

HISTORY: 62-year-old man with new-onset chest pain

IMAGING FINDINGS: Horizontal long-axis (4-chamber) (Figure 13.21.1) and vertical long-axis (2-chamber) (Figure 13.21.2) MDE images demonstrate transmural enhancement of the left ventricular apex. Note the prominent nonenhancing filling defect in the apical cavity adjacent to the enhancing infarct.

DIAGNOSIS: Left apical infarct with layering thrombus

COMMENT: Infarct imaging was the application that made cardiac MRI a viable clinical tool. It had long been recognized that myocardial infarctions showed hyperenhancement on T1-weighted images obtained several minutes after injection of standard extracellular gadolinium contrast agents; however, the image quality was often marginal and the contrast between infarct and normal myocardium was not striking. This situation was markedly improved by the addition of an inversion recovery pulse to the standard ECG-gated 2D SPGR T1-weighted acquisition, which allowed the user to choose a TI that optimized contrast between normal myocardium, infarct, and blood pool. This is the MDE or LGE technique.

The concept of an enhancing infarct is counterintuitive but is explained by the increased extravascular volume in acute or chronic infarcts. In the acute infarct, myocyte cell membrane integrity is lost, and gadolinium freely diffuses into the damaged cells; in the chronic infarct, myocytes have been replaced by predominantly acellular fibrotic tissue, greatly increasing the extravascular extracellular space. Gadolinium therefore encounters a larger extravascular space in an infarct and takes longer to wash in and wash out. If image acquisition is delayed long enough so that most of the gadolinium has washed out of normal myocardial tissue (usually 10-20 minutes), the infarct with its retained gadolinium is then seen as an enhancing structure.

The size and extent of an infarct correlates with prognosis, and the extent of transmural involvement reflects the likelihood of functional recovery. If less than 25% of the myocardial thickness is involved, cardiac function will likely return to normal, whereas if the transmural extension is 75% to 100%, functional recovery is unlikely. This distinction gives MRI an advantage over nuclear medicine techniques, which generally lack the spatial resolution to distinguish partial thickness from transmural involvement.

MDE images distinguish viable from nonviable tissue but do not tell you anything about the status of viable myocardium (ie, whether it is ischemic and at risk of infarction). Various supplemental techniques, including T2-weighted images (triple inversion recovery FSE), can be useful in this regard to identify myocardial edema in acute infarction. Stress testing can also be performed with a gadolinium-enhanced myocardial perfusion sequence in coordination with administration of a vasodilator, such as adenosine, or with a cine SSFP wall motion sequence and incremental doses of an inotropic agent, such as dobutamine. The idea is to carefully induce myocardial ischemia, which then becomes evident as a perfusion defect or a focal wall motion abnormality.

Infarct protocols, in addition to delayed enhancement acquisitions, also include long- and short-axis SSFP images for functional assessment of the ventricles and, usually, perfusion images to detect first-pass perfusion defects that would indicate resting ischemia. As seen in this case, MDE images are ideal for visualizing atrial or ventricular thrombus in patients with large infarcts and poorly functioning ventricles.

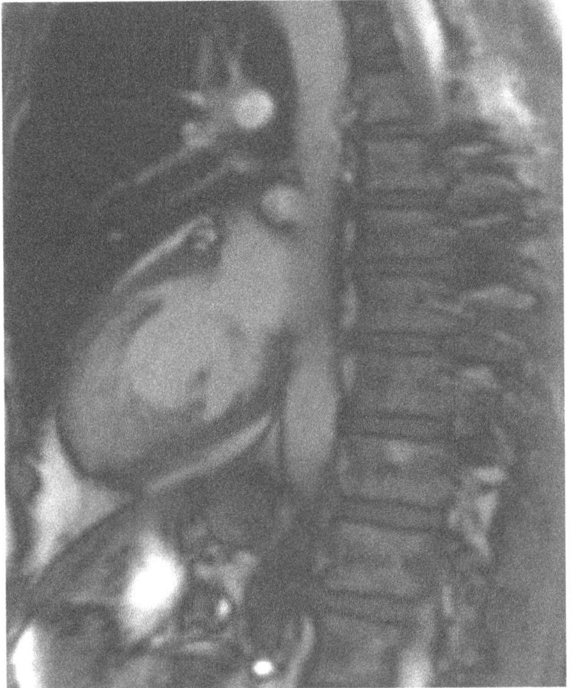

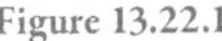

Figure 13.22.1

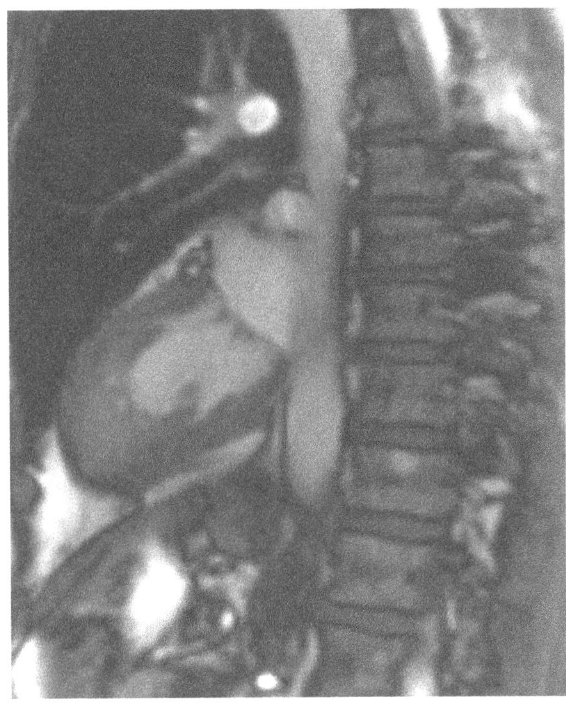

Figure 13.22.2

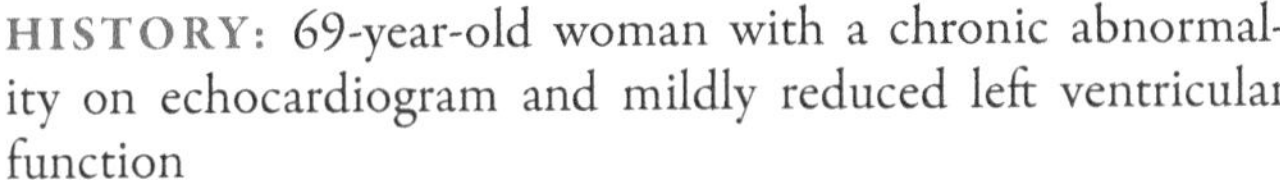

HISTORY: 69-year-old woman with a chronic abnormality on echocardiogram and mildly reduced left ventricular function

IMAGING FINDINGS: Two-chamber end-diastolic (Figure 13.22.1) and end-systolic (Figure 13.22.2) frames from a cine SSFP acquisition demonstrate thinning of the mid-apical left ventricular myocardium with extensive trabeculations within the left ventricular cavity.

DIAGNOSIS: Left ventricular noncompaction

COMMENT: Noncompaction is a congenital abnormality categorized by the American Heart Association as a primary cardiomyopathy and is thought to result from an arrest of the normal process of myocardial compaction during the fifth through the eighth weeks of gestation. Noncompaction was first described in 1990, and early reports usually discussed pediatric patients presenting with cardiac failure and severely reduced systolic function, often in association with additional cardiac abnormalities. As familiarity with this entity grew, reports of affected adults became more frequent, and associations with neuromuscular disorders were noted, including muscular dystrophy, myotonic dystrophy, Pompe disease, and Friedreich ataxia.

Noncompaction is characterized by prominent trabeculations within the ventricular cavity, most often in the midventricle to the apex, which connect to the more compacted myocardium. Normally, a few trabeculations are observed in the left ventricle; they are much more common in the right ventricle, often in association with papillary muscles, but extensive trabeculation (a somewhat subjective distinction) is abnormal and indicates noncompaction. Right ventricular involvement is thought to be less common, occurring in less than half of patients, although this may be related to the more prominent normal trabeculation of the right ventricle and to its limited visualization on transthoracic echocardiography.

The diagnostic criteria for noncompaction on echocardiography include visualization of a 2-layer myocardium with a noncompacted to compacted ratio greater than 2:1 measured at end systole. MRI descriptions of noncompaction are a more recent phenomenon, but it is probably true that diagnosis with MRI is slightly more reliable than echocardiography and that right ventricular involvement can be more readily assessed with MRI. The most widely referenced MRI article describes criteria for noncompaction based on an end-diastolic noncompacted to compacted ratio greater than 2.3:1 and is remarkable mainly for its success in establishing a widely accepted diagnostic standard based on measurements from only 7 patients.

Defects in coronary microcirculation have been reported from patients with noncompaction and might be partly responsible for some of the functional impairment. These defects might also explain the association of noncompaction with myocardial fibrosis or scarring on postgadolinium delayed enhancement imaging. Small case series have reported myocardial scarring in as many as 70% of patients with noncompaction, although some caution regarding this finding is warranted, since some of the published images likely depict gadolinium in the blood pool trapped within the trabeculations during systole rather than true myocardial injury.

The true incidence of noncompaction is uncertain. It is generally considered a rare entity; however, cases are detected with increasing frequency as incidental findings on MRI, and an autopsy study has reported that some degree of noncompaction can be found in 70% of normal hearts. Noncompaction probably includes a broad spectrum ranging from severely debilitated patients presenting early in life to asymptomatic adults in whom the finding is best considered a normal variant with no prognostic implications.

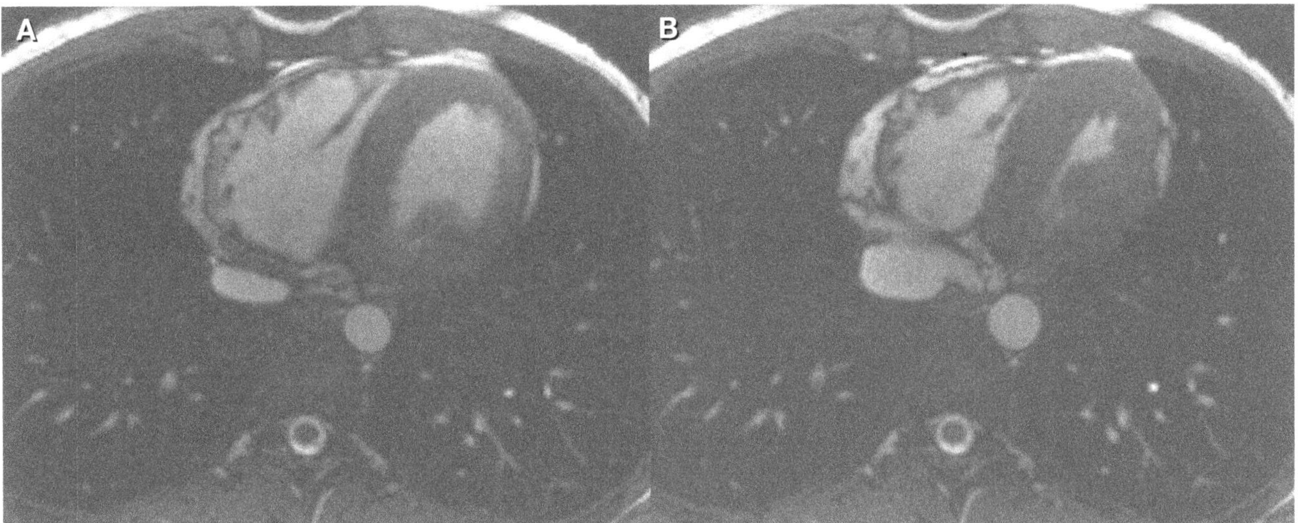

Figure 13.23.1

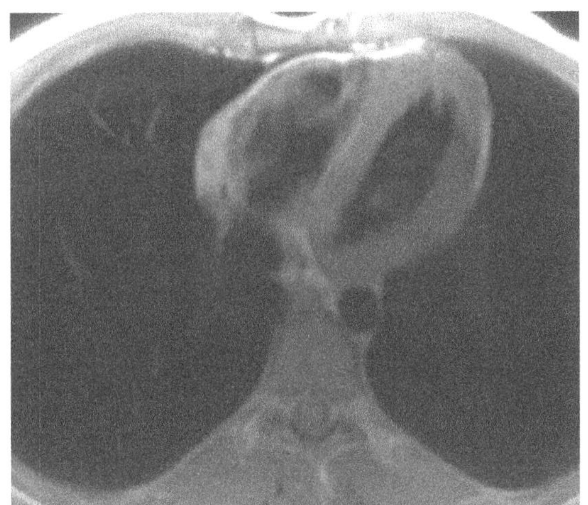

Figure 13.23.2

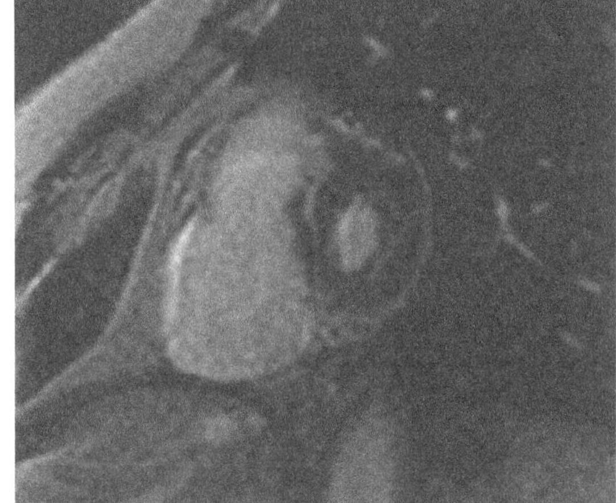

Figure 13.23.3

HISTORY: 16-year-old male adolescent with an arrhythmia during elective surgery

IMAGING FINDINGS: Axial end-systolic SSFP images (Figure 13.23.1) demonstrate small focal outpouchings along the free wall of the right ventricle. Axial double inversion recovery proton density-weighted FSE image (Figure 13.23.2) reveals minimal fatty replacement in the right side of the ventricular septum. Short-axis MDE image (Figure 13.23.3) after gadolinium administration shows focal enhancement of the right ventricular free wall.

DIAGNOSIS: Arrhythmogenic right ventricular dysplasia

COMMENT: ARVD was once the most common indication for cardiac MRI, a situation that undoubtedly drove many talented residents and fellows away from cardiac imaging as a subspecialty. The diagnostic criteria were nebulous, many of the recognized ARVD experts were notoriously inaccurate in their interpretations, and the patients' arrhythmias led to image quality that was often marginal at best.

The situation is somewhat improved today, mostly because ARVD cases are a much smaller percentage of the total cardiac MRI volume, but also because some progress has been made in the technical and diagnostic aspects of these examinations.

ARVD is a cardiomyopathy primarily affecting the right ventricle and is characterized by fibrofatty replacement of the myocardium, myocyte loss, ventricular arrhythmias, and right-sided heart failure. It can exist in both sporadic and familial forms, most often with autosomal dominant inheritance. ARVD is typically diagnosed after puberty and before the age of 50 in patients who have symptoms ranging from palpitations to syncope to sudden cardiac death. The prevalence is estimated to be 1 in 5,000 in the United States, and ARVD is thought to account for as many as 5% of sudden deaths in young adults.

Diagnosis of ARVD requires documentation of 2 major criteria, 1 major and 2 minor criteria, or 4 minor criteria as specified by a task force on cardiomyopathies (recently modified with much ensuing controversy). Only 1 major criterion is MRI based: 1) regional right ventricular akinesia or dyskinesia *or* dyssynchronous right ventricular contraction *and* 2) a right ventricular ejection fraction less than 40% *or* a ratio of right ventricular end-diastolic volume to body surface area greater than or equal to 110 mL/m^2 for male patients or 100 mL/m^2 for female patients. Other major criteria are not imaging related: inverted T waves or epsilon waves in right precordial leads, nonsustained or sustained ventricular tachycardia of left bundle branch morphology, and ARVD confirmed in a first-degree relative.

An interesting feature of the task force criteria is that many of the classic MRI findings of ARVD are not mentioned. The presence of fat in the right ventricular free wall, probably the best example, was described in several early papers because it was found in nearly all patients who had ARVD and almost never in normal controls; subsequently, the search for fat became the holy grail of the ARVD protocol. However, 15% to 20% of normal adults have fatty infiltration of the right ventricular free wall, and the presence of right ventricular fat, real or imagined, has led to many false-positive diagnoses on MRI. Focal thinning of the right ventricular free wall is another feature often mentioned, but in practice, it is difficult to identify in any but the most severe cases. Since the normal right ventricular free wall is only 2 to 3 mm thick, visualization of focal thinning on axial or oblique images with a typical slice thickness of 5 to 8 mm is an optimistic proposition at best.

In our practice, we rely primarily on the following findings to suggest the diagnosis: right ventricular dilatation, decreased right ventricular function, and focal right ventricular dyskinesis, often with the small aneurysmal outpouchings seen in this case. Approximately 50% of ARVD patients show late enhancement of the right ventricular myocardium following gadolinium administration, usually associated with focal wall motion abnormalities. This finding is not specific to ARVD and can be seen in right ventricular infarcts, myocarditis, sarcoidosis, amyloidosis, and other cardiomyopathies.

It's important to remember that MRI alone can never confirm the diagnosis of ARVD. Additional clinical and physiologic data are required as specified by the task force criteria.

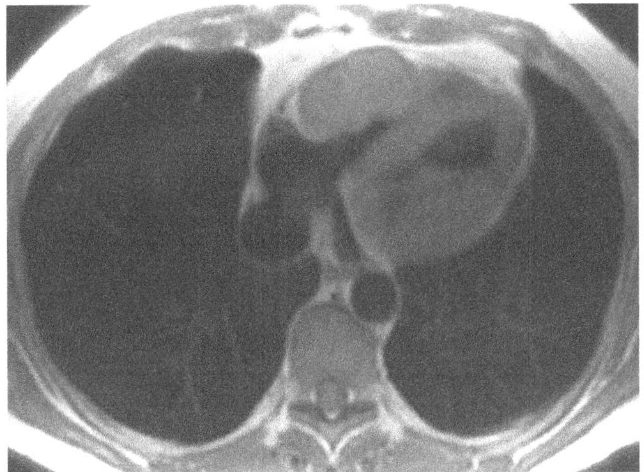

Figure 13.24.1

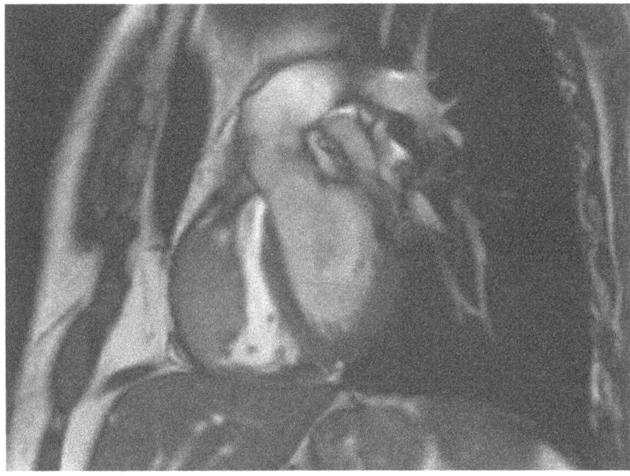

Figure 13.24.2

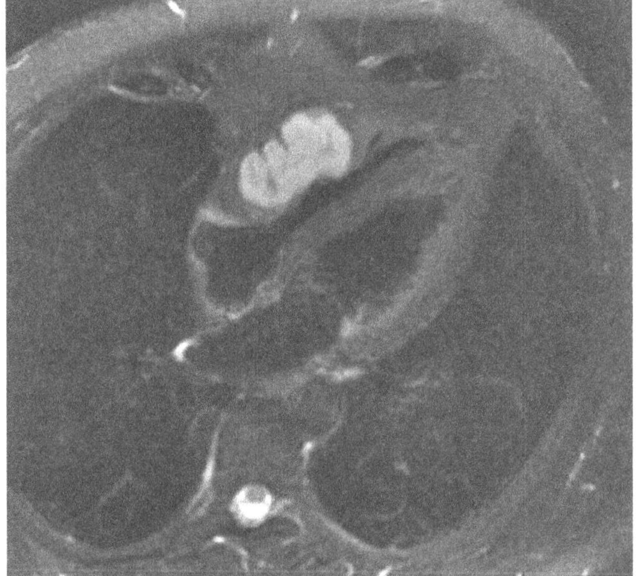

Figure 13.24.3

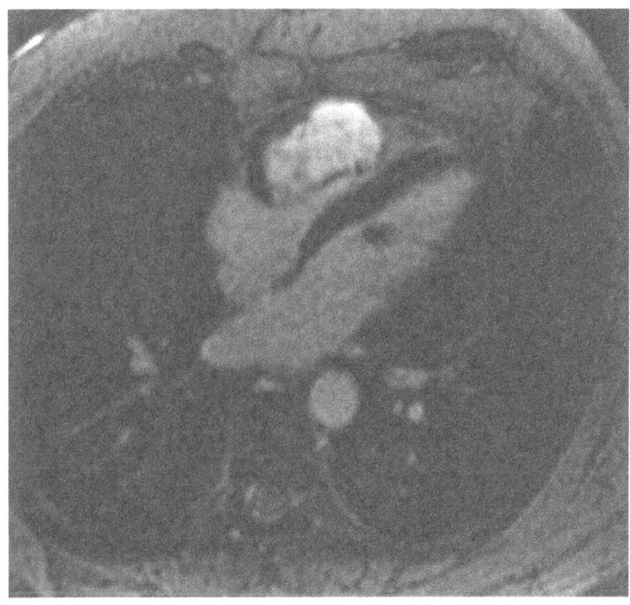

Figure 13.24.4

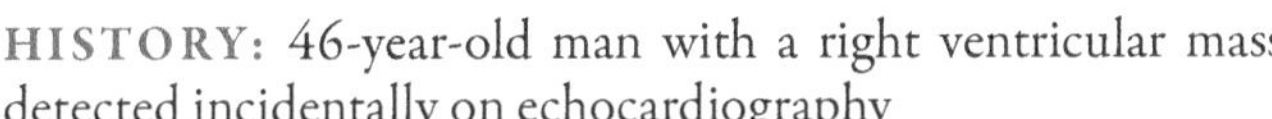

HISTORY: 46-year-old man with a right ventricular mass detected incidentally on echocardiography

IMAGING FINDINGS: A lobulated, well-defined mass in the right ventricular free wall demonstrates mild hyperintensity relative to myocardium on axial double inversion recovery proton density-weighted FSE (Figure 13.24.1) and short-axis SSFP (Figure 13.24.2) images. The lesion is markedly hyperintense on a horizontal long-axis T2-weighted triple inversion recovery FSE image (Figure 13.24.3) and shows contrast retention above the level of the blood pool on an 8-minute horizontal long-axis MDE image (Figure 13.24.4).

DIAGNOSIS: Hemangioma

COMMENT: Hemangiomas are rare cardiac tumors, accounting for 2% to 3% of all benign cardiac neoplasms. They are classified according to the size of their vascular channels as capillary, cavernous, and arteriovenous, with mixed tumors accounting for a large percentage of lesions. Hemangiomas can involve any cardiac chamber but seem to occur more commonly in the ventricles. They occur in all age groups without an obvious sex predilection.

These lesions are often asymptomatic; however, when large enough, they may cause symptoms related to outflow obstruction. Arrhythmias, pericardial effusion, congestive heart failure, thromboembolism, and sudden death have all been reported in association with hemangiomas.

Cardiac hemangiomas have characteristics on MRI similar to their appearance in other organs: sharply demarcated lesions with high and generally uniform signal intensity on T2-weighted images. Hemangiomas may be mildly hypointense to mildly hyperintense on T1-weighted or proton density-weighted double inversion recovery images. The other defining feature is rapid and persistent enhancement after gadolinium administration. Enhancement is visible on first-pass perfusion images and should persist at levels near the signal intensity of the blood pool on T1-weighted or delayed enhancement images. Nodular peripheral enhancement has been described in some lesions but is probably more difficult to discern in cardiac lesions than in hepatic hemangiomas.

Hemangiomas are benign tumors with no malignant potential. Symptomatic lesions are usually resected when possible; however, surgery for incidentally discovered lesions is controversial, and they are often left alone. Depending on the location of the lesion, the differential diagnosis may include angiosarcoma, myxoma, paraganglioma, and metastasis. Angiosarcomas appear most often in the right atrium and right ventricle and generally have a more aggressive, infiltrative, and heterogeneous appearance. Despite their name, enhancement is usually less intense than in hemangiomas. Myxomas may also have high T2-signal intensity, but generally they have much less prominent enhancement. Paragangliomas can have high T2-signal intensity and intense early enhancement; however, their classic location in the right atrioventricular groove is not typical of hemangiomas, and patients are usually symptomatic.

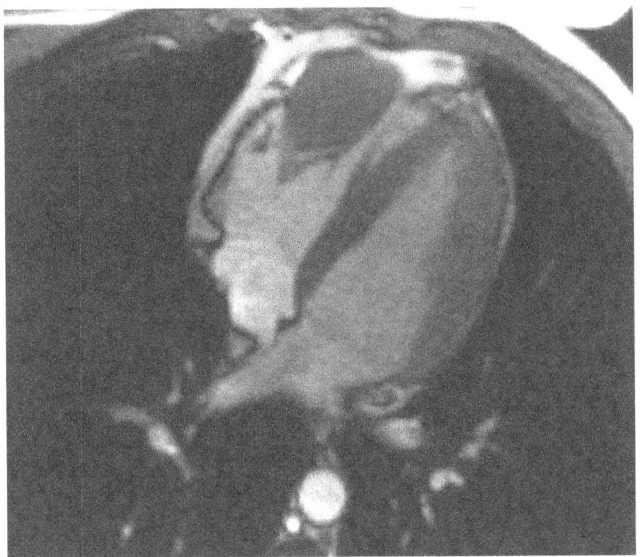

Figure 13.25.1

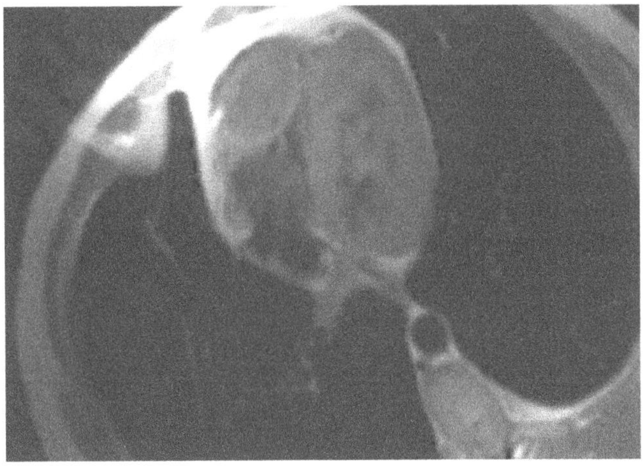

Figure 13.25.2

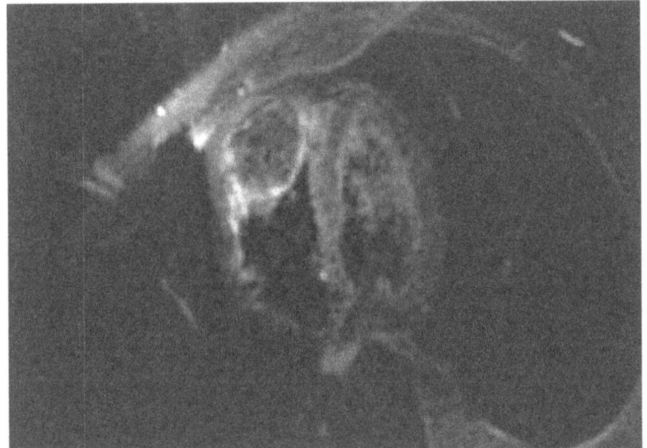

Figure 13.25.3

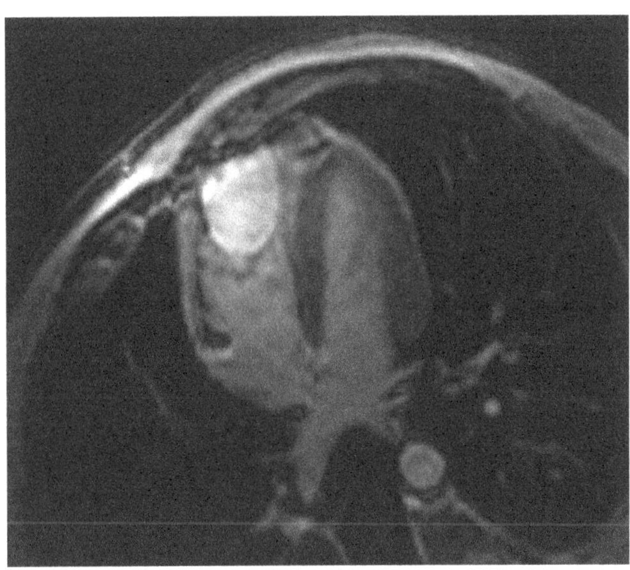

Figure 13.25.4

HISTORY: 27-year-old man with a 3-month history of chest pain and mild shortness of breath

IMAGING FINDINGS: Four-chamber SSFP image (Figure 13.25.1) demonstrates a large well-defined mass in the right ventricular free wall. Four-chamber double (Figure 13.25.2) and triple (Figure 13.25.3) inversion recovery FSE images with proton density- and T2-weighting reveal mildly decreased signal intensity relative to myocardium. Four-chamber MDE image (Figure 13.25.4) obtained approximately 15 minutes after gadolinium injection reveals intense uniform enhancement of the right ventricular mass.

DIAGNOSIS: Right ventricular fibroma

COMMENT: Primary cardiac neoplasms are uncommon, and as is true in many other organs, metastases are much more frequent, probably by a factor of 20 to 100. Cardiac fibromas are rare, but they are the most commonly resected tumor in the pediatric population (hamartomas have a higher incidence but do not have to be resected since they almost always regress with time). Most fibromas occur in children and adolescents, and most are located in the free wall of the left ventricle. This case is therefore atypical on at least 2 counts, but its appearance on MRI is so classic that it's worth including. Fibromas are benign neoplasms that are generally well-circumscribed solitary lesions composed of fibroblasts, collagen, and a fibromyxoid stroma. In children, fibromas are more cellular; in adults, fibromas tend to be nearly acellular and composed primarily of collagen. Calcification is a useful sign on CT and can be seen in 25% to 50% of fibromas. The presence of calcium, while not absolutely specific to fibromas, is uncommon in most other primary or metastatic tumors and therefore often helps to narrow the differential diagnosis. Definitive identification of focal calcification on MRI requires either luck or cheating; however, the constellation of uniform low signal intensity on T2-weighted triple inversion recovery images and intense enhancement on MDE images is even more suggestive of the diagnosis.

Most fibromas are resected if possible, not because of any potential for malignancy but because they may cause symptoms related to their location (in this case, near the RVOT) and because they are thought to induce significant arrhythmias in some patients.

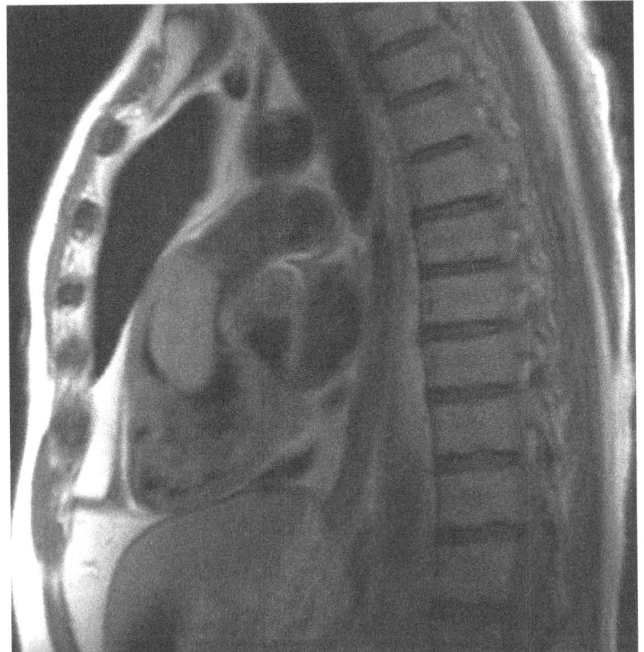

Figure 13.26.1

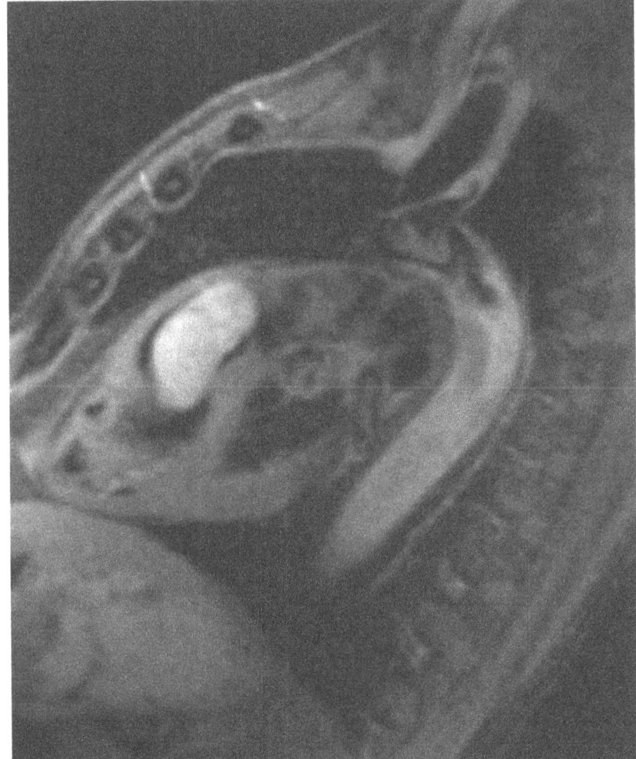

Figure 13.26.2

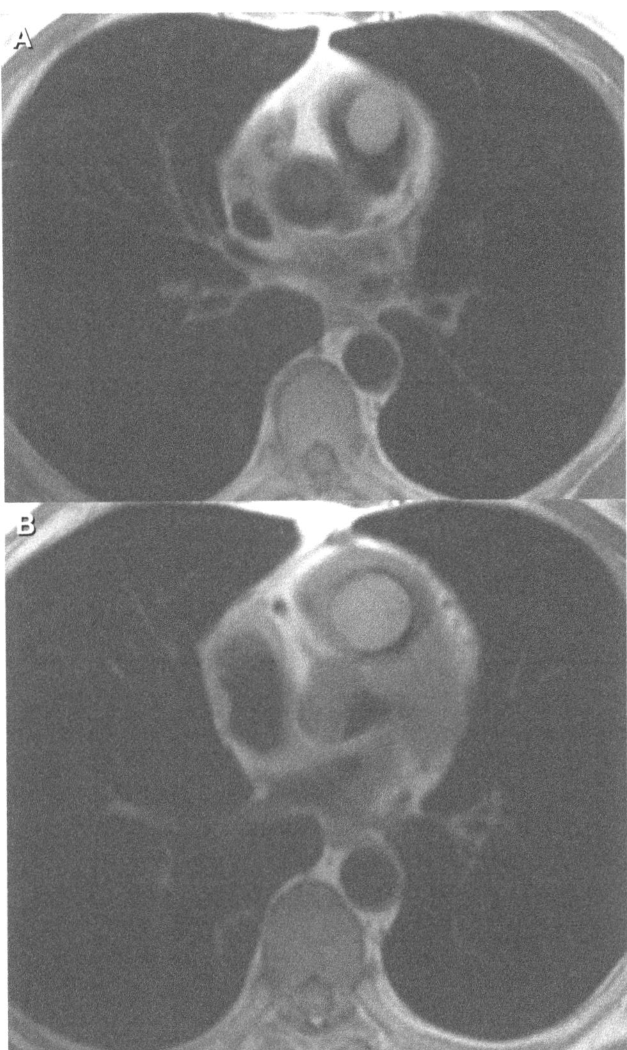

Figure 13.26.3

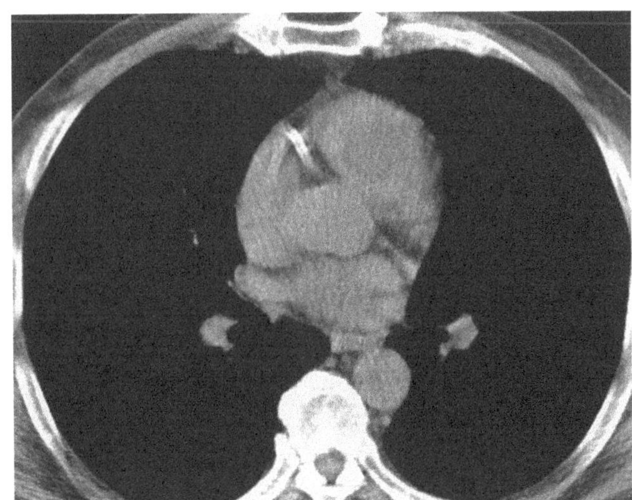

Figure 13.26.4

HISTORY: 62-year-old asymptomatic man with a heart murmur on physical examination; echocardiography revealed a cardiac mass, and MRI was requested for further characterization

IMAGING FINDINGS: Sagittal oblique black-blood double (Figure 13.26.1) and triple (Figure 13.26.2) inversion recovery FSE images through the RVOT demonstrate a well-circumscribed ovoid mass with markedly increased signal intensity on the T2-weighted triple inversion recovery image. Axial proton density-weighted double inversion recovery images (Figure 13.26.3) again reveal a round mass projecting into the RVOT. Axial image from low-dose noncontrast chest CT (Figure 13.26.4) performed for pulmonary nodule surveillance also demonstrates the mildly hypointense mass outlined by the blood pool in the RVOT.

DIAGNOSIS: RVOT myxoma

COMMENT: The major project of 1 of our fellow residents was collecting egregious misses of staff radiologists. He had no trouble finding examples and had assembled a collection that was quite substantial by the time he graduated. This case is a good illustration of 3 principles about radiologists: 1) The only radiologists who don't regularly make significant mistakes are those who are retired or dead. 2) When a finding has been missed, it is much more likely to be missed again on a follow-up examination. 3) Most radiologists don't like to look at the heart.

In this case, the patient had a noncalcified pulmonary nodule and participated in a Mayo Clinic longitudinal study that necessitated low-dose chest CT at regular intervals. His various CTs were read at one time or another by nearly all of our chest radiologists, none of whom reported the round mass in his RVOT. His primary care physician detected a murmur on a routine physical examination, which led to an echocardiogram and then to an MRI for further characterization of the mass.

Myxomas are the most common primary cardiac neoplasm, with an incidence of approximately 0.5 per million per year, and account for more than half of benign cardiac tumors. Approximately 75% are located in the left atrium, usually attached to the atrial septum in the region of the fossa ovalis, and most of the remaining tumors are in the right atrium; however, approximately 5% occur in the ventricles, as in this case. Multiple myxomas may occur in patients with Carney syndrome (which consists of myxomas of the heart and skin, hyperpigmented skin lesions, and endocrine hyperactivity and is different from Carney triad). Myxomas are thought to develop from primitive endothelial or subendocardial cells, and they consist of uniform polygonal cells lying in a myxomatous stroma rich in mucopolysaccharides.

The clinical presentation and symptoms depend on the location and size of the tumor. Patients with left atrial myxomas may present with dyspnea on exertion, orthopnea, or pulmonary edema resulting from obstruction at the level of the mitral valve and left-sided heart failure. Symptoms may change depending on position, and systemic embolization may occur in 20% of patients. Patients with a rare myxoma in the RVOT may have signs of right-sided heart failure, including peripheral edema, ascites, and shortness of breath.

Myxomas typically show high signal intensity on T2-weighted images. In cardiac MRI, these are usually obtained with ECG-gated fast-spin echo sequences with 2 pulses to null the signal from blood and an optional third inversion pulse for fat suppression (chemical fat suppression also works). Myxomas may show mild enhancement after gadolinium administration, but some lesions have only minimal enhancement. Since thrombus is the main differential diagnosis, particularly for an atrial lesion, a minimally enhancing myxoma must be distinguished from a nonenhancing thrombus. Another helpful clue is that a thrombus rarely has high T2-signal intensity.

Most myxomas are benign; however, a few reports describe malignant degeneration. Even if all lesions were benign, the treatment would remain surgical because they have a high potential for thrombogenesis and embolization.

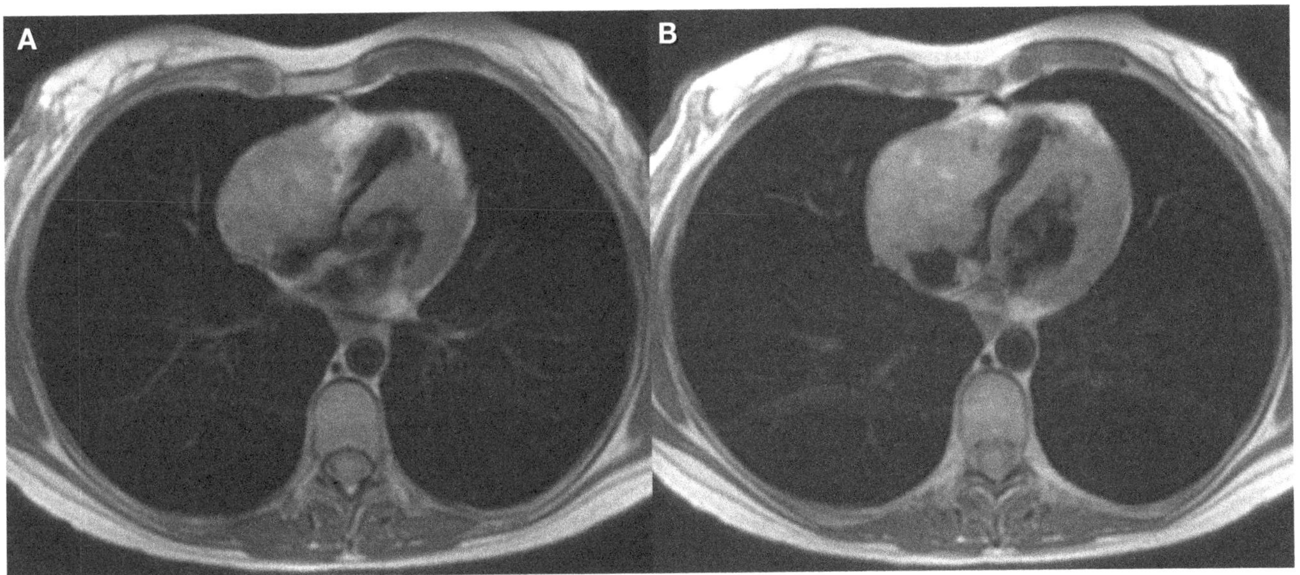

Figure 13.27.1

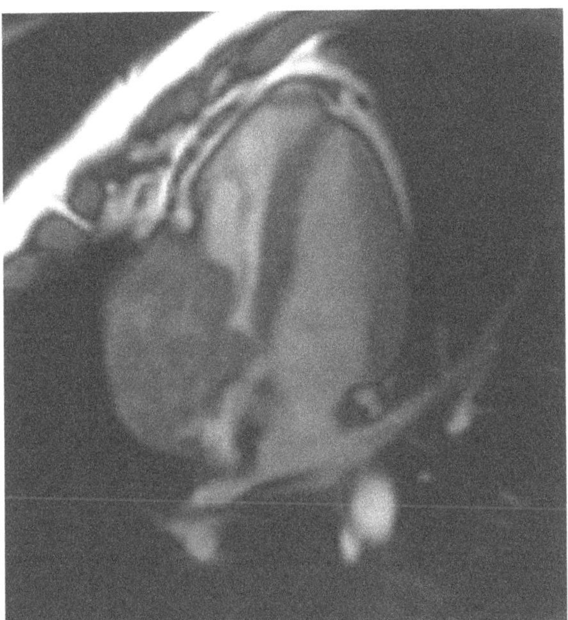

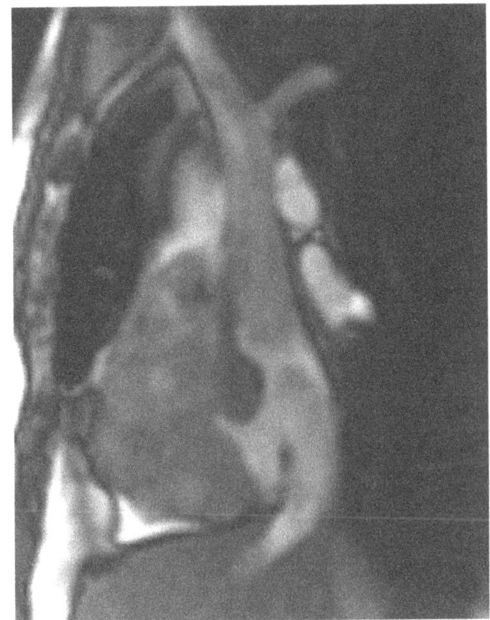

Figure 13.27.2

Figure 13.27.3

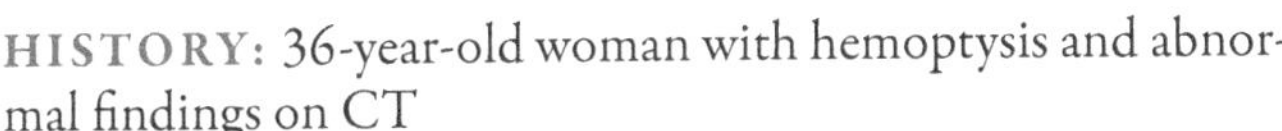

HISTORY: 36-year-old woman with hemoptysis and abnormal findings on CT

IMAGING FINDINGS: Axial proton density-weighted double inversion recovery FSE images (Figure 13.27.1) demonstrate a heterogeneous mass infiltrating the right atrium, the right atrioventricular groove, and the base of the right ventricle. Horizontal long-axis (Figure 13.27.2) and short-axis (Figure 13.27.3) SSFP images also show the heterogeneous nature of the lesion and its extension into the right atrial cavity.

DIAGNOSIS: Angiosarcoma

COMMENT: Angiosarcoma is the most common malignant primary cardiac tumor, which of course means that it's very rare and occurs much less frequently than metastatic disease involving the heart. Lesions are composed of irregular vascular channels lined by anaplastic epithelial cells with intermixed regions of necrosis and hemorrhage.

Angiosarcomas are more common in men and have a peak incidence in the third to fifth decades. The right atrium is the site of origin in 75% of cases, but lesions have been reported in all chambers and the pericardium. Patients may present with symptoms related to right-sided heart failure; obstruction of the superior vena cava, inferior vena cava, or tricuspid

thmias or pericardial effusion with tamponade; embolism (ie, bland or tumor thrombus).

omas are usually highly aggressive tumors, and % of patients have metastatic disease at presenta- Complete surgical resection is the treatment of choice ut is rarely possible, and even in this patient population the median survival is generally less than 1 year.

Angiosarcomas appear as heterogeneous infiltrative masses centered in the right atrium and often extend across the atrioventricular groove along the free wall of the right ventricle. Many residents expect angiosarcomas (because of their name) to show intense early enhancement and will sometimes exclude the diagnosis if early enhancement is not apparent (usually while exhibiting the unfortunate tendency to discuss a case by first mentioning all the lesions they have excluded from the differential diagnosis). Angiosarcomas typically have mild to moderate heterogeneous enhancement in contrast to lesions such as paragangliomas, hemangiomas, and hypervascular metastases that do have intense early enhancement. Scattered regions of necrosis are a frequent finding and appear as regions of high T2-signal intensity and hypoenhancement.

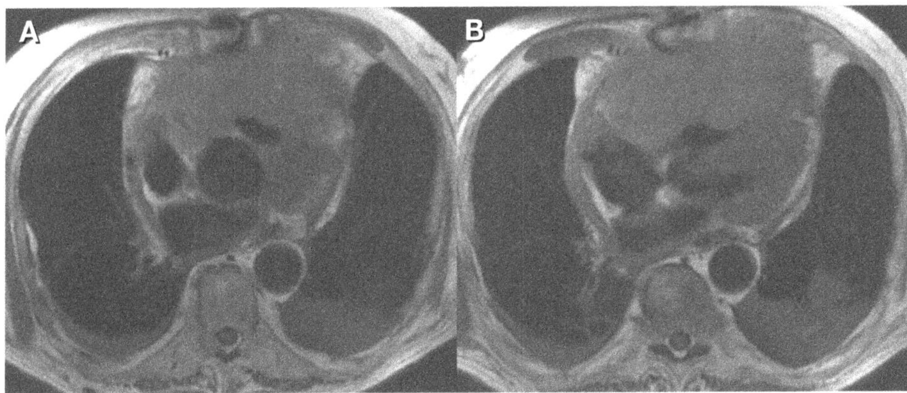

Figure 13.28.1

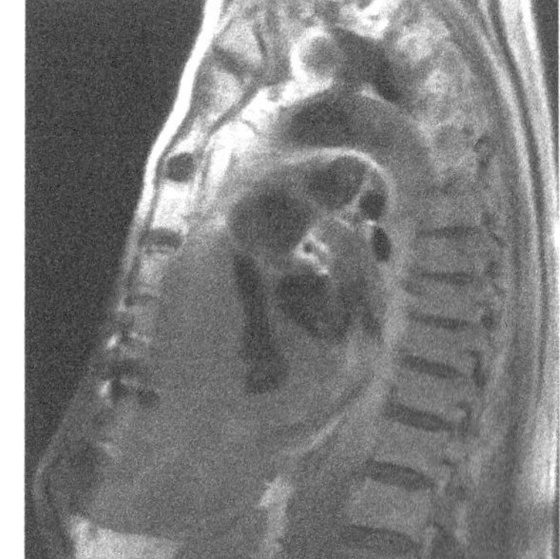

Figure 13.28.2

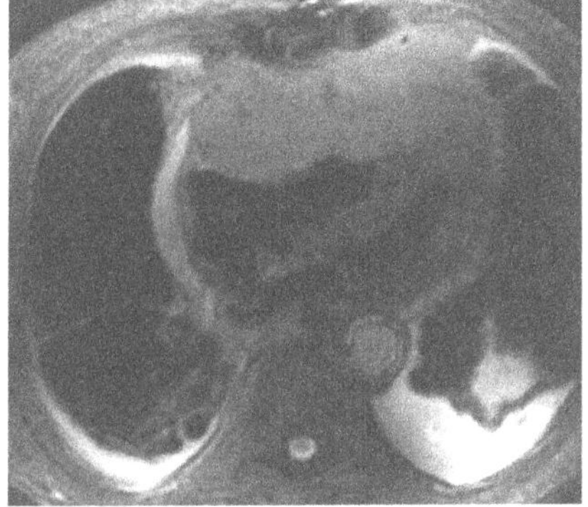

Figure 13.28.3

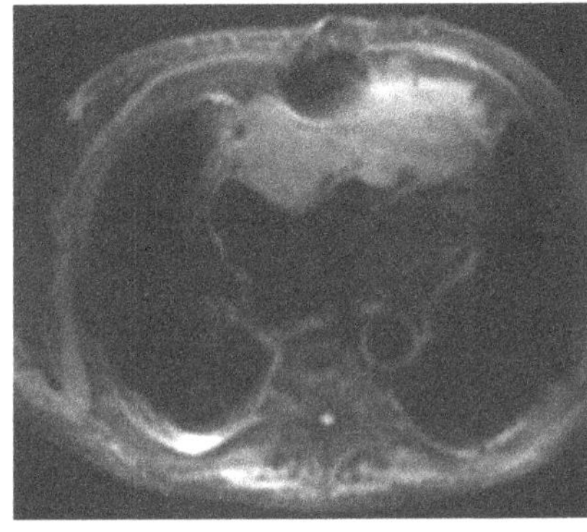

Figure 13.28.4

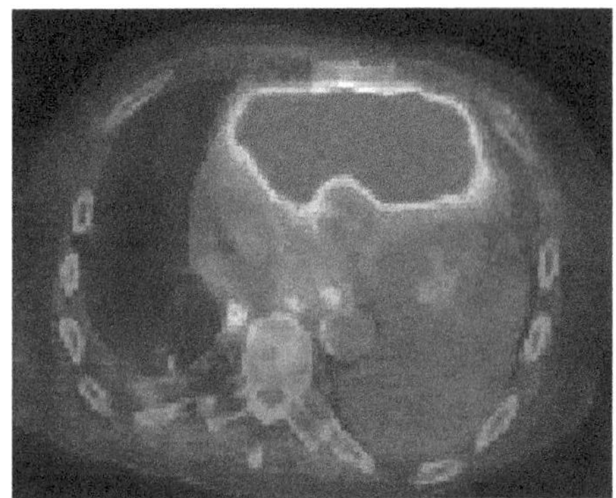

Figure 13.28.5

HISTORY: 73-year-old man with nausea and epigastric pain; echocardiography showed a large mass in the epicardial space

IMAGING FINDINGS: Axial (Figure 13.28.1) and sagittal (Figure 13.28.2) double inversion recovery proton density-weighted FSE images reveal an infiltrative, fairly homogeneous mass involving the pericardium and right ventricular free wall and extending inferiorly to the diaphragm. Note thickening of the pericardium overlying the posterior right and left atria. The mass shows mildly increased signal intensity relative to myocardium on an axial T2-weighted triple inversion recovery FSE image (Figure 13.28.3) and markedly increased signal intensity on a low b-value diffusion-weighted image (b=100 s/mm^2) (Figure 13.28.4). Bilateral pleural effusions are also present. Fusion image from a PET-CT scan (Figure 13.28.5) shows hypermetabolism that corresponds to the mass.

DIAGNOSIS: Cardiac lymphoma

COMMENT: This case is an example of primary cardiac lymphoma. Initial criteria for the diagnosis specified that no extracardiac involvement could be present; however, this definition has been extended to include patients who have extracardiac disease that is less prominent than their cardiac disease (in this patient, a few mediastinal lymph nodes were involved).

Primary cardiac lymphoma is a rare entity, with fewer than 100 reported cases. It is thought to account for approximately 2% of all primary cardiac tumors and less than 1% of extranodal lymphomas. Secondary cardiac involvement in patients with systemic lymphoma is more common; it is present at autopsy in approximately 10% of patients who died from lymphoma, although cardiac imaging is rarely performed in this patient population. Cardiac lymphoma is generally a B-cell lymphoma of the large cell type; a few reports describe T-cell lymphoma in immunocompromised patients.

The right atrium and right ventricle are the most commonly involved cardiac chambers, and the presenting symptoms, while nonspecific, are often related to the site of involvement.

As is true of most cardiac masses, the appearance of lymphoma on MRI is nonspecific, and the diagnosis can rarely be made with absolute confidence, although if a patient has systemic lymphoma and a homogeneous infiltrative cardiac mass, lymphoma should certainly be at the top of the list. Lymphoma tends to have a more homogeneous appearance sarcoma, another lesion that favors the right ght ventricle, and is less likely to have regions . Enhancement following gadolinium adminis- is generally less in lymphomas than in normal myo- ium, another feature that distinguishes lymphoma from angiosarcoma but not from some cardiac metastases. The high signal intensity on the low b-value diffusion-weighted image is probably a reflection of both T2 and diffusion effects. DWI is a somewhat tricky technique in the heart, but when it is performed successfully, it can be useful in detecting subtle masses.

The prognosis for patients with primary or secondary cardiac lymphoma is poor, although a few patients have achieved long-term survival.

CASE 13.29

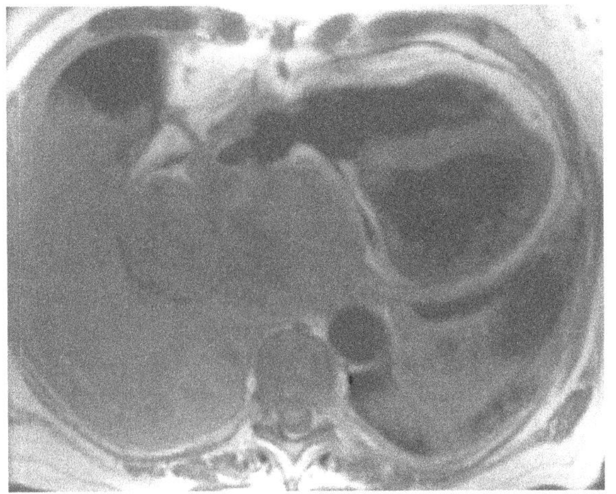

Figure 13.29.1

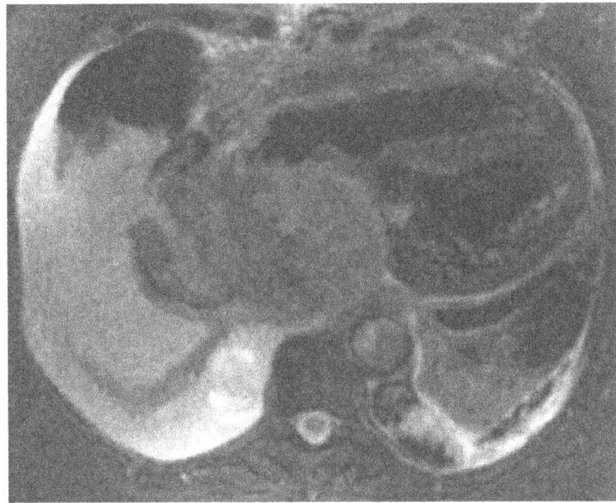

Figure 13.29.2

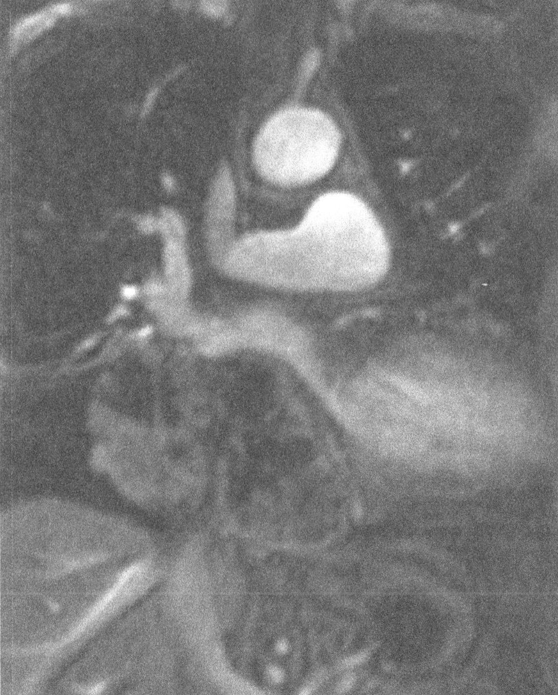

Figure 13.29.3

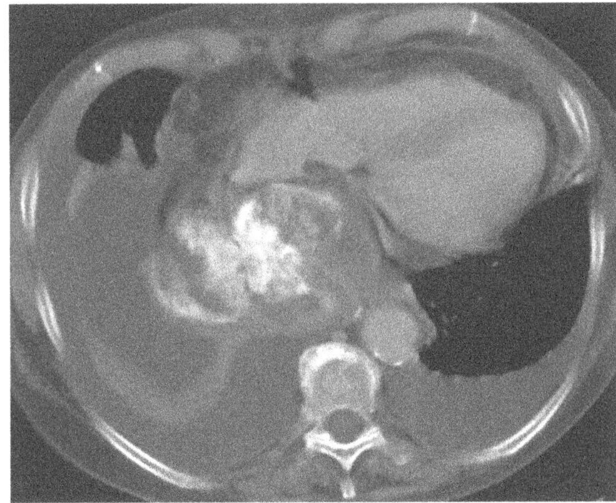

Figure 13.29.4

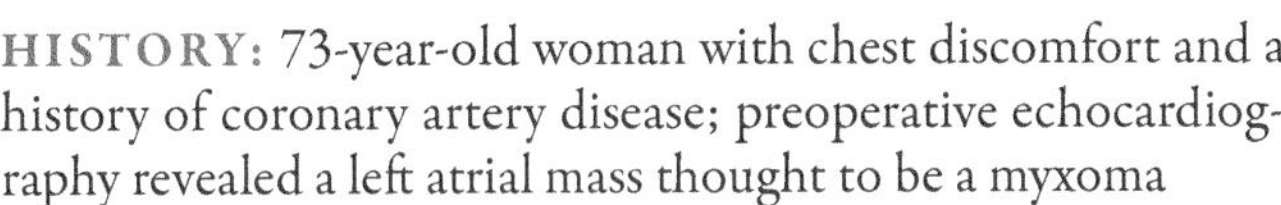

HISTORY: 73-year-old woman with chest discomfort and a history of coronary artery disease; preoperative echocardiography revealed a left atrial mass thought to be a myxoma

IMAGING FINDINGS: Axial double (Figure 13.29.1) and triple (Figure 13.29.2) inversion recovery FSE images with proton density- and T2-weighting reveal a large mass with very low T2-signal intensity occupying the entire left atrium, a prominent right pleural effusion, and right base atelectasis. Coronal postgadolinium 3D SPGR image (Figure 13.29.3) demonstrates heterogeneous enhancement of the mass. Axial contrast-enhanced CT image (Figure 13.29.4) shows extensive irregular calcification in the center of the left atrial mass.

DIAGNOSIS: Primary osteogenic sarcoma of the left atrium

COMMENT: Malignant tumors constitute approximately 10% of all primary cardiac neoplasms, and osteosarcoma is one of the more uncommon varieties, accounting for 3% to 9% of cardiac sarcomas. Approximately 40 cases have been reported; most of them arose in the left atrium and were accompanied by signs and symptoms of left-sided heart failure. Osteosarcomas have been reported in all cardiac chambers; however, right-sided tumors are more likely to be metastatic than primary lesions.

Primary cardiac osteosarcomas are generally aggressive lesions that carry a poor prognosis similar to other cardiac sarcomas; however, a few patients have had successful resection and long-term survival.

Because of their predominant left atrial location, the main differential diagnosis is often myxoma, as in this case. Distinguishing features of osteosarcomas include an origin distinct from the atrial septum, a broad base of attachment, relatively low signal intensity on T2-weighted images, and extension into pulmonary veins or invasion into atrial walls. The presence of calcification within cardiac osteosarcomas is variable, but extensive calcification (as seen in this case) can suggest the diagnosis and is definitely a feature that CT is much better suited to detect. On the basis of MRI alone, it's very difficult to be definitive about the presence of calcification (or even to suggest that it might be present).

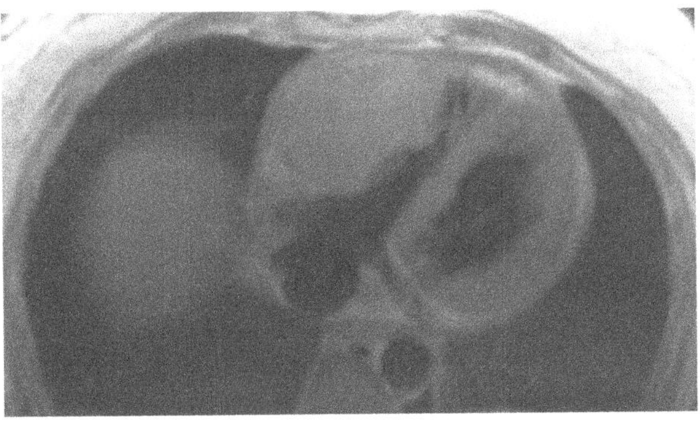

Figure 13.30.1

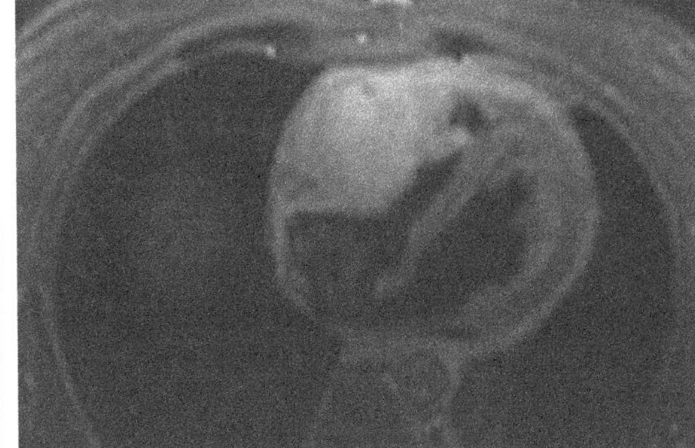

Figure 13.30.2

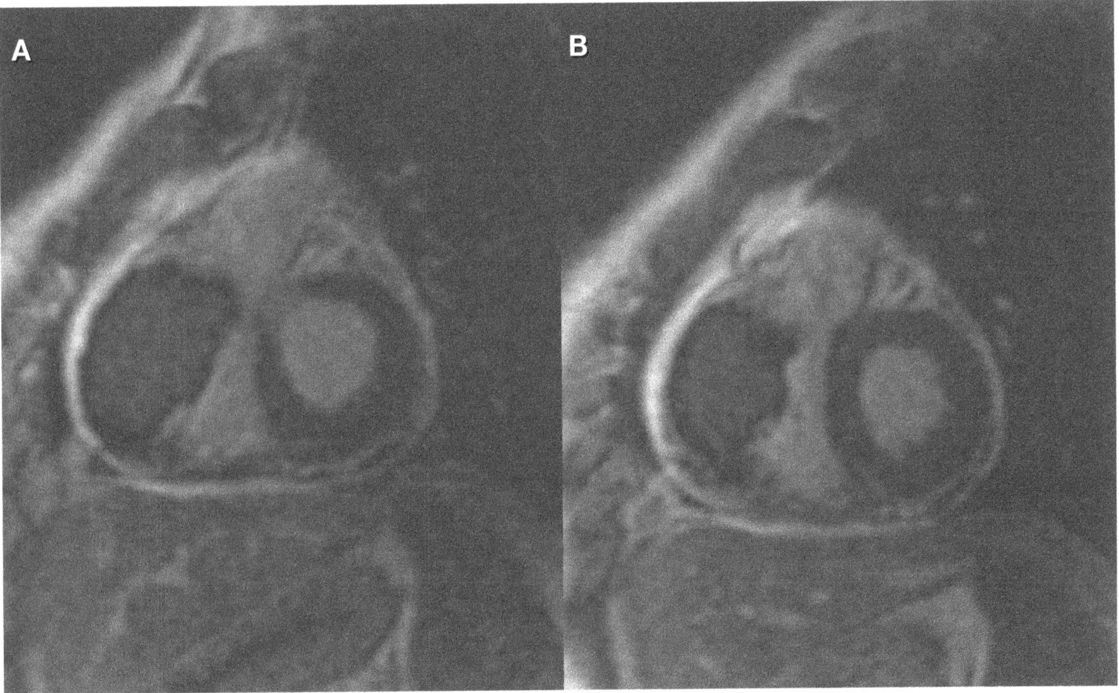

Figure 13.30.3

HISTORY: 46-year-old woman receiving chemotherapy and radiotherapy for cervical carcinoma diagnosed 6 months ago; she now has new-onset chest pain

IMAGING FINDINGS: Axial double (Figure 13.30.1) and triple (Figure 13.30.2) inversion recovery FSE images with proton density- and T2-weighting demonstrate a poorly defined mass involving the anterior wall of the right atrium and free wall of the right ventricle. Short-axis contrast-enhanced LGE images (Figure 13.30.3) reveal minimal enhancement of the mass. Note diffuse enhancement of the pericardium, likely reactive.

DIAGNOSIS: Cardiac metastasis from cervical carcinoma

COMMENT: Cardiac metastases are 20 to 100 times more common than primary cardiac neoplasms, depending on whose autopsy study you read; however, most cardiac metastases are not detected or imaged before death, whereas primary cardiac tumors often elicit great interest and are frequently evaluated with multiple imaging modalities. Nevertheless, it is important to remember these statistics and to appreciate that even when the diagnosis is less clinically obvious than in this case, the possibility of metastasis should be strongly considered.

Cervical carcinoma is the third most common gynecologic malignancy in the United States. When the tumor is confined to the uterus, patients have an excellent prognosis, with 5-year survival rates exceeding 80%; however, metastatic disease is a poor prognostic sign, and survival for patients with cardiac metastases is generally measured in weeks or months.

Approximately 20 cases of metastatic cervical carcinoma to the heart have been reported. The interval between the initial diagnosis of cervical cancer and the identification of cardiac metastasis ranged from a few days to 43 months. Several different treatments were described; however, most patients died within a few months.

Autopsy studies have demonstrated the presence of cardiac metastases in 10% to 15% of patients with metastatic malignancy. The neoplasms most often associated with cardiac metastases include melanoma (48% of metastases), lung cancer, lymphoma, and breast cancer. The incidence of cardiac metastasis from cervical carcinoma has been reported as ranging from 1% to 7%. The most common sites for cardiac metastases are the epicardium and pericardium, although any site or cardiac chamber may be involved. The right side of the heart is more frequently involved, probably because of direct seeding from venous and lymphatic microemboli.

The appearance of cardiac metastases on MRI is highly variable. Pericardial metastases may take the form of nodular thickening and effusion, while myocardial metastases may be well-defined discrete lesions or have a more infiltrative appearance, as seen in this case. The differential diagnosis for an infiltrative lesion involving the right atrium and ventricle would include angiosarcoma, which usually has more prominent enhancement, and lymphoma. The right atrioventricular groove is a classic site for metastatic melanoma lesions; however, they are generally hypervascular and show intense early enhancement.

ABBREVIATIONS

ADC	apparent diffusion coefficient
AICD	automatic implantable cardioverter-defibrillator
ARVD	arrhythmogenic right ventricular dysplasia
AVM	arteriovenous malformation
CABG	coronary artery bypass graft
CT	computed tomography
CTA	computed tomographic angiography
DWI	diffusion-weighted imaging
ECG	electrocardiography
FDG	fluorodeoxyglucose F18
FRFSE	fast-recovery fast-spin echo
FSE	fast-spin echo
HCM	hypertrophic cardiomyopathy
HHT	hereditary hemorrhagic telangiectasia
LGE	late gadolinium enhancement
LHIAS	lipomatous hypertrophy of the interatrial septum
LVOT	left ventricular outflow tract
MDE	myocardial delayed enhancement
MRA	magnetic resonance angiography
MRI	magnetic resonance imaging
PET	positron emission tomography
PIOPED III	Prospective Investigation of Pulmonary Embolism Diagnosis III
PNET	primitive neuroectodermal tumor
RVOT	right ventricular outflow tract
SPGR	spoiled gradient recalled
SSFSE	single-shot fast-spin echo
SSFP	steady-state free precession
TE	echo time
3D	3-dimensional
TI	inversion time
TR	repetition time
2D	2-dimensional
US	ultrasonography
VENC	velocity-encoding
VR	volume-rendered

14.

MUSCULOSKELETAL SYSTEM

CASE 14.1

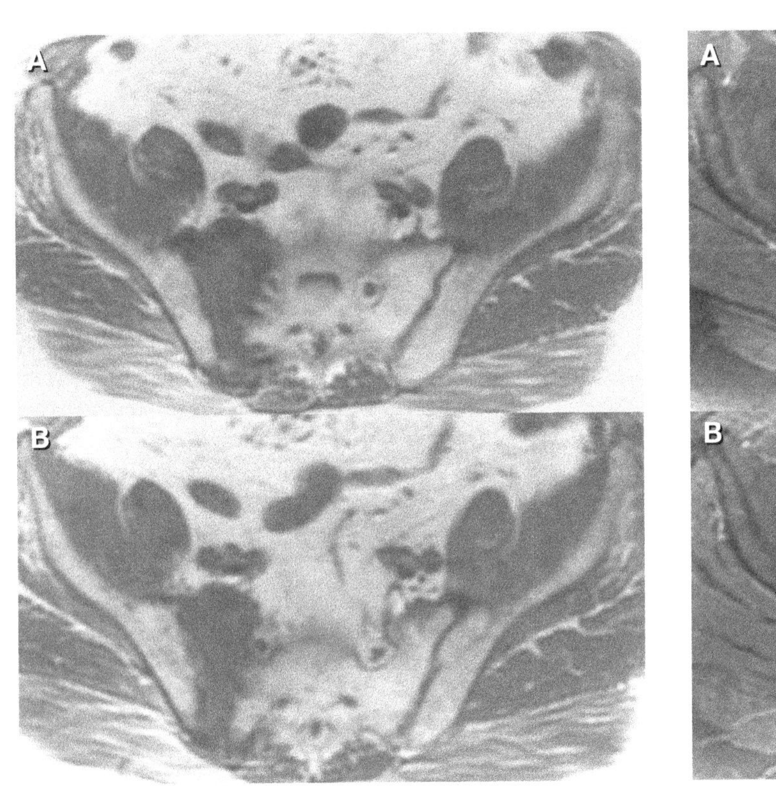

Figure 14.1.1

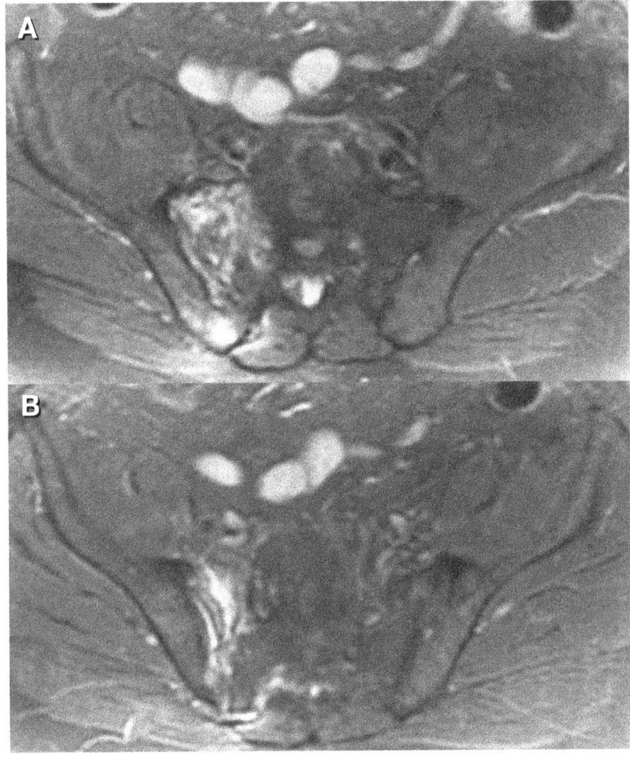

Figure 14.1.3

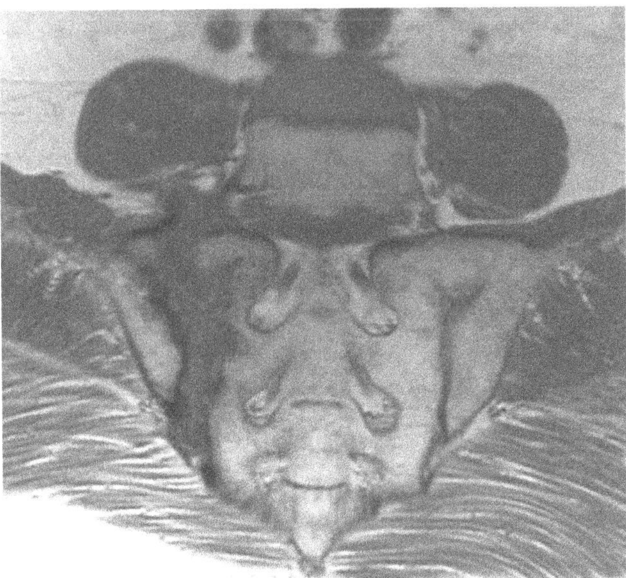

Figure 14.1.2

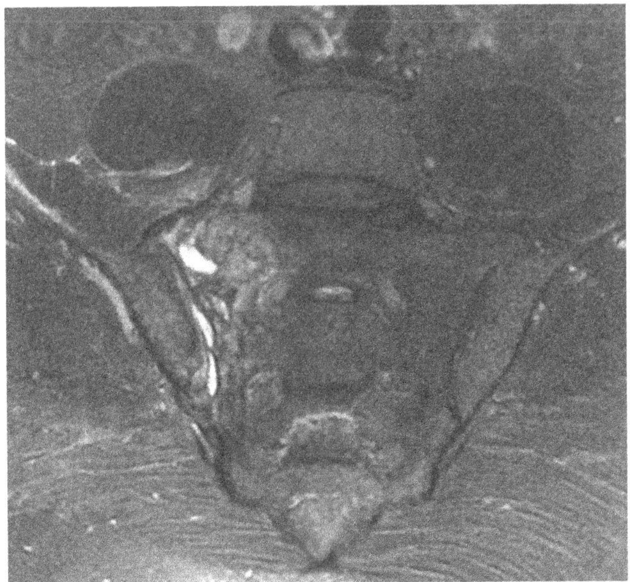

Figure 14.1.4

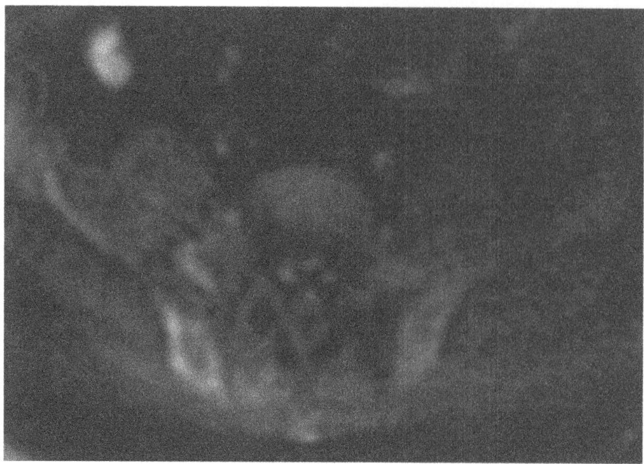

Figure 14.1.5

HISTORY: 72-year-old man with a history of prostate cancer and new posterior right buttock pain

IMAGING FINDINGS: Axial (Figure 14.1.1) and coronal oblique (Figure 14.1.2) T1-weighted images and axial (Figure 14.1.3) and coronal oblique (Figure 14.1.4) fat-suppressed T2-weighted FSE images demonstrate a linear defect in the right side of the sacrum with low signal intensity on T1-weighted images and mildly increased T2-signal intensity. Axial diffusion-weighted image (b=800 s/mm^2) (Figure 14.1.5) reveals only minimally increased signal intensity.

DIAGNOSIS: Sacral insufficiency fracture

COMMENT: This is not a particularly subtle case; however, sacral insufficiency fractures can be important incidental findings in abdominopelvic examinations performed by body imagers and are easily overlooked by those of us who rapidly glance at the bones and muscles on our way to an evaluation of the truly important anatomy.

Sacral stress fractures are an uncommon cause of low back pain, but they are seen fairly regularly in our practice because of the nearly universal presence of this symptom in persons older than 40 years. Sacral stress fractures have been classified into fatigue fractures and insufficiency fractures. The distinction is that fatigue fractures occur in normal bone exposed to abnormal or repetitive stresses (eg, long-distance runners), and insufficiency fractures occur in abnormal bones exposed to normal stresses. Risk factors for insufficiency fractures include osteoporosis, rheumatoid arthritis, prolonged corticosteroid therapy, pelvic radiotherapy, fibrous dysplasia, Paget disease, and osteomalacia. Most pelvic insufficiency fractures occur in elderly osteoporotic women.

The clinical presentation is variable and nonspecific. Patients usually complain of intractable low back or pelvic pain associated with reduced mobility and occasionally radiation to the leg.

Sacral fractures have been classified into 3 zones according to their location. Zone 1 fractures occur in the most lateral portion of the sacrum and include most insufficiency fractures. These injuries seldom involve the exiting nerves and are usually not associated with neurologic symptoms. Zone 2 fractures involve the sacral foramina, and zone 3 fractures involve the sacral canal. Fractures in zone 2 or 3 are generally accompanied by nerve injuries, which are unilateral in zone 2 fractures and often bilateral in zone 3 fractures. As with traumatic pelvic fractures, several authors have reported a high incidence of coexisting pubic rami fractures in patients with sacral stress fractures.

The appearance of sacral insufficiency fractures on MRI is usually fairly straightforward. They tend to be vertically oriented, with linear regions of low T1-signal intensity and high T2-signal intensity extending through the sacral ala. Occasionally in early or mild injuries, a fracture line cannot definitely be identified, but the diagnosis may be suggested in the absence of an obvious mass on diffusion-weighted or postgadolinium images. If you or your technologist routinely checks images before discharging the patient (once a universal policy in our practice, but now discouraged because of a belief that this reduces patient throughput), a supplementary T1- or T2-weighted acquisition in a coronal oblique orientation along the sacrum prescribed from a sagittal view can be very helpful in demonstrating the linear nature of the lesion.

The major differential diagnosis is often metastatic disease. The patient in this case had prostate cancer, prior radiotherapy (notice the lack of red marrow on the T1-weighted images), and mildly elevated levels of prostate-specific antigen. Visualization of a linear defect in the lateral sacrum without a focal mass and without significant abnormality on the diffusion-weighted images confirms the diagnosis of sacral insufficiency fracture.

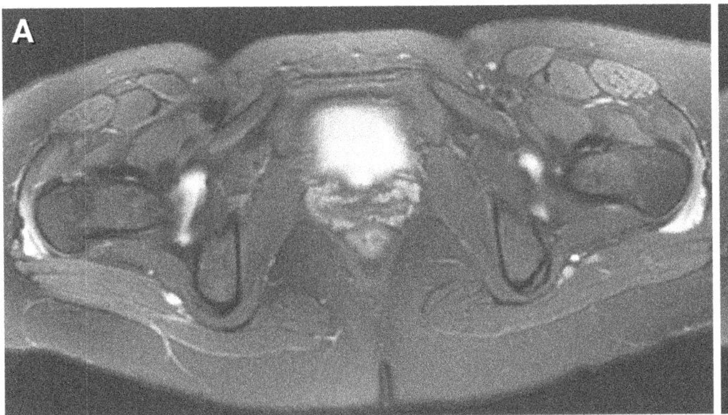

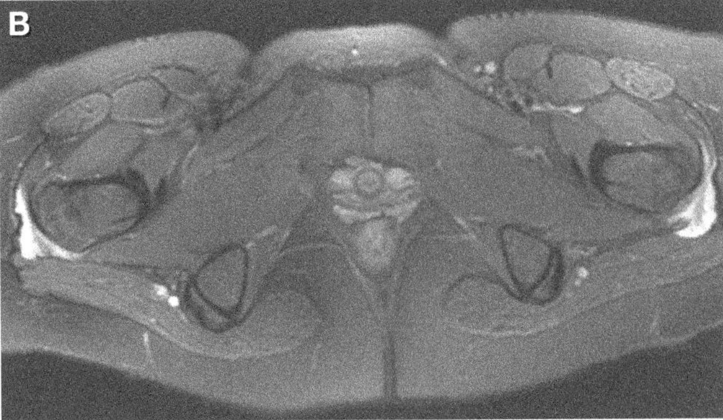

Figure 14.2.1

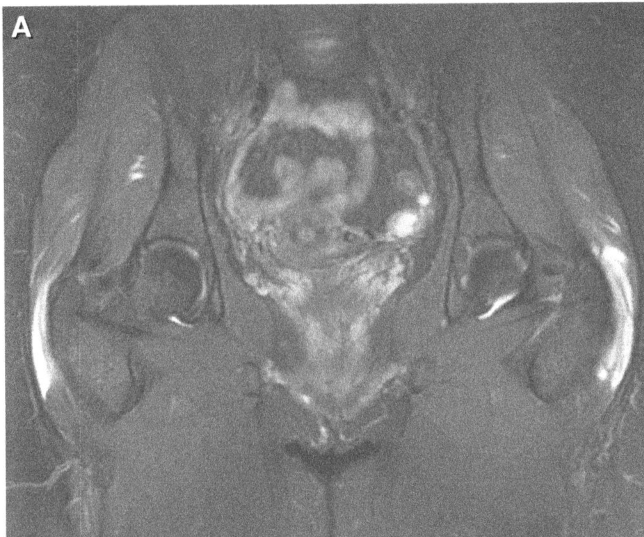

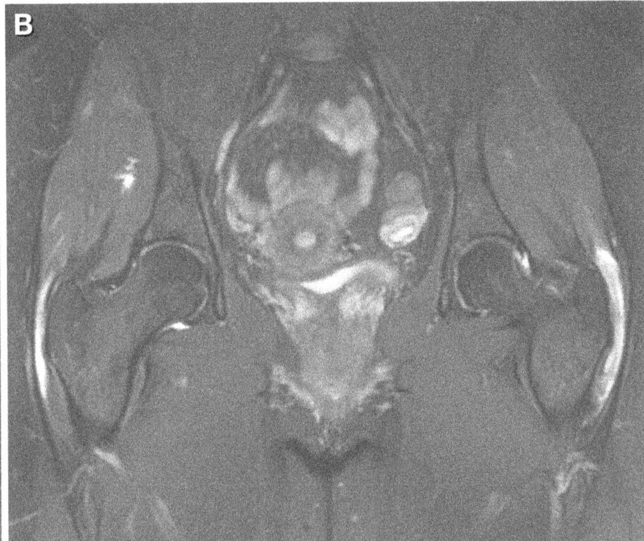

Figure 14.2.2

HISTORY: 42-year-old woman with bilateral hip pain

IMAGING FINDINGS: Axial (Figure 14.2.1) and coronal (Figure 14.2.2) fat-suppressed FSE T2-weighted images reveal crescentic fluid collections adjacent to the greater trochanters bilaterally.

DIAGNOSIS: Trochanteric bursitis

COMMENT: Greater trochanteric pain syndrome is a clinical diagnosis made in the setting of lateral hip pain exacerbated by movement of the leg or lying on the affected hip, with associated tenderness on palpation of the greater trochanter. *Trochanteric bursitis* is often used interchangeably in describing this syndrome, although there is much controversy regarding the significance of the traditional imaging findings associated with bursitis (ie, fluid-filled bursa or peribursal edema).

Bursal inflammation or injury has been invoked as the explanation for the symptomatology of trochanteric pain syndrome. More recently, impingement of the iliotibial band on the greater trochanter has been proposed as a cause of trochanteric bursitis (along with a corresponding corrective arthroscopic procedure).

None of these explanations are supported by the literature. One paper, for example, stated that only 40% of patients with greater trochanteric pain syndrome actually had bursal fluid collections. Many authors have reported that gluteus medius and gluteus minimus muscle tears or tendinopathy are more strongly associated with greater trochanteric pain syndrome (the gluteus medius tendon attaches to the superior posterior and lateral facets, and the gluteus minimus tendon inserts on the anterior facet of the greater trochanter). Peritrochanteric fluid or increased T2-signal intensity is a very common finding, particularly in older patients—1 investigation reported a prevalence of 88% for patients referred for hip MRI but without greater trochanteric pain syndrome.

All of this is interesting and perhaps an inevitable consequence of our tendency to image anyone for nearly any indication, but it does raise the question of what to say about the incidental finding of trochanteric fluid on a pelvic MRI performed for another reason. Our recommendation is to downplay (or ignore) the presence of minimal fluid or edema, particularly if it is bilateral and symmetrical in an older patient. Larger amounts of fluid (as in this case) should merit discussion and perhaps prompt the clinician to evaluate the hips more closely. It is also worth examining the gluteal muscles and tendons for signs of tears or tendinopathy (if you can find them).

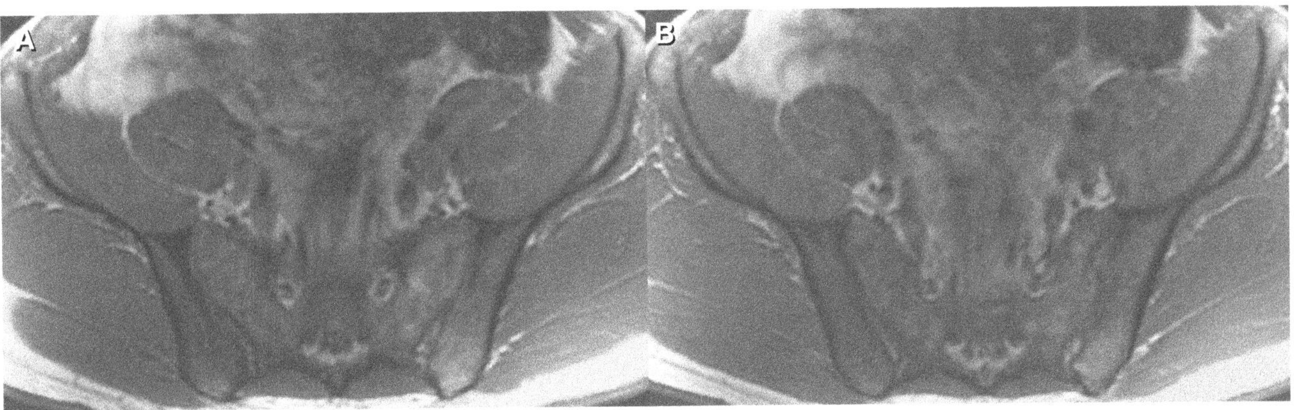

Figure 14.3.1

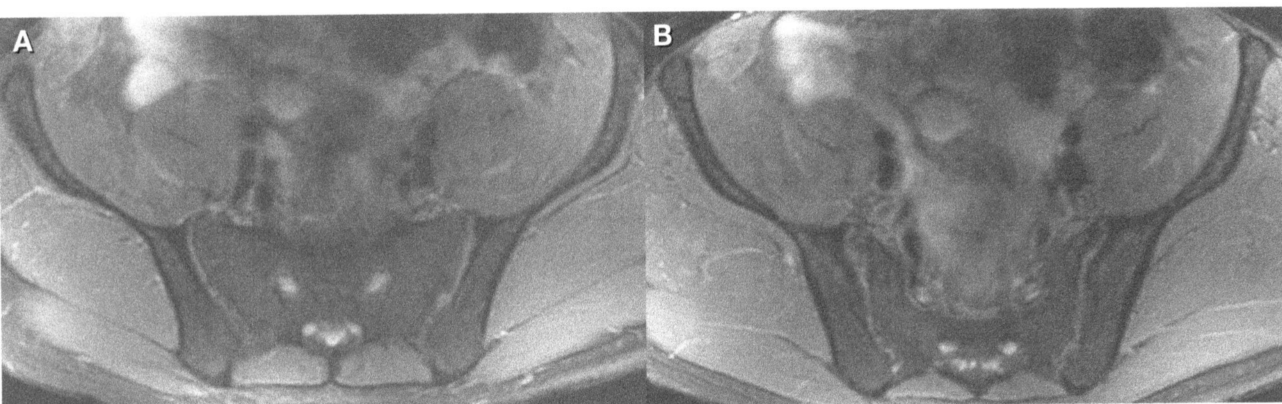

Figure 14.3.2

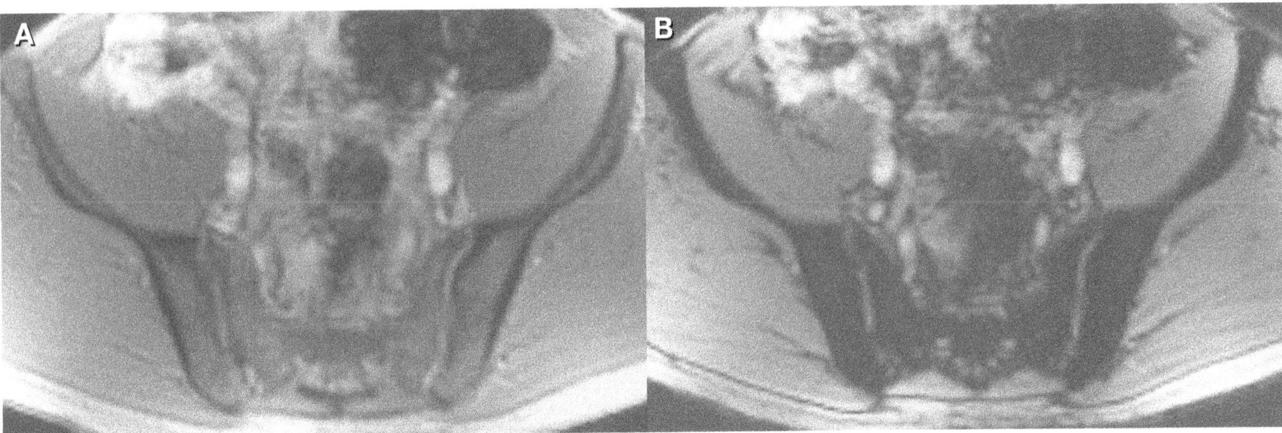

Figure 14.3.3

HISTORY: 31-year-old man with chronic midline back pain; recent spinal MRI suggested a marrow infiltrative disorder

IMAGING FINDINGS: Axial FSE T1-weighted images (Figure 14.3.1) demonstrate diffuse decreased signal intensity within the marrow of the iliac bones, with some regions slightly hypointense to adjacent skeletal muscle. Axial fat-suppressed FSE T2-weighted images (Figure 14.3.2) reveal no regions of increased signal intensity within the iliac marrow. Axial IP-OP images (Figure 14.3.3) show diffuse marrow signal dropout between the IP and OP images, consistent with the presence of fat.

DIAGNOSIS: Red marrow hyperplasia

COMMENT: Bone marrow has a fairly wide range of appearances within the nonpathologic spectrum and is a frequent source of confusion for residents in their first week on the body

MRI rotation (after the first week, they usually stop looking at bones, modeling the behavior of the staff radiologists).

One of the largest organs, bone marrow accounts for 5% of body weight. The cellular composition of marrow is complex. The most important elements are stem cells that are responsible for production of erythrocytes, granulocytes, and monocytes. Additional cells, including macrophages, adipocytes, osteoblasts, osteoclasts, and reticular cells, provide nutrients and cytokines that regulate hematopoiesis. A rich vascular supply of venous sinuses provides nutrients and allows release of blood cells into the circulation. Bone marrow is classified as yellow or red marrow according to its structure and function. In the adult, approximately 50% of the medullary cavity is occupied by yellow marrow and 50% by red marrow. Yellow marrow is found predominantly in the appendicular skeleton and consists of 80% fat, 15% water, and 5% protein; red marrow is most common in the axial skeleton and is 40% fat, 40% water, and 20% protein.

In general, yellow marrow poses no diagnostic dilemmas. It has high signal intensity on T1-weighted images, reflecting its high fat content and correspondingly low signal intensity on fat-suppressed T2-weighted images. Red marrow is more cellular and has lower signal intensity on T1-weighted images, but it generally has higher signal intensity than adjacent skeletal muscle, and it may have mild hyperintensity on fat-suppressed T2-weighted images. If you're looking at the spine, another rule of thumb for T1-weighted images is that the marrow signal should be higher than that of adjacent nondesiccated intervertebral disks.

These guidelines are sufficient for arbitrating the majority of cases of red marrow hyperplasia in which the marrow looks diffusely abnormal; however, occasionally, as in this case, the marrow signal intensity on T1-weighted images is lower than adjacent skeletal muscle, raising the possibility of marrow replacement disorders such as multiple myeloma, leukemia, lymphoma, myelofibrosis, and diffuse metastatic disease. The finding of no significant hyperintensity on fat-suppressed T2-weighted images is helpful in excluding most malignant causes (with the possible exception of myelofibrosis), and additionally, the significant signal dropout from IP to OP images demonstrates a diffuse background of fat-containing elements, which would be very unusual in an infiltrative marrow replacement disorder. Diffusion-weighted images can also be helpful on occasion. Restricted diffusion and high signal intensity suggest an infiltrative process; however, red marrow hyperplasia occasionally manifests as moderately high signal intensity on diffusion-weighted images.

Red marrow hyperplasia occurs when the hematopoietic capacity of existing marrow is exceeded and may be associated with chronic illness, heavy smoking, long-distance running, obesity, and anorexia.

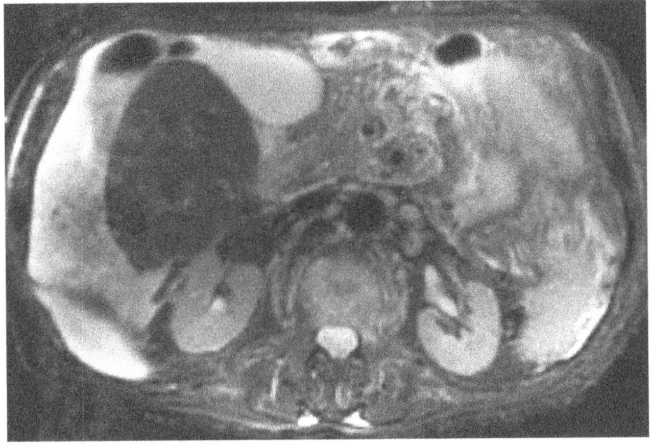

Figure 14.4.1

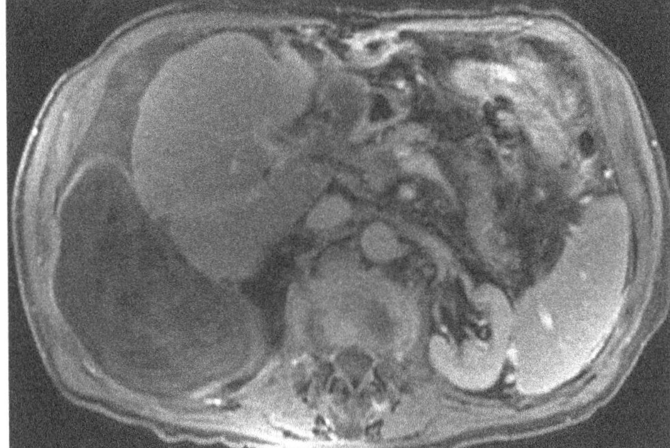

Figure 14.4.2

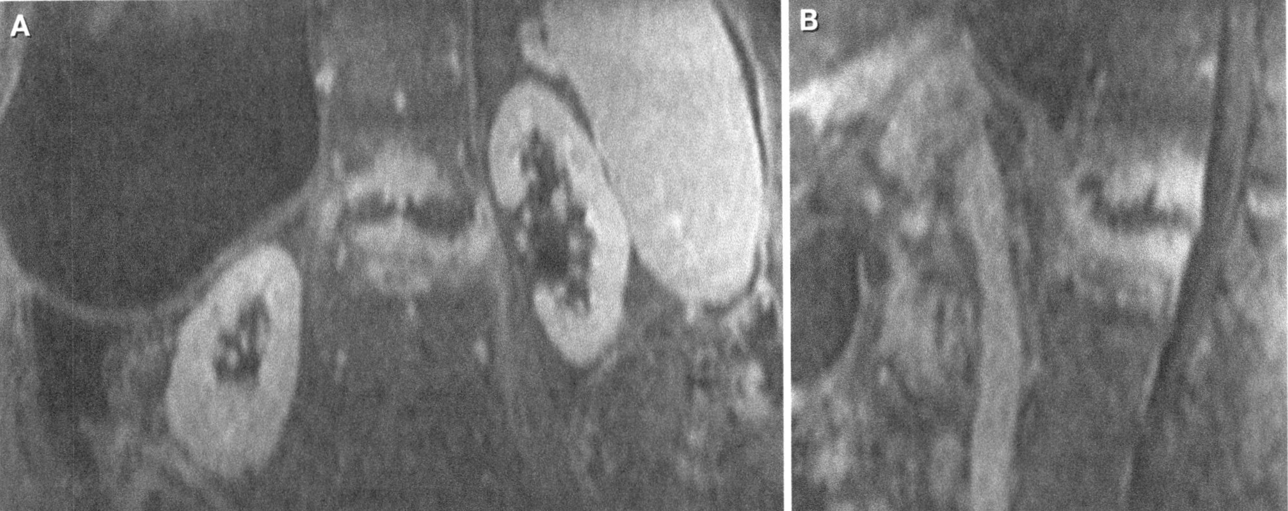

Figure 14.4.3

HISTORY: 80-year-old man with primary sclerosing cholangitis and end-stage liver disease

IMAGING FINDINGS: Axial fat-suppressed FSE T2-weighted image (Figure 14.4.1) demonstrates increased signal intensity in a lumbar vertebral body. There is corresponding enhancement on a postgadolinium 2D SPGR image (Figure 14.4.2). Note also abdominal ascites, peritoneal enhancement, and a cirrhotic liver. Coronal and sagittal reformatted views (Figure 14.4.3) from portal venous phase postgadolinium 3D SPGR acquisition reveal intense enhancement of vertebral end plates adjacent to the L1-2 disk, with expansion of the disk space.

DIAGNOSIS: Diskitis and vertebral osteomyelitis

COMMENT: Vertebral osteomyelitis is rarely discussed in the context of cross-sectional abdominal imaging, but the symptoms can be sufficiently vague so that the diagnosis is not suspected for weeks or months after onset. We have seen a few instances, such as this case, in which the diagnosis was first suggested on abdominal MRI.

The affected vertebral bodies are clearly abnormal on the axial T2-weighted FSE and postgadolinium SPGR images; however, the destructive end plate changes and disk-centered vertebral enhancement are much more apparent on the sagittal reformatted images from the venous phase 3D SPGR acquisition. The concept of reformatting dynamic 3D SPGR images is often lost on our residents (and staff) but can be helpful in confirming suspected vascular pathology (eg, mesenteric or renal artery stenosis) or a vertebral abnormality.

Vertebral osteomyelitis is an uncommon condition, with an estimated incidence of 2.4 cases per 100,000 population. Incidence increases with age, and vertebral diskitis and osteomyelitis are more common in patients with diabetes mellitus, coronary artery disease, immunosuppressive disorders, cancer, intravenous drug abuse, or renal failure requiring dialysis. Vertebral osteomyelitis usually occurs as a result of hematogenous seeding, direct inoculation during spinal surgery, or contiguous spread from an infection in adjacent soft tissue.

Complications include seeding of adjacent compartments, resulting in epidural abscess (17%), paravertebral abscess (27%), and disk space abscess (5%). Neurologic complications are common and have been reported in 38% of patients. Mortality ranges from 2% to 20%.

MRI has a high accuracy (>90% in most series) for diagnosing vertebral osteomyelitis. Typical features include high signal intensity within the disk on T2-weighted images. The vertebral end plates are irregular or partially destroyed, and there is often marrow edema and enhancement involving the 2 vertebral bodies adjacent to the affected disk. The earlier the diagnosis is made, the better; however, the MRI findings can be much more subtle in early disease and may be mistaken for degenerative end plate changes, which occasionally manifest with increased T2-signal intensity within the disk.

Treatment of vertebral osteomyelitis consists of intravenous antibiotics for 4 to 6 weeks and is successful in approximately 80% of patients. In difficult cases, surgery may be required for removal of hardware, drainage of abscesses, or débridement with additional stabilization or reconstruction.

CASE 14.5

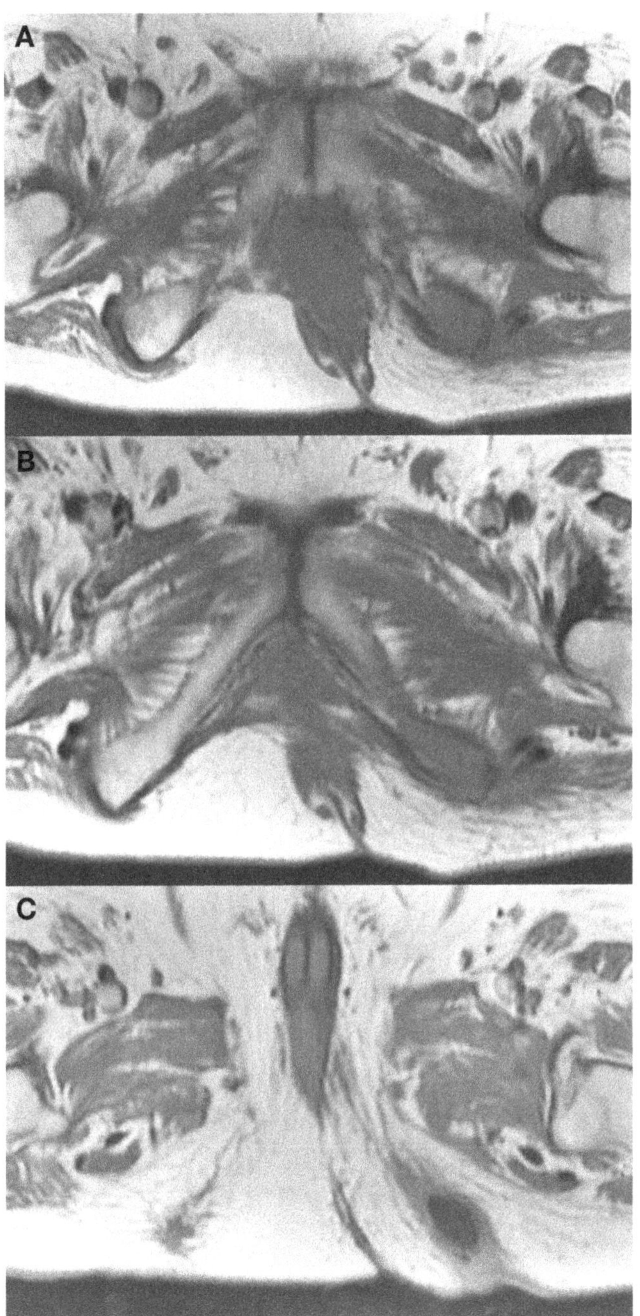

Figure 14.5.1

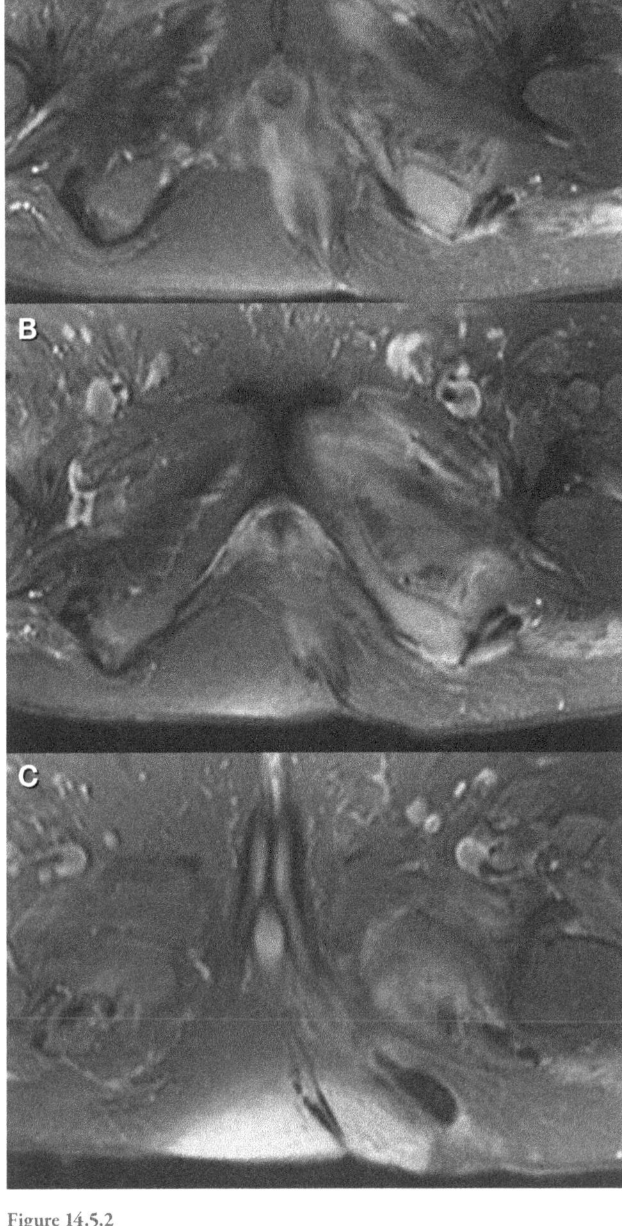

Figure 14.5.2

HISTORY: 31-year-old man with quadriplegia after a motor vehicle accident now has a draining decubitus ulcer

IMAGING FINDINGS: Axial FSE T1-weighted images (Figure 14.5.1) and fat-suppressed T2-weighted images (Figure 14.5.2) demonstrate a large soft tissue defect in the left lower buttock extending to the ischial tuberosity. The ischial tuberosity shows abnormally decreased T1-signal intensity and increased T2-signal intensity. Note also the abnormally increased signal intensity in the adjacent left obturator externus muscle.

DIAGNOSIS: Pelvic osteomyelitis

COMMENT: In the past, body MRI on-call cases in our practice were shared by the musculoskeletal and abdominal MRI groups, which meant that on weekends abdominal radiologists were asked to read images of diabetic feet with potential osteomyelitis, and musculoskeletal imagers scanned pregnant women with abdominal pain and suspected appendicitis. Which group had the better deal was a question that was never answered to anyone's satisfaction, and after many complaints from both sides, the on-call responsibilities were separated into abdominal and musculoskeletal components. This means that diabetic foot ulcers have largely disappeared from the abdominal practice, but osteomyelitis is still occasionally seen, as demonstrated by this case where MRI was requested to assess for an intrapelvic abscess.

The 3 basic mechanisms responsible for osteomyelitis and septic arthritis are hematogenous seeding, spread from adjacent soft tissue infection (the most likely cause in this case), and direct inoculation from penetrating trauma or surgery. The appearance of osteomyelitis on MRI includes abnormal marrow signal intensity on both T1-weighted and T2-weighted images, hyperenhancement after gadolinium administration, destructive changes, periosteal reaction, and adjacent soft tissue edema or a soft tissue mass.

Occasionally the important differential diagnosis is neoplasm, but most often the clinical question centers on whether the visualized marrow changes reflect actual osteomyelitis or reactive marrow edema. In the absence of gross bony destruction, the answer is not always definitive; however, as a rule of thumb, when the marrow signal intensity is lower than adjacent muscle on T1-weighted images, the balance has probably tipped in favor of osteomyelitis. Abnormal increased signal intensity on fat-suppressed T2-weighted images and abnormal marrow enhancement are probably more sensitive signs than changes on T1-weighted images, but they are also less specific. Some of our musculoskeletal colleagues are adamant that postgadolinium images add nothing of value to the osteomyelitis examination, but we have seen enough cases in which subtle soft tissue abscesses, myonecrosis, fasciitis, and deep vein thrombosis become apparent on postcontrast images that we almost always give contrast unless there is a contraindication.

Advances in multidisciplinary therapy have led to increased life expectancy for patients with spinal cord injury, but pressure ulcers remain a common problem. Nearly one-third of all patients with spinal cord injury have a pressure ulcer; of these, nearly 70% have more than one. These ulcers are responsible for considerable morbidity; they are quite costly to treat; and the presence of underlying osteomyelitis has significant implications for antibiotic therapy, surgical planning, and overall prognosis.

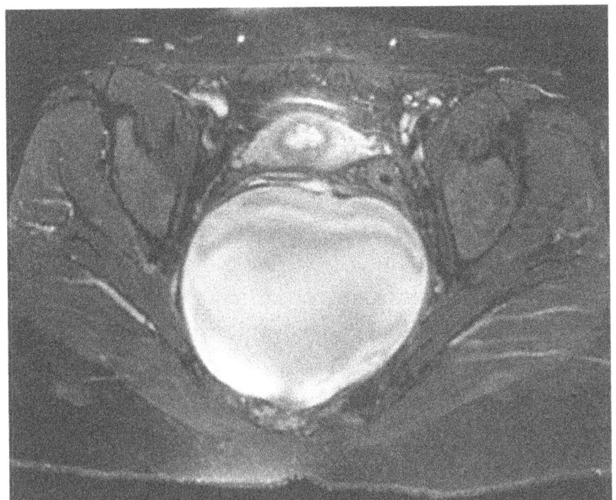

Figure 14.6.1

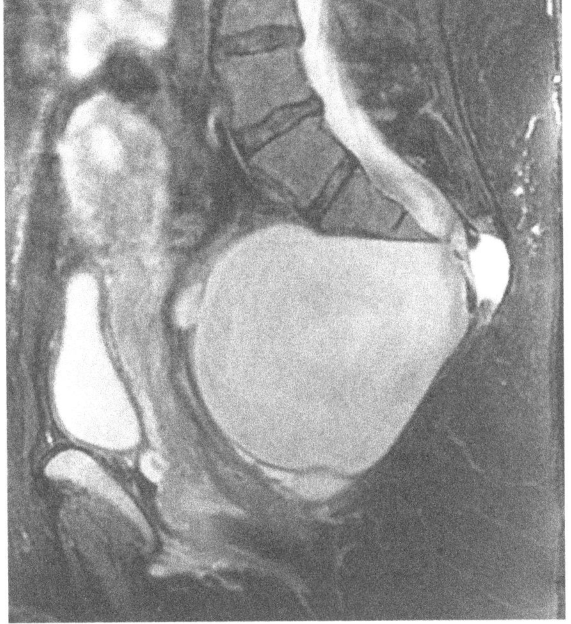

Figure 14.6.2

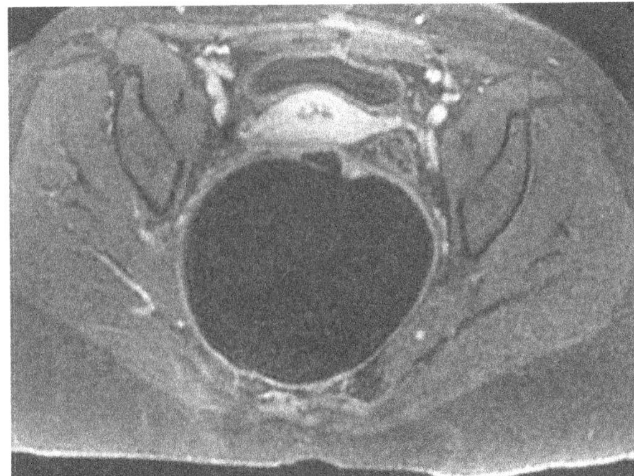

Figure 14.6.3

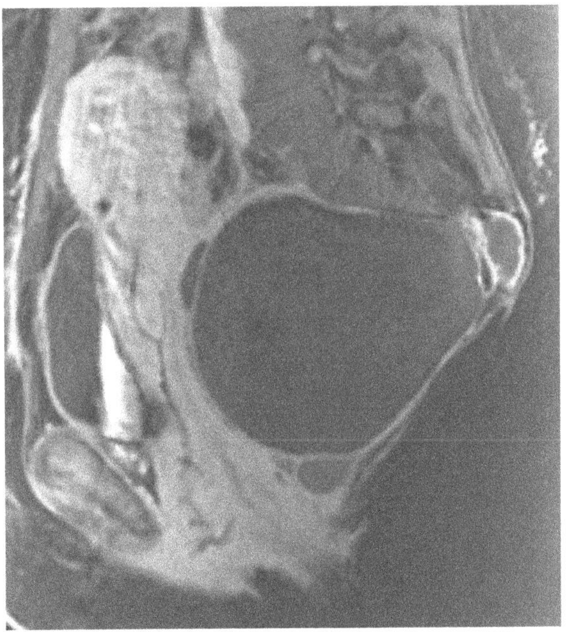

Figure 14.6.4

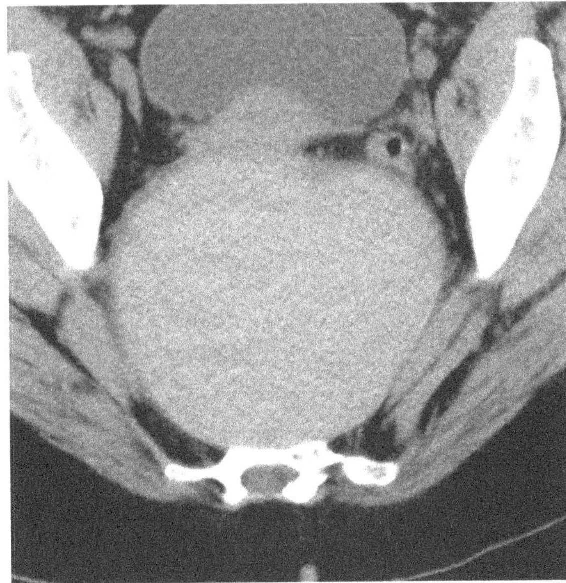

Figure 14.6.5

HISTORY: 26-year-old woman with a large presacral mass discovered on prenatal US during a recent pregnancy

IMAGING FINDINGS: Axial (Figure 14.6.1) and sagittal (Figure 14.6.2) fat-suppressed FSE T2-weighted images demonstrate a large cystic mass in the posterior pelvis. On the sagittal image there is communication with the spinal canal through a small neck. Note also a second small cystic lesion extending inferiorly from the spinal canal. Axial postgadolinium 3D SPGR image (Figure 14.6.3) and sagittal postgadolinium 2D SPGR image (Figure 14.6.4) demonstrate minimal rim enhancement of the presacral cystic lesion. Note also partial agenesis of the sacrum and coccyx. Axial image from a CT myelogram (Figure 14.6.5) demonstrates contrast enhancement within the presacral lesion.

DIAGNOSIS: Anterior meningocele

COMMENT: Anterior sacral meningoceles are herniations of the meninges through defects in the sacrum, coccyx, or adjacent disk spaces to form a cerebrospinal fluid–filled cystic mass within the pelvis. They may occur as an isolated defect or as part of the caudal regression syndromes, which include various degrees of lumbosacral agenesis in combination with other anomalies, such as imperforate anus, genital malformations, renal dysplasia or aplasia, and fused lower extremities. Meningoceles also occur in association with generalized mesenchymal dysplasia, such as in NF1 or Marfan syndrome.

The differential diagnosis for cystic lesions in the pelvis is fairly long and includes ovarian cyst, duplication cysts, tailgut cyst, dermoid or epidermoid cyst, lymphocele, and abscess. The key to the diagnosis is recognizing that the lesion communicates with the spinal canal. Sometimes the finding is subtle and is best appreciated on high-resolution 3D acquisitions. If you're not absolutely certain, confirmation can be obtained with a myelogram, as in this case.

Meningoceles are in a family of lesions occasionally shown on board examinations to unsuspecting radiologists, who if unsure of the diagnosis are then asked whether they would like to biopsy the lesion. Although biopsying a meningocele would be less catastrophic than biopsying a pseudoaneurysm, the answer is still no.

CASE 14.7

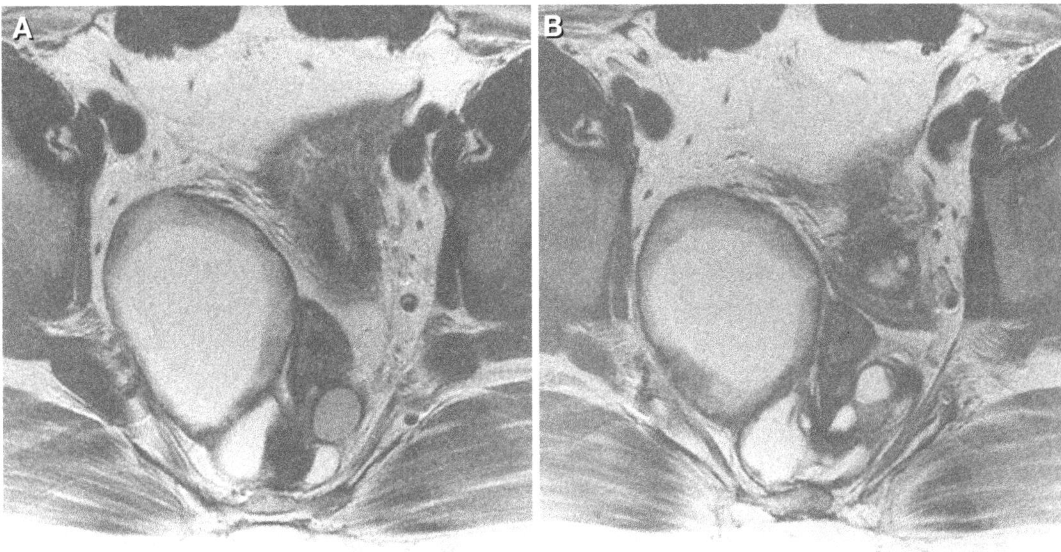

Figure 14.7.1

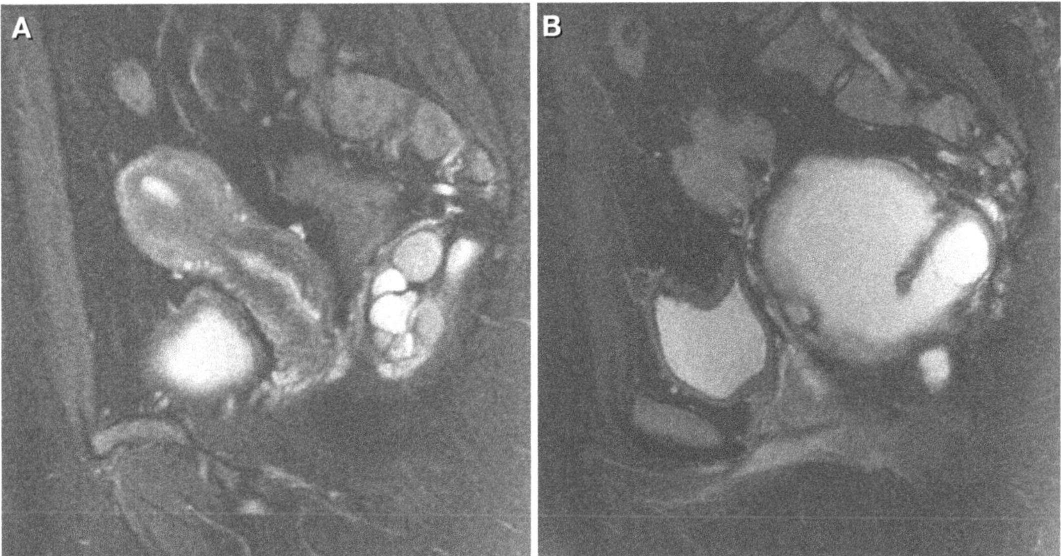

Figure 14.7.2

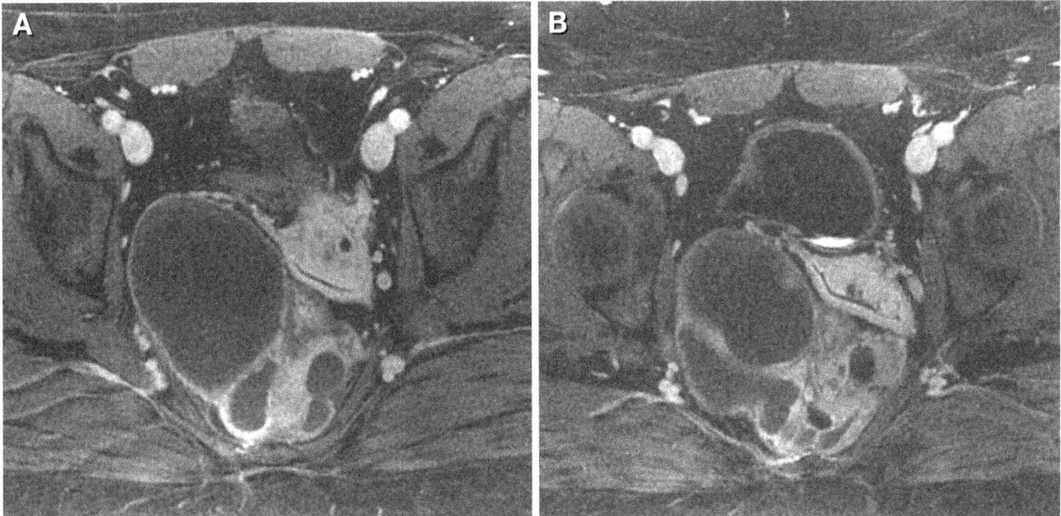

Figure 14.7.3

HISTORY: 40-year-old woman with previously resected ileal gastrointestinal stromal tumor; CT performed for postoperative surveillance demonstrated a complex mass in the pelvis

IMAGING FINDINGS: Axial FSE T2-weighted images (Figure 14.7.1) and sagittal fat suppressed FSE images (Figure 14.7.2) demonstrate a complex cystic lesion posterior to the rectum. There is a large dominant cyst with additional adjacent smaller cysts. Axial postgadolinium 3D SPGR images (Figure 14.7.3) reveal prominent enhancing soft tissue between the small cystic components.

DIAGNOSIS: Tailgut cyst

COMMENT: Inclusion of a tailgut cyst in the musculoskeletal chapter is somewhat arbitrary since it's not clear exactly where it belongs. It was placed in this chapter because many of the other lesions in the differential diagnosis of a sacral or presacral mass belong in the musculoskeletal category.

The tailgut is the most caudal part of the hindgut, distal to the future anus, and normally involutes by the eighth week of embryonic development. If a tailgut remnant persists, it may give rise to a tailgut cyst, typically appearing as a multicystic lesion in the retrorectal space. Tailgut cysts are thought to be more common in women and usually present in middle-aged patients.

Histologically, tailgut cysts are multicystic lesions lined by various epithelial cell types. Columnar or transitional epithelium must be present to exclude dermoid or epidermoid cysts, and the absence of a myenteric plexus and serosa must be documented to exclude a duplication cyst.

Malignant transformation of tailgut cysts is rare, but various neoplasms have been described, including adenocarcinoma, carcinoid, neuroendocrine carcinoma, and sarcoma. The small malignant potential of tailgut cysts means that surgical resection is usually performed when these lesions are discovered, and that it is useful to make the distinction between a tailgut cyst and lesions that are always benign (eg, duplication cyst, dermoid, or epidermoid cyst). Most tailgut cysts are multicystic; duplication cysts, dermoids, and epidermoids are usually unilocular. The presence of fat within a cystic lesion should lead to the diagnosis of dermoid or epidermoid. Signal intensity within the cysts can be variable. Although simple fluid and corresponding high T2- and low T1-signal intensity is the predominant finding, proteinaceous or hemorrhagic fluid can alter the appearance. Regardless of the cyst content, only rim enhancement should be seen after gadolinium administration. Large enhancing solid components projecting into the cysts should raise concerns about malignant degeneration.

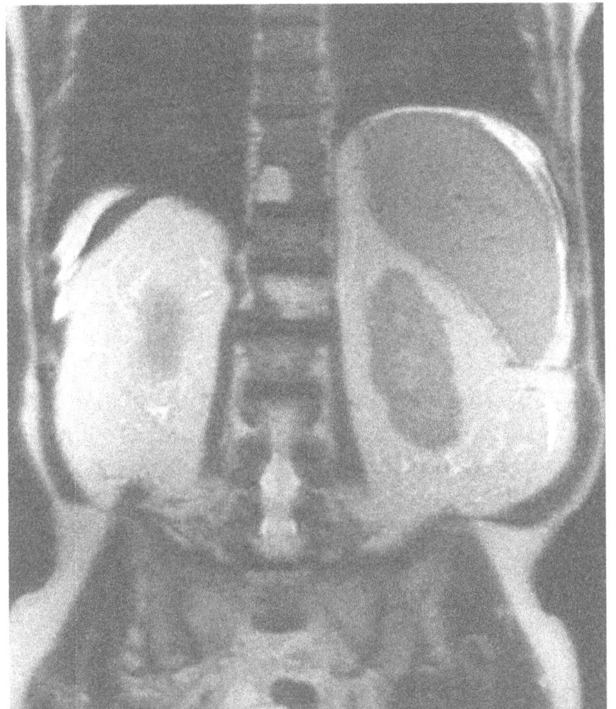

Figure 14.8.1

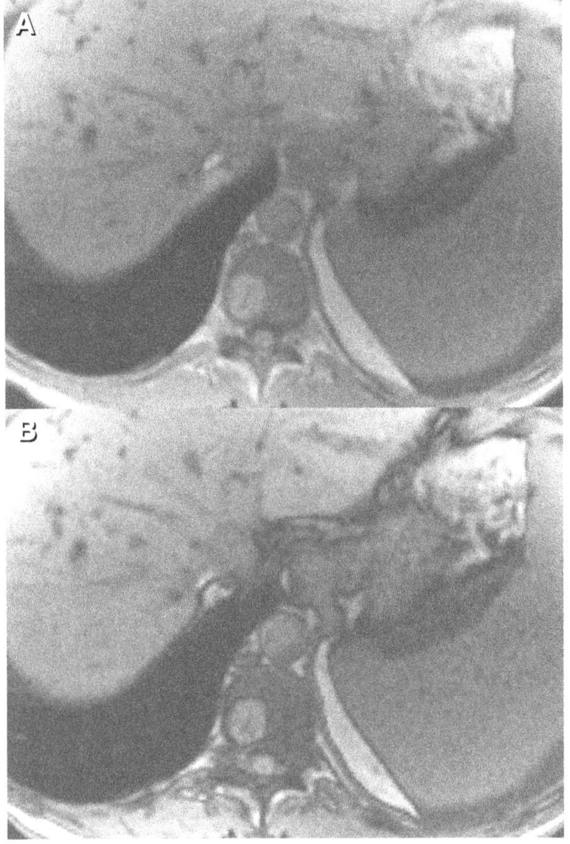

Figure 14.8.2

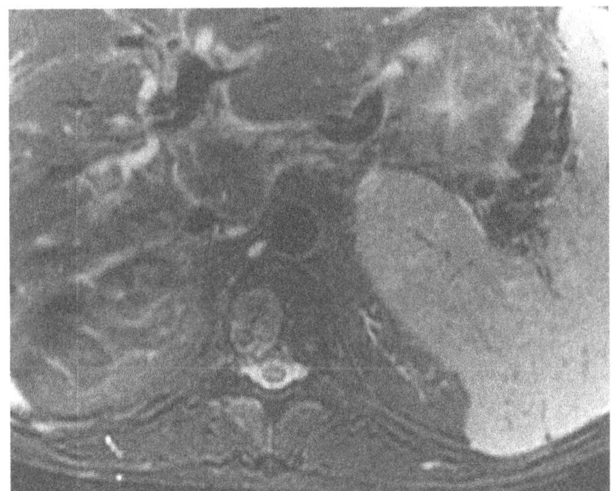

Figure 14.8.3

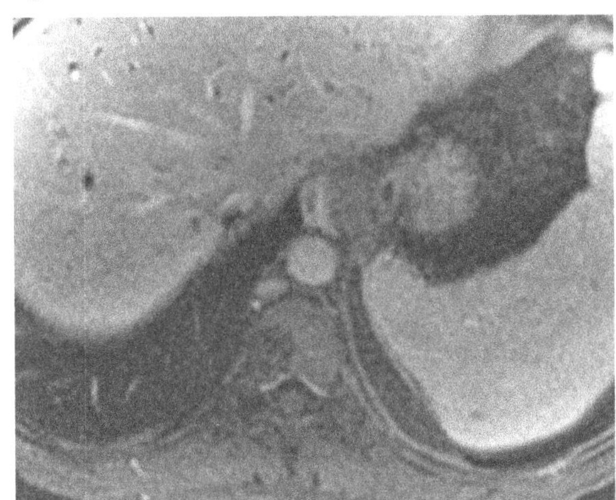

Figure 14.8.4

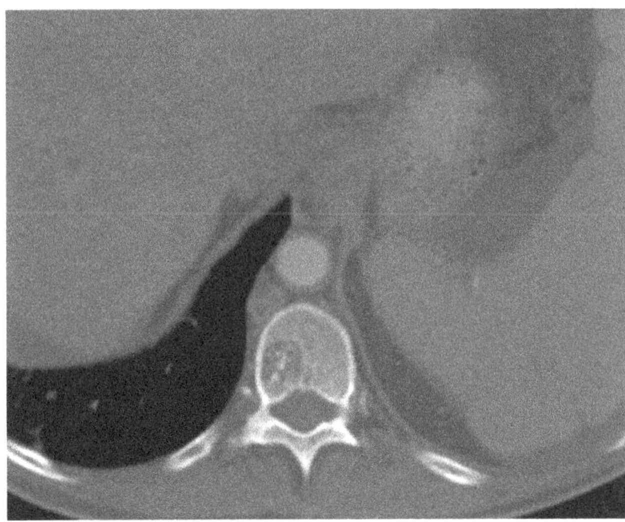

Figure 14.8.5

HISTORY: 69-year-old man with a hepatic lesion that was detected on CT

IMAGING FINDINGS: Coronal SSFSE image (Figure 14.8.1) demonstrates 2 hyperintense lesions in lower thoracic and upper lumbar vertebral bodies. Axial IP-OP 2D SPGR images (Figure 14.8.2) show that the superior-most lesion has increased signal intensity relative to adjacent bone marrow without significant dropout on the OP image. The lesion shows mild hyperintensity on an axial fat-suppressed FSE T2-weighted image (Figure 14.8.3) and appears hypoenhancing relative to marrow on a portal venous phase postgadolinium 3D SPGR image (Figure 14.8.4). Image from CT with bone window settings (Figure 14.8.5) demonstrates prominent punctuate trabeculations within the lesion.

DIAGNOSIS: Vertebral hemangiomas

COMMENT: The incidentally discovered focal vertebral lesion is an unpleasant but all too frequent problem for the body imager reading abdominal MRI. Although most of these lesions are benign, a fairly high percentage of our patient population has a known or suspected malignancy; therefore, bone metastases must be excluded. The option of recommending dedicated thoracic or lumbar spine MRI for "further characterization" has the virtue of tossing the ball into a colleague's court (who admittedly may be more likely to make the correct diagnosis), but it can be somewhat demoralizing if done on a regular basis, and so it's worth being able to recognize the classic appearance of benign bone lesions.

Vertebral hemangiomas are extremely common and have been found in as many as 11% of patients at autopsy. Multifocal lesions are present in 25% to 30% of cases. Hemangiomas are more common in the thoracic spine than in the lumbar spine, but they may occur at any level. Lesions typically involve the vertebral body but may extend into the pedicle or lamina. Most vertebral hemangiomas are asymptomatic incidental findings, but epidural expansion or fracture may cause cord compression and result in neurologic signs and symptoms. Hemangiomas consist of thin-walled blood vessels interspersed between nonvascular components, including fat, muscle, fibrous tissue, and bone.

The prominent, vertically oriented, mildly sclerotic trabeculae are best appreciated on CT, as in this case, but they can be seen with MRI as well. Hemangiomas are often hyperintense on T1-weighted images, reflecting fatty overgrowth. On abdominal MRI, this can usually be appreciated with IP-OP images, which are often the only sequence acquired with T1 weighting and without fat suppression. Hemangiomas are typically hyperintense on T2-weighted images, reflecting the vascular components of the lesions and fat (with non–fat-suppressed SSFSE images), although this is not a particularly helpful distinguishing feature. Contrast enhancement is somewhat variable, again reflecting the relative amount of vascular stroma. The nodular peripheral enhancement of hepatic hemangiomas is generally not seen; however, persistent enhancement on delayed images can sometimes be appreciated.

Our general approach to the incidentally detected vertebral lesion includes inspection of IP-OP images, since not many malignant lesions have T1 hyperintensity. When hyperintensity is present, the differential diagnosis includes hemangiomas, lipoma, or focal fatty proliferation. One caveat to keep in mind is that in the presence of diffuse marrow infiltration, a lesion may appear relatively hyperintense on T1-weighted images without actually containing a significant amount of fat. If T1-weighted images aren't helpful, we inspect for persistent enhancement, which is a good sign, versus the more worrisome pattern of early hyperenhancement and rapid washout. Fortunately, a high percentage of patients have prior MRIs or CTs (or both) for comparison: The coarse trabeculations of hemangiomas are often more easily seen on CT, and an indeterminate lesion that has been stable over several years is very likely benign.

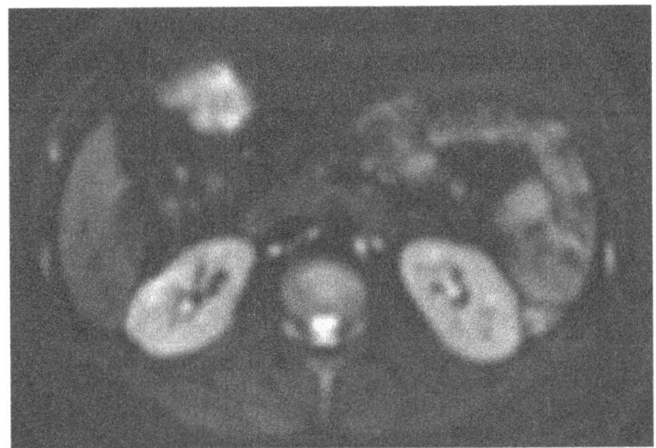

Figure 14.9.1

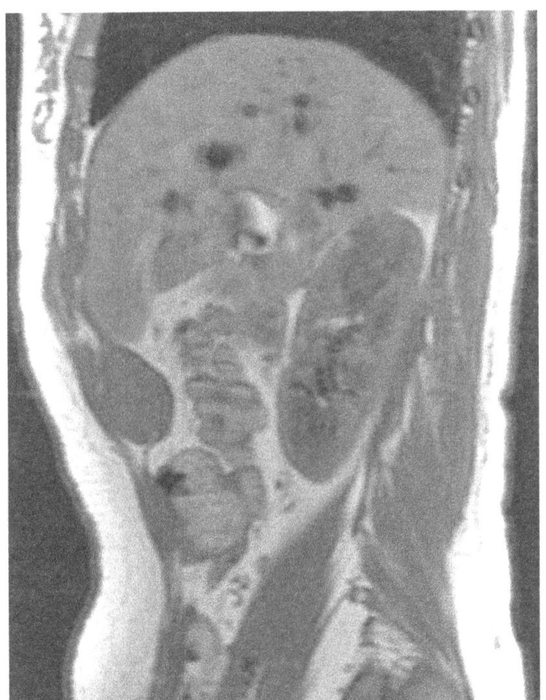

Figure 14.9.2

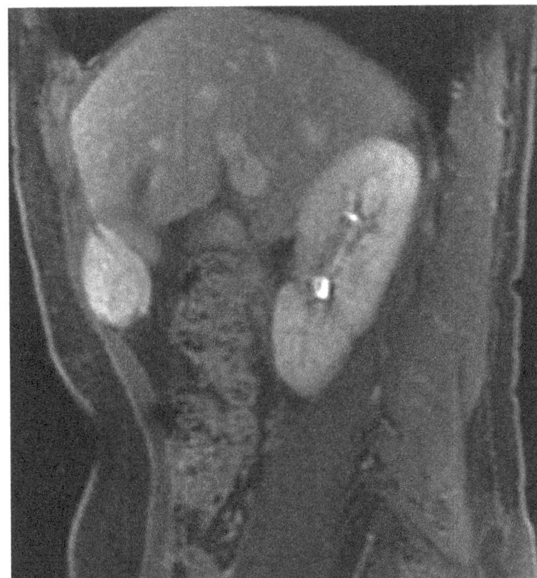

Figure 14.9.4

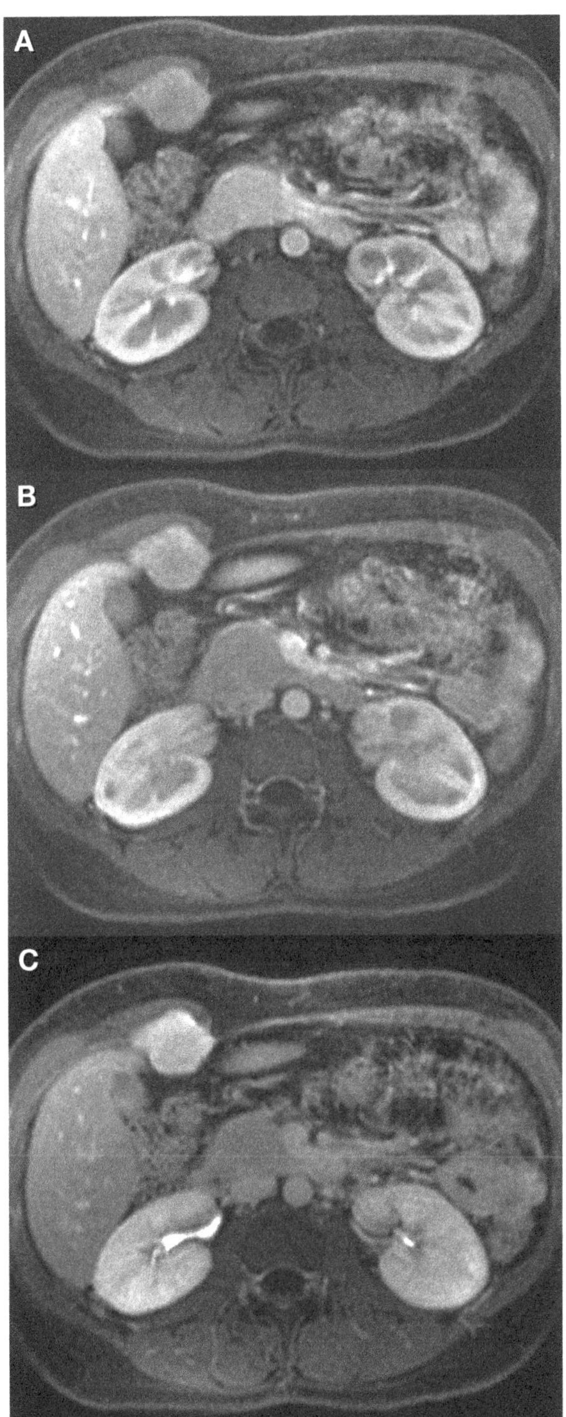

Figure 14.9.3

HISTORY: 29-year-old woman who noted an abdominal wall mass during the third trimester of her pregnancy

IMAGING FINDINGS: Axial diffusion-weighted image (b=600 s/mm^2) (Figure 14.9.1) and sagittal T1-weighted FSE image (Figure 14.9.2) demonstrate a fairly well-defined mass within the rectus muscle with high signal intensity on the diffusion-weighted image and mild hypointensity relative to skeletal muscle on the T1-weighted image. Axial arterial (Figure 14.9.3A), portal venous (Figure 14.9.3B), and equilibrium-phase (Figure 14.9.3C) postgadolinium 3D SPGR images demonstrate gradual enhancement of the lesion, with diffuse hyperenhancement seen on the equilibrium-phase image and an additional sagittal 3D SPGR equilibrium-phase image (Figure 14.9.4).

DIAGNOSIS: Abdominal wall desmoid

COMMENT: Desmoids are uncommon mesenchymal tumors consisting of elongated spindle cells separated by dense bands of collagen. The term *desmoid* was introduced by Muller in 1838 and is derived from the Greek word *desmos* for *tendon*. Desmoids account for approximately 0.03% of all neoplasms and less than 3% of all soft tissue tumors, with an estimated 900 new cases annually in the United States.

Most desmoid tumors arise spontaneously; however, they have a strong association with familial adenomatous polyposis (Gardner syndrome): 10% to 15% of patients with familial adenomatous polyposis syndrome have desmoid tumors at some point during their lives, and the risk in this group is increased more than 800% relative to the general population.

Many desmoids (28%-69%) occur in the abdomen or pelvis, either within the mesentery (which is more common in association with familial adenomatous polyposis) or within the abdominal wall. Additional sites include the shoulder, upper extremity, gluteal region, chest wall, and head and neck. Trauma, prior surgery, pregnancy, and oral contraceptive use are also predisposing factors for development of desmoid tumors.

The appearance of desmoid tumors on MRI can be variable: Signal intensity on T2-weighted images depends on the relative amounts of cellular tissue and collagen; in general, they are mildly hyperintense relative to skeletal muscle on T2-weighted images and more hyperintense on diffusion-weighted images. A fairly reliable feature is their increasing enhancement on equilibrium and delayed-phase postgadolinium acquisitions, a characteristic shared by many fibrotic tumors and nicely seen in this case. The differential diagnosis is broad and includes soft tissue sarcomas, lymphoma, metastases, neurogenic tumors, and endometriosis in the proper clinical context; however, desmoid can often be suggested as the most likely choice in patients with a history of polyposis or other predisposing factors.

Desmoids have no metastatic potential, but they are often locally aggressive, with high recurrence rates (19%-77%) that necessitate frequent surveillance examinations after surgery. The high incidence of recurrence is no doubt linked to the infiltrative nature of these lesions, which means that complete resection with wide surgical margins is often difficult. Desmoids also respond well to radiotherapy, which can be used for unresectable lesions or as adjuvant therapy to reduce the risk of local recurrence.

CASE 14.10

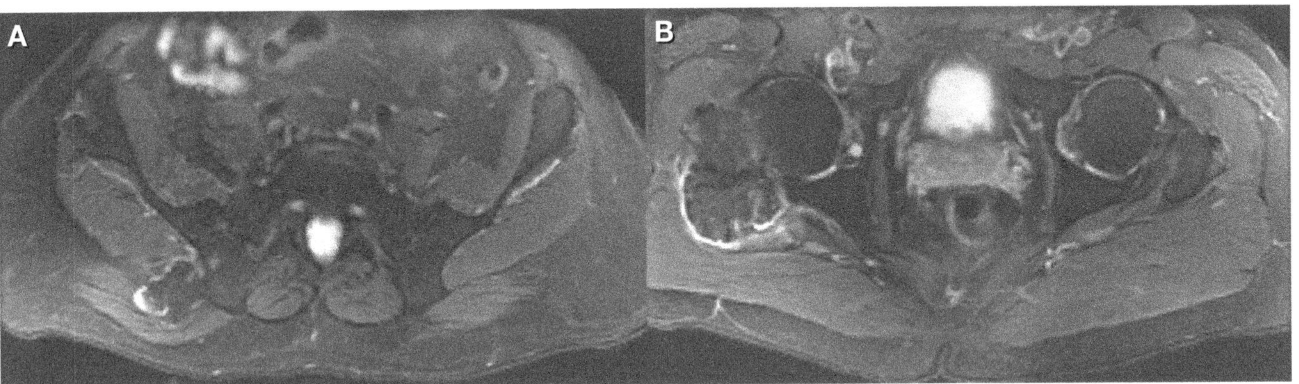

Figure 14.10.1

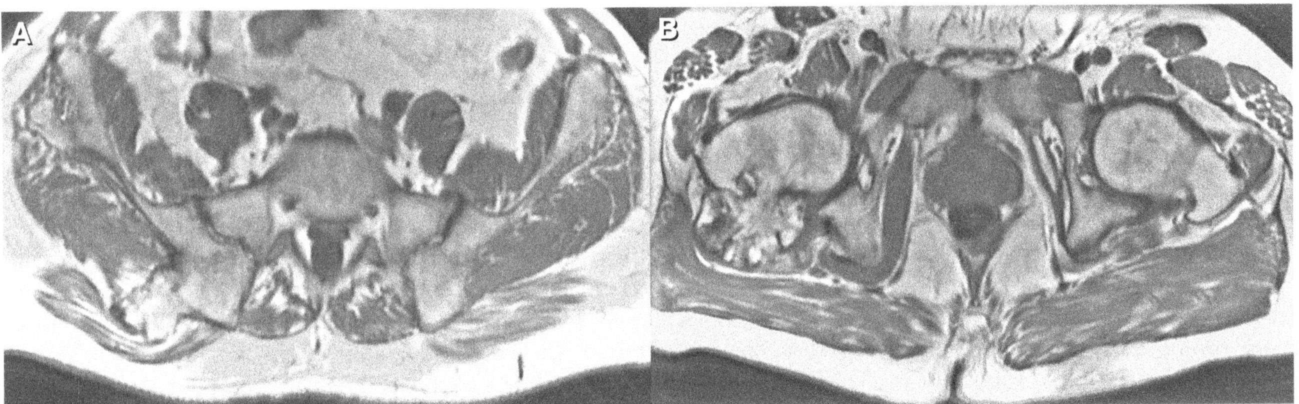

Figure 14.10.2

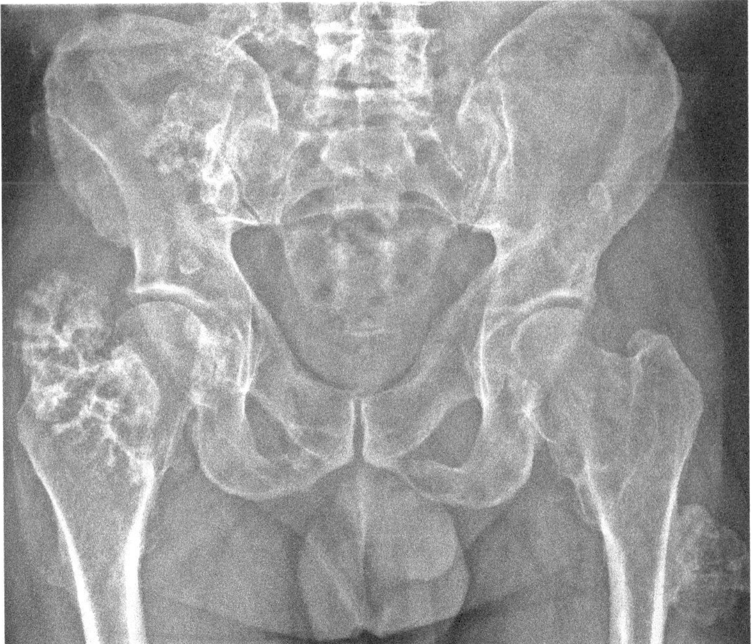
Figure 14.10.3

HISTORY: 52-year-old man with a hereditary disorder

IMAGING FINDINGS: Axial fat-suppressed FSE T2-weighted images (Figure 14.10.1) demonstrate multiple exophytic lesions extending from the right and left iliac bones and the right femoral neck. All the lesions have a thin outer margin with high signal intensity. Axial T1-weighted FSE images (Figure 14.10.2) reveal continuity of the underlying medullary cavity with the lesions. Plain radiograph of the pelvis (Figure 14.10.3) demonstrates multiple exophytic lesions with chondroid matrix projecting from the pelvic bones and from the proximal part of each femur.

DIAGNOSIS: Hereditary multiple exostoses (osteochondromas)

COMMENT: Osteochondroma is the most common bone tumor, accounting for 10% to 15% of all lesions and present in 1% to 2% of the population. Considered a developmental lesion rather than a true neoplasm, osteochondroma results when a fragment of the epiphyseal growth plate cartilage herniates through the periosteal bone cuff that normally surrounds the growth plate. Persistent growth of this fragment creates a subperiosteal osseous excrescence with a cartilage cap projecting from the bone surface. In a true osteochondroma, the stalk of the protruding lesion must be in direct continuity with the underlying cortex and medullary canal. Osteochondromas enlarge from growth of the cartilage cap, which is identical to a normal physeal plate; likewise, no further growth should occur after skeletal maturity. Osteochondromas are associated with radiation and Salter-Harris fractures.

Most solitary lesions are asymptomatic and are detected incidentally. Symptomatic lesions generally manifest as a painless cosmetic deformity, with additional symptoms related to fracture, vascular or nerve compromise, and malignant transformation.

Hereditary multiple exostoses, first described in 1786, is an autosomal dominant disorder characterized by the development of multiple osteochondromas. The estimated prevalence is 1 in 50,000 to 1 in 100,000. Genetic studies have linked the syndrome to genes on chromosomes 8, 11, and 19, which may function as tumor suppressor sites. In contrast to solitary osteochondromas, hereditary multiple exostoses is usually diagnosed at a young age (nearly always by 12 years) as a result of a combination of multiple skeletal deformities and a positive family history. Involvement of nearly every bone (except the skull) has been described, with hip involvement in 30% to 90% of patients and pelvic involvement in 5% to 15%.

Malignant degeneration is the most serious complication of osteochondroma; it occurs in approximately 1% of solitary lesions and in approximately 3% to 5% of patients with hereditary multiple exostoses. The malignant transformation is almost invariably the result of chondrosarcoma arising in the cartilage cap of the lesion.

Diagnosis of 1 or more osteochondromas is usually not difficult, particularly in hereditary multiple exostoses, and can usually be accomplished with a plain radiograph, which demonstrates an exophytic lesion with a broad or narrow stalk in continuity with the underlying bone. Similar findings can be appreciated on MRI. T1-weighted images are useful for documenting continuity of the lesion with the medullary cavity of native bone, and T2-weighted images reveal markedly high signal intensity within the cartilage cap. Thickness of the hyaline cartilage cap is an important criterion for assessing malignant degeneration: The average cap thickness in benign osteochondromas is approximately 0.6 to 0.8 cm and in patients with secondary chondrosarcomas, 5.5 to 6.0 cm. Cutoff values of 1.5 to 2.0 cm have been proposed for distinguishing benign from malignant lesions and have been shown to have high sensitivity and specificity.

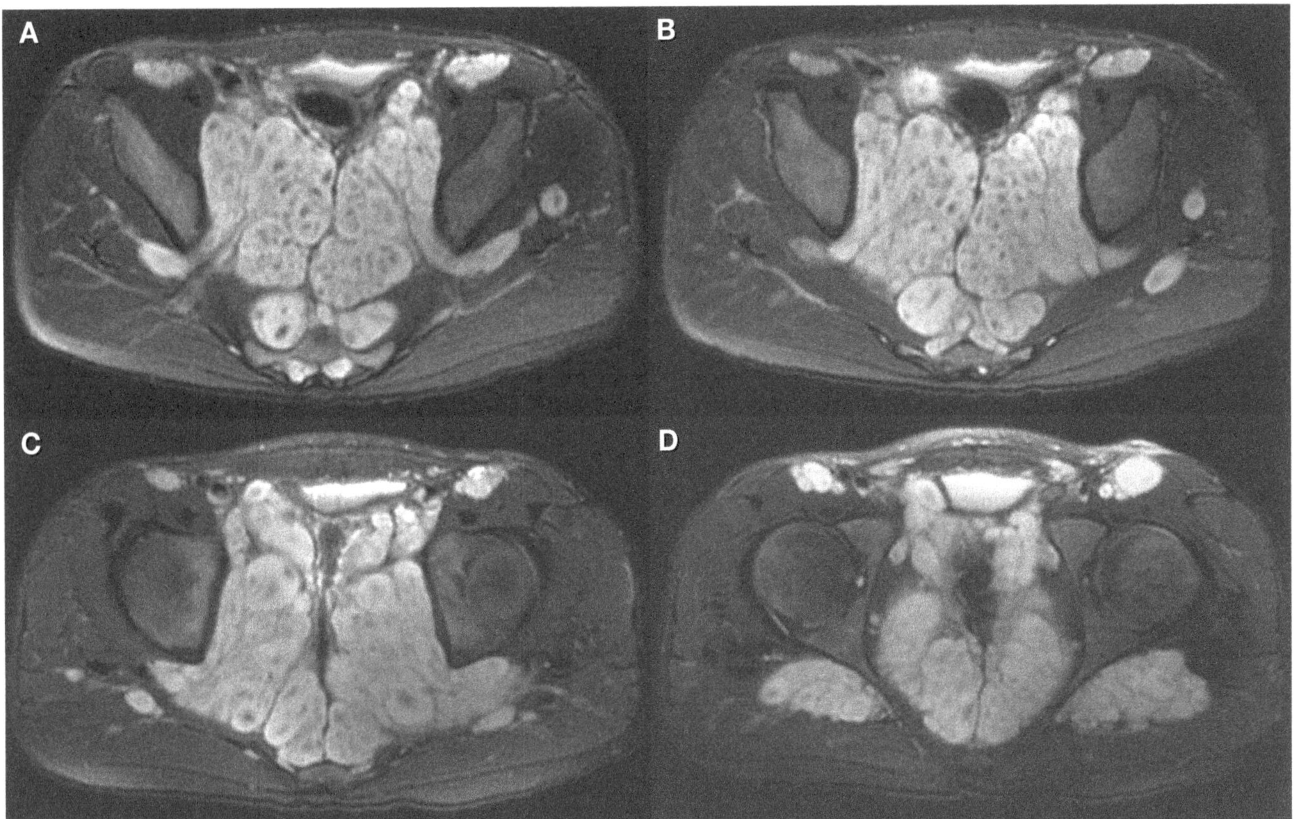

Figure 14.11.1

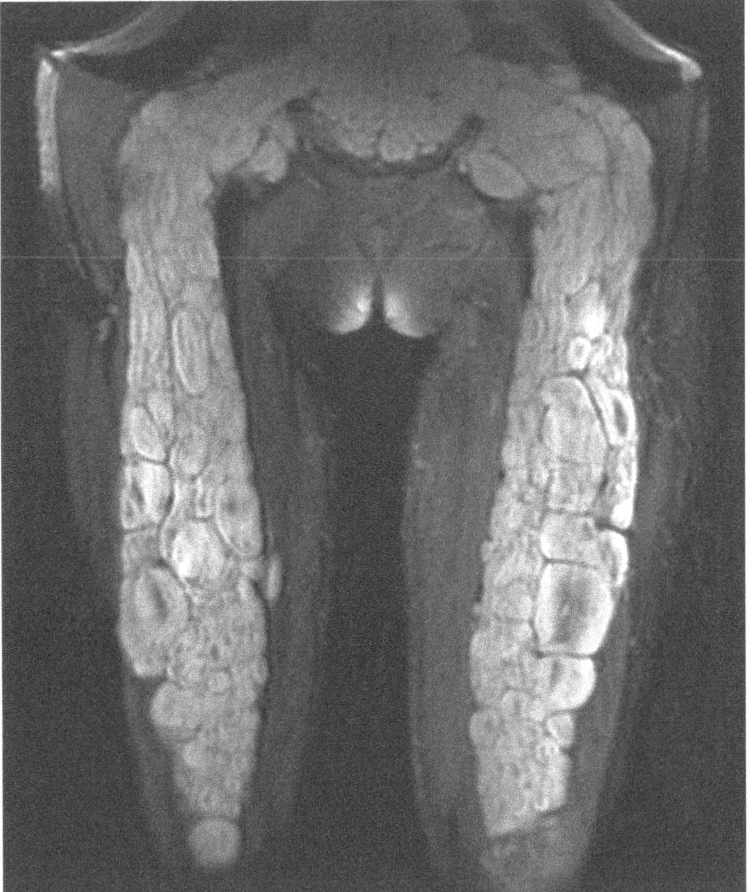

Figure 14.11.2

HISTORY: 17-year-old adolescent male with lower extremity numbness

IMAGING FINDINGS: Axial fat-suppressed FSE T2-weighted images (Figure 14.11.1) demonstrate innumerable hyperintense lesions containing central low-signal-intensity foci along the course of virtually all nerves in the pelvis. Coronal FSE T2-weighted image (Figure 14.11.2) through the posterior thighs reveals diffuse expansion of the sciatic nerves with lesions similar to those in the pelvis.

DIAGNOSIS: NF1 with plexiform neurofibromas

COMMENT: NF1 is an autosomal dominant neurocutaneous syndrome with an estimated prevalence of 1 in 4,000 to 1 in 5,000. Diagnostic criteria have been developed by a National Institutes of Health consensus conference. Diagnosis requires 2 or more of the following: 6 or more café au lait macules, 2 or more cutaneous or subcutaneous neurofibromas or 1 plexiform neurofibroma, axillary or groin freckling, optic glioma, 2 or more Lisch nodules (iris hamartomas), bony dysplasia (sphenoid wing dysplasia or bowing of long bones), or a first-degree relative with NF1.

A wide spectrum of clinical abnormalities is associated with NF1. Café au lait patches, Lisch nodules, and cutaneous neurofibromas are present in more than 95% of patients. An association with many additional tumors in addition to neurofibromas is well known, including optic glioma (15%), cerebral glioma (2%-3%), gastrointestinal stromal tumor, and pheochromocytoma. NF1 patients have a 7% to 13% lifetime risk of developing MPNST from an existing neurofibroma.

The gene for NF1 is located on chromosome 17 and contains 3 embedded genes, the function of which has not yet been determined.

This case provides an excellent illustration of plexiform neurofibromas. They are detected clinically in 27% of patients and by imaging in 50% of patients, and they consist of a network of neurofibroma tissue growing along the length of nerves, often involving multiple nerve fascicles, branches, and plexi. Plexiform neurofibromas are usually congenital or appear in childhood and often have rapid enlargement during adolescence. They may persist for years without causing significant symptoms; however, when they do cause neurologic deficits, medical or surgical treatment is difficult.

Neurofibromas typically demonstrate very high signal intensity on T2-weighted images, often with a central region of lower signal intensity (the target appearance); low T1-signal intensity; and mild to moderate enhancement after gadolinium administration. Development of MPNST may be suspected with rapid focal enlargement of a neurofibroma and development of a more heterogeneous appearance; however, the diagnosis is not always certain, and detecting the bad actor among innumerable benign lesions is occasionally very challenging.

CASE 14.12

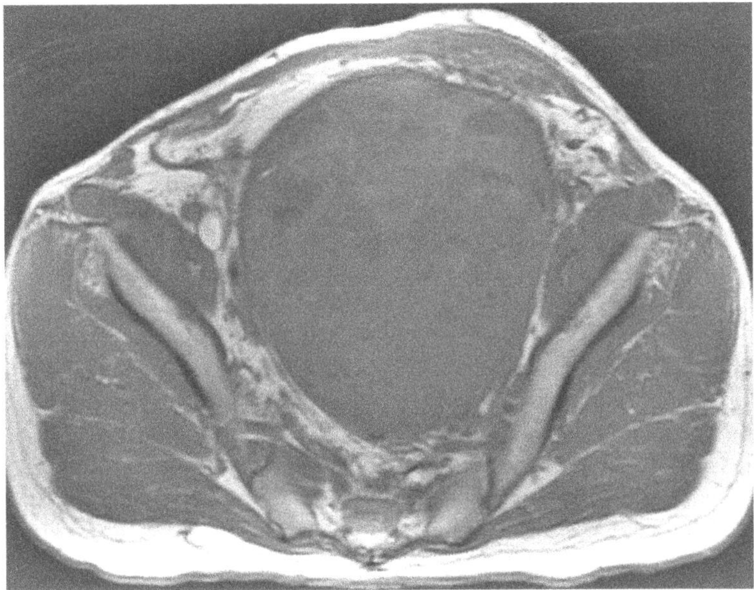

Figure 14.12.1

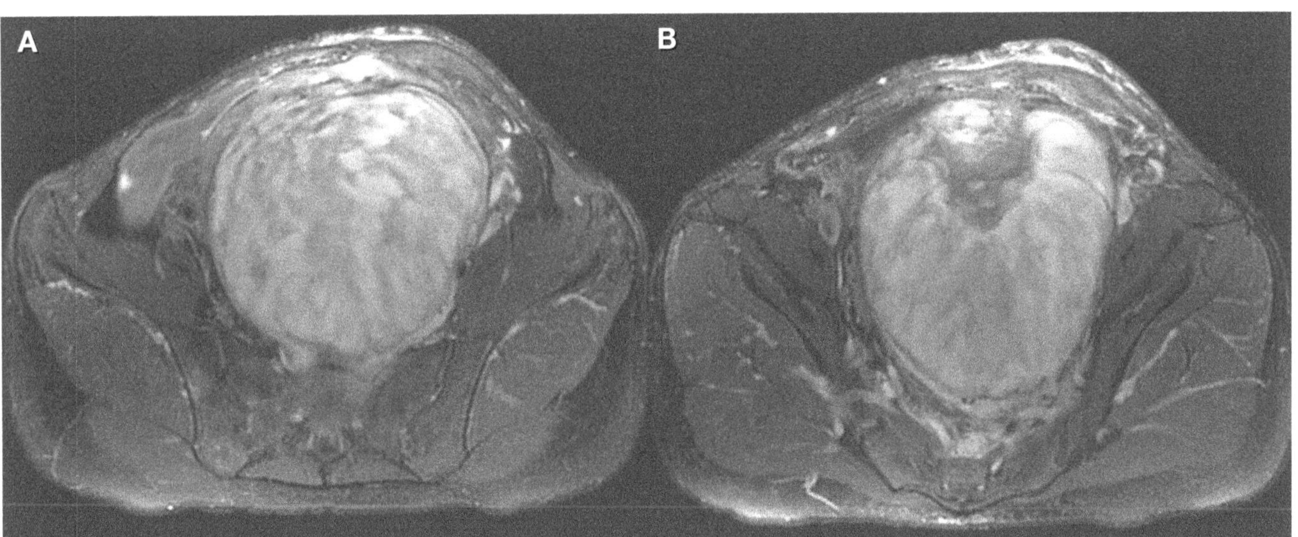

Figure 14.12.2

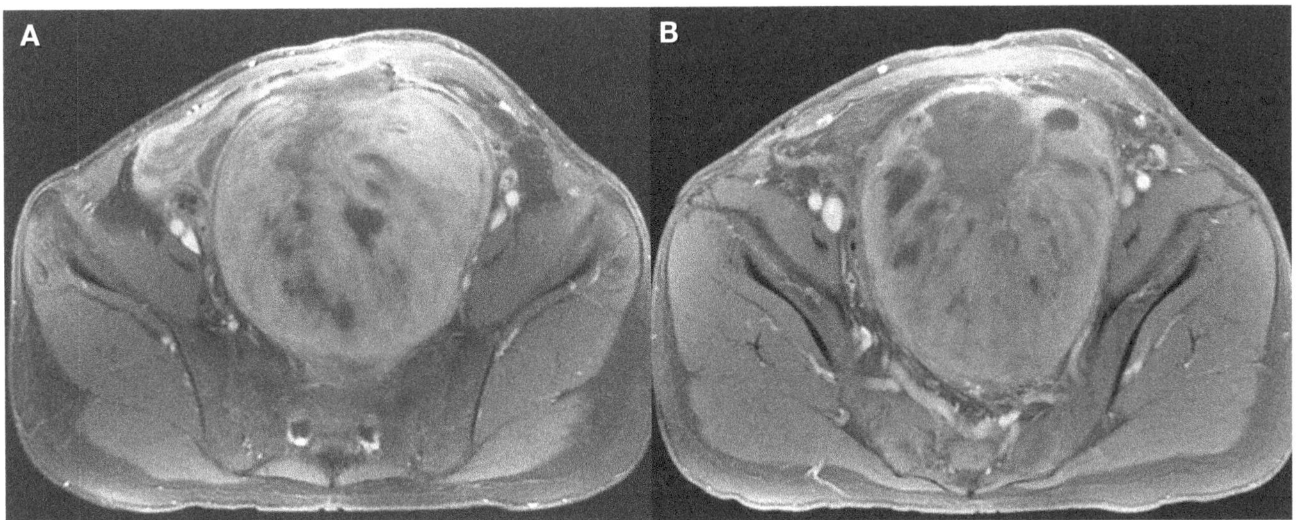

Figure 14.12.3

HISTORY: 52-year-old woman with an enlarging mass in her lower abdomen

IMAGING FINDINGS: Axial FSE T1-weighted image (Figure 14.12.1) and fat-suppressed T2-weighted images (Figure 14.12.2) reveal a large pelvic mass that is mildly hypointense relative to skeletal muscle on the T1-weighted image and heterogeneously hyperintense on the T2-weighted images with a region of focal scarring anteriorly. Axial post-gadolinium 2D SPGR images (Figure 14.12.3) demonstrate heterogeneous enhancement with scattered regions showing little or no enhancement.

DIAGNOSIS: Pelvic schwannoma

COMMENT: Schwannomas originate from Schwann cells, which are found in the nerve sheath of peripheral nerves, and can develop in any nerve except the first and second cranial nerves, which don't contain Schwann cells. Schwannomas occur most often in cranial nerves and peripheral nerves of the upper limb. Pelvic and retroperitoneal schwannomas represent 0.3% to 3% of all lesions; however, they are the most common benign soft tissue tumor of the retroperitoneum. Malignant retroperitoneal tumors are more common than benign varieties, and schwannomas account for approximately 4% of all retroperitoneal neoplasms.

Schwannomas are encapsulated tumors with areas of dense cellularity and aggregated spindle cells arranged in parallel configurations termed Antoni A regions. Hypocellular areas of predominantly myxoid matrix are Antoni B regions, which likely account for the cystic nonenhancing regions on MRI. Immunohistochemistry is positive for S-100 protein, vimentin, and neuron-specific enolase.

Pelvic schwannomas are almost always solitary and benign, and they are frequently large at diagnosis (reported average diameter, 8-14 cm), probably because of the lack of specific symptoms. Malignant transformation and local recurrence after resection are extremely rare.

While the appearance of small peripheral schwannomas or neurofibromas is often diagnostic on MRI, large pelvic schwannomas are usually difficult to distinguish from malignant tumors, such as liposarcoma, leiomyosarcoma, malignant fibrous histiocytoma, and other sarcomas in the differential diagnosis of a large pelvic mass. Typically, schwannomas appear as a smooth, well-marginated lesion with heterogeneous hyperintense signal intensity on T2-weighted images, heterogeneous enhancement, and occasional cystic changes.

CASE 14.13

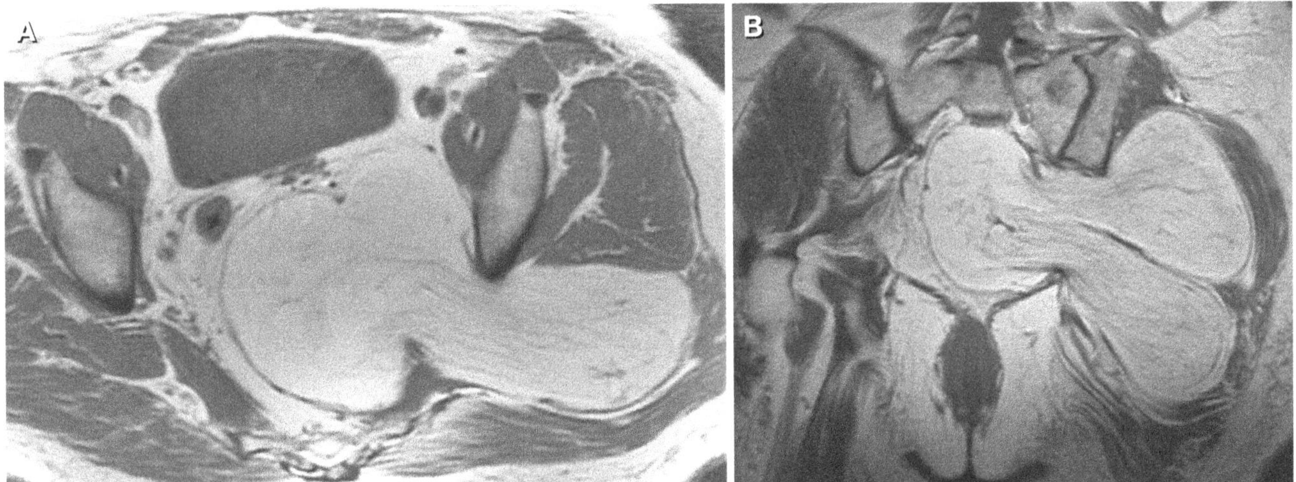

Figure 14.13.1

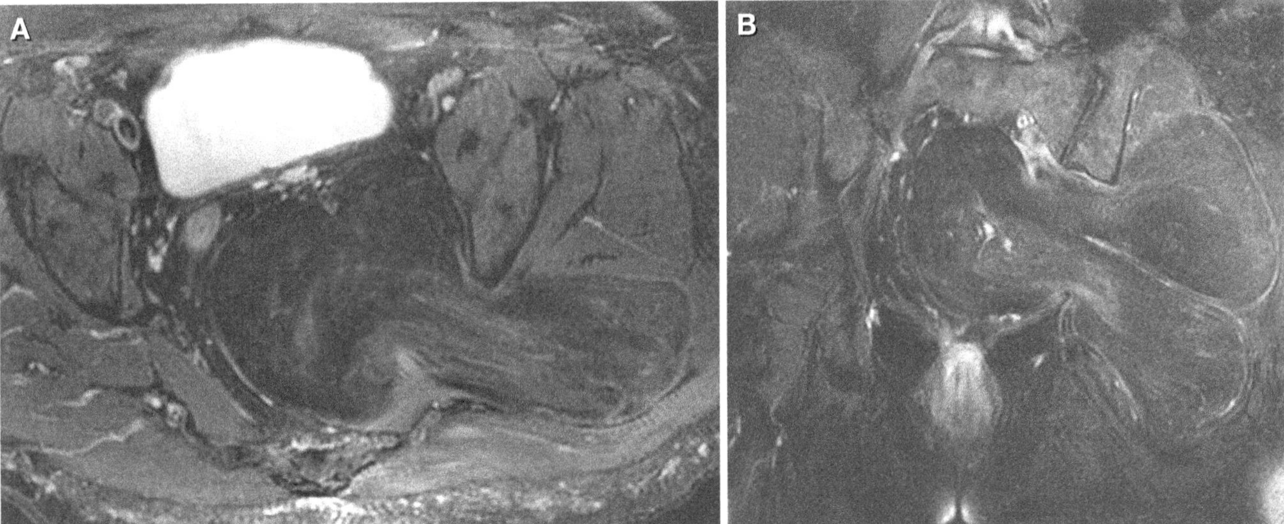

Figure 14.13.2

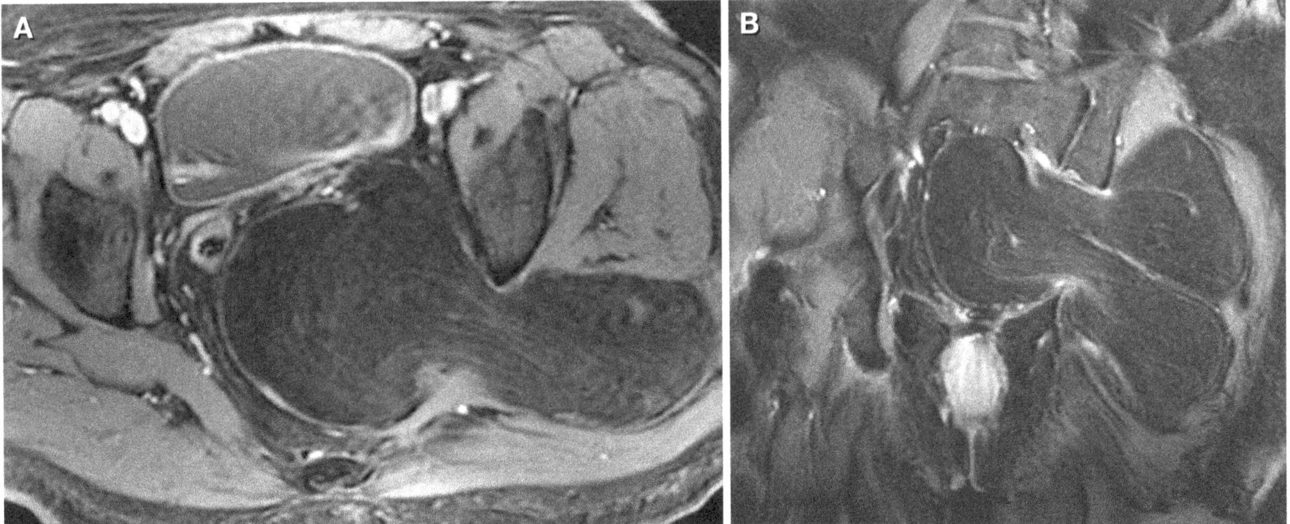

Figure 14.13.3

HISTORY: 65-year-old woman with a pelvic mass

IMAGING FINDINGS: Axial (Figure 14.13.1A) and coronal (Figure 14.13.1B) T1-weighted FSE images and axial (Figure 14.13.2A) and coronal (Figure 14.13.2B) fat-suppressed T2-weighted FSE images demonstrate a dumbbell-shaped lesion extending from the pelvis through the left sciatic notch. The mass consists almost entirely of fat but does have several thin septations. Axial and coronal postgadolinium 2D SPGR images (Figure 14.13.3) reveal minimal enhancement of a few septations within the lesion.

DIAGNOSIS: Pelvic lipoma

COMMENT: Lipomas are the most common soft tissue tumors and are composed of mature adipocytes. Lesions are often classified as superficial (subcutaneous) or deep. Superficial lipomas are usually small, homogeneous fatty lesions and are fairly easy to classify as benign without waking up in the middle of the night and wondering whether you missed a liposarcoma. In the ideal case, a lipoma is composed entirely of homogeneous fat without any additional components, has no regions of increased signal intensity on fat-suppressed T2-weighted images, and demonstrates no enhancement after gadolinium administration.

Deep lesions, as in this case, are often more challenging to characterize. They tend to be much larger, they often have thin septations or internal vessels, and the distinction between lipoma and liposarcoma can be extremely difficult. Several authors have described signs they use to distinguish lipomas from liposarcomas with nearly 100% accuracy, while subsequent papers have reported much less successful results and instead propose new criteria. The proposed distinguishing features include size, indistinct or infiltrative margins, soft tissue nodules, and internal components with high signal intensity on short TI inversion recovery or fat-suppressed T2-weighted images.

Our strategy is to look for obvious features that suggest something more than a simple lipoma (eg, the presence of thick, enhancing septations or prominent nonfatty soft tissue nodules within the lesion). When 1 or more of these features is present, the lesion is suspicious and probably should be resected if possible. You won't be right all the time, but you will be reasonably accurate. For larger lipomas with minor inhomogeneities, as in this case, we generally hedge in our report and recommend follow-up examinations. In this patient, for example, the lesion has not changed significantly over approximately 10 years.

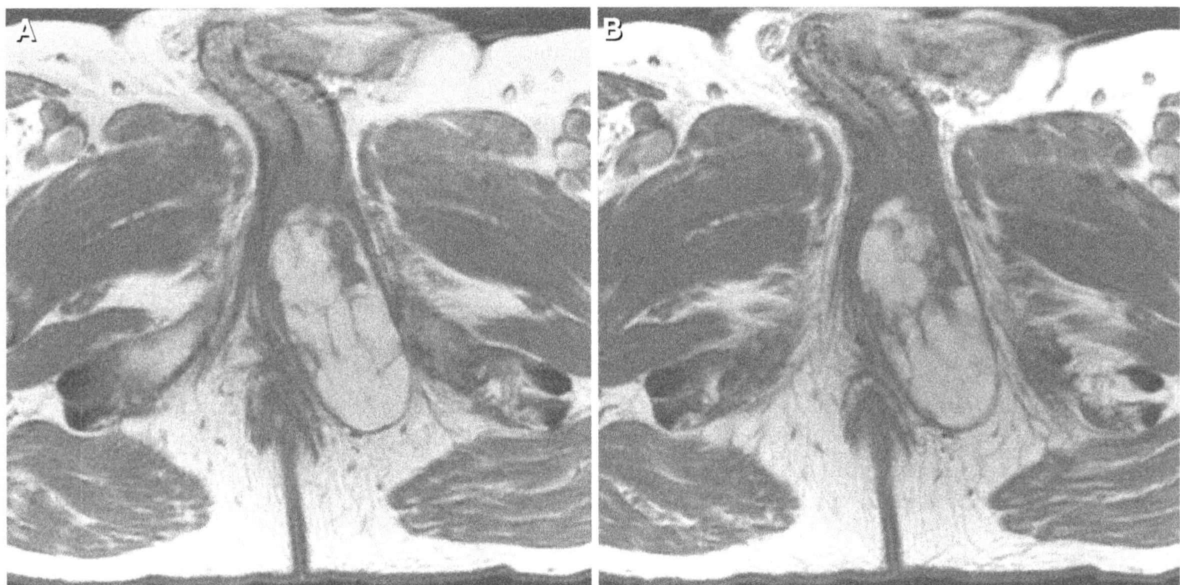

Figure 14.14.1

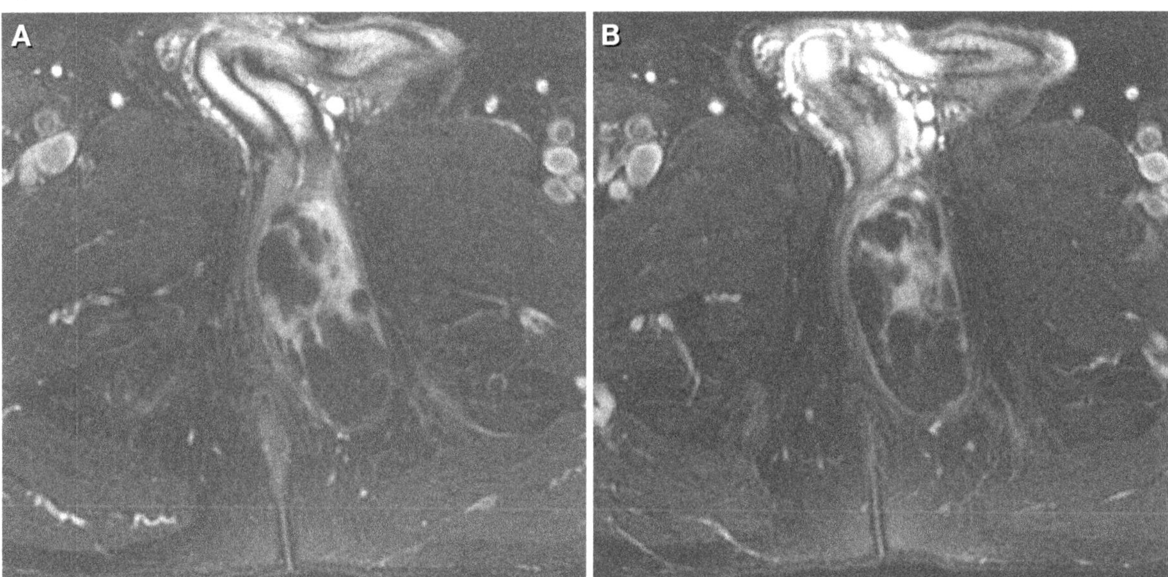

Figure 14.14.2

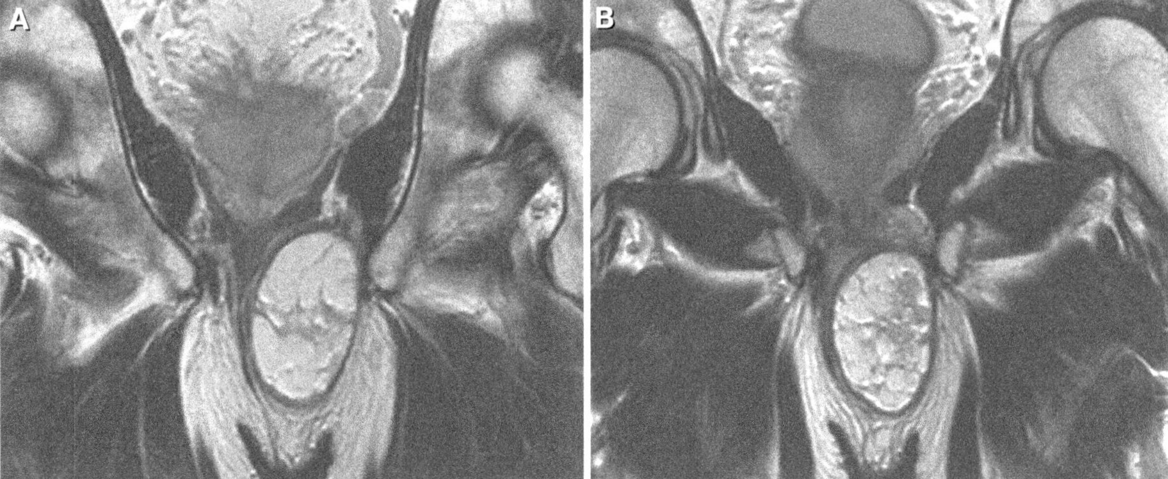

Figure 14.14.3

HISTORY: 59-year-old man with a history of lymphoma; a presacral mass was noted on a recent CT

IMAGING FINDINGS: Axial FSE T1-weighted images (Figure 14.14.1), fat-suppressed FSE T2-weighted images (Figure 14.14.2), and coronal FSE T2-weighted images (Figure 14.14.3) demonstrate an ovoid mass in the left perineum predominantly composed of fat. The mass has multiple septations and a more nodular component near the anterior margin.

DIAGNOSIS: Spindle cell lipoma

COMMENT: Spindle cell lipomas are uncommon benign mesenchymal tumors first described by Enzinger and Harvey in 1975. They account for approximately 1.5% of all lipomatous neoplasms and occur most frequently as subcutaneous lesions in the upper back, shoulder, or posterior neck of men who are middle-aged or older. Histologically, they are characterized by a mixture of mature fat, bland spindle cells, and collagen in a variably myxoid background. Immunohistochemical studies show spindle cells positive for vimentin and CD34.

The imaging characteristics of spindle cell lipoma may mimic those of liposarcoma; in fact, the original description of the lesion was in the context of its frequent misdiagnosis as myxoid liposarcoma. This case illustrates a lesion composed predominantly of fat but with enough unusual features to raise the possibility of a liposarcoma.

Only a relatively small number of spindle cell lipomas have been described in the literature, and most have been located in the neck, shoulder, and upper back. A few case reports have also noted lesions in unusual locations, including the face, oral cavity, bronchus, orbit, breast, scrotum, spermatic cord, perianal region, and space of Retzius. The lesion in this case fits this category of unusual locations and suggests that the original reports may not have encompassed the true extent of this unusual neoplasm.

CASE 14.15

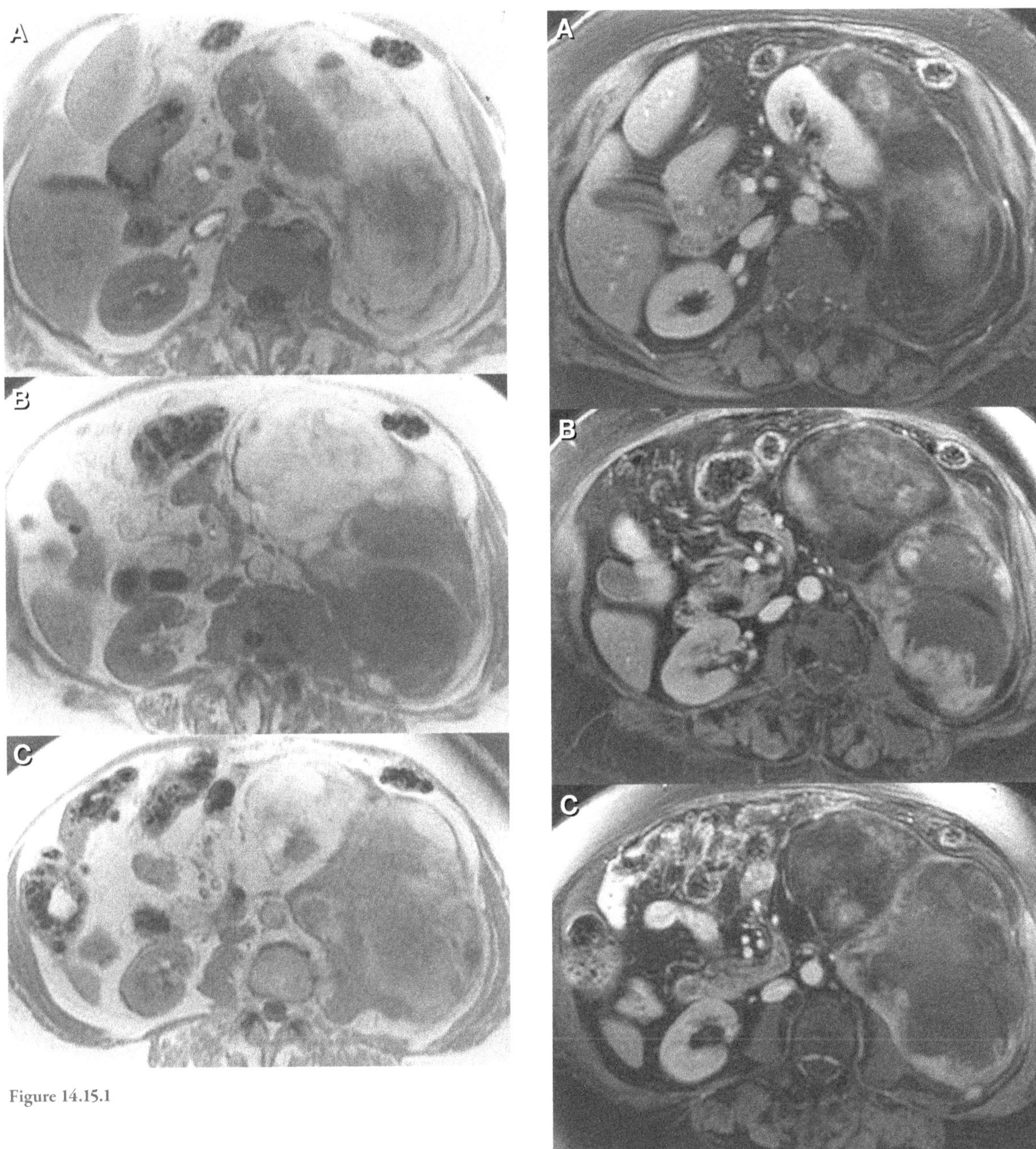

Figure 14.15.1

Figure 14.15.2

HISTORY: 78-year-old woman with a large retroperitoneal mass discovered on a preoperative CT performed before ventral hernia repair

IMAGING FINDINGS: Axial IP 2D SPGR images (Figure 14.15.1) demonstrate a large heterogeneous mass in the left abdomen abutting and displacing the left kidney anteriorly. Note that the anterior portion of the mass has high signal intensity. Axial postgadolinium 2D SPGR images (Figure 14.15.2) reveal patchy heterogeneous enhancement of the posterior portion of the lesion, with predominantly low signal intensity anteriorly.

DIAGNOSIS: Liposarcoma

COMMENT: Lipomas are the most common soft tissue tumors, occurring in superficial and deep locations and characterized by the presence of mature adipose tissue that is unavailable for systemic metabolism. In contrast, liposarcomas are relatively rare; nevertheless, they are the second most common soft tissue sarcoma in adults after malignant fibrous histiocytoma, and they account for 20% to 25% of all soft tissue sarcomas. The peak age at onset is in the fifth to seventh decades. Liposarcomas can occur anywhere in the body, but they are most frequently found in the extremities and retroperitoneum.

The World Health Organization has categorized liposarcomas into subtypes, including well-differentiated liposarcoma, dedifferentiated liposarcoma, myxoid liposarcoma, pleomorphic liposarcoma, and mixed-type liposarcoma.

Well-differentiated liposarcoma is the most common subtype, representing approximately 50% of all liposarcomas; it is a low-grade malignancy that almost never metastasizes unless there is a focus of dedifferentiation. Well-differentiated liposarcomas most commonly occur in the lower extremities (50%) and retroperitoneum (20%-33%). Retroperitoneal lesions are often large at presentation and are difficult to resect, with reported local recurrence rates of 90% to 100%. On MRI, well-differentiated liposarcoma typically appears as a mass composed of more than 75% adipose tissue with thick septations. Internal soft tissue nodules are also commonly seen, although dedifferentiated liposarcoma should be suggested when these components are larger than 2 to 3 cm in diameter. Metastases, most often to the liver and lungs, occur in 15% to 20% of patients who have dedifferentiated liposarcoma.

Myxoid liposarcoma is an intermediate- to high-grade neoplasm and is the second most common subtype. The peak age at diagnosis is in the fourth and fifth decades, about a decade younger than other liposarcoma subtypes. Most myxoid liposarcomas (75%-80%) occur in the lower extremities and are characterized by components with high T2-signal intensity and a relatively small amount of macroscopic fat. Compared with well-differentiated and dedifferentiated subtypes, myxoid liposarcomas have a more aggressive course, with frequent metastases and reduced survival.

Pleomorphic liposarcoma is the least common subtype and most often occurs in the deep soft tissue of the extremities in elderly patients. These are aggressive, high-grade lesions with a high incidence of recurrence and metastases.

This case illustrates a fairly common appearance of a retroperitoneal liposarcoma: a large lesion with prominent fatty and soft tissue components and an overall heterogeneous appearance. Given the large amount of nonfatty tissue, a simple lipoma would not be in the differential diagnosis, and a dedifferentiated subtype could be suggested. This lesion abuts and displaces the left kidney, a not uncommon occurrence with a large retroperitoneal mass, and therefore raises the possibility of an exophytic renal angiomyolipoma, but the lack of a claw sign in the kidney and an epicenter inferior to the kidney suggest that it is not.

More difficulties arise with a well-differentiated liposarcoma composed almost entirely of fat, where the distinction between lipoma and liposarcoma is not trivial. Although large size, poorly defined margins, the presence of septations with increased T2-signal intensity, or thick and nodular septations all favor the diagnosis of liposarcoma, it is not always possible to be absolutely certain of the diagnosis.

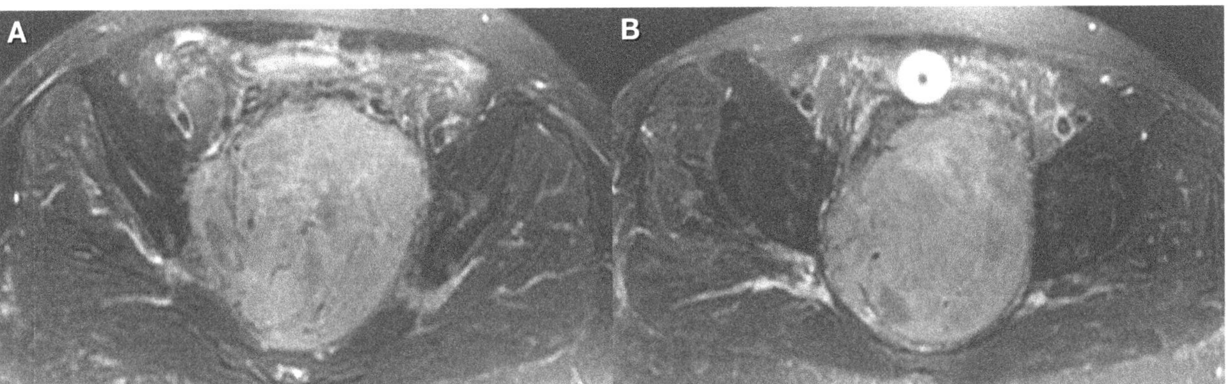

Figure 14.16.1

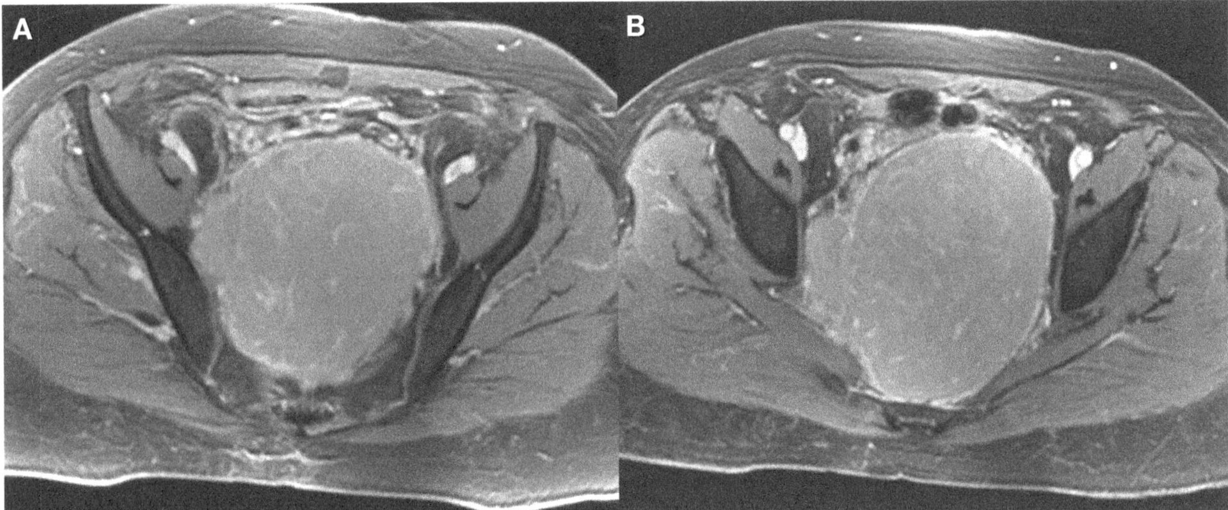

Figure 14.16.2

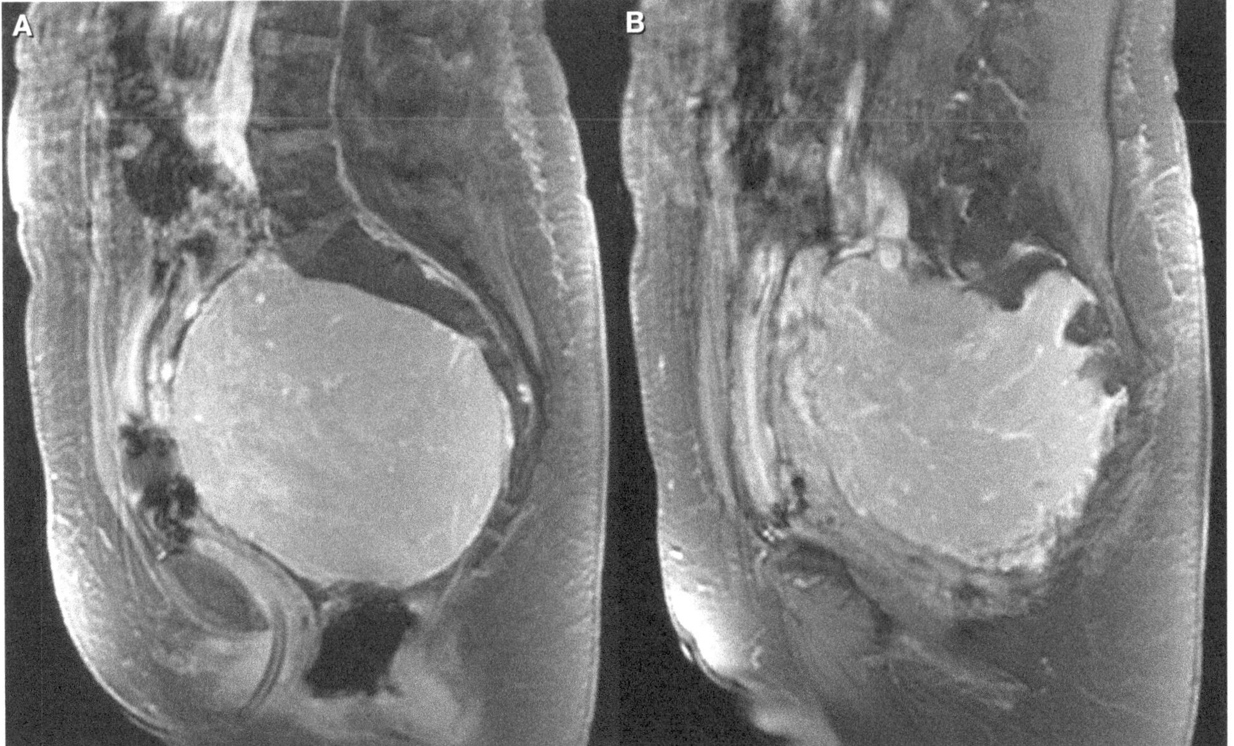

Figure 14.16.3

HISTORY: 57-year-old woman with leg numbness, hip pain, and diminished energy

IMAGING FINDINGS: Axial fat-suppressed FSE T2-weighted images (Figure 14.16.1) demonstrate a large pelvic mass displacing the bladder anteriorly with heterogeneous mildly increased signal intensity. Note also several small serpiginous flow voids within the lesion as well as a Foley catheter balloon in the collapsed bladder. Axial (Figure 14.16.2) and sagittal (Figure 14.16.3) post-gadolinium 2D SPGR images demonstrate fairly homogeneous enhancement of the mass with multiple small internal vessels and septations as well as extension into a sacral neuroforamen.

DIAGNOSIS: Hemangiopericytoma

COMMENT: Hemangiopericytomas arise from the pericytes of Zimmerman, which are contractile cells providing mechanical support to capillaries. The lower extremities, pelvis, and retroperitoneum are the most common locations, and most lesions occur in adults aged 40 to 50 years, although approximately 10% arise in children.

Hemangiopericytomas are almost always solitary lesions. Pelvic tumors are typically painless or associated with vague urinary or gastrointestinal tract symptoms and therefore are often quite large at diagnosis. Insulinlike growth factors have been found in tumor cells and cause hypoglycemia in some patients.

Histologically, hemangiopericytomas consist of spindle-shaped cells arranged in multiple layers surrounding thin-walled capillary channels lined with normal epithelial cells.

As is true for many of the lesions in this chapter, the MRI findings are relatively nonspecific. This example is fairly homogeneous; however, regions of necrosis and hemorrhage have been described, particularly in malignant neoplasms, and the differential diagnosis could include pelvic schwannoma and soft tissue sarcomas. Most hemangiopericytomas have high signal intensity on T2-weighted images and demonstrate intense enhancement, reflecting their vascular nature. One author has noted that the presence of prominent internal vascularity, as seen in this case, suggests the diagnosis, although this is not a very specific finding and can be seen in many varieties of sarcoma.

Metastases, most commonly to lungs and bone, have been identified in 10% to 60% of patients, with malignancy suggested by 4 or more mitoses per high-power field, foci of necrosis, and large size. Treatment is surgical excision; adjuvant radiotherapy and chemotherapy are of uncertain value.

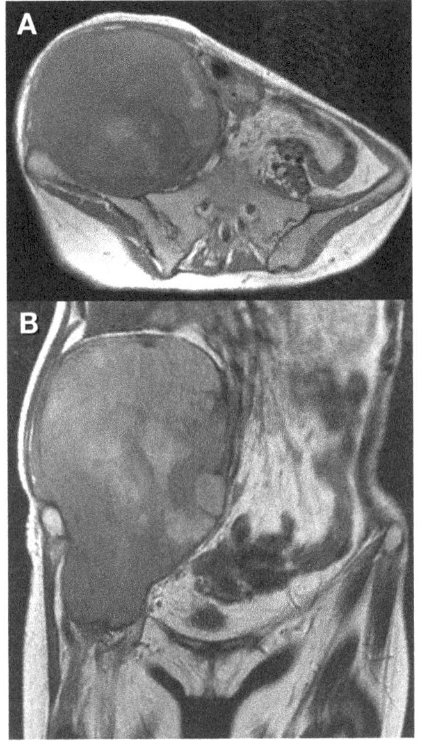

Figure 14.17.1

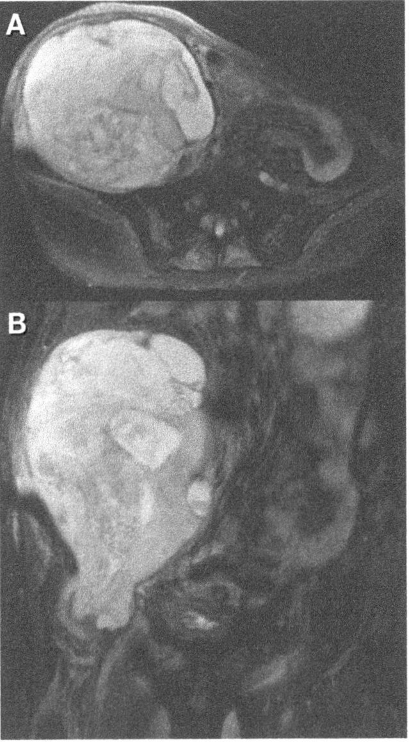

Figure 14.17.2

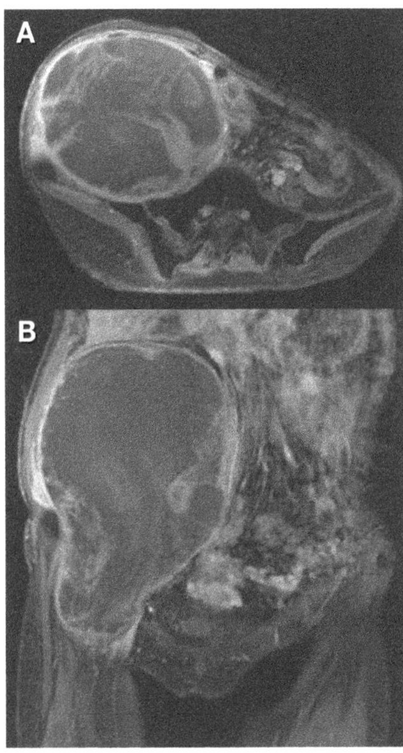

Figure 14.17.3

HISTORY: 30-year-old woman with a history of neurofibromatosis and a painful right thigh mass

IMAGING FINDINGS: Axial (Figure 14.17.1A) and coronal (Figure 14.17.1B) FSE T1-weighted images and axial (Figure 14.17.2A) and coronal (Figure 14.17.2B) fat-suppressed FSE T2-weighted images reveal a large heterogeneous mass in the right pelvis extending into the groin with high signal intensity on T2-weighted images and regions of low and high signal intensity on T1-weighted images. Axial (Figure 14.17.3A) and coronal (Figure 14.17.3B) postgadolinium 2D SPGR images demonstrate peripheral enhancement of the lesion and enhancement of septations and nodules centrally.

DIAGNOSIS: Malignant peripheral nerve sheath tumor

COMMENT: MPNSTs account for 3% to 10% of all soft tissue sarcomas; 25% to 50% of cases are associated with NF1, and 4% to 10% develop as late sequelae of radiotherapy. Although NF1 accounts for a significant percentage of MPNST cases, only 4% of patients with NF1 will develop MPNST during their lives. Most MPNSTs occur in major nerve trunks, such as the brachial plexus, lumbosacral plexus, or sciatic nerve. Patients are typically between 20 and 50 years of age and present with pain, paresthesias, neurologic dysfunction, and a palpable mass.

The large, dominant, heterogeneous mass in this case is obviously worrisome, but the distinction between MPNST and a benign neurofibroma is not always straightforward. Several authors have proposed signs more frequently associated with malignant lesions, including large size, intratumoral cystic or necrotic regions, peripheral enhancement or perilesional edema, infiltrative margin, and lack of continuity with a nerve.

The appearance of MPNSTs on MRI is similar to that of many other soft tissue sarcomas: heterogeneous increased T2-signal intensity with regions of cystic degeneration or necrosis and irregular enhancement after gadolinium administration. Histologically, the cellular elements of MPNSTs resemble Schwann cells, with densely cellular areas alternating with hypocellular myxoid regions. Perineural and intraneural extension suggests neurogenic origin and therefore MPNST. The immunohistochemical markers S-100 protein, Leu-7, and myelin basic protein also indicate a neurogenic origin but are not specific for MPNST.

MPNSTs are highly aggressive, with rapid invasive growth and early hematogenous dissemination. Even after surgery, the prognosis is limited, with 5-year survival rates of 20% to 50%.

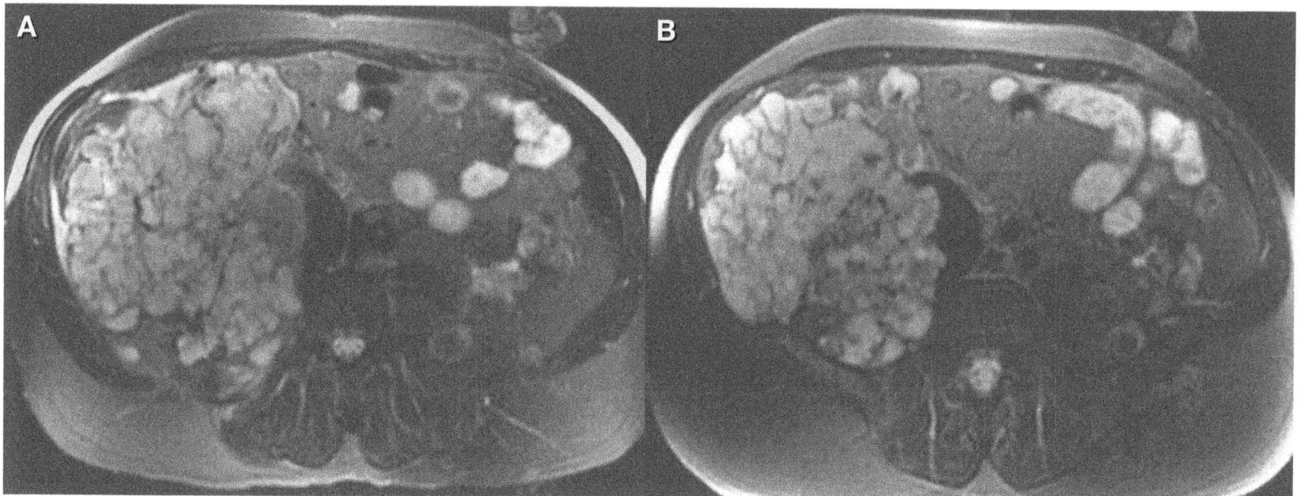

Figure 14.18.1

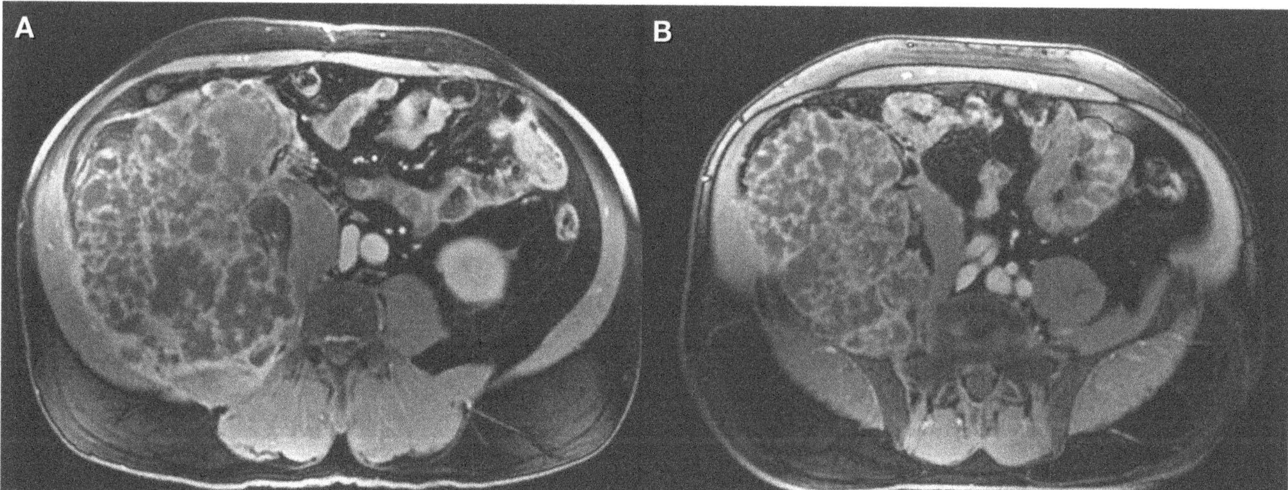

Figure 14.18.2

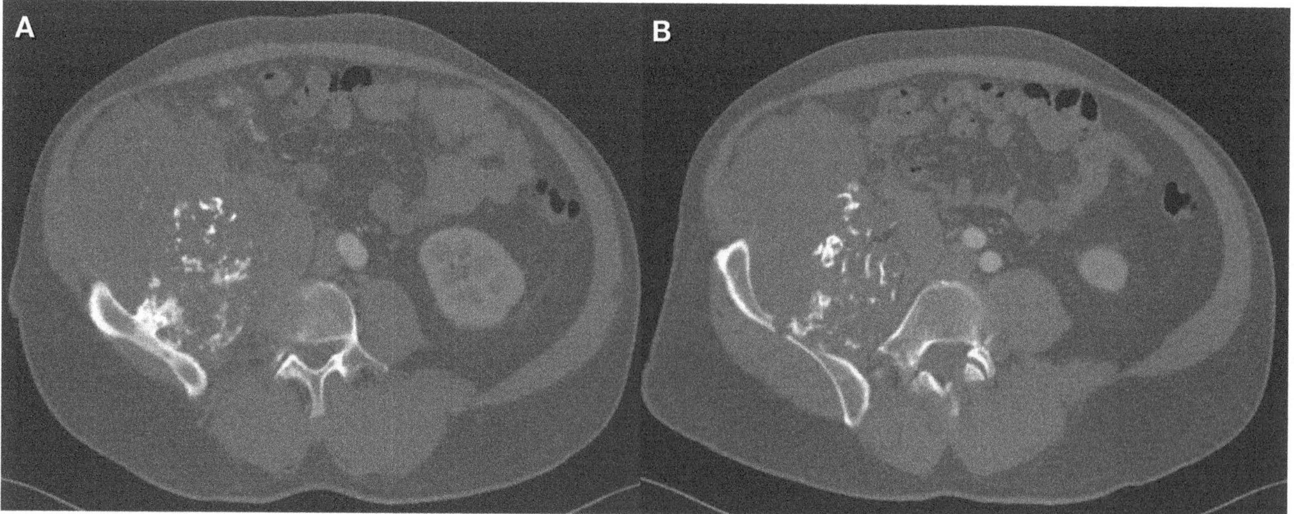

Figure 14.18.3

HISTORY: 52-year-old man with right upper quadrant pain and a right abdominal mass

IMAGING FINDINGS: Axial fat-suppressed FSE T2-weighted images (Figure 14.18.1) demonstrate a large, hyperintense lobulated mass arising from the right iliac bone. Axial postgadolinium 3D SPGR images (Figure 14.18.2) reveal mild enhancement of the multiple septations within the lesion. Note the prominent mass effect and distortion involving the adjacent psoas muscle. Axial CT images (Figure 14.18.3) demonstrate destructive changes in the right ilium and chondroid matrix within the lesion.

DIAGNOSIS: Conventional chondrosarcoma

COMMENT: Chondrosarcoma is the third most common primary malignant tumor of bone after multiple myeloma and osteosarcoma, and it is also the most common primary malignant tumor of the pelvic bones, accounting for 32% of cases. Chondrosarcoma is characterized by malignant proliferation of cells that produce chondroid matrix and is classified in several ways, including origin (primary or secondary; ie, from enchondromas or osteochondromas), location (central, peripheral, or juxtacortical), and histology (clear cell, myxoid, or mesenchymal).

The appearance on MRI depends to some extent on the grade of the lesion: Low-grade lesions have well-defined margins, cortical expansion, and chondroid matrix; high-grade tumors have a more aggressive permeative pattern of destruction with ill-defined margins and prominent soft tissue components. Pelvic chondrosarcomas are usually low grade, as in this case, and the prominent lobules of chondroid matrix with high T2-signal intensity separated by low-signal-intensity fibrovascular septations are fairly typical. The "rings and arcs" terminology used to describe the pattern of mineralization seen on plain radiographs and CT could apply just as well to the pattern seen on MRI, although it represents unmineralized rather than mineralized chondroid matrix.

Clear cell chondrosarcoma is characterized by cells with clear, vacuolated cytoplasm containing large amounts of glycogen and, unlike conventional chondrosarcoma, frequently contains large areas of hemorrhage or cyst formation. Myxoid chondrosarcoma may occur both in bone and in soft tissue and contains abundant myxoid stroma. Mesenchymal chondrosarcoma is characterized by regions of small uniform cells resembling those of Ewing sarcoma. Conventional intramedullary chondrosarcoma is the most common variant and usually manifests in the fourth to fifth decades of life. The long tubular bones are the most common sites of origin; however, as noted above, the pelvis is frequently involved, with the innominate bone accounting for 25% of cases.

Pelvic chondrosarcomas are often quite large at diagnosis because the associated symptoms are frequently minor and nonspecific and the lesions tend to be surprisingly inconspicuous on plain radiographs. The differential diagnosis includes metastasis, myeloma, Ewing sarcoma, osteosarcoma, fibrosarcoma, and malignant fibrous histiocytoma. Mineralization, particularly the presence of chondroid matrix, is a key distinguishing feature that is generally absent in Ewing sarcoma, myeloma or plasmacytoma, metastasis, malignant fibrous histiocytoma, and fibrosarcoma. Although MRI is not the ideal technique for visualizing mineralized chondroid matrix, it is very useful for defining the extent of the tumor and for detecting invasion of adjacent structures and distant metastases.

The prognosis for patients with pelvic chondrosarcoma is moderate, with an overall 5-year survival rate of 59%.

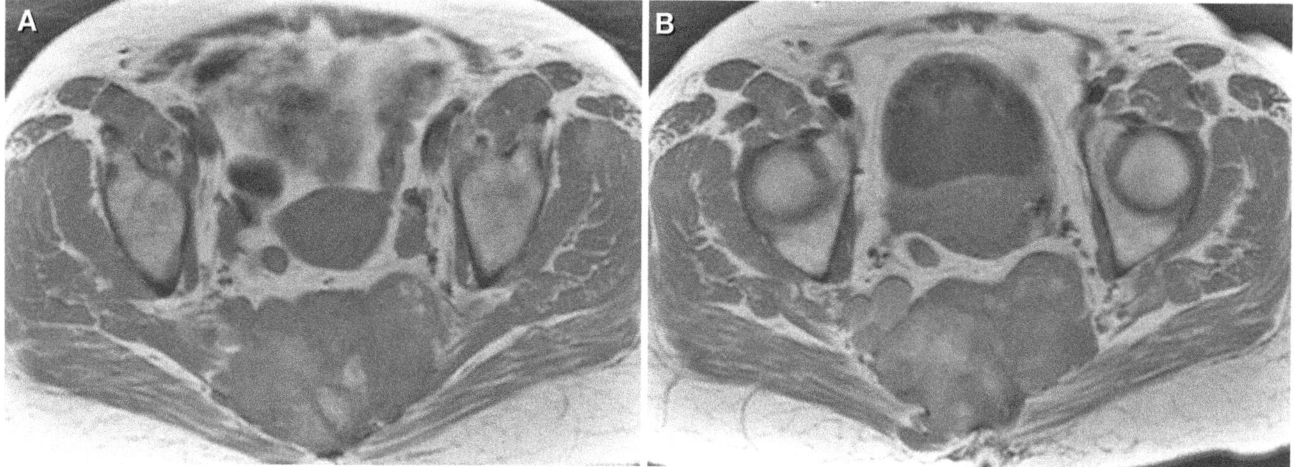

Figure 14.19.1

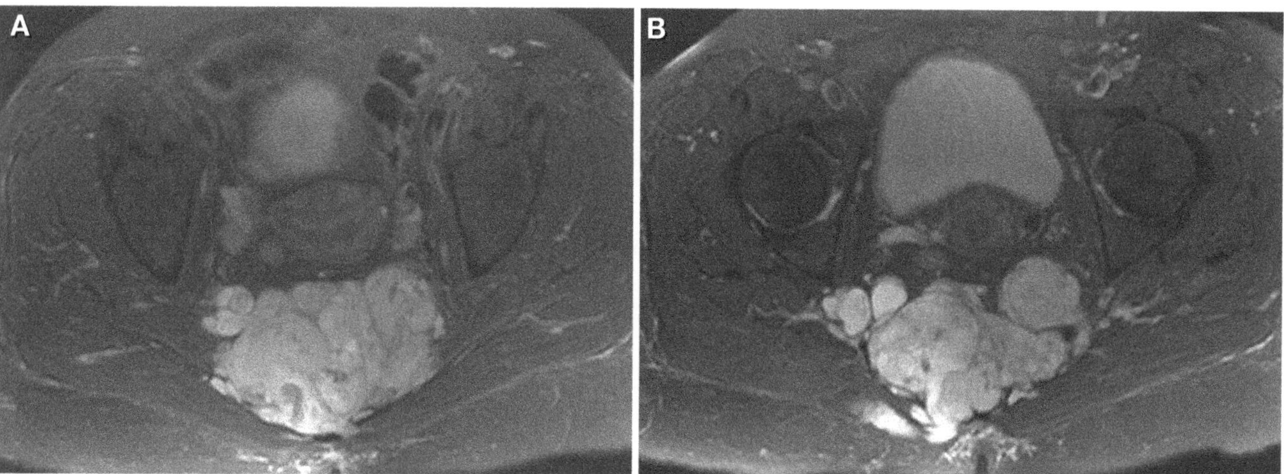

Figure 14.19.2

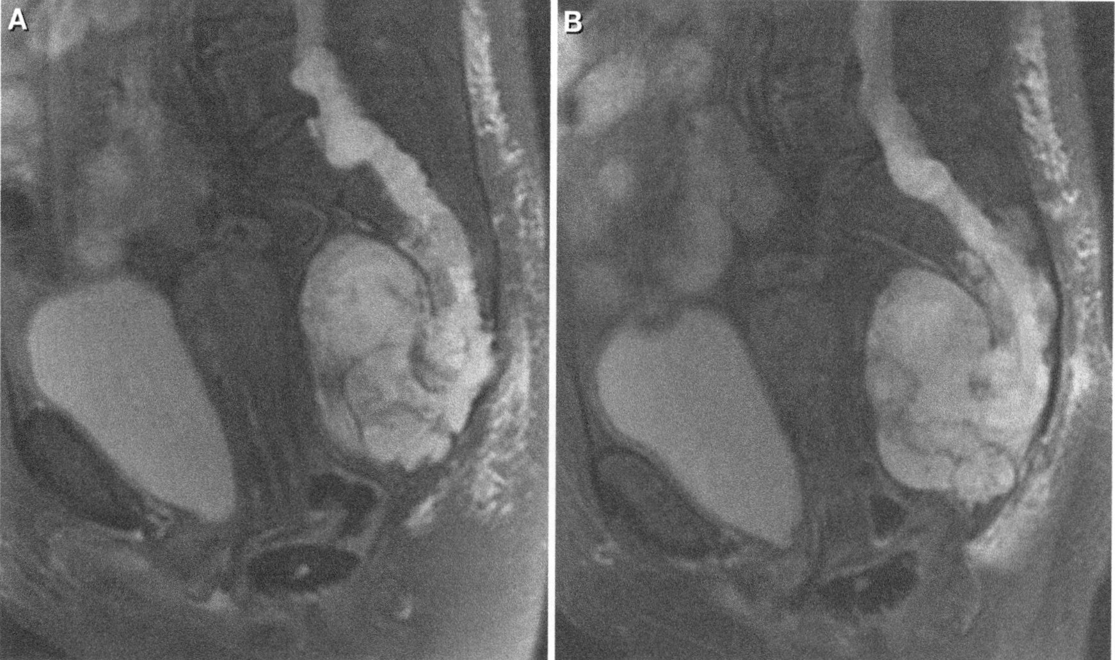

Figure 14.19.3

HISTORY: 52-year-old woman with a sacral mass that was incidentally identified after minor trauma

IMAGING FINDINGS: Axial T1-weighted FSE images (Figure 14.19.1) and fat-suppressed T2-weighted FSE images (Figure 14.19.2) reveal a lobulated mass with marked T2 hyperintensity originating in the sacrum and having a large anterior soft tissue component. The mass is predominantly hypointense to skeletal muscle on the T1-weighted images, with smaller regions of increased signal intensity. Sagittal fat-suppressed T2-weighted FSE images (Figure 14.19.3) demonstrate similar findings as well as extension of the tumor superiorly along the spinal canal.

DIAGNOSIS: Sacral chordoma

COMMENT: Chordoma is a rare neoplasm accounting for 2% to 4% of all primary malignant bone tumors, but it is the most common primary malignant sacral tumor. Chordomas were first characterized in 1857 by Virchow, who described unique intracellular bubble-like vacuoles, which he termed physaliphorous. These vacuoles remain a distinguishing pathologic feature of chordomas. Chordomas are derived from undifferentiated notochord remnants (hence the name) that reside in vertebral bodies and the axial skeleton. Historically, the sacrum has been considered the most common location; however, more recent data suggest an equal distribution in the sacrum, spine, and skull base.

Chordomas have a male predominance, and patients typically present between 50 and 60 years of age. The tumors are often large at diagnosis because the symptoms are mild and nonspecific; they include pain, numbness, constipation, incontinence, and weakness. The nonspecific symptoms of pelvic bone tumors also explain why the diagnosis is occasionally made by an abdominal radiologist on an examination performed to assess for intra-abdominal disease.

Chordomas usually appear as a large destructive midline sacral mass, often with prominent soft tissue extension. Regions of punctate calcification may be seen on CT. The most striking feature of chordomas on MRI is high signal intensity on T2-weighted images. T1-weighted images typically show signal intensity hypointense or isointense to skeletal muscle; however, regions of hemorrhage or mucinous degeneration may show focal hyperintensity. Modest enhancement is seen after gadolinium administration.

The differential diagnosis of destructive sacral tumors includes giant cell tumor, chondrosarcoma, ependymoma, plasmacytoma, and metastasis. Giant cell tumors are the second most common primary sacral neoplasm and tend to involve the upper sacrum, often with an eccentric location that may extend across the sacroiliac joint. They may have low to intermediate signal intensity on T2-weighted images, in contrast to the high signal intensity seen with chordomas, although this is not universally true. Chondrosarcomas are also more likely to have an eccentric location; they often demonstrate a chondroid matrix; and they are only rarely hemorrhagic.

The prognosis for patients with chordoma is generally determined by local recurrence rather than metastatic disease, although 5% of patients have metastatic disease at presentation, and as many as 65% with advanced disease may have metastases. Overall survival rates are 68% at 5 years and 40% at 10 years. Clinical management of sacral chordoma is often difficult because of the frequently large tumor burden at presentation and the involvement of adjacent structures. Complete surgical excision is often not possible, and although adjuvant radiotherapy does improve disease-free survival, chordomas are fairly resistant to radiotherapy.

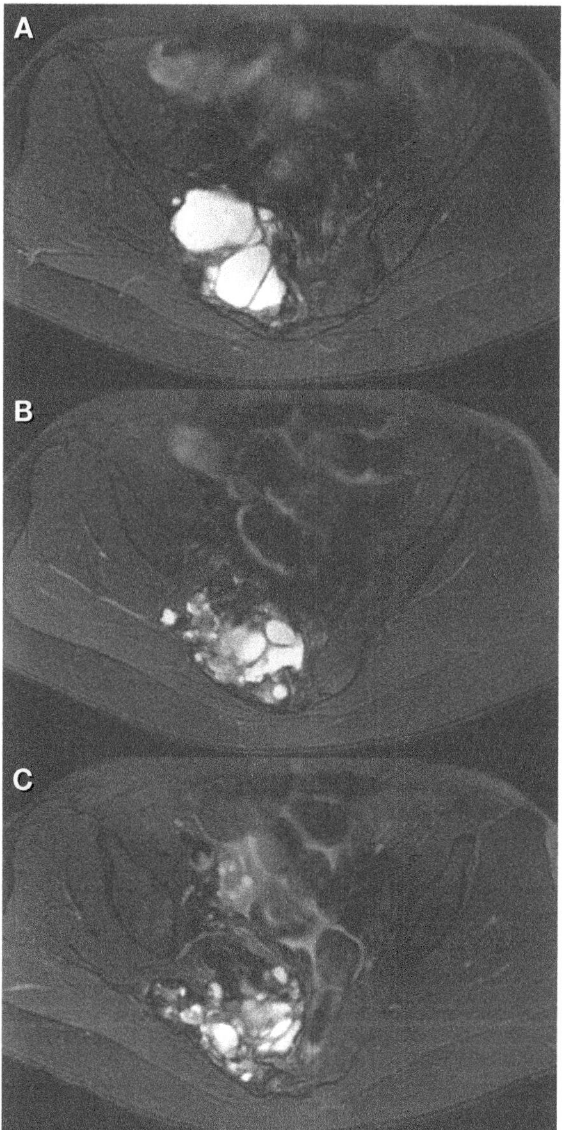

Figure 14.20.1

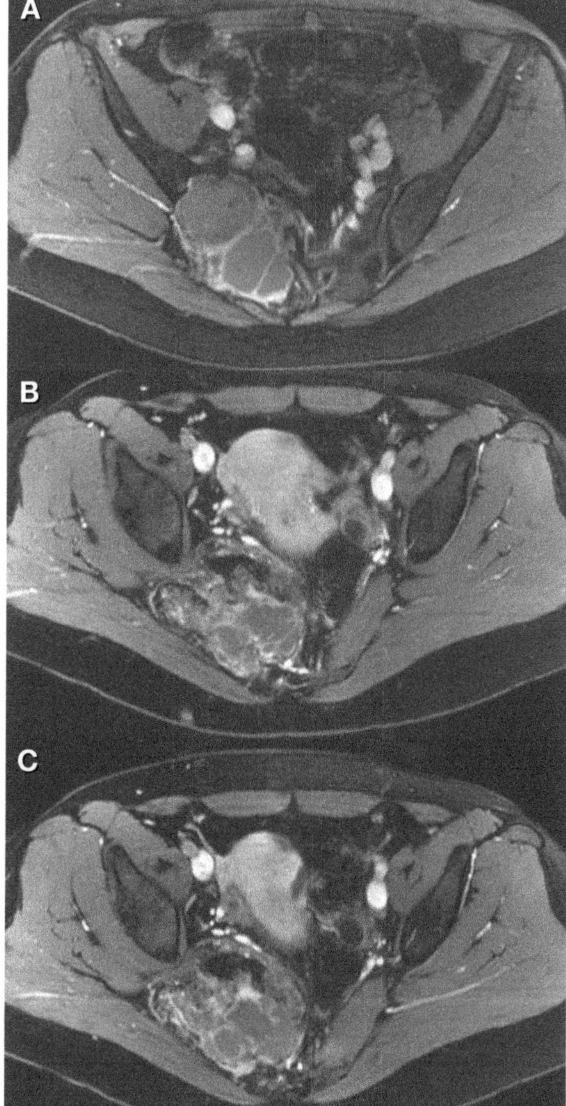

Figure 14.20.2

HISTORY: 29-year-old woman with gradually increasing intermittent back pain

IMAGING FINDINGS: Axial fat-suppressed FSE T2-weighted images (Figure 14.20.1) demonstrate a complex multicystic mass involving the right sacrum, sacroiliac joint, and iliac bone. Axial postgadolinium 2D SPGR images (Figure 14.20.2) reveal similar findings, with prominent enhancement of the septations separating the cystic components of the lesion.

DIAGNOSIS: Giant cell tumor

COMMENT: Giant cell tumors are uncommon neoplasms that account for approximately 5% of all primary bone tumors in adults and occur most frequently in the ends of long bones. They most commonly manifest in patients aged 20 to 45 years. The sacrum is an unusual location (2%-8% of all lesions), and in the classic description the tumors tend to involve the cephalad portion of the sacrum, often in a peripheral location.

The majority of these tumors are benign but locally aggressive lesions; recurrence after initial therapy is 2.3% to 57%, depending on the location, surgical accessibility, and mode of treatment. Malignant transformation may occur, however, and has been reported in 16% of primary lesions and in as many as 30% of recurrent lesions. Most malignant lesions arise after radiotherapy. Pulmonary metastases, reported in 3% of cases, may arise from either benign or malignant tumors (seeding is thought to occur in benign lesions during surgical manipulation of the primary tumor).

Giant cell tumors are osteolytic lesions that lack sclerotic margins and usually any periosteal reaction on plain radiographs and CT. MRI often demonstrates multilobulated lesions that may contain cystic components (with or without fluid-fluid levels) related to internal hemorrhage or aneurysmal bone cyst elements as well as solid components. Imaging characteristics depend on whether cystic or solid components are predominant and on the content of the cystic elements (simple fluid or hemorrhagic material). The differential diagnosis for a sacral giant cell tumor includes plasmacytoma, metastasis, chordoma, and chondrosarcoma. The eccentric location, multicystic appearance, and lack of previous history of malignancy helped to suggest the diagnosis in this case.

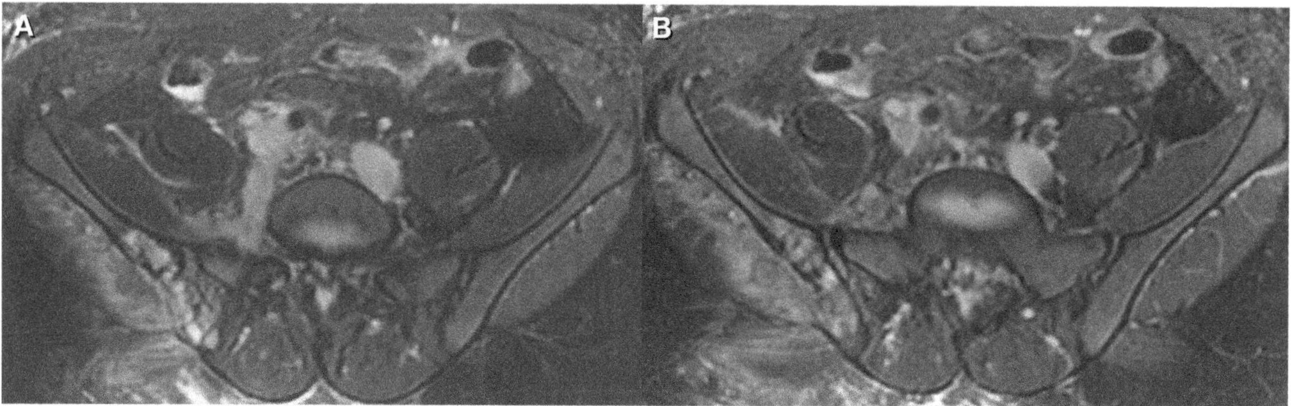

Figure 14.21.1

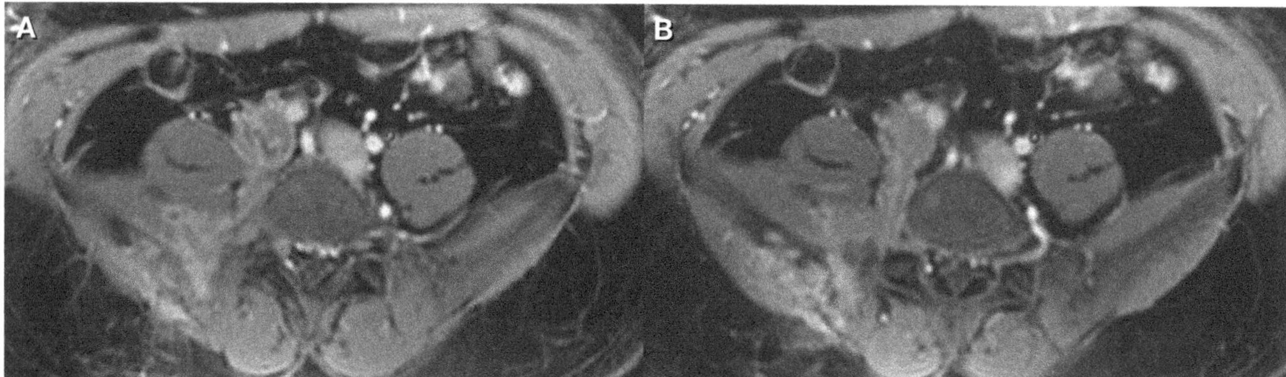

Figure 14.21.2

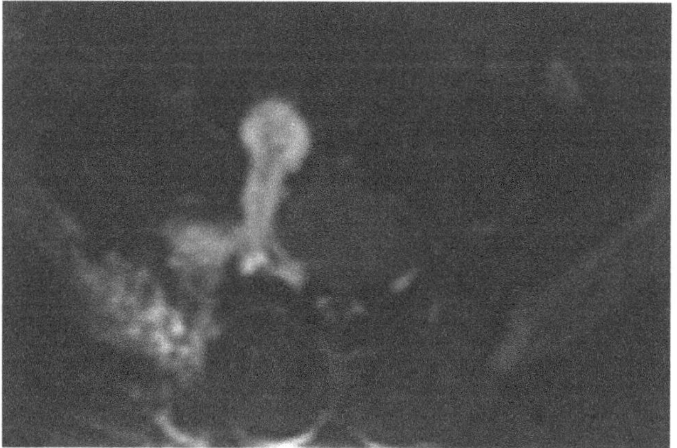

Figure 14.21.3

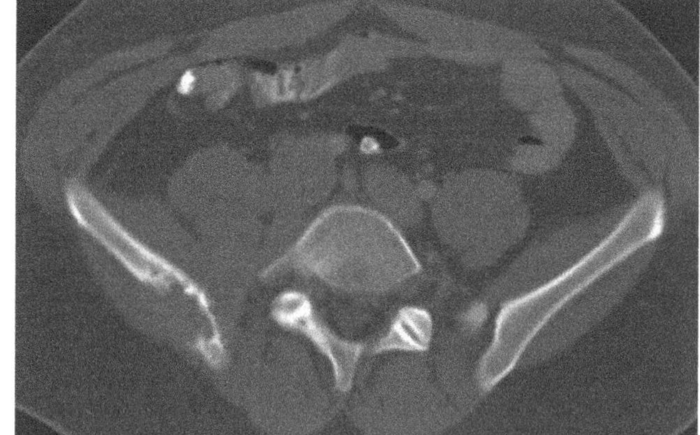

Figure 14.21.4

HISTORY: 26-year-old man with an acute onset of right leg redness and swelling

IMAGING FINDINGS: Axial fat-suppressed FSE T2-weighted images (Figure 14.21.1) demonstrate expansion of the right common and internal iliac veins by a heterogeneous tumor thrombus that extends toward the right ilium, where infiltrative increased signal intensity involves bone and the adjacent muscle. Axial postgadolinium 2D SPGR images (Figure 14.21.2) reveal the iliac vein tumor thrombus and irregular enhancement in the right iliac bone and adjacent gluteal muscle, corresponding to the region of heterogeneous increased signal intensity on T2-weighted images. Axial diffusion-weighted image (b=600 s/mm^2) (Figure 14.21.3) also demonstrates the tumor thrombus in the right iliac vein extending toward an ill-defined lesion in the iliac bone. Axial CT image (Figure 14.21.4) confirms the presence of a lytic lesion in the upper right ilium.

DIAGNOSIS: Ewing sarcoma with iliac vein tumor thrombus

COMMENT: Ewing sarcoma is a malignant tumor characterized by small round cells arranged in a sheetlike configuration. It accounts for 5% of all primary bone malignancies and is the second most common primary bone tumor in children. The pelvis is the second most common site of origin after the femur, accounting for 18% of cases in a Mayo Clinic series, and Ewing sarcoma comprises 22% of the primary pelvic bone malignancies in children. Ewing sarcoma has a peak incidence in patients aged 10 to 20 years and has a slight male predominance.

The classic appearance on radiographs is a permeative destructive lesion with ill-defined margins. Findings on MRI are nonspecific and can be difficult to distinguish from other malignancies: low signal intensity on T1-weighted images and heterogeneous increased T2-signal intensity, often with regions of necrosis and a prominent soft tissue mass. The differential diagnosis includes osteomyelitis (which usually has a more rapid clinical onset and less prominent soft tissue component), osteosarcoma (distinguished by mineralized matrix, not well seen on MRI), lymphoma, and metastases.

The prognosis for patients with pelvic Ewing sarcoma is guarded, with 5-year survival of approximately 45%. Survival is lower than for patients with lesions involving the extremities, probably because of delayed detection and greater difficulty in achieving complete resection and local control. The patient in this case, for example, had venous invasion with tumor thrombus extending into the iliac vein; the thrombus was seen well on the diffusion-weighted, FSE T2-weighted, and postgadolinium images and was responsible for his presenting symptoms. (The question of venous thrombosis was also what moved this case from musculoskeletal to body MRI jurisdiction.)

Extraskeletal Ewing sarcoma is fairly common and probably accounts for 30% of all lesions. These tumors are even more difficult to classify and generally have an appearance on MRI similar to that of other soft tissue sarcomas (eg, Case 14.22). A large study demonstrated that survival for patients with localized extraskeletal Ewing sarcoma was slightly better than survival for patients with skeletal lesions but found little difference in prognosis for patients with locally advanced or metastatic disease.

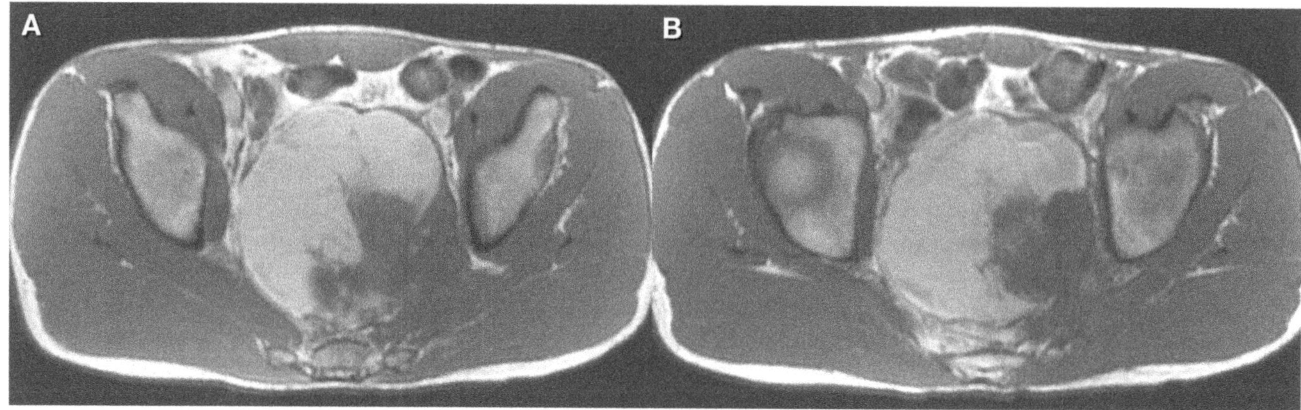

Figure 14.22.1

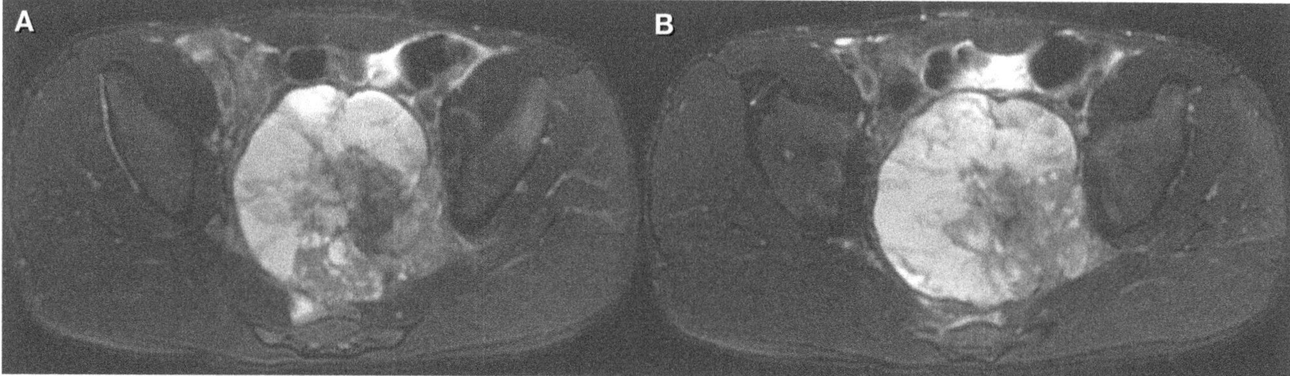

Figure 14.22.2

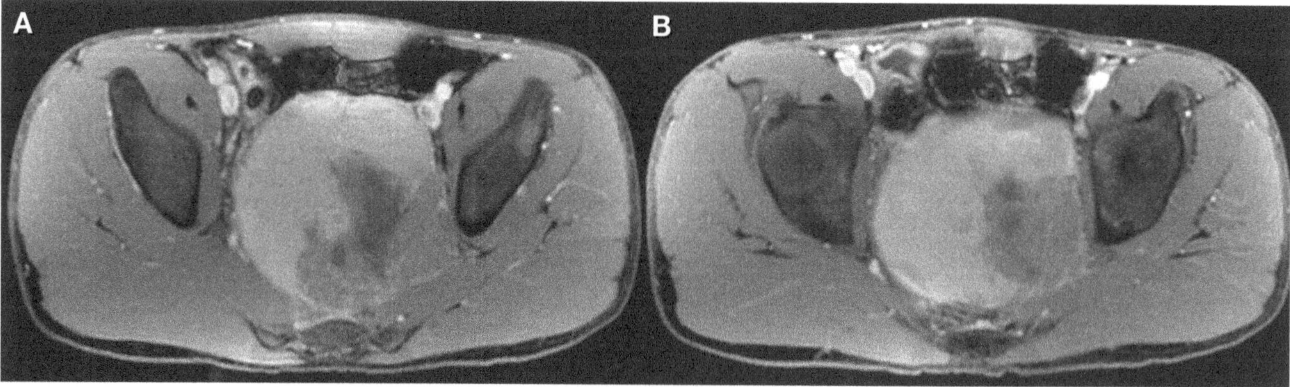

Figure 14.22.3

HISTORY: 17-year-old male adolescent with intermittent testicular pain; CT from another medical facility demonstrated a pelvic mass

IMAGING FINDINGS: Axial FSE T1-weighted images (Figure 14.22.1) and fat-suppressed FSE T2-weighted images (Figure 14.22.2) demonstrate a large heterogeneous pelvic mass with regions of high signal intensity on both T1- and T2-weighted images and a more solid-appearing component posteriorly. Axial postgadolinium 2D SPGR images (Figure 14.22.3) reveal increased signal intensity corresponding to the regions of high T2-signal intensity (likely nonenhancing hemorrhagic or proteinaceous material) and mild enhancement of the posterior solid component.

DIAGNOSIS: Extraskeletal Ewing sarcoma

COMMENT: This case is a companion to the case of skeletal Ewing sarcoma (Case 14.21). Extraskeletal Ewing sarcoma is less common but not extremely rare and, as noted previously (Comment section, Case 14.21), is thought to account for approximately 30% of all cases. The appearance on MRI is often heterogeneous, as in this case. The regions of high signal intensity on T1-weighted images might raise the possibility of liposarcoma; however, they remain very bright on fat-suppressed T2-weighted images and have moderately high signal intensity on the fat-suppressed postgadolinium SPGR images and therefore indicate proteinaceous or hemorrhagic material rather than fat. This mass is more heterogeneous than the previous examples of pelvic schwannoma (Case 14.12) and hemangiopericytoma (Case 14.16). Because of this appearance, one could reasonably assume that this lesion is malignant rather than benign; however, the differential diagnosis certainly includes most soft tissue sarcomas.

CASE 14.23

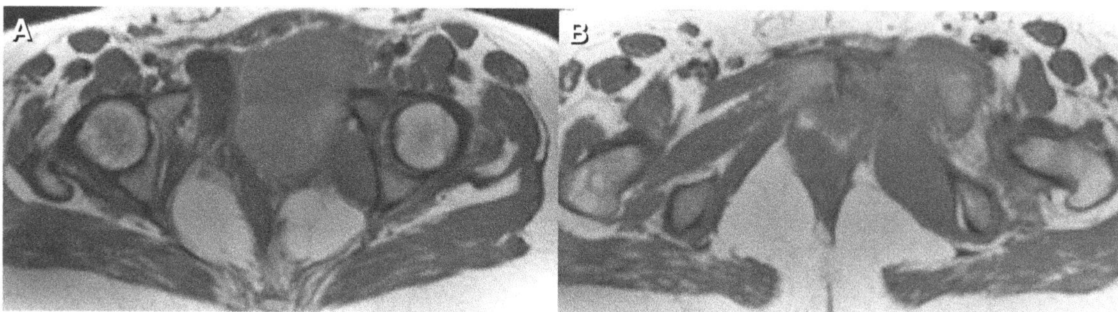

Figure 14.23.1

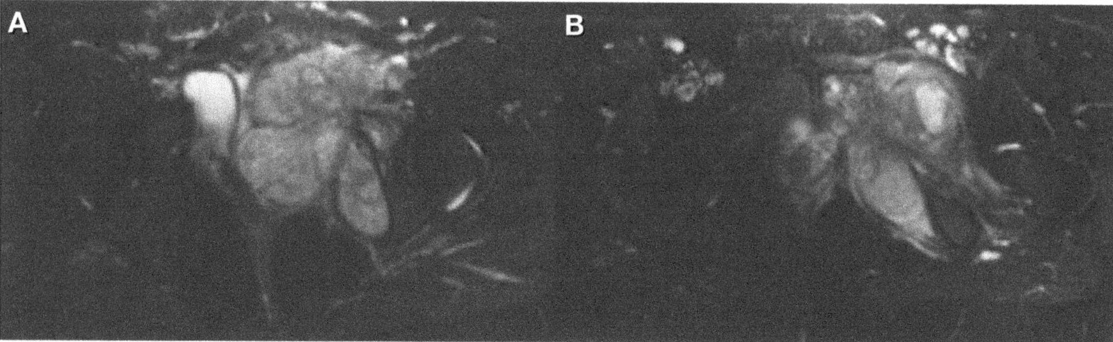

Figure 14.23.2

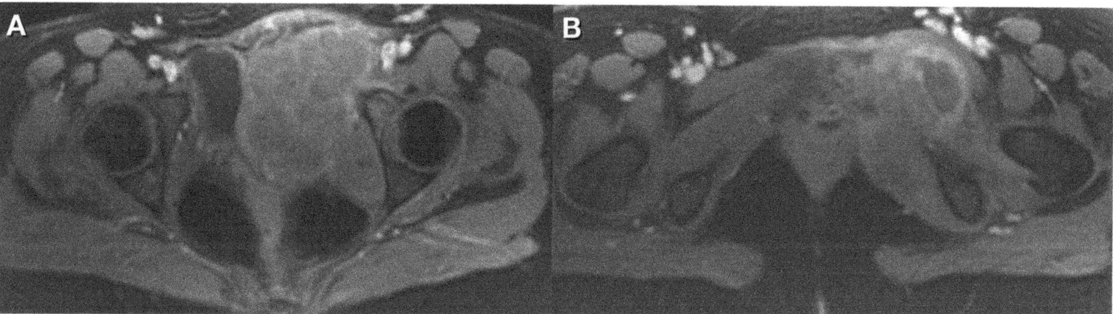

Figure 14.23.3

HISTORY: 32-year-old woman with a complex pelvic mass that was incidentally detected on prenatal US

IMAGING FINDINGS: Axial FSE T1-weighted images (Figure 14.23.1) and fat-suppressed FSE T2-weighted images (Figure 14.23.2) demonstrate a heterogeneous mass with moderately high T2-signal intensity and low T1-signal intensity originating from the left superior pubic ramus. Prominent soft tissue components extend both anteriorly and posteriorly from the epicenter of the lesion. Axial postgadolinium 2D SPGR images (Figure 14.23.3) reveal heterogeneous enhancement of the mass.

DIAGNOSIS: Osteosarcoma

COMMENT: Osteosarcoma is the second most common primary bone malignancy after multiple myeloma and is characterized by proliferation of neoplastic osteoid matrix with various amounts of cartilage, fibrous tissue, and other connective tissue components. Depending on the dominant cell type, osteosarcomas can be classified as osteoblastic (50%-80%), fibroblastic (7%-25%), chondroblastic (5%-25%), telangiectatic (2%-12%), or small cell (1%).

Approximately 8% of osteosarcomas occur in the pelvis, and osteosarcoma accounts for 2% of all pelvic primary bone malignancies. Most osteosarcomas occur in the second or third decade of life; a second incidence peak includes older patients who have tumors that generally are complications of prior radiotherapy or occur with Paget disease.

The appearance of osteosarcoma on MRI is nonspecific and depends partly on the classification. Lesions are often fairly large, with a prominent soft tissue component. Osteoid matrix exhibits low signal intensity on all imaging sequences; however, many lesions (including this case) show intermediate T1-signal intensity, high T2-signal intensity, and heterogeneous enhancement.

The prognosis is worse with pelvic osteosarcoma than with lesions in the extremities; the 5-year survival rate is approximately 20%. This is probably related to the relatively large size of most lesions at diagnosis and to the difficulty in achieving complete surgical resection.

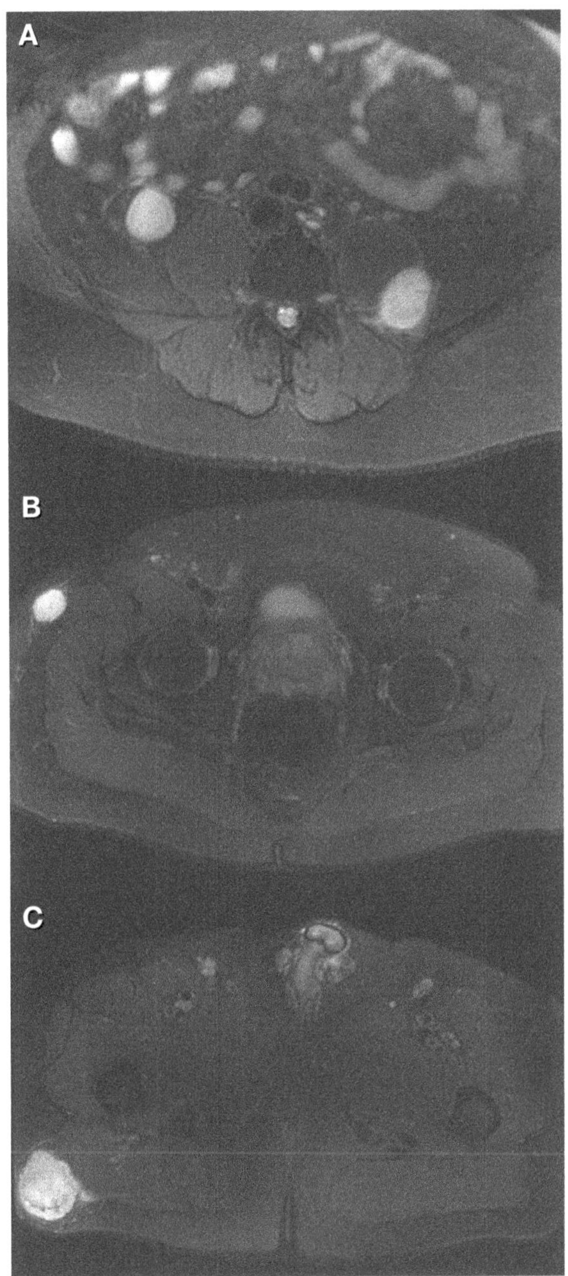

Figure 14.24.1

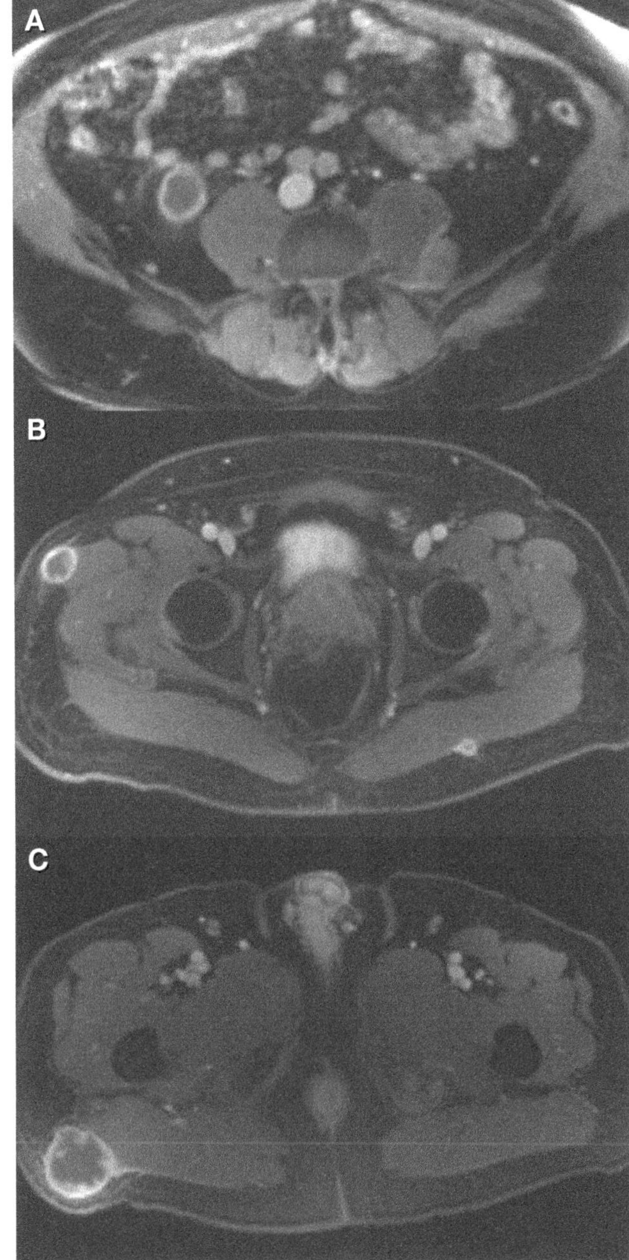

Figure 14.24.2

HISTORY: 64-year-old man with right buttock pain and lower extremity weakness

IMAGING FINDINGS: Axial fat-suppressed FSE T2-weighted images (Figure 14.24.1) demonstrate multiple markedly hyperintense masses involving the paraspinous regions bilaterally and the anterior and posterior right lower pelvis. Axial postgadolinium 2D SPGR images (Figure 14.24.2) reveal similar findings, with prominent ring enhancement of the lesions. Note the additional small enhancing lesion in the left gluteal muscle.

DIAGNOSIS: Metastatic melanoma

COMMENT: Melanoma is the least common but most lethal skin cancer. The worldwide incidence of melanoma is increasing, and this is thought to be related to a combination of increased exposure to UV radiation and improved detection through screening. In the United States, the lifetime risk of developing malignant melanoma increased from 1 in 1,500 in 1930 to 1 in 75 in 2000.

Melanoma confined to the epidermis is curable; 5-year survival for patients with thin lesions is greater than 98%. For patients with lesions more than 4 mm thick, however, 5-year survival is less than 50%.

Melanoma metastases are famous in the radiology community for 2 properties: They can be found anywhere, and when they contain abundant amounts of melanin they may appear as bright lesions on T1-weighted images. Nearly every radiologist has overlooked a subcutaneous or muscular melanoma metastasis at least once (and likely several times), usually on CT, because the metastases can blend into the adjacent tissues without much contrast unless they are imaged during the arterial phase. Subcutaneous and muscular melanoma metastases are generally easier to detect on MRI, where they appear as hyperintense lesions on fat-suppressed T2-weighted images or on diffusion-weighted images and as hyperenhancing lesions after gadolinium administration. It's worth remembering that you have to image a metastasis in order to see it (body protocols not uncommonly cut off the uninteresting subcutaneous and muscular margins of the abdomen and pelvis) and that you have to inspect the bones, muscles, and subcutaneous tissues to find all the lesions.

Lymph nodes are the most common site for melanoma metastases, and lung and liver lesions are also very common; however, autopsy studies have shown that soft tissue metastases are present in more than two-thirds of patients who die of melanoma.

The issue of T1 hyperintensity usually arises in discussions of hepatic metastases. Melanin-rich lesions can occur anywhere, however, and therefore, a T1-hyperintense soft tissue lesion, particularly if it enhances and is bright on diffusion-weighted and T2-weighted images, should not be an unexpected finding in a patient with malignant melanoma.

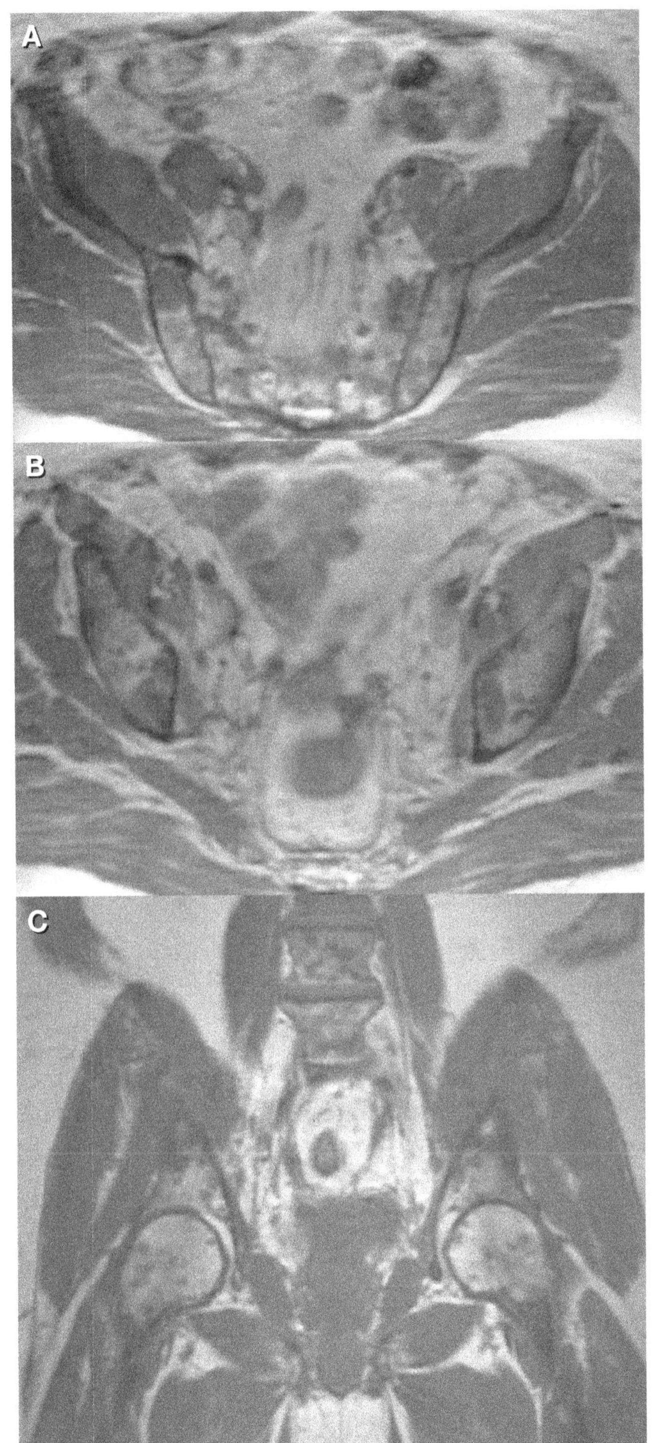

Figure 14.25.1

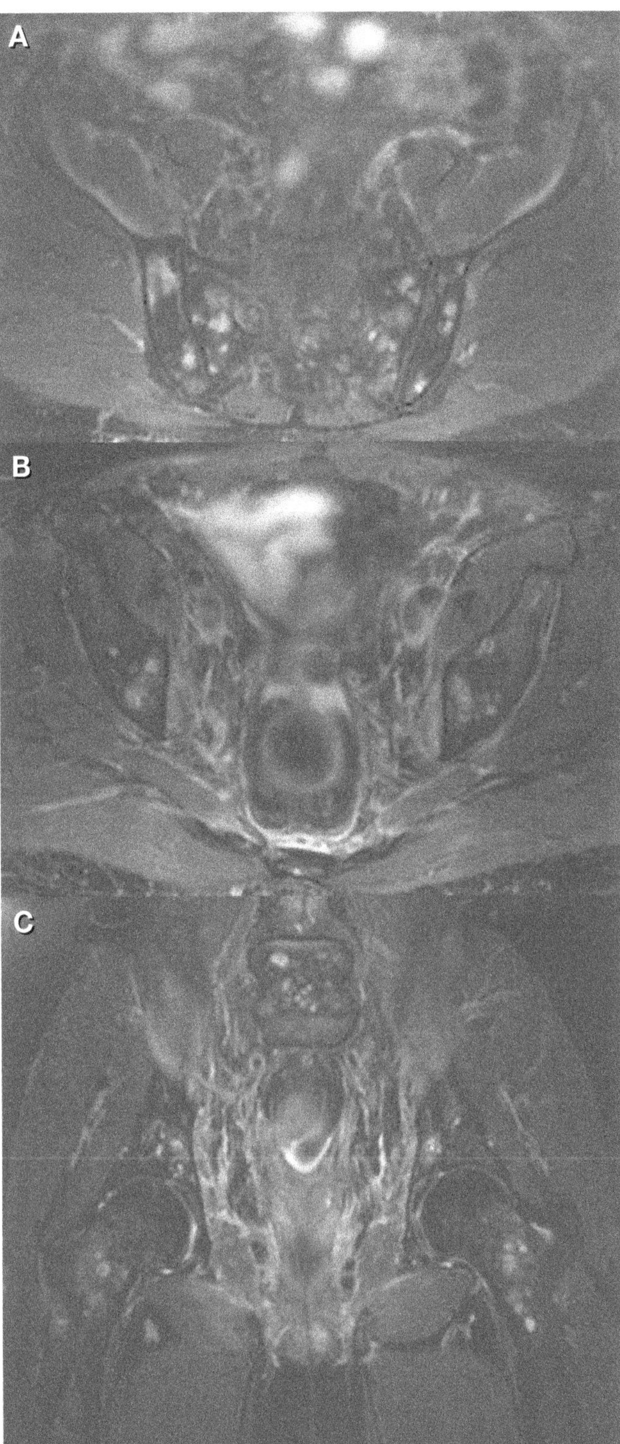

Figure 14.25.2

HISTORY: 60-year-old man with a history of prostate carcinoma

IMAGING FINDINGS: Axial (Figure 14.25.1A and 14.25.1B) and coronal (Figure 14.25.1C) T1-weighted FSE images and axial (Figure 14.25.2A and 14.25.2B) and coronal (Figure 14.25.2C) fat-suppressed T2-weighted FSE images reveal innumerable small lesions involving the lumbar spine, pelvic bones, and proximal femurs, which show decreased T1-signal intensity and increased T2-signal intensity relative to normal marrow.

DIAGNOSIS: Bone metastases from prostate cancer

COMMENT: Prostate carcinoma is the most common non-skin cancer in men in the United States, with approximately 200,000 new cases diagnosed annually and 28,000 deaths per year. Although prostate-specific antigen screening is controversial, it is widely used in the United States and has resulted in the diagnosis of more early-stage disease. Patients with early-stage disease can be offered potentially curative therapy such as radical prostatectomy, external beam radiotherapy, or radiation seed placement.

In most screening trials, metastatic disease is present at diagnosis in less than 10% of patients, and algorithms based on the prostate-specific antigen value and Gleason score are typically used to determine which patients are at high risk for metastatic disease and require additional imaging. Since the most common metastatic sites are bone and lymph nodes, assessment of the skeletal system is an important part of the workup: Skeletal metastases develop in approximately 70% of patients with advanced local disease. Most guidelines still recommend technetium Tc 99m bone scintigraphy, whose major virtue is its wide availability. Technetium 99m bone scans detect bone metastases at a relatively advanced stage of tumor infiltration, when osteoblastic reaction to tumor deposits occurs. It is well known that bone scans have relatively low sensitivity and specificity for detection of metastases. FDG PET is also relatively insensitive for detection of bone metastases; however, more specific markers, such as FDG-fluoride, and carbon C 11- or FDG-labeled choline and acetate have shown very high sensitivity and specificity for detection of bone metastases in limited trials.

MRI with standard T1-weighted and fat-suppressed T2-weighted imaging, as in this case, is fairly effective and has outperformed bone scintigraphy in most investigations. Metastases generally appear as focal lesions with decreased T1- and increased T2-signal intensity. Difficulties may arise, however, with diffusely heterogeneous bone marrow (red marrow hyperplasia, iron deposition, etc) or with more diffuse, nonfocal metastatic marrow infiltration. Rib imaging with MRI is also notoriously difficult; consequently, detection of a solitary rib metastasis as part of a screening examination is problematic. The addition of gadolinium-enhanced 2D or 3D SPGR images is helpful and can improve both sensitivity and specificity. Bone islands, for example, show decreased T1-signal intensity and are usually (but not always) isointense on T2-weighted images. This appearance is similar to sclerotic metastases; however, bone islands, unlike more avidly enhancing metastases, typically show little if any enhancement after gadolinium administration. Dynamic gadolinium-enhanced perfusion imaging has been advocated by some authors as an effective technique for identifying and characterizing bone metastases, although this is difficult to implement in a screening examination.

Whole body DWI has stimulated much interest in the past few years as an alternative to PET-CT or bone scintigraphy in screening cancer patients for metastatic disease. This entails acquisition of diffusion-weighted images, typically with high b values (b=800-1,000 s/mm^2), over the entire body (obtained in several separate stations). The apparent diffusion coefficient maps can then be joined together and displayed in 3D rotating images that resemble single-photon emission CT reconstructions from bone scan and PET acquisitions. DWI is exquisitely sensitive for detection of focal marrow lesions, and preliminary studies have shown that whole body DWI compares favorably with bone scintigraphy in detection of bone metastases from prostate cancer. Limitations include a lack of specificity because not all lesions with restricted diffusion are malignant, and although DWI is a sensitive technique for identification of lymph nodes, the ability to distinguish positive from negative lymph nodes is poor. The protocols are also somewhat unclear about how to deal with hepatic, renal, and other parenchymal lesions that may be visible on DWI (either with b=0 s/mm^2 or standard DWI), many of which are benign but need further characterization, often with dynamic gadolinium-enhanced imaging. Case 14.26 is an example of DWI in a second prostate cancer patient with less advanced metastatic disease.

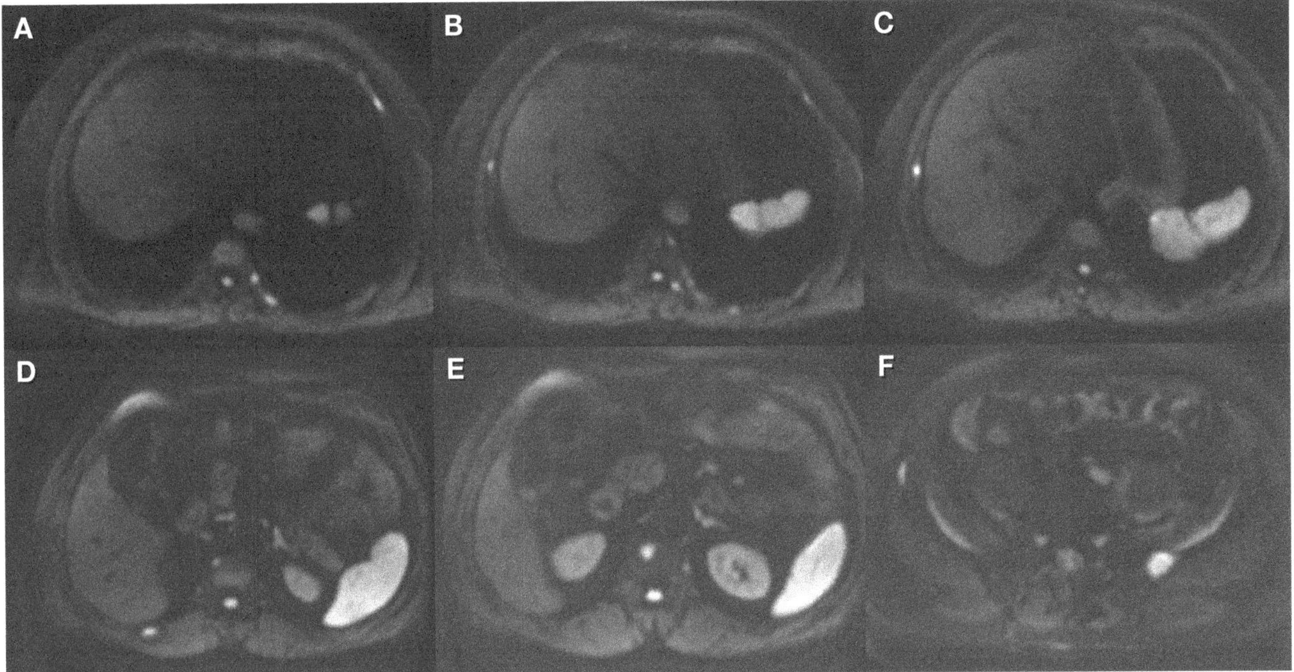

Figure 14.26.1

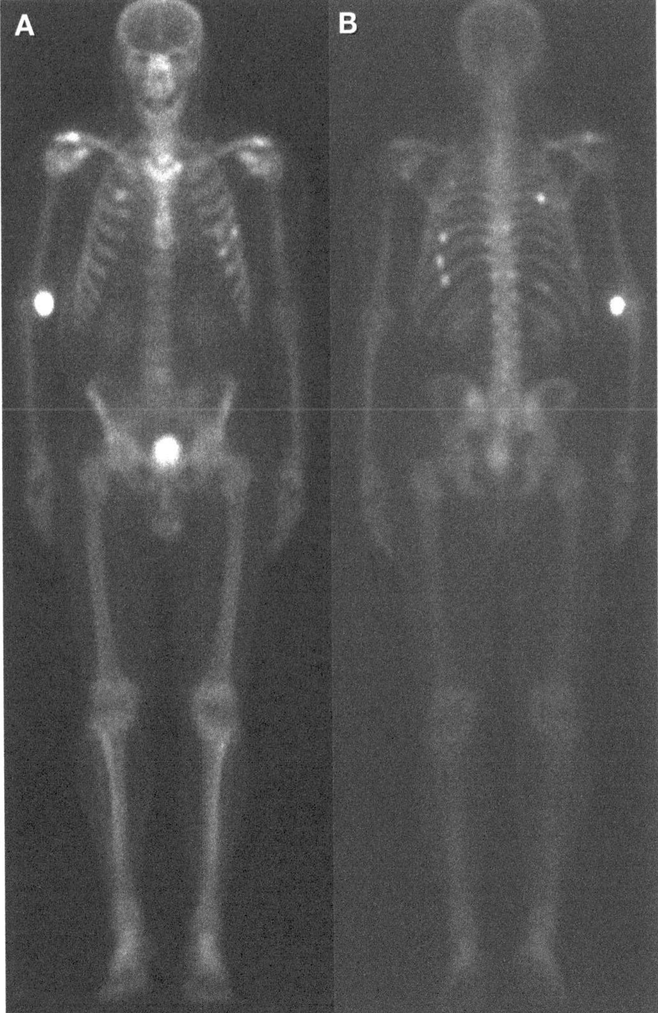

Figure 14.26.2

HISTORY: 64-year-old man with recently diagnosed prostate carcinoma and elevated alkaline phosphatase level; abdominal pelvic MRI was requested to screen for metastases in this patient with a severe allergy to iodinated CT contrast

IMAGING FINDINGS: Axial diffusion-weighted images (b=800 s/mm^2) (Figure 14.26.1) reveal multiple small hyperintense lesions involving lower thoracic and lumbar vertebral bodies, bilateral ribs, and the left iliac bone. Anterior and posterior views from bone scintigraphy (Figure 14.26.2) reveal fewer lesions. Notice also the vertically aligned lesions involving the left lower ribs on the posterior view consistent with prior trauma. These lesions did not show restricted diffusion and were therefore not visible on diffusion-weighted images.

DIAGNOSIS: Bone metastases from prostate cancer

COMMENT: This case, a companion to the previous example of bone metastases from prostate cancer (Case 14.25), illustrates the utility of DWI. The multiple small bone metastases involving the spine, ribs, and pelvic bones in Figure 14.26.1 are easily distinguished by their high contrast, which could be further accentuated by increasing the b value to 900 to 1,000 s/mm^2 to reduce the background signal. Whole body DWI with multiple sets of coils and parallel imaging can be performed fairly efficiently, usually in 20 to 30 minutes, and the resulting images displayed as a 3D rotation, similar to our favorite nuclear medicine examinations.

This case illustrates the increased sensitivity of DWI compared to standard technetium Tc 99m scintigraphy. An additional benefit is that if the healing rib fractures are old enough, you won't be able to see them and therefore won't have to worry about this differential diagnosis. Whole body DWI is very much in a developmental stage, and it is not clear what else will need to be included in standard protocols to address the parenchymal lesions, benign or malignant, that will inevitably appear on these examinations.

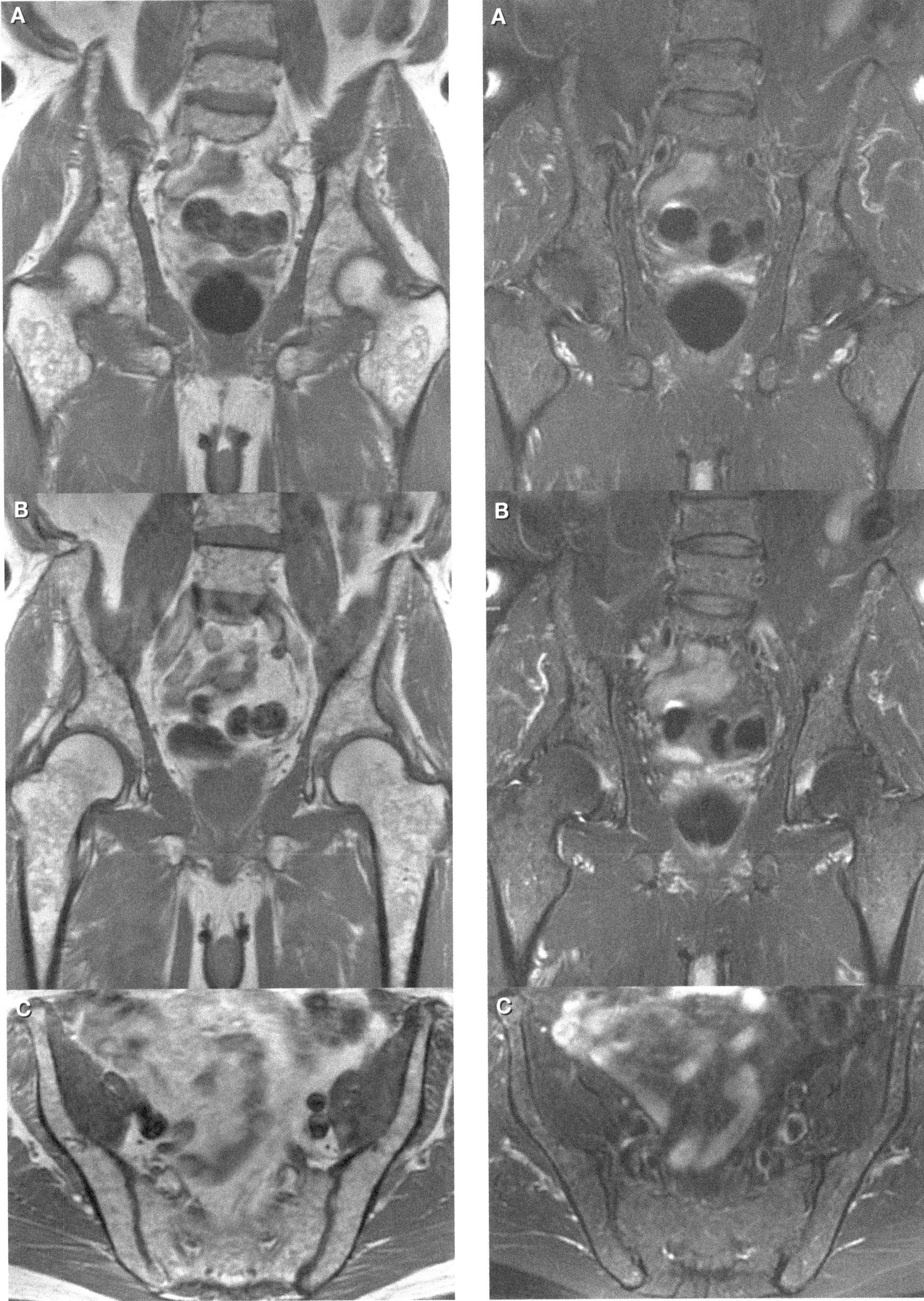

Figure 14.27.1

Figure 14.27.2

HISTORY: 70-year-old man with lumbar and sacral pain

IMAGING FINDINGS: Coronal (Figure 14.27.1A and 14.27.1B) and axial (Figure 14.27.1C) T1-weighted FSE images and coronal (Figure 14.27.2A and 14.27.2B) and axial (Figure 14.27.2C) fat-suppressed T2-weighted FSE images demonstrate diffuse heterogeneous marrow replacement, most prominently on T1-weighted images, which show innumerable hypointense lesions. The lesions are mildly hyperintense on T2-weighted images.

DIAGNOSIS: Multiple myeloma

COMMENT: Multiple myeloma is the most common primary bone tumor, accounting for approximately 10% of all hematologic malignancies. Myeloma, one of the plasma cell disorders, is a malignant proliferation of plasma cells derived from a single clone. The etiology is uncertain, but genetic factors have been identified, and exposure to radiation also increases risk. The annual incidence is approximately 4 per 100,000, with most patients initially receiving a diagnosis between the ages of 60 and 70 years.

Patients typically present with bone pain involving the back and ribs. This is associated with lytic lesions caused by proliferation of tumor cells and activation of osteoclasts that destroy bone. As marrow elements are replaced by proliferating myeloma cells, patients become susceptible to infections; 25% of patients present with recurring infections. Renal failure also occurs in 25% of patients and is related to several factors, including hypercalcemia, glomerular deposits of amyloid, recurrent infections, and tubular damage associated with light chain excretion. Diagnosis of multiple myeloma requires fulfillment of 3 criteria: 1) more than 10% atypical marrow plasma cells or plasmacytoma, 2) serum or urine monoclonal protein or paraprotein, and 3) myeloma-related organ dysfunction.

Myeloma initially involves active red marrow, with common sites including the skull, spine, pelvis, ribs, and proximal long bones. On plain radiographs, multiple myeloma is characterized by multiple small, well-circumscribed lytic lesions or diffuse inhomogeneous osteopenia. Bone surveys are still useful in diagnosis and monitoring disease progression, but they often yield false-negative results, particularly in the spine and pelvis, and may understage disease in as many as one-third of patients.

Multiple myeloma has various appearances on MRI. The most common is focal marrow-replacing lesions that are dark on T1-weighted images and bright on T2-weighted images. Alternatively, there may be diffuse marrow replacement, again with low T1- and high T2-signal intensity. A salt-and-pepper pattern has also been described in which the marrow appears patchy and inhomogeneous but without discrete lesions on fat-suppressed T2-weighted images. This pattern is generally associated with mild disease. The Durie-Salmon PLUS staging system, which correlates fairly well with survival, describes the imaging appearance of the spine and long bones as follows:

- Stage I: normal skeletal survey (stage IA) or <5 focal lesions (stage IB)
- Stage II: 5-20 lesions or moderate diffuse marrow disease
- Stage III: >20 focal lesions or severe diffuse marrow disease

Survival of patients with multiple myeloma is highly variable. Within the first 3 months after diagnosis, 15% of patients die; the subsequent yearly mortality is approximately 15%. The 5-year survival is 30% for patients with abnormal findings on MRI and 80% for patients with normal MRI. Most patients receive chemotherapy, and promising results have been achieved after stem cell transplant in selected patients.

ABBREVIATIONS

CT	computed tomography
DWI	diffusion-weighted imaging
FDG	fluorodeoxyglucose F18
FSE	fast-spin echo
IP	in-phase
MPNST	malignant peripheral nerve sheath tumor
MRI	magnetic resonance imaging
NF1	neurofibromatosis 1
OP	out-of-phase
PET	positron emission tomography
SPGR	spoiled gradient recalled
SSFSE	single-shot fast-spin echo
3D	3-dimensional
TI	inversion time
2D	2-dimensional
US	ultrasonography
UV	ultraviolet

15.

BREAST

CASE 15.1

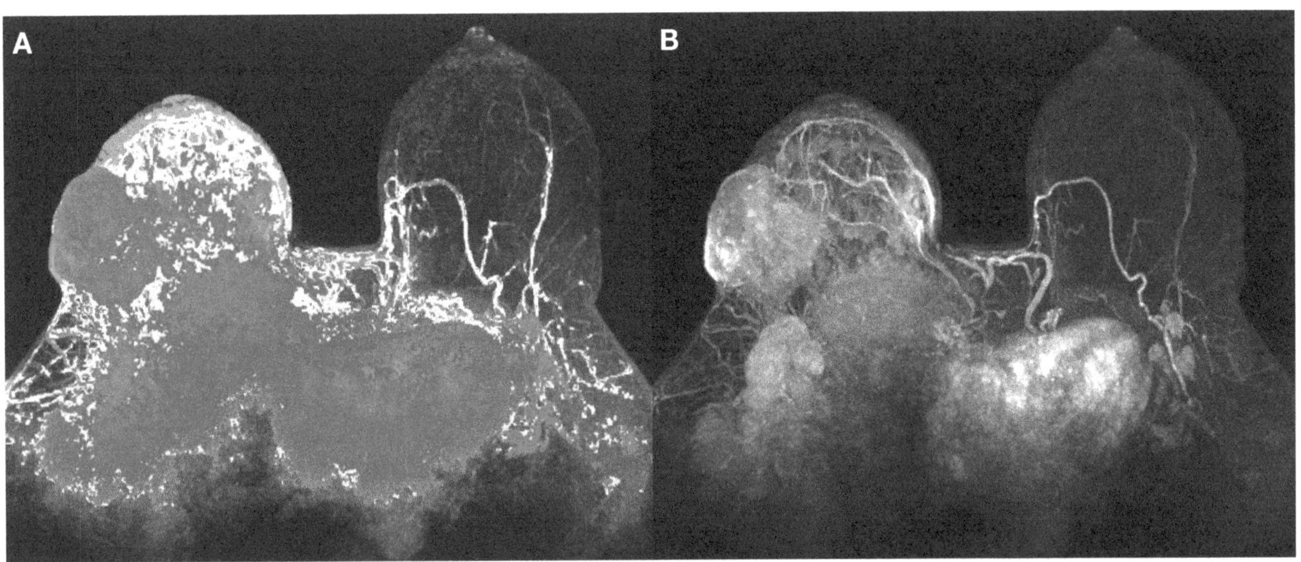

Figure 15.1.1

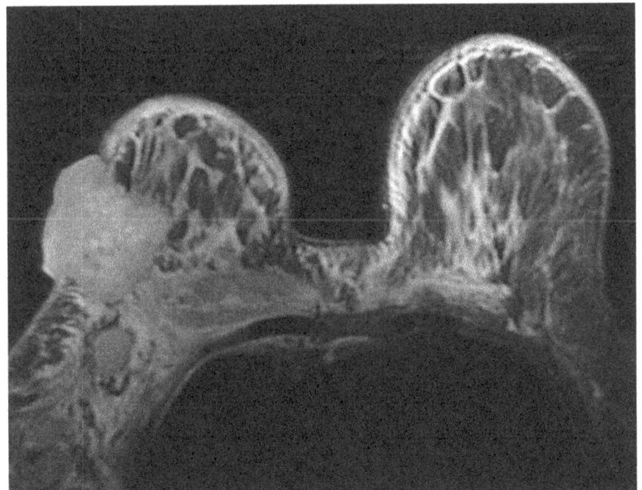
Figure 15.1.2

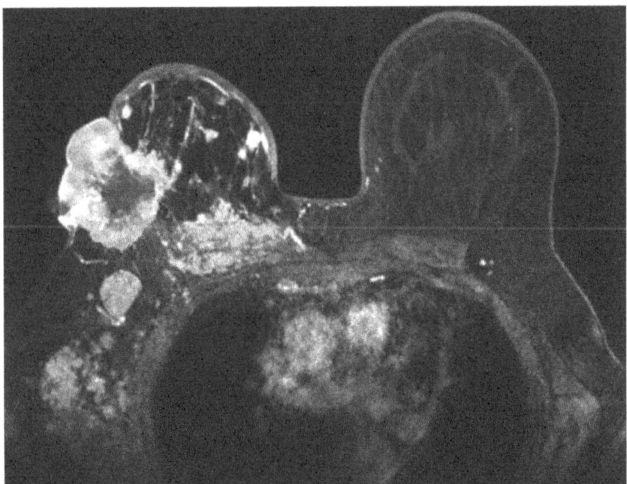
Figure 15.1.3

HISTORY: 71-year-old woman with a right breast mass and trouble using her right arm

IMAGING FINDINGS: The MIP image at peak enhancement with CAD color overlay (Figure 15.1.1A) demonstrates a large fungating mass in the right breast that has marked enhancement and involves the right side of the chest wall and right axilla. These findings are also evident on the MIP image without the CAD color overlay (Figure 15.1.1B). Axial water image (Figure 15.1.2) from a T2-weighted FSE acquisition using a modified 3-point Dixon (IDEAL) method for fat suppression demonstrates intermediate signal intensity of the fungating right breast mass and the muscles of the chest wall, as well as axillary and internal mammary chain adenopathy.

Note also cutaneous edema in the contralateral breast. A postgadolinium 3D SPGR image (Figure 15.1.3) acquired 60 to 90 seconds (*first postgadolinium*) after contrast injection demonstrates heterogeneous enhancement of the right breast and chest wall masses, as well as adenopathy and skin thickening.

DIAGNOSIS: Invasive ductal carcinoma

COMMENT: This case is not so much an exercise in detection as it is a search for extent of disease. It is also a quiet reminder that even in developed countries, tragic, advanced disease can be found all too frequently. Evaluation of breast MRI in a patient with suspected or known breast malignancy usually includes an assessment of the ipsilateral breast, looking for multifocal (≥2 cancers in the same quadrant) or multicentric (≥2 cancers in different quadrants and usually >5 cm apart) disease, as well as inspection of the contralateral breast, the chest wall, the mediastinum, axillae, lymph nodes, bones, liver, and skin. Subsequent imaging determined that this patient had brachial plexus involvement.

It is not surprising that the exquisite soft tissue characterization of MRI offers high sensitivity for breast cancer detection, with reported sensitivities ranging from 94% to 100%. The high sensitivity of breast MRI for cancer detection is tempered by its less impressive specificity and negative predictive value. In the diagnostic setting of a suspicious or indeterminate mammographic or sonographic finding, the most optimistic studies report negative predictive values of about 85%, which means that when MRI is considered, it is important for clinicians and patients to recognize the potential for false-positive results and the occasional need for additional work-up, such as a second-look US or even biopsy. The ACR, American Cancer Society, and Society of Breast Imaging all agree on the utility of MRI for indications that include screening of high-risk patients, cancer staging, assessment of implant integrity, and image-guided biopsy. High-risk patients are defined as those who have a lifetime risk of 20% to 25%, are *BRCA1* or *BRCA2* carriers or are untested first-degree relatives of a carrier, have a strong family history of breast cancer or ovarian cancer, or have had chest radiotherapy at 10 to 30 years of age. Very dense breasts and prior mammographically occult breast cancer are considered indicative of intermediate risk and are addressed on a case-by-case basis. MRI is used for cancer staging to evaluate extent of disease, treatment response, and positive margins in patients after lumpectomy.

In earlier days of breast MRI, at least in our practice, most examinations were performed and read by body imagers, and the relatively small number of cases were generally requested for evaluation of suspected breast implant rupture. Little emphasis was placed on cancer detection, and gadolinium-enhanced acquisitions were rare. Breast MRI is very different today, with most examinations performed for cancer detection or cancer staging, or both. Interpretation of these cases is greatly aided by the ability to incorporate information from mammography, breast US, and clinical history—skills that are generally lacking in most abdominal imagers, who, for the most part, have been happy to relinquish these cases to the breast imaging practice.

Breast MRI protocols can vary considerably in acquisition planes, spatial and temporal resolutions of dynamic postgadolinium images, use of fat suppression on dynamic postgadolinium images or T2-weighted images, and inclusion of functional imaging techniques, such as DWI. In 2010, the ACR launched an accreditation program for breast MRI aligned with similar programs for mammography, breast US, and stereotactic breast biopsy. This was an effort to establish a set of minimal performance standards (and was facilitated by phantoms, available for purchase only from the ACR). The existence of a low barrier to prevent true amateurs from performing breast MRI is in general a good idea; however, it can create a sense of complacency in which all efforts concerning quality control and improvement are centered on ACR qualification and then are abandoned after the certificate arrives in the mail.

Our own breast MRI protocol has changed a few times during the past 7 or 8 years, but the cases shown in this chapter all follow the same basic format:

- Axial acquisition
- Water and fat images from a T2-weighted FSE acquisition using a modified 3-point Dixon (IDEAL) method for fat suppression
- Fat-suppressed pregadolinium and postgadolinium 3D SPGR images acquired at 60 to 90 seconds (*first postgadolinium*), 2 to 3 minutes (*second* or *peak postgadolinium*), and about 7 to 8 minutes (*delayed postgadolinium*) after contrast injection. Between 3 and 7 minutes after contrast injection, a higher-resolution 3D SPGR (*third postgadolinium*) image is acquired that has sufficient resolution to perform reformatted sagittal and coronal views. The first postgadolinium image is acquired 27 seconds after contrast injection
- Single-dose gadobenate dimeglumine (Multihance) (1 mmol/kg) is injected at a rate of 3 mL per second
- Diffusion-weighted images are acquired in the sagittal plane with a b value of 800 s/mm^2

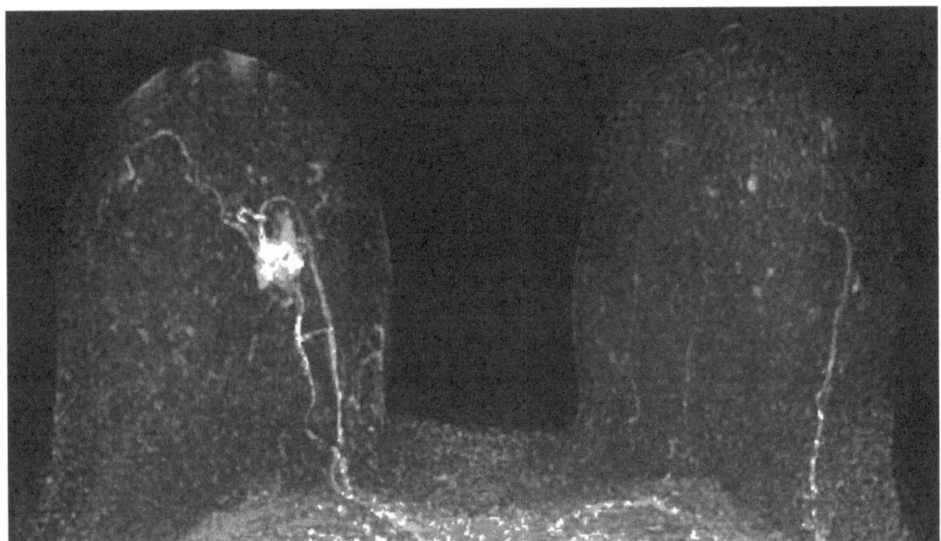

Figure 15.2.1

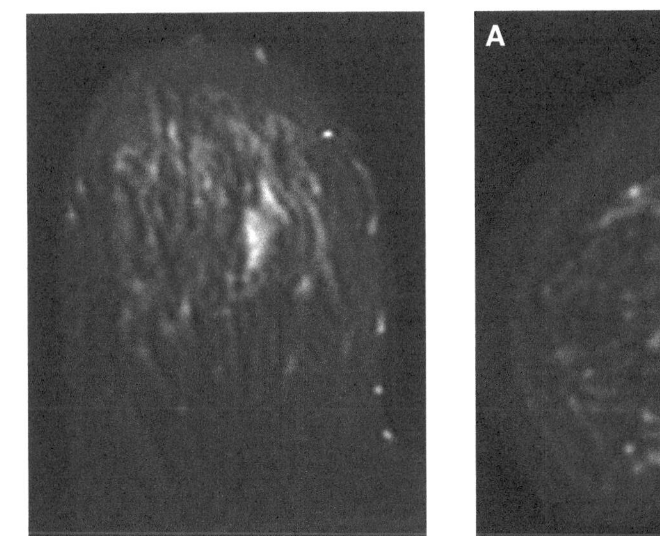

Figure 15.2.2

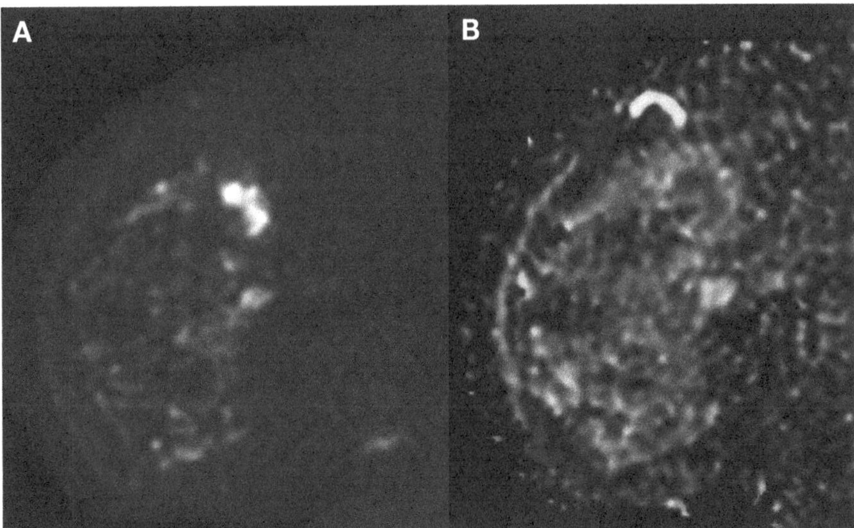

Figure 15.2.3

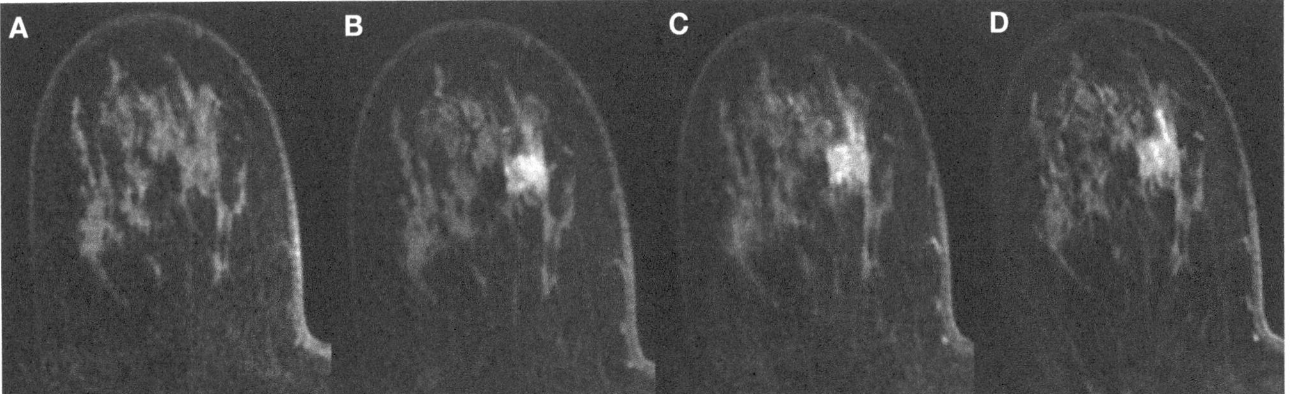

Figure 15.2.4

HISTORY: 61-year-old woman on postmenopausal hormone replacement therapy with 1-year persistent, asymmetrical fullness in the left upper outer breast. Clinical examination and diagnostic mammography were unremarkable

IMAGING FINDINGS: The MIP image at peak enhancement with CAD color overlay (Figure 15.2.1) demonstrates mild background enhancement and a mass in the right breast. Axial water image (Figure 15.2.2) from a T2-weighted FSE acquisition using a modified 3-point Dixon (IDEAL) method for fat suppression demonstrates an irregular mass with intermediate signal intensity in the right breast. Diffusion-weighted image (b=800 s/mm^2) (Figure 15.2.3A) and the corresponding ADC map (Figure 15.2.3B) show restricted diffusion of the mass. Axial pregadolinium (Figure 15.2.4A) and first postgadolinium (Figure 15.2.4B), second or peak postgadolinium (Figure 15.2.4C), and delayed postgadolinium (Figure 15.2.4D) dynamic 3D SPGR images demonstrate an irregular, enhancing mass in the upper inner quadrant of the right breast.

DIAGNOSIS: Invasive lobular carcinoma

COMMENT: This case does not technically fit an indication for breast MRI as discussed in Case 15.1; however, the negative diagnostic mammogram is not completely reassuring, particularly given the negative clinical findings in a symptomatic patient taking postmenopausal hormone therapy. Use of MRI for trouble shooting a clinical question that cannot be resolved by mammogram or US is generally recommended after a discussion of the possibility of false positives with the patient. Sometimes the imaging is challenging and sometimes not so much, as in this case where cancer was serendipitously discovered in the contralateral breast on MRI.

MRI has been helpful in staging breast cancers, particularly the invasive ones. For example, invasive lobular carcinomas, which can be mammographically and sonographically occult, are sometimes more apparent on MRI despite their varied manifestations, with some appearing as a mass with spiculated margins, some as a mass with satellite lesions, some as multiple foci, and others as normal parenchyma. The sensitivity of MRI has been reported to be 93% to 96% for invasive lobular carcinoma and 99% for evaluation of extent of disease in newly diagnosed breast cancer when combined with mammography and physical examination. If second-look US is performed, you may find a correlating vague, hypoechoic mass with indistinct margins or an echogenic rim. In this case, the morphologic characteristics of the mass (ie, irregular margins) and the mostly plateau enhancement kinetics, with areas of rapid washout, made this case worrisome for malignancy. These features are also concerning for invasive disease rather than in situ disease. Trying to differentiate between ductal and lobular subtypes is generally more of a gamble than an art—and that is with the benefit of knowing the mammographic and clinical findings.

Kinetic enhancement curves in breast MRI are obtained by plotting signal intensity for each pixel over time before and after gadolinium injection. For each pixel of breast parenchyma, the signal behavior can therefore be qualitatively characterized both before and after peak enhancement, which occurs typically within 2 to 3 minutes. *Initial enhancement* is the enhancement pattern of the kinetic curve before peak enhancement and is described as slow, medium, or rapid. Analogously, *delayed enhancement* refers to the enhancement behavior after peak enhancement and is described as persistent, plateau, or washout. The delayed enhancement pattern is more often used as a clue to malignancy and is emphasized in this chapter.

CAD software is widely used in breast MRI to automate the analytical process and generate parametric color maps. Most of these programs rely on some user-specified values, which generally include the time delay from gadolinium injection to the first image acquisition, designation of the peak enhancement series, the percentage of signal increase between pregadolinium and initial enhancement acquisitions, which will identify those pixels with kinetic curves (and thus a color on the overlay), and the percentage signal decrease between delayed enhancement and initial enhancement to assign either a washout, plateau, or persistent pattern. Default values tend to be 50% for percent signal increase between pregadolinium and initial enhancement. By default, blue indicates persistent contrast kinetics; yellow, plateau kinetics; and red, washout kinetics.

Qualitative assessment of gadolinium uptake and washout that is used to evaluate hepatic masses, for example, is facilitated by timing clues provided by adjacent arteries, portal veins, and hepatic veins. Similar clues are not available in the breasts, however, where the use of enhancement kinetic analysis has been shown to improve specificity of lesion characterization when combined with morphologic information. Some breast imaging practices, including ours, have decided that if a patient cannot receive gadolinium, then breast MRI is not performed. Although the gadolinium dose is generally constant from practice to practice (ie, set to the dose recommended by the vendor and the FDA), there is considerable variability in the injection rate, the time delay between injection and first image acquisition, and the time of peak enhancement—all of which affect CAD analysis of enhancement kinetics. Because these variables are generally not self-evident, reading breast MRIs performed at another medical facility is not as straightforward as one might think, and you would be wise to verify that the CAD parametric images actually make sense.

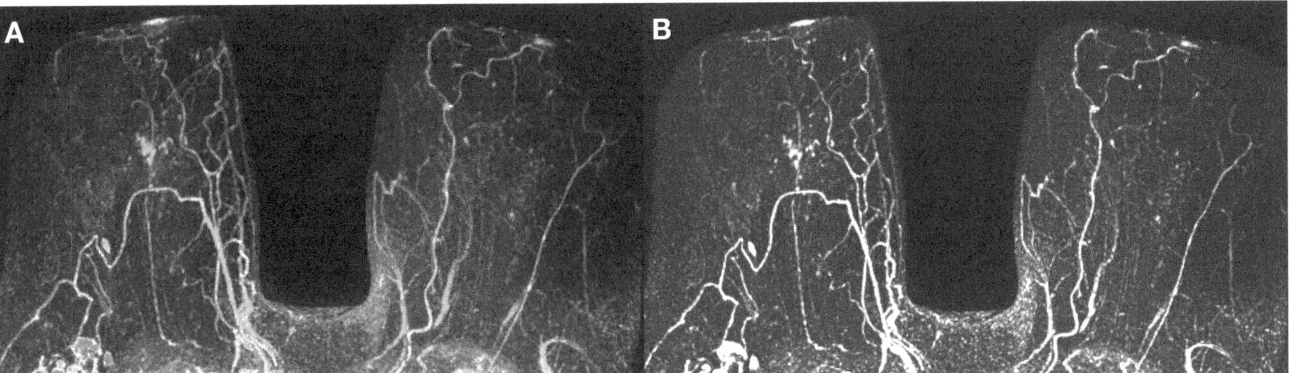

Figure 15.3.1

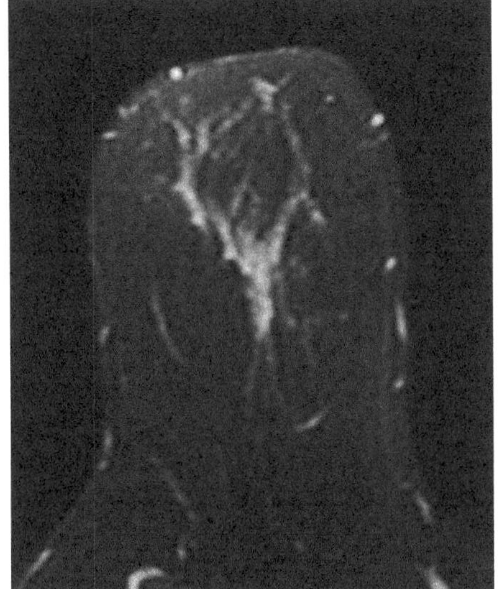

Figure 15.3.2

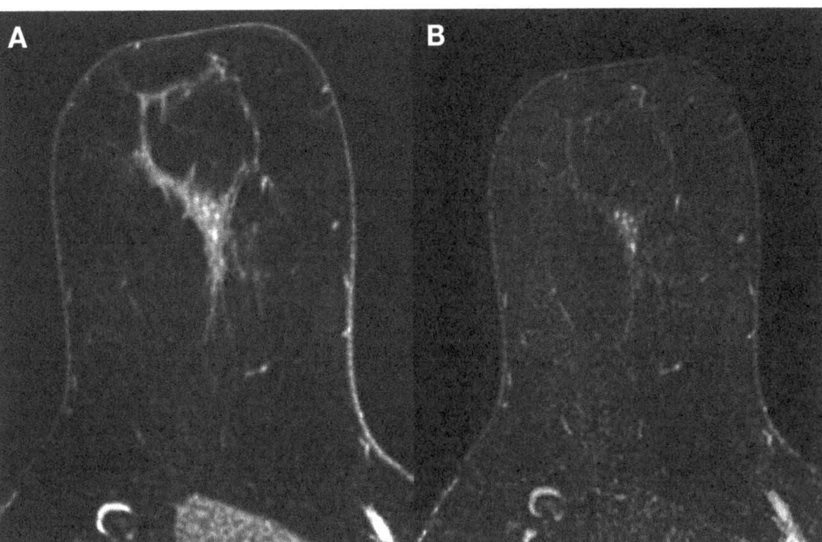

Figure 15.3.3

HISTORY: 47-year-old woman with a *BRCA1* mutation and recent negative mammogram and US

IMAGING FINDINGS: The MIP images at peak enhancement with (Figure 15.3.1A) and without (Figure 15.3.1B) CAD color overlay demonstrate a small nonmass enhancement with persistent enhancement kinetics in the middle-depth right breast. This nonmass enhancement has intermediate to increased signal intensity on the T2-weighted water image (Figure 15.3.2) and clumped linear enhancement on the peak postgadolinium image (Figure 15.3.3A), which is more evident on the subtraction image (peak enhancement minus pregadolinium) (Figure 15.3.3B).

DIAGNOSIS: Ductal carcinoma in situ

COMMENT: It can be difficult to diagnose DCIS radiologically: Approximately 15% are mammographically occult, and the sensitivity of MRI for detecting DCIS ranges from 68% to 97%. On MRI, DCIS generally appears as nonmass enhancement with clumped features that can have a ductal, linear, segmental, or regional distribution. The BIRADS lexicon defines a mass as a 3D space-occupying lesion and a nonmass enhancement as an area that is not a mass. The BIRADS lexicon further characterizes a mass through its shape, margins, and enhancement pattern and characterizes a nonmass enhancement through its distribution and enhancement pattern. Sometimes, there is an overlap in the appearance of an irregular mass with irregular margins and a focal area of nonmass enhancement, and the distinction between the two is not always straightforward. But both could conceivably connote the same level of suspicion. All 3 kinetic enhancement patterns—persistent, plateau, and washout—have been described for DCIS, and the distribution is typically segmental or linear.

Nonmass enhancement can be difficult to diagnose and manage clinically. It is not unique to DCIS or malignancy and can be seen in benign entities such as focal adenosis, fibrocystic changes, and inflammatory changes. Sometimes, in cases of minimal or mild background parenchymal enhancement, the contralateral breast can serve as an internal control, making the clumped nature of the finding more apparent, as in this case. Ambiguity on reformatted sagittal and coronal views should not dissuade you from considering the diagnosis. When there is moderate or marked background enhancement, differentiating nonmass enhancement, particularly small lesions, from background can be more problematic, as can be seen in later cases in this chapter. Enhancement kinetics can be just as confounding, and when lesions are small, DWI may not be able to provide additional information, which was the case here. Because of the asymmetry of the finding compared with the left breast, second-look US was recommended.

Although evaluation of enhancement kinetics has clear diagnostic value in the interpretation of breast MRI, it's important to realize that the appearance of lesions on a particular vendor's CAD software depends on the algorithms used, the user-specified threshold settings, and the imaging parameters chosen for the dynamic acquisitions. "Red is bad" may be a useful first approximation, but it's very likely that some adjustment of the software will be needed to achieve optimal results for a particular practice. For example, there is considerable variability in contrast agents, contrast injection rates, and time delays before acquisition of the first postcontrast series and peak enhancement series across different practices, all of which can have small effects on the enhancement properties of various lesions. Similar variation in technique can be seen in MRI protocols for other organs; however, the breast is unique in its reliance on CAD software for interpretation (although the prostate may not be far behind). Therefore, internal validation that the user-defined variables applied to every case actually reflect what is happening on the kinetic enhancement curve for most of the cases is probably a good exercise to perform at least a few times every year, if for no other reason than to remind radiologists that every time they read a breast MRI, they are taking a leap of faith that the software is providing the correct answer most of the time.

Targeted US was unremarkable in this patient. Given the negative US, the relatively benign appearance of the MRI, the negative mammogram, and the absence of a palpable abnormality, this case would normally lead to a benign or probably benign BIRADS assessment. BIRADS is a collaborative effort by the ACR and several other medical disciplines, as well as the FDA, to standardize reporting and facilitate outcome monitoring. An assessment category of BIRADS 0 means incomplete and additional imaging is needed; BIRADS 1, negative (no abnormal enhancement and no lesion found); BIRADS 2, benign findings; BIRADS 3, a probably benign finding; BIRADS 4, a suspicious abnormality; BIRADS 5, highly suggestive of malignancy; and BIRADS 6, a known cancer or biopsy-proven malignancy. Each BIRADS assessment has recommendations for management. BIRADS 1 and 2 recommend routine follow-up; BIRADS 3, short-interval follow-up; BIRADS 4, consideration of biopsy; BIRADS 5 and 6, appropriate action. In this case, however, the patient's additional history of a *BRCA1* mutation raised our level of suspicion, and therefore MRI-guided biopsy was performed, revealing DCIS. The question of whether we would have biopsied this nonmass enhancement if the patient was not high risk is, fortunately for us, a more rhetorical one, since we would hopefully not be performing an MRI on such a patient without a reasonable indication; the honest answer in this hypothetical case is "We don't know."

Given the patient's history (*BRCA1* positivity and a mother who had breast cancer at age >50 years), she opted for right mastectomy and left prophylactic mastectomy. Pathology at that time was consistent with the findings at biopsy and was not upgraded; lymph nodes were negative for malignancy.

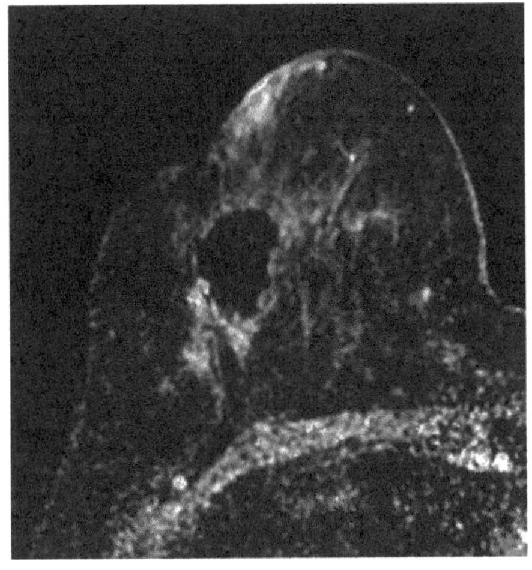

Figure 15.4.1

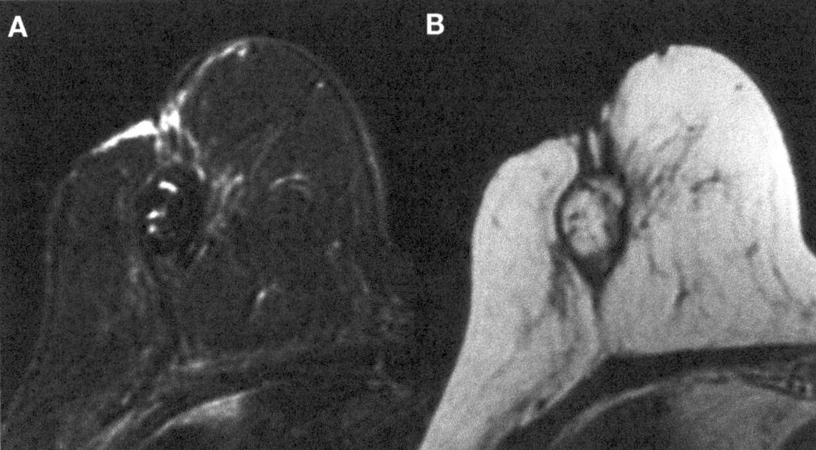

Figure 15.4.2

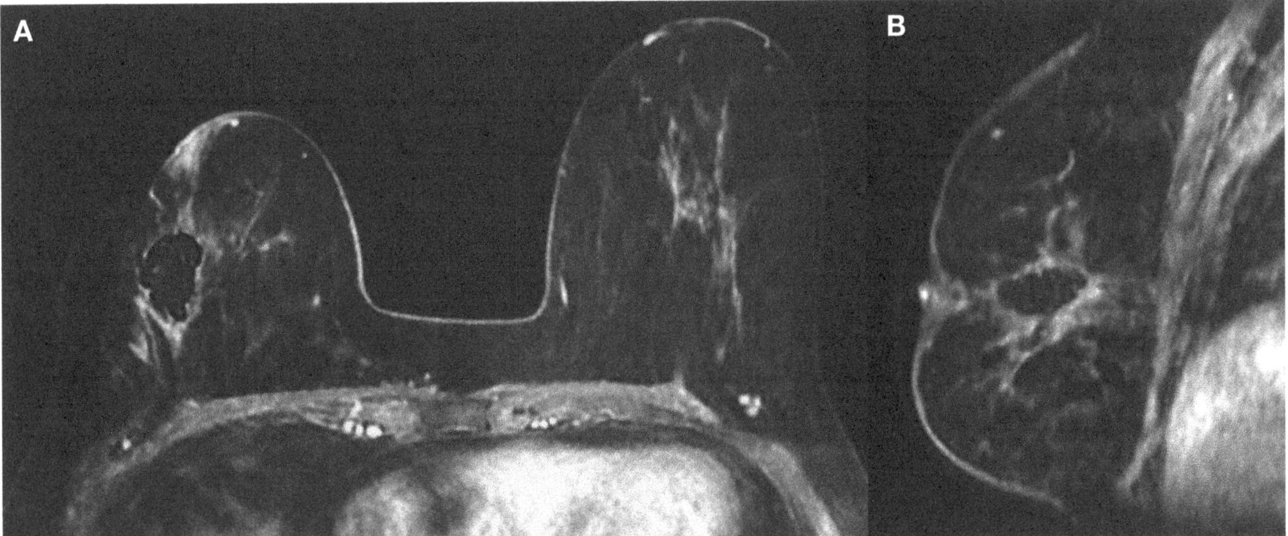

Figure 15.4.3

HISTORY: 66-year-old woman with invasive lobular carcinoma and LCIS of the right breast status post wide local excision about 15 months ago followed by radiation therapy

IMAGING FINDINGS: The axial subtracted image at peak enhancement with CAD color overlay (Figure 15.4.1) demonstrates postoperative and postradiation changes in the right breast without any worrisome kinetic enhancement. Axial noncontrast water (Figure 15.4.2A) and fat (Figure 15.4.2B) images from a T2-weighted FSE acquisition using a modified 3-point Dixon (IDEAL) method for fat suppression show an oval mass with irregular, somewhat thickened margins and tethering of the adjacent parenchyma at the operative site. Axial postgadolinium 3D SPGR image (Figure 15.4.3A) and sagittal reformatted view (Figure 15.4.3B) demonstrate slight heterogeneous internal enhancement of the lesion and mild peripheral enhancement.

DIAGNOSIS: Fat necrosis

COMMENT: The varied MRI features of fat necrosis are well described in the literature. Fat necrosis is a relatively common sequela of trauma to the fat cells of the breast, usually resulting from blunt trauma such as a seat-belt injury, a fall, or an overexcited pet dog (true case), but also from iatrogenic causes, such as biopsy, surgery, and radiation. Fortunately, the mammographic appearances of fat necrosis often correlate with what you might expect to see on MRI.

Fat necrosis can look like almost anything—coarse calcifications, microcalcifications, focal asymmetries, and even spiculated masses. Perhaps the least ambiguous manifestation of fat necrosis is a lipid cyst, which appears mammographically as a circumscribed radiolucent mass with a thin opaque rim, reflecting the pathophysiologic process of compromised vascular integrity to the fat cells with an inflammatory response by histiocytes, lymphocytes, and plasma cells. The necrotic fat cells are then walled off by a fibrotic response, ultimately resulting in an apparent rim or capsule. On MRI, lipid cysts reflect the fatty nature of the mass: a focal round or oval mass with signal characteristics consistent with fat and a rim that may or may not enhance. The Dixon-based FSE acquisition shown in this case is a convenient method for demonstrating the presence of fat (and the absence of water) in a single acquisition; however, any combination of T1- or T2-weighted images with and without fat suppression will work just as well. A fat-fluid level is another classic sign of fat necrosis and, when present, can provide increased confidence in the diagnosis. The intensity of rim enhancement can be variable in fat necrosis and should not deter its diagnosis, particularly when the clinical history is suggestive and there is mammographic correlation.

The remaining spectrum of the appearance of fat necrosis is often more challenging. In particular, diagnostic dilemmas often arise in the setting of a palpable area of concern or an examination performed to rule out recurrent malignancy. Just as the margins of fat necrosis can become spiculated on mammography, the morphologic appearance on MRI may be analogously worrisome. In these difficult cases, it becomes even more important to correlate the MRI findings with mammography, sonography, and the clinical examination.

This patient did not have a palpable area of concern, and her surgery was 15 months ago. Findings correspond to a fat-containing mass on mammogram.

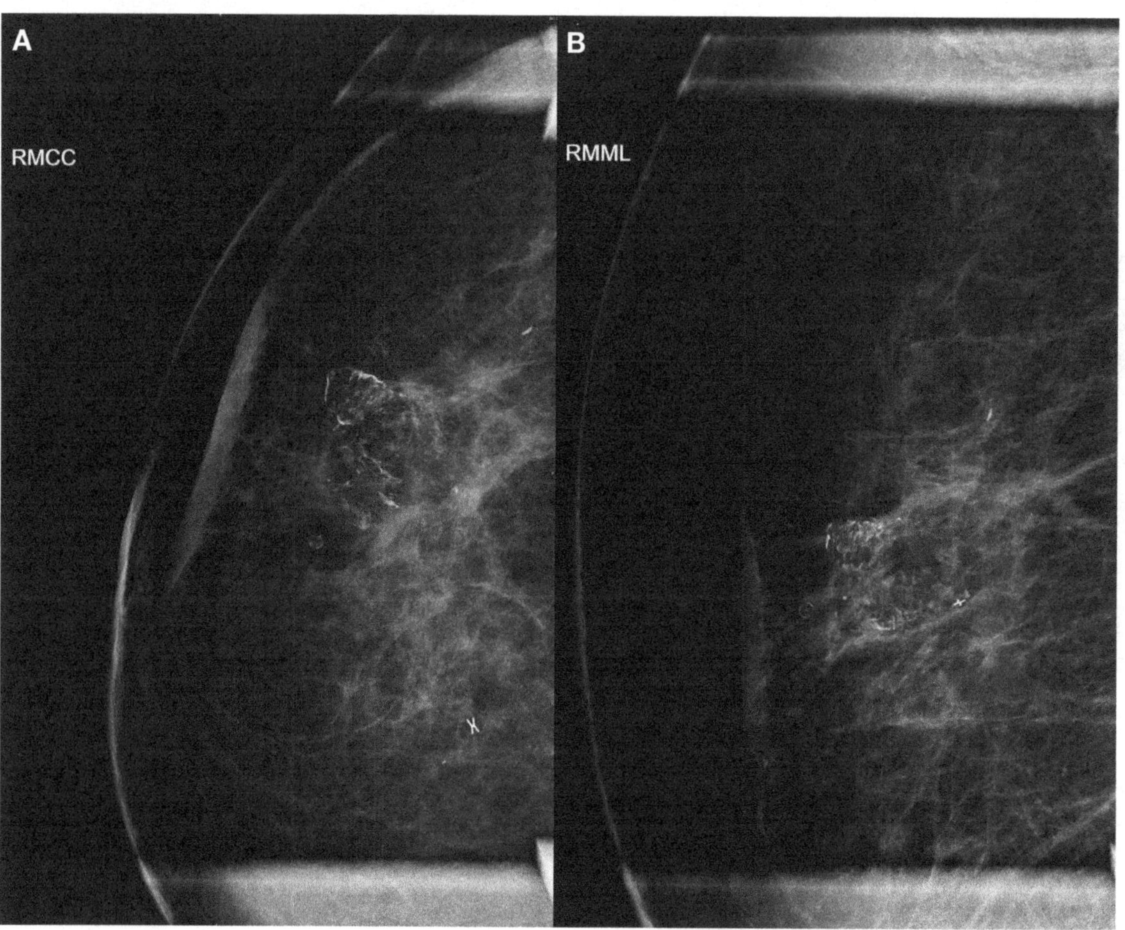

Figure 15.4.4

Craniocaudal (Figure 15.4.4A) and mediolateral (Figure 15.4.4B) magnification mammographic views and MRI are concordant, with both providing convincing evidence of fat necrosis...this time. Subsequent follow-up examinations may not be so straightforward, particularly if a palpable abnormality develops or calcifications appear on the mammogram. Sometimes, a biopsy is the only way to obtain a definitive answer.

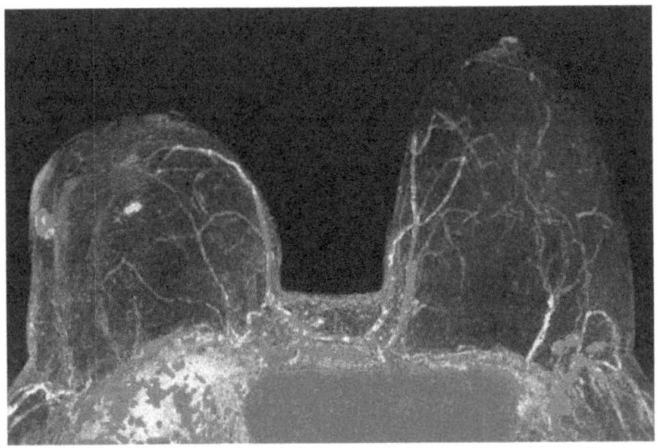

Figure 15.5.1

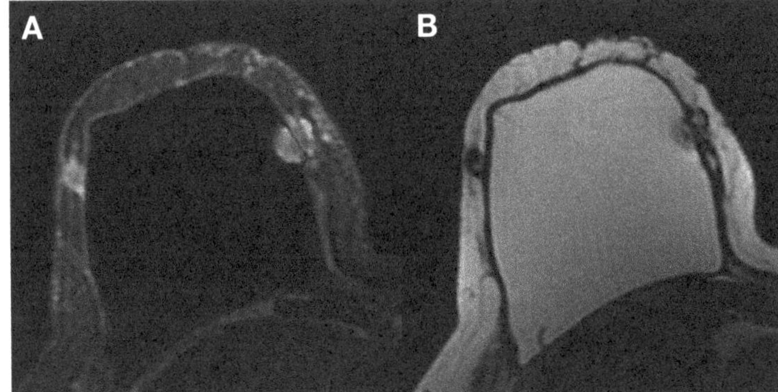

Figure 15.5.2

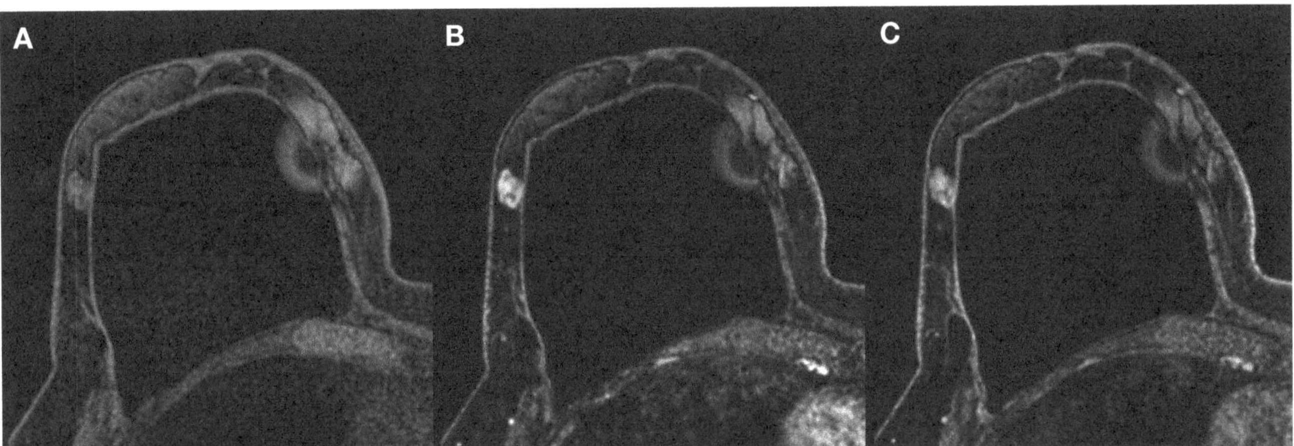

Figure 15.5.3

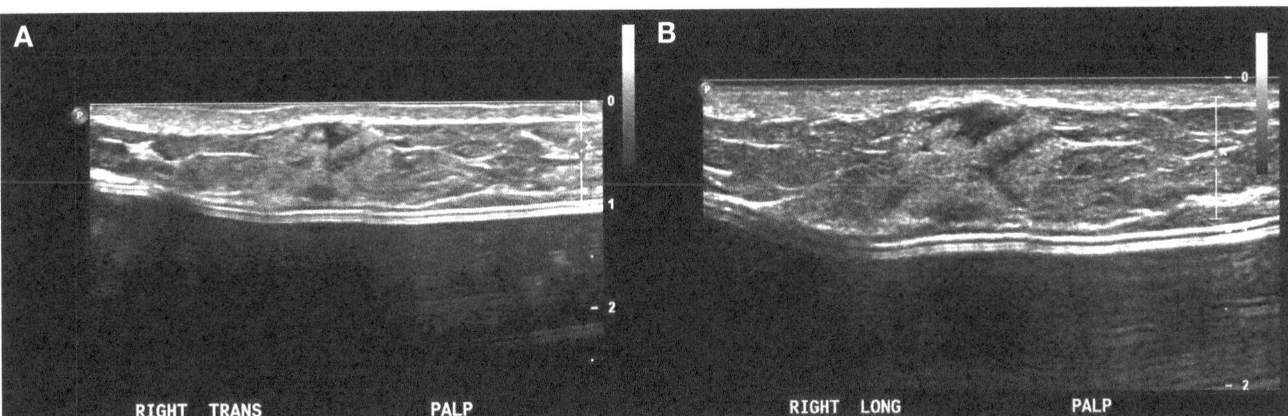

Figure 15.5.4

HISTORY: 49-year-old woman with a history of invasive ductal carcinoma and DCIS of the right breast status post right mastectomy with bilateral subpectoral silicone implants and left mastopexy and currently taking tamoxifen; a screening breast MRI was requested

IMAGING FINDINGS: The MIP image at peak enhancement with CAD color overlay (Figure 15.5.1) demonstrates a round mass with rapid washout enhancement kinetics in the lateral right breast. There is an additional, small oval mass with persistent enhancement kinetics in the middle-depth right breast that was near the fibrous capsule and thought to be fat necrosis. Water (Figure 15.5.2A) and fat (Figure 15.5.2B) images from a T2-weighted FSE acquisition using a modified 3-point Dixon (IDEAL) method for fat suppression demonstrate a heterogeneous mass immediately lateral to the silicone implant on the right. Pregadolinium (Figure 15.5.3A), first postgadolinium (Figure 15.5.3B), and delayed postgadolinium

(Figure 15.5.3C) 3D SPGR images reveal rapid enhancement of the lesion with washout on the delayed postgadolinium image. Note susceptibility artifact from surgical clips in the medial right breast.

Four months before the MRI, targeted US was performed to further evaluate a palpable area of concern. US images (Figure 15.5.4) demonstrate a heterogeneous, but predominantly hyperechoic, mass at this location. The sonographic features were described as being most consistent with benign fat necrosis.

DIAGNOSIS: Recurrent invasive ductal carcinoma

COMMENT: This case illustrates potential pitfalls in the diagnosis of fat necrosis. The sonographic features 4 months earlier in the clinical setting of a palpable mass were suggestive of fat necrosis, likely resulting from recent mastectomy and reconstruction. The MRI (which was performed for screening) is much less convincing, however. Even though the fat image from the 3-point Dixon T2-weighted FSE acquisition depicts a small amount of fat in the center of the lesion, the majority of the mass has relatively high signal intensity on the water image and shows intense enhancement following gadolinium administration. The natural evolution of fat necrosis includes not only liquefied fat, but also an inflammatory reaction and eventual fibrosis. When the inflammatory component is dominant, it can demonstrate washout contrast kinetics, and when there is fibrosis, fat necrosis can appear as a spiculated mass. Where there is enhancement, contrast kinetics may not be particularly helpful in distinguishing fat necrosis from malignancy. Therefore, biopsy may be warranted, which is what happened here.

This case generated some controversy in our breast practice, with US-oriented radiologists favoring a diagnosis of fat necrosis, while those more comfortable with MRI being suspicious of a recurrent neoplasm (the cases where MRI was wrong will, of course, appear in the US teaching file). It's also likely that the appearance of the lesion evolved in the 4 months between US and MRI, with postoperative changes regressing and the recurrent lesion becoming more obvious. Nevertheless, this is a good example of the utility of discussions (or arguments) within the imaging group, allowing those with more experience in a particular modality to share their expertise.

CASE 15.6

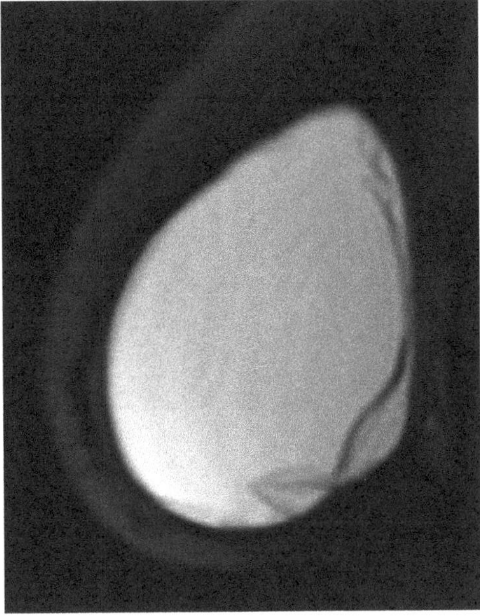

Figure 15.6.1

HISTORY: 55-year-old woman with bilateral augmentation mammoplasties 30 years ago, now with a palpable asymmetry in the right breast

IMAGING FINDINGS: Sagittal 2D IR image with fat suppression and selective water suppression of the right breast (Figure 15.6.1) demonstrates a well-circumscribed area of silicone signal and the linguine sign. *Linguine sign* is used to describe the layering, low-signaling curvilinear lines, or *noodles*, indicating rupture of the implant shell, leakage of silicone gel into the space within the fibrous capsule, which is intact here, and collapse of the implant shell on itself, thereby giving the noodlelike appearance.

DIAGNOSIS: Intracapsular implant rupture

COMMENT: When water, fat, and silicone are all present, the peak resonant frequencies are, from left to right: water, fat, and silicone, with silicone about 320 Hz lower than water and about 100 Hz lower than fat at 1.5 T. Silicone imaging is performed by suppressing the water and fat signals, which is generally accomplished by using a 2D IR sequence with the TI set to fat suppression, which is about 100 ms, and applying a spectral water suppression pulse. Good images are dependent on excellent field homogeneity and the ability to identify the water resonance peak for suppression, which is not always straightforward.

There are also silicone-selective sequences, which use a 3-point Dixon technique that separates water and fat images but which, in this case, can allow for calculation of a silicone-only image. Both silicone imaging techniques often have long acquisition times (>5 minutes), and it is often helpful to obtain these silicone images in 2 planes. We typically acquire the silicone images in both the axial and sagittal planes. The axial acquisitions generally take about 3 to 4 minutes and the sagittal acquisitions take about 8 minutes.

Intracapsular rupture in this case is demonstrated by the linguine sign. After breast implant surgery, a fibrous capsule forms around the implant shell. The "linguine" represents a completely ruptured implant shell that is free-floating within the silicone gel inside the fibrous capsule. The linguine sign has been shown to have 96% sensitivity and 94% specificity for intracapsular rupture. Incomplete collapse of the implant shell is sometimes difficult to distinguish from normal radial folds that typically occur peripherally, but a few signs have been described to facilitate diagnosis of incomplete intracapsular rupture. These are the *subcapsular line sign*, the *teardrop sign*, and the *keyhole sign*, which are all signs of the implant shell regressing from the fibrous capsule because of silicone leak and invaginating on itself to various degrees, with silicone appearing outside of the shell.

CASE 15.7

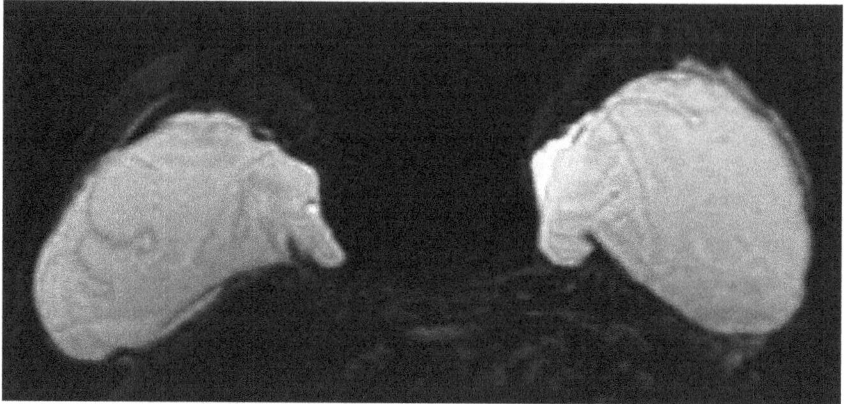

Figure 15.7.1

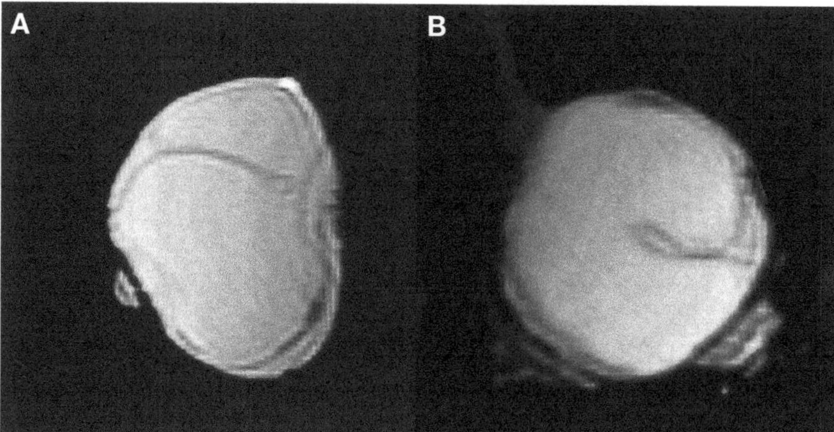

Figure 15.7.2

HISTORY: 65-year-old woman with bilateral breast implants placed 25 years ago presents with increasing capsular contracture

IMAGING FINDINGS: Axial (Figure 15.7.1) and bilateral sagittal (right, Figure 15.7.2A; left, Figure 15.7.2B) IR images with fat suppression and selective water suppression demonstrate silicone outside of the fibrous capsule bilaterally. Intracapsular rupture of both implants is indicated by the teardrop signs and subcapsular line signs in both breasts.

DIAGNOSIS: Extracapsular implant ruptures

COMMENT: In general, the life expectancy of a breast implant is 10 to 15 years, with rupture occurring in about 50% of implants that are 12 years old. A clinical diagnosis, capsular contraction involves contraction of the fibrous capsule, which can occur at any time after surgery. Correct interpretation of MRIs performed to assess for implant rupture relies on an accurate clinical history, which may be important—if not critical—for obtaining the correct diagnosis. We have encountered cases with very little clinical history where a small amount of extracapsular silicone was called an *extracapsular rupture*, only to find out later that the patient had had a known ruptured implant, which was explanted and replaced, making the current extracapsular silicone just a vestige from the prior rupture. In this case, this implant was the patient's first.

More often than not, subtle—and sometimes, not-so-subtle—silicone signal is identified in the pericardium, anterior mediastinum, or internal mammary regions on silicone imaging. This is almost always artifactual and is probably related to suboptimal shimming or suboptimal localization of the water peak at the time of image acquisition. Extracapsular extravasation of silicone is an occasional real finding; however, the presence of silicone in the mediastinum or pericardial space is extremely unlikely.

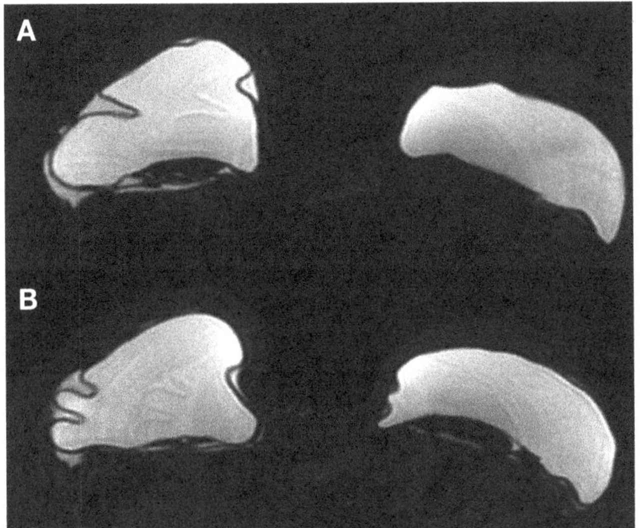

Figure 15.8.1

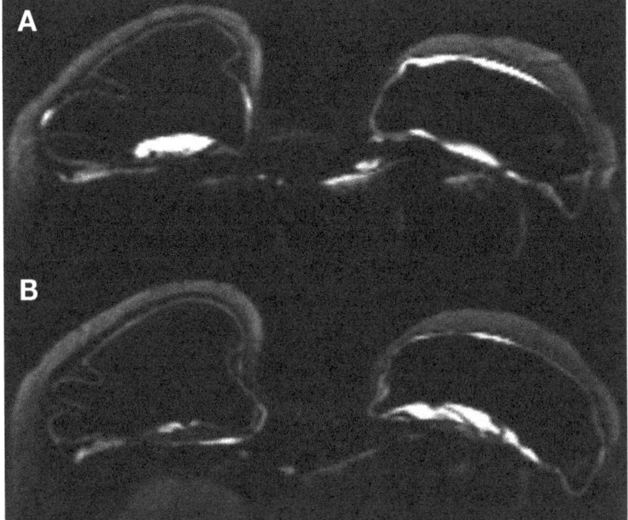

Figure 15.8.2

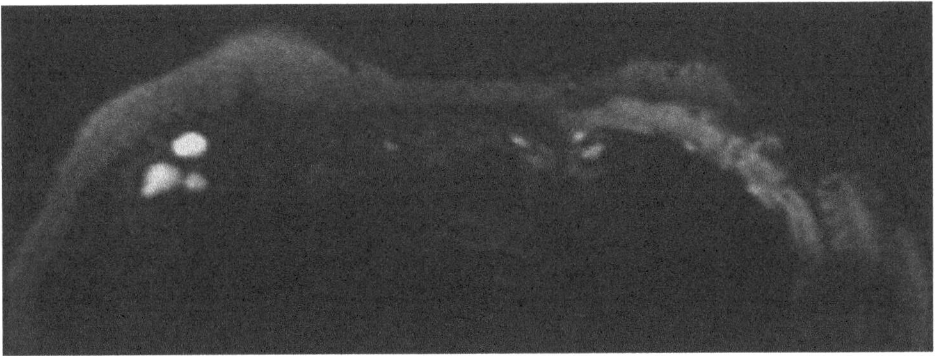

Figure 15.8.3

HISTORY: 46-year-old woman with a history of metachronous bilateral breast cancers status post bilateral mastectomies with implant reconstruction; her physician detected an area of palpable concern in the 12 o'clock position of the right breast

IMAGING FINDINGS: Water images (Figure 15.8.1) from a T2-weighted FSE acquisition using a modified 3-point Dixon (IDEAL) method for fat suppression demonstrate features suggestive of dual-lumen implants. Corresponding T2-weighted IR images with water suppression (Figure 15.8.2) confirm that there are bilateral dual-lumen implants (silicone outer lumen and saline inner lumen). Notice phase ghosting artifacts within the lumen of the saline implants, more noticeable on the right. No expected silicone signal is seen in the lateral aspect of the right outer lumen, and there is slightly decreased water signal in this area relative to the inner saline lumen (Figure 15.8.1A). A more superior image (Figure 15.8.3) demonstrates silicone within enlarged right axillary lymph nodes.

DIAGNOSIS: Extracapsular rupture of the silicone outer lumen of the right Becker implant (silicone outer lumen and saline inner lumen) and silicone lymph nodes, or siliconomas; the left implant is intact

COMMENT: Sometimes, patients are unaware of the type of implant they have, and because there is the possibility of a history of prior silicone implants with subsequent explantation and reimplantation of saline implants, we always perform the silicone series whenever there is an implant. Ruptured saline implants are generally a clinical diagnosis with rapid decompression of the involved breast; MRI is not needed and mammography can show the residual shell wrinkled on itself.

Silicone lymph nodes, free silicone, or silicone granulomas (ie, siliconomas) are signs of extracapsular implant rupture with silicone extending into the surrounding soft tissues. This finding can be related either to the current implant or, possibly, to a remotely ruptured implant. At the time of surgery in this patient, a posterior separation of the seam of the right outer gel shell was noted.

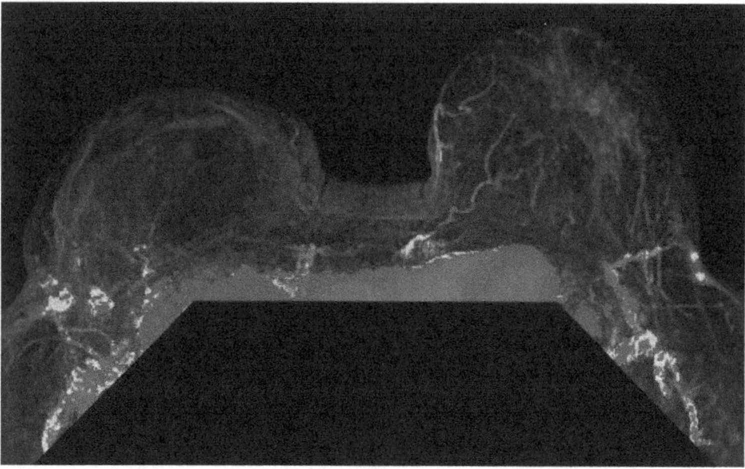

Figure 15.9.1

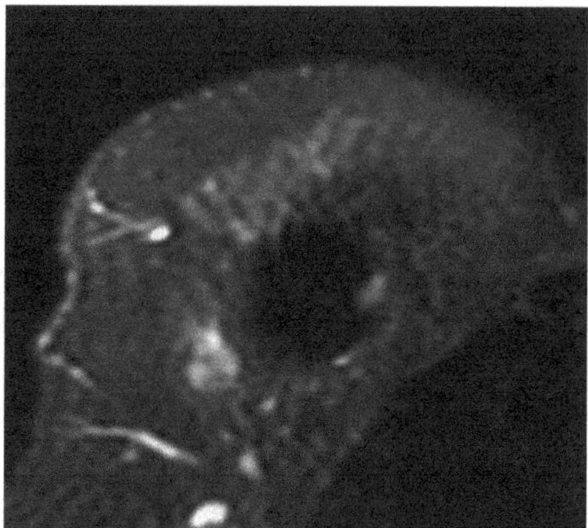

Figure 15.9.2

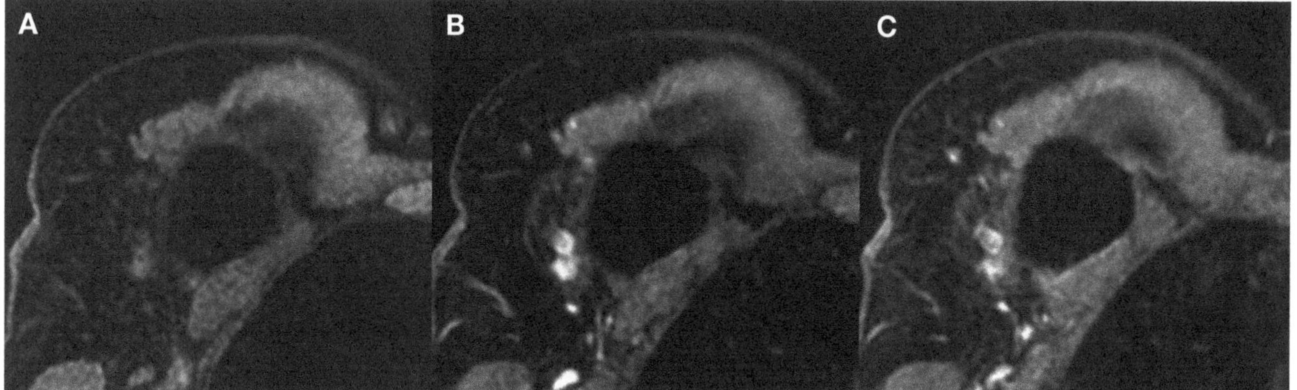

Figure 15.9.3

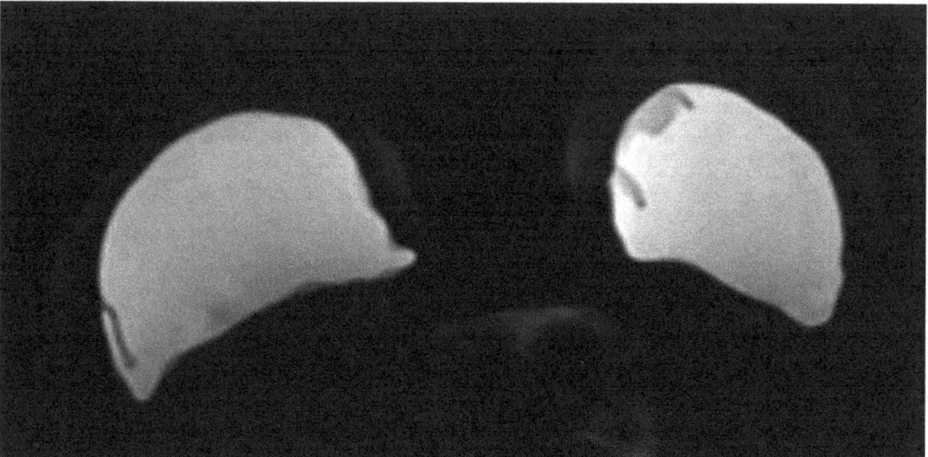

Figure 15.9.4

HISTORY: 61-year-old woman with a history of a ruptured left silicone implant 12 to 15 years ago. At that time, the ruptured implant and as much free silicone as possible were removed and a new silicone implant was placed. Recently, the patient was called back after screening mammography for a dense left axillary lymph node that on subsequent US was thought to contain silicone. Etiologic considerations included residual silicone from the prior implant rupture vs rupture of the current silicone implant. MRI was recommended for evaluation of implant integrity

IMAGING FINDINGS: The MIP image at peak enhancement with CAD color overlay (Figure 15.9.1) demonstrates enhancing right-sided peri-implant masses that have heterogeneous increased signal intensity (Figure 15.9.2) on T2-weighted FSE acquisition using a modified 3-point Dixon (IDEAL) method for fat suppression. Note the more homogeneous signal associated with a lymph node located more posteriorly. Pregadolinium (Figure 15.9.3A), first postgadolinium (Figure 15.9.3B), and delayed postgadolinium (Figure 15.9.3C) fat-suppressed axial 3D SPGR images demonstrate an enhancing focus and 2 small enhancing nodules with rapid washout adjacent to the right implant. Not shown are additional, similar-appearing, smaller peri-implant masses. Silicone imaging (Figure 15.9.4) demonstrates intact bilateral subpectoral silicone implants.

DIAGNOSIS: Invasive ductal carcinoma

COMMENT: The question of whether contrast should be administered for breast MRI performed to evaluate implant integrity arises once or twice a year in our practice and always generates mixed opinions. Deciding whether an implant is intact or ruptured does not require gadolinium, and in fact, this assessment can be performed in a few minutes using fast 2D or 3D T2-weighted FSE (or SSFP) acquisitions. On the other hand, many implants are placed after previous breast cancer surgery, and therefore it might be reasonable to consider screening this population for residual or recurrent disease, particularly given that physical examination, mammography, and sonography all become more difficult and less reliable following implant placement.

The benefits of a short, noncontrast breast implant protocol include higher patient throughput and easier, less stressful interpretation from the radiologist's perspective; the patient would also appreciate a shorter, less expensive examination with fewer false-positive findings requiring an invasive and expensive work-up. On the other hand, as illustrated in this case, cancer does occur in breasts with or without implants, and you're much more likely to find it when gadolinium is administered.

This patient had atypical ductal hyperplasia and DCIS in the right breast 12 years ago and underwent lumpectomy, which showed an invasive low-grade adenocarcinoma with areas of lymphatic invasion; she subsequently had a simple right mastectomy with reconstruction and was treated with tamoxifen for 5 years. Given this history, a comprehensive gadolinium-enhanced examination was a reasonable choice, and it revealed multiple suspicious, enhancing nodules, which proved malignant at biopsy.

CASE 15.10

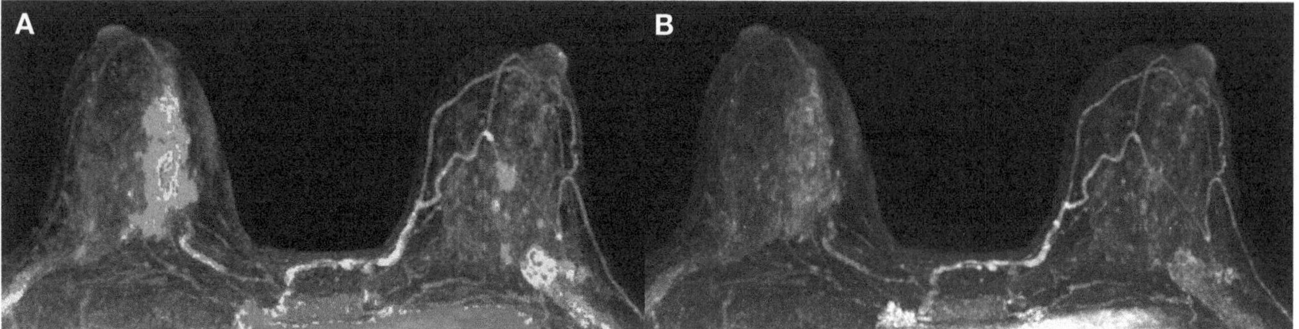

Figure 15.10.1

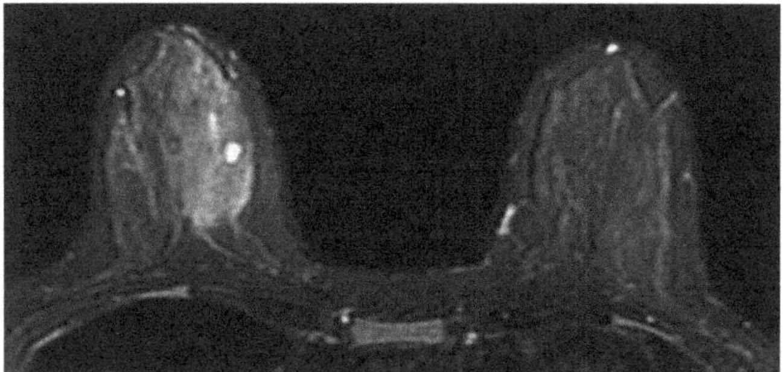
Figure 15.10.2

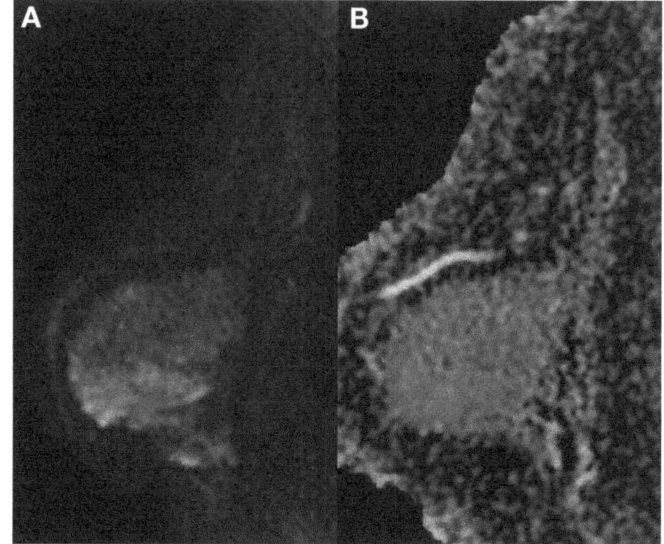

Figure 15.10.3

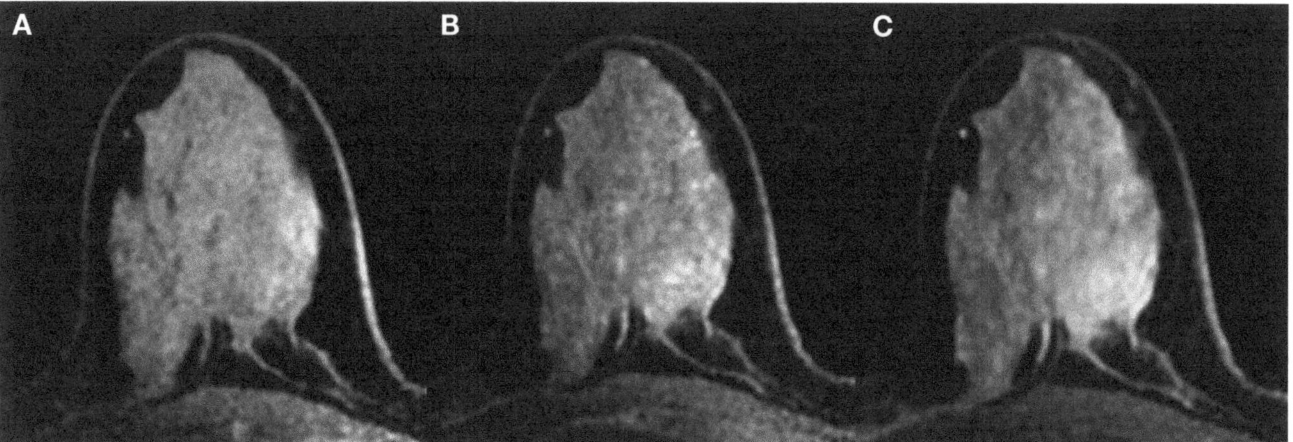

Figure 15.10.4

HISTORY: 36-year-old woman with biopsy-proven left-sided infiltrating ductal carcinoma; MRI was ordered for staging purposes

IMAGING FINDINGS: The MIP images at peak enhancement with (Figure 15.10.1A) and without (Figure 15.10.1B) CAD color overlay demonstrate a left-sided irregular mass with predominantly plateau and scattered washout enhancement corresponding to known malignancy. More anteriorly in the left breast, there is a small area of nonmass enhancement that was attributed to background and, possibly, some motion.

In the medial right breast, which is the focus of this case, there is a segmental nonmasslike enhancement that corresponds to relatively increased signal intensity (Figure 15.10.2) on T2-weighted FSE acquisition using a modified 3-point Dixon (IDEAL) method for fat suppression. Sagittal diffusion-weighted image (b=800 s/mm^2) (Figure 15.10.3A) and corresponding ADC map (Figure 15.10.3B) of the right breast do not demonstrate appreciable restricted diffusion. Pregadolinium (Figure 15.10.4A), first postgadolinium (Figure 15.10.4B), and delayed postgadolinium (Figure 15.10.4C) fat-suppressed axial 3D SPGR images demonstrate a somewhat vague, segmentally distributed nonmass enhancement in the lower inner quadrant of the right breast.

DIAGNOSIS: Benign breast parenchyma with nonproliferative fibrocystic changes (from right breast biopsy)

COMMENT: The satisfaction of detecting breast cancer on MRI is often overshadowed by the more difficult job of determining the extent of disease and "clearing the contralateral breast," a point that radiology residents learn rather quickly. The somewhat notorious low specificity of breast MRI can be exacerbated by the effects of estrogen and progesterone on background parenchymal enhancement during the menstrual cycle. In the ideal case, MRI is performed during the second week of the cycle, when hormonal levels are lowest. As estrogen and progesterone levels rise, there is increasing background parenchymal enhancement, as well as increasing stromal edema and lobular development, all of which contribute to what has been termed *nonmasslike enhancement*.

Of course, the timing of a particular patient's breast MRI is not solely determined by her menstrual cycle, but is much more frequently dependent on the next available open appointment, the patient's work schedule, the clinician's schedule, and the radiology administrator's need to fill as many open slots as possible. In this case, for example, the patient was on day 18 of her menstrual cycle, the luteal phase, where both estrogen and progesterone are at near-peak levels.

When the timing of the menstrual cycle with MRI is suboptimal, there are a few things that might help you favor background enhancement over a suspicious lesion. First, look at the other breast; even if it has a biopsy-proven cancer, as in this case, it can still serve as a comparison. Although the breasts are not perfectly symmetrical, the similarity of apparent nonmass enhancement in both breasts is more typical of background enhancement.

Second, remember to review the case at least once without any CAD postprocessing color overlays. Parametric images are only as good as the input data, and since analysis of enhancement kinetics is based on detecting signal intensity changes in individual voxels over 4 sets of images acquired over several minutes, relatively small changes in position or artifacts introduced into a particular acquisition can lead to significant errors in the color overlay map, some of which may present a very convincing appearance for malignancy. A linearly distributed red area of enhancement at a glandular fat interface, for example, may result from motion artifact rather than from DCIS, and sometimes the artifact cannot be appreciated until the images are reformatted in another plane.

And third, an evaluation and discussion of radiologic-pathologic concordance can help to narrow the differential diagnosis. Fibrocystic changes often present as prominent areas of glandular parenchyma, and in fact, many patients associate fibrocystic breasts with "lumpy bumpy" breasts. Fibrocystic changes respond to hormonal influences from estrogen and progesterone. Histologically, fibrocystic changes are divided into nonproliferative fibrocystic changes and proliferative fibrocystic changes. *Nonproliferative fibrocystic changes* describe cystic dilation of terminal ducts, stromal fibrosis, and apocrine metaplasia, all benign with no increased risk of malignancy. Proliferative fibrocystic changes are associated with an increased number of cells of the epithelium of the terminal duct lobular unit and, compared with their nonproliferative counterpart, are associated with an increased risk of malignancy in age-matched populations. Because US and MRI cannot definitely distinguish nonproliferative fibrocystic changes from proliferative ones, biopsy is almost always performed. Although not definitive, features that can sometimes provide reassurance that you are looking at background parenchyma are scattered fluid-filled cysts, similar-appearing enhancing foci, and normal or increased ADC values on DWI in a region of nonmass enhancement.

CASE 15.11

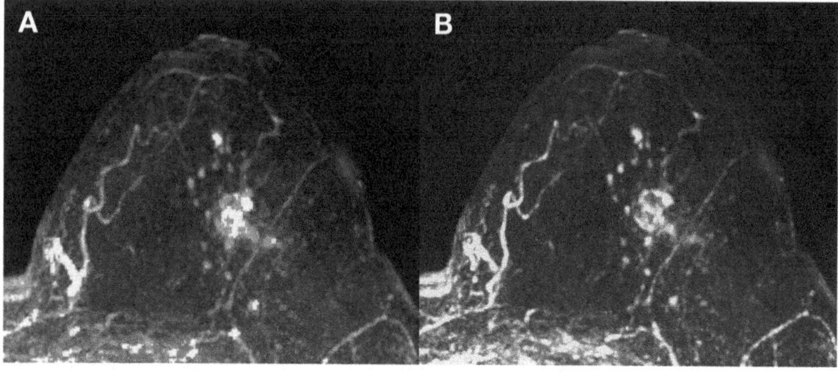

Figure 15.11.1

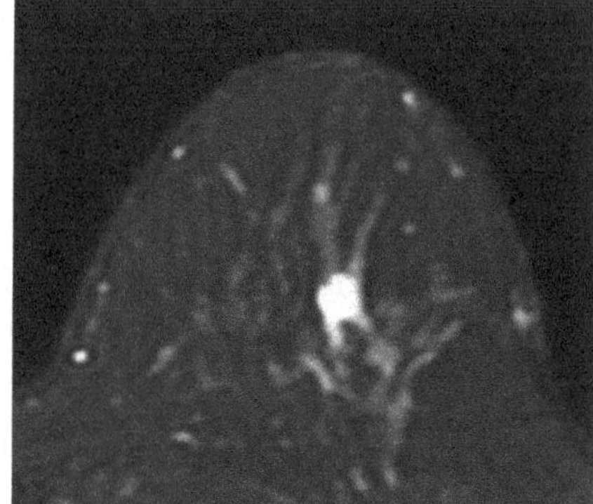

Figure 15.11.2

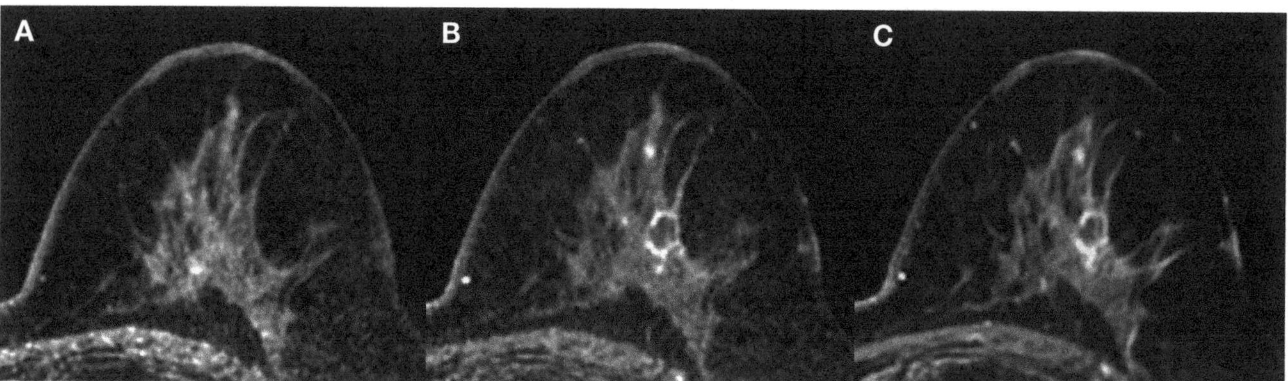

Figure 15.11.3

HISTORY: 58-year-old woman status post stereotactic-guided biopsy of grouped pleomorphic calcifications in the left breast with pathology indicating DCIS. Mammographically in this region, there were scattered parenchymal densities with areas of relatively greater density associated with the known cancer; MRI was performed 8 days after the biopsy to exclude other areas of disease

IMAGING FINDINGS: The MIP images of the left breast at peak enhancement with (Figure 15.11.1A) and without (Figure 15.11.1B) CAD color overlay demonstrate mild stippled background enhancement, clumped nonmass enhancement corresponding to DCIS and recent biopsy changes, and a focus of enhancement with plateau contrast kinetics more anteriorly. Water image (Figure 15.11.2) from a T2-weighted FSE acquisition using a modified 3-point Dixon (IDEAL) method for fat suppression reveals increased signal intensity in the left breast at the biopsy site and intermediate signal intensity corresponding to the focus. Pregadolinium (Figure 15.11.3A), first postgadolinium (Figure 15.11.3B), and third postgadolinium (Figure 15.11.3C) fat-suppressed 3D SPGR images show rim enhancement at the biopsy site and enhancement of the focus anteriorly.

DIAGNOSIS: CSL, or radial scar, in a background of proliferative fibrocystic changes, including usual ductal hyperplasia, apocrine metaplasia, and fibrosis

COMMENT: One of the benign lesions that can mimic cancers on all imaging modalities is the radial scar, or CSL. In grossly simplified pathology-speak, a radial scar is an idiopathic, benign fibroelastic lesion with radiating or stellate ducts and lobules that is entirely unrelated to a scar and is not a sequela of prior surgery or trauma. The term *complex sclerosing lesion* is sometimes reserved for lesions that are larger than 10 mm. The stellate morphology of CSLs makes them difficult to distinguish from the spiculated morphology of cancers, particularly tubular carcinomas, which are often small, slow-growing spiculated masses, similar to a radial scar. Current speculation (albeit conflicting) suggests that CSL may represent a premalignant condition, and therefore these lesions are typically surgically excised. With the use of large-gauge vacuum-assisted biopsy devices, it is possible to remove the entire mass at biopsy, depending on the individual circumstances. If this occurs, follow-up imaging rather than additional surgery could be a reasonable option.

The relative importance and subsequent management of an isolated focus (<5 mm of enhancement) with plateau contrast kinetics are uncertain and generally need to be considered in context with the clinical situation, degree of background parenchymal enhancement, and stability of the lesion in comparison with any prior MRIs. In this case, the focus is near a recent biopsy-proven cancer, warranting further evaluation to exclude a satellite lesion, which would be included in the total extent of disease. This provides information to our surgeons and breast clinicians, who can then make a decision with the patient about disease management. In this case, if breast conservation therapy is desired, presurgical bracket localization could be performed.

A second-look US was recommended for the MRI focus, which demonstrated no correlative findings, and therefore this patient proceeded to MRI-guided biopsy. Given the adjacent biopsy-proven DCIS, concern for upstaging of the CSL led to excision of this lesion at the time of surgical excision of the known DCIS.

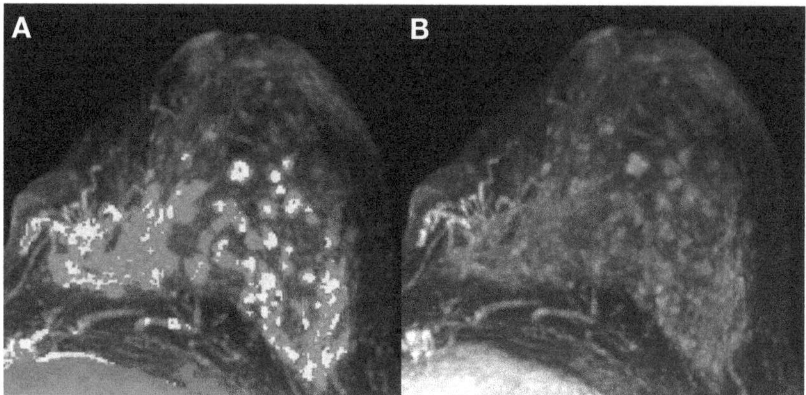

Figure 15.12.1

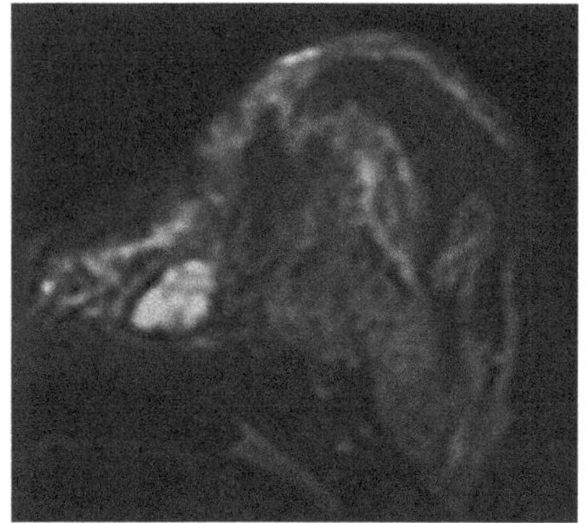

Figure 15.12.2

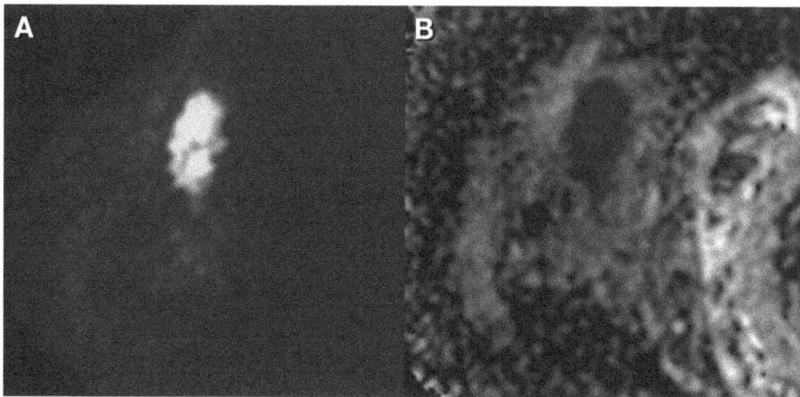

Figure 15.12.3

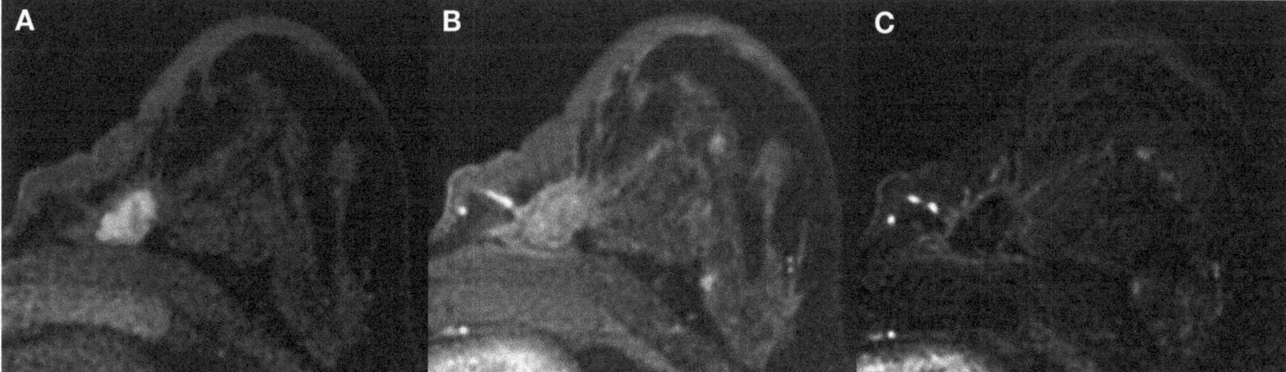

Figure 15.12.4

HISTORY: 43-year-old woman status post wide local excision of infiltrating ductal carcinoma in the left breast 7 weeks before this MRI, which was performed to rule out residual disease

IMAGING FINDINGS: The MIP images of the left breast at peak enhancement with (Figure 15.12.1A) and without (Figure 15.12.1B) CAD color overlay demonstrate moderate, stippled background enhancement. Water image (Figure 15.12.2) from a T2-weighted FSE acquisition using a modified 3-point Dixon (IDEAL) method for fat suppression reveals a heterogeneous, hyperintense mass with restricted diffusion, as seen on DWI (b=800 s/mm^2) (Figure 15.12.3A) and the ADC map (Figure 15.12.3B). Pregadolinium (Figure 15.12.4A) and first postgadolinium (Figure 15.12.4B) fat-suppressed 3D SPGR images and their subtraction image (Figure 15.12.4C) demonstrate nonenhancing increased T1 signal associated with this mass.

DIAGNOSIS: Postoperative hematoma in the left breast

COMMENT: This case illustrates the principle that hematomas look like hematomas regardless of location: Subacute hematomas show increased T1-signal intensity and variable T2-signal intensity and should not enhance after gadolinium administration. Subtraction images, if free from artifact, are particularly useful for demonstrating the absence of enhancement in a complex lesion. Clinical history is also helpful because most patients with a hematoma should have a reason for it, such as recent surgery in this case. The most important consideration is to exclude an underlying lesion or, in this recent postoperative case, a residual tumor.

DWI in breast MRI has sparked much interest scientifically and clinically. Lesion detection with DWI had a reported sensitivity of 92.5% in a study of 67 tumors ranging in size from 0.3 to 1.1 cm (median size, 0.7 cm). Currently, investigations into lesion characterization (including benign vs malignant, distinction of cancer types and subtypes, and prognosis) with mean ADC values indicate substantial variability, and further investigation is needed. The resident's first approximation that dark signal (low values) on an ADC map equates to restricted diffusion, which equates to cancer, is not particularly helpful in this case, and the occasional confounding appearance of hematomas on DWI has been noted by several authors. Perhaps the best way to regard DWI in the breast is as an occasionally helpful tool that provides information which must always be interpreted within the context of the entire examination.

Note the moderate background enhancement and the nonmass enhancement in the outer right breast that was attributed to background enhancement. There are also scattered cysts in the left breast.

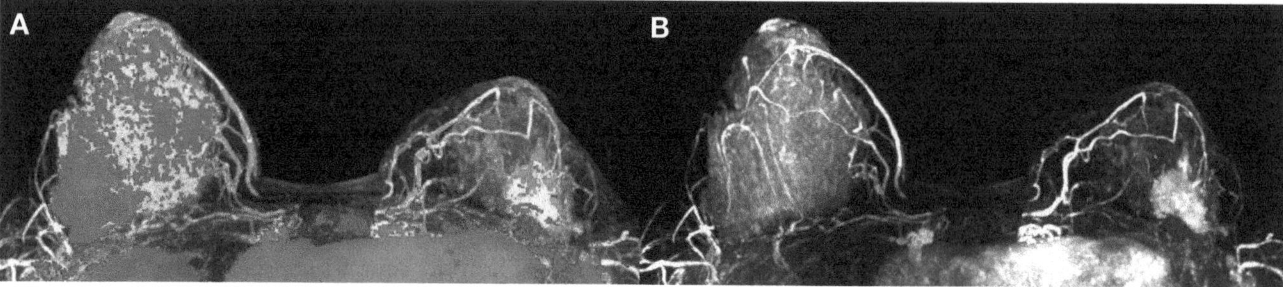

Figure 15.13.1

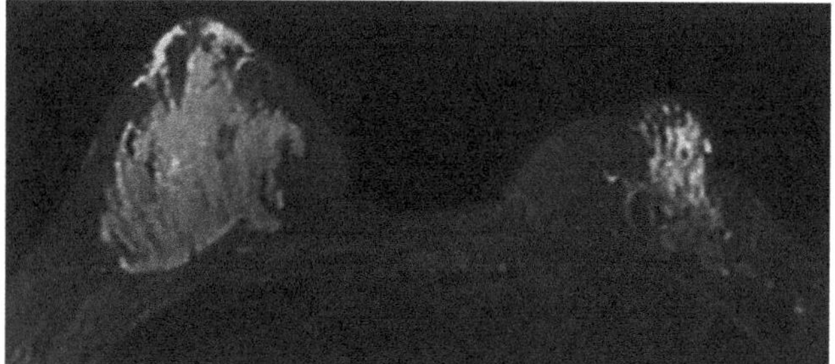

Figure 15.13.2

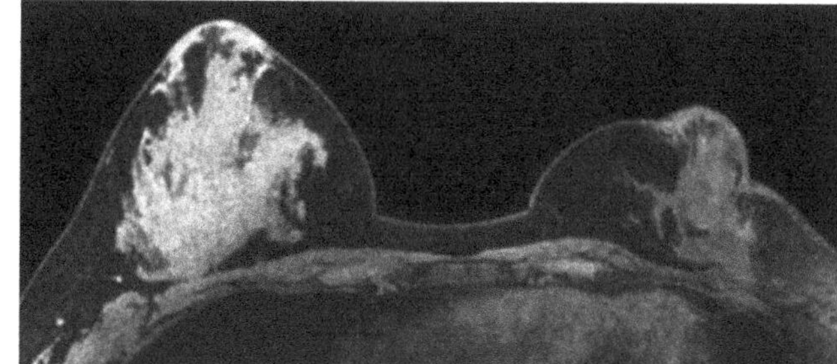

Figure 15.13.3

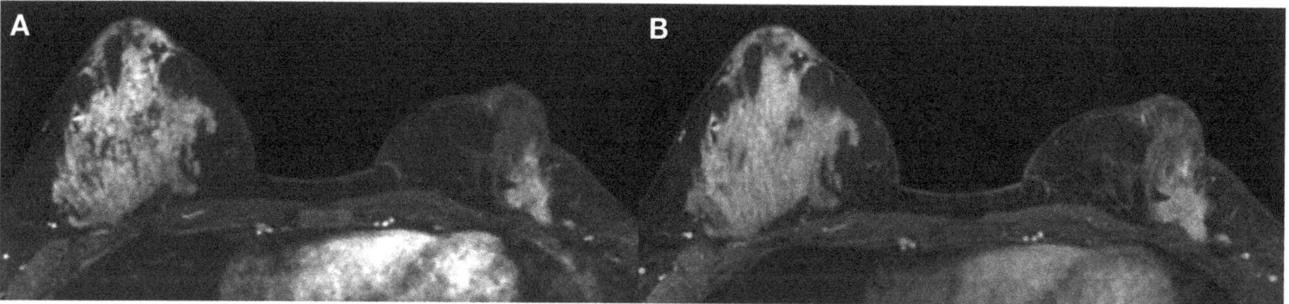

Figure 15.13.4

HISTORY: 35-year-old woman who during the ninth month of pregnancy noticed some nipple deviation of the left breast. After she gave birth to a healthy baby, the breast abnormality persisted along with a palpable area of concern; an MRI was ordered

IMAGING FINDINGS: The MIP images at peak enhancement with (Figure 15.13.1A) and without (Figure 15.13.1B) CAD color overlay demonstrate marked background enhancement, particularly on the right. Water image (Figure 15.13.2) from a T2-weighted FSE acquisition using a modified 3-point Dixon (IDEAL) method for fat suppression demonstrates asymmetrical breasts with a smaller left breast. There is a region of parenchyma in the posterior left breast with relative decreased signal intensity compared with the anterior tissue, which corresponds to a heterogeneously enhancing mass on dynamic pregadolinium (Figure 15.13.3) and peak (Figure 15.13.4A) and delayed (Figure 15.13.4B) postgadolinium 3D SPGR images. The larger right breast demonstrates diffuse high-T2-signal-intensity parenchyma and extensive diffuse enhancement following gadolinium administration without a discrete mass.

DIAGNOSIS: Invasive ductal carcinoma in the left breast. Nonneoplastic right breast parenchyma with lactational changes

COMMENT: Diagnostic evaluation of the lactating breast is one of the most difficult tasks of the breast imager. Even though we almost always try to postpone the examination until the patient has finished lactation, the answer to this request, particularly when involving a known or suspected cancer, is often no, since pregnancy-associated breast cancer is usually more advanced than breast cancer in age-matched nonpregnant patients. *Pregnancy-associated breast cancer* is defined as cancer diagnosed either during pregnancy, the first 12 months postpartum, or anytime while lactating. It is a rare diagnosis with an incidence of about 0.3 per 1,000 pregnancies and is generally associated with a more advanced histopathology and relatively poor prognosis, at least in part a result of the delay in diagnosis given the challenges of radiologic evaluation of the lactating breast.

Mammographically, the lactating breast is very difficult to evaluate, and most radiologists closely review the history and clinical indication before actually getting the mammogram. During lactation, the breasts are extremely dense, reducing the conspicuity of small masses and limiting the visibility of microcalcifications. For mammograms, it is sometimes helpful to ask the patient to use a lactation pump before the examination, but for US—and even more so for MRIs—the nature of the scans does not make the interpretation any easier. The hormonally induced changes of background breast parenchyma associated with lactation make MRI highly challenging.

As this case demonstrates, it is easy to be distracted by the extensive nonmass enhancement in the right breast. The lactating breast has increased vascular permeability with enhancement characteristics very similar to invasive cancers, which means that interpretation of the CAD-generated parametric images based on enhancement kinetics can be problematic. On the other hand, there is a striking discrepancy between the appearance of the 2 breasts and, given the lactating background, the left breast is actually the more abnormal one, lacking the expected extensive enhancing parenchyma. Anecdotally, this is an appearance occasionally seen in pregnancy-associated breast cancer, presumably because the infant does not nurse well on the side of the cancer.

Few references are available on MRI of the lactating breast or pregnancy-associated breast cancers. Small case series have described cancers with decreased signal intensity on T2-weighted images relative to background parenchyma and rapid enhancement on postgadolinium images. Although the background changes of lactation are problematic with any imaging modality, MRI remains a reasonable option when you are faced with a pregnant or lactating patient with suspected breast cancer. In this case, the left breast mass was biopsied.

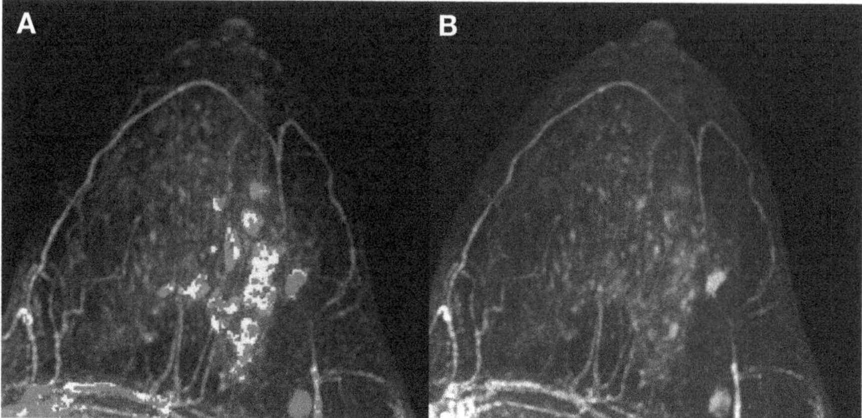

Figure 15.14.1

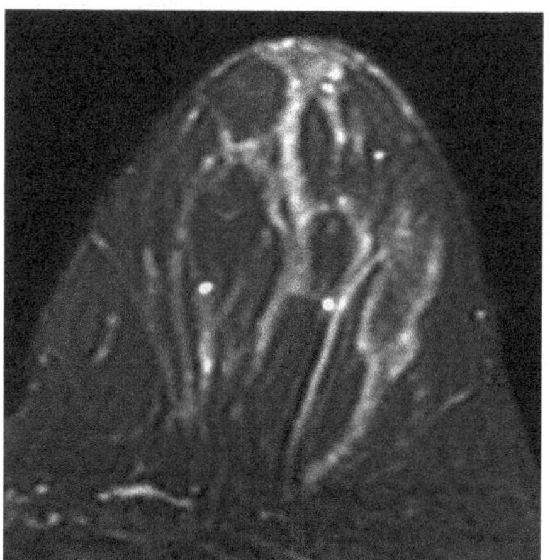

Figure 15.14.2

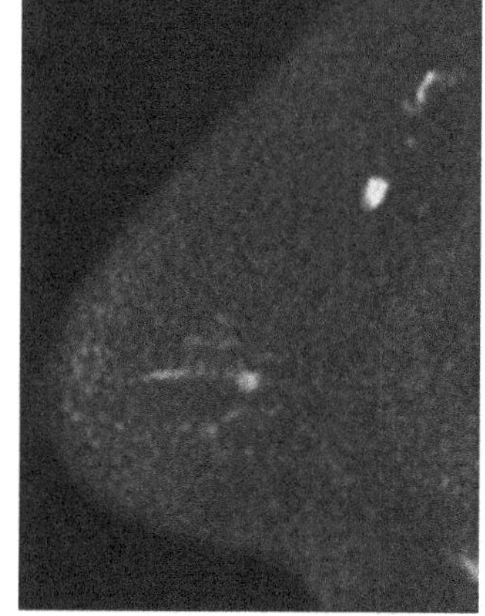

Figure 15.14.3

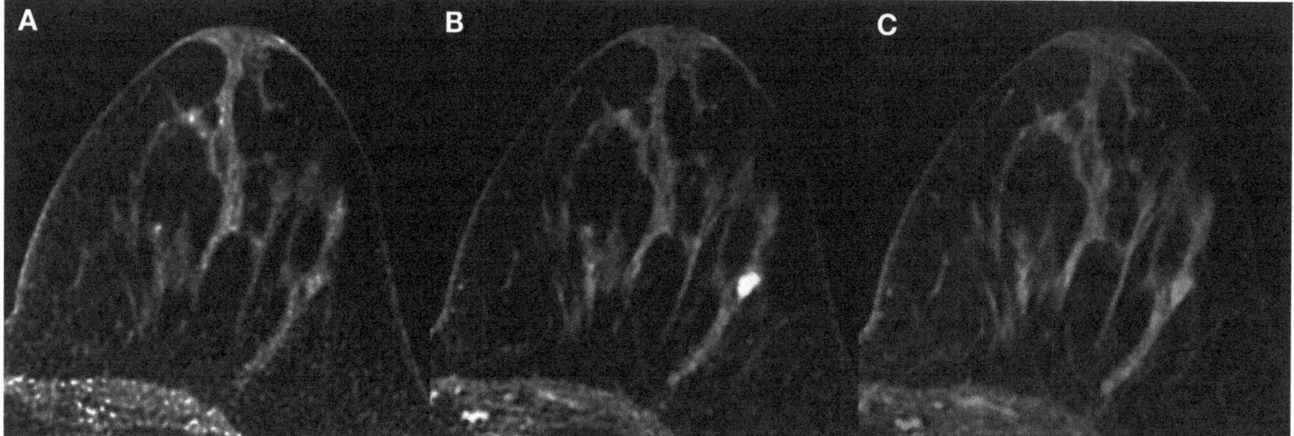

Figure 15.14.4

HISTORY: 36-year-old woman with a strong family history of breast cancer and a remote history of surgical excision of a 3-cm fibroadenoma at 16 years of age; this examination was performed as a baseline screening MRI

IMAGING FINDINGS: The MIP images of the left breast at peak enhancement with (Figure 15.14.1A) and without (Figure 15.14.1B) CAD color overlay demonstrate moderate stippled background enhancement. There is a nodule in the lateral left breast at middle depth with slightly heterogeneous, intermediate-to-high signal intensity on T2-weighted FSE image (Figure 15.14.2) using a modified 3-point Dixon (IDEAL) method for fat suppression. The nodule demonstrates mildly increased signal intensity compared with an axillary lymph node on a sagittal diffusion-weighted image (b=800 s/mm^2) (Figure 15.14.3). Pregadolinium (Figure 15.14.4A), peak postgadolinium (Figure 15.14.4B), and delayed post-gadolinium (Figure 15.14.4C) fat-suppressed 3D SPGR images show mixed plateau and rapid washout enhancement kinetics of the mass. The contrast-enhanced fat-suppressed 3D SPGR images also demonstrate a small enhancing mass within the outer left breast.

DIAGNOSIS: Fibroadenoma

COMMENT: Fibroadenomas are benign breast tumors with a reported incidence of 7% to 13% in adolescent girls and young women up to the third decade of life. The prevalence in this age-group in the general population is 2.2% and decreases with increasing age. These lesions are hormonally stimulated and often present as a palpable area of concern. Histologically, fibroadenomas are comprised of both stromal and epithelial components and are included in the set of fibro-epithelial lesions that also include phyllodes tumors, which can be benign or malignant depending on histologic features. Fibroadenomas can have a neoplastic component depending on the cellularity and mitotic activity, so sometimes, if the imaging features are not classically benign, core-needle biopsy is performed or a short-interval follow-up is performed to ensure there is no increase in size.

Fibroadenoma is a diagnosis encountered with some frequency in our weekly radiology-pathology conferences when reviewing biopsies. Other benign diagnoses commonly encountered include fibroadenomatoid nodule, sclerosing adenosis, cluster of microcysts, apocrine metaplasia, and dense stromal fibrosis. All of these contribute to the less-than-perfect specificity of MRI, which has been reported to range from 81% to 97%, with negative predictive values from 92% to 100% in selected populations.

The practical implication of this case is that your biopsy statistics will include a small percentage of benign lesions. In our practice, we seldom classify lesions as BIRADS 3 on MRI (more on BIRADS in Case 15.3). In part, this is because we strive to perform as thorough a targeted second-look US as possible, so that if there are no associated worrisome sonographic features, we would have no reservations in recommending a return to routine screening mammography. If, however, the MRI is worrisome and the lesion is sonographically occult, then we generally recommend an MRI-guided biopsy.

Evaluation of fibroadenomas that were recommended for biopsy on MRI has taught us several things. The classic finding of nonenhancing septations is often difficult to appreciate, particularly for masses less than 1.5 cm in diameter, which is a direct reflection of the MR acquisition technique. Similarly, the presence of smooth or lobulated borders is also difficult to appreciate with certainty in small lesions. These issues emphasize the need for high-spatial-resolution T2- and T1-weighted postgadolinium images, which can be helpful for resolving subtle morphologic features. The classic fibroadenoma has high signal intensity on T2-weighted images; however, many lesions have intermediate signal intensity that is difficult to distinguish from a malignant lesion. The enhancement characteristics of fibroadenomas show predominately persistent or plateau washout kinetics, but this is not universally true, and a small, but significant, percentage of lesions demonstrate rapid washout. DWI also may provide useful information; a lesion with little restricted diffusion is usually benign, and there are a few papers attempting to classify lesions as benign or malignant on the basis of ADC values. Keep in mind, however, that DWI pulse sequences vary from vendor to vendor and ADC values also depend on field strength, b value, and choice of imaging parameters, so the use of a cutoff ADC value to discriminate benign from malignant lesions is not a good idea unless the cutoff is based on data from your own equipment.

While the imaging appearance of a lesion is of course important, the level of suspicion should also reflect the clinical history. A fibroadenoma or fibroadenomatoid-appearing mass in the ipsilateral breast of a patient with a biopsy-proven malignancy would be a little more worrisome than one found on a screening examination in a young patient.

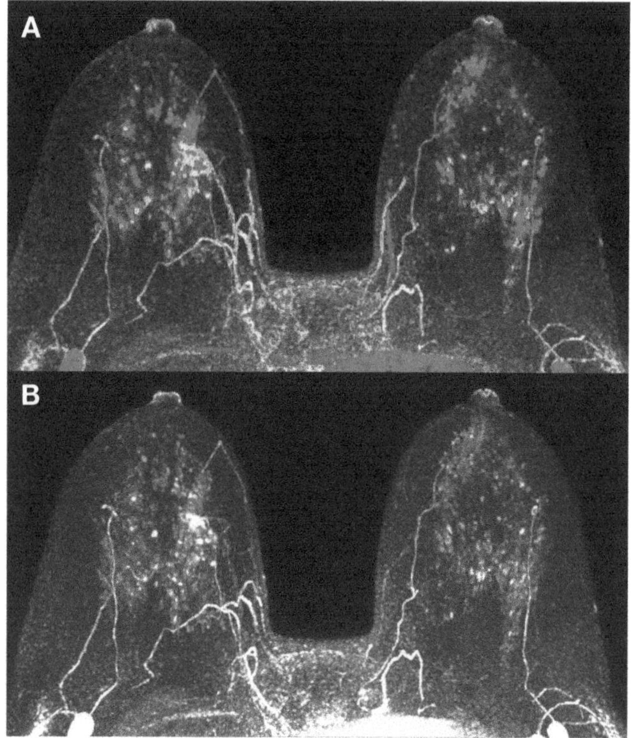

Figure 15.15.1

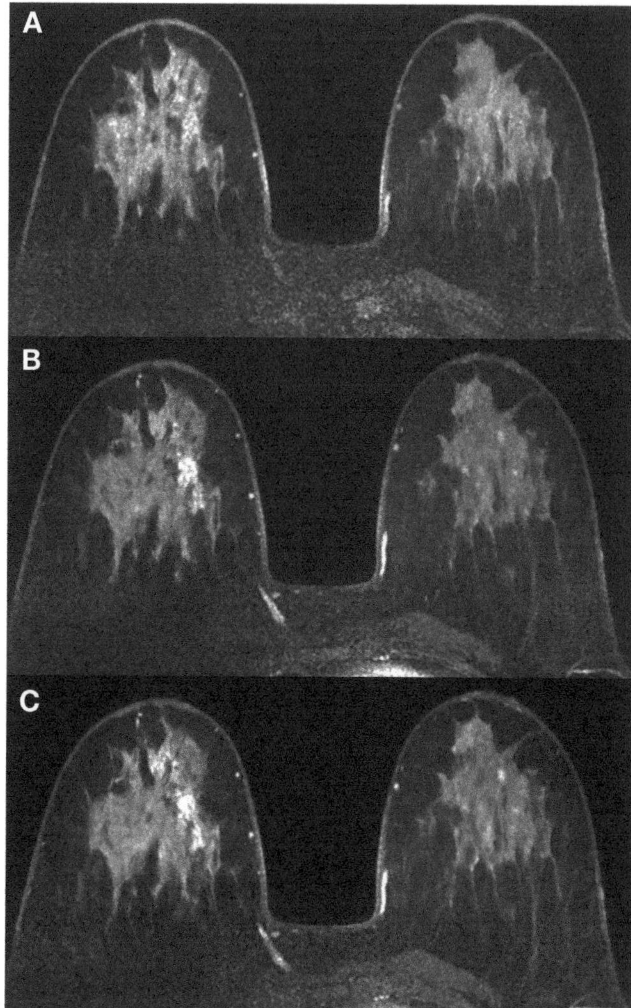

Figure 15.15.3

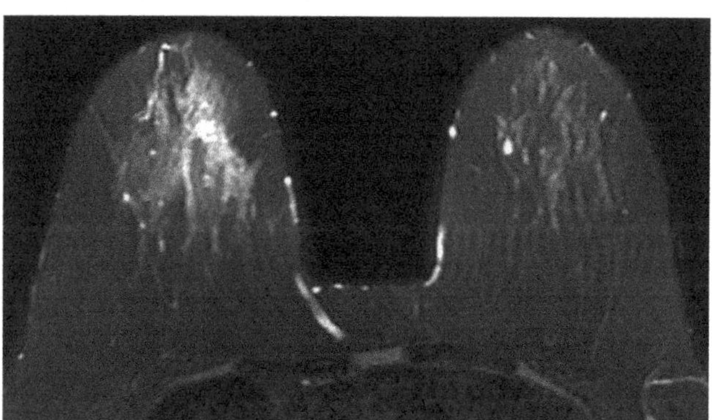

Figure 15.15.2

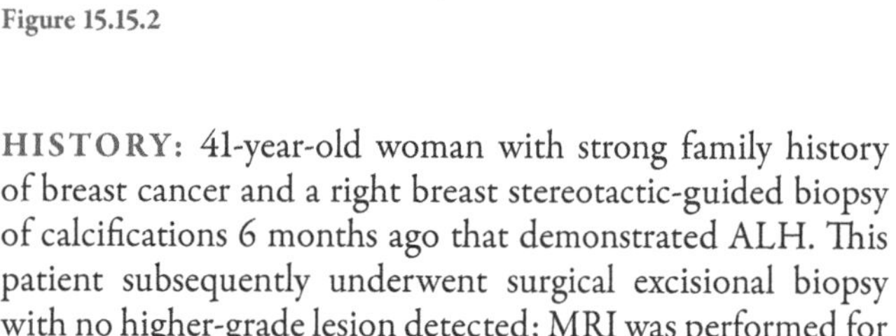

HISTORY: 41-year-old woman with strong family history of breast cancer and a right breast stereotactic-guided biopsy of calcifications 6 months ago that demonstrated ALH. This patient subsequently underwent surgical excisional biopsy with no higher-grade lesion detected; MRI was performed for screening purposes in this high-risk patient

IMAGING FINDINGS: The MIP images at peak enhancement with (Figure 15.15.1A) and without (Figure 15.15.1B) CAD color overlay demonstrate moderate stippled background enhancement. In the medial right breast, there is segmental, clumped nonmass enhancement with predominantly plateau and rapid washout kinetics. This area is associated with hyperintensity on T2-weighted FSE acquisition (Figure 15.15.2) using a modified 3-point Dixon (IDEAL) method for fat suppression. Pregadolinium (Figure 15.15.3A), peak postgadolinium (Figure 15.15.3B), and delayed postgadolinium (Figure 15.15.3C) fat-suppressed axial 3D SPGR images illustrate the clumped internal enhancement pattern of the nonmasslike enhancement. Findings are more prominent than background enhancement in the contralateral breast.

DIAGNOSIS: Focal ALH, involving a sclerosing papillary lesion with usual ductal hyperplasia

COMMENT: ALH is not a high-grade lesion but has a 4 to 5 times increased relative risk of cancer at 10 to 15 years postbiopsy. Management of these lesions usually includes a surgical consultation where excision is performed to exclude upstaging to an in situ or invasive cancer. One study reports an upstaging to DCIS or invasive carcinoma in 8% of surgically excised ALHs at core-needle biopsy, and other authors report an upstaging of 25% to DCIS or invasive lobular carcinoma.

When an MIP demonstrates moderate stippled background enhancement, as in this case, the first thing we tend to do is look at the case without the color overlay. The description of the finding as "segmental clumped nonmass enhancement with predominantly plateau and rapid washout kinetics" in and of itself connotes a suspicious finding. It cannot be distinguished from ductal carcinoma, and second-look US was recommended with the additional comment that should this be sonographically occult, an MRI-guided biopsy is recommended.

This particular patient went to second-look US and the area was sonographically occult, so MRI-guided biopsy was performed. Patients with biopsy-proven atypical hyperplasia, whether lobular or ductal, do not have cancer but have an entity that may develop into carcinoma in situ or invasive cancer. Because of the possibility of sampling error at biopsy and the possibility of in situ or invasive cancer that was not sampled at biopsy, patients are generally referred for wide local excision or lumpectomy to ensure there is no upstaging at pathologic assessment, which is what happened for this patient. Patients with atypical hyperplasia usually undergo more aggressive surveillance. This patient did not want to undergo additional surveillance and opted for bilateral mastectomies.

ABBREVIATIONS

ACR	American College of Radiology
ADC	apparent diffusion coefficient
ALH	atypical lobular hyperplasia
BIRADS	Breast Imaging Reporting and Data System
CAD	computer-aided detection
CSL	complex sclerosing lesion
DCIS	ductal carcinoma in situ
DWI	diffusion-weighted imaging
FDA	US Food and Drug Administration
FSE	fast-spin echo
IDEAL	iterative decomposition of water and fat with echo asymmetry and least-squares estimation
IR	inversion recovery
LCIS	lobular cancer in situ
MIP	maximum intensity projection
MR	magnetic resonance
MRI	magnetic resonance imaging
SPGR	spoiled gradient-recalled echo
SSFP	steady-state free precession
3D	3-dimensional
TI	inversion time
2D	2-dimensional
US	ultrasonography

16.

VASCULAR SYSTEM

CASE 16.1

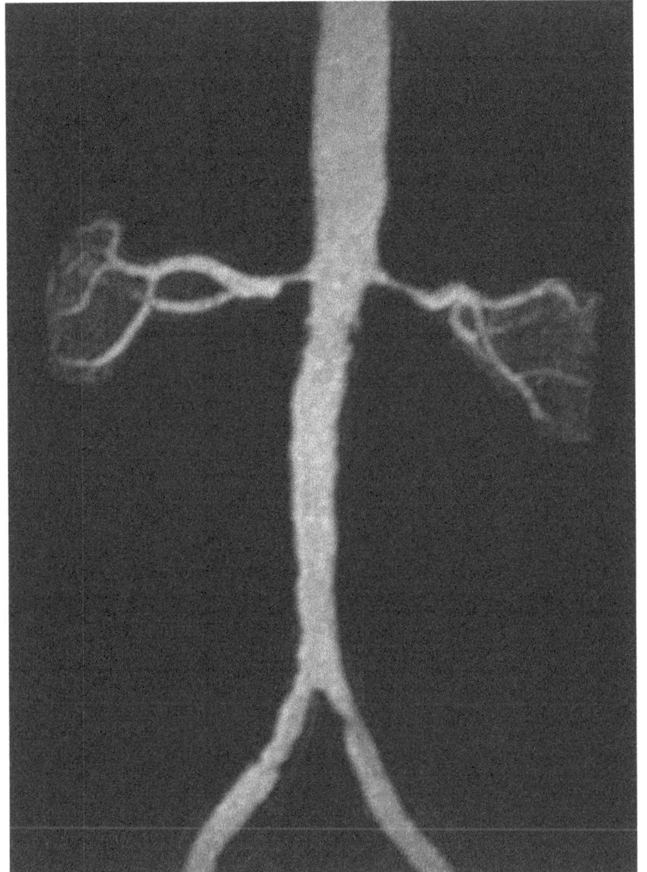

Figure 16.1.1

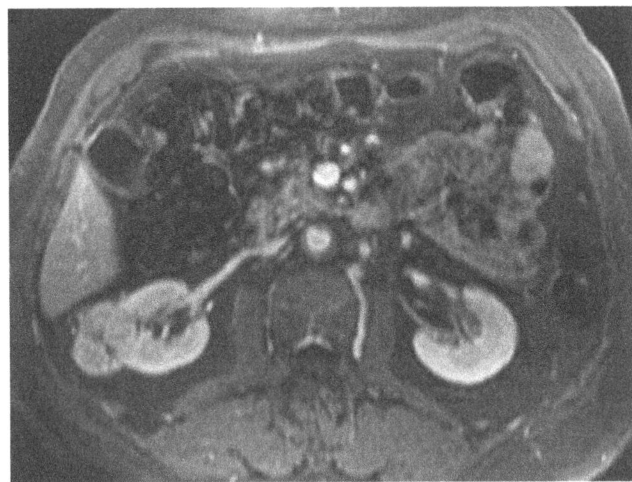

Figure 16.1.2

HISTORY: 75-year-old man with drug-resistant hypertension

IMAGING FINDINGS: MIP image from 3D CE MRA of the abdomen (Figure 16.1.1) demonstrates severe stenosis of the right and left renal arteries. Axial postgadolinium fat-suppressed 3D SPGR image (Figure 16.1.2) reveals an enhancing right renal mass consistent with renal cell carcinoma.

DIAGNOSIS: Renal artery stenosis

COMMENT: Renal MRA for detection of renal artery stenosis was one of the earliest applications of 3D CE MRA, and many studies support the widely held (and likely correct) belief that this technique is highly accurate for detection of significant renal artery stenosis. As is true of much of the radiology literature, however, most of the studies are relatively small and come from single institutions. One of the few prospective multicenter trials compared renal MRA (and CTA) with the gold standard of conventional angiography (the RADISH trial). Results were much less favorable, prompting the authors to conclude that neither technique was accurate enough to use for screening in patients with suspected renovascular hypertension (interestingly, another study with the same first author was a meta-analysis demonstrating the high accuracy of renal MRA). The truth probably lies somewhere between the 99% accuracy rates of some of the single-institution studies and the disappointing results of the RADISH trial. Good results depend on good technique (unfortunately, there were no standard protocols in the RADISH trial), but even good technique won't prevent suboptimal results if patients cannot hold their breath.

The key to accurate renal MRA is adequate spatial resolution. Generally, this means an in-plane resolution of less than 1 mm and a through-plane resolution of less than 2 mm, which is most efficiently accomplished with a coronal oblique acquisition plane. Since acquisition time is proportional to the spatial resolution in the phase encoding direction and to the number of phase encoding steps in the through-plane direction, there is obviously a trade-off between resolution and acquisition time. It's almost always better to acquire an MRA with slightly less than ideal spatial resolution but no motion artifact than one with higher resolution that is uninterpretable because patients could not hold their breath. Parallel imaging (1-dimensional or 2D) can be useful for improving spatial resolution without significantly increasing acquisition time, but it does come at a cost in signal to noise ratio and it can generate significant image artifacts. One simple and underappreciated technique to improve spatial resolution is to minimize the FOV while keeping the phase and frequency matrix constant: After patients raise their arms above their head, crop the FOV to 26 to 28 cm, rather than to 35 to 45 cm as favored by many practices, and carefully prescribe anteroposterior coverage to minimize extraneous coverage that doesn't include the aorta or renal arteries. This approach provides high spatial resolution without using parallel imaging or other cutting-edge techniques.

It should go without saying that accurate assessment of the degree of renal artery stenosis requires viewing the source data within a 3D viewer that allows reformatted or MIP views of arbitrary thickness and orientation. It is unacceptable to view only the 3D reconstructions generated by your technologist and make the diagnosis solely on the basis of those images.

In many practices, ours included, the volume of renal MRA examinations decreased dramatically following the initial reports linking NSF to gadolinium contrast agents. To some extent, this change reflects the extensive publicity about NSF in the medical literature (there are more articles about NSF than reported cases) and in the nonmedical literature (ie, legal advertisements) and the reluctance of referring physicians to expose patients with even mild renal insufficiency to gadolinium. However, no documented cases of NSF have occurred in patients who have an estimated glomerular filtration rate greater than 30 mL/min/1.73 m^2, and no new cases have occurred at our institution for several years. In addition, there is increasing controversy regarding the efficacy of renal artery revascularization in patients with renovascular hypertension in light of 2 prospective randomized trials that compared medical therapy with endovascular revascularization (the ASTRAL and STAR trials). They failed to show significant benefits for patients who had endovascular treatment of renal artery stenosis (although both studies had significant limitations in the study design and implementation). A third prospective randomized trial (CORAL) is underway, and if it does not produce the results expected by interventional radiologists and endovascular surgeons, there will probably be a fourth trial.

One of the implications of recent research in renovascular hypertension is that the kidneys are remarkably effective at autoregulation over a wide range of perfusion pressures and that it takes a relatively severe stenosis (70%-80% cross-sectional diameter) to generate a significant hemodynamic effect (which may partially explain the negative results of the ASTRAL and STAR trials). So keep in mind when reading these cases that there is a real difference between a 55% stenosis and a 75% stenosis.

Renal artery stenosis is highly correlated with systemic atherosclerosis (a study of screening renal angiography in patients having clinically indicated coronary angiography demonstrated a 30% prevalence of renal artery atherosclerosis and a 10%-18% incidence of >50% stenosis in patients with significant coronary artery disease). Moreover, patients with renal artery stenosis and coexisting systemic atherosclerosis have higher morbidity and mortality for subsequent cardiovascular events.

Recognition of the link between NSF and gadolinium contrast agents has had the positive effect of stimulating renewed interest in noncontrast MRA techniques for the abdomen and lower extremities. The most common technique currently available is a 3D fat-suppressed SSFP sequence with a form of arterial spin labeling (the imaging slab is suppressed with an inversion pulse, while nonsuppressed blood flowing into the slab is bright). The images have excellent background suppression and allow very nice 3D reconstructions. In our hands (and in most of the published literature), these techniques are as accurate or nearly as accurate as 3D CE MRA. They do have a couple of limitations to keep in mind, however: 1) Acquisition times are fairly long (4-6 minutes); therefore, some form of respiratory gating is required, and this can be problematic in patients with irregular respiration. 2) Visualization of the renal arteries depends on unsuppressed blood flowing into the imaging slab between the initial inversion pulse and image acquisition. This limits the superior-inferior coverage (which means that some accessory renal arteries may be missed) and can be problematic in patients with slow arterial flow (eg, those with heart failure or abdominal aortic aneurysms).

The incidental renal cell carcinoma also deserves mention. It is obviously an important finding that could easily be missed if only a scout series and MRA were performed. For this reason, every renal MRA protocol must include parenchymal imaging of the kidneys (at a minimum, in-phase and out-of-phase imaging for identification of adrenal adenomas and 2D or 3D postcontrast fat-suppressed SPGR imaging for identification of renal masses). Incidental nonvascular findings in renal MRA are quite common, and even significant findings are not rare.

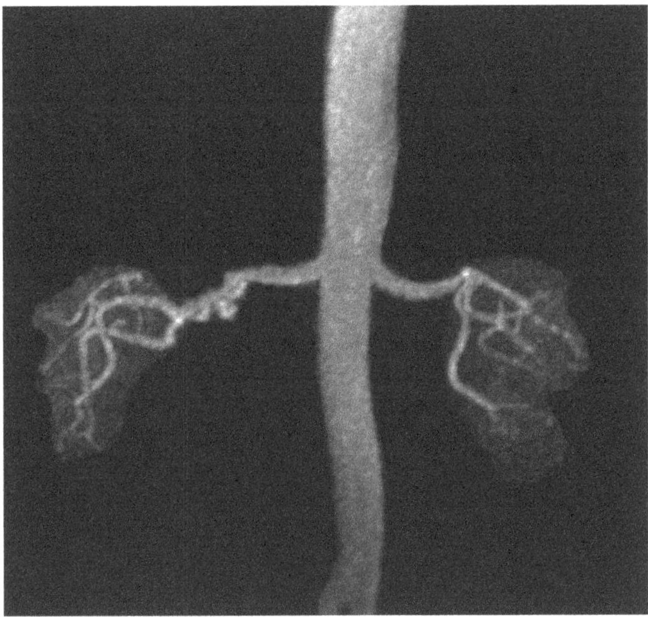

Figure 16.2.1

HISTORY: 59-year-old man with a history of hypertension

IMAGING FINDINGS: MIP image from 3D CE MRA (Figure 16.2.1) reveals prominent beading of the mid-distal right main renal artery.

DIAGNOSIS: Fibromuscular dysplasia

COMMENT: FMD, first reported by Leadbetter and Burkland in 1938, is a nonatherosclerotic, noninflammatory vascular disorder that occurs most often in women aged 20 to 60 years. It commonly involves the renal and extracranial carotid arteries, although any vascular territory can be affected. The renal arteries are affected in 75% of FMD patients, with bilateral involvement in more than 35%. Renal artery aneurysms are a fairly common complication of renal FMD and have been reported in 9% of patients. The incidence of FMD in the extracranial carotid arteries is uncertain. It was long accepted that carotid artery FMD occurred in 25% to 30% of patients with FMD; however, a much higher incidence of 70% has been identified for the first 200 patients enrolled in the FMD international registry. Vertebral arteries are less commonly involved than the carotid arteries. The etiology of FMD is unknown, but speculation has centered on hormonal and genetic factors.

FMD is classified into 3 categories on the basis of the location of anatomical involvement in the arterial wall: intimal fibroplasia, medial fibroplasia, and adventitial (or perimedial) fibroplasia. Medial fibroplasia, involving the middle layer of the arterial wall, is by far the most common type, accounting for 80% to 90% of FMD lesions. It is characterized by alternating layers of thinned media and thickened collagen containing medial ridges, giving rise to the classic string-of-beads appearance seen in this case. Intimal fibroplasia, involving the inner layer, accounts for 10% of lesions and results from intimal collagen deposition. The classic lesion of intimal fibroplasias is a focal bandlike stenosis in the mid-distal main renal artery. Perimedial fibroplasia occurs rarely. It also has a string-of-beads appearance, but the "beads" are fewer and smaller. (Medial disease is further classified into 3 additional subcategories, 2 of which are extremely rare and probably not worth remembering.)

The typical clinical manifestation of renal FMD is hypertension in a young woman, although as renal MRA and CTA have become more common, FMD is detected with increasing frequency as an incidental finding in male patients and older patients. In addition to the classic string-of-beads appearance in the mid-distal renal artery, other features to look for are the classic complications: renal artery dissection, aneurysm, and thrombosis. After you've identified FMD, it's always tempting to rate the severity of the disease, but there isn't really much documentation in the literature suggesting that this can be done accurately, even with conventional angiography. Measurements of pressure gradients across individual stenoses are required to identify significant lesions.

The question of whether MRA is an adequate test to screen for FMD in a young patient with hypertension is controversial. Early in the use of 3D CE MRA, the consensus seemed to be that cases with extensive disease could occasionally be identified, but the lesions were often too subtle to detect. More recent articles describe successful identification of renal FMD in nearly all patients using conventional angiography as a gold standard. For good results, attention to technique is very important: Spatial resolution should be as high as possible within the constraints of the patient's breath-hold capacity (which may be a little longer in younger patients). This may be one of the few instances when CTA has a slight advantage over MRA since the spatial resolution of CTA is usually significantly higher.

Pseudo-FMD lesions can also be seen with CE MRA. You might notice a subtle beaded appearance in normal arteries, which is probably the result of limited spatial resolution in the slice-encoding direction in combination with slight motion artifact. If you're not sure whether the lesion is real, look at other arteries in the abdomen. If you see the same appearance, it's most likely artifact.

Little data have been published assessing the ability of the newer noncontrast renal MRA techniques to detect FMD. Sensitivity and specificity for identification of FMD are likely good to excellent, since visualization of the distal main renal arteries and segmental arteries is often better with the noncontrast 3D SSFP pulse sequences than with conventional 3D CE MRA, but, of course, this is dependent on good respiratory triggering and minimal motion artifact.

Differential diagnosis is usually not difficult. Renal atherosclerosis is much more common than FMD, but it occurs in older patients, and most atherosclerotic lesions are located at the renal artery ostia or in the proximal arteries (or in both locations). Vasculitis affecting the kidneys typically results in elevated acute-phase reactants, which are not seen in noninflammatory FMD.

Renal FMD causing significant hypertension is treated initially with pharmacologic management, and angioplasty is performed if FMD is resistant to medical management. Angioplasty generally has excellent results if complications such as dissection, embolus, and arterial rupture are avoided. The restenosis rate ranges from 7% to 27%.

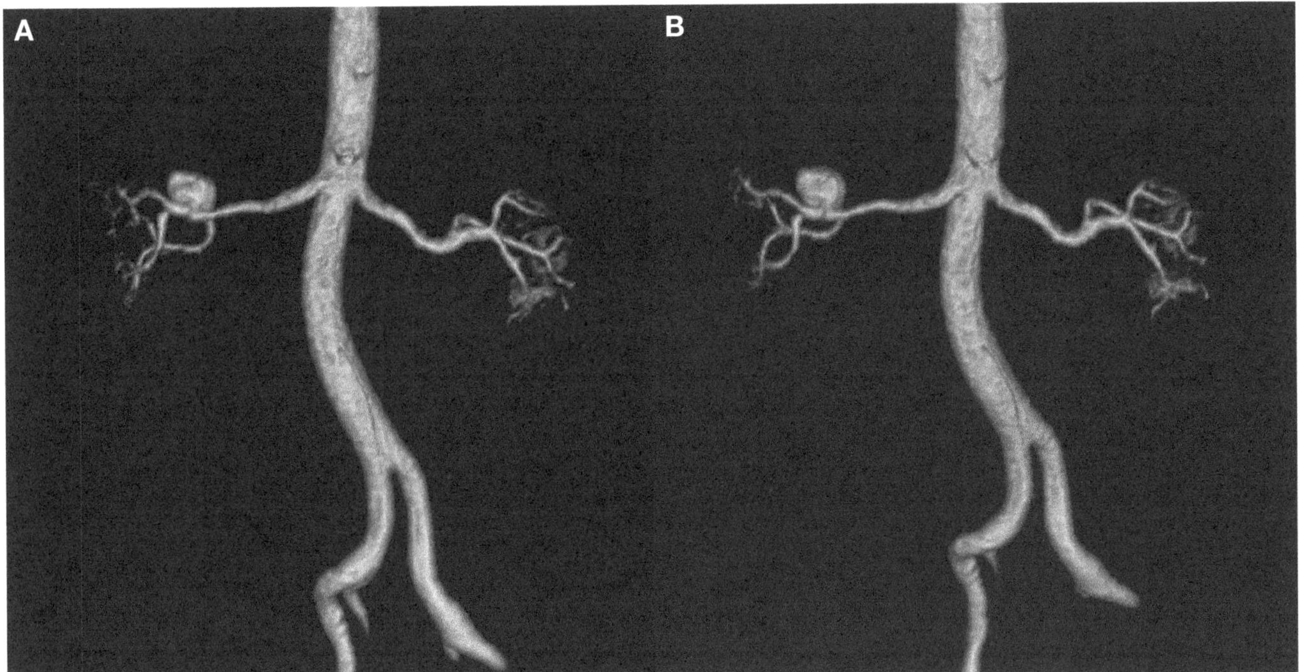

Figure 16.3.1

HISTORY: 43-year-old man with hypertension resistant to medical therapy

IMAGING FINDINGS: Focal dilatation of the right renal artery at its bifurcation is seen on VR images from 3D CE MRA (Figure 16.3.1).

DIAGNOSIS: Renal artery aneurysm

COMMENT: Renal artery aneurysms are relatively infrequent, but nevertheless they are the second most common visceral artery aneurysm after splenic artery aneurysms. The estimated incidence on autopsy studies is approximately 0.01%, while an incidence of 0.3% to 1% has been reported for patients undergoing renal angiography. Renal artery aneurysms are most often detected in middle age and are more common in women. Patients are typically asymptomatic. The aneurysms are associated with hypertension in as many as 73% of cases, but it is not always clear whether the aneurysm is the result or the cause of hypertension. Certainly poststenotic dilatation can result from severe renal artery stenosis, and distal embolization from renal artery aneurysms could result in parenchymal loss and activation of the renin-angiotensin cascade. Renal artery aneurysms have several potential causes, but the 2 most common are atherosclerosis and FMD. Both tend to occur most frequently in the main renal artery, at its bifurcation, or in the proximal branches. Aneurysms due to arteritis, such as polyarteritis nodosa, Wegener granulomatosis, and necrotizing angiitis, as well as most posttraumatic aneurysms and pseudoaneurysms, occur within intrarenal arteries. Additional causes include EDS, neurofibromatosis, infection (mycotic), and iatrogenic causes. FMD is discussed more completely in Case 16.2; however, FMD occurs most frequently in young hypertensive patients, most often women.

There is no clear consensus on when renal artery aneurysms require treatment, although a 2-cm diameter is a common cutoff. Special note should be made of patients who are pregnant or are contemplating pregnancy because pregnant women have a higher incidence of renal artery aneurysm rupture and an accompanying high mortality with rupture (up to 80%). Treatment options include embolization, covered stent placement, nephrectomy, or surgical bypass.

MRA is an ideal technique for diagnosis and follow-up of renal artery aneurysms: It is accurate, reproducible, and fairly straightforward, and it also avoids the cumulative radiation exposure of multiple CTAs. US is a less expensive alternative, but visualization of the aneurysm and accurate measurement are much more user dependent. In virtually all radiology practices, 3D CE renal MRA is a standard technique, but it has a few pitfalls to keep in mind. Adequate spatial resolution is important but probably to a lesser extent than for renal artery stenosis; it is almost always better to err on the side of slightly lower resolution and a shorter breath-hold than to ruin the examination with an acquisition time exceeding the patient's breath-hold capacity. As with aneurysms in any vascular bed, it is important to 1) look at source images, not only the 3D reconstructions, and 2) perform fat-suppressed 3D SPGR imaging after MRA to ensure that the measurements include the entire aneurysm and not just the nonthrombosed portion.

Noncontrast renal MRA techniques also work well for detection of aneurysms. Most of these are respiratory triggered and therefore depend to some extent on fairly even and reproducible respirations. The same problem exists with visualization of the thrombosed portion of the aneurysm, but the extent of the aneurysm can usually be seen well with conventional axial 2D or 3D SSFP images.

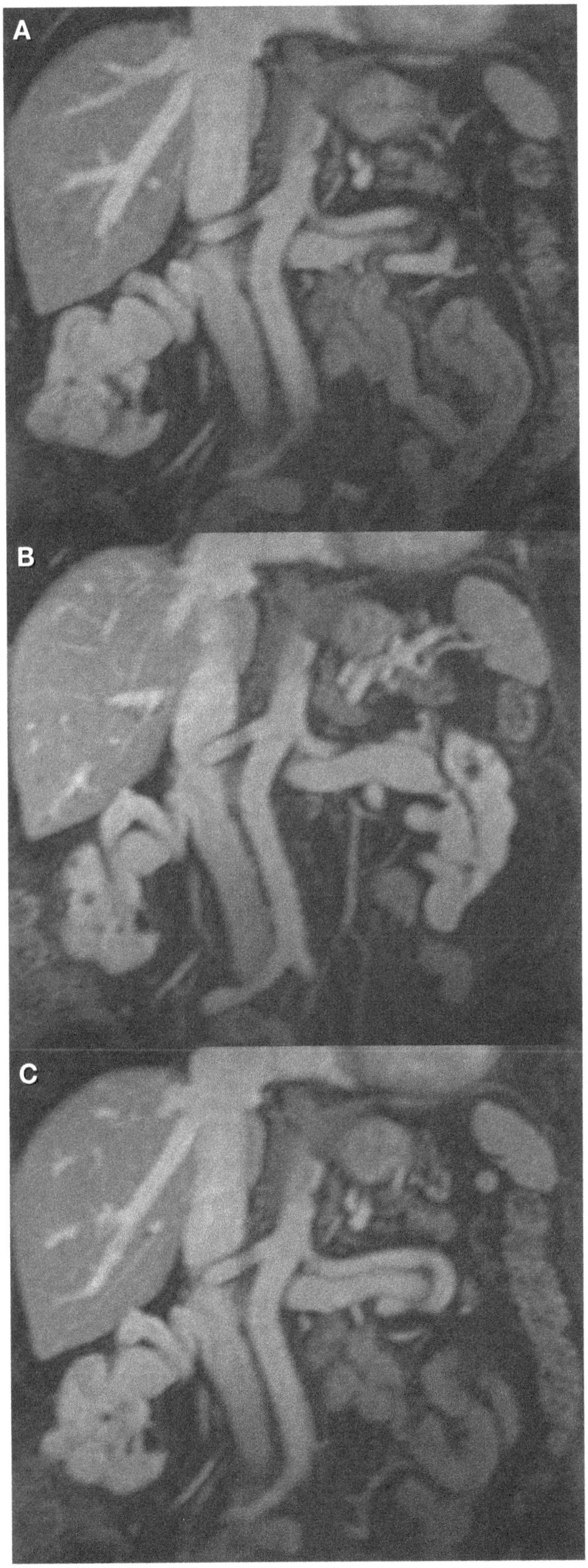

Figure 16.4.1

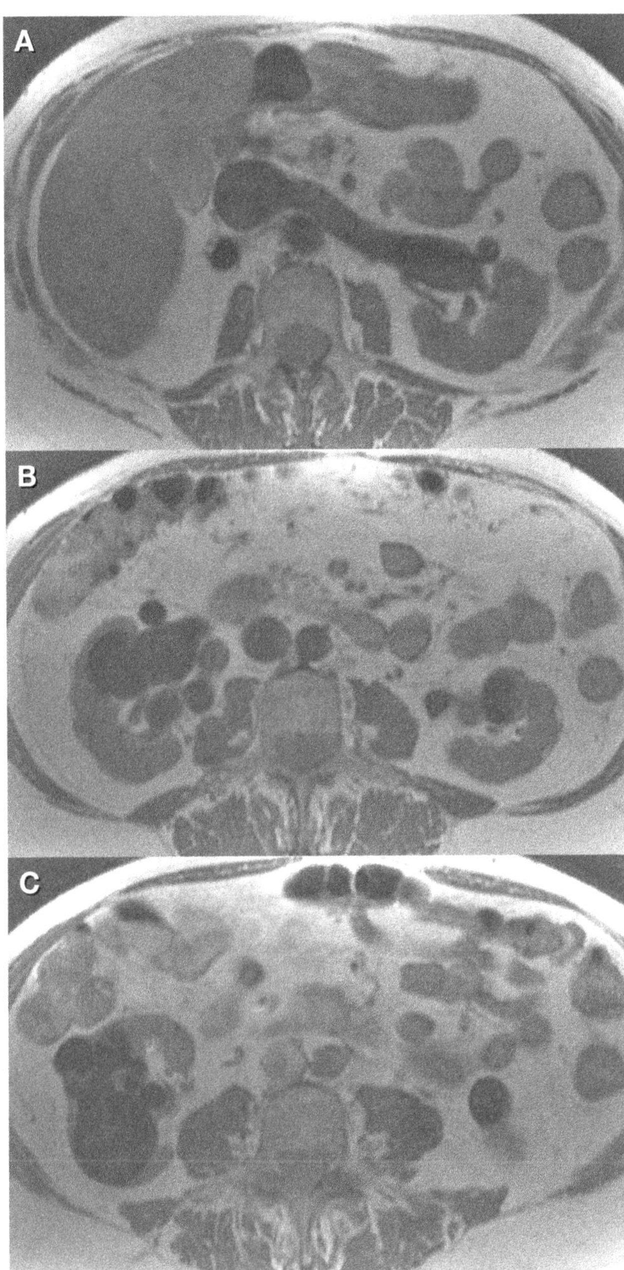

Figure 16.4.2

HISTORY: 71-year-old woman with gradually increasing dyspnea, atrial fibrillation, and pulmonary hypertension

IMAGING FINDINGS: Coronal fat-suppressed postgadolinium 3D SPGR images (Figure 16.4.1) reveal large varicosities replacing much of the right kidney. Note the enlarged left renal artery and vein and varicosities in the lower pole of the left kidney. Axial T1-weighted FSE images (Figure 16.4.2) demonstrate large vessels with flow voids in both kidneys.

DIAGNOSIS: Renal AVF

COMMENT: Renal AVFs are uncommon, with a prevalence of less than 1% of the general population, and large congenital AVFs of the type seen in this case are quite rare (this is 1 of 2 cases we've seen). Iatrogenic (ie, related to biopsy) or traumatic causes of renal AVFs are likely the most common. A distinction is generally made in the literature between AVF and AVM. AVFs have a single direct communication between a renal artery and a renal vein; AVMs have an abnormal communication between the renal arteries and veins through a vascular nidus.

Tortuous dilated arteries and veins are the hallmark of renal AVFs, and MRA or conventional angiography shows early intense venous opacification. In about 72% of cases, the large vessels adjacent to urothelium lead to hematuria, which is the most common presenting symptom. A flank bruit can often be heard. The arteriovenous shunt bypasses renal parenchyma and may result in renal vascular hypertension, which has been reported in 50% of cases. High-output cardiac failure, which was present in this case, is not uncommon and has been reported in 5% to 32% of patients with congenital renal AVF or AVM.

The patient in this case was told that she had renal AVMs as a young adult, about 40 years before the images shown above. Because symptomatic high-output cardiac failure developed, she had embolization of the left kidney AVF with improved symptoms and improved cardiac function. A few years after that, the right-sided AVF acutely ruptured (another reported complication) and the patient required emergent nephrectomy.

This case is not a diagnostic dilemma (at least after you're aware of the entity and have seen 1 or 2 examples). Occasionally more problematic is distinguishing a small AVM or AVF from a true hypervascular lesion. The AVM should have higher flow; therefore, it is much more likely to have enlarged vessels with flow voids. Most important, however, is the lack of a definable mass in an AVM, which requires standard T1- and T2-weighted imaging with postcontrast 2D or 3D SPGR images.

The preferred treatment of these lesions is embolization, since this offers the best chance to preserve unaffected renal parenchyma.

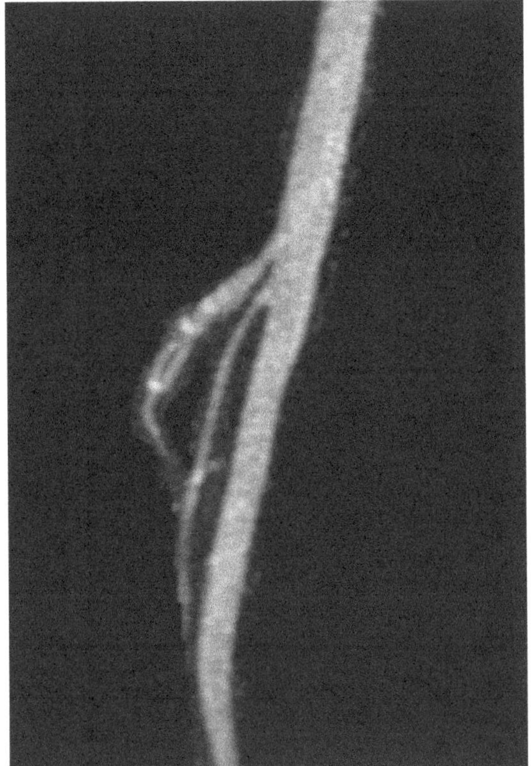

Figure 16.5.1

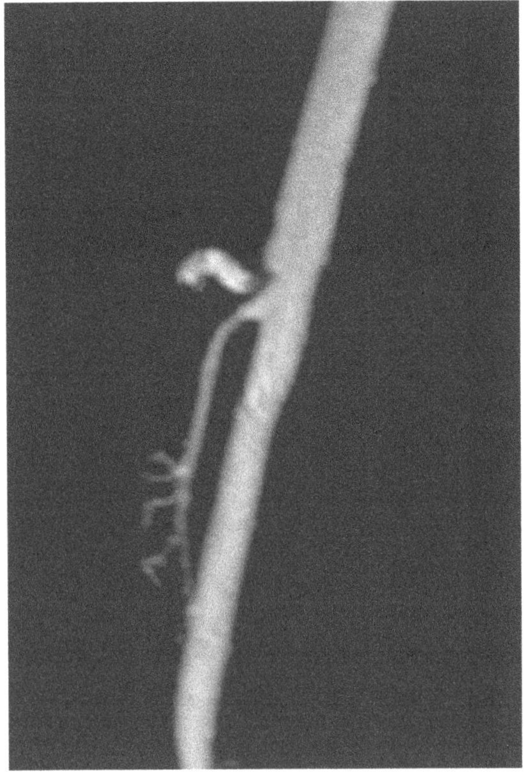

Figure 16.5.2

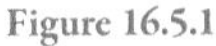

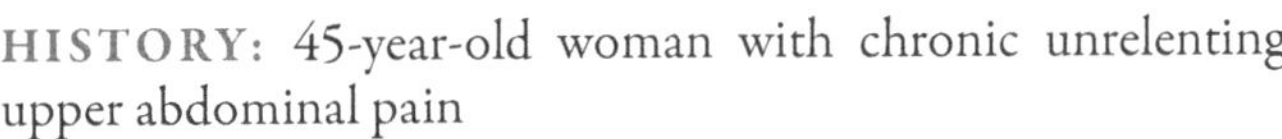

HISTORY: 45-year-old woman with chronic unrelenting upper abdominal pain

IMAGING FINDINGS: Sagittal oblique partial volume MIP images from 3D CE MRA of the abdomen performed at end inspiration (Figure 16.5.1) and end expiration (Figure 16.5.2) demonstrate mild to moderate proximal narrowing of the celiac artery on the inspiratory view with severe stenosis on the expiratory view.

DIAGNOSIS: MAL syndrome

COMMENT: MAL syndrome, also known as celiac axis compression syndrome, is characterized by the clinical triad of postprandial abdominal pain, epigastric bruit that increases with expiration, and anatomical narrowing of the celiac artery demonstrated by vascular imaging. The syndrome is most common in young women with a thin body habitus.

The mechanism of abdominal pain is not well understood. Intestinal ischemia resulting from celiac compression and reduced blood flow is the most popular theory, but this explanation is at odds with the conventional wisdom that loss of flow in at least 2 mesenteric arteries is required for development of mesenteric ischemia. Other theories include irritation of the celiac plexus leading to splanchnic vasoconstriction and ischemia.

Diagnosis of MAL syndrome is often difficult because symptoms are usually nonspecific and other causes of chronic abdominal pain are much more common. Also, there is some controversy in the surgical literature as to whether this is a real disease, and it does raise a red flag when surgeons are reluctant to operate for any reason. In our experience, narrowing of the celiac artery origin is a fairly common incidental finding in abdominal MRI and MRA, and most of these patients have no corresponding symptoms. Some authors have emphasized the importance of demonstrating severe stenosis on both inspiratory and expiratory views. This should improve the specificity of the diagnosis, although it is not a universally accepted criterion.

The MAL of the diaphragm is formed by fibrous bands connecting the left and right crura and bordering the aortic hiatus. Its shape, consistency, and location are highly variable, and it sometimes compresses the origin of the celiac artery superiorly. Dynamic studies have demonstrated variation in the degree of compression with respiration: The celiac artery origin and the MAL move apart on inspiration and come closer together on expiration, leading to the classic finding of expiratory compression in MAL syndrome.

Because of the controversies regarding this syndrome (and even its existence), we do not make an absolute diagnosis of MAL syndrome from the MRA findings alone, but in the proper clinical setting, MRA can be very helpful. We perform a sagittal oblique 3D CE MRA on expiration first (which is most likely to be abnormal) and then on inspiration. A 10-minute wait between injections is usually sufficient to return the background vascular signal to a low level in patients with normal renal function. CE MRA is probably the easiest way to perform this examination, but it is not absolutely necessary. A breath-held 3D SSFP technique would also work, but you probably won't be able to generate the nice 3D reconstructions beloved by clinicians. Another option (but one that is not ideal) is to use a single dose of an intravascular gadolinium agent, perform the expiratory acquisition first, and then acquire an inspiratory MRA when convenient. The second acquisition will have enough arterial signal to be diagnostic, but there will be even more signal in the veins, which again will prevent generation of 3D reconstructions.

Treatment of MAL syndrome consists of surgical division of the constrictive fibers of the celiac plexus and release of the celiac trunk up to its origin from the aorta.

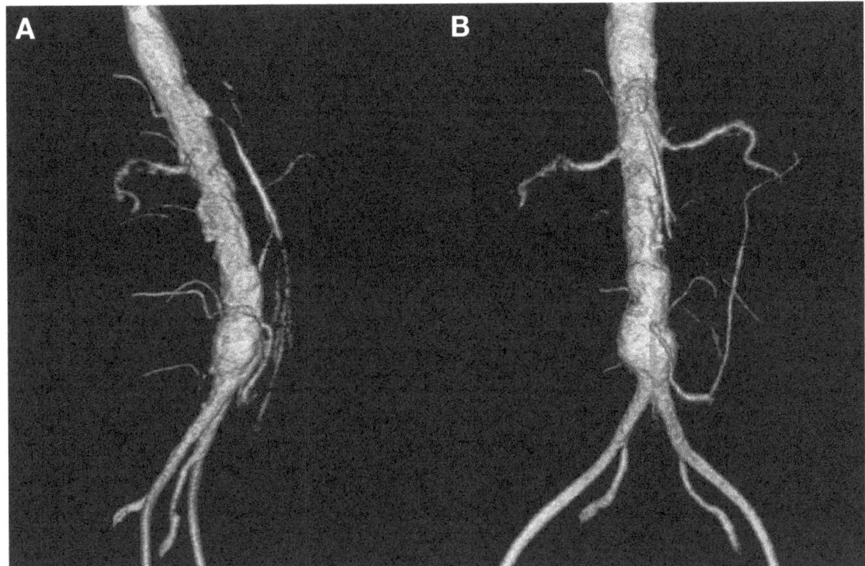

Figure 16.6.1

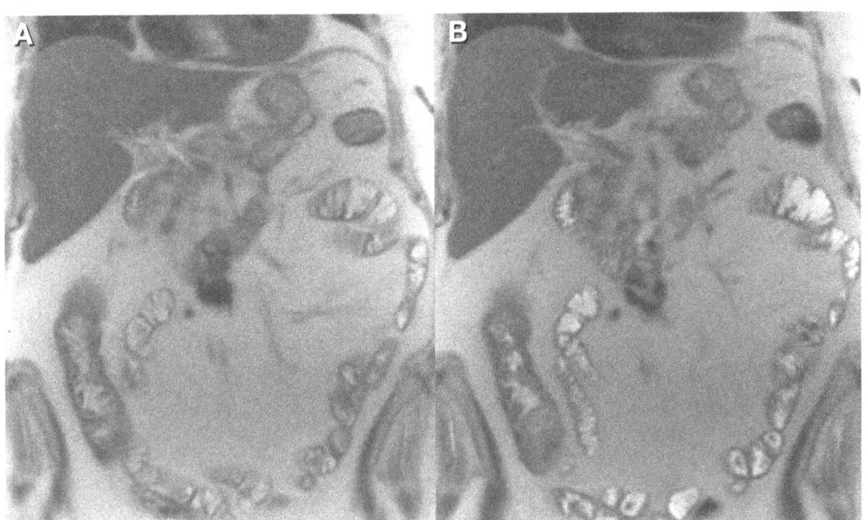

Figure 16.6.2

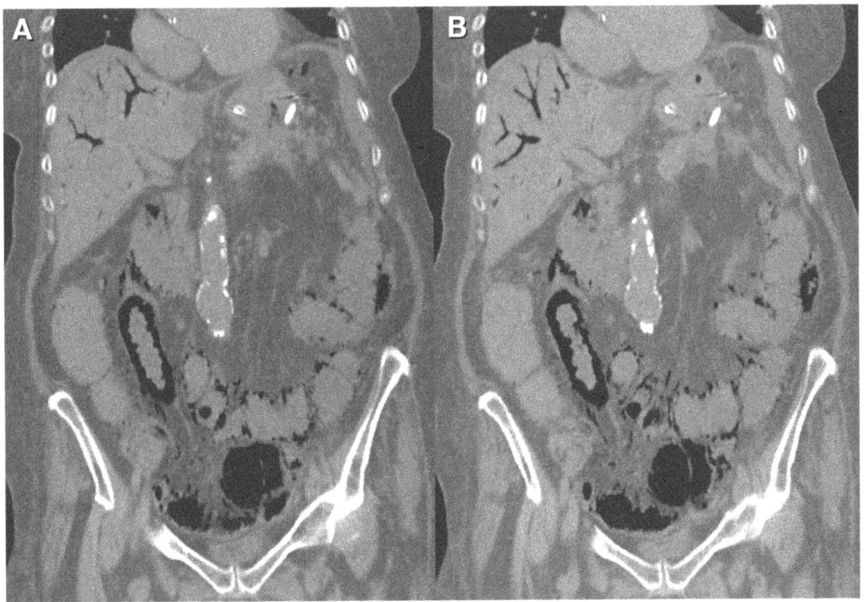

Figure 16.6.3

HISTORY: 79-year-old with abdominal pain and nausea

IMAGING FINDINGS: VR images from 3D CE MRA (Figure 16.6.1) demonstrate occlusion of the celiac artery, severe stenosis of the superior mesenteric artery origin, and a patent inferior mesenteric artery with a prominent arc of Riolan. Coronal SSFSE images (Figure 16.6.2) reveal thickening of the cecum and ascending colon. Coronal reformatted images from abdominal CT performed 1 week later (Figure 16.6.3) show extensive gas within intrahepatic portal veins and pneumatosis involving multiple small bowel loops.

DIAGNOSIS: Mesenteric ischemia

COMMENT: Mesenteric ischemia is generally categorized as either acute or chronic. AMI is uncommon, accounting for less than 1 in every 1,000 hospital admissions. Women are more commonly affected, perhaps because of their greater longevity, and patients are typically older than 60 years and have multiple comorbidities. Risk factors include any conditions predisposing to development of thrombus, including atrial fibrillation, recent myocardial infarction, and congestive heart failure.

Arterial embolism, usually in the superior mesenteric artery, is probably the most common cause of AMI, accounting for 40% to 50% of cases, with arterial thrombosis responsible for 25% to 30% of cases. Symptoms are nonspecific. The classic manifestation is abdominal pain, often greater than expected from the physical examination findings. Mortality is high (60%-80%).

CMI is also more common in women, and is probably even more difficult to diagnose than AMI. The classic symptom of CMI is postprandial abdominal pain resulting in significant weight loss. CMI classically requires significant stenosis or thrombosis of at least 2 of the 3 mesenteric arteries, and atherosclerosis is thought to be responsible for more than 95% of cases.

Diagnosis of either AMI or CMI can be problematic because of the lack of specificity of the vascular findings. Asymptomatic patients with stenosis or occlusion of 2 or 3 mesenteric arteries are not uncommonly encountered when performing abdominal MRA for other reasons (eg, renal artery stenosis or abdominal aortic aneurysm). In the actively symptomatic patient, finding an acute thrombus in an artery (the artery is expanded by thrombus rather than being atretic) should be relatively specific for the diagnosis. Nevertheless, it is important to look for ancillary findings, particularly bowel wall thickening or abnormal enhancement. Pneumatosis or gas in the mesenteric and portal veins is much easier to appreciate on CT but can sometimes be seen on MRI as signal void, most notably on 2D or 3D SPGR images (Case 2.14). Pneumoperitoneum is similarly important to look for but much more difficult to detect on MRI than on CT.

Several papers have evaluated functional assessment of CMI with MRI. This usually involves measuring blood flow in the mesenteric vein or artery before and after a functional challenge. Our protocol involves cine phase-contrast flow measurement in the superior mesenteric vein just proximal to the portal confluence at baseline (ie, fasting) and then immediately after a fatty meal (a liquid nutritional supplement [Ensure]). Normally, mesenteric venous flow increases by a factor of 3 to 4, whereas patients with CMI typically show only minimally increased flow (less than a factor of 2) or no increase in flow. Good results have been reported with this technique, although in our experience, the change in flow often seems to fall into the indeterminate range.

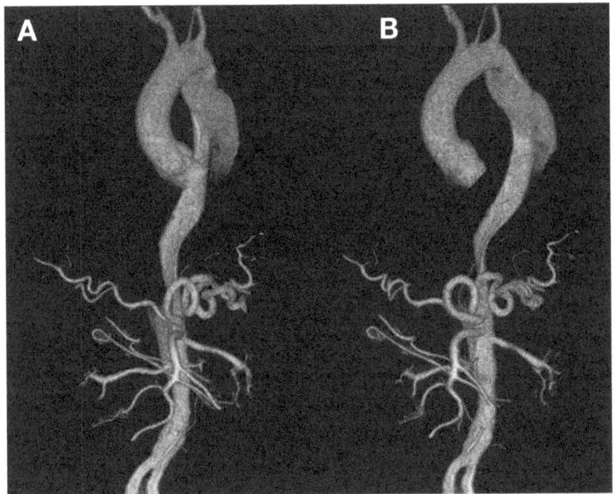

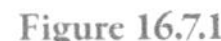
Figure 16.7.1

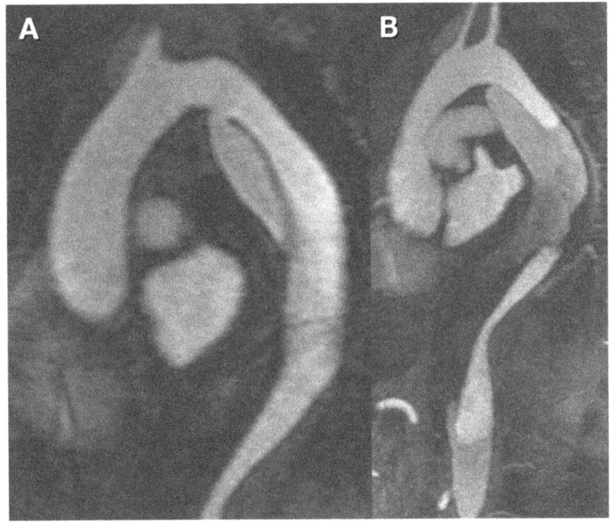

Figure 16.7.2

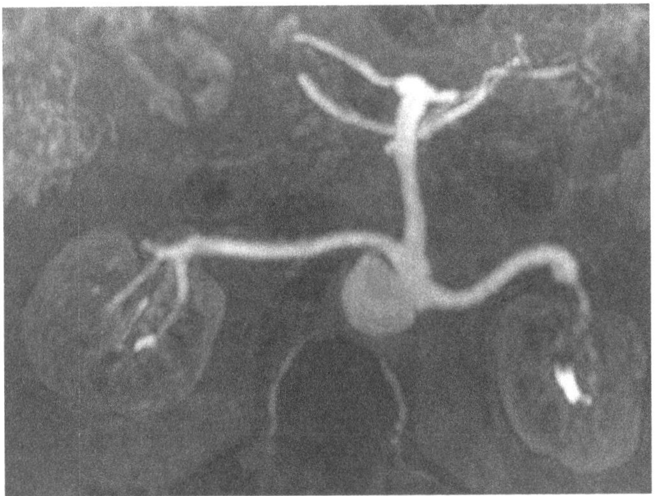

Figure 16.7.3

HISTORY: 60-year-old man with a history of hypertension and intermittent back and flank pain

IMAGING FINDINGS: Coronal oblique VR images from 3D CE MRA of the thoracoabdominal aorta (Figure 16.7.1) demonstrate compression and distortion of the lumen of the descending thoracic and upper abdominal aorta. Sagittal oblique reformatted images from MRA (Figure 16.7.2) demonstrate a flap originating in the posterior arch with less contrast enhancement than the true lumen. Axial oblique partial volume MIP image from postgadolinium 3D SPGR acquisition (Figure 16.7.3) shows a flap in the abdominal aorta with both renal arteries and the superior mesenteric artery filling from the true lumen.

DIAGNOSIS: Type B aortic dissection

COMMENT: *Aortic dissection* is defined as a disruption of the intimal layer of the aorta with propagation of a false lumen within the media. An acute dissection is a true emergency and must be diagnosed quickly and accurately. Men are affected twice as often as women. With the relatively straightforward Stanford classification of aortic dissections, 60% are type A (involving the ascending aorta) and 40% are type B (not involving the ascending aorta). The DeBakey classification categorizes aortic dissections as type I (involving the ascending aorta and the descending aorta), type II (involving only the ascending aorta), and type III (involving only the descending aorta). Patients with type A dissections have a mortality rate of 1% to 2% per hour in the first 24 hours and a cumulative mortality of 50% to 75% in the acute phase. Patients with acute type B dissections have a much lower mortality, with a 5-year survival rate of 80%. Patients with type A dissections have a higher mortality because of the risk of inferior extension into the pericardium, with bleeding and subsequent tamponade, or extension into the coronary arteries. Dissections can also extend superiorly into the carotid arteries and cause stroke. Type B dissections may involve the renal and mesenteric vessels (resulting in bowel ischemia, renal infarction, or splenic infarction) or the iliac arteries (potentially causing lower extremity ischemia). Both type A and type B dissections have an increased risk of aortic rupture. Risk factors for aortic dissection include hypertension, connective tissue disease (Marfan syndrome, EDS, etc), aneurysm, coarctation, vasculitis, cocaine use, and pregnancy.

MRI in aortic dissection should generally be reserved for follow-up of known type B dissections or for screening of patients at higher risk for aneurysms and dissections (eg, patients with Marfan syndrome or EDS). The hemodynamically unstable patient with tearing chest pain does not need to spend 40 minutes unmonitored in a magnet when CE CTA can be performed in a few minutes. Generally, 3D CE MRA is the best technique for imaging hemodynamically stable dissection patients by virtue of its speed, simplicity, and ability to cover a large FOV with reasonably good spatial resolution.

Dissections frequently extend from the posterior aortic arch into the iliac arteries, and in a large person, the FOV may be too large to cover with a single acquisition. In that case, alternative strategies include a stepping table acquisition or a second injection of contrast for the abdomen and pelvis (our preference). If the 2-injection technique is used, it is usually better to start with the abdomen and pelvis, where venous contamination (and residual organ enhancement) is a little more problematic than in the chest. The abdominal-pelvic acquisition should be in a coronal oblique plane; the thoracic MRA can be performed in the more efficient sagittal oblique ("candy cane") view if you're sure that you don't need to see very far into the subclavian arteries. Stepping table acquisitions are usually fine but occasionally can be problematic because vessel transit times, in general, scale inversely with the size of the artery. Therefore, the contrast bolus travels fairly quickly in the descending aorta, and if you're not very efficient you may miss the bolus in the abdomen. Also, running the MRA sequence at least twice in each station is a good practice for any MRA but is particularly applicable for a dissection because the false lumen often opacifies much more slowly than the true lumen, and you may only see both lumens enhancing during the second run.

The examination should conclude with axial fat-suppressed 3D SPGR acquisitions to provide transverse images through the dissection. In this case, for example, the false lumen has not filled in on the initial MRA acquisition but is well seen on the 3D SPGR images. We also obtain a precontrast axial 2D fat-suppressed SSFP series through the aorta, which not only nicely demonstrates the true and false lumens in a very time-efficient manner (<1 second per slice) but also helps in prescribing the 3D MRA volume. If intravenous contrast cannot be given, 2D SSFP images are usually more than adequate for diagnostic purposes. A few papers have demonstrated the efficacy of ECG-gated and respiratory-gated 3D SSFP sequences for imaging the aorta. This is essentially the same technique routinely used for coronary MRA. It is generally an effective method, except that the acquisition times can be very long (6-10 minutes) and image quality is heavily dependent on the regularity of the patient's breathing. ECG-gated 2D cine SSFP images are occasionally a useful supplement to demonstrate cyclical changes in the size of the true and false lumens or to obtain clear, motion-free views of the aortic root and proximal ascending aorta. These can be fairly time-consuming procedures, however, with single-slice acquisition times of 10 to 15 seconds, so it is not a first-line method for imaging the entire aorta.

Time-resolved MRA can show temporal differences between filling of true lumens and false lumens, and several papers have extolled the virtues of this method (particularly 1 vendor's pulse sequence). These are clever techniques, but they are not really necessary for imaging dissections, and they force you to make some compromises in spatial resolution that are not required with conventional MRA acquisitions. What generally happens is that the time-resolved MRA is run with a small dose of contrast, generating a series of low-resolution MRAs (and collapsed 3D views, which can be shown in conferences and meetings), and then the conventional MRA is performed to actually read the case.

The subject of IMH is always linked to dissection. An IMH is thrombus within the medial layer of the aorta with an intact intima and is thought to result from spontaneous rupture of the vasa vasorum. The current thinking is that IMH is a distinct entity from dissection, with its own natural history. Traditional management has dictated treating IMH in essentially the same way as dissection: early surgery or intervention for patients with IMH in the ascending aorta and medical management of patients in stable condition who have descending aorta IMH. IMH can progress to classic dissection or to aortic rupture, or it may be reabsorbed. A significant percentage of lesions do not progress, and 30% to 50% resolve within 6 months. Poor prognostic signs include an associated aneurysm larger than 5 cm and an associated penetrating ulcer.

Diagnosis of IMH has been emphasized (somewhat obsessively) in the MRI literature for many years. After the entity was discovered, MRI was considered to be highly sensitive for detecting IMH and to compare favorably with CT (diagnosis was made by visualizing focal crescentic thickening of the aortic wall with high T1-signal intensity indicating subacute hemorrhage but no communication with the lumen). This is probably no longer true in the era of high-resolution multidetector CT, especially if you remember to include a precontrast acquisition to help detect the hyperdense IMH.

Unfortunately, the classic techniques of the early MRI era are still used today at some institutions, so you may occasionally hear speakers recommend gated spin echo T1 pulse sequences to demonstrate the high signal intensity of subacute hemorrhage within the aortic wall. These acquisitions are unnecessary; they're long (up to 10 minutes) and have terrible image quality at least half the time (although once in a while the images are spectacular, thereby providing intermittent positive reinforcement—the most powerful kind). Most importantly, they may prevent you from obtaining a diagnostic examination; these images need to be acquired before contrast administration, and a patient with significant pain, claustrophobia, or other complicating factors may not tolerate a long examination and will want to quit before you get to the CE MRA. This fundamental principle of body MRI—obtain the most important information as quickly as possible and as soon as possible—is unfortunately one that is frequently forgotten.

Diagnosis of IMH can be made with precontrast MRA (high T1-signal intensity in a T1-weighted 3D SPGR acquisition), with precontrast axial fat-suppressed 3D SPGR images, or with a breath-held ECG-gated FSE (double inversion recovery) acquisition. Noncontrast 3D SPGR images have an inherently low signal to noise ratio, so it's not a bad idea to decrease the spatial resolution somewhat to make the images more pleasant to look at. If you see an intramural hematoma on the 3D SPGR acquisition, you can prescribe a few double IR FSE slices through the region to obtain more photogenic images. This is much more efficient than acquiring spin echo or FSE images through the entire chest. Remember that the high T1-signal intensity appearance holds true only for subacute hemorrhage and not for hyperacute blood or for old blood.

Another entity usually lumped into discussions of aortic dissection is penetrating atheromatous ulcer, in which ulceration in an atherosclerotic plaque disrupts the intimal layer of the aortic wall and extends into the media. This can subsequently lead to IMH or dissection, focal saccular aneurysm, or aortic rupture. Penetrating atheromatous ulcer occurs most frequently in elderly patients who have extensive atherosclerotic disease. The natural history of these lesions is uncertain. Some authors have found the prognosis to be worse than that for aortic dissection, with a higher incidence of aortic rupture, but others have reported slow disease progression with a relatively low incidence of catastrophic complications. The imaging appearance on MRI is that of focal ulceration in a nonenhancing plaque that extends into or beyond the aortic wall. We have typically found these lesions in relatively asymptomatic patients who are undergoing scanning for assessment of known aneurysms or atherosclerotic disease. It is then important to try to determine whether the lesion is new or old: Look for IMH or adjacent inflammatory changes as indications of a new or active lesion.

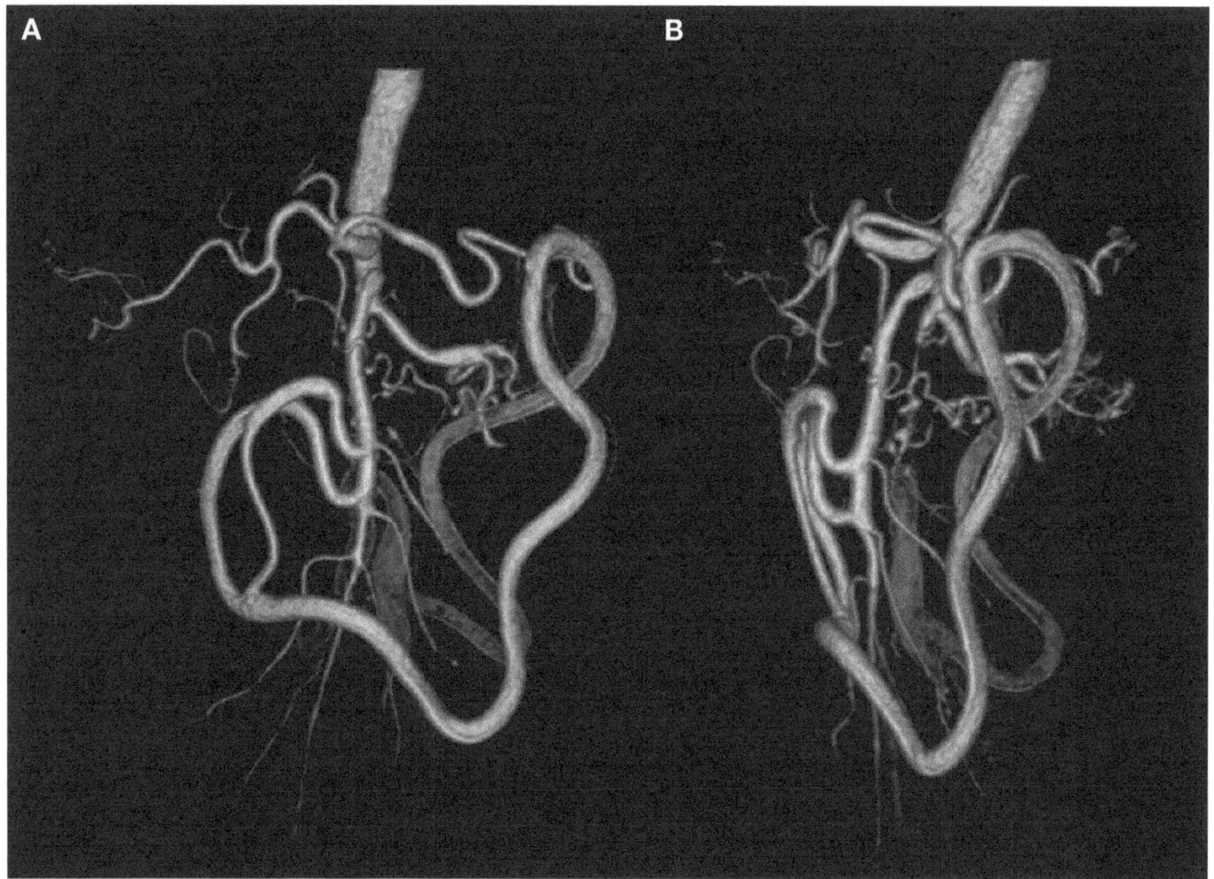

Figure 16.8.1

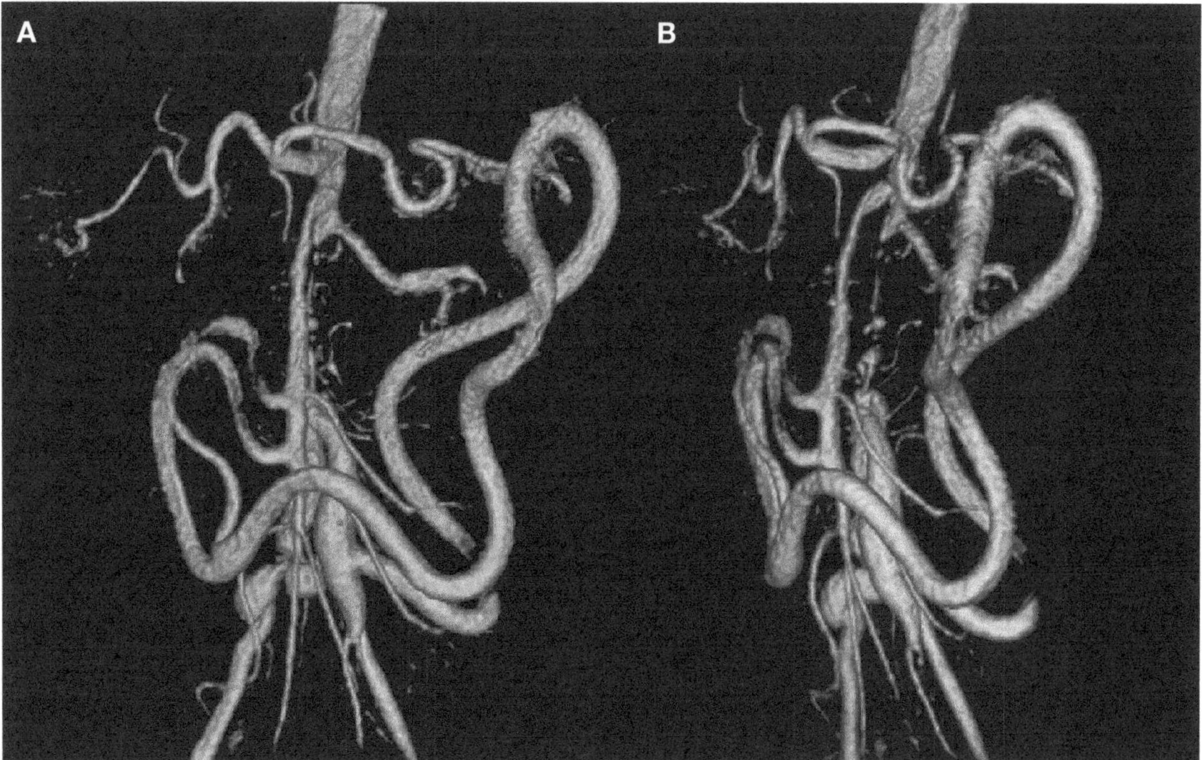

Figure 16.8.2

HISTORY: 67-year-old woman with mild abdominal discomfort after eating

IMAGING FINDINGS: Anterior (Figure 16.8.1A) and oblique (Figure 16.8.1B) VR images from 3D CE MRA and anterior (Figure 16.8.2A) and oblique (Figure 16.8.2B) images from an immediate delayed acquisition demonstrate near occlusion of the abdominal aorta just below the renal artery origins with massive dilatation of the superior mesenteric artery and the inferior mesenteric artery and a large arc of Riolan supplying the infrarenal aorta.

DIAGNOSIS: Abdominal aortic coarctation with collateralization via the arc of Riolan

COMMENT: This case is a nice example of the collaterals that develop between the superior and inferior mesenteric arteries with slow occlusion of the aorta (these collaterals also may develop with stenosis or occlusion of a mesenteric artery). There are 3 major collateral pathways between the superior mesenteric artery and the inferior mesenteric artery: 1) The marginal artery of Drummond lies within the mesentery of the colon and gives rise to the vasa recta. It consists of branches from the ileocolic, right colic, middle colic, and left colic arteries. 2) The arc of Riolan is more centrally located within the mesentery and usually joins the middle and left colic arteries. The arc of Riolan was first described by the 17th century French anatomist Jean Riolan, who served as physician to King Henry IV and King Louis XIII and was an opponent of Harvey's theory of the circulation of blood. 3) The wandering mesenteric artery may in fact be a dilated arc of Riolan or a discrete vessel within the mesentery. We think this case involves a dilated arc of Riolan. There is also an arc of Barkow (between omental branches of the superior mesenteric artery and branches of the celiac axis) and an arc of Buhler (direct communication between the celiac artery and the superior mesenteric artery).

This patient had an abdominal aortic coarctation (a rare location compared to the usual location in the juxtaductal descending thoracic aorta), which eventually reached the point of occlusion. The tiny vessels bridging the occluded aorta have been described variously as collaterals (our view) or as severe coarctation of the native aorta.

The term *Leriche syndrome* is commonly used to describe any occlusion of the abdominal aorta, although it refers to a more specific triad of claudication, impotence, and decreased peripheral pulses with thrombotic occlusion. Leriche's index case was a young truck driver from Paris who had a successful outcome after surgery.

MRA for mesenteric ischemia (the indication for the examination in this case) can be performed in either the sagittal plane or the coronal plane. In theory, thrombosis or stenosis can occur anywhere in the mesenteric arteries and cause symptoms of mesenteric ischemia; in practice, thrombosis or stenosis is most common in the proximal arteries. A coronal acquisition plane encompasses a greater percentage of the peripheral mesenteric arteries; however, even under nearly ideal circumstances it may be difficult to distinguish real disease from motion artifact in distal branch vessels. Coronal images do require longer acquisition times, and they are best acquired with patients' arms above their heads; therefore, if patients are frail or have difficulty with breath-holding, we favor a sagittal approach.

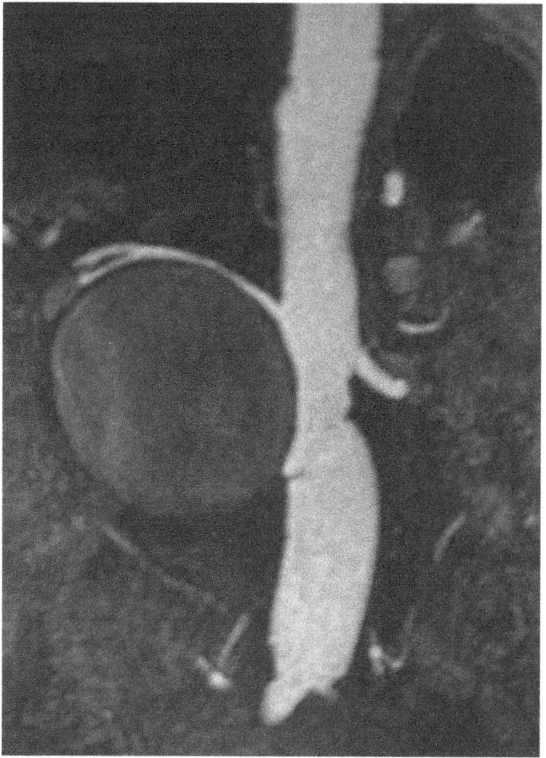

Figure 16.9.1

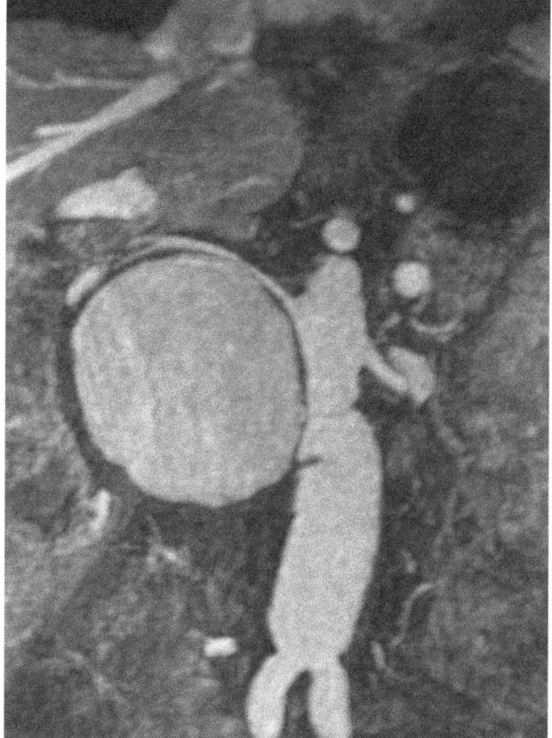

Figure 16.9.2

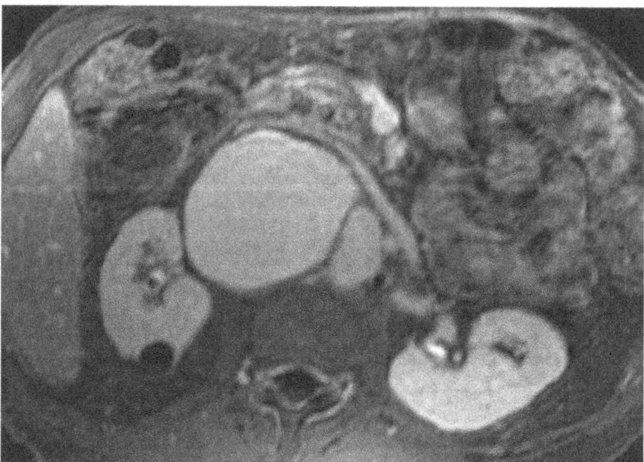

Figure 16.9.3

HISTORY: 80-year-old man with a thoracoabdominal aortic aneurysm repaired 1 year ago; noncontrast CT showed a periaortic mass in the upper abdomen

IMAGING FINDINGS: Partial volume MIP image from coronal 3D CE MRA of the abdomen (Figure 16.9.1) demonstrates a large hypointense round lesion adjacent to the aorta and right kidney without contrast enhancement. Venous phase partial volume MIP image from the same location (Figure 16.9.2) reveals that this structure now has diffuse homogeneous enhancement similar to the adjacent aorta. Axial fat-suppressed 3D SPGR image (Figure 16.9.3) also shows the periaortic structure displacing the IVC and renal veins anteriorly and enhancing with an intensity similar to that of the aorta.

DIAGNOSIS: Aortic pseudoaneurysm after abdominal aortic aneurysm repair

COMMENT: This finding is not subtle, but the slight delay in diagnosis does have an interesting history. The patient had a mild allergy (hives) to CT contrast dye, and so the first few follow-up studies after his aneurysm repair were CTs done without contrast (the vascular surgeon was not a fan of MRI). The initial report mentioned the pseudoaneurysm and noted that it was probably a hematoma, but without contrast a pseudoaneurysm could not be excluded. The next follow-up report said that the "hematoma" was about the same size and deleted pseudoaneurysm from the differential diagnosis. Two examinations later, the "hematoma" had enlarged, so a contrast-enhanced examination was recommended.

With contrast, the diagnosis is easy as long as you remember to acquire delayed images. In this case, an immediate venous phase MRA acquisition shows rapid filling of the pseudoaneurysm. An intravascular contrast agent (eg, gadofosveset trisodium [Ablavar]) would have also been good for this case had it been available when the examination was performed. For such a large pseudoaneurysm, an intravascular contrast agent is not really necessary, but its long intravascular half-life is well suited for identifying slow or subtle extravasation (it is very good for identifying endoleaks after endovascular stent graft repair of an aneurysm).

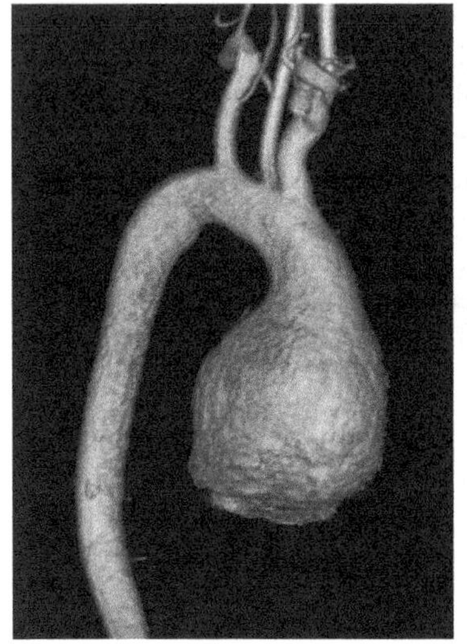

Figure 16.10.1

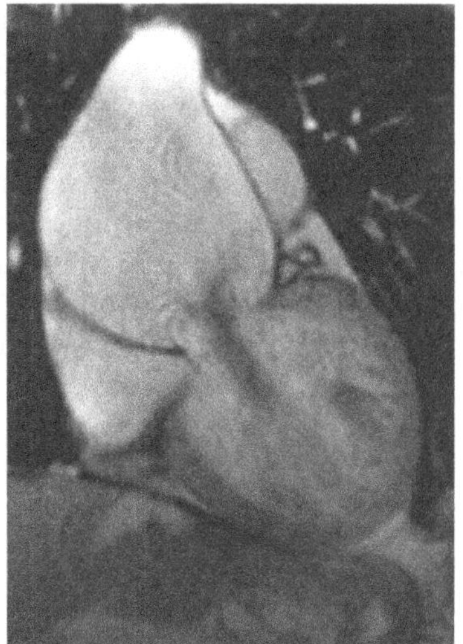

Figure 16.10.2

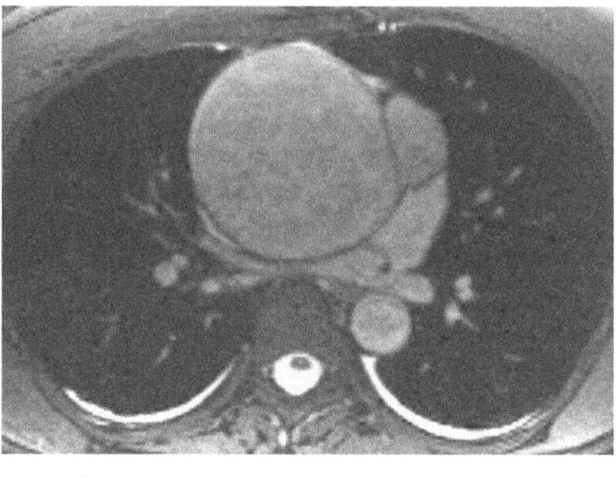

Figure 16.10.3

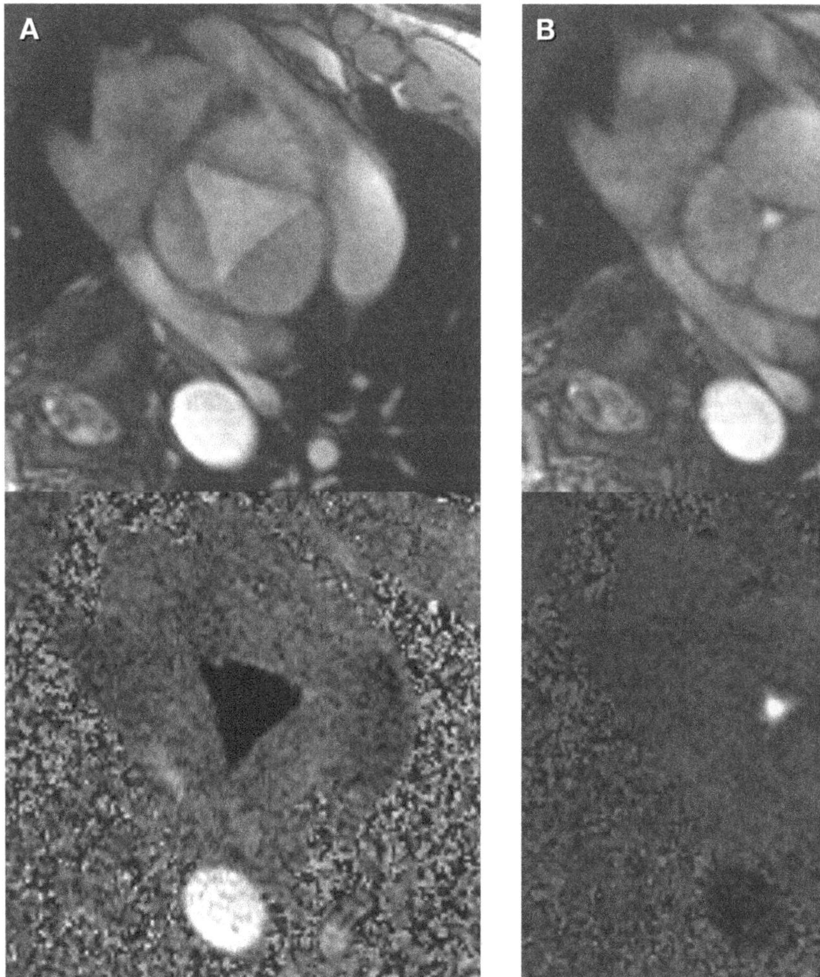

Figure 16.10.4

HISTORY: 50-year-old man with a gradually increasing exercise limitation and a cardiac murmur on examination; he has a family history of aortic aneurysm and coronary artery dissection

IMAGING FINDINGS: VR image from 3D CE MRA (Figure 16.10.1) reveals marked dilatation of the aortic root, extending to the sinotubular junction. Coronal oblique SSFP image through the aortic valve and root (Figure 16.10.2)

shows a prominent flow void at the valve level, which represents aortic regurgitation. Axial SSFP image through the proximal aorta (Figure 16.10.3) reveals massive aneurysmal dilatation. Transverse magnitude and phase images from cine phase-contrast acquisition through the aortic valve at end systole (Figure 16.10.4A) and at end diastole (Figure 16.10.4B) demonstrate a tricuspid aortic valve with central aortic regurgitation on the diastolic image resulting from a lack of coaptation of the valve leaflets.

DIAGNOSIS: Marfan syndrome with aortic root aneurysm and aortic regurgitation

COMMENT: Marfan syndrome, first described by the French pediatrician Antoine Marfan in 1896, is a systemic connective tissue disorder inherited in an autosomal dominant pattern with variable penetrance. The prevalence is 2 to 3 in 10,000, and approximately 27% of patients present without a previous family history. Clinical diagnosis with the Ghent criteria requires identification of 2 major criteria in 2 different body systems. The criteria include skeletal abnormalities (disproportionate overgrowth of long bones of the arms and legs, arachnodactyly, joint laxity, and pectus deformity), ocular findings (lens dislocation, early and severe myopia, and retinal detachment), central nervous system manifestations (dural ectasia), and cardiovascular abnormalities (annuloaortic ectasia, dilatation of the aortic root, aortic aneurysms and dissections, and prolapse of the mitral and tricuspid valves, often with regurgitation). Most of the time, you'll be looking for cardiovascular abnormalities when MRI is requested (although we occasionally receive telephone calls from referring physicians who are surprised that we didn't comment on the presence or absence of lumbosacral dural ectasia on the thoracic MRA they had ordered). By age 21, more than half of Marfan syndrome patients have cardiovascular involvement.

The primary genetic defect in Marfan syndrome involves the fibrillin 1 gene on chromosome 15, which generates a primary component of elastin fibers in the aorta. This defect is thought to result in weakened and disordered elastic fiber formation and in disruption of the microfibril network in the extracellular matrix.

Patients with untreated Marfan syndrome have a mean survival of 40 years, and most die of catastrophic aortic dissection or rupture. The most common site of vascular involvement in Marfan syndrome is the aortic root. Disruption of the elastic media leads to cystic medial necrosis and consequent dilatation of the aortic annulus and aortic root (annuloaortic ectasia), resulting in the classic tulip-shaped aorta seen in this case. Note that this appearance on its own is not pathognomonic of Marfan syndrome; however, this finding in a relatively young patient without any other reason for an ascending aortic aneurysm (aortic valve disease most commonly) should prompt inclusion of Marfan syndrome high in the differential diagnosis.

The most common technique for evaluating the aorta in patients with Marfan syndrome is 3D CE MRA. In general, it works well but can be limited in assessing the aortic root because of motion artifacts from cardiac pulsation, and it's not uncommon to have such severe blurring and stepping artifacts that you can't really be sure that there isn't an aortic root dissection (which is often the whole point of the examination).

What are your options? One alternative technique is ECG-gated 3D CE MRA, which is like a regular MRA, except that the acquisition is gated to the ECG tracing (obtained by applying cardiac leads or peripheral gating from a finger). Data are typically acquired during diastole, when the heart is relatively still. This method effectively eliminates pulsation artifact, but keep in mind that essentially what you're doing is vastly decreasing the efficiency of the sequence by sampling data for only a fraction of the cardiac cycle, and therefore, the acquisition time is much longer. For that reason, ECG-gated MRA generally requires 1-dimensional or 2D parallel imaging, and even so, the acquisition times are often longer than standard nongated sequences. Also remember that as the heart rate increases, diastole decreases as a relative percentage of the cardiac cycle, and artifacts will appear unless some of the acquisition parameters are adjusted (ie, shortening the data acquisition window).

A second useful alternative (which we always include when evaluating the aortic root) is ECG-gated cine SSFP. These images are typically acquired in a coronal oblique view through the aortic root, and in the corresponding orthogonal view, to generate a 3-chamber cardiac or left ventricular outflow tract view. These 2 views are subsequently used to prescribe a stack of cine images along the transverse axis of the aorta from the valve through the sinotubular junction. This technique usually adds about 5 minutes to the examination, but if you always acquire these views you will almost never worry about missing an aortic root dissection, and you'll always be able to provide accurate and reproducible measurements of the aortic root.

The advent of ECG-gated MRI raised the question of which phase of the cardiac cycle should be used when measuring the aortic diameter. We were surprised to learn that our echocardiographic colleagues measure diameters during diastole (ie, the smallest diameter) and measure the diameter from the outer edge of the anterior vessel wall to the inner edge of the posterior wall instead of from outer edge to outer edge. Since the average aortic wall is less than 1 mm thick and the average error in aortic diameter measurement is probably 2 to 3 mm, it is doubtful that these measurement discrepancies present a real problem. Systolic versus diastolic measurement is likely a more important issue: The difference in aortic dimension between systole and diastole is a measurement of vascular compliance, which decreases with age and is a prognostic indicator for future cardiovascular events. Young patients typically have higher compliance and are therefore more likely to show a significant difference in diameter between systolic and diastolic measurements. The solution to this issue is to be consistent in the techniques that you use to follow these patients or to provide both measurements.

Another technique used in this case is cine phase-contrast imaging through the aortic valve. Marfan patients with annuloaortic ectasia often have aortic insufficiency because the valve leaflets are stretched by the dilated annulus and do not coapt centrally. The magnitude image has a central hole, and the corresponding velocity-encoded image shows high-velocity backward flow. These same images can be used to measure the amount of regurgitant flow per heartbeat and to determine the forward flow across the valve, which corresponds to the cardiac stroke volume. The ratio of regurgitant volume to stroke volume is the *regurgitant fraction*, and there are guidelines for relating the severity of aortic regurgitation to the regurgitant volume and regurgitant fraction. Significant aortic regurgitation can almost always be seen on the cine SSFP images as well, where it appears as a flow void, most likely the result of intravoxel dephasing during the acquisition.

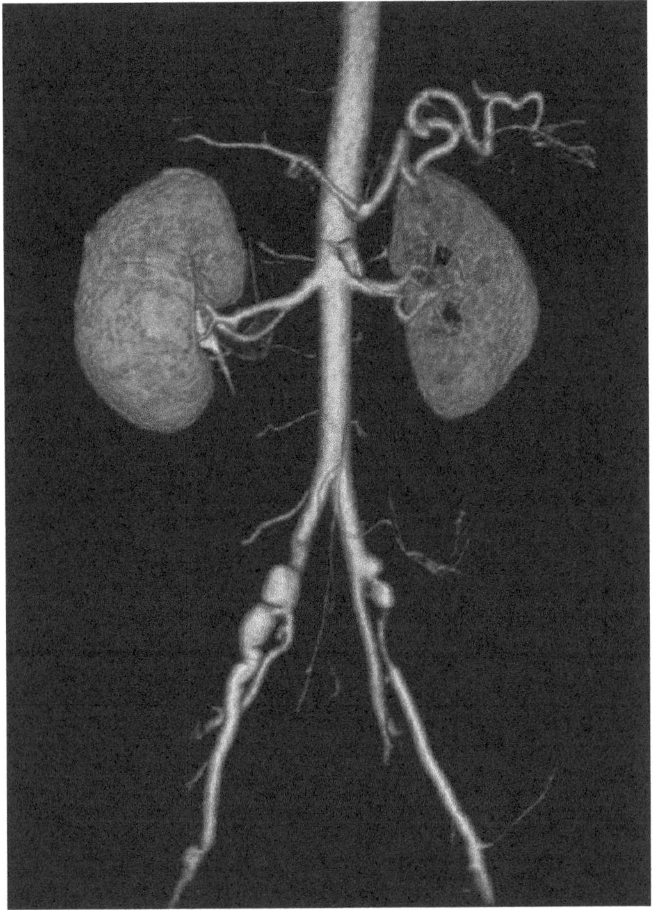

Figure 16.11.1

HISTORY: 22-year-old man with a history of multiple episodes of bleeding, bruising, and hematomas

IMAGING FINDINGS: Coronal VR image from 3D CE MRA of the abdomen and pelvis (Figure 16.11.1) reveals lobulated aneurysms of both external iliac arteries and the right common femoral artery. Note the severe stenosis of the left external iliac artery distal to the aneurysm.

DIAGNOSIS: EDS with iliac and common femoral artery aneurysms

COMMENT: EDS is a connective tissue disorder with an estimated incidence of 1 in 25,000 births. Classic signs include joint hypermobility, increased skin elasticity, and tissue fragility. Of the several distinct inherited subtypes, the most serious is the vascular subtype, EDS type IV, with autosomal dominant inheritance. This subtype is rare, comprising less than 4% of EDS patients, and results from mutations in the gene *COL3A1* encoding for type III procollagen synthesis. By age 40, patients with EDS type IV have generally experienced at least 1 vascular complication, such as spontaneous arterial rupture or dissection, and are also prone to intestinal and uterine rupture. Vascular complications do occur in other subtypes of EDS but at a much lower frequency. The diagnosis of EDS type IV can be difficult because of its rarity and variability in some of its phenotypic features. The skin and musculoskeletal features of EDS type IV are slightly different and more subtle than in the classic, more common forms of EDS. In a Mayo Clinic review, only 26% of patients were aware of their diagnosis when they presented with a serious complication. Survival is reduced among patients with EDS type IV. In the Mayo Clinic series, the average age at death was 54 years. Death results from catastrophic vascular complications, including dissections, aneurysms, arterial tears resulting in pseudoaneurysms, contained hematomas, and intracavitary bleeding.

Management of EDS type IV is controversial. A conservative approach to vascular lesions has been advocated because of the fragility of the underlying connective tissue and the concern that complications during elective repair would result in higher mortality. Recent studies have advocated a more aggressive approach, noting that surgical and endovascular morbidity and mortality can be reduced with careful technique. This shift in the management approach emphasizes the importance of routine vascular screening. In our practice, vascular EDS patients are surveyed annually. Since many of them are young, MRA is favored over CTA with its concomitant cumulative radiation exposure. Aneurysms and dissections can occur in any vascular territory, and the frequency of occurrence at particular locations is not known. We typically perform MRA of the chest, abdomen, and pelvis, usually with 2 injections and 2 separate acquisitions. The appearance of the lesions on MRA alone is not sufficient to make the diagnosis, but in a young patient, the finding of an aneurysm or dissection without a known cause should suggest a connective tissue disorder such as EDS, Marfan syndrome, or Loeys-Dietz syndrome.

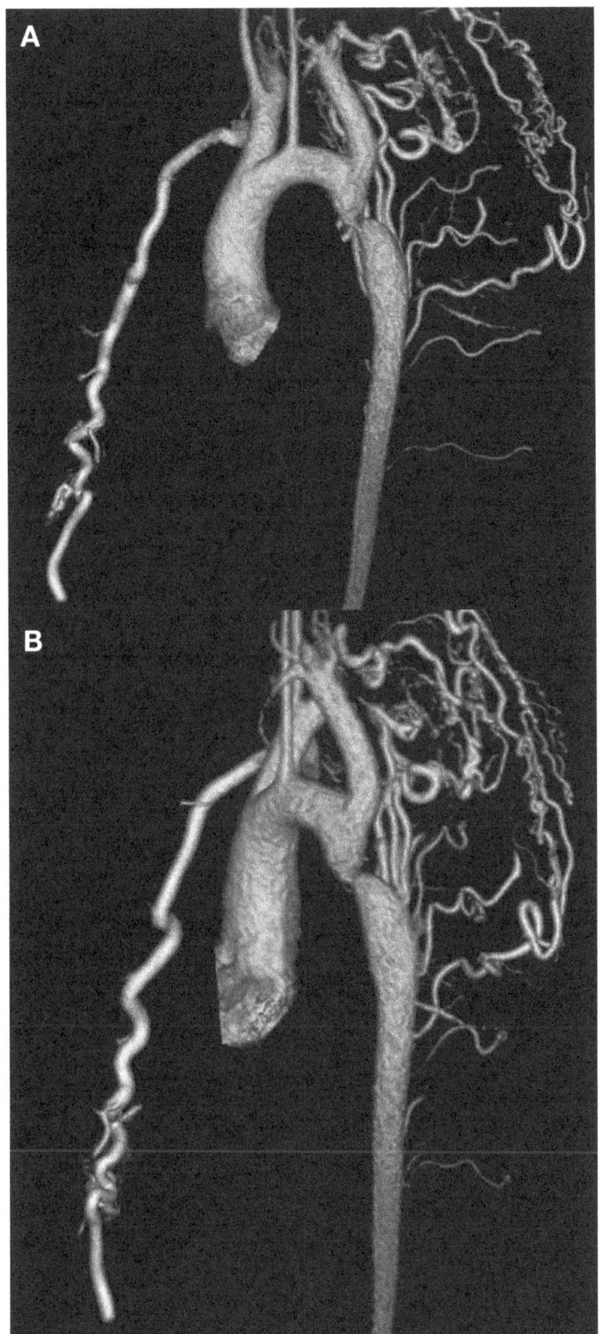

Figure 16.12.1

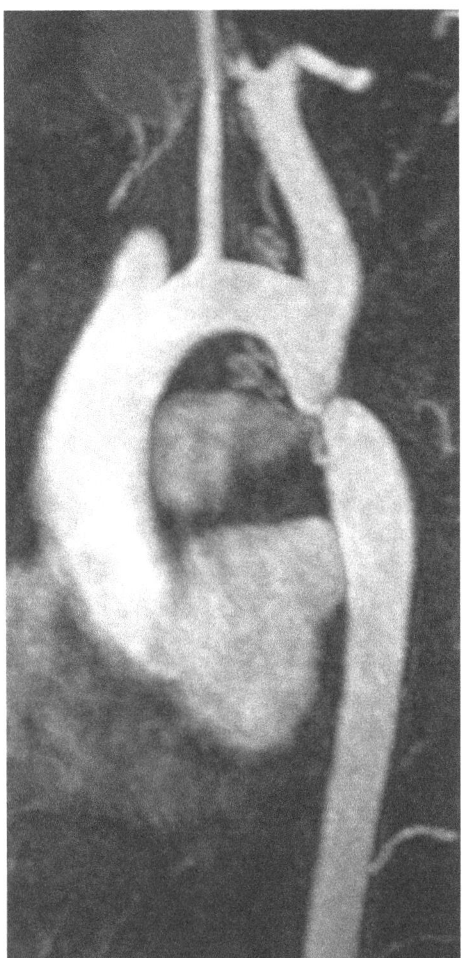

Figure 16.12.2

HISTORY: 31-year-old man with a history of hypertension that was diagnosed at age 10

IMAGING FINDINGS: Sagittal oblique VR images (Figure 16.12.1) and a partial volume MIP image (Figure 16.12.2) from 3D CE MRA reveal severe focal narrowing of the proximal descending thoracic aorta just distal to the origin of the left subclavian artery. Note also enlarged internal mammary and intercostal arteries representing sources of collateral blood flow to the descending aorta.

DIAGNOSIS: Coarctation

COMMENT: Coarctation is a congenital narrowing of the aorta. It usually occurs in the region of the ligamentum arteriosum, occurs more frequently in males, and is associated with a bicuspid aortic valve in up to 50% of cases and with Turner syndrome. The incidence of coarctation is 4 in 10,000 live births, which accounts for 5% to 8% of congenital heart defects. When the coarctation occurs proximally to the ductus arteriosus, symptoms develop early because of the lack of collateral vessel formation in utero. When the coarctation occurs at or distal to the ductus, collateral flow develops early, and patients can remain asymptomatic until well into adulthood, when they present with heart failure, aortic rupture, or complications related to hypertension in the upper body. Late detection of coarctation has significant implications for survival: The mean life expectancy of patients without repair is 35 years, and 90% of these patients die before age 50.

Rib notching is the classic radiographic finding (usually a retrospective diagnosis) that is bilateral when the stenosis is distal to the left subclavian artery and unilateral (on the right) when the stenosis is proximal to the left subclavian artery origin. An extremely meticulous MRI protocol might show rib notching, but the vascular findings are much more apparent.

The easiest way to make the diagnosis is with 3D CE MRA. If the examination is requested to rule out coarctation, a sagittal oblique (or candy cane) acquisition probably makes the most sense since it is more efficient (ie, faster) than a coronal acquisition.

Diagnosis of coarctation is usually straightforward: severe stenosis of the aorta, typically in the region of the isthmus, with prominent collateral vessels (internal mammary and intercostals) supplying the descending thoracic aorta below the coarctation. If the stenosis is only moderate, the question of functional significance arises. The term *pseudocoarctation* is unfortunately sometimes applied to these cases or to redundant, tortuous thoracic aortas. To us, this term is an oxymoron because *coarctation* means narrowing—either the aorta is narrow or it isn't.

A similar problem can arise if patients have had previous coarctation repairs. It's not uncommon to see relative narrowing in the region of the repair, raising the question of whether the pressure gradient across the lesion is large enough to warrant additional correction. The decision is not always straightforward, but a few imaging findings may indicate a functionally significant aortic narrowing. The presence of prominent collaterals in a patient with a native coarctation is a good indication that the coarctation is severe, but this sign is less useful if patients have already had a repair, since dilated collaterals can persist even when there is no longer a significant stenosis. This is particularly true if patients have had subclavian patch grafts, in which case the proximal left subclavian artery is sacrificed and the distal vessel is supplied via collaterals. Cine phase-contrast imaging, an ECG-gated velocity-encoded acquisition allowing measurement of flow in the aorta, can be helpful in these difficult patients. Probably the simplest method is to measure flow in the aorta proximally and distally to the coarctation. Normally flow diminishes distally in the aorta, since multiple intercostal arteries supplied by the aorta all reduce the net flow by a small amount. When the stenosis is significant and collateral flow is present, the situation may be reversed (ie, the collateral vessels have retrograde flow into the descending aorta), and the net flow may increase in the descending aorta below the coarctation.

Other techniques include directly measuring the peak velocity through the site of maximal narrowing with cine phase-contrast imaging. The peak velocity can then be converted to a pressure gradient (in millimeters of mercury) by use of the modified Bernoulli equation: $\Delta P=4v^2$, where v is peak velocity (in meters per second). A gradient of more than 20 mm Hg is considered significant. This technique is more difficult since the plane of acquisition must be oriented exactly in the correct direction and the temporal resolution must be high enough to capture the peak velocity (higher temporal resolution corresponds to a longer acquisition time).

Another approach is to find a prominent collateral adjacent to the descending aorta and then assess the relative direction of flow. If the flow is directed toward the descending aorta, the collateral is active and the stenosis is significant; if the flow is in the opposite (ie, normal) direction, a significant stenosis is not present.

In our practice, we spend more time imaging patients who have had prior coarctation repairs to assess for restenosis or other complications rather than looking for de novo coarctation. Patients with coarctation have lower mortality if the coarctation is repaired earlier; however, rates of restenosis are correspondingly higher for earlier repairs (44% in neonates vs 0%-9% in adult patients). Aneurysm or pseudoaneurysm at the site of coarctation repair is also a well-recognized complication, with an estimated incidence of 10%. The risk is higher after subclavian flap and patch graft repair than after end-to-end anastomosis.

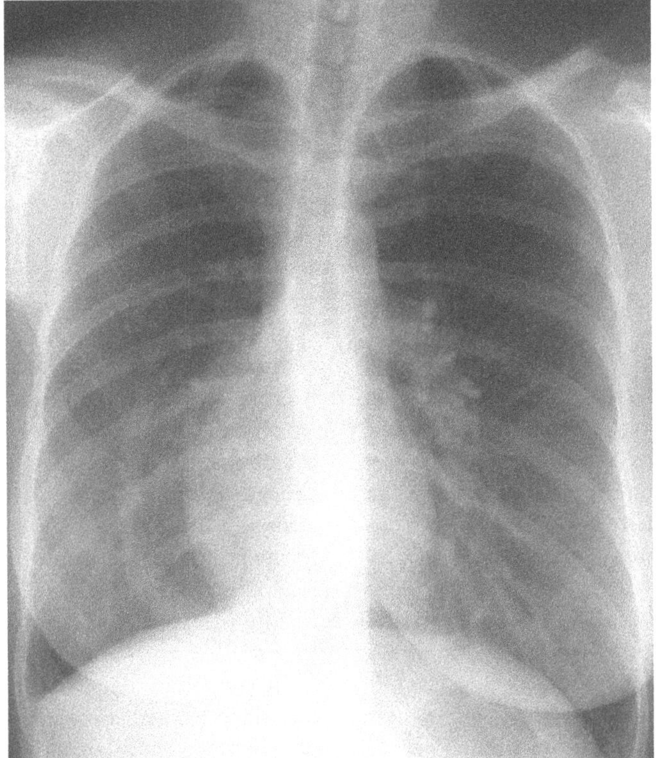

Figure 16.13.1

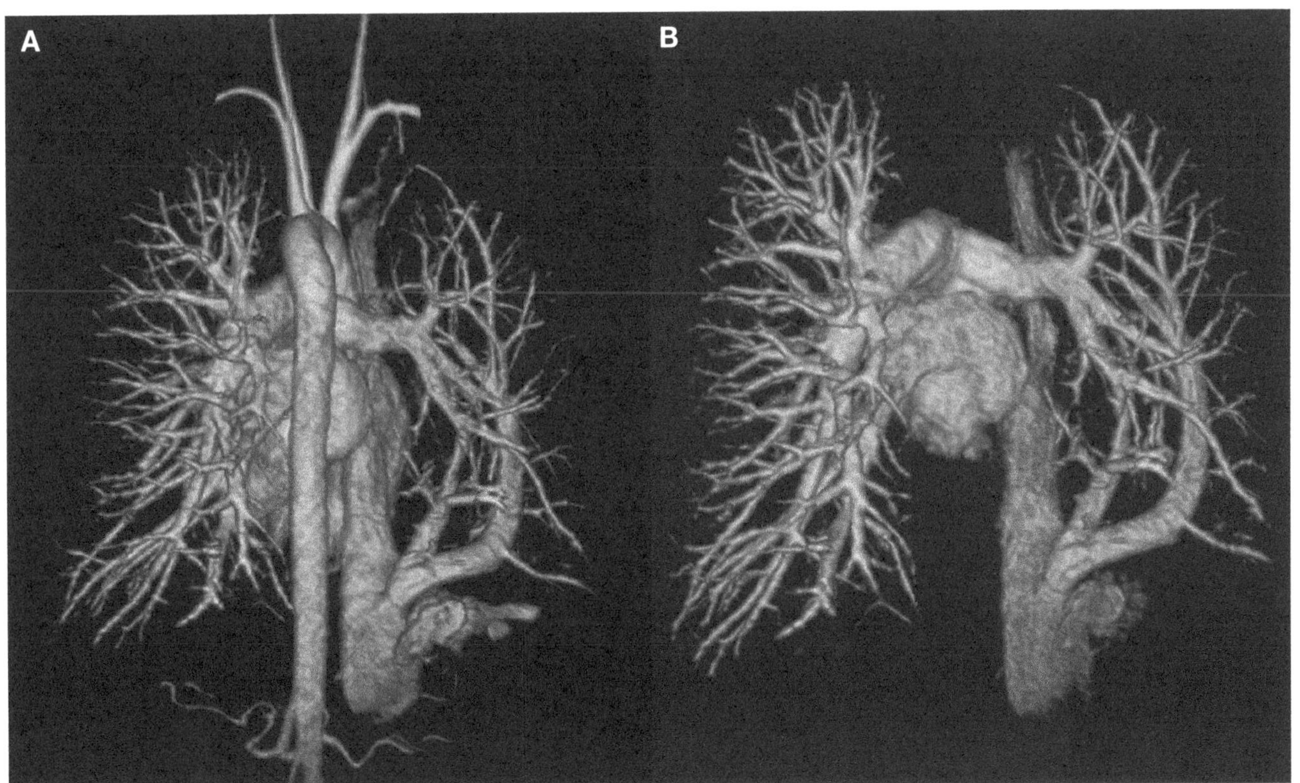

Figure 16.13.2

HISTORY: 35-year-old asymptomatic woman with a history of an abnormality on chest radiograph that was diagnosed when she was an infant

IMAGING FINDINGS: Chest radiograph (Figure 16.13.1) reveals a curvilinear density in the right lung extending toward the diaphragm. Note the enlargement of the right heart border. Posterior VR images from 3D CE MRA (Figure 16.13.2) demonstrate an enlarged anomalous pulmonary vein draining all of the right lung into the suprahepatic IVC.

DIAGNOSIS: Scimitar syndrome (partial anomalous pulmonary venous return)

COMMENT: Scimitar syndrome is usually presented as a classic plain film diagnosis in radiology resident conferences. In fact, very few radiologists have ever made a de novo diagnosis, partly because the scimitar vein may not be obvious on a chest radiograph, especially when you're not looking for it, and also because this anomaly is so rare (incidence, 2 per 100,000 births).

Scimitar syndrome involves partial anomalous pulmonary venous return to the IVC or cavoatrial junction via an abnormal vein. In two-thirds of cases (and in this case), the scimitar vein provides drainage for the entire right lung; in the other cases, it drains only the lower portion of the lung. The scimitar vein varies considerably in its location and course. It may insert below or above the diaphragm, it may be stenotic at its junction with the IVC in 10% of cases, and multiple veins have been described. Additional abnormalities are frequently associated with the anomalous vein, including right lung hypoplasia (virtually always present), hypoplasia of the right pulmonary artery (in 60% of cases), systemic arterial supply to the right lower lung from the infradiaphragmatic aorta (in 60%), and secundum atrial septal defect (in 40%). In addition, the infantile form is associated with multiple cardiovascular anomalies, including ventricular septal defect, patent ductus arteriosus, hypoplastic aortic arch, coarctation of the aorta, tetralogy of Fallot, truncus arteriosus, and anomalous origin of the coronary arteries.

The 2 distinct forms of scimitar syndrome are the infantile form and the pediatric or adult form. The infantile form is almost always more serious, with mortality estimated at 45%. Patients present within the first few months of life with symptoms including failure to thrive, tachypnea, heart failure, and significant left-to-right shunting with pulmonary hypertension.

Symptoms are mild or absent in the adult form, although many patients have a history of recurrent pulmonary infections. In some patients, atrial fibrillation develops from chronic right heart overload.

In our practice, most of the patients are referred for MRI because anomalous pulmonary venous return is suspected from echocardiography. Coronal 3D CE MRA usually shows the abnormal pulmonary vein if the acquisition is timed to the arrival of the contrast bolus in the pulmonary veins or left atrium (not the aorta). A time-resolved MRA can also be performed with the hope of obtaining distinct pulmonary arterial, pulmonary venous, and aortic phase images. ECG-gating for the MRA generally is not necessary and adds additional time to the breath-hold.

If you're familiar with the basics of cardiac MRI, a couple of additional acquisitions may help with the decision of whether surgical repair is indicated. Cine SSFP images through the ventricles can be used to assess right ventricular size and function—a dilated and hypofunctional right ventricle might be an indication for surgery. These images can also be used to look for an atrial septal defect. Cine phase-contrast acquisitions through the ascending aorta and main pulmonary artery can be used to determine the shunt ratio, Qp/Qs, or the ratio of pulmonary artery blood flow to aortic (systemic) blood flow. Normally, Qp/Qs=1. With anomalous pulmonary venous return and a left-to-right shunt, Qp/Qs will be elevated. A high shunt ratio (Qp/Qs >1.5) may also indicate a significant shunt and the need to correct the anomalous pulmonary venous return.

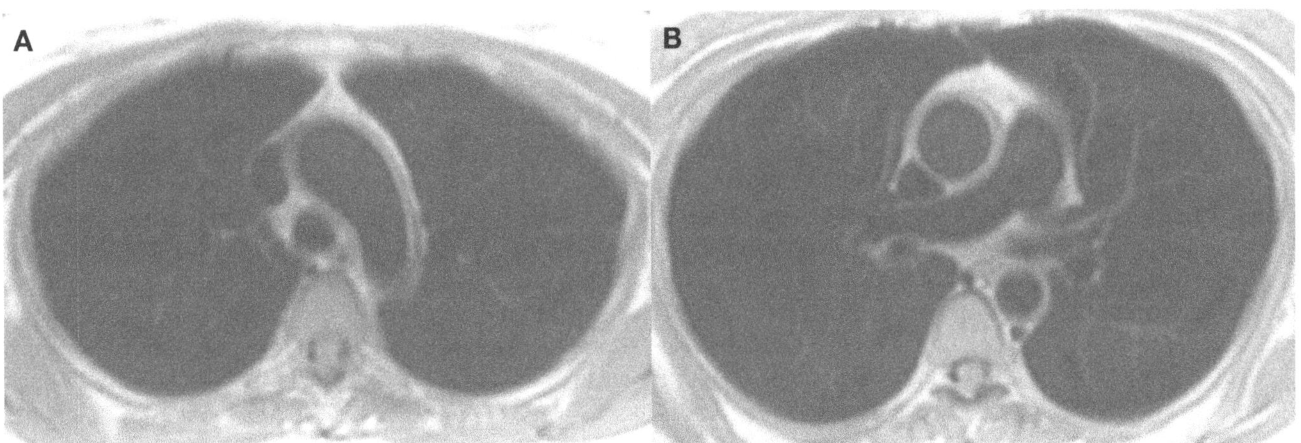

Figure 16.14.1

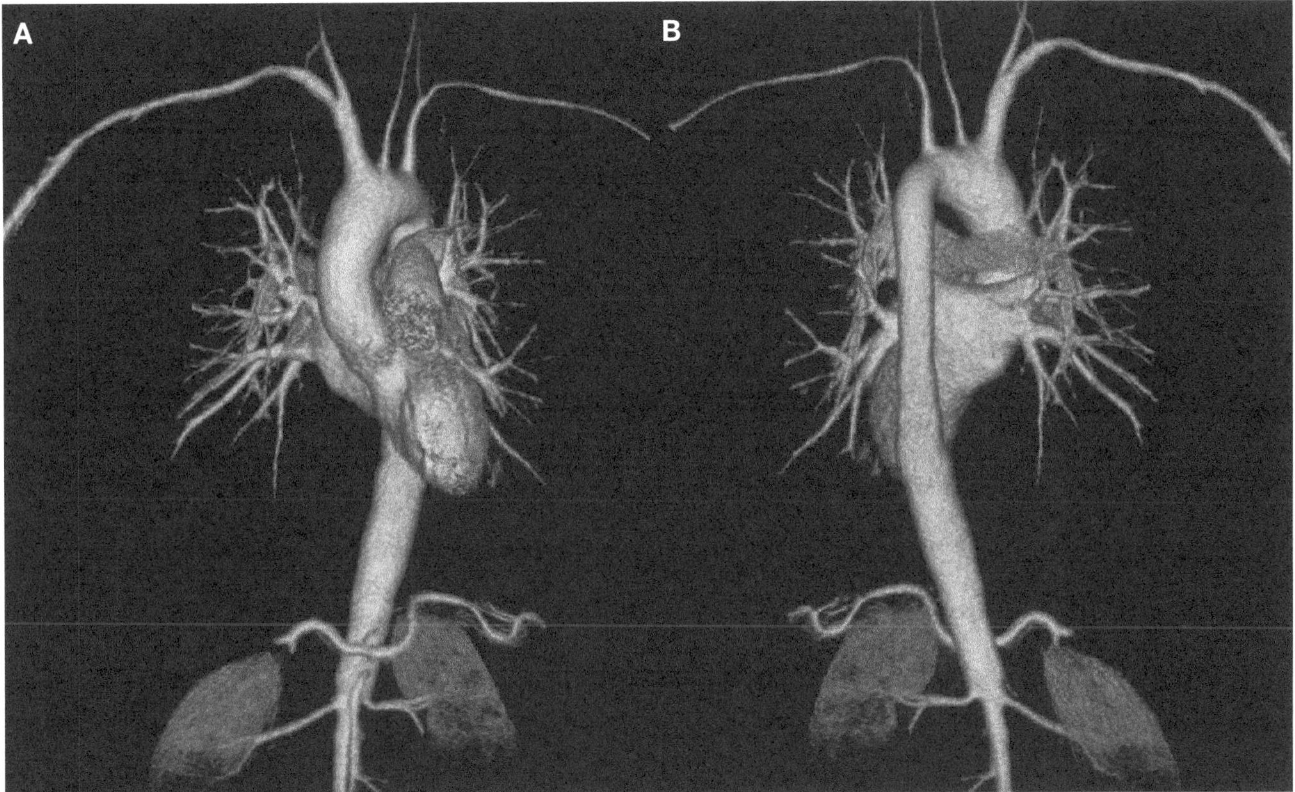

Figure 16.14.2

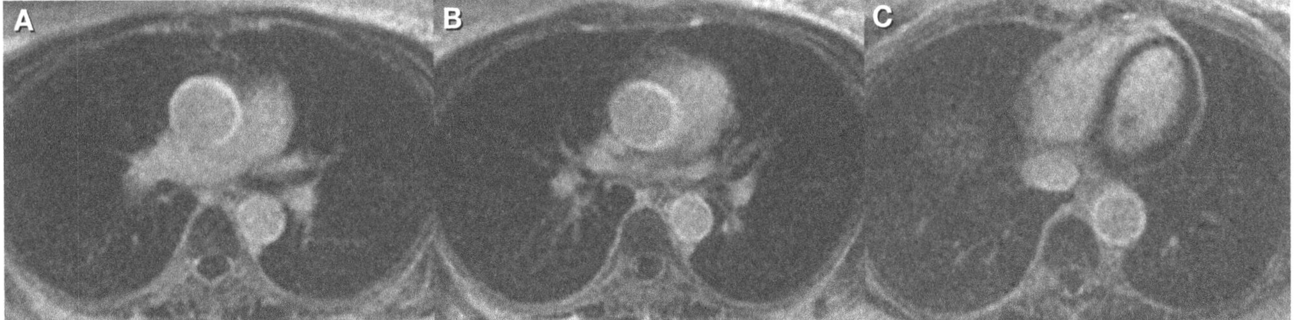

Figure 16.14.3

HISTORY: 25-year-old woman with a history of high fevers and joint aches developing 1 week after childbirth; values for erythrocyte sedimentation rate and C-reactive protein are elevated

IMAGING FINDINGS: Axial ECG-gated black-blood proton density-weighted FSE images (Figure 16.14.1) show diffuse mild thickening of the aortic arch and ascending and descending aorta. Anterior (Figure 16.14.2A) and posterior (Figure 16.14.2B) VR images from 3D CE MRA demonstrate segmental narrowing of the mid-distal left subclavian artery, mild diffuse narrowing of the descending thoracic aorta, and significant narrowing of the infrarenal abdominal aorta. Axial 2D late gadolinium enhancement images of the thoracic aorta (Figure 16.14.3) demonstrate mild mural thickening and significant mural enhancement in the ascending thoracic aorta and, to a lesser extent, in the descending aorta.

DIAGNOSIS: Takayasu arteritis

COMMENT: TA was first described in 1908 by Mikito Takayasu, who noted a wreathlike appearance of retinal blood vessels in patients without wrist pulses. TA has a striking female preponderance (9:1) and typically affects young women from age 10 to 40, with an incidence of 1 to 2 per million. Initial symptoms are typically nonspecific and related to systemic inflammation, including weight loss, low-grade fever, joint pain, and muscle weakness. Symptoms develop eventually in relation to specific sites of arterial involvement and include hypertension, vascular bruits, asymmetrical arm blood pressure, and ischemic phenomena such as extremity claudication, stroke, and myocardial infarction.

MRI and MRA offer a wide range of techniques for assessment of patients with known or suspected vasculitis. Conventional CE MRA is effective for making an initial diagnosis of vasculitis based on findings such as luminal narrowing or occlusion or aneurysm formation. This technique is sensitive only if the disease is relatively advanced, however, and does not provide information about disease activity.

MRI also allows assessment of the vessel wall, and findings that have been demonstrated to correlate with the presence of vasculitis include vessel wall thickening of more than 3 mm, increased mural signal intensity or edema on T2-weighted images, and enhancement of the vessel wall on postcontrast T1-weighted images.

Whether MRI findings accurately reflect disease activity in TA is uncertain. Some authors have found good correlation between disease activity and vessel wall edema, thickening, or enhancement, but others have noted the persistence of some of these findings when the disease is in clinical remission. Some of the discrepancies may be related to the wide variation in techniques used by different authors. Vessel wall enhancement, for example, may represent active inflammation if it is apparent within a few minutes after contrast injection, or it may indicate chronic fibrosis if it appears after a longer delay following contrast administration.

Our standard protocol for imaging TA patients includes MRA of the chest, abdomen, and pelvis. We use 1 injection with a large FOV acquisition in short patients and 2 injections with separate chest and abdominal pelvic acquisitions in everyone else. Thoracic imaging should include a coronal acquisition with wide right-to-left coverage since the distal subclavian and axillary arteries are often affected and occasionally are the only sites of obvious involvement (we don't worry about complete coverage of the carotid arteries since they are usually evaluated in a separate examination of the head and neck).

As noted above, vessel wall imaging is very important. We obtain axial fat-suppressed 2D SSFP images covering the entire aorta and a few ECG-gated T1-weighted or proton density-weighted double IR FSE images through the thoracic aorta (and anywhere else that looks suspicious on the SSFP images). T2-weighted images through the thoracic aorta, and sometimes through the abdominal aorta, are acquired with respiratory triggered fat-suppressed FSE images (triple IR ECG-gated FSE images are an alternative, but the acquisition time for extended coverage is problematic). Double IR FSE black-blood images are useful for visualizing mural thickening, and the T2-weighted images demonstrate increased mural signal intensity in the presence of edema. Diffusion-weighted images are an interesting alternative technique for visualizing vessel wall edema—a breath-held acquisition is fast, blood suppression is automatic with diffusion weighting, and edematous thickened walls show increased signal intensity on acquisitions with a low b value (b=50-100 s/mm^2). Older patients with significant atherosclerosis may also have increased mural signal intensity on diffusion-weighted images, but this is much less problematic for younger TA patients.

After performing 3D CE MRA (always with an additional venous phase acquisition), we acquire immediate axial fat-suppressed 3D SPGR images of the entire aorta. Mural enhancement within the first few minutes after contrast injection is a good sign of active inflammation. With a significant delay between contrast injection and axial 3D SPGR imaging, mural scarring within the aorta may also enhance; for that reason, we try to finish the axial imaging as quickly as possible. ECG-gated myocardial delayed enhancement sequences can increase the conspicuity of vessel wall enhancement, but with longer acquisition times, we usually reserve this technique for evaluating regions of obvious thickening or questionable enhancement on 3D SPGR images.

The imaging appearance of TA is almost identical to that of giant cell arteritis; however, the distinction between the 2 entities can almost always be made on the basis of age. TA affects young patients, and giant cell arteritis generally affects elderly patients.

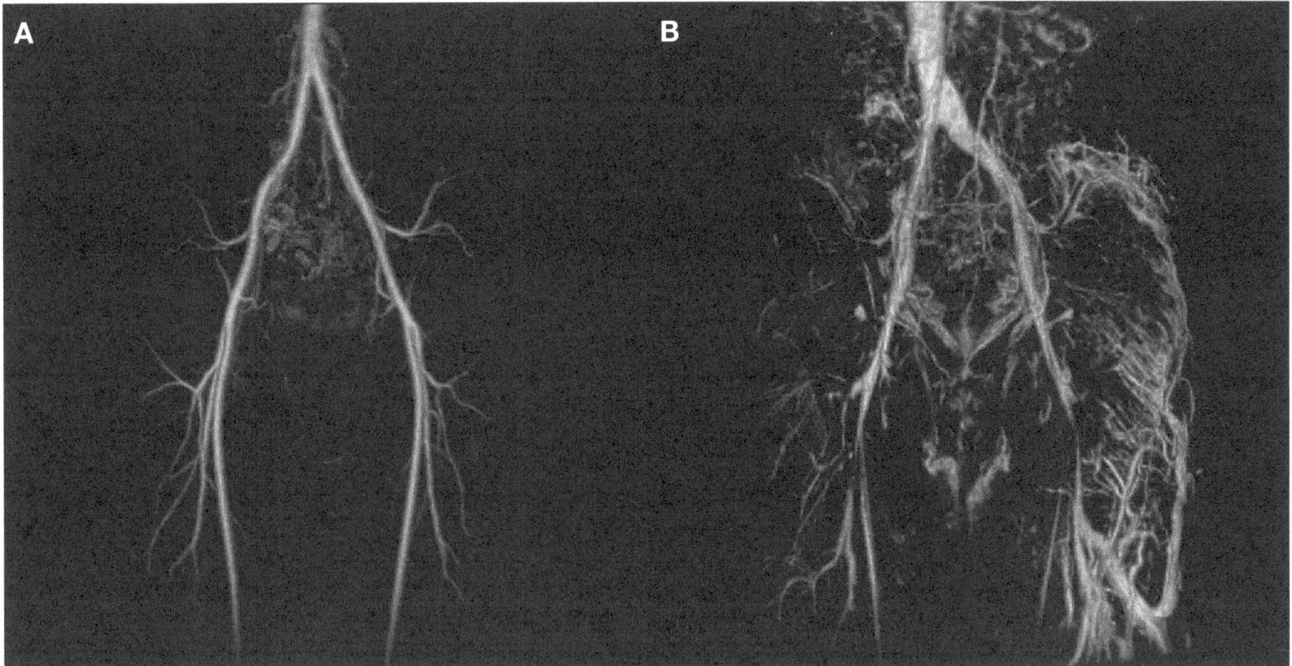

Figure 16.15.1

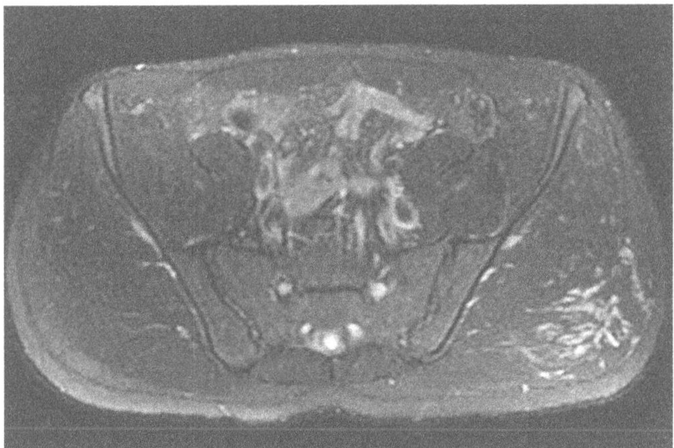

Figure 16.15.2

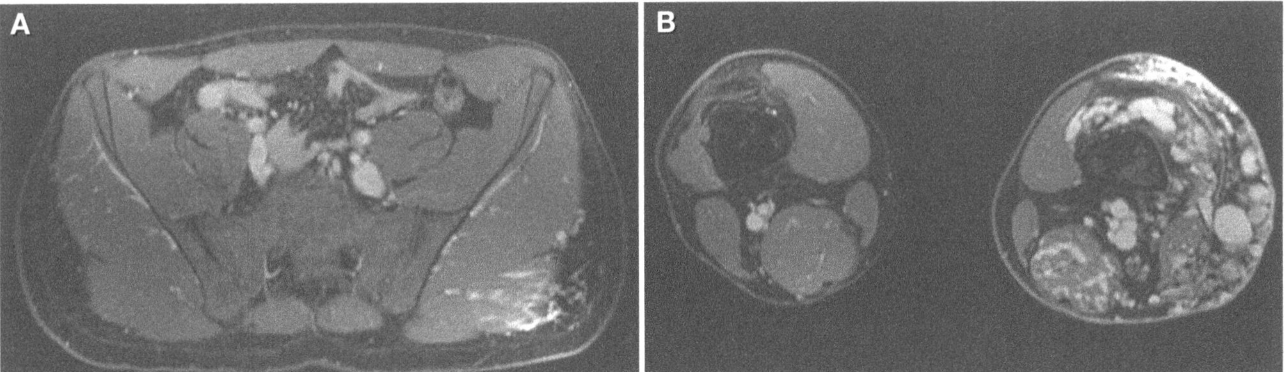

Figure 16.15.3

HISTORY: 32-year-old man with an abnormal left leg, multiple varicose veins, and a history of multiple prior deep vein thromboses and pulmonary emboli

IMAGING FINDINGS: Arterial phase (Figure 16.15.1A) and venous phase (Figure 16.15.1B) MIP images from time-resolved 3D MRA with a gadolinium blood pool contrast agent (gadofosveset trisodium [Ablavar]) demonstrate normal arterial anatomy with prominent varicosities posteriorly in the left pelvis and upper thigh on the venous phase image. Pseudostenosis of the common femoral veins bilaterally is likely a subtraction artifact. Axial FSE T2-weighted (Figure 16.15.2) and postcontrast 3D SPGR (Figure 16.15.3A) images demonstrate corresponding venous malformation in the left gluteal muscle with high T2-signal intensity and enhancement. An additional axial 3D SPGR image from the mid thighs (Figure 16.15.3B) shows extensive superficial and deep varicosities in the left leg.

DIAGNOSIS: Klippel-Trénaunay syndrome

COMMENT: Klippel-Trénaunay syndrome, first described in 1900 by the French physicians Klippel and Trénaunay, is characterized by a combination of capillary malformations (usually port-wine stains), hypertrophy of soft tissue or bone (or both), and varicose veins or venous malformations, often with persistent lateral embryologic veins. In addition, patients frequently have associated deep venous anomalies, such as hypoplasia, aplasia, or venous incompetence, and lymphatic malformations. The constellation of Klippel-Trénaunay syndrome in association with arteriovenous malformations is known as Klippel-Trénaunay-Weber syndrome, or Parkes Weber syndrome. (During my residency, the chief of body MRI showed a case of Klippel-Trénaunay syndrome in a conference. A resident described the findings and made the diagnosis and was then asked what distinguished this syndrome from Klippel-Trénaunay-Weber syndrome, to which he replied that he didn't know. This didn't go over well, and the chief's final comment was, "This is the kind of knowledge that distinguishes an excellent radiologist from an average one." The judgment seemed somewhat harsh, particularly since our future chairman had mixed up the syndromes himself, although no one was bold enough to mention it at the time.)

MRI is an ideal technique for diagnosis of Klippel-Trénaunay syndrome because limb hypertrophy, proliferation of subcutaneous fat in the affected extremity, and muscle enlargement are easily appreciated. Venous malformations are clearly visualized as serpiginous infiltrative lesions that have high T2-signal intensity and gradually enhance after contrast administration.

MRV is probably not necessary for the diagnosis of Klippel-Trénaunay syndrome. It can be important, however, if surgical or interventional therapy for a venous malformation or varicose veins is being considered and the location and venous supply of the lesions need to be delineated. More importantly, MRV is used to document the patency of the underlying deep veins because resection or embolization of a vascular malformation in a patient without a patent deep venous system can have catastrophic consequences.

We favor 3D SPGR contrast-enhanced multiphase acquisitions with the blood pool contrast agent gadofosveset trisodium (Ablavar). An arterial phase acquisition is always a good idea (and you can subtract this from subsequent venous phase acquisitions to generate a pure venogram, as shown in Figure 16.15.1B) but not absolutely necessary unless the patient has Klippel-Trénaunay-Weber syndrome and arteriovenous malformations with rapid early filling. Contrast accumulates throughout the venous system and venous malformations, and images with high spatial resolution and high signal to noise ratios can be obtained without the time constraints imposed by renal clearance of the standard gadolinium agents. After MRA or MRV images have been obtained, usually in the coronal plane, we then acquire axial fat-suppressed 3D SPGR images through the pelvis and involved extremity. These are often the most useful in confirming the patency of the deep venous system.

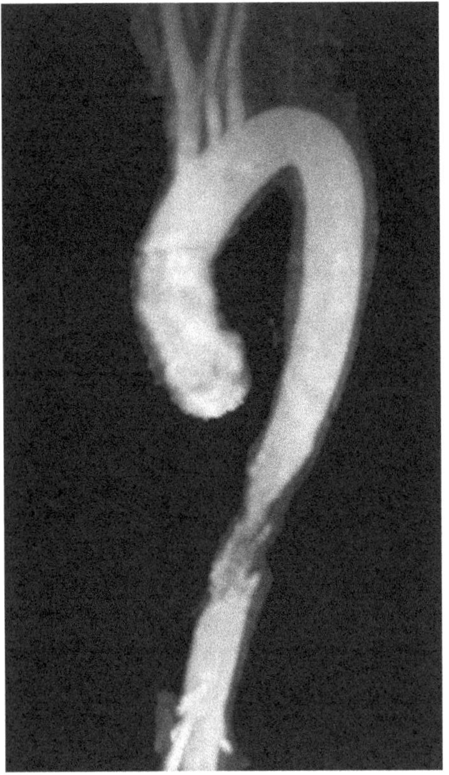

Figure 16.16.1

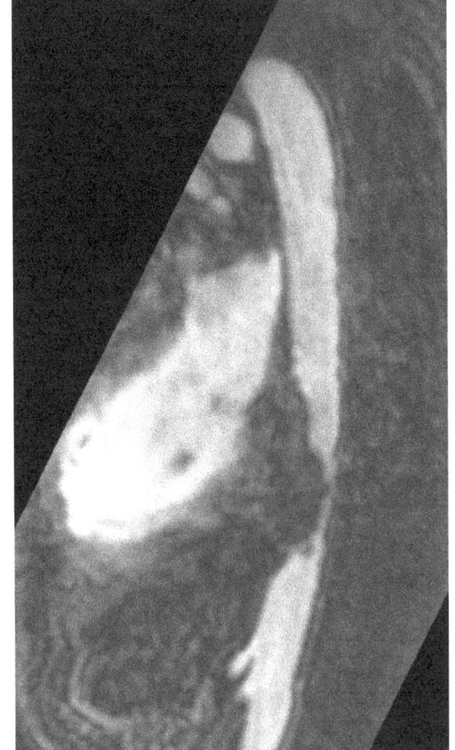

Figure 16.16.2

HISTORY: 82-year-old woman with drug-resistant hypertension and a blood pressure discrepancy between upper and lower extremities

IMAGING FINDINGS: MIP image from 3D CE MRA of the thoracic aorta (Figure 16.16.1) shows an irregular filling defect in the distal thoracic aorta, which causes significant narrowing of the aorta. Coronal oblique reformatted image from the 3D CE MRA (Figure 16.16.2) also demonstrates a large focal filling defect in the distal thoracic aorta causing severe focal narrowing of the aorta.

DIAGNOSIS: Aortic sarcoma

COMMENT: Aortic sarcomas are very rare, with fewer than 200 reported cases. The clinical presentation of these lesions is variable, depending to some extent on location and whether widespread metastatic disease is present. Typical symptoms include claudication, pain, and end-organ ischemia. Metastatic disease is common at diagnosis, occurring in more than 70% of patients in most series. The prognosis is poor, with 5-year survival of about 8%.

These lesions are often misdiagnosed initially (as was this case) as focal atherosclerosis (ie, an atypical appearance of a common entity). In this case, the rest of the aorta looks remarkably free of atherosclerosis, especially given the patient's age; this observation should probably have raised some red flags. Another problem in this case was that post-MRA SPGR images showed no enhancement of the lesion. On pathologic evaluation, the sarcoma was nearly completely necrotic, making the correct diagnosis even more difficult to determine. It is worth noting that a decision on whether a lesion enhances should never be based on MRA source images alone. The MRA should be acquired when the contrast bolus peaks in the arterial lumen; therefore, you won't see enhancement of anything but lesions with brisk arterial phase enhancement. This is yet another reason to always acquire a set of axial 3D SPGR images after MRA. Other important reasons include visualization of aneurysms (including the thrombosed portions), complex atherosclerotic plaques, enhancement patterns of true and false lumens in dissection, mural enhancement in vasculitis, endoleaks after endovascular aneurysm repair, slow-filling pseudoaneurysms or penetrating ulcers, and incidental lesions in the liver, kidneys, and other organs.

Case 16.17 illustrates a more typical appearance (if such a thing can be said to exist for such a rare entity) of an aortic sarcoma.

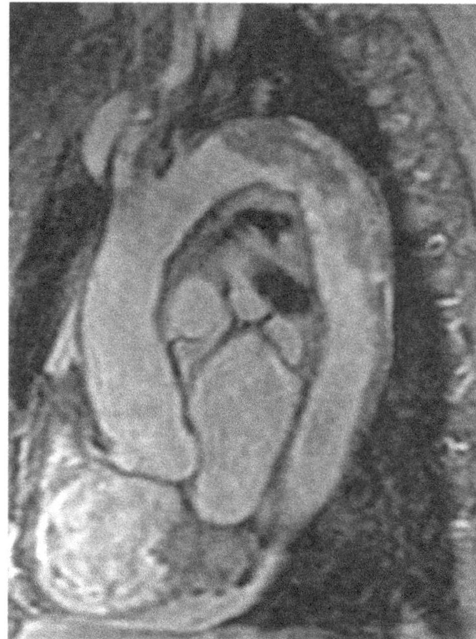

Figure 16.17.1

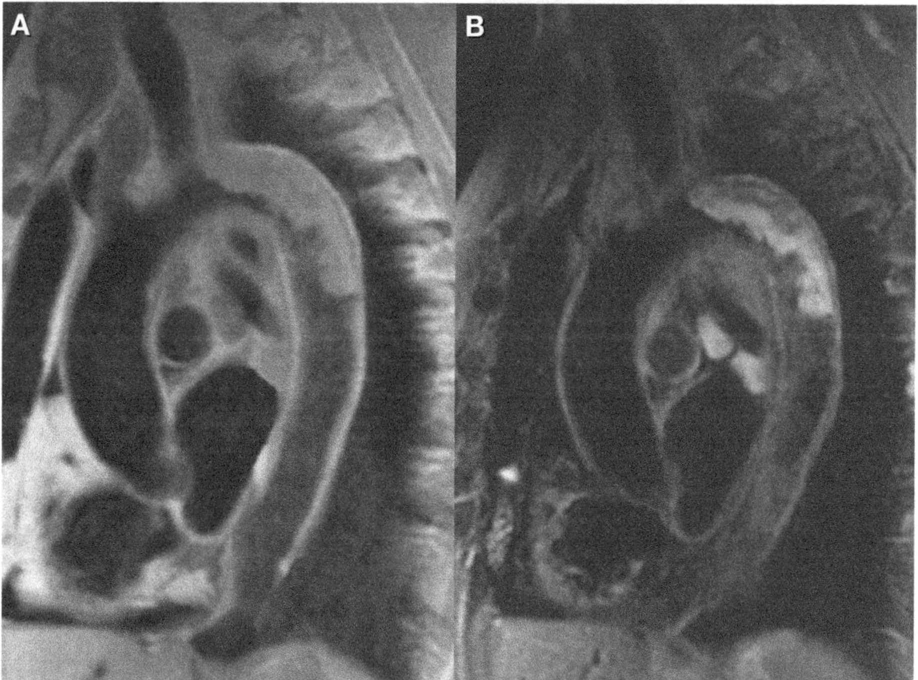

Figure 16.17.2

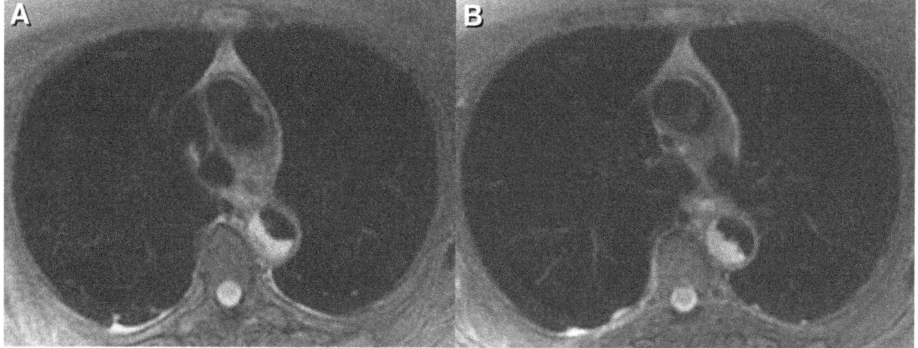

Figure 16.17.3

HISTORY: 66-year-old woman with new-onset hypertension and weight loss; laboratory investigations revealed anemia, an elevated erythrocyte sedimentation rate, and an increased C-reactive protein level

IMAGING FINDINGS: Sagittal oblique image from navigator-gated, ECG-gated, fat-suppressed 3D SSFP acquisition of the thoracic aorta (Figure 16.17.1) reveals a large irregular filling defect in the posterior arch and proximal descending aorta. Sagittal oblique ECG-gated double (Figure 16.17.2A) and triple (Figure 16.17.2B) IR FSE (proton density-weighted and T2-weighted) images and axial triple IR FSE images (Figure 16.17.3) show the lesion to have heterogeneous increased signal intensity, most notably on the triple IR images. Note also the enlarged left hilar lymph nodes.

DIAGNOSIS: High-grade pleomorphic aortic sarcoma

COMMENT: This case should not really be a diagnostic dilemma, at least on MRI. The lesion is large and has markedly abnormal signal intensity on proton density-weighted and T2-weighted black-blood images and therefore should not be mistaken for an unusual atherosclerotic plaque. Also, as noted in Case 16.16, this patient does not really have significant atherosclerosis anywhere else, so it's a bit of a stretch to call this a large focal plaque. Postcontrast 3D SPGR images (not shown) also demonstrated mild enhancement within the lesion, which again is highly suggestive of an aortic tumor. The case was interesting in that several other initial tests yielded ambiguous results before MRI and MRA gave the correct answer.

Mostly on the basis of the patient's elevated inflammatory markers, she was thought to have vasculitis, and a PET-CT scan was performed. This is arguably a reasonable decision because a few papers have shown that PET is more sensitive and specific than MRI for detection of large-vessel vasculitis, and the examination should detect occult malignancy, which could also account for the symptoms. Unfortunately, in this case, the extent of the lesion was not appreciated on the noncontrast CT portion of the examination, and the mild activity in the thoracic aorta was interpreted as evidence of vasculitis. The patient was subsequently treated with corticosteroids without improvement. At some point, transthoracic and transesophageal echocardiography were performed, mostly because a cardiologist was consulted, and these revealed thickening or plaque in the aortic arch, which was incompletely imaged. CTA was then performed, and the findings were interpreted as most consistent with aortic sarcoma. Apparently, the report lacked enough strength of conviction to convince all the attending physicians, who then ordered MRI and MRA.

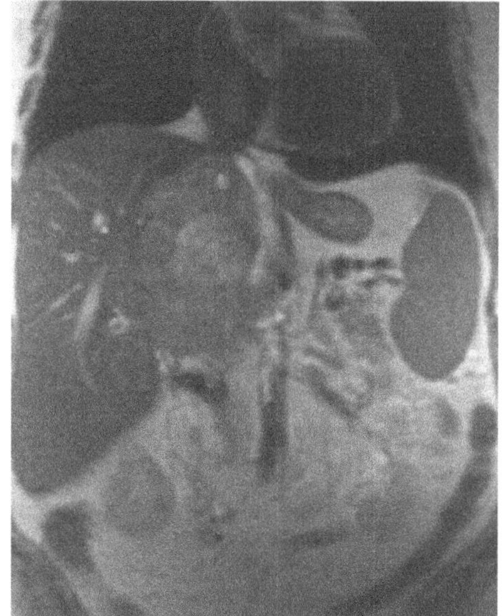

Figure 16.18.1

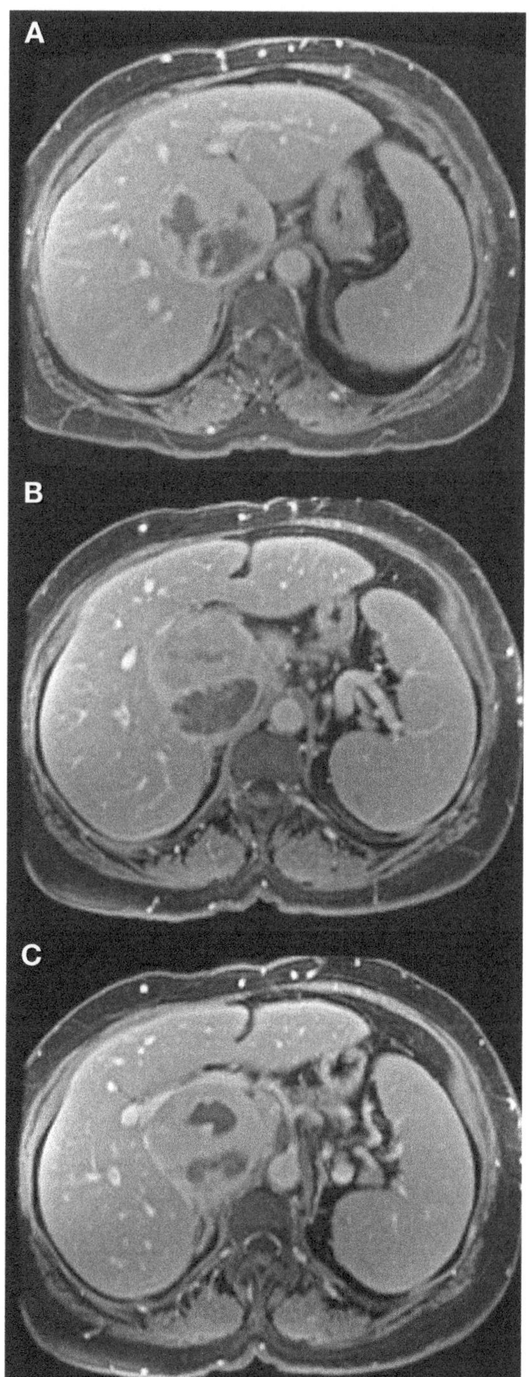

Figure 16.18.4

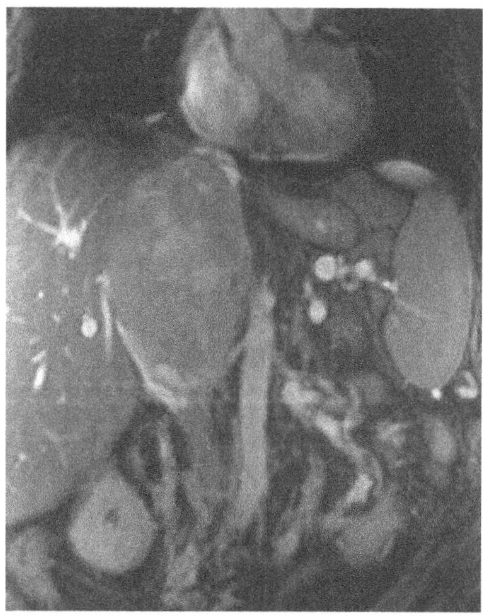

Figure 16.18.2

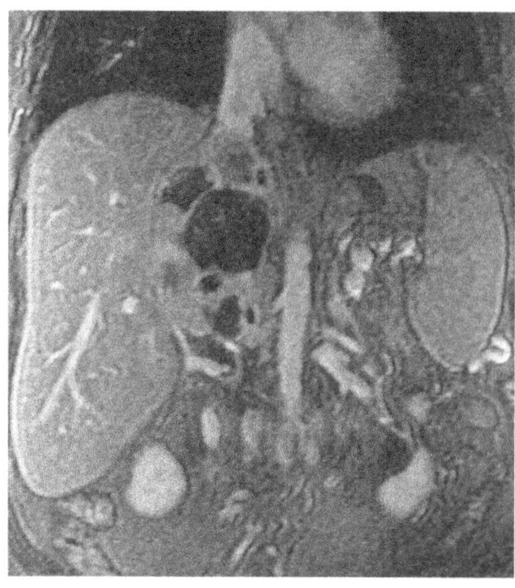

Figure 16.18.3

HISTORY: 64-year-old woman with a history of fevers and anemia

IMAGING FINDINGS: Coronal SSFSE (Figure 16.18.1) and fat-suppressed SSFP (Figure 16.18.2) images demonstrate a heterogeneous mass expanding the intrahepatic IVC. Coronal source image from venous phase acquisition of a 3D CE MRA (Figure 16.18.3) reveals heterogeneous enhancement of the lesion with multiple necrotic foci. Axial post-gadolinium 2D SPGR images (Figure 16.18.4) also reveal a heterogeneously enhancing mass expanding the intrahepatic IVC. Note the prominent enhancing collateral veins in the anterior and posterior subcutaneous tissues.

DIAGNOSIS: IVC leiomyosarcoma

COMMENT: IVC sarcoma is a rare entity first described in 1871; approximately 300 cases have been reported. Diagnosis of IVC sarcoma at imaging is usually fairly straightforward. The presenting symptoms, however, are quite vague, and often diagnosis is made at a relatively late stage when the IVC has been completely obstructed and patients present with symptoms such as lower extremity edema, massive ascites, or deep vein thrombosis. If the tumor involves the intrahepatic IVC, the hepatic veins may become occluded, and the patient can present with Budd-Chiari syndrome.

The imaging appearance is that of a complex mass centered in the IVC. Typically, the IVC is expanded, and the lesion shows significant enhancement after gadolinium administration, unlike a bland thrombus, which should not enhance. If contrast cannot be administered, the diagnosis generally remains simple and is based on heterogeneously increased T2-signal intensity, restricted diffusion, and clear distinction from the lumen on black-blood and bright-blood images.

IVC leiomyosarcomas are malignant tumors that develop in the smooth muscle of the tunica media. An initial period of mural growth is followed by intraluminal or extraluminal extension (or both). Optimal treatment consists of complete resection of the tumor with reconstruction of the IVC, which is often not possible. Survival rates are low even with successful surgery (after complete resection, 5-year survival is 30%).

Differential diagnostic dilemmas can occur if the tumor has grown beyond the IVC into an adjacent organ, so that it is difficult to determine the primary origin of the lesion. We have seen 1 case of an IVC sarcoma exclusively confined to the intrahepatic IVC and hepatic veins, with the bulk of the tumor in the hepatic veins, that was misdiagnosed initially as hepatocellular carcinoma partly because the heterogeneous enhancement pattern of the liver parenchyma on dynamic images (from hepatic vein obstruction) simulated an infiltrative mass.

ABBREVIATIONS

AMI	acute mesenteric ischemia
ASTRAL	Angioplasty and Stenting for Renal Artery Lesions
AVF	arteriovenous fistula
AVM	arteriovenous malformation
CE	contrast-enhanced
CMI	chronic mesenteric ischemia
CORAL	Cardiovascular Outcomes in Renal Atherosclerotic Lesions
CT	computed tomography
CTA	computed tomographic angiography
ECG	electrocardiographic
EDS	Ehlers-Danlos syndrome
FMD	fibromuscular dysplasia
FOV	field of view
FSE	fast-spin echo
IMH	intramural hematoma
IR	inversion-recovery
IVC	inferior vena cava
MAL	median arcuate ligament
MIP	maximum intensity projection
MRA	magnetic resonance angiography
MRI	magnetic resonance imaging
MRV	magnetic resonance venography
NSF	nephrogenic systemic fibrosis
PET	positron emission tomography
Qp/Qs	ratio of pulmonary artery blood flow to aortic (systemic) blood flow
RADISH	Renal Artery Diagnostic Imaging Study in Hypertension
SPGR	spoiled gradient recalled
SSFP	steady-state free precession
SSFSE	single-shot fast-spin echo
STAR	Stent Placement and Blood Pressure and Lipid-Lowering for the Prevention of Progression of Renal Dysfunction Caused by Atherosclerotic Ostial Stenosis of the Renal Artery
TA	Takayasu arteritis
3D	3-dimensional
2D	2-dimensional
US	ultrasonography
VR	volume-rendered

17.

ARTIFACTS

CASE 17.1

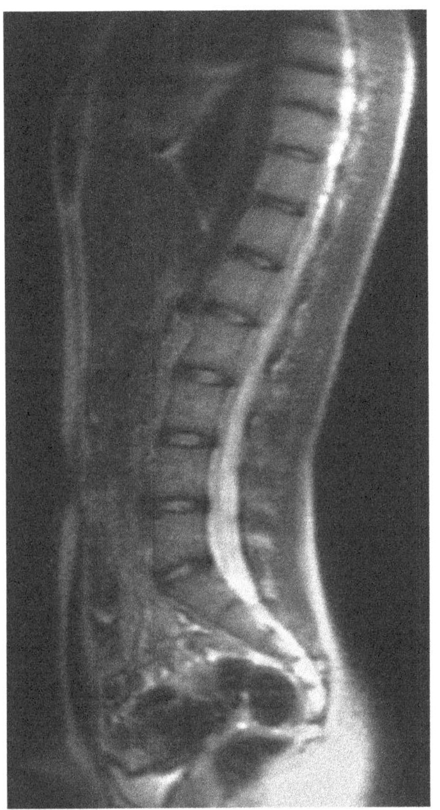

Figure 17.1.1

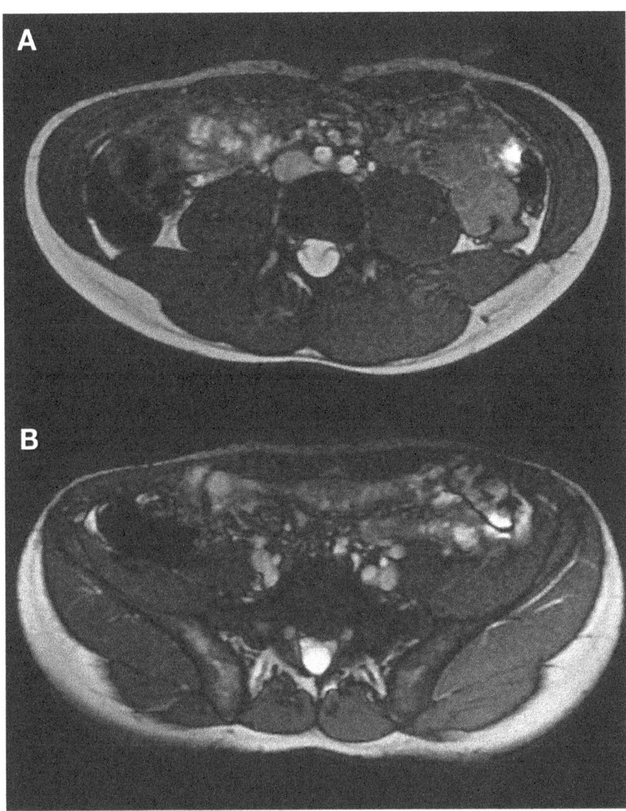

Figure 17.1.2

HISTORY: 20-year-old man with abdominal pain and possible Crohn disease

IMAGING FINDINGS: Sagittal image from 3-plane SSFSE scout series (Figure 17.1.1) demonstrates diffuse signal loss over the anterior abdomen and pelvis in comparison to the spine and paraspinous muscle. Axial SSFP images from the mid abdomen (Figure 17.1.2A) and upper pelvis (Figure 17.1.2B) demonstrate similar findings.

DIAGNOSIS: Anterior phased array coil not plugged in

COMMENT: This case is an example of an easily correctable mistake that wasn't recognized by the technologist and led to an entire examination acquired with marginal image quality. The only saving grace was that the patient was very thin, so that some anterior signal could be provided by the posterior coil.

Scout series are frequently ignored by radiologists, and while technologists have to look at them in order to prescribe subsequent series, they don't always remember to inspect the images from a quality control perspective. This is a habit that should be continually reinforced: It's unrealistic to expect your technologists to pay more attention to the images than you do, and if no one reminds them about technical errors or complains about poor image quality, they will eventually conclude (justifiably) that either you don't care or you're not capable of distinguishing good images from bad and will cease to spend much effort on quality control.

Scout images serve a number of functions and should always be inspected for the following:

1) Technical problems—Are all the coil elements working? That is, are there regions of absent or reduced signal intensity in areas that will be imaged during the examination?
2) Coil positioning—Determining the location of the superior margin of the liver from external anatomy is not easy, and it is not uncommon for the anterior coil to be positioned too low, leading to low signal intensity and reduced image quality in the dome of the liver.
3) Undisclosed metal—Patients may forget or not realize that their clothing has metallic elements (underwire bras, metallic snaps, zippers, etc), or they may assume that it doesn't really matter. Images should be inspected for metallic susceptibility artifact; if it originates from the patient's clothing or skin, the metal should be removed whenever possible.
4) Clinical findings—Uncomfortable or claustrophobic patients may not be able to continue much beyond the scout series, and an important finding visualized on scout images can help to salvage some of these examinations. Scout images also provide views of the pelvis and thorax often not obtained in subsequent series of an abdominal examination. Even if you aren't able to change your protocol in light of an unexpected finding, it is preferable to describe a large pelvic mass in your report rather than have it pointed out to you by a curious clinician. Sagittal views are relatively rare in most abdominal protocols, and therefore scout images may provide the best opportunity for noticing a compression fracture or narrowing of the spinal canal.

Our department is a strong proponent of structured reports, and even though they have a tendency to stifle independent thought, they do contain some interesting elements, one of which is a line in our enterography report rating the quality of the examination (poor, fair, good, or excellent). This is a useful exercise for our residents, since it encourages them to look at the images from a quality control perspective. It's a passive assessment, though, and we're almost always met with blank stares when, after reading residents' descriptions of poor or fair image quality, we ask them what they did to fix it.

The solution in this case is, of course, trivial—plug in the anterior coil. It's also possible that this appearance could represent a more serious problem with the coil, and that it might need to be repaired or replaced. Recognizing when only 1 or 2 elements of a phased array coil fail can be much more challenging, and we have seen several instances where both technologists and radiologists became accustomed to the appearance of the degraded images and failed to recognize that the coil needed to be replaced. Most MRI systems allow the signal from individual coil elements to be checked during prescanning, and this is a useful exercise if you notice that the SNR is consistently asymmetric across the FOV.

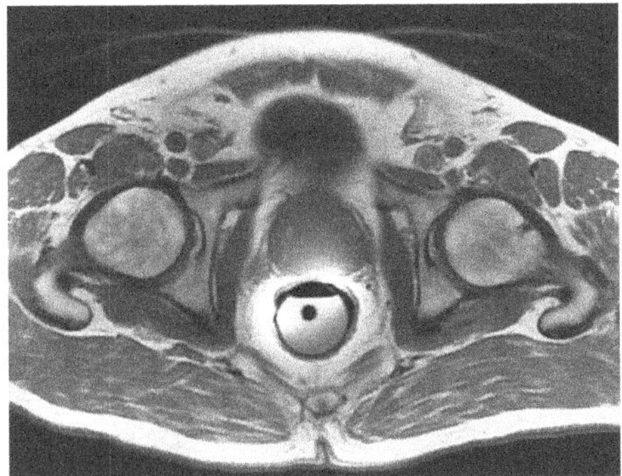

Figure 17.2.1

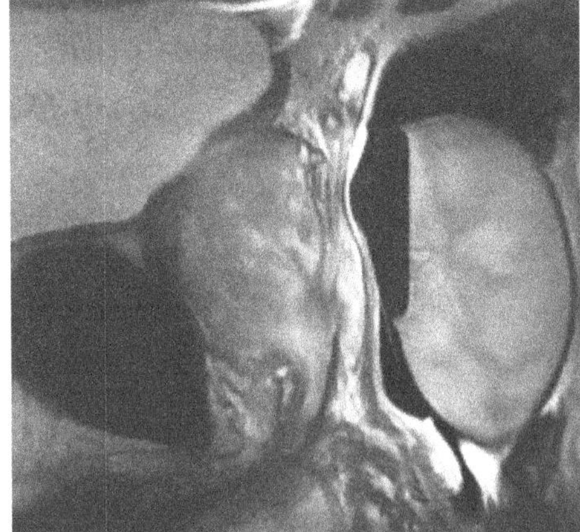

Figure 17.2.2

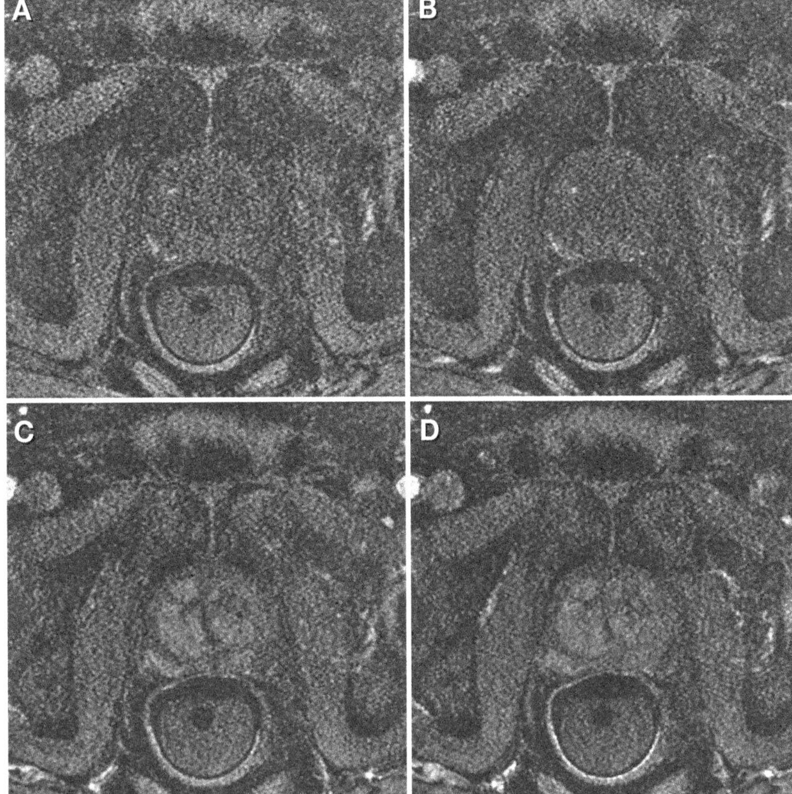

Figure 17.2.3

HISTORY: 70-year-old man with newly diagnosed prostate cancer; prostate MRI was requested for preoperative staging

IMAGING FINDINGS: Axial FSE T1-weighted image (Figure 17.2.1) and sagittal FSE T2-weighted image (Figure 17.2.2) demonstrate a normally functioning endorectal prostate coil with high signal intensity along the margin of the coil, dropping off as the distance from the coil increases. Axial pregadolinium (Figures 17.2.3A and 17.2.3B) and dynamic postgadolinium (Figures 17.2.3C and 17.2.3D) 3D SPGR images are much noisier, without the signal intensity gradient near the endorectal coil margin.

DIAGNOSIS: Failure of an endorectal coil

COMMENT: This problem is more difficult to notice and correct than in Case 17.1, where an obvious signal intensity gradient was present on the scout series and persisted throughout the examination. In this case, the endorectal coil was initially functional and failed only on the precontrast small FOV 3D SPGR acquisition. The precontrast images from the dynamic gadolinium-enhanced series are usually noisy, but not to this degree, and the technologist should have noticed that the normal gradient of high signal intensity emanating from the endorectal coil was no longer present. The end result was a set of nondiagnostic postcontrast images.

Many authors believe that prostate MRI performed at 3 T does not require the use of an endorectal coil, since improved SNR at the higher magnetic field strength compensates for the stronger signal provided by the endorectal coil. This is true in many cases, although an endorectal coil examination at 3 T is probably the optimal technique when the clinical question concerns the presence or absence of extracapsular extension of known prostate carcinoma. In this case, the examination was performed in a large-bore 1.5-T magnet on a claustrophobic patient, and the endorectal coil was necessary to achieve adequate SNR.

When an endorectal coil fails in the middle of an examination, there are no good options: The patient should have been removed from the magnet and the deficient coil replaced with a functional one, even though this would have required extra time and an additional set of scout images, not to mention duplication of the unpleasant task of endorectal coil insertion.

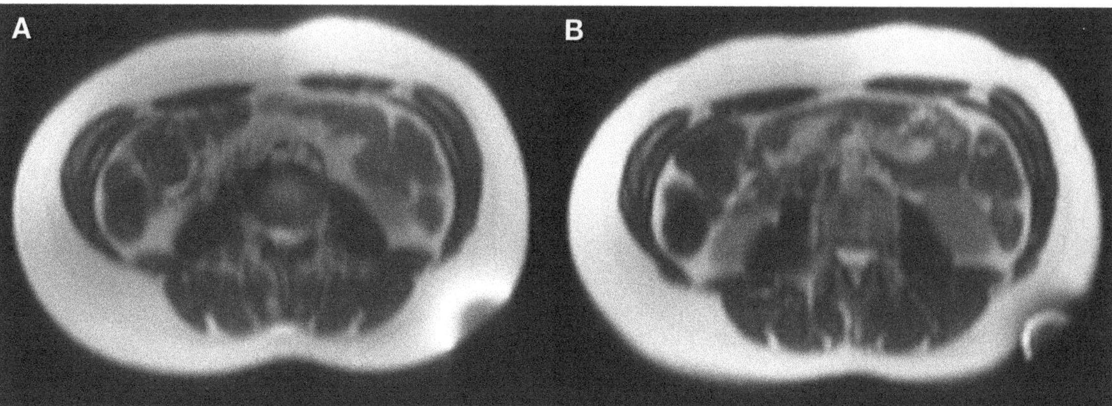

Figure 17.3.1

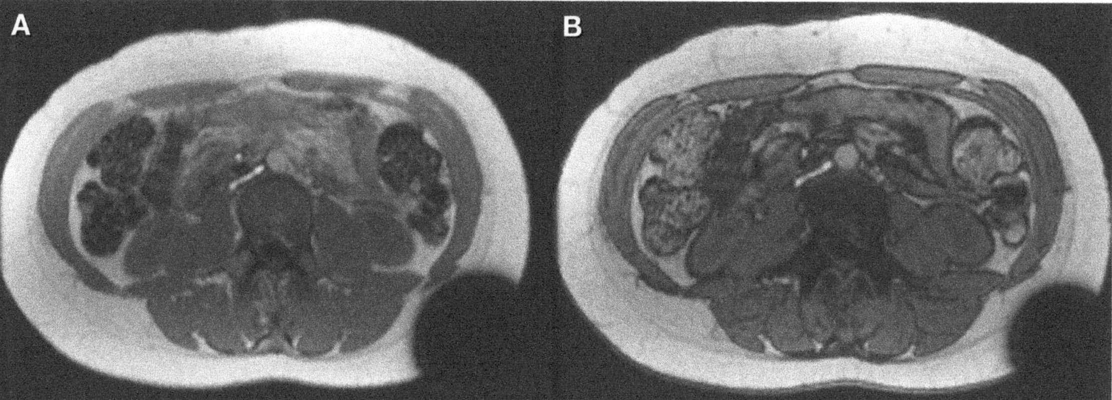

Figure 17.3.2

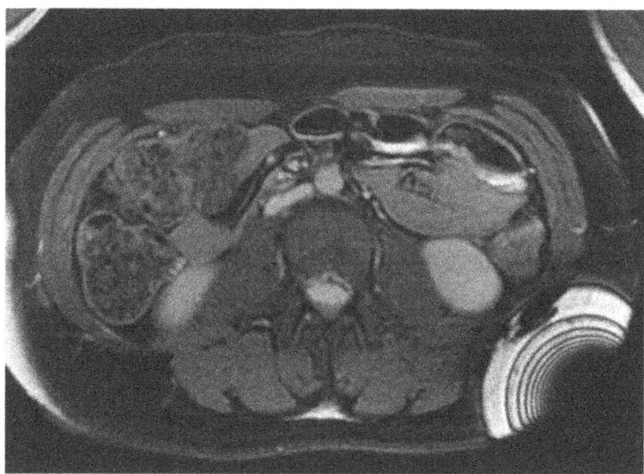

Figure 17.3.3

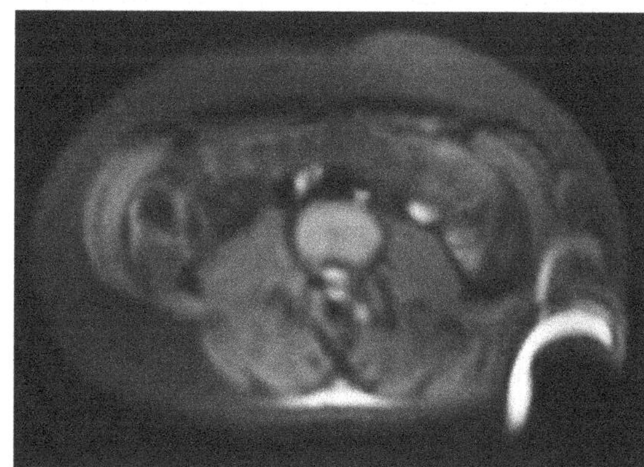

Figure 17.3.4

HISTORY: 24-year-old woman with suspected renal abscess

IMAGING FINDINGS: Axial images from SSFSE 3-plane scout sequence (Figure 17.3.1) show localized artifact in the posterior left lower abdomen. The artifact is much more prominent on axial IP (Figure 17.3.2A) and OP (Figure 17.3.2B) SPGR images as well as on an axial fat-suppressed SSFP image (Figure 17.3.3) and a diffusion-weighted image (b=600 s/mm^2) (Figure 17.3.4).

DIAGNOSIS: Susceptibility artifact from metal snap in a patient gown

COMMENT: *Susceptibility* refers to the ability of a substance to become magnetized in the presence of a magnetic field, generating a small contribution that can augment the static field (paramagnetic materials, such as gadolinium, platinum, and titanium) or oppose it (diamagnetic materials, including water and most biological substances). Ferromagnetic materials (iron, cobalt, nickel) have strongly positive nonlinear susceptibility.

Materials with high susceptibility (eg, metallic objects) distort the B_0 field and the linearity of the frequency-encoding gradient next to the object, leading to shifts in the resonant frequency of protons that are unrelated to their spatial location, which in turn causes geometric distortion of the resultant images. Frequency shifts also mean that precession frequencies vary around the metal object, leading to dephasing and alternating bright and dark bands of signal.

Some of the effects of susceptibility can be mitigated by FSE or SSFSE pulse sequences, which provide 180° refocusing pulses to partially correct the sources of dephasing. In contrast, gradient echo sequences use gradient reversal to realign spins rather than 180° refocusing RF pulses. This does not account for local dephasing effects and thereby leads to accentuation of susceptibility artifacts—notice the much more prominent artifact in the gradient echo IP-OP and SSFP images. Longer echo times provide greater opportunity for dephasing, which is why the artifact blooms on the IP image with a TE of 4.2 ms and is smaller on the OP image with a TE of 1.2 ms. Echo planar sequences are commonly used in DWI because of their short acquisition times and resistance to motion artifact. They fare poorly in the presence of metal, however, since all of k-space is filled following a single RF pulse without refocusing, allowing phase errors to accumulate throughout the readout.

Strategies for minimizing susceptibility artifact in gradient echo images primarily rely on minimizing TE (thereby minimizing time available for dephasing), accomplished through fractional echo sampling and increased receiver bandwidth.

The solution to the problem in this case is once again simple: The technologist looks at the scout images, sees the artifact, and then rechecks the patient and removes the offending metal. It's possible that the artifact was subtle enough on the scout series that it wasn't noticed, but it's easy to appreciate that there's something wrong with the SPGR, SSFP, and diffusion-weighted images. The appearance of the artifact on 1 or more of these series should have prompted the technologist to take action to correct it.

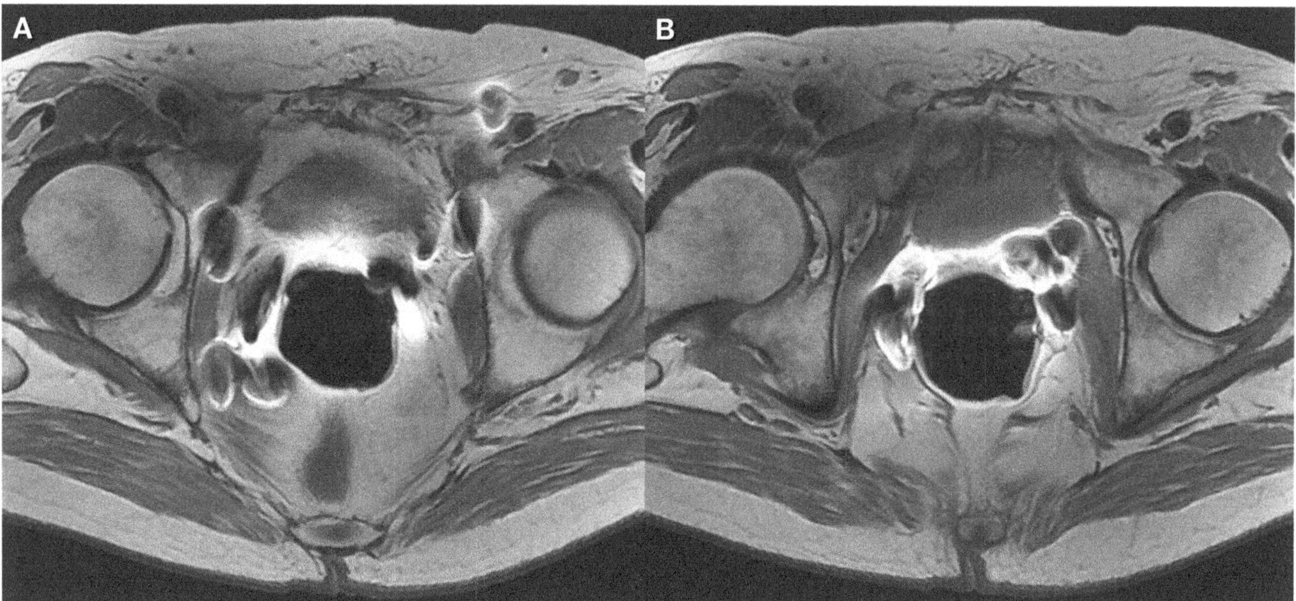

Figure 17.4.1

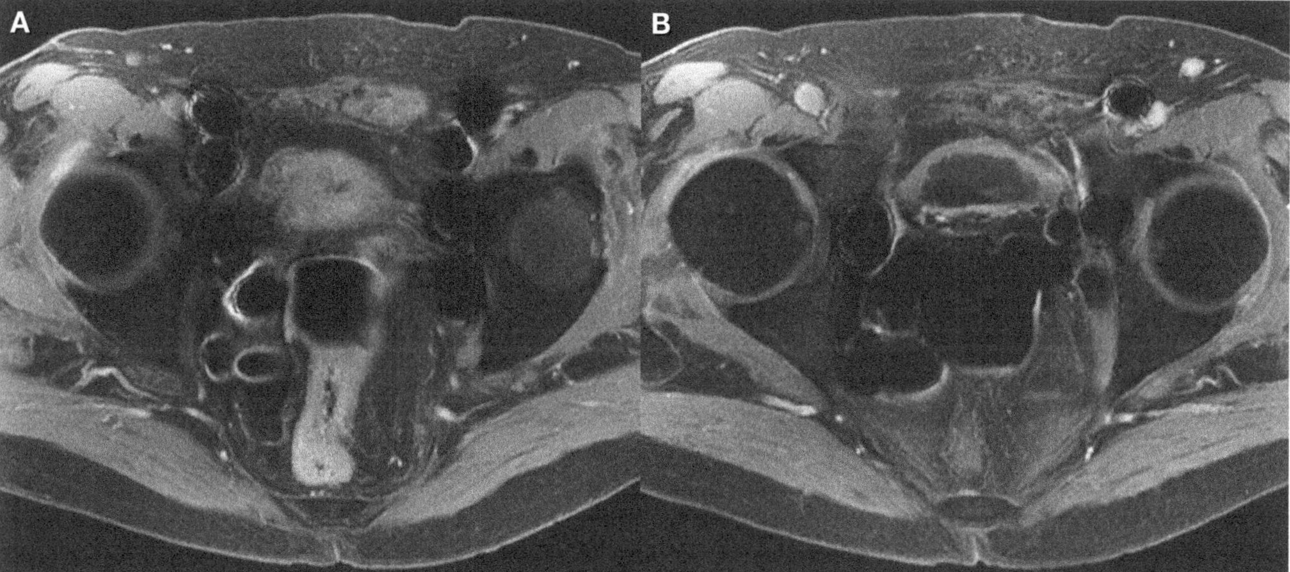

Figure 17.4.2

HISTORY: 82-year-old man with increasing prostate-specific antigen following prostatectomy

IMAGING FINDINGS: Axial FSE T1-weighted images performed on a 3-T system (Figure 17.4.1) demonstrate prominent artifact arising from surgical clips in the pelvis. This artifact is accentuated on corresponding axial 3D SPGR images (Figure 17.4.2).

DIAGNOSIS: Prominent susceptibility artifact from surgical clips at 3 T

COMMENT: Three-tesla magnets are more expensive than 1.5-T systems, typically by a factor of 1.5 to 2, and this cost is borne primarily by imagers rather than their patients, since insurance providers do not base their reimbursement on magnetic field strength. It's not unreasonable, then, to expect that examinations performed at 3 T should provide significant benefits over 1.5-T studies, whether in image quality, diagnostic accuracy, or reduced examination times.

There is surprisingly little evidence in the MRI literature in support of the proposition that 3-T MRI is better than 1.5-T MRI in any meaningful (ie, clinically significant) way.

This is in part because clinical 3-T systems supporting body MRI are still relatively new and because the kinds of experiments that need to be done to demonstrate added benefit are difficult, not particularly exciting, and problematic from the patient recruitment standpoint. It's also true that the manufacturers' initial forays into 3-T body MRI were plagued by artifacts, which were exacerbated by their tendency to adapt existing pulse sequences to higher field strengths by recompiling them after changing the resonant frequency, rather than by undertaking a more sophisticated redesign based on different physical and engineering considerations.

The situation is improving; however, there remain some fundamental limitations of 3-T MRI, illustrated in this case by metallic susceptibility artifact. Obviously, the most important consideration with regard to metal and MRI is patient safety. Metal objects that become magnetized in the presence of a large magnetic field are potentially dangerous as a result of the strong forces exerted on them (which is why wheelchairs, oxygen tanks, and scissors are not MRI friendly and why welders are carefully screened so that the small metallic fragments some of them accumulate are not pulled out of their eyes during the examination). Another potential problem is RF heating, which typically occurs in leads and guidewires of the appropriate length in relation to the RF wavelength so that they act like antennae.

Once safety concerns are alleviated, metal is then problematic on the basis of artifact generation. The large susceptibility gradients from a tissue-metal interface can induce large local variation in the static magnetic field, and this in turn means that there are large variations in resonant frequency around metal devices. This rapid variation in magnetic field leads to significant dephasing of the signal, which in turn causes signal loss in the resultant images. The remaining signal is subjected to variations in resonant frequency, which are not spatially correlated and therefore lead to displacement artifacts, generally appearing as signal loss or pile-up as well as geometric distortion of the image. In addition, chemical fat suppression techniques routinely fail in regions of significant metallic artifact, since differences in resonant frequencies of fat and water may be overwhelmed by the susceptibility effects.

Susceptibility artifacts unfortunately scale with magnetic field strength and therefore represent one of the significant limitations of 3-T imaging. In this case, the best solution is for the technologist to recognize that the extensive metallic artifact obscures visualization of important anatomy and to move the patient to a 1.5-T system. If this is not a possibility, there are a number of steps that can be taken to minimize susceptibility artifact, including the following:

1) Use FSE rather than gradient echo pulse sequences whenever possible. FSE sequences include 180° refocusing pulses that reverse static field dephasing; these are absent in gradient echo acquisitions.
2) Perform gradient echo sequences with the minimum allowable TE, which minimizes the allowable time for dephasing.
3) Maximize the bandwidth used during slice selection and readout—spatial distortion is inversely proportional to the gradient strength, which scales with the bandwidth. Increased RF bandwidth also increases power deposition, however, which can become a limiting factor, particularly at 3 T. Increased readout bandwidth reduces displacement artifact in the readout direction, but at a cost in SNR.
4) Avoid chemical fat suppression techniques—IR and Dixon-based fat suppression techniques are more resistant to susceptibility gradients generated by metal.

More sophisticated metal artifact reduction techniques are becoming available, including MAVRIC and SEMAC. These use multiple RF pulses to excite the imaging volume and apply a 3D spin echo acquisition to resolve through-plane distortion, and they generally achieve superior results in comparison to conventional FSE pulse sequences, at a cost in longer acquisition times.

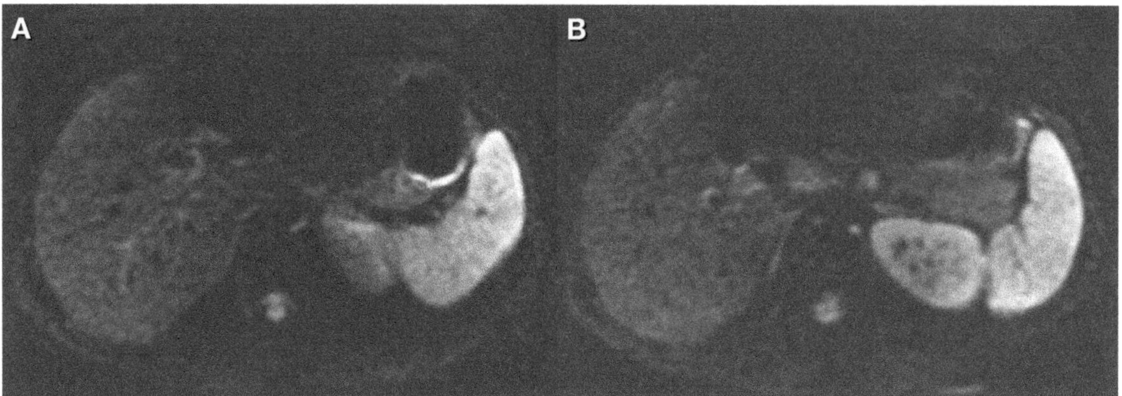

Figure 17.5.1

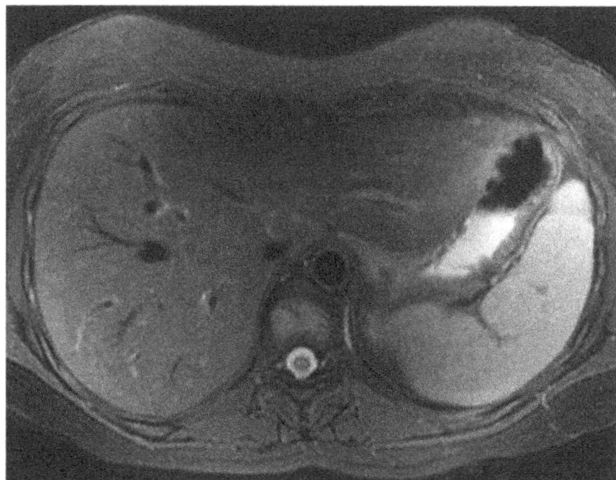

Figure 17.5.2

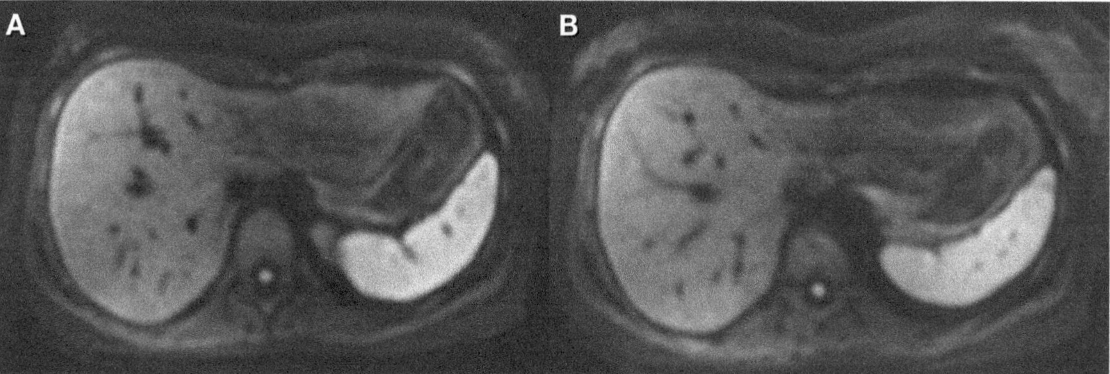

Figure 17.5.3

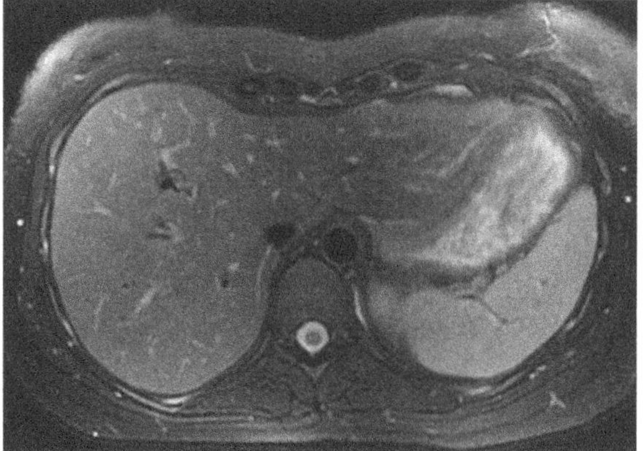

Figure 17.5.4

HISTORY: 26-year-old woman with elevated liver function tests

IMAGING FINDINGS: Axial diffusion-weighted images (b=400 s/mm^2) (Figure 17.5.1) from an examination performed with a 3-T magnet demonstrate marked signal loss in the left hepatic lobe as well as a generally reduced SNR. Axial respiratory-triggered FSE T2-weighted image (Figure 17.5.2) demonstrates mild signal loss in the left lobe. Axial diffusion-weighted images (b=600 s/mm^2) (Figure 17.5.3) from an examination performed the following year on a 1.5-T system show improved SNR and less prominent signal loss in the left lobe. Respiratory-triggered FSE image (Figure 17.5.4) shows similar improvement in the left lobe signal loss.

DIAGNOSIS: DWI susceptibility, standing wave, and cardiac pulsation artifact accentuated on a 3-T system

COMMENT: DWI can be somewhat problematic at 3 T since the susceptibility-related phase errors that accumulate in an EPI readout scale with the magnetic field strength. Minimizing echo spacing, echo train length, and TE are all important considerations in limiting artifact at 3 T, and this case illustrates what happens when you don't pay attention to these factors. The TE was actually twice as long for the 3-T acquisition (100 ms vs 50 ms), which was related to adjustments of other parameters in order to maximize the number of available slices. A longer TE for a 1.5-T DWI acquisition isn't necessarily bad, particularly at low b values and in patients without significant hepatic iron deposition—this increases the T2-weighting of the acquisition, which in turn often increases lesion conspicuity. In contrast, long TEs are almost always a bad idea at 3 T, where the signal loss can be dramatic. Parallel imaging should always be employed at 3 T to minimize the length of the echo train, and some manufacturers also recommend a reduction in the phase encode matrix.

Both standing wave and cardiac pulsation artifacts probably contribute to the striking signal loss in the left hepatic lobe in this case. Standing wave artifacts result from a reduction in soft tissue wavelengths of the RF excitation pulses at 3 T, which approach values similar to the spatial dimensions of many patients. This in turn can result in patterns of constructive and destructive interference in the B_1 field and in corresponding regional variation in signal intensity. This effect can also be seen by comparing the FSE images from the 1.5-T and 3-T studies, where the signal dropout in the left lobe anteriorly remains noticeable but less prominent in comparison to the diffusion-weighted images. Standing wave effects can be reduced by the application of dielectric pads, which are placed anteriorly and posteriorly to the patient and contain an encapsulated gel with a high dielectric constant. This material shortens the wavelength of the RF pulses, thereby mitigating some of the interference artifacts.

The effects of cardiac pulsation can also be appreciated at 1.5 T, but they appear accentuated at 3 T. Cardiac pulsation is transmitted to the liver, with the largest effects seen in the left hepatic lobe, which lies directly beneath the heart. These transmitted pulsations can induce additional phase shifts in liver voxels during application of the motion probing gradients of the DWI sequence, which may lead to signal loss as well as artificial elevation of measured ADC values in the liver. Perhaps the most obvious solution to this problem is to add electrocardiographic gating to the DWI acquisition, thereby acquiring data when cardiac motion is frozen in end diastole; however, this greatly increases the acquisition time and is not commercially available from most manufacturers. Additional strategies include the addition of velocity compensation to the diffusion gradients and simultaneous application of the X, Y, and Z diffusion gradients to minimize the directional impact of the transmitted pulsations.

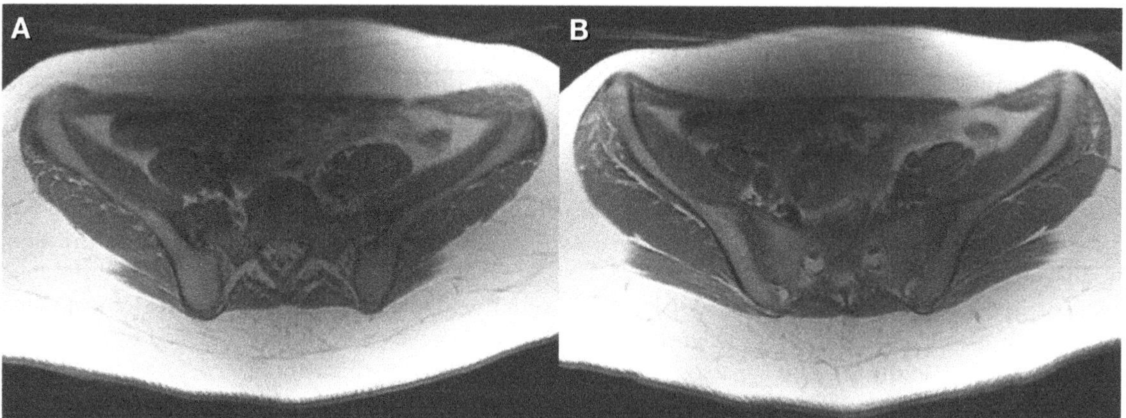

Figure 17.6.1

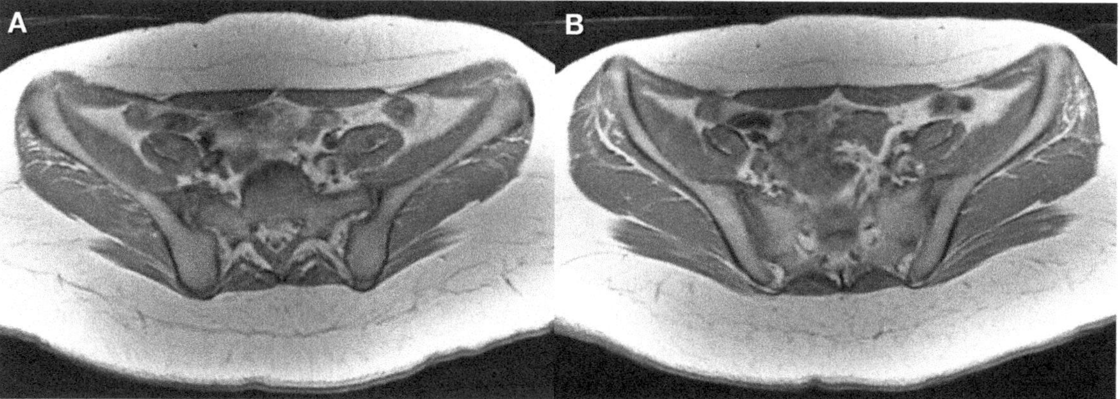

Figure 17.6.2

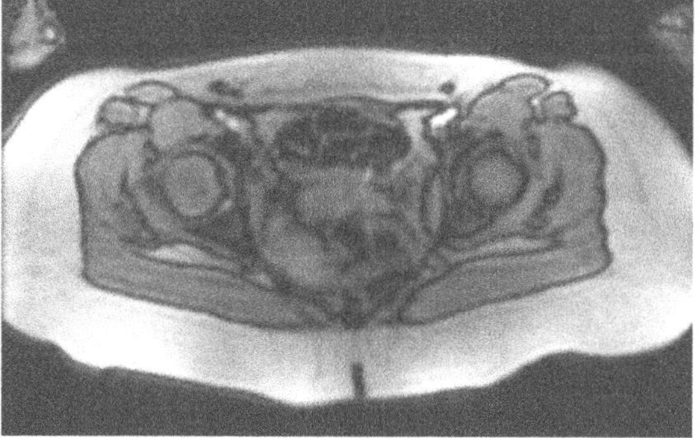

Figure 17.6.3

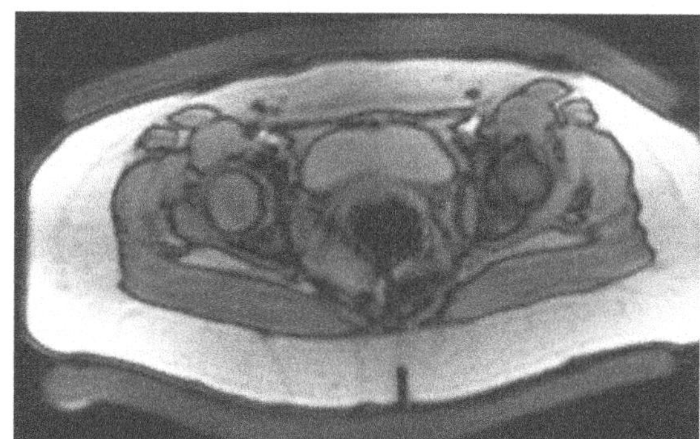

Figure 17.6.4

HISTORY: 17-year-old woman with chronic pelvic pain

IMAGING FINDINGS: Axial FSE T1-weighted images (Figure 17.6.1) demonstrate intense signal loss along the anterior pelvis. Axial FSE T1-weighted images from an examination performed the year before (Figure 17.6.2) show much less prominent signal dropout. Axial images from the 3-plane localizers from each examination demonstrate anterior and posterior dielectric pads absent on the current examination (Figure 17.6.3) and present on the prior one (Figure 17.6.4).

DIAGNOSIS: Shading artifact related to 3-T standing wave artifact, significantly improved by the use of dielectric pads

COMMENT: Image shading is one of the more commonly encountered artifacts at 3 T and is thought to result from destructive interference generated by the RF waves travelling through tissue. The resonant frequency of water protons is doubled at 3 T relative to 1.5 T, since according to the Larmor equation it's proportional to the strength of the external magnetic field. This means that the wavelengths of the RF pulses travelling through tissue are shorter, because wavelength is inversely proportional to frequency. The spatial dimensions of these RF waves at 3 T are similar to the dimensions of many patients and can induce resonance phenomena leading to standing waves and patterns of constructive and destructive interference in the B_1 field, which in turn generates regional variation in signal intensity across the resulting image.

This artifact can be quite impressive and, as seen in the initial images, can easily negate any intrinsic advantages in SNR provided by increasing the static magnetic field strength. The dielectric pad is a low-tech but often surprisingly effective solution. The pads contain gel with a very high dielectric constant, which shortens the wavelength of the traversing RF pulses, thereby reducing the standing wave effect and reducing the variation in signal intensity across the image. More sophisticated approaches involve mapping and then correcting spatial variations in the B_1 field. This can be accomplished by using multielement transmit coils to modulate the phase and frequency of the RF pulses; phased array transmit coils are currently novel and expensive, but they also offer some interesting opportunities in image generation and may become standard technology within a few years.

The reason why the dielectric pads were used for the first examination but not the second is unclear—perhaps the patient objected, or the pads were missing, or the technologist forgot, but whatever the cause, it's an unfortunate example of quality control progressing in the wrong direction.

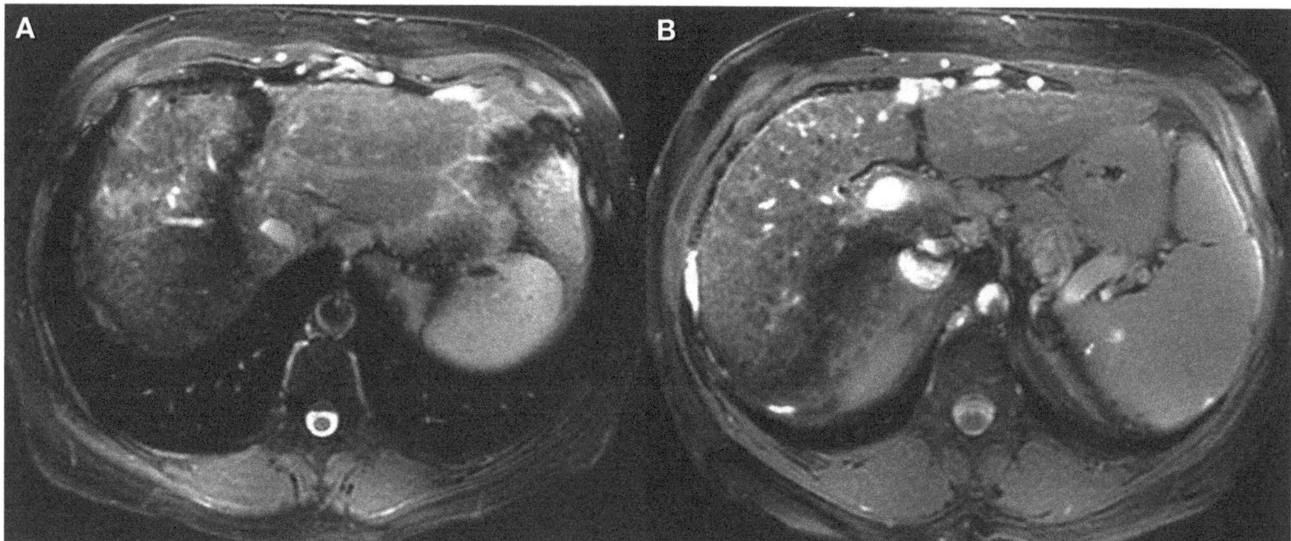

Figure 17.7.1

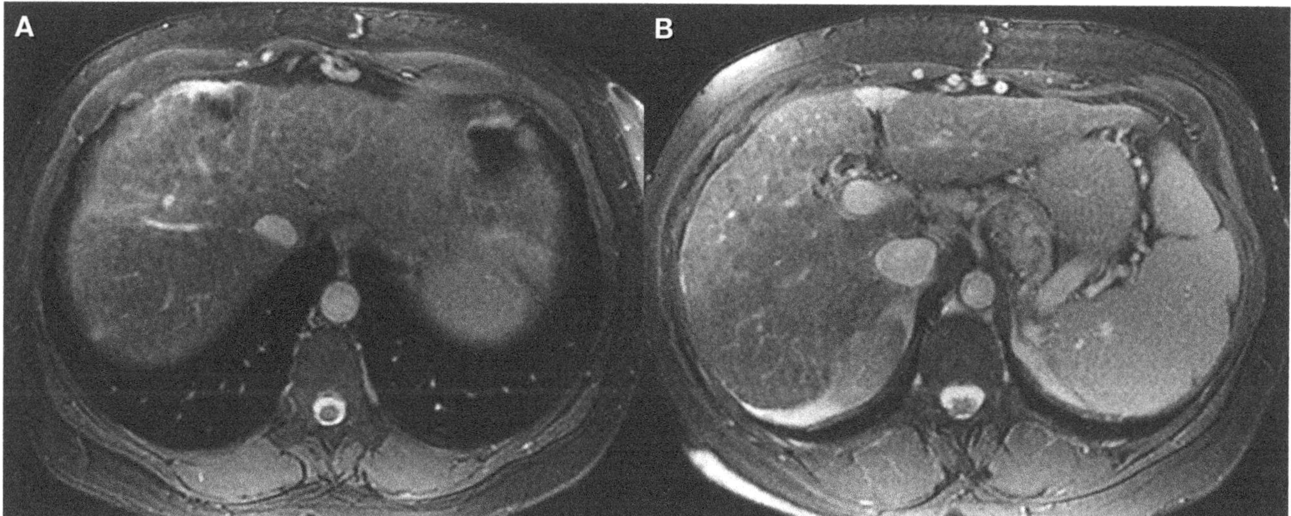

Figure 17.7.2

HISTORY: 59-year-old woman with chronic hepatitis B infection and cirrhosis

IMAGING FINDINGS: Axial fat-suppressed 2D SSFP images acquired on a 3-T system (Figure 17.7.1) demonstrate a cirrhotic liver, splenomegaly, and periumbilical varices. Note also the prominent banding artifact crossing the liver on both images. Similar fat-suppressed 2D SSFP images obtained during the previous examination with a 1.5-T system (Figure 17.7.2) demonstrate similar findings but without significant artifact.

DIAGNOSIS: Balanced SSFP banding artifact accentuated on a 3-T system

COMMENT: The concept of balanced SSFP was initially described by Carr in 1958, but its practical application was long delayed by hardware limitations, and this technique has only recently become popular and widely available. Balanced SSFP (incorrectly referred to by us and many others as SSFP) describes a gradient echo pulse sequence in which the gradient-induced dephasing within each TR is exactly zero. This is achieved by virtue of the fact that all gradient pulses are compensated by pulses of opposite polarity, so that the net area under the time-gradient curve is zero.

Balanced SSFP pulse sequences have several unique and beneficial features, including an SNR independent of TR, T2/T1 contrast weighting, short acquisition times, and relative insensitivity to flow artifacts. Balanced SSFP has become the dominant technique for assessing cardiac wall motion and also has a prominent role in noncontrast MRA. Abdominal radiologists have taken longer to appreciate the virtues of balanced SSFP techniques, partly because FSE and diffusion-weighted images provide superior soft tissue contrast for detection of solid parenchymal lesions. However, the soft tissue contrast in fat-suppressed balanced SSFP images is at least as good as in SSFSE images; the acquisition times are just as fast if not faster; the images are less susceptible to motion artifact and image blurring; and they also provide excellent visualization of major veins and arteries. Our philosophy, then, is that balanced SSFP images can be used either as a replacement or as a supplement in any situation where you would ordinarily acquire SSFSE images, including enterography and MRCP. They are also very helpful in assessing the patency of veins, particularly if gadolinium contrast is contraindicated or if postgadolinium images are degraded because of poor breath-holding or some other reason.

A major limitation of balanced SSFP techniques, however, is their propensity for artifact generation. Banding artifacts are very common and are caused by signal nulling resulting from off-resonance effects, which appear at intervals of 1/TR in resonant frequency. A simple method for reducing this artifact is to increase the separation between bands by minimizing the TR. Minimal values of TR are sometimes limited by gradient performance and tissue energy deposition considerations, particularly at 3 T. It's also worth noting that for very short values of TR, the spatial resolution may be compromised, since the duration of the frequency readout is reduced.

Because banding artifacts appear as a consequence of off-resonance spins, local shimming is also very important to minimize their appearance, and this helps to explain their increased prominence at 3 T. Recall that susceptibility effects (eg, at the lung-liver interface) are proportional to the strength of the static field and that therefore maintaining magnetic field homogeneity at 3 T is considerably more difficult than at 1.5 T.

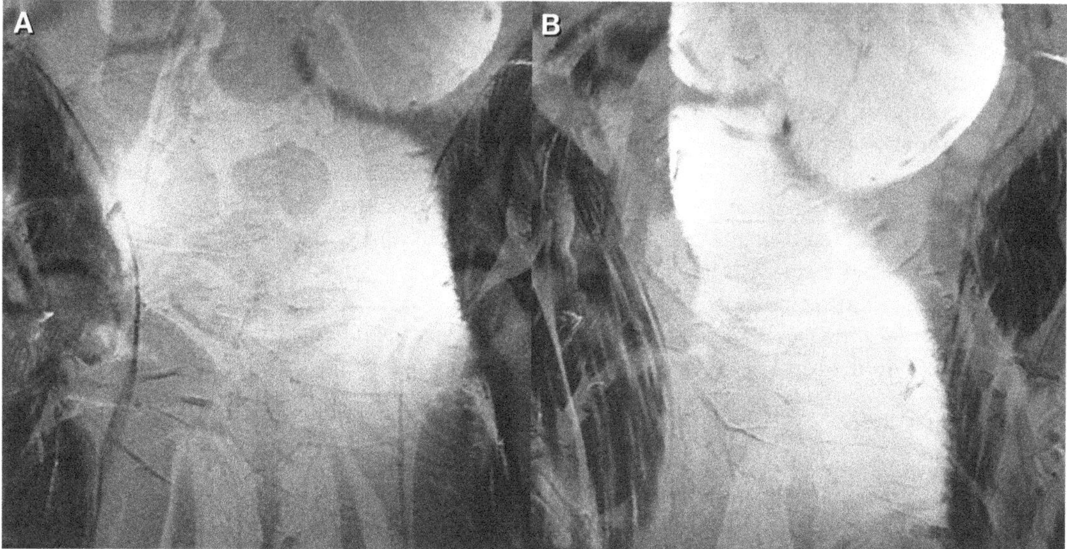

Figure 17.8.1

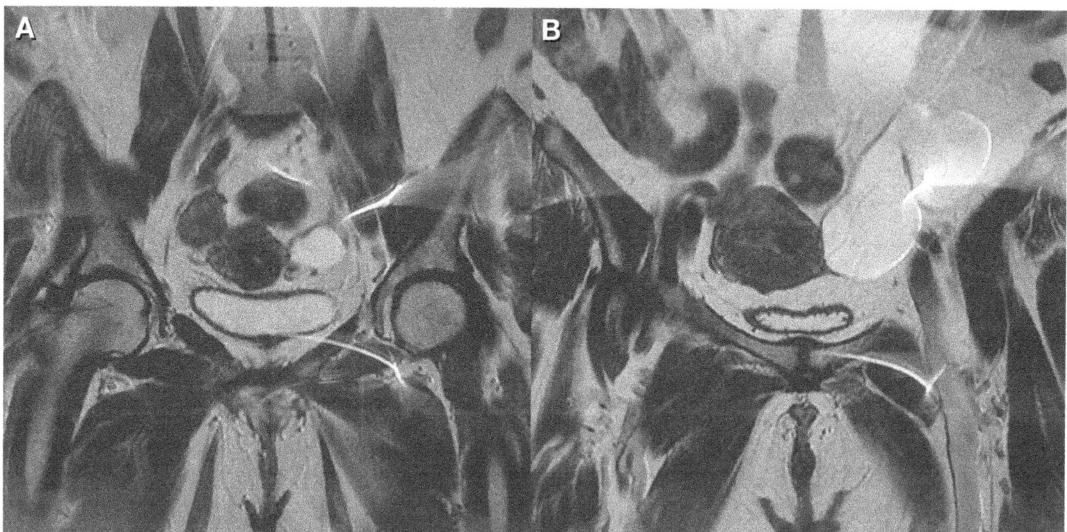

Figure 17.8.2

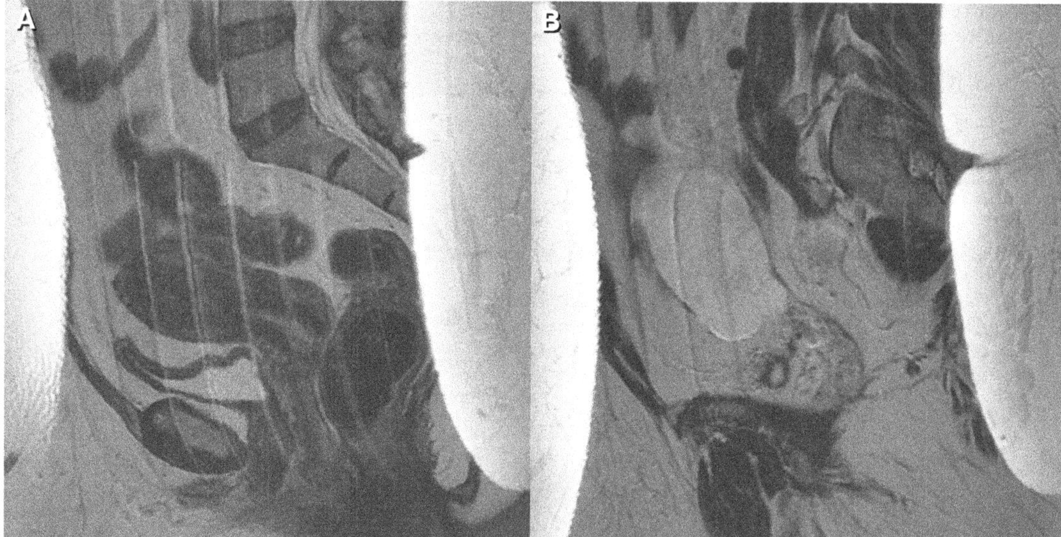

Figure 17.8.3

HISTORY: 57-year-old woman with an adnexal mass seen on pelvic US

IMAGING FINDINGS: Coronal FSE T2-weighted images (Figure 17.8.1) reveal abnormal signal superimposing the interior of the pelvis. A second set of coronal FSE images (Figure 17.8.2) demonstrates improved visualization of the pelvis but with persistent linear artifacts. Bright signal from subcutaneous fat superimposes the anterior and posterior margins of sagittal FSE images (Figure 17.8.3). A tubular cystic lesion in the left adnexa represents a dilated fallopian tube.

DIAGNOSIS: Aliasing artifact

COMMENT: This case illustrates the problem of an inexperienced technologist trying to rigidly adhere to a default protocol, in this case for an adnexal mass. The protocol specifies small FOV T2-weighted images of the pelvis, and new technologists who have just spent several months training with our neuroradiology colleagues have learned that the worst mistake they can make is to deviate even slightly from any of the parameters prescribed in their protocols. The merits of this philosophy are debatable, particularly in body MRI, where the range of body sizes and types encountered is much wider and the number of different organs examined on a regular basis is much larger in comparison to neuroradiology.

The initial coronal FSE images provide an extreme example of aliasing, which results when the specified FOV in the phase encoding direction is too small, and therefore the data outside of the FOV wraps around to the opposite side of the image. This occurs because spatial position in the phase encoding direction is mapped to particular phase shift values, and the phase FOV determines the spatial limits of the maximal phase shift (ie, a 360° shift corresponds to the edge of the FOV). Tissue outside of the specified FOV, which is nevertheless close enough to the receiver coil to generate significant signal, experiences a larger phase shift that is no longer unique. For instance, a 365° shift is exactly the same as a 5° shift, and so tissue in this location is mapped back to the other edge of the image, generating aliasing, or wraparound artifact.

The only way to avoid this problem of ambiguous phase measurement is to specify an FOV that is large enough in the phase encoding direction so that the range of phases sampled is not greater than 360°. The NPW option offered by some manufacturers doubles the FOV in the phase encoding direction while also doubling the phase encoding matrix, so that the spatial resolution (and SNR) is not changed. The resulting image is reconstructed with the initial FOV, thereby eliminating or greatly reducing aliasing artifact. The major limitation of this technique is that the acquisition time is doubled for pulse sequences acquired without signal averaging; the technique is therefore not a viable option for dynamic CE series or for most breath-held acquisitions. A similar technique is known as phase oversampling, in which the user specifies the degree of oversampling in the phase encoding direction.

The NPW option should have been selected for our default adnexal mass protocol; however, a quirk of our manufacturer's software makes it relatively easy for this option to be inadvertently turned off, resulting in the massive artifact seen in this case. After recognizing the artifact, the technologist tried to fix the problem by swapping the phase and frequency direction and making the FOV slightly larger but did not remember to turn on the NPW option. This resulted in a significant improvement in image quality but with persistent aliasing artifact, this time in the superior-inferior direction.

The final set of sagittal FSE images demonstrates that our technologist remained wedded to the FOV specified in the default protocol, and again the result is significant aliasing artifact as well as prominent phase ghosting. This time, the default protocol does not specify the NPW option, since in most patients a smaller phase FOV can be used in the anterior-posterior direction. Again, potential solutions to this problem include using a larger FOV (or phase FOV) or turning on the NPW option. Anterior saturation bands would help to reduce the prominent phase ghosting artifacts, as would the addition of respiratory triggering.

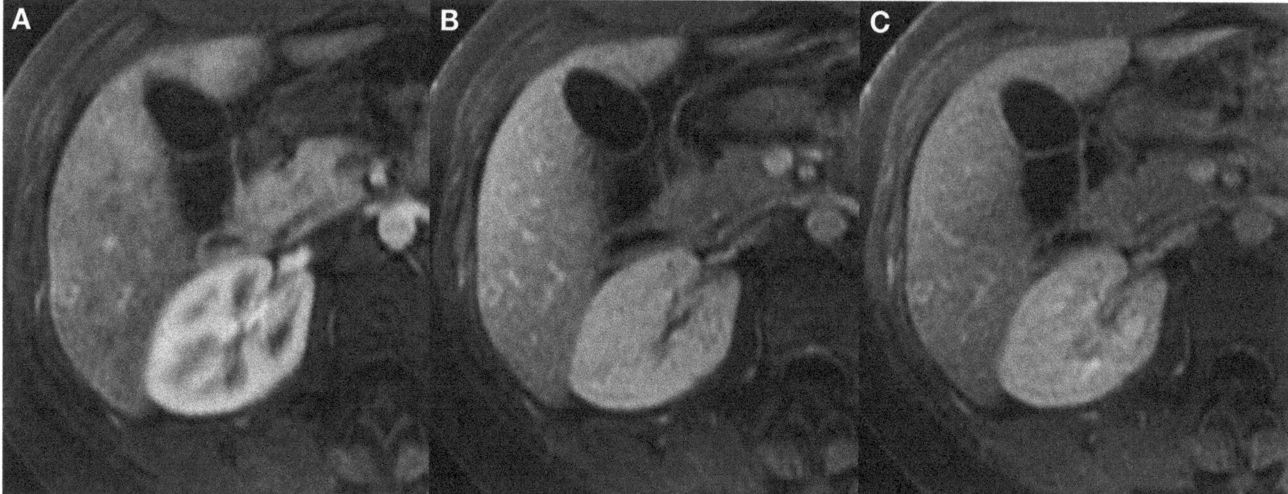

Figure 17.9.1

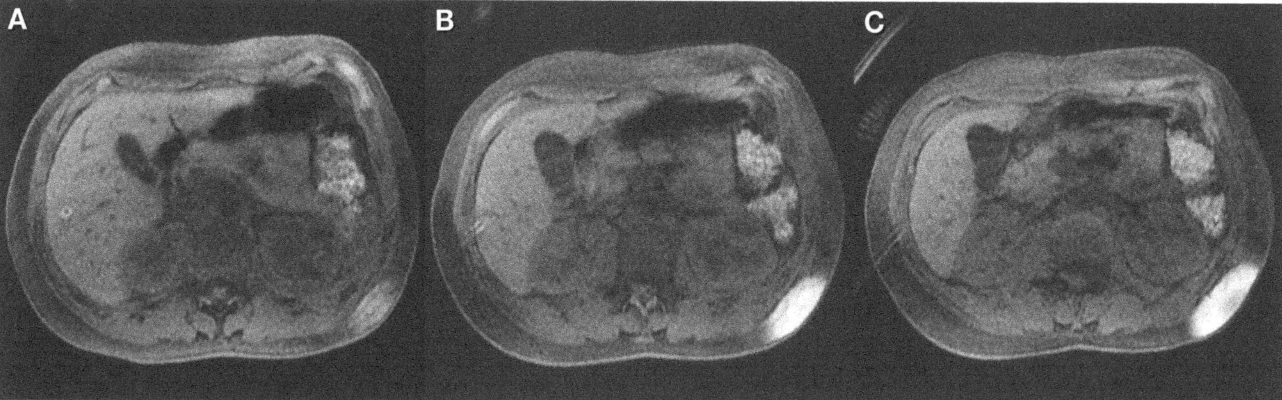

Figure 17.9.2

HISTORY: 24-year-old woman with suspected renal abscess

IMAGING FINDINGS: Axial arterial (Figure 17.9.1A), portal venous (Figure 17.9.1B), and equilibrium phase (Figure 17.9.1C) postgadolinium 3D SPGR images demonstrate an apparent small ring-enhancing lesion in the posterior right hepatic lobe. Axial precontrast 3D SPGR images (Figure 17.9.2) demonstrate a similar appearance but also show that on subsequent inferior images the artifact has a tubular appearance and crosses the liver into the subcutaneous fat. Notice also the artifact overlying the patient anteriorly on the most inferior image as well as the focal loss of fat suppression in the left inferior lateral abdomen.

DIAGNOSIS: Aliasing and ghosting artifact from intravenous tubing

COMMENT: Astute observers will notice that this clinical history is identical to that of a previous case of susceptibility artifact resulting from metal snaps in a patient gown (Case 17.3), and, in fact, this is the same patient, illustrating the general principle that errors tend to accumulate when technologists aren't paying attention.

In this case, the problem results from intravenous tubing for the gadolinium injection crossing over the patient from left to right—the injector is on the left side of the patient, and the intravenous catheter is in the right arm. The obvious solution is to move the injector to the right side, so that the tubing rests along the side of the patient rather than crossing in front of the liver. Since the phase encoding direction for most acquisitions in an abdominal examination is anterior-posterior rather than right-left, this eliminates the possibility of aliasing or ghosting artifact. The caveat to this is a coronal series, in which the frequency encoding direction is superior-inferior and the phase encoding direction right-left. Even in this case, as long as the tubing lies immediately adjacent to the patient rather than crossing several inches in front of her, aliasing artifact will rarely occur.

Artifact caused by tubing in cross section can generate a fairly convincing simulation of a ring-enhancing lesion on individual images, as in this case; however, careful inspection of precontrast and postcontrast images generally reveals the true nature of the artifact, and often visualization of the overlying tubing is possible on 1 or more series.

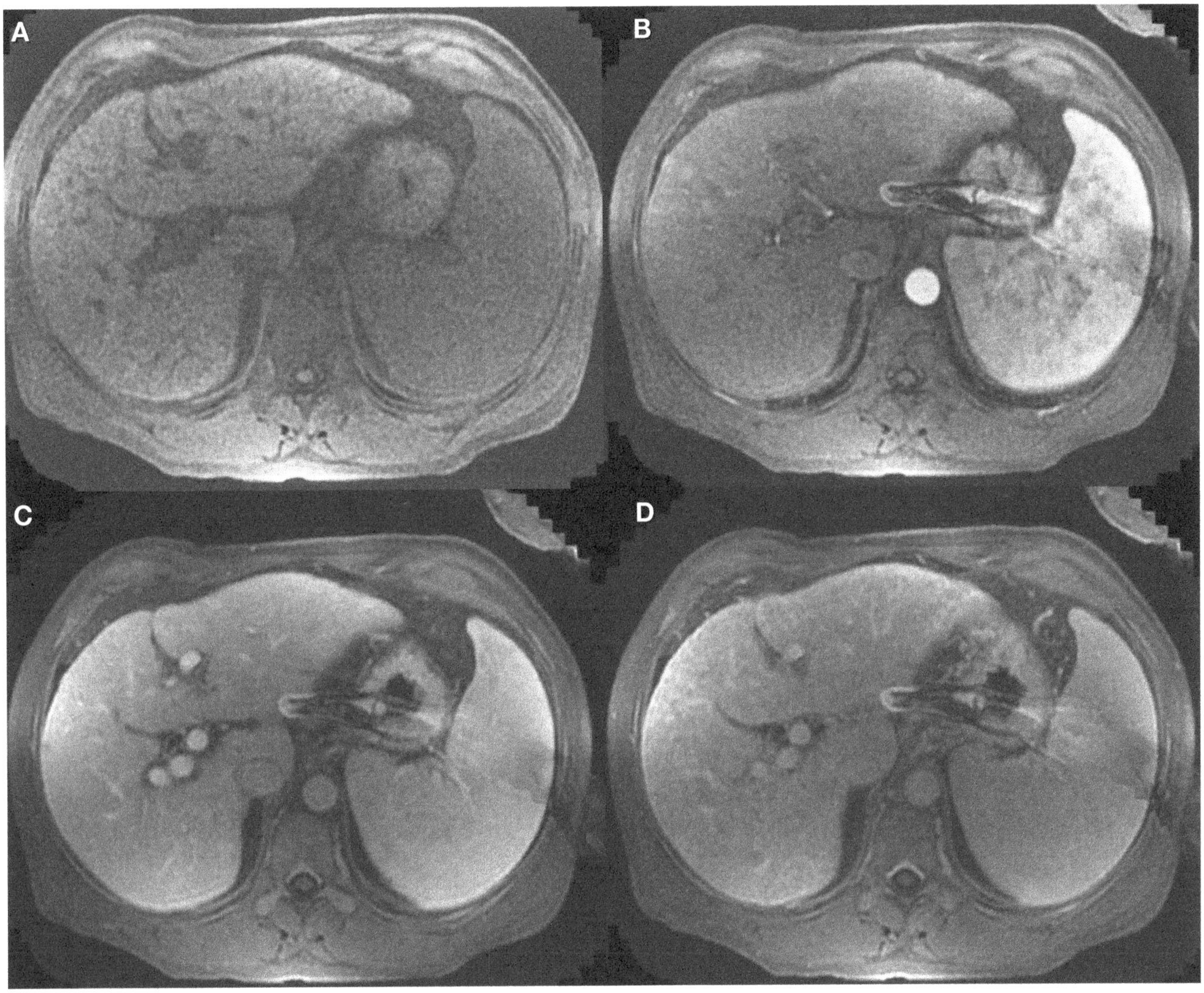

Figure 17.10.1

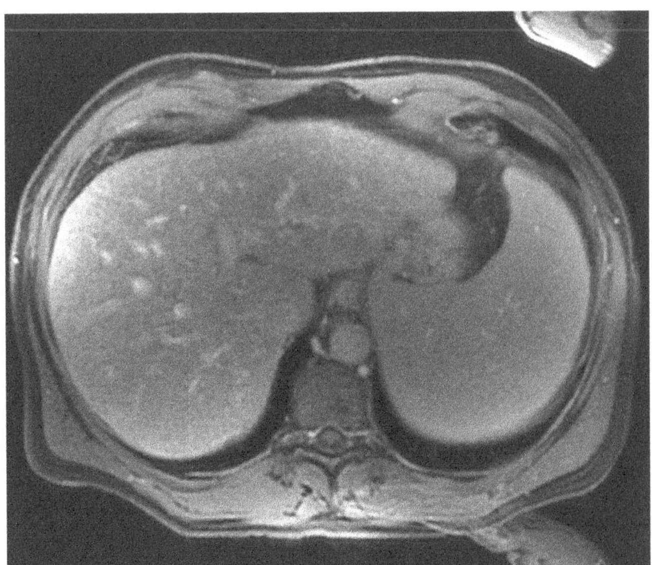

Figure 17.10.2

HISTORY: 54-year-old man with cirrhosis

IMAGING FINDINGS: Axial precontrast 3D SPGR image (Figure 17.10.1A) demonstrates a nodular hepatic contour and moderate splenomegaly. Postgadolinium arterial (Figure 17.10.1B), portal venous (Figure 17.10.1C), and equilibrium phase (Figure 17.10.1D) images reveal a finger superimposing the left side of the abdomen (and pointing toward 2 arterial phase enhancing nodules in the periphery of the right hepatic lobe). Axial 2D SPGR image (Figure 17.10.2) shows the artifact along the posterior margin of the image.

DIAGNOSIS: Aliasing artifact related to sensitivity encoded parallel imaging

COMMENT: This artifact arose because the patient decided to place his left hand on his abdomen between the precontrast and postcontrast dynamic 3D SPGR images. Normally this would generate a slightly annoying aliasing artifact propagated to the posterior margin of the image (as seen in the 2D SPGR image); however, the addition of parallel imaging makes the situation much worse.

Parallel imaging is a technique in which the number of phase encoding steps is reduced by a factor of 2 or more. This is done by increasing the separation between the lines of k-space, and this in turn means that the FOV is reduced, since FOV is inversely related to Δk. For a parallel imaging acquisition with an acceleration factor of 2, for example, the FOV is halved, and for an acceleration factor of 3, the resultant FOV is one-third of the original size. This results in an aliased image with extensive wraparound artifact, since the spatial location of points not included in the FOV is no longer uniquely determined.

This problem is solved by using the spatial sensitivity profile of each phased array coil element to aid in reconstructing the aliased image, essentially turning the reconstruction process into a matrix inversion problem whose complexity increases as the acceleration factor rises. This inversion can be performed in k-space (prior to Fourier transformation), with techniques including SMASH, GRAPPA, and ARC, or in image space following the Fourier transformation, with techniques including SENSE and ASSET. The k-space–based parallel imaging techniques are also known as autocalibrating methods, since measurement of the phased array coil element spatial sensitivity profile is included within the clinical pulse sequence (by the addition of a few extra lines of k-space), whereas the image space reconstruction techniques rely on a separate low spatial resolution calibration scan. The autocalibrating techniques are probably the most popular clinical applications of parallel imaging, since they are simpler to use and generate fewer artifacts.

This case is an example of an aliasing artifact that arises with SENSE or ASSET but is much less problematic with a k-space–based reconstruction technique. When the FOV in the phase encoding direction is too small (ie, when aliasing would occur without parallel imaging), the wraparound artifact is propagated to the center of the image rather than merely to the posterior margin. This doesn't occur with GRAPPA or ARC, where the potential artifact is distributed over the entire image. Similar ghosting artifacts can occur when the calibration scan and the parallel imaging acquisition are not obtained in the same position (eg, when the breath-holding is slightly different). One limitation of the autocalibration techniques is that the acquisition times are slightly longer, since extra lines of k-space are included in the acquisition. When speed is of the essence, then, SENSE-based parallel imaging may be preferable.

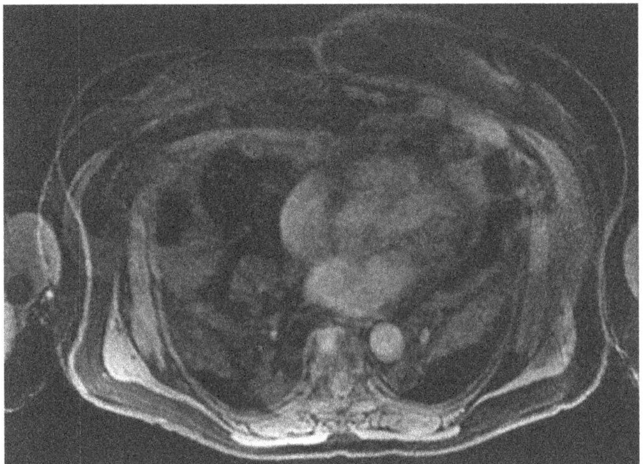

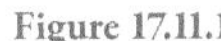

Figure 17.11.1

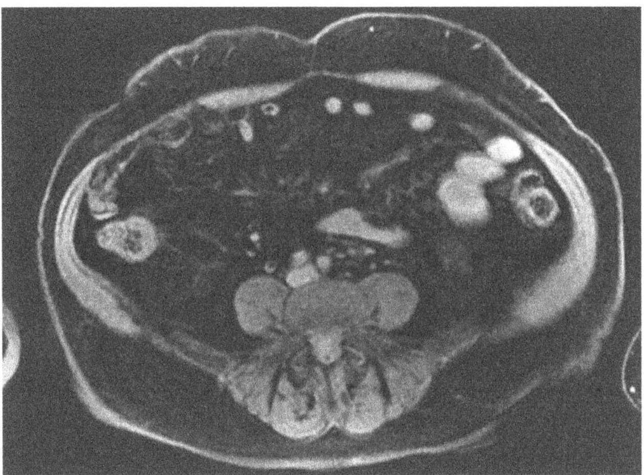

Figure 17.11.2

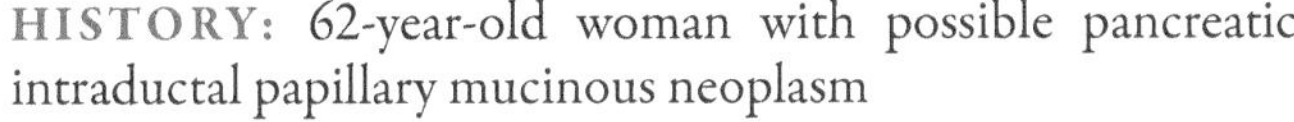

HISTORY: 62-year-old woman with possible pancreatic intraductal papillary mucinous neoplasm

IMAGING FINDINGS: Superiormost image from a venous phase postgadolinium 3D SPGR acquisition (Figure 17.11.1) shows artifact superimposing the lower thorax as well as a possible enhancing lesion in a lower thoracic vertebral body. The inferiormost image is relatively artifact-free (Figure 17.11.2). Notice how the location of the ascending and descending colon corresponds fairly well with the location of the artifacts on the upper image.

DIAGNOSIS: Slice wrap on a 3D SPGR acquisition

COMMENT: It's easy to forget that 3D pulse sequences have 2 axes of phase encoding, which explains why without using very short TRs in comparison to standard FSE (and 2D SPGR) pulse sequences, the acquisition times would be prohibitive. (The T1 weighting of a 3D SPGR sequence is more a function of flip angle than TR, but even flip angles are kept relatively low in order to minimize saturation effects, since you're exciting the entire volume rather than a single slice with every RF pulse. This means that the actual T1 weighting of a 3D SPGR sequence isn't as strong as that of a 2D SPGR sequence with a higher flip angle. This in turn has led a small and diminishing percentage of radiologists to persist in performing dynamic gadolinium-enhanced imaging with 2D rather than 3D acquisitions, while the rest have accepted this minor limitation as a small price to pay for the many advantages of 3D dynamic imaging.)

In a standard axial 3D SPGR acquisition, the frequency encoding direction is in the usual right-left direction, with 1 phase encoding in the anterior-posterior direction, and the second along the slice encoding axis (ie, superior-inferior direction). The Nyquist theorem also applies in the slice encoding direction, and the only reason aliasing isn't a more significant problem is the substantial signal drop-off provided by the use of surface coils (so that there isn't slice wrap from the head during an abdominal examination). Slice wrap actually occurs very frequently, and the reason you usually don't notice it is that the manufacturers build an extra 4 to 8 sections into their 3D acquisitions and then discard the first few slices at the top and bottom of the data set. Even so, if you look carefully, it's often possible to identify subtle signs of slice wrap. This is a more frequent observation at 3 T, because the SNR, even near the edge of a surface coil, is relatively high (and again illustrates the problem of converting 1.5-T pulse sequences to 3 T by simply changing the resonant frequency of the RF pulse).

Slice wrap rarely causes diagnostic difficulties, unless you're interested in something very high in the dome of the liver and there's also a very bright object at the bottom of your acquisition volume that can wrap into the upper images. The pseudolesion in the thoracic vertebral body is a consequence of aliasing from the relatively bright signal from the IVC, but the presence of artifact throughout the image should suggest that this might also not be real and should lead to a careful examination of the precontrast images for the same artifact and to verification of its absence on all other sequences.

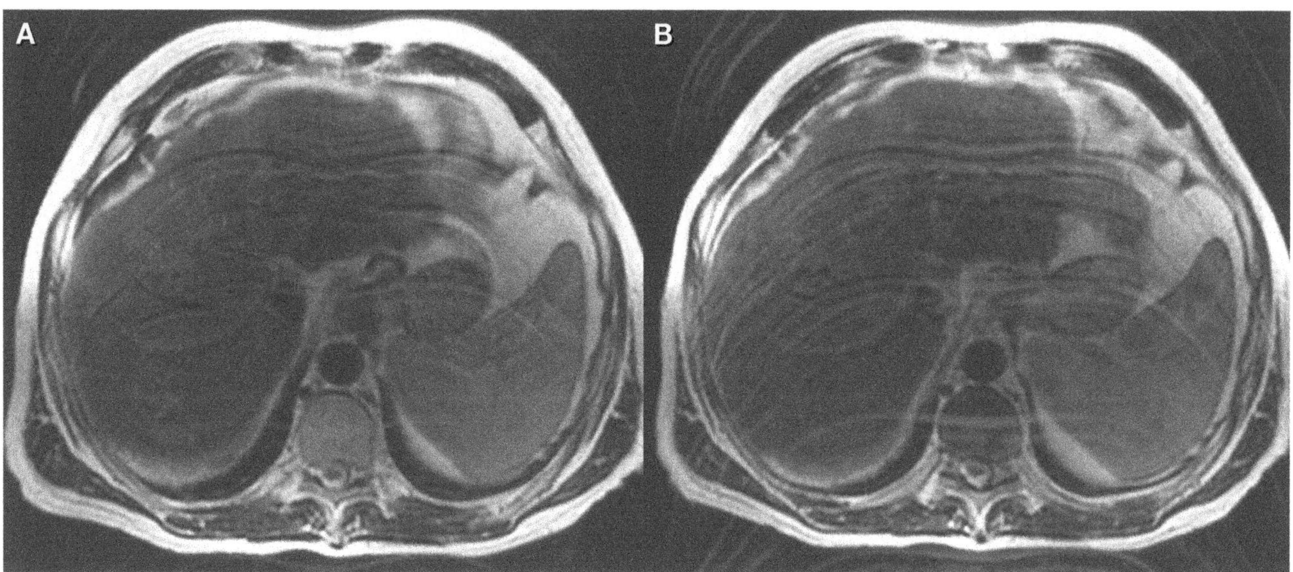

Figure 17.12.1

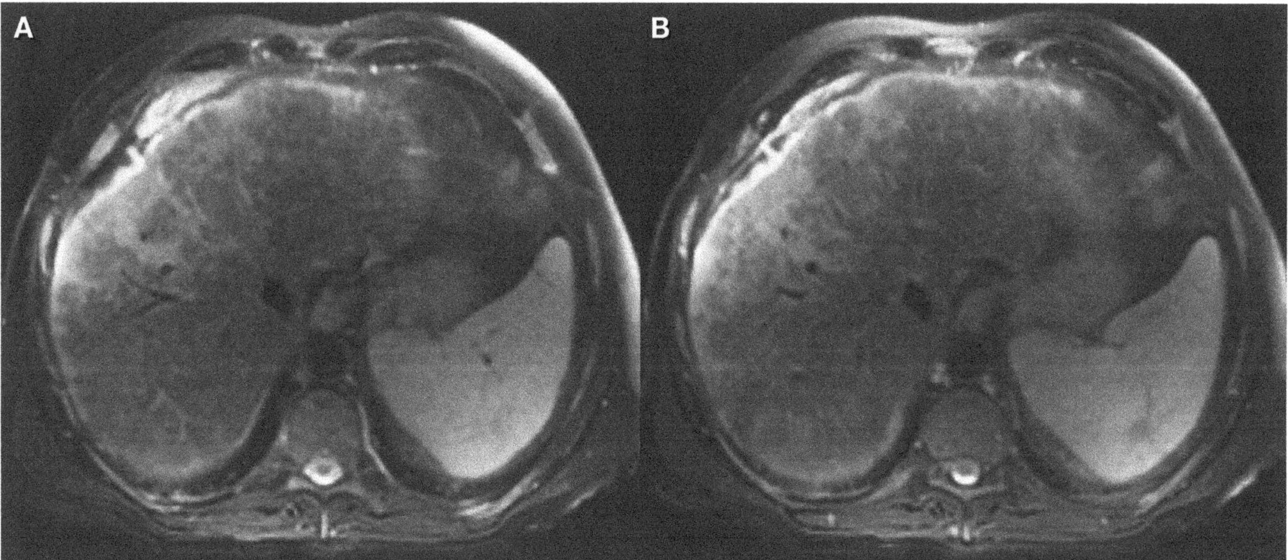

Figure 17.12.2

HISTORY: 56-year-old man with cirrhosis and suspected hepatocellular carcinoma

IMAGING FINDINGS: Axial respiratory-triggered T2-weighted FSE images obtained without fat suppression (Figure 17.12.1) demonstrate extensive phase ghosting artifact. T2-weighted images obtained with fat suppression (Figure 17.12.2) reveal minimal ghosting artifact and also allow improved visualization of confluent peripheral fibrosis.

DIAGNOSIS: Phase ghosting artifact minimized by chemical fat suppression

COMMENT: As far as we're concerned, there's never a good reason to acquire respiratory-triggered (or navigator-gated) T2-weighted images of the liver without fat suppression, and there's certainly no reason to acquire both sets of images, since this effectively doubles the length of the most time-intensive sequence in the standard liver protocol without any appreciable benefit. (This case was performed as part of a multicenter trial whose protocol included both fat-suppressed and non–fat-suppressed T2-weighted acquisitions.)

Phase ghosting artifact occurs when the signal from periodically moving structures is erroneously rendered in different locations along the phase encoding direction. Ghosting artifact is usually much more prominent in the phase encoding axis, since the opportunity for errors (in a voxel's position and signal amplitude) essentially encompasses all phase encoding steps, while artifact along the frequency encoding direction must occur within the short duration of the readout along the x-axis in k-space. The intensity of the ghosting artifact is related to the motion amplitude, the particular pulse sequence, and the choice of sequence parameters in a fairly complex manner, but it is also strongly dependent on the signal intensity of the moving structure (ie, bright structures generate bright ghosting artifacts).

This is nicely illustrated in this case, where the application of an imperfect and somewhat inhomogeneous chemical fat suppression pulse (notice the poor fat suppression along the anterior left abdomen) greatly reduces the ghosting artifact. By comparison, in the non–fat-suppressed images, subcutaneous fat is intensely bright by virtue of its intrinsically long T2 as well as its location immediately beneath the anterior phased array coil. (Signal intensity in the simplest model is inversely proportional to the square of the distance from the voxel to the center of the coil, although the falloff is less steep with multielement phased array coils.)

A second benefit of fat suppression in abdominal imaging is a reduction in the dynamic range of contrast. Notice how much easier it is to appreciate the signal intensity differences between the peripheral hepatic fibrosis and the more normal central hepatic parenchyma on the fat-suppressed images. By comparison, the intensely bright signal from subcutaneous fat on the non-fat-suppressed images renders the relatively subtle distinction between gradations in hepatic signal intensity nearly impossible. This situation can be improved by application of signal intensity correction algorithms, which correct for the expected geometric variation in signal intensity; however, these techniques can't get rid of phase ghosting artifact and won't alter its relative brightness.

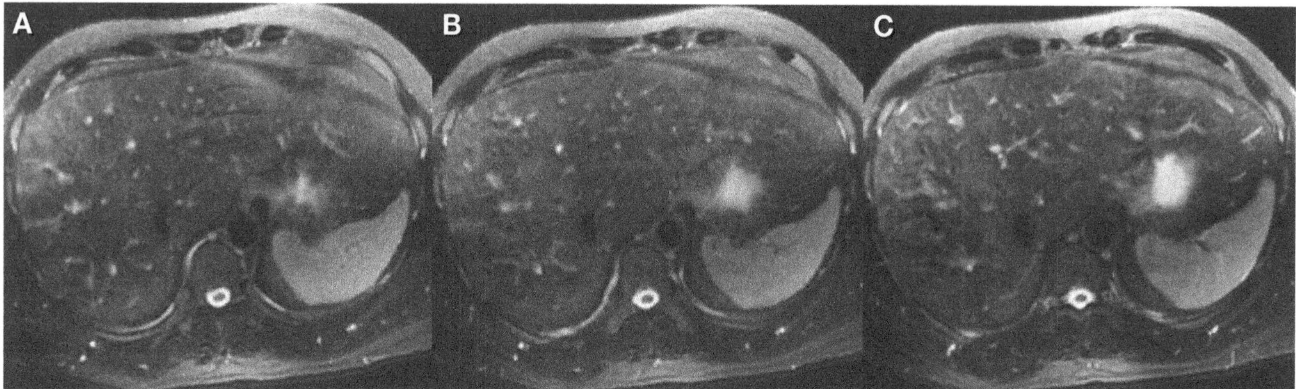

Figure 17.13.1

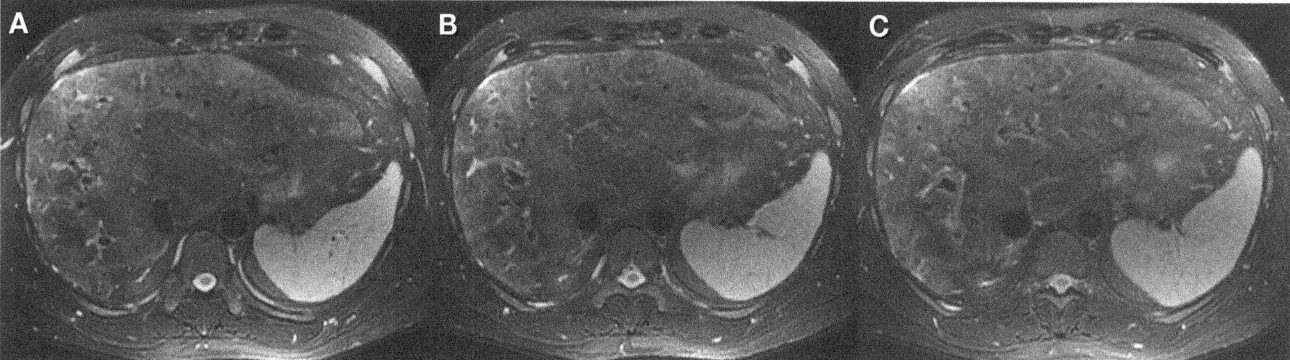

Figure 17.13.2

HISTORY: 43-year-old man with primary sclerosing cholangitis

IMAGING FINDINGS: Axial respiratory-triggered fat-suppressed FSE T2-weighted images (Figure 17.13.1) demonstrate inhomogeneous fat suppression and mild motion blurring throughout the liver. FSE T2-weighted images performed with parallel imaging (Figure 17.13.2) and otherwise identical imaging parameters demonstrate sharper images with no significant motion artifact.

DIAGNOSIS: Reduction in respiratory motion artifact with parallel imaging

COMMENT: Parallel imaging is most often discussed in the context of a technique allowing significant reductions in acquisition time, but at a cost in reduced SNR and occasionally in the introduction of additional artifacts.

It is less widely appreciated, however, that parallel imaging can also have a role in artifact reduction, and this case is a good illustration of that principle. Respiratory-triggered or navigator-gated FSE pulse sequences acquire a number of phase encoding steps, specified by the ETL, during every breath, ideally at end expiration when the diaphragm is maximally elevated and there is no significant respiratory motion. Since this flat part of the cycle often represents a relatively small percentage of the total respiratory interval (or RR interval), there is a tension between the need to maximize the efficiency of the acquisition by acquiring as much data as possible during every breath and the requirement that data acquisition should not occur when the diaphragm is moving rapidly. This is usually played out by adjusting the ETL according to the respiratory rate—as the rate increases, the flat part of the curve becomes shorter, and the ETL should be correspondingly lowered to reduce the amount of data acquired during each breath. Reducing the ETL means that the acquisition time is longer, since a smaller percentage of k-space is sampled during each respiration, and this can sometimes be problematic in patients who fall asleep and develop irregular respirations, variable triggering, and consequently increased motion artifact. If, however, the ETL is too high, data are sampled during the end of expiration and the beginning of inspiration while the diaphragm is moving, again introducing motion artifact. Another problem with long ETLs is that the total number of slices that can be excited during each breath is reduced, sometimes requiring 2 or 3 breaths to excite enough slices to cover the entire liver. This represents the worst of both worlds—the potential for motion artifact related to a long ETL but without the expected time savings.

Parallel imaging can be helpful in this situation because it reduces the total number of sampled lines of k-space. For an acceleration factor of 2, for example, only half of the usual number of samples is acquired, which means that for a given ETL you could in theory be finished twice as quickly. In practice, we typically shorten the ETL to minimize motion artifact within each breath and also to increase the number of slices acquired per breath, and this often allows us to cover the entire liver with an RR interval of 1 or 2 rather than 3 or 4. In this case, for example, the initial acquisition was performed with an ETL of 12 and RR interval of 3, resulting in an acquisition time of approximately 6 minutes, while the parallel imaging series was obtained with an ETL of 8, RR interval of 1, and acquisition time of just over 2 minutes.

It's rare in MRI to simultaneously reduce the acquisition time and improve image quality, and so we try to take advantage of these opportunities whenever they arise. However, it is also possible to make things worse with parallel imaging: If your baseline SNR is low (eg, poorly positioned coils not adequately covering the dome of the liver), the loss of signal accompanying a parallel imaging acquisition could easily negate any small reduction in motion artifact. Similarly, very large patients often generate significant parallel imaging reconstruction artifacts that overwhelm the benefits of motion artifact reduction.

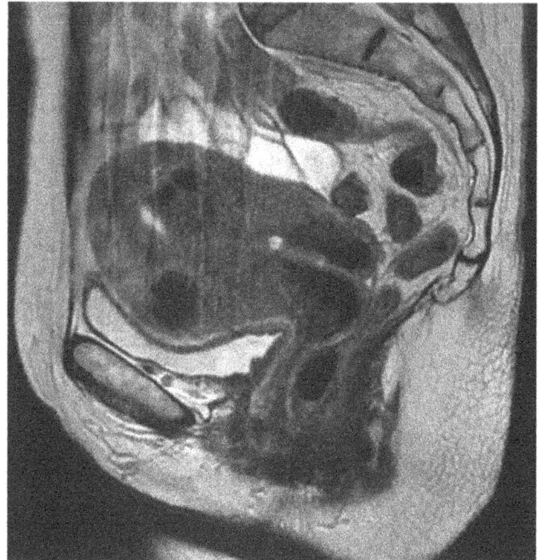

Figure 17.14.1

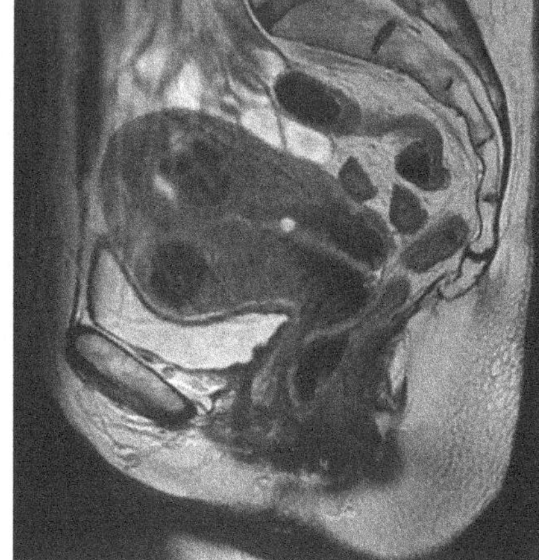

Figure 17.14.2

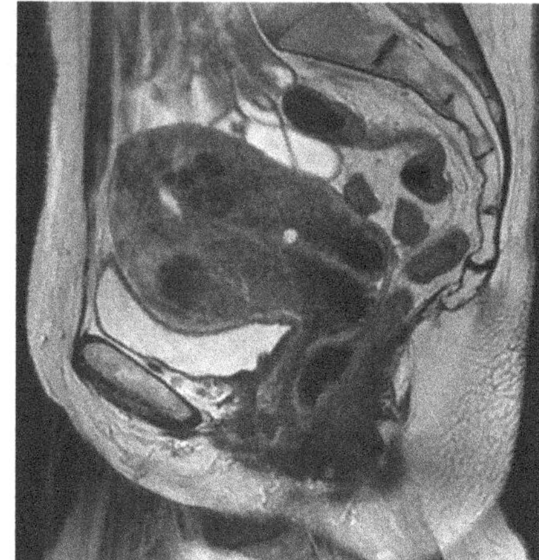

Figure 17.14.3

HISTORY: 65-year-old woman with endometrial carcinoma

IMAGING FINDINGS: Sagittal FSE T2-weighted image (Figure 17.14.1) demonstrates prominent phase ghosting artifacts superimposing the uterus. The series was repeated with an anterior saturation band (Figure 17.14.2) (notice the low signal intensity of the subcutaneous fat) with significant reduction in artifact. The series was repeated again with the phase and frequency directions swapped (ie, the phase encoding direction is now superior-inferior) (Figure 17.14.3). This also results in reduction but not elimination of phase ghosting artifacts across the uterus but with new aliasing artifact along the inferior margin of the image. Notice also multiple uterine fibroids as well as a small cystic lesion in the endometrium adjacent to the cervix.

DIAGNOSIS: Phase ghosting artifact in the pelvis related to breathing motion and peristalsis

COMMENT: In this case, the technologist recognized that there was significant artifact on the initial acquisition and that the artifact was a result of phase ghosting, primarily from the bright anterior subcutaneous fat. An anterior saturation band is a fairly simple solution and almost always does result in some reduction in artifact: The idea is that the signal intensity of the artifact is proportional to the signal of the ghosting tissue and that by suppressing the tissue with a spatial saturation band, the corresponding artifact will be reduced. Subcutaneous fat is bright both by virtue of its intrinsic physical properties as well as by its location immediately beneath the anterior surface coil elements (as a first approximation, signal intensity falls off as the square of the distance from the center of the coil).

There are a few limitations of spatial saturation bands: First, it's sometimes difficult to achieve a balance between obtaining adequate saturation of the subcutaneous fat while avoiding saturation of signal from adjacent tissue that you're interested in (eg, the uterine fundus in this case). Second, anterior saturation bands without respiratory triggering won't eliminate motion-induced blurring and won't eliminate artifact from peristalsis.

If the anterior saturation band is not completely successful in eliminating motion artifact, a second alternative is to swap the phase and frequency encoding directions, so that the phase direction is superior-inferior rather than anterior-posterior. This typically results in a longer acquisition time, since the rectangular FOV can no longer be applied to reduce the phase matrix along the shorter direction. In fact, to prevent aliasing artifact, it will be necessary to extend the phase FOV, either by applying NPW, which automatically doubles the phase FOV while maintaining the same spatial resolution, or by manually adjusting the phase FOV (phase oversampling). A superior saturation band, again placed just above the area of interest, is also a good idea to suppress potential artifact from irrelevant anatomy. This strategy probably resulted in the highest quality, although not completely artifact-free, images.

The case deserves a few additional comments: This exercise in artifact reduction required 3 fairly long acquisitions, and it's almost certainly true that a single respiratory-triggered sequence would have been more efficient and may have successfully eliminated the phase ghosting artifact. A second point to remember is that fat suppression, applied alone or in addition to the strategies discussed above, would help to minimize the signal intensity of the phase ghosts. Finally, motion artifact from peristalsis is a very common problem in evaluation of the pelvis, and, for that reason, we always use an antiperistaltic agent (subcutaneous glucagon) for these examinations unless there is a compelling contraindication.

CASE 17.15

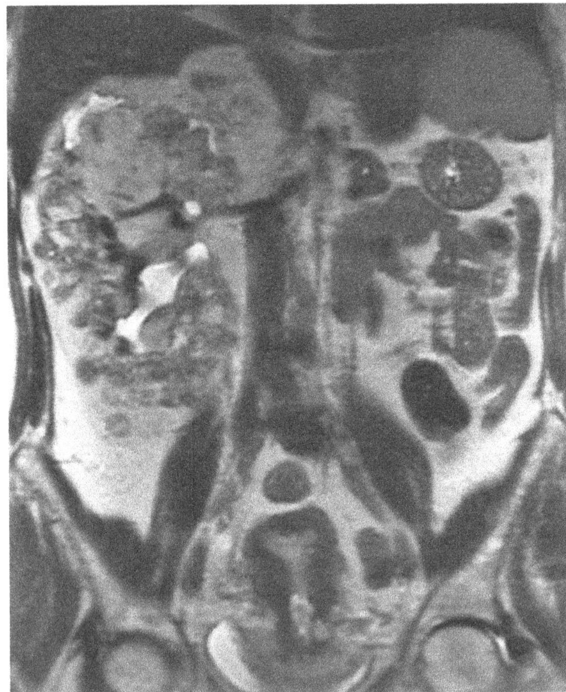

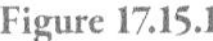

Figure 17.15.1

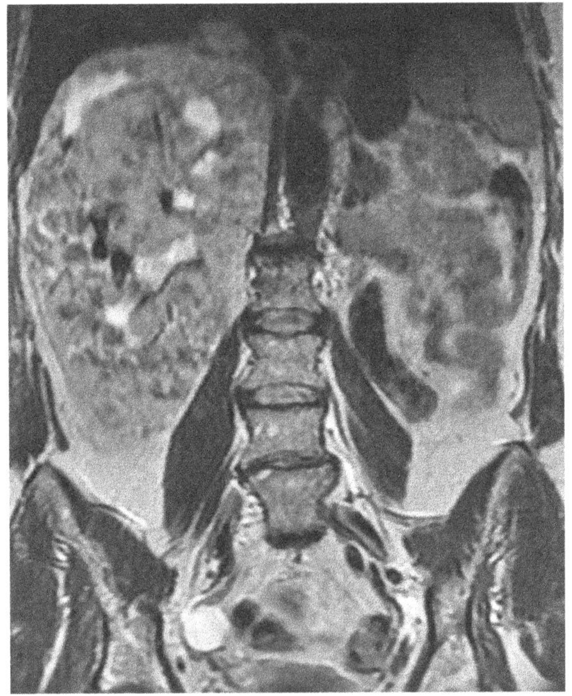

Figure 17.15.2

HISTORY: 53-year-old woman with chronic kidney disease

IMAGING FINDINGS: Coronal SSFSE image (Figure 17.15.1) demonstrates massive enlargement of the right kidney, which contains multiple fatty lesions as well as several round nodules. The left kidney is surgically absent. Coronal respiratory-triggered FSE T2-weighted image (Figure 17.15.2) reveals similar findings but with image blurring related to motion artifact.

DIAGNOSIS: Reduction in respiratory motion artifact with SSFSE images in comparison to respiratory-triggered FSE images

COMMENT: While it is true that both the SSFSE and the FSE series contained diagnostic images from this patient with tuberous sclerosis, multiple angiomyolipomas, and massive enlargement of the right kidney, significant motion artifact can be seen on the FSE image which is notably absent on the SSFSE image.

Coronal FSE series with high spatial resolution and without fat suppression have achieved a substantial following in our practice, particularly for patients with renal or adrenal masses. When acquired without motion artifact, the resulting images can indeed be spectacular. This is unfortunately a relatively infrequent occurrence—the phase encoding direction is usually right-left, and when small bowel loops begin to appear in the images (typically about halfway through the kidneys), the resulting motion artifact from peristalsis is substantial. This case is probably a somewhat extreme example, since in the absence of the left kidney, small bowel loops fall posteriorly and generate artifact affecting nearly the entire right kidney.

One bad series is not a great tragedy, and the thought and effort involved in making a decision to deviate from a standard protocol should be applauded, but it is worth noting that the acquisition time of the respiratory-triggered sequence was nearly 10 minutes, while the SSFSE series was obtained in two 15-second breath-holds.

The decision to embark on a long acquisition with marginal advantages over a much shorter one should be approached with caution, particularly when patients are in pain, are mildly claustrophobic, or are otherwise inclined to stop the examination. In general, it's a good idea to acquire the most important sequences at the beginning of the examination, although an occasionally contradictory rule states that all the respiratory or navigator-gated acquisitions should be performed at the beginning of the examination, since multiple breath-holds over a relatively short period of time can lead to irregular breathing in some patients and result in poor triggering, long acquisitions, and greater motion artifact.

If nevertheless you are determined to obtain high spatial resolution coronal FSE images, consider the following suggestions:

1) Parallel imaging (with k-space–based reconstruction) along with a slightly shorter echo train length can reduce the total acquisition time and may also help to minimize motion artifact.
2) Even though this isn't the pelvis, subcutaneous glucagon can substantially reduce artifact from peristalsis.
3) Remind your technologist that when imaging a renal mass, the coverage does not need to extend through the anterior margin of the liver.
4) Remember that fat suppression is your friend (except perhaps in this case, where the angiomyolipomas would be better appreciated without it).

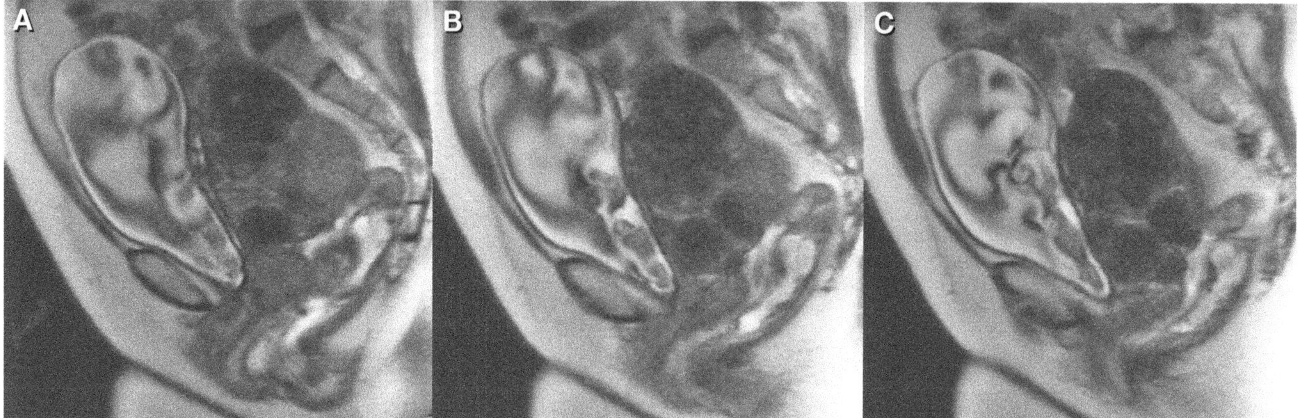

Figure 17.16.1

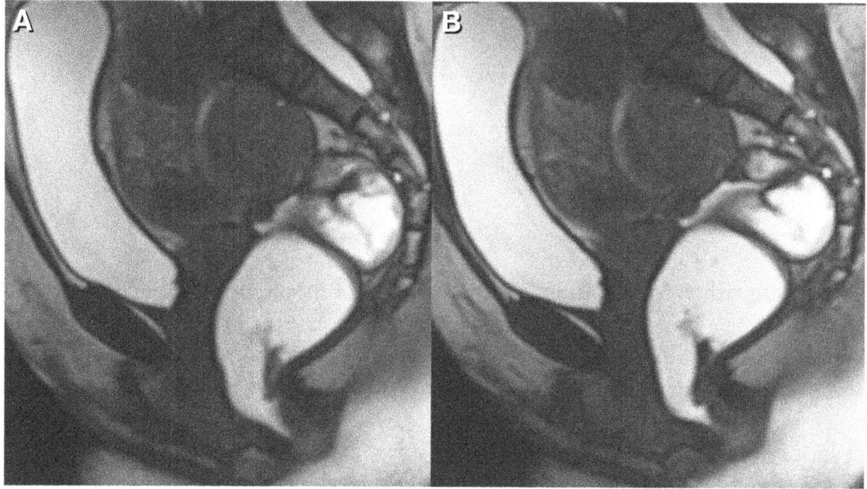

Figure 17.16.2

HISTORY: 55-year-old woman with fecal incontinence

IMAGING FINDINGS: Sagittal SSFSE images from a dynamic proctography examination (Figure 17.16.1) demonstrate heterogeneous abnormal signal throughout the bladder. Sagittal SSFP images (following administration of rectal contrast) (Figure 17.16.2) show no abnormality within the bladder.

DIAGNOSIS: Motion artifact in SSFSE images related to ureteral peristalsis

COMMENT: Even though both 2D SSFSE and SSFP images are obtained using a rapid sequential acquisition, SSFSE images are much more susceptible to the effects of bulk motion, as illustrated by this case, where regions of low signal intensity reflect motion and dephasing occurring during acquisition of central lines of k-space.

This artifact is rarely as apparent as it is in this case and is usually recognized fairly easily (by its absence on most other pulse sequences), but it can occasionally be problematic in MRCP examinations, particularly if your protocol is heavily invested in breath-held thin-section SSFSE acquisitions as a backup for a failed or motion-degraded 3D FSE series. Flow-related artifact in the biliary tree may appear as a central region of variable low signal intensity and can at times provide a fairly convincing simulation of a stone. For this reason, we have replaced the thin section SSFSE acquisition with overlapping fat-suppressed 2D SSFP images in our MRCP protocol, with the caveat that the presence of multiple surgical clips or extensive adjacent bowel gas may force us to return to SSFSE images.

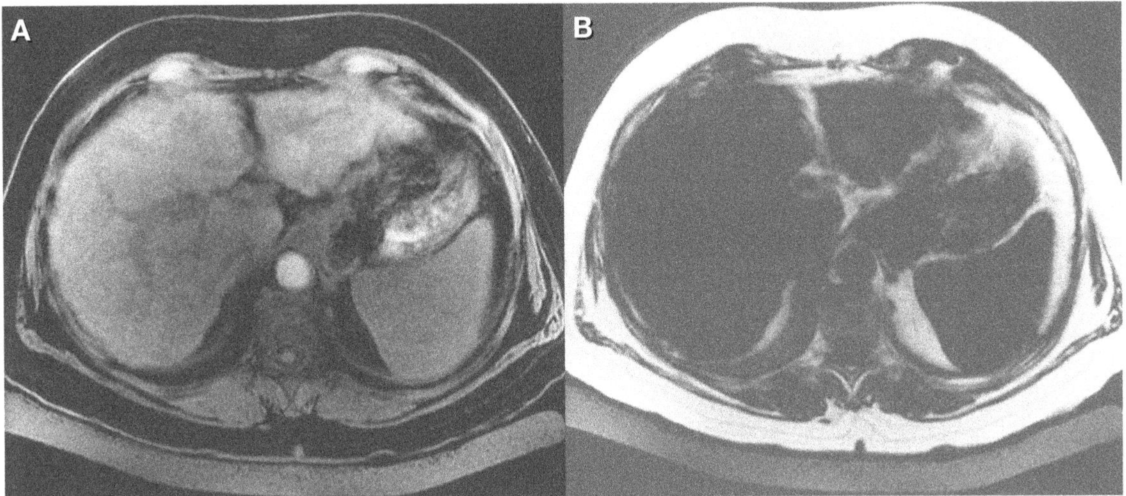

Figure 17.17.1

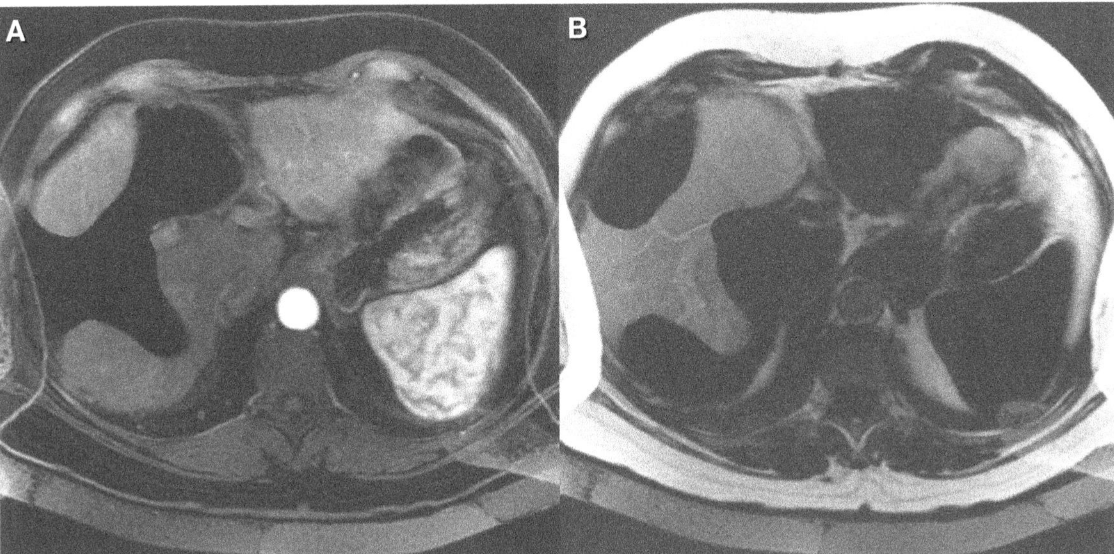

Figure 17.17.2

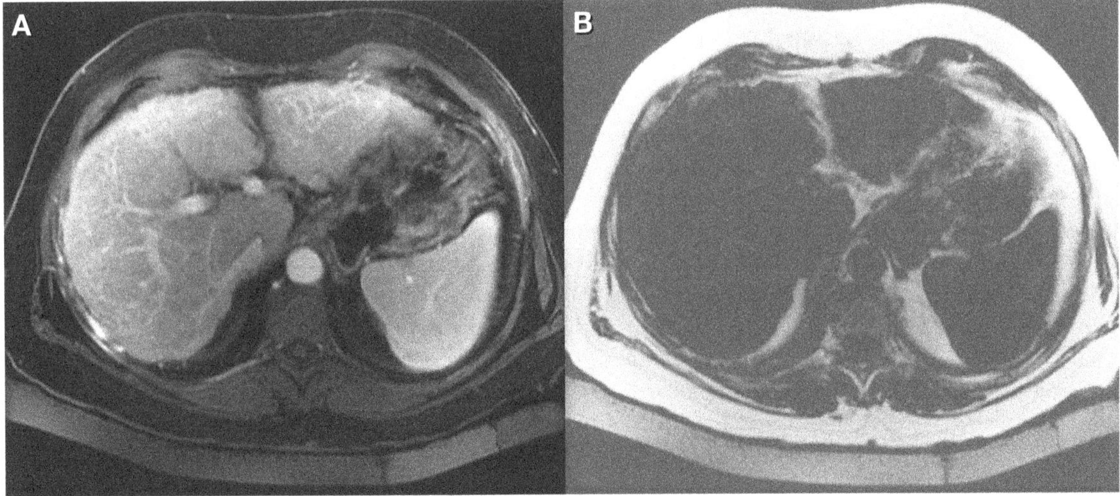

Figure 17.17.3

HISTORY: 58-year-old woman with cirrhosis

IMAGING FINDINGS: Axial precontrast (Figure 17.17.1) and arterial phase (Figure 17.17.2) and portal venous phase (Figure 17.17.3) postgadolinium water and fat images from a 3D SPGR Dixon acquisition. Notice that the phase and frequency directions have been swapped on the arterial phase acquisition and that there is a large geographic signal void in the middle of the liver on the water image, with the missing anatomy appearing on the corresponding fat image. All artifacts have been corrected on the portal venous phase images.

DIAGNOSIS: Fat-water swap on a 3D SPGR Dixon acquisition

COMMENT: Few if any radiologists would dispute the occasional benefits of fat suppression, most frequently used in T2- and postgadolinium T1-weighted imaging. Although several approaches have been introduced over the years, the most popular remains chemical fat suppression, in which a frequency selective RF pulse and a spoiler gradient pulse are used to excite and then saturate fat magnetization before water is excited for image formation. An alternative approach is to use a frequency selective RF pulse to directly excite only water protons.

Chemical fat suppression is a simple and generally very effective technique, but it does have a few limitations, including slightly longer acquisition times to accommodate the suppression pulses. Another limitation is that the fat suppression pulse requires an accurate 90° flip angle, which can vary if the B_1 field is inhomogeneous. Similarly, the B_0 magnetic field must also be uniform, since the inhomogeneity must be substantially less than the chemical shift between water and fat (3.5 parts per million, or 220 Hz at 1.5 T) in order for the frequency selective fat suppression pulse to achieve adequate fat suppression while avoiding water suppression. These effects become much more prevalent as the distance from the magnet isocenter increases and in regions of rapidly varying susceptibility, such as near metallic objects or near gas in the lung or bowel.

STIR is a technique used less commonly, but it does have some advantages over chemical fat suppression. This technique uses an initial 180° inversion pulse followed by a short delay, in which the longitudinal magnetization is allowed to partially relax toward its equilibrium state. When the fat magnetization crosses its null point, the standard RF excitation and image acquisition is then applied. This captures the signal from water since the T1 relaxation time for water is much longer than for fat, and its signal has only partially relaxed when the fat magnetization crosses the null point. STIR techniques are relatively insensitive to both B_0 and B_1 inhomogeneities; however, their limitations include significantly longer acquisition times (to account for the TI), reduced SNR (since the water magnetization is allowed to partially decay), and poor performance as postgadolinium T1-weighted pulse sequences (since gadolinium shortens the T1 relaxation time of water protons to values similar to those of fat, in which case their signal is also suppressed by the STIR inversion pulses).

A third, more recent approach was initially described by Dixon. In this technique, the chemical shift difference between water and fat is encoded into the signal phase, and then fat-water separation is achieved through postprocessing manipulation of the data. In the original implementation, images were acquired with the fat and water protons in-phase and 180° out-of-phase (by acquiring 2 TE values), and fat and water images were obtained by summation and subtraction of the signal from the 2 different TEs (it should be obvious that this method also allows generation of IP and OP images from the same data set). This initial approach was just as limited by B_0 and B_1 inhomogeneity effects as the chemical fat suppression techniques and generally required longer acquisition times. Recent developments have focused on improvements in phase correction as a result of improved postprocessing algorithms as well as more sophisticated data acquisition. All major manufacturers now offer versions of Dixon techniques in a variety of pulse sequences, and these often achieve fat-water separation that is superior to standard chemical fat suppression techniques.

This case demonstrates a pitfall of relying on a postprocessing algorithm to achieve fat-water separation: Small (or large) phase errors introduced into 1 or more voxels can propagate an incorrect solution to many adjacent voxels, or even to the entire slice, and then tissue signal from water is erroneously attributed to fat and vice versa. This is illustrated by the large geographic signal void in the liver on the arterial phase postgadolinium image, with the appropriate water signal appearing in the corresponding fat image. Fat-water swaps are more likely to occur in regions of rapidly varying susceptibility (such as near the diaphragm) as well as in regions where significant aliasing has occurred, and both risk factors were present in this case. (The technologist reduced the inferior coverage of the imaging volume between the precontrast and postcontrast acquisitions to shorten the breath-hold but, in the course of making this adjustment, managed to swap the phase and frequency directions, and this introduced enough phase ambiguities to generate the erroneous reconstruction.) Fortunately, this problem was immediately recognized and corrected before a minimally delayed portal venous phase acquisition, which was reconstructed correctly.

As Dixon techniques have evolved and improved, the incidence of fat-water swap has significantly declined, but it remains occasionally problematic; for that reason, fat and water images are always reconstructed (in a perfect world you might want to be able to turn off the fat reconstruction, particularly during postgadolinium dynamic acquisitions). If there is a complete fat-water swap of 1 or more images, it is relatively straightforward (although tedious) for the technologist to swap the images and generate a corrected series. When only parts of the image contain a fat-water swap, as in this case, there isn't really any solution other than looking at both images simultaneously and trying to piece them together in your head.

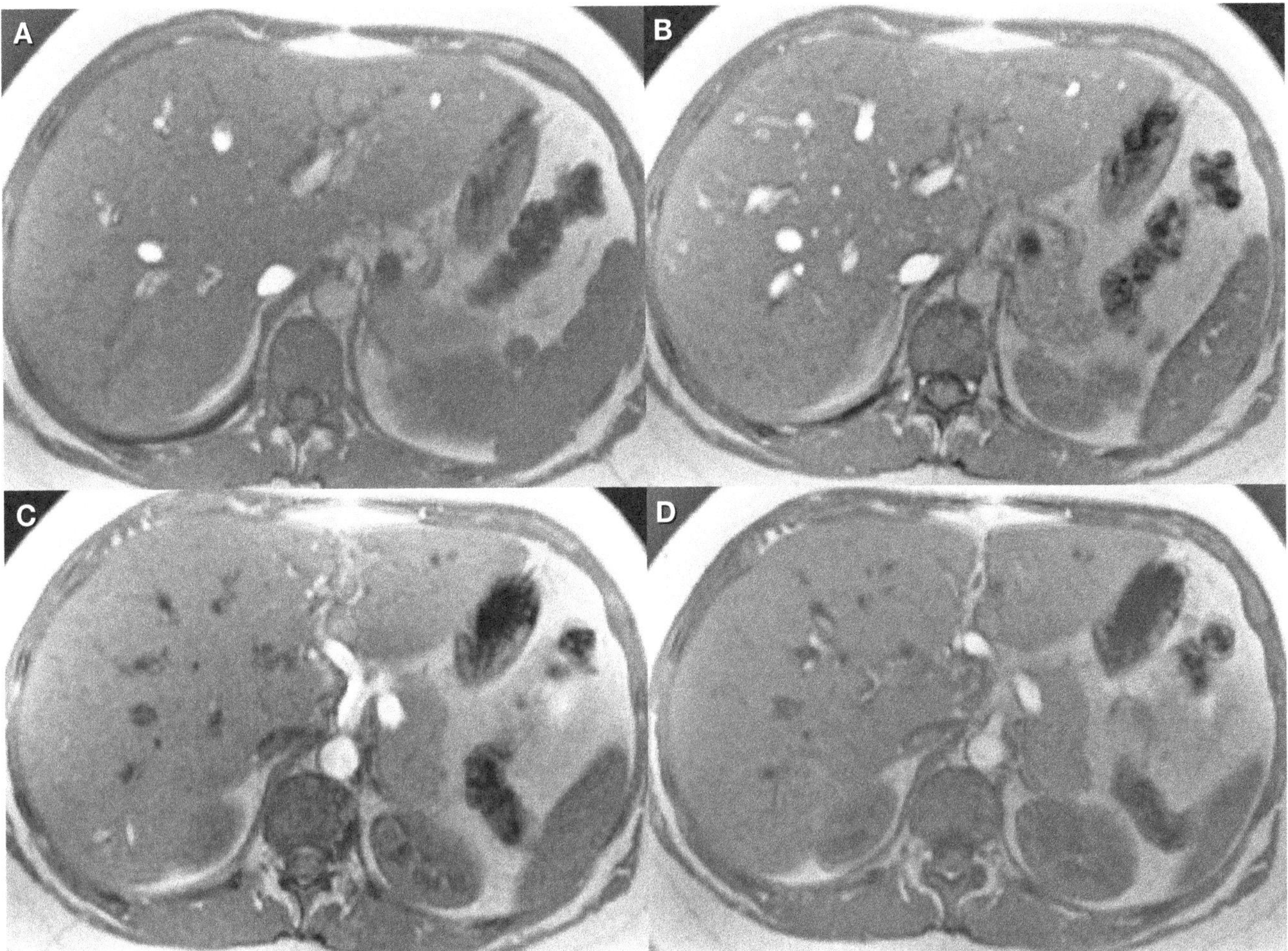

Figure 17.18.1

HISTORY: 39-year-old woman with Crohn disease and suspected primary sclerosing cholangitis

IMAGING FINDINGS: Consecutive IP images from a 2D SPGR IP-OP acquisition (Figure 17.18.1) demonstrate high signal intensity within the IVC and hepatic veins on the superior 2 images which disappears on the bottom images. Note the appearance of high signal intensity within the aorta and celiac artery on the inferior images.

DIAGNOSIS: Vascular inflow effects in arteries and veins

COMMENT: The vascular inflow effect depicted in this case usually isn't noticed by residents or fellows, who have trained their eyes to ignore the presence of high signal intensity in an artery or vein that disappears on the next slice. The explanation involves acquisitions that are divided into 2 or more breath-holds (or concatenations).

The slice acquisition order is arbitrary to some extent but is often broken down into packs of consecutive slices: During the first breath-hold, all the slices in the upper half of the liver are acquired, and in the second breath-hold, the remaining inferior slices are obtained. The value of TR determines how many slices can be acquired for each acquisition, since the dead time between the initial RF excitation and the readout of each slice can be used to acquire data from other slices. So, essentially all slices within the pack are subjected to multiple RF pulses within a short period of time, resulting in some mild in-plane saturation. This saturation effect is magnified for moving spins travelling perpendicular to the acquisition plane. Arterial blood entering the top slice, for example, has experienced no saturation effects and consequently has high signal intensity. As these spins travel inferiorly, however, they are subjected to repeated RF pulses, become saturated, and lose signal intensity. Therefore, the aorta at the top of the liver shows high signal intensity, which progressively fades inferiorly until the bottom slice of the first pack is reached, where the signal reaches its minimal value. The next slice is the first slice of the second pack, and so the process repeats itself, and this explains the abrupt transition from low to high signal intensity. The situation is reversed for the IVC and hepatic veins, where flow is in the opposite direction: The bottom slice represents the peak signal intensity of unsaturated blood, and in the top slice the IVC and hepatic veins have experienced maximal saturation and therefore have their lowest signal intensity.

This artifact is often not noticed, and therefore only rarely causes difficulties in interpretation, although the abrupt transition from low to high signal intensity, particularly in veins, has tempted the unwary into suspecting subacute thrombosis.

This phenomenon is also the basis of TOF MRA, except that TOF acquisitions are performed sequentially; that is, all phase encoding steps are played out in 1 slice before moving on to the next slice. This maximizes the in-plane saturation and thereby maximizes vascular contrast but at a cost in acquisition time, since this is a much less efficient strategy than exciting multiple slices simultaneously.

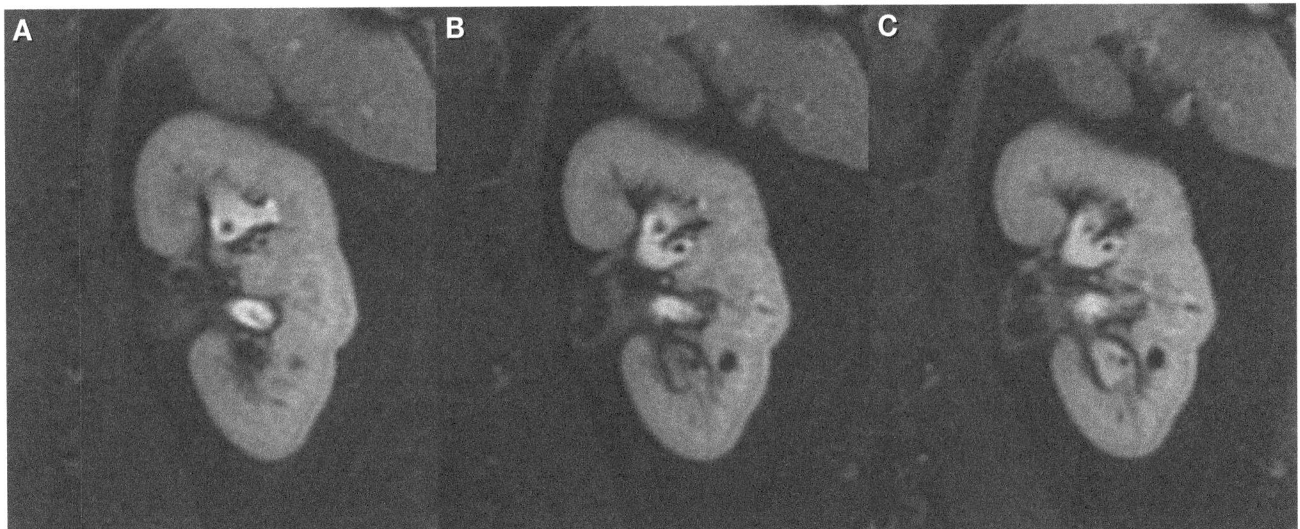

Figure 17.19.1

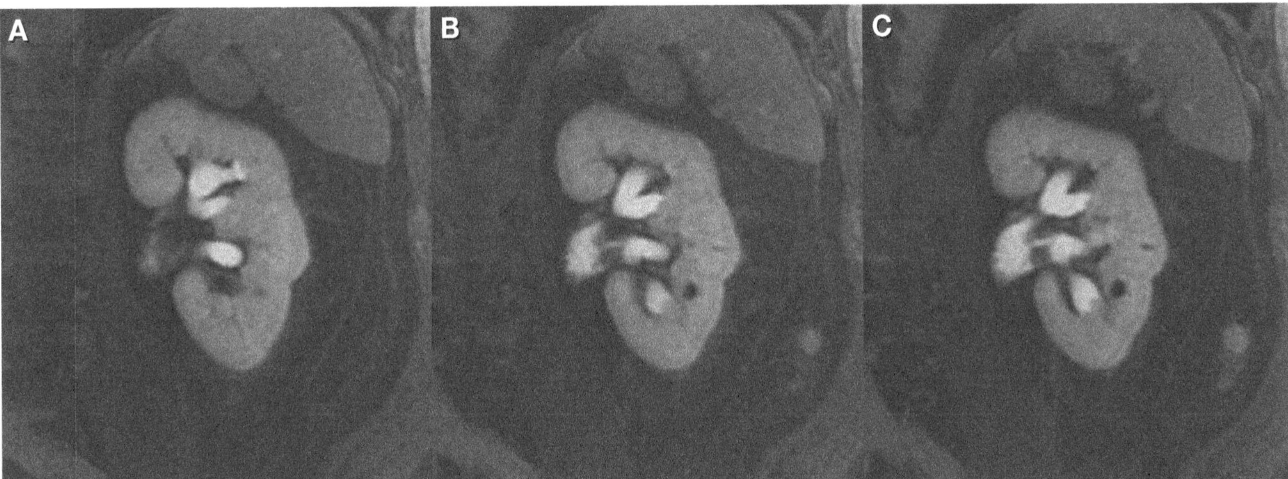

Figure 17.19.2

HISTORY: 60-year-old man with history of urothelial carcinoma

IMAGING FINDINGS: Coronal oblique early excretory phase images from gadolinium-enhanced 3D SPGR MR urogram (Figure 17.19.1) demonstrate multiple small filling defects within the left renal pelvis, with incomplete filling of the renal pelvis. Delayed images (Figure 17.19.2) reveal that most of the small filling defects have not persisted; however, a lesion along the inferior margin of the renal pelvis is more apparent.

DIAGNOSIS: Susceptibility artifact related to excretion of concentrated gadolinium in the renal pelvis in a patient with recurrent urothelial carcinoma

COMMENT: Signal void in the renal collecting system seen on postgadolinium 2D or 3D SPGR images is a fairly well-known phenomenon and has occasionally provided an excuse for missing lesions in the renal pelvis. The artifact arises because gadolinium excreted by the kidney into the collecting system may have a higher concentration than the levels reached within blood vessels and tissue following intravenous injection, to the extent that the T2* properties of the contrast agent become dominant, resulting in susceptibility artifact and signal void.

This is a minor consideration for most abdominal examinations, even for many of those performed to characterize renal masses, but it does pose a significant problem for CE MR urography. The issue hasn't been completely solved, but administration of a diuretic (typically furosemide [Lasix]) prior to gadolinium injection is helpful and has become a standard element of most urography protocols. The diuretic leads to increased production of more dilute urine, which has 2 beneficial effects: reducing urinary gadolinium concentration and distending the renal collecting system so that small lesions are more conspicuous.

The rate of urine production and gadolinium excretion is highly variable from person to person (and sometimes from kidney to kidney); therefore, a urography protocol should never have a prescribed set of acquisitions, which when completed, signifies the end of the examination. Instead, the technologist should keep repeating the 3D SPGR acquisition until the calyces, renal pelvis, and ureters of both kidneys have been filled with contrast and are well visualized. This allows the kinds of artifacts seen in this case to resolve and the real lesions to be found. A similar rationale would advise caution in interpreting the incidentally detected small filling defect in the renal pelvis seen on a single postgadolinium 3D SPGR series as a stone without confirmation on other sequences.

CASE 17.20

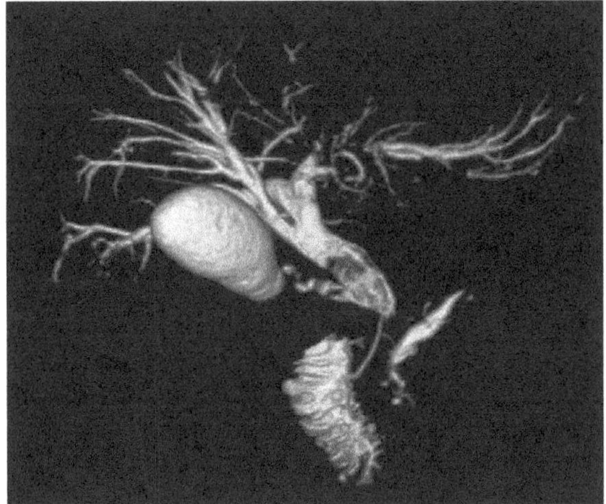

Figure 17.20.1

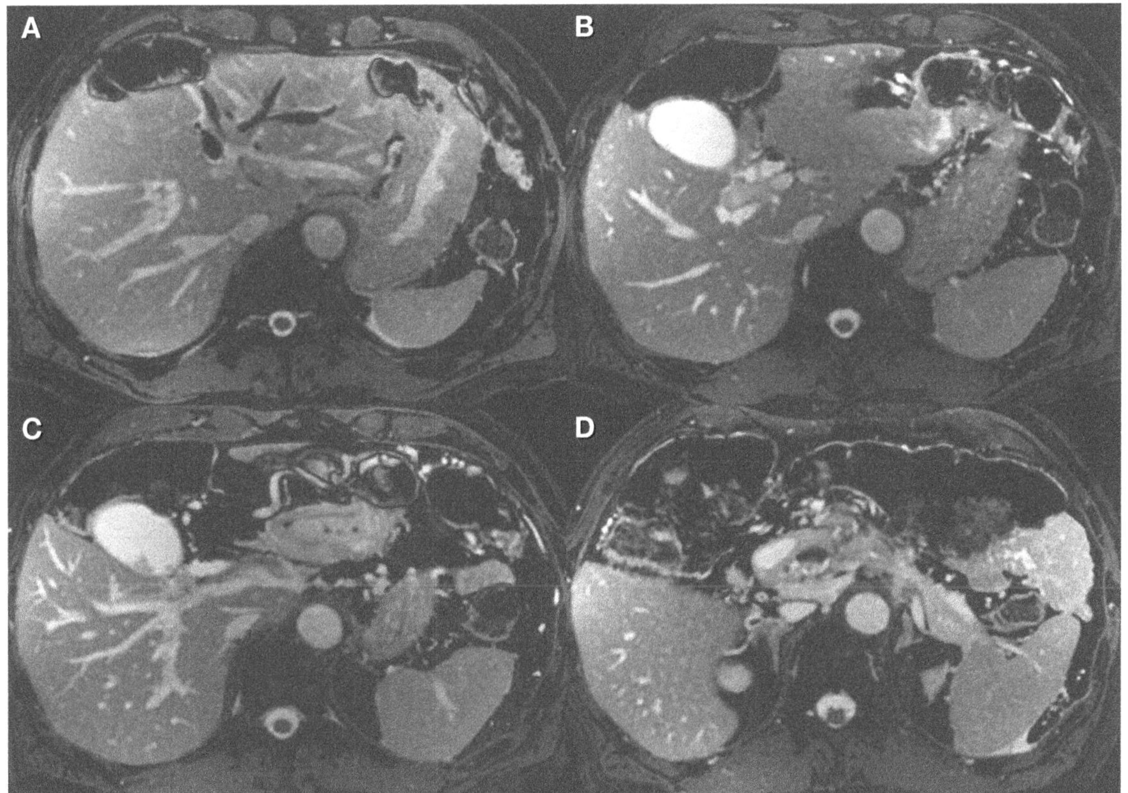

Figure 17.20.2

HISTORY: 72-year-old man with cholangiocarcinoma in the distal common bile duct

IMAGING FINDINGS: VR image from 3D FRFSE MRCP (Figure 17.20.1) demonstrates moderately dilated intrahepatic ducts in the central right hepatic lobe, poorly visualized ducts in the medial left lobe, and dilated ducts in the lateral left lobe. There is an abrupt cutoff of the common bile duct near the pancreatic head, with a stent extending into the duodenum, and an apparent filling defect proximal to the obstruction. Notice also the dilated pancreatic duct. Axial fat-suppressed 3D SSFP images (Figure 17.20.2) demonstrate signal void in the left hepatic lobe ducts as well as an air-fluid level in the common bile duct.

DIAGNOSIS: Pneumobilia

COMMENT: Pneumobilia can generate some interesting artifacts, particularly on 3D reconstructions of heavily T2-weighted MRCPs, as in this case, where the presence of a signal void gives the appearance of either absent ducts or a filling defect within the duct. The heavy T2 weighting of 3D FRFSE acquisitions and consequent excellent background suppression mean that sorting out low signal intensity within the ducts can be somewhat difficult, since these regions tend to blend into the background, and it's often easier to see what's going on by examining the precontrast SPGR or SSFP images, where the signal void within the biliary ducts is more easily visualized against the prominent background signal intensity of the liver. (The advantage of SSFP images in this regard is that the high signal intensity of bile is preserved in comparison to SPGR images, where bile is relatively dark; however, the observation of blooming artifact when switching from OP to IP SPGR images, by virtue of the longer TE of the IP acquisition, is occasionally helpful for identifying small foci of gas within the biliary tree.)

When pneumobilia is as prominent as it is in this case, the diagnosis is obvious. If only a few bubbles of gas are present, however, particularly in a nondilated system where an air-fluid level may not be apparent, the distinction between gas and an intraductal stone is more difficult. Always remember that gas should rise to the highest (nondependent) available point and therefore should always rest along the anterior margin of the duct. Susceptibility artifact from gas is almost always more prominent than any artifact generated by a stone or other filling defect, and therefore obvious blooming of artifact on IP images is highly suggestive of pneumobilia rather than choledocholithiasis.

Remember also that the presence of gas does not exclude additional real filling defects. Did you notice, for example, the small cluster of stones in the gallbladder and in the distal common bile duct?

CASE 17.21

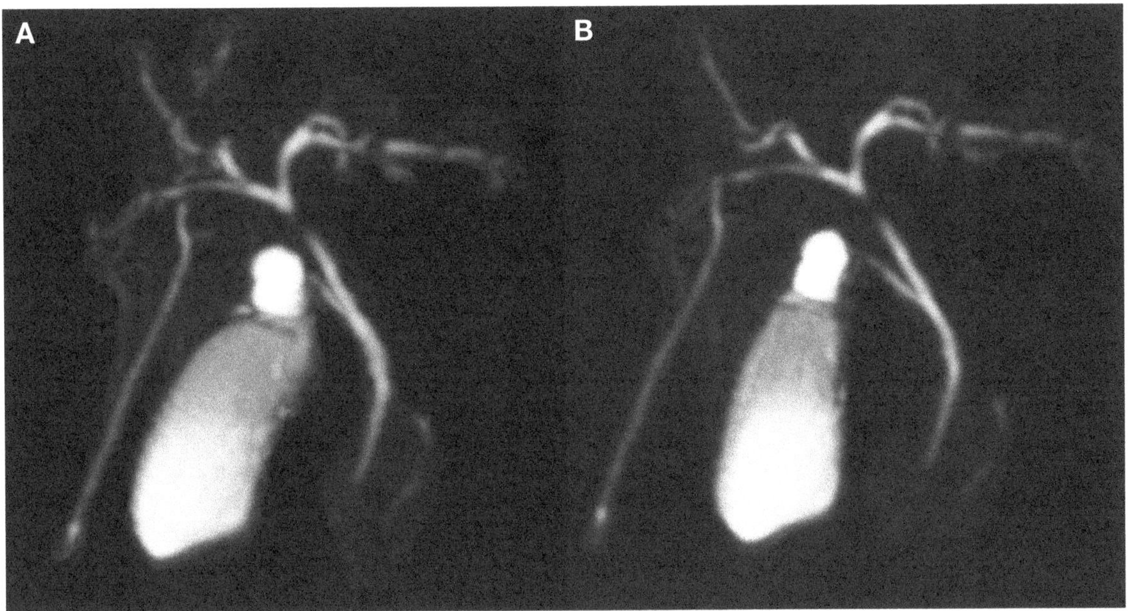

Figure 17.21.1

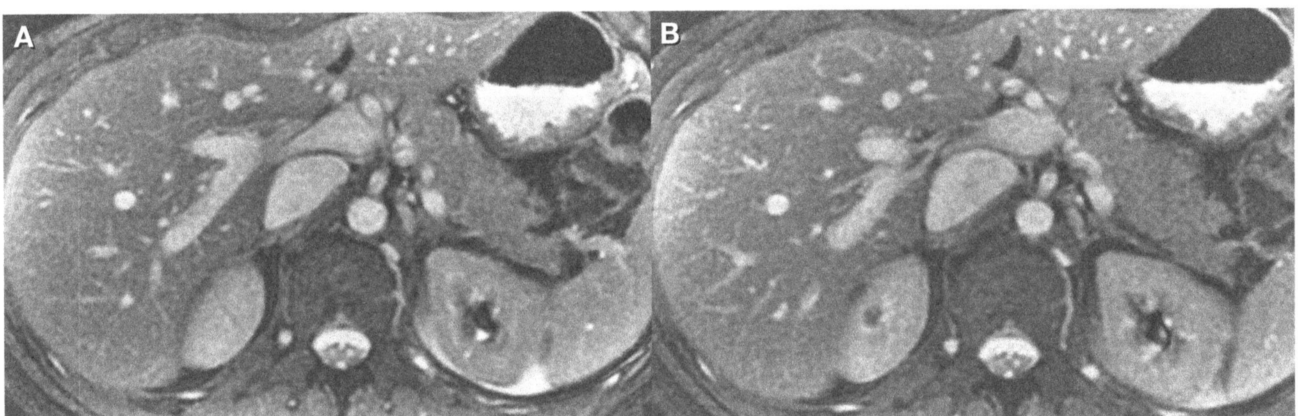

Figure 17.21.2

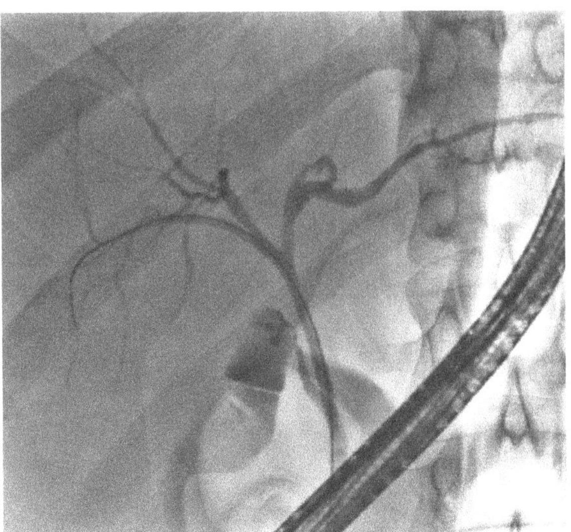

Figure 17.21.3

HISTORY: 23-year-old man with ulcerative colitis and elevated liver function test results

IMAGING FINDINGS: MIP images from 3D FRFSE MRCP (Figure 17.21.1) demonstrate focal stricture of the common bile duct at its bifurcation in the hepatic hilum. Focal beading of a mildly prominent duct in the left hepatic lobe is also noted. Axial fat-suppressed 2D SSFP images (Figure 17.21.2) show a prominent hepatic artery crossing the small common bile duct. Image from subsequent ERCP (Figure 17.21.3) shows no biliary abnormality in the hepatic hilum and questionable mild irregularity of the left lobe duct.

DIAGNOSIS: Pseudostricture of the common bile duct resulting from hepatic artery pulsation artifact

COMMENT: This is a difficult case to interpret because the abnormalities in the minimally prominent left hepatic biliary duct are probably real but accentuated by artifact. There are some subtle corresponding irregularities in the duct on the ERCP image; however, the ERCP was read as negative, probably because the MRCP report had emphasized the finding of the prominent hilar stricture, which turned out to be completely artifactual.

FSE pulse sequences (particularly SSFSE varieties) are well known to be exquisitely sensitive to flow and pulsation effects. Even though some protection is offered by 3D acquisitions (which have 2 sets of phase encoding steps to help average out signal irregularities related to flow), flow-related artifact is a recognized feature of 3D MRCP pulse sequences, particularly in the hepatic hilum where the hepatic artery often crosses in front of the common bile duct near its bifurcation.

Distinguishing a true common bile duct stricture from hepatic artery pulsation artifact can be very difficult, and often the decision is based on identifying additional abnormalities that might confirm the presence of a significant stricture, such as upstream ductal dilatation, stones or debris within the ducts, mural thickening and enhancement of the common duct, or a hilar mass. It is also helpful to try to confirm the abnormality on 2D or 3D SSFP acquisitions, which are less sensitive to flow artifacts. This will often convince us one way or another, although when the ducts are small, as in this case, the results may be ambiguous.

It should also be noted that a similar pseudostricture can result from susceptibility artifact generated by surgical clips in the gallbladder fossa following cholecystectomy. In this case, the artifact is more prominent on gradient echo SSFP acquisitions and less prominent on 2D and 3D FSE images. Since the presence of surgical clips is difficult to discern on long TE 3D FSE source images (with excellent background suppression), their presence and location can be more easily appreciated on the gradient echo acquisitions included in most standard liver-MRCP protocols.

The artifacts seen in the left hepatic lobe accentuating the subtle ductal abnormalities are likely related to motion and phase ghosting artifacts. The left lobe lies immediately beneath the heart and adjacent to the stomach, which are both potential sources of artifact, particularly if the stomach contains a significant amount of fluid. These anatomical relationships probably explain why blurred MRCP images are more frequently encountered in the left hepatic lobe than in the right.

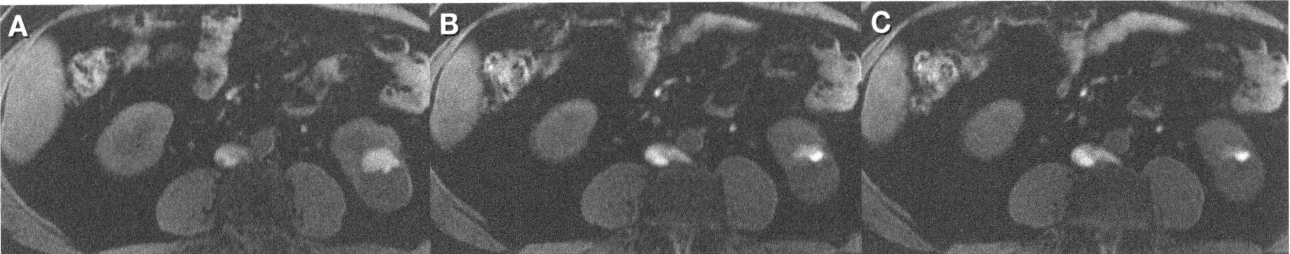

Figure 17.22.1

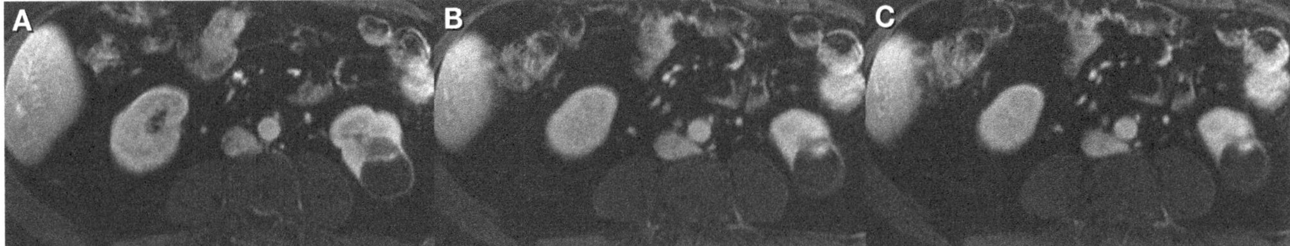

Figure 17.22.2

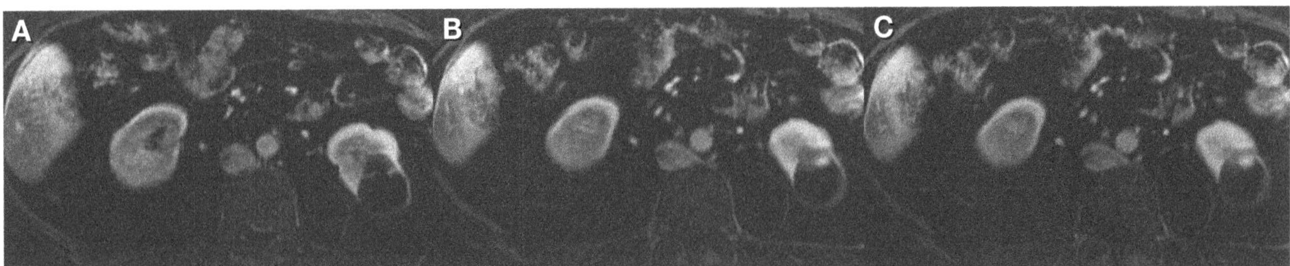

Figure 17.22.3

HISTORY: 51-year-old woman with a complex cystic lesion in the left kidney

IMAGING FINDINGS: Axial precontrast 3D SPGR images (Figure 17.22.1) reveal an exophytic lesion in the lower pole of the left kidney containing a posterior region with low signal intensity, a thin septation encompassing a small lateral nodule with markedly high signal intensity, and an anterior component with moderately high signal intensity. Axial venous phase postgadolinium images in the same location (Figure 17.22.2) show mild enhancement of the rim of the lesion as well as the septation. Axial subtracted images (Figure 17.22.3) demonstrate increased signal intensity within the small septal nodule and within the anterior component, suggesting that these regions enhance.

DIAGNOSIS: Subtraction artifact

COMMENT: The benefits of subtraction images when evaluating a complex lesion in the liver or kidneys are well known, and most manufacturers now include software that will automatically subtract precontrast images from postcontrast images to generate subtracted series.

Even though every resident and fellow in our department knows that subtraction artifacts can lead to errors in interpretation, this is an admonition more often appreciated in theory than in practice, and we have seen several mistakes made by radiologists swayed by the appearance of subtracted images.

In this case, a careful evaluation of the precontrast images and venous phase postcontrast images reveals that the patient's breath-holding had significantly deteriorated between the 2 acquisitions—notice the sharpness of the precontrast images in comparison to the mild blurring of the margins of the liver and kidneys on the corresponding postcontrast images. This means that the edges of enhancing tissue will be slightly wider and less distinct and that a residual rim of spurious enhancement could be generated on the subtracted series. Notice, for example, how much wider the rim of cortical enhancement is along the anterior margin of the right kidney.

Slight blurring and subtle shifts in position are especially problematic for objects that are already bright on the precontrast images—even if there is no real enhancement, a slight change in position can generate the appearance of enhancement. This effect is apparent in this case, where the very bright focus of septal hemorrhage and the moderately hyperintense blood products in the anterior component of the lesion have slightly shifted between the 2 views, thereby generating spurious enhancement on the subtracted image.

It is generally true that renal lesions demonstrating intense uniform high signal intensity on precontrast fat-suppressed T1-weighted images are hemorrhagic cysts; therefore, their internal components do not enhance. A few papers have attempted to elevate this general guideline to an absolute truth, but the numbers reported are far too small to be taken seriously. The best way to convince yourself that a complex lesion does or does not show internal enhancement is to place small ROIs on the relevant components of the lesion and then copy them to the precontrast images, always remembering to avoid ROIs at the blurred margin of a lesion—signal intensity differences less than the standard deviation of the measurements are convincing evidence of a lack of enhancement.

A final problem occasionally arises when the auto prescan is repeated between the precontrast and postcontrast acquisitions. The prescan makes small adjustments in the shim fields, flip angle, and receiver gain, all of which can lead to changes in the acquired signal intensity (remember that there is no absolute signal intensity measurement scale in MRI), and repeating the prescan may lead to significant differences in acquired signal, thereby generating diffuse subtraction artifacts. These artifacts are fairly easy to recognize if you're aware of them. What looks like a simple cyst will show uniform low-level enhancement. If you're in the unfortunate position of evaluating a complex partially cystic lesion when this happens, an effective solution is to perform ROI measurements on 3 (or more) postcontrast phases. A real mass (as opposed to a hemorrhagic cyst) will generally show some washout (or, less often, wash-in) by the time of the final phase; therefore, you should expect to see changes in the signal intensity of a mass from phase to phase following contrast administration.

Another point worth remembering is that it's much more difficult to generate a subtraction artifact showing uniform nonenhancement than one with spurious enhancement of a lesion; therefore, you should be more suspicious of subtraction artifact when the result is positive for enhancement rather than negative.

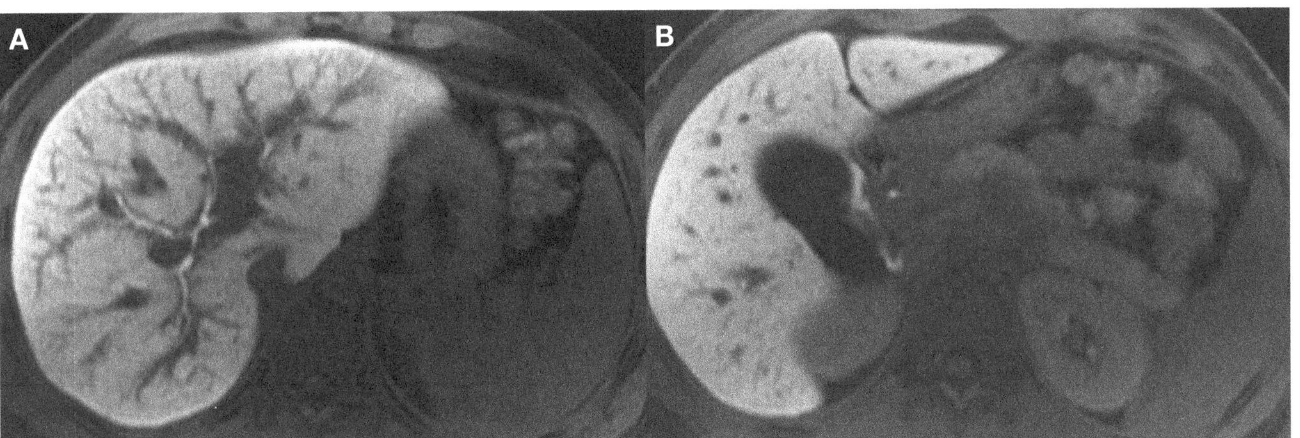

Figure 17.23.1

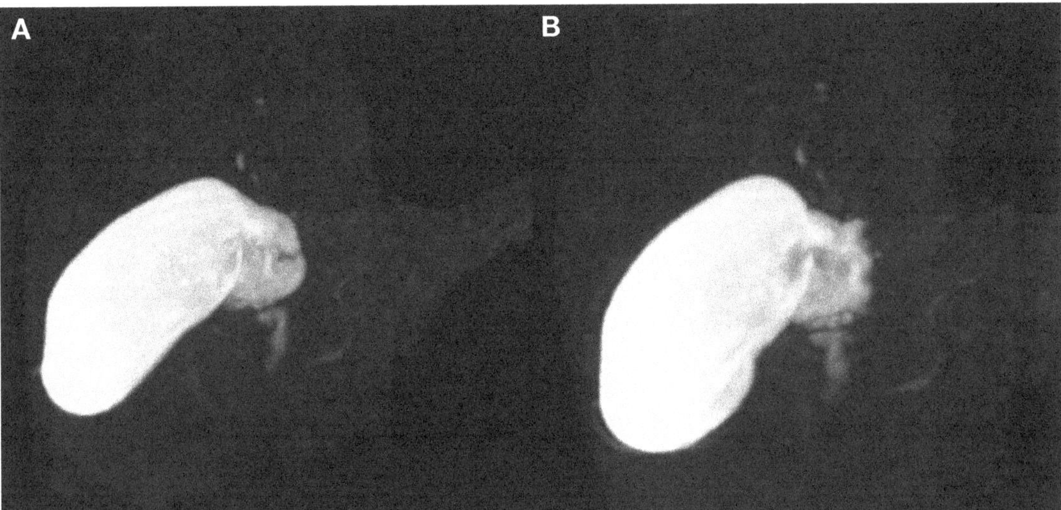

Figure 17.23.2

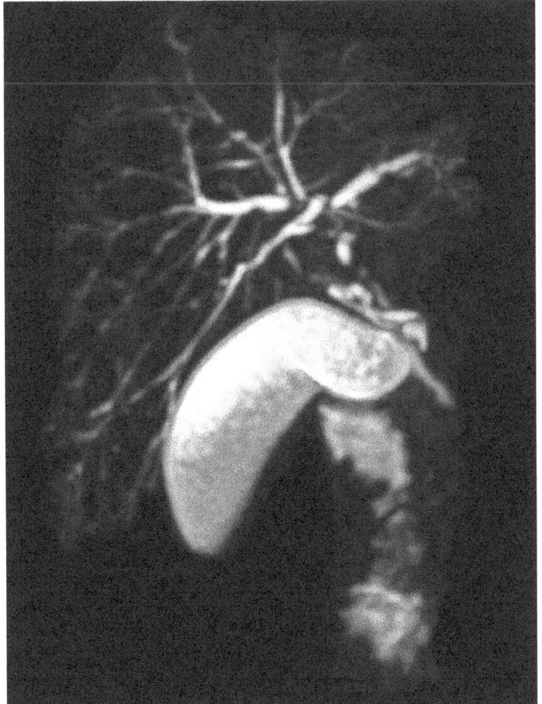

Figure 17.23.3

HISTORY: 22-year-old man with history of primary sclerosing cholangitis

IMAGING FINDINGS: Axial hepatobiliary phase post-gadolinium 3D SPGR images obtained following gadoxetate disodium (Eovist) administration (Figure 17.23.1) demonstrate mild irregularity of intrahepatic biliary ducts, consistent with primary sclerosing cholangitis. MIP images from 3D FRFSE MRCP obtained between contrast injection and hepatobiliary phase acquisition (Figure 17.23.2) reveal markedly limited visualization of the biliary tree, with only the gallbladder clearly seen. MIP image from an MRCP performed during the previous examination (Figure 17.23.3) shows mild dilatation and multiple strictures of intrahepatic bile ducts.

DIAGNOSIS: Susceptibility artifact from gadolinium excreted into the biliary tree

COMMENT: The question of which pulse sequences can be acquired during the 15-minute delay between initial Eovist injection and acquisition of the hepatobiliary phase images has generated some mild controversy in the literature. Most authors agree that FSE T2-weighted images are a reasonable choice, and a few articles have even suggested that postgadolinium acquisition is always preferred, regardless of which contrast agent is used. This is based on the idea that T1 and T2 contrast is generally complementary in the liver and tends to make lesions more conspicuous. (A similar argument was made in favor of fast IR images over FSE images, although this technique was eventually abandoned by most users as a result of the poor quality, low SNR, and long acquisition times relative to FSE images.) A second argument in favor of postgadolinium FSE images is that the susceptibility or T2* effect of gadolinium reduces the signal intensity of normal liver, thereby increasing the conspicuity of lesions that don't accumulate gadolinium.

The fact that gadolinium is an effective T2* contrast agent is often not appreciated by residents and fellows, who can occasionally be goaded into seeing renal stones when the dark signal intensity in the renal collecting system generated by concentrated gadolinium excreted into urine is pointed out to them on postcontrast SPGR or SSFP images. While a 3D FRFSE MRCP pulse sequence has less intrinsic susceptibility weighting than a gradient-echo-based acquisition, it also has an extremely long TE. Therefore, anything that even slightly reduces the T2 of bile may well have a detrimental effect on resultant images as illustrated in this case, where the biliary tree cannot be visualized on the 3D MRCP projection images because the T2 has been shortened by excreted gadolinium. The gallbladder, however, is clearly visualized, since only a small amount of excreted contrast has reached this structure.

There is at least 1 paper in the literature asserting that 3D FSE MRCP performed after Eovist administration has identical image quality and no higher incidence of artifacts when compared to acquisitions performed prior to gadolinium administration. We suspect this means that the MRCP images were acquired immediately after contrast administration and that the authors were fortunate not to encounter a significant percentage of patients with rapid biliary excretion of Eovist. Our preference is to avoid this gamble, and so our MRCP series is always performed before contrast is injected. (This case resulted from a radiologist who read the above paper and decided that he could improve the efficiency of our Eovist protocol.)

Many authors have pointed out that a positive-contrast MRCP can be obtained following Eovist administration using a 3D SPGR pulse sequence. We have not found this application particularly compelling, except with a suspected bile leak. The image quality of the resultant MRCP is usually much lower than the standard heavily T2-weighted acquisitions, generally with limited visualization of peripheral intrahepatic ducts. But if you are considering this technique, a higher flip angle can help to reduce some of the intrinsic background signal intensity of the liver.

CASE 17.24

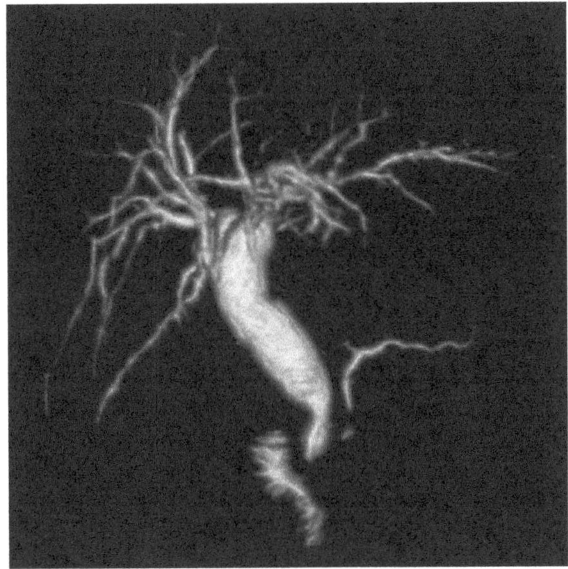

Figure 17.24.1

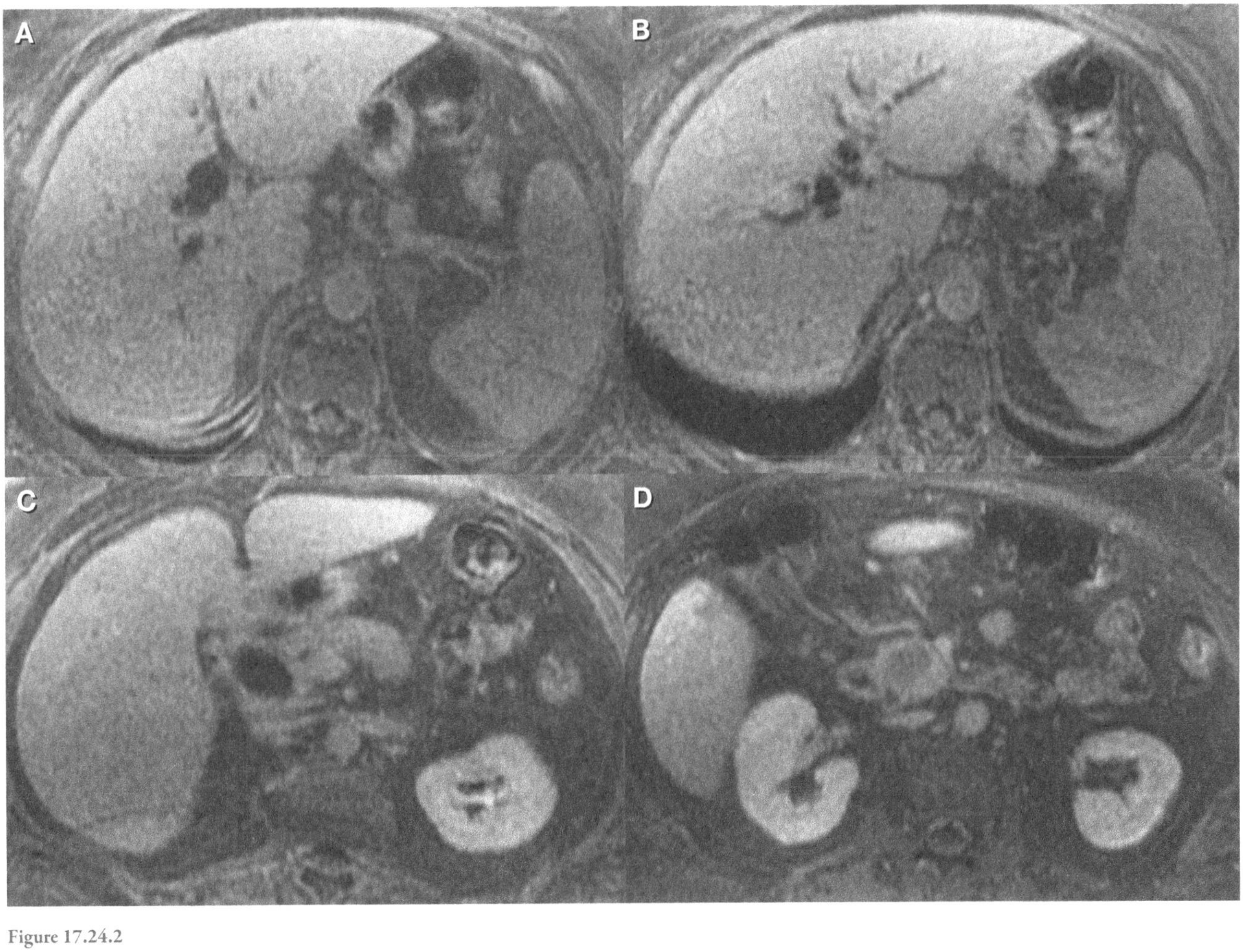

Figure 17.24.2

HISTORY: 64-year-old woman with pancreatic cancer and suspected hepatic metastases

IMAGING FINDINGS: VR image from 3D MRCP (Figure 17.24.1) demonstrates moderate dilatation of intrahepatic ducts and marked extrahepatic biliary dilatation extending to the pancreatic head, where there is also obstruction of the pancreatic duct. Axial hepatobiliary phase 3D SPGR images obtained 20 minutes following gadoxetate disodium (Eovist) injection (Figure 17.24.2) reveal poor enhancement of the liver and no excretion of contrast into the biliary tree. The hypoenhancing pancreatic head mass can be seen on the most inferior image.

DIAGNOSIS: Improper administration of Eovist in a patient with biliary obstruction

COMMENT: In defense of our colleague who performed this examination, it is unusual in our practice to encounter a patient with biliary obstruction diagnosed elsewhere but not already relieved by stent or percutaneous drainage before the patient is referred to Mayo Clinic. In this case, however, the obstruction was not treated, and the patient's bilirubin measured on the day before the MRI was 21 mg/dL, considerably above the recommended cutoff value of 6.0 mg/dL for administration of Eovist.

The problem with using Eovist in this situation is that while all the standard limitations of the agent still apply (ie, the reduced quality of the dynamic phase acquisitions related to the small total contrast dose), none of the usual benefits are available. In a patient with biliary obstruction or poor hepatic function, most of the contrast is excreted by the kidneys rather than the liver, so there isn't enough contrast in the liver for an effective hepatobiliary phase acquisition (no matter how long you wait).

This case occurred relatively early in our experience with Eovist, before we had approved a standard protocol in which the nurse routinely checks the patient's bilirubin level. Even so, it behooves the prudent radiologist considering Eovist administration to determine whether the patient has biliary obstruction or whether hepatic function is significantly depressed by parenchymal disease (eg, severely cirrhotic patients may not be good candidates).

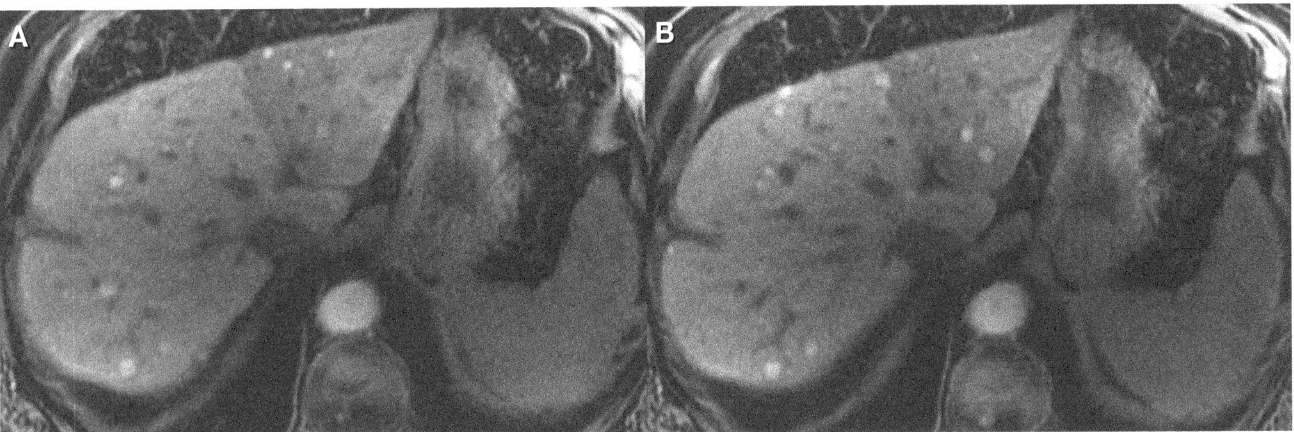

Figure 17.25.1

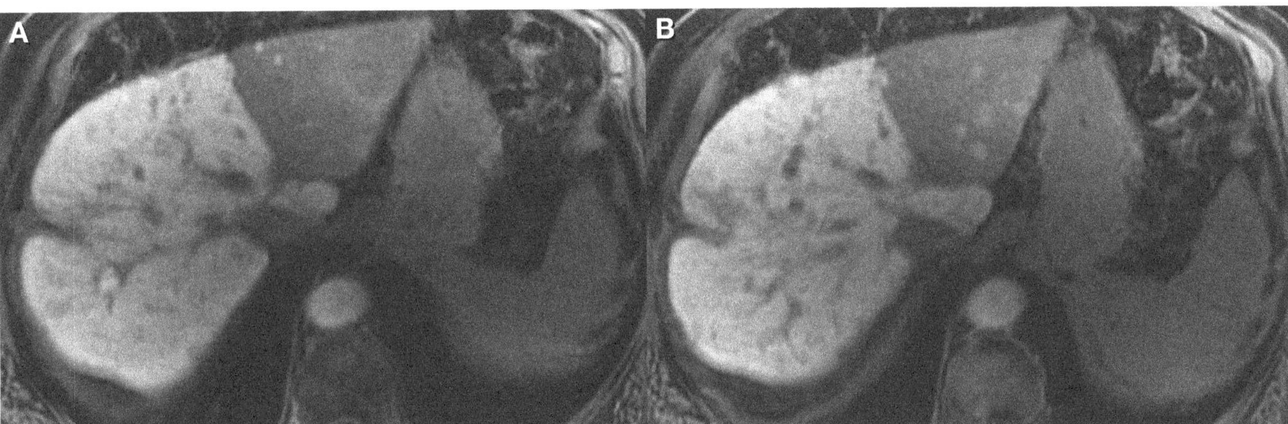

Figure 17.25.2

HISTORY: 51-year-old man with a history of metastatic melanoma

IMAGING FINDINGS: Axial precontrast 3D SPGR images (Figure 17.25.1) reveal multiple T1 hyperintense lesions throughout the liver, representing melanoma metastases. Note also geographic decreased signal intensity in the left hepatic lobe, likely representing fibrotic changes from previous radiotherapy. Many of the lesions are more difficult to visualize on equilibrium phase images obtained 20 minutes after gadoxetate disodium (Eovist) administration (Figure 17.25.2), since their signal intensity is now approximately equivalent to that of normal liver.

DIAGNOSIS: Reduced lesion conspicuity following Eovist administration in a patient with metastatic melanoma

COMMENT: This is a final example of artifacts occasionally encountered when imaging with Eovist. Metastatic melanoma is a rare diagnosis in our practice, and contrary to the prevalent mythology, many metastases do not contain enough melanin to appear hyperintense on precontrast T1-weighted images. This does occasionally happen, however, and may lead to the unusual occurrence of hepatic metastases that are better visualized on pregadolinium images, since in the hepatobiliary phase the retained contrast in hepatocytes reduces the T1 of normal liver, thereby lowering the contrast between lesions and liver.

Of course, one might argue that there's no point in using gadolinium at all in a case such as this; however, not all the lesions were T1 hyperintense, and it is sometimes useful to evaluate the extent of lesion enhancement when assessing therapeutic response. A conventional extracellular agent would probably have been a better choice in this case, since the arterial phase images are generally better and in the equilibrium phase the background enhancement is lower. Subtraction images are a good idea in theory, but in practice they can be quite difficult to interpret, especially with very small multiple nodules in a patient who isn't a particularly good or consistent breath-holder.

A similar (and more common) situation can occur in patients with severe cirrhosis and multiple T1-hyperintense regenerative or dysplastic nodules. Again, the hepatobiliary phase images are potentially confounding, in that suspicious lesions without contrast retention but with high signal intensity on precontrast acquisitions may appear benign in the hepatobiliary phase on the basis of signal intensity that is similar to adjacent liver. Subtraction images (equilibrium phase minus precontrast) can be very helpful in sorting this out, but in our experience the consistency of breath-holding in the cirrhotic population is probably lower than average, and the additional delay (15-20 minutes) between precontrast and hepatobiliary phase acquisitions provides greater opportunity for small shifts in position that degrade the quality of the subtraction. In general, we prefer using standard extracellular gadolinium contrast agents in this population and relying on the superior arterial and portal venous phase images rather than hoping that the hepatobiliary phase images will provide the most useful information.

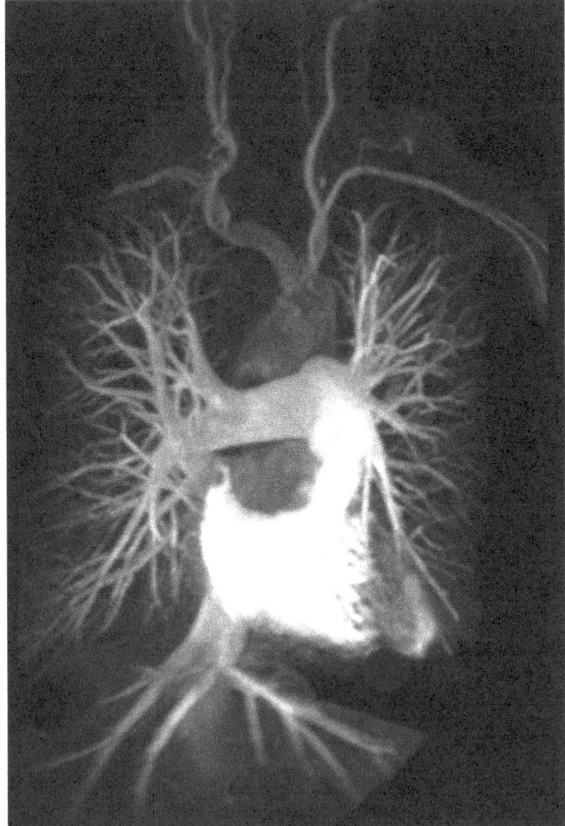

Figure 17.26.1

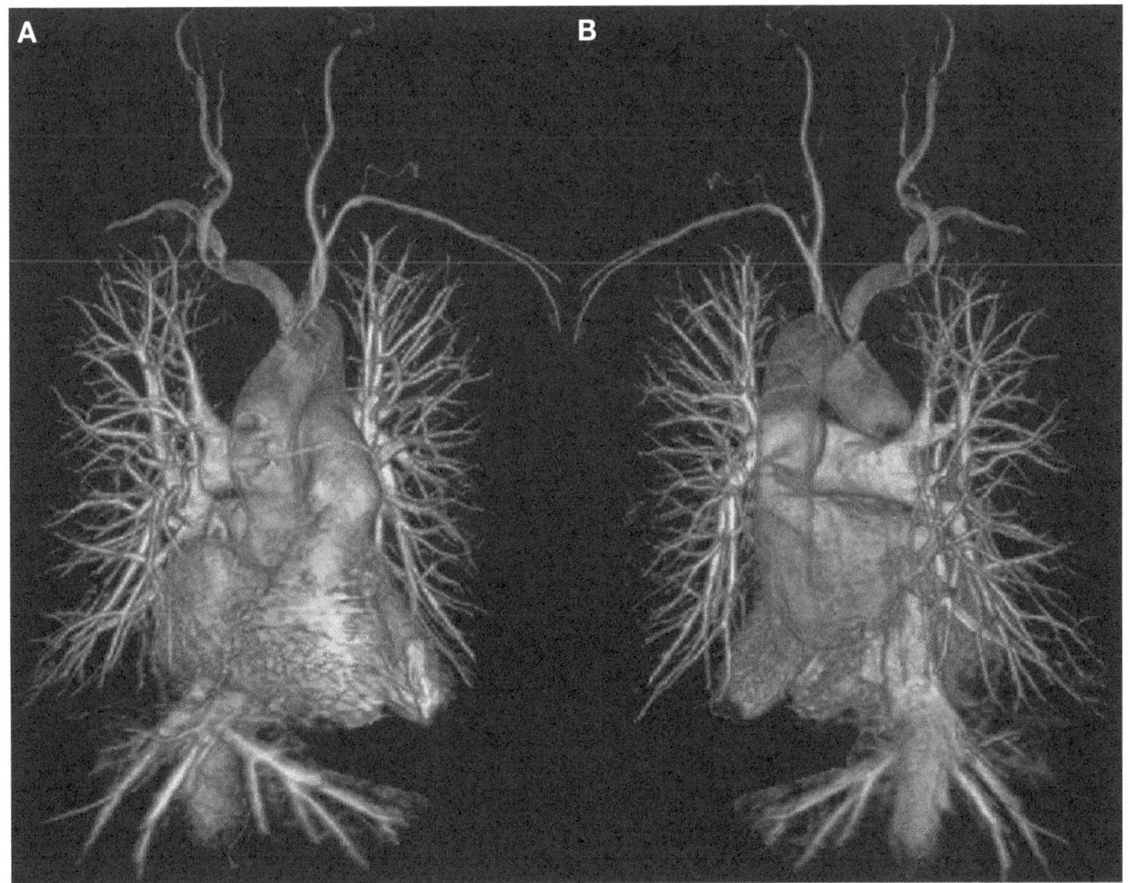

Figure 17.26.2

HISTORY: 82-year-old woman with giant cell arteritis

IMAGING FINDINGS: Coronal MIP image from 3D CE MRA (Figure 17.26.1) demonstrates poor bolus timing (for the requested examination of the thoracic aorta). Anterior (Figure 17.26.2A) and posterior (Figure 17.26.2B) VR images show slightly improved visualization of the thoracic aorta.

DIAGNOSIS: Error in bolus timing related to linear versus elliptical centric phase encoding

COMMENT: At first glance, this looks like a beautiful pulmonary MRA rather than a mistake, except that the examination requested was actually of the thoracic aorta. This acquisition was mistimed by several seconds, which usually doesn't happen unless a mechanical problem with the intravenous line arises between the test bolus and the MRA.

In this case, the error resulted from confusion about the particular k-space acquisition scheme of the MRA. The vast majority of CE MRAs in our practice are obtained using an elliptical centric acquisition (or a variant). This means that the center of k-space is sampled at the beginning of the acquisition, and then the coverage of k-space spirals outward to sample more peripheral lines. This is different from the linear phase encoding of many standard pulse sequences, in which initially peripheral lines are sampled, the center of k-space is acquired in the middle of the acquisition, and gradually increasing negative values are obtained at the end.

Elliptical centric ordering has the virtue of simplicity when performing CE MRA using a test bolus technique—the scan delay is equal to the contrast arrival time plus 2 or 3 seconds (to ensure that a stable high plateau of contrast has been reached). However, with linear phase encoding, the concentration of gadolinium in the artery of interest should peak just prior to the middle of the acquisition (ie, when the central lines of k-space are acquired), and therefore half of the scan time is subtracted from the contrast arrival time to calculate the scan delay. A somewhat more esoteric, but equally important, benefit of elliptical centric phase ordering is that the sampling of central k-space is more compact, so that the acquisition is less susceptible to venous contamination (ie, the venous signal arrives when more peripheral lines of k-space with lower signal intensity are being sampled and after the central lines have been acquired).

In this case, the radiologist thought that linear phase encoding would be performed, but actually elliptical centric ordering was selected, and therefore the calculated scan delay was several seconds too short (but it did correspond almost exactly to the arrival of gadolinium in the pulmonary arteries). This example illustrates 1 of the many reasons why at least 2 acquisitions should be performed for every MRA—to have a backup if something bad happens during the initial acquisition. A mistimed bolus and poor breath-holding are the usual culprits for substandard MRAs, and the additional acquisition provides a second chance to fix the problem, although if the initial scan delay was too long rather than too short, the second run may not look any better.

Fluoroscopic triggering of MRAs is preferred by many radiologists. It has the virtue of eliminating the test bolus, thereby simplifying and shortening the examination as well as eliminating the possibility of discrepancies between contrast travel times during the test bolus and MRA (which might occur if a patient performs a Valsalva maneuver or flexes an arm and compresses a vein for 1 but not both acquisitions). However, performing a rapid breath-hold is difficult for many patients, who may need 10 or more seconds to actually stop breathing, and it's also true that an infiltrated intravenous line is more problematic if you've just injected 15 or 20 mL of gadolinium into the subcutaneous tissues rather than 1 mL.

Notice how the VR reconstructions provide better visualization of the thoracic aorta and how these images would make the bolus timing error less apparent if an immediate second acquisition had not been obtained. This is because volume rendering allows greater flexibility in adjusting intensity thresholds at both low and high ends, so that the apparent contrast and signal intensity discrepancies between the aorta and pulmonary arteries can be somewhat reduced (although this works only if there is sufficient contrast in the aorta and if there is relatively low background signal intensity).

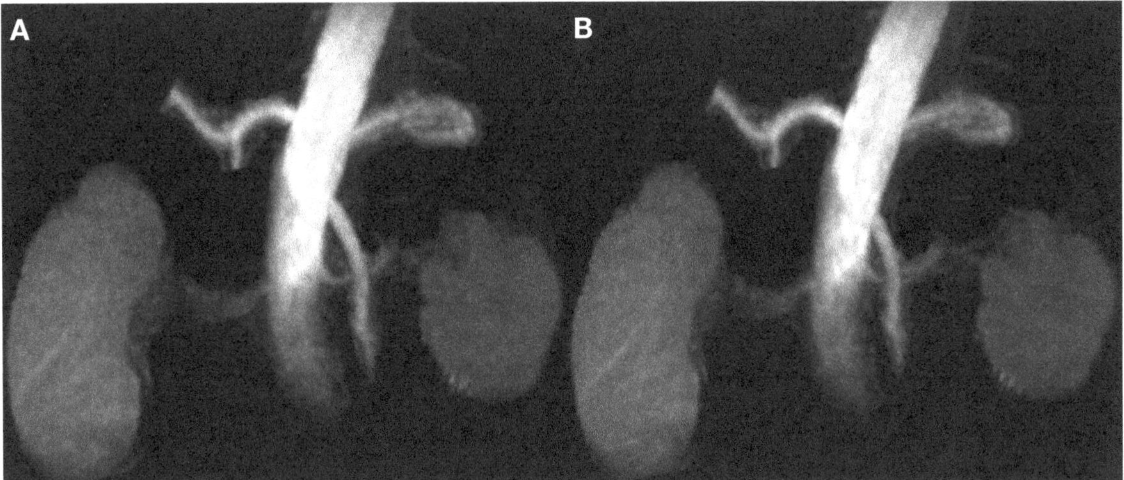

Figure 17.27.1

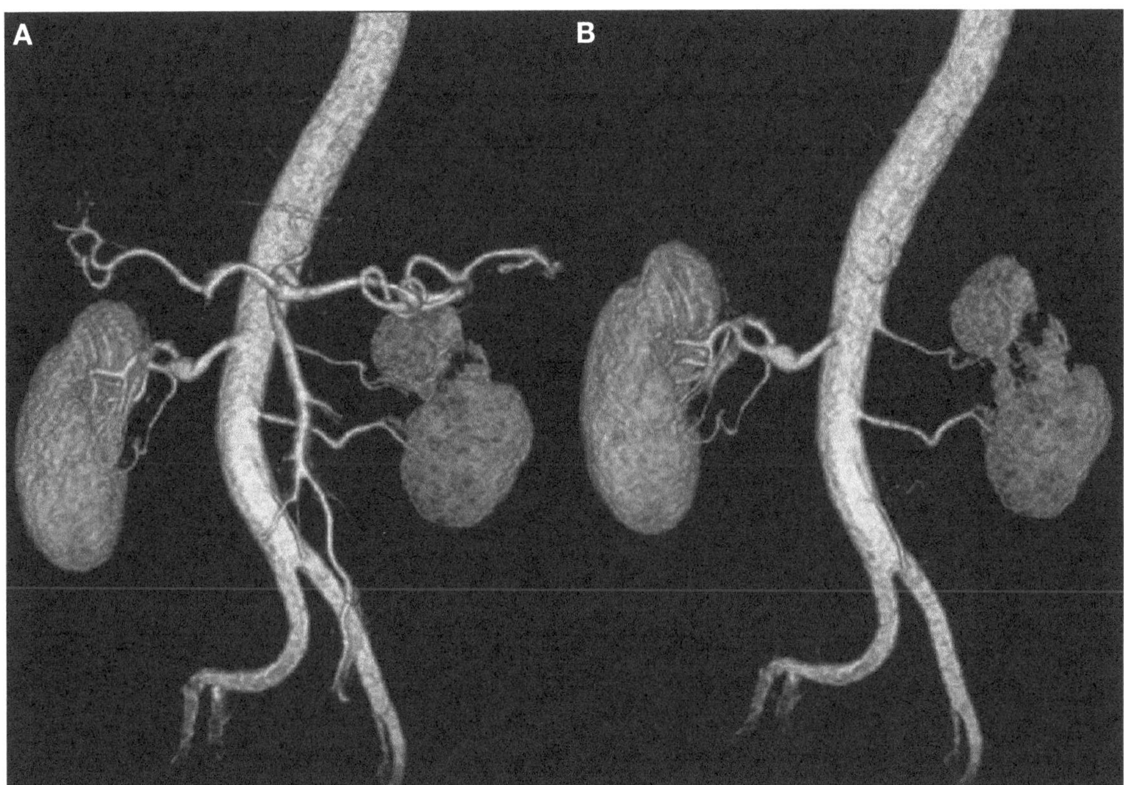

Figure 17.27.2

HISTORY: 60-year-old man with hypertension resistant to medical therapy

IMAGING FINDINGS: MIP images from noncontrast 3D SSFP renal MRA (Figure 17.27.1) demonstrate poor visualization of the renal arteries, with low contrast and low SNR. VR images from CE 3D MRA (Figure 17.27.2) reveal 2 left renal arteries and aneurysmal dilatation of the distal right main renal artery.

DIAGNOSIS: Artifact on noncontrast 3D SSFP renal MRA related to poor slab positioning

COMMENT: This case illustrates a fairly common artifact encountered with noncontrast 3D SSFP MRA: The inversion slab is too large or its leading edge is positioned too far above the origins of the renal arteries, so that bright blood never reaches the renal arteries.

The noncontrast 3D SSFP MRA sequence involves the addition of a spatially selective IR prepulse to a standard respiratory-gated 3D SSFP acquisition. The inversion slab encompasses the imaging volume and also extends several centimeters inferiorly in order to null the signal from venous blood entering the slab. The TI is selected to minimize the signal intensity of static background tissue and is typically 1,200 to 1,400 ms. The TI also defines the transit time for nonsuppressed arterial blood to flow into the slab, which imposes limits on the extent of superior-inferior coverage. In this case, for example, fresh blood flowing into the imaging volume during the TI has just barely reached the origin of the renal arteries, and therefore visualization of the renal arteries is poor. This problem is exacerbated in patients with slow arterial flow (eg, aortic aneurysms or heart failure).

There are several potential solutions to this problem. The simplest approach is to make sure that you can identify the renal artery origins (by performing adequate scout acquisitions), and then position the superior margin of the imaging volume slightly above them (rather than at the inferior margin of the slab, as in our example). This is even more straightforward if you don't care about visualizing the mesenteric arteries (although you probably should care most of the time). A second solution is to increase TI. This will lead to increased background signal intensity, but small increments in TI are generally well tolerated and can provide a noticeable improvement in the extent of superior-inferior coverage. A third technique is to perform 2 overlapping acquisitions, but for us this is usually a last resort because of the associated problems in generating 3D reconstructions.

Notice also on the CE MRA that there is an inferior accessory left renal artery. The prevalence of multiple renal arteries is fairly high, and this again emphasizes the importance of identifying the presence and location of the renal arteries prior to prescribing the imaging volume. (Also remember that since data acquisition in most respiratory-gated series occurs at end expiration, breath-held scout images should be obtained during expiration rather than inspiration.)

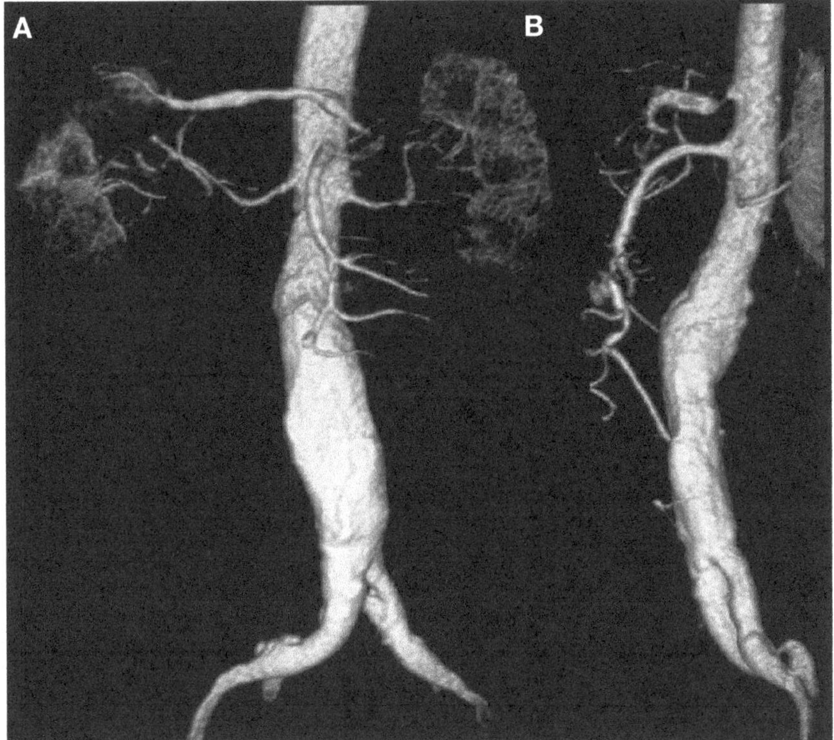

Figure 17.28.1

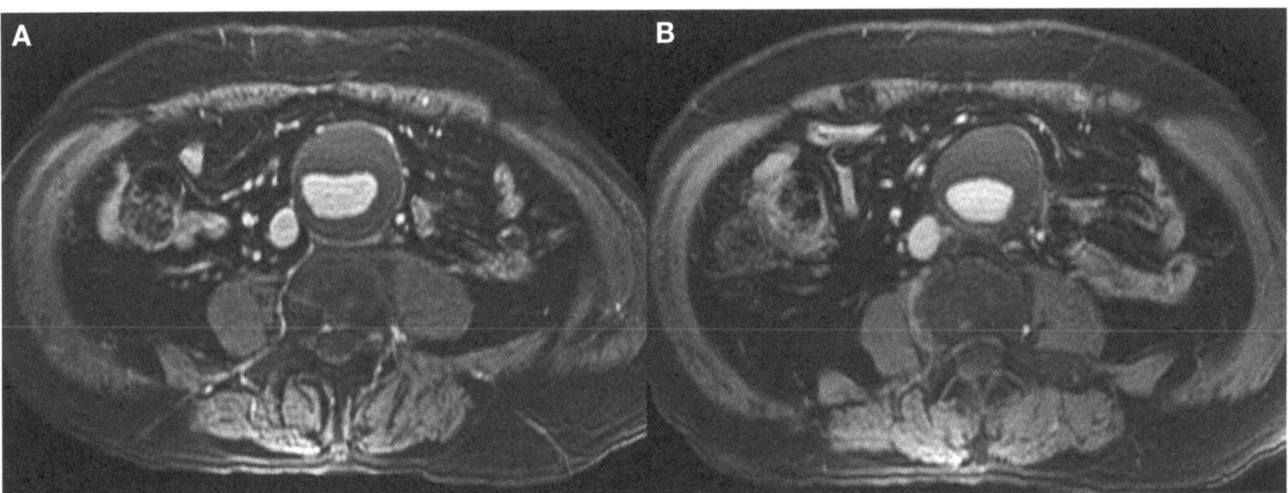

Figure 17.28.2

HISTORY: 68-year-old man with abdominal aortic aneurysm

IMAGING FINDINGS: Anterior and lateral VR images from 3D CE MRA (Figure 17.28.1) reveal diffuse atherosclerosis of the abdominal aorta, severe stenosis of the proximal celiac artery, and mild dilatation of the infrarenal aorta. Axial postgadolinium 2D SPGR images (Figure 17.28.2) demonstrate extensive peripheral thrombus in the aneurysm, with a true diameter much larger than what is seen on the VR images.

DIAGNOSIS: Underestimation of the true aneurysm size on 3D reconstructed images from CE MRA

COMMENT: While the vast majority of radiologists recognize that it's a bad idea to make a diagnosis based solely on assessment of 3D reconstructions, this is a difficult concept for many clinicians, who understandably gravitate to the prettiest images and don't want to spend their time inspecting hundreds or even thousands of source images—this has led to many long conversations with vascular surgeons convinced that we can't be trusted with a ruler or its electronic equivalent.

Although the benefits of acquiring delayed images in CT must always be balanced against the cost of additional radiation, no such considerations apply in MRI. Therefore, an immediate second acquisition is obtained for every CE 3D MRA performed in our practice, followed by post-MRA axial fat-suppressed 3D SPGR acquisition. The immediate delayed MRA can be valuable if there was an error in selection of the scan delay following contrast injection (Case 17.26), or if there is also an interest in visualizing mesenteric or systemic veins. Delayed images are also important in patients with aneurysms, particularly if the MRA covers a large FOV (such as the entire aorta and iliac arteries), since large aneurysms often fill slowly and visualization of vascular territories below the aneurysm may be limited. Similarly, in patients with dissections, a delayed acquisition may be necessary to appreciate filling of the false lumen.

The image contrast of typical 3D CE MRA pulse sequences is deliberately poor (high flip angles are used to suppress signal from background tissues not containing gadolinium, and most MRAs are performed without fat suppression), and therefore, post-MRA fat-suppressed 3D SPGR images are often very helpful, as in this case, for clearly visualizing the margin of a partially thrombosed aneurysm. We prefer 3D SPGR images to 2D SPGR acquisitions, since they can be more easily reformatted to provide accurate measurements of eccentric or tortuous aneurysms.

Important incidental findings are not uncommonly encountered in thoracic or abdominal MRA, since these examinations are most often performed in older patients who may have multiple medical problems. Here again, the post-MRA 3D SPGR images can be valuable for detection and characterization of a serendipitous renal cell carcinoma or hepatic mass.

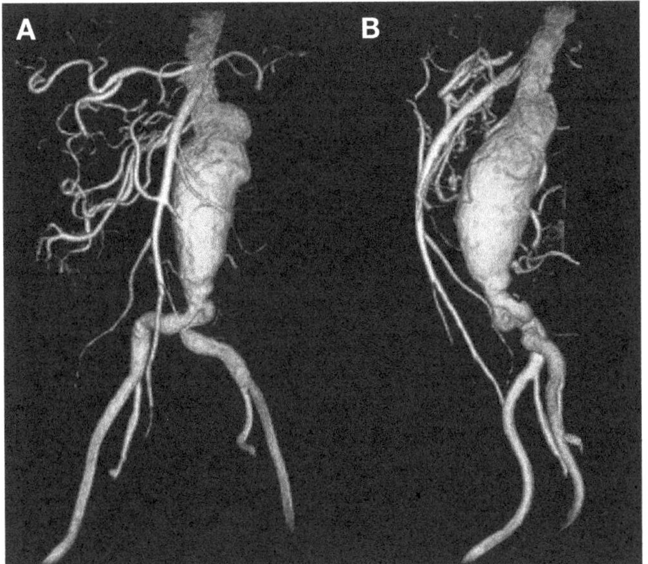

Figure 17.29.1

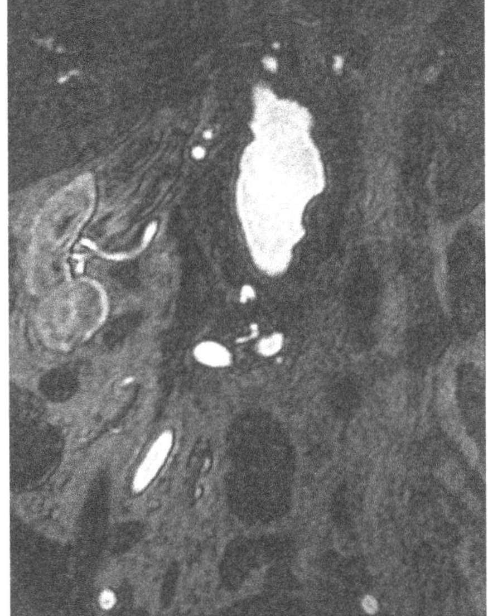

Figure 17.29.2

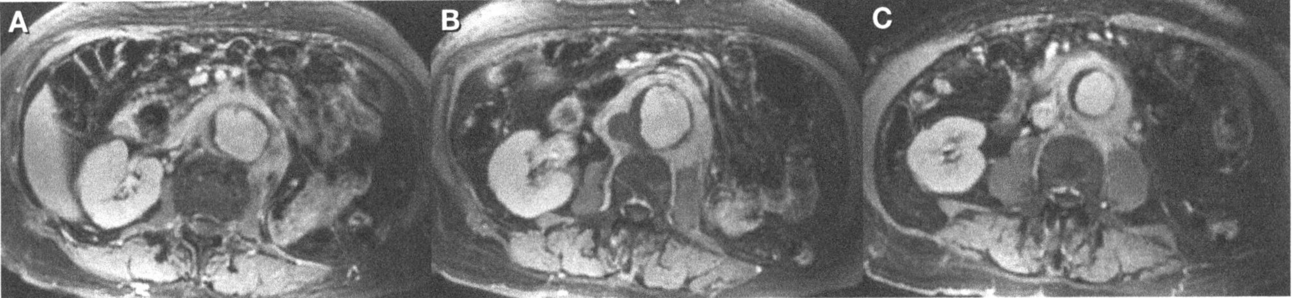

Figure 17.29.3

HISTORY: 79-year-old woman with abdominal aortic aneurysm

IMAGING FINDINGS: Anterior and lateral VR images from 3D CE MRA (Figure 17.29.1) reveal a large aneurysm involving much of the abdominal aorta as well as severe stenosis or focal occlusion of the proximal celiac artery. Source image from the 3D CE MRA (Figure 17.29.2) shows relatively subtle mural thickening throughout the visualized aorta. Axial postgadolinium 2D SPGR images (Figure 17.29.3) demonstrate marked mural thickening and enhancement of the wall of the aneurysm along with a thrombosed focal outpouching adjacent to the right kidney.

DIAGNOSIS: Inflammatory aneurysm not appreciated on 3D reconstructed views and thrombosed penetrating ulcer

COMMENT: This companion to Case 17.28 illustrates another pitfall of 3D reconstructions: They provide little if any visualization of the vessel wall, an important consideration in patients with known or suspected vasculitis.

This case is a particularly florid example, with marked thickening and enhancement of the aortic wall and periaortic soft tissue; even so, it's a relatively subtle finding on the MRA source images. Vasculitis is usually much more subtle, and mild mural thickening or enhancement may be impossible to detect on the MRA source images alone, particularly if only a single phase was acquired. This is related both to the intrinsically poor soft tissue contrast of the MRA pulse sequence as well as to the fact that maximal enhancement of the aortic wall, supplied by the vasa vasorum, usually occurs several seconds to minutes after the contrast bolus arrives in the vessel lumen. This again illustrates the necessity of a post-MRA 3D SPGR series: These acquisitions require little time or effort but are not included in the standard MRA protocols of all practices. We have a small collection of cases from other practices where, in retrospect, fairly obvious vasculitis was missed because the only archived series from the MRA examination were the scout sequence, the subtracted MRA source images, and the 3D reconstructions.

CASE 17.30

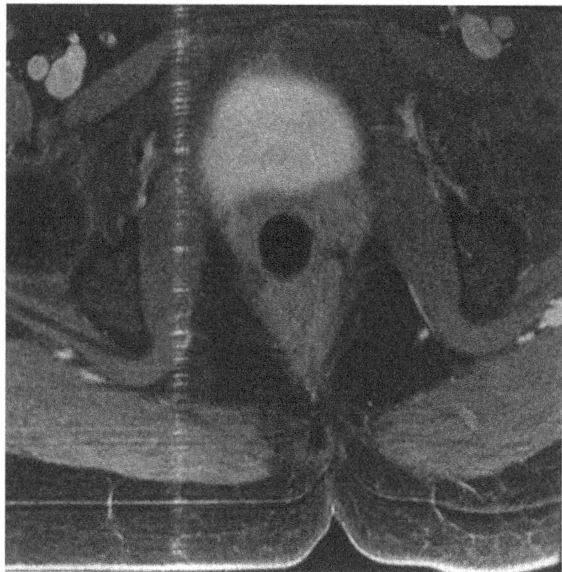

Figure 17.30.1

HISTORY: 19-year-old woman with inflammatory bowel disease and suspected perianal fistula

IMAGING FINDINGS: Axial postgadolinium 2D SPGR image (Figure 17.30.1) demonstrates a prominent artifact extending across the right side of the pelvis along the phase encoding direction.

DIAGNOSIS: Zipper artifact

COMMENT: Zipper artifacts most often occur as a result of a frequency leak—this is just extraneous RF radiation detected by the receiver coil. Notice that the line of artifact is off-center, indicating that the fundamental frequency is different from the Larmor frequency of the MRI system, which is what you would expect from an extraneous source.

In our practice, this artifact usually appears because the technologist or nurse went into the room between series to give contrast or another medication, or to encourage the patient to continue with the examination, and then forgot to close the door completely prior to continuation of the scan, thereby allowing nearby sources of RF radiation (eg, computers or other electronics) a pathway to enter the magnet and be detected by the receiver coil.

If closing the door to the magnet room does not solve the problem, the next most likely source is an electronic device within the room. In our practice, this is usually an anesthesia-related machine.

If you're really unlucky, the artifact could signify a leak in the radiation shielding surrounding the magnet room, which is typically a lengthy and expensive repair.

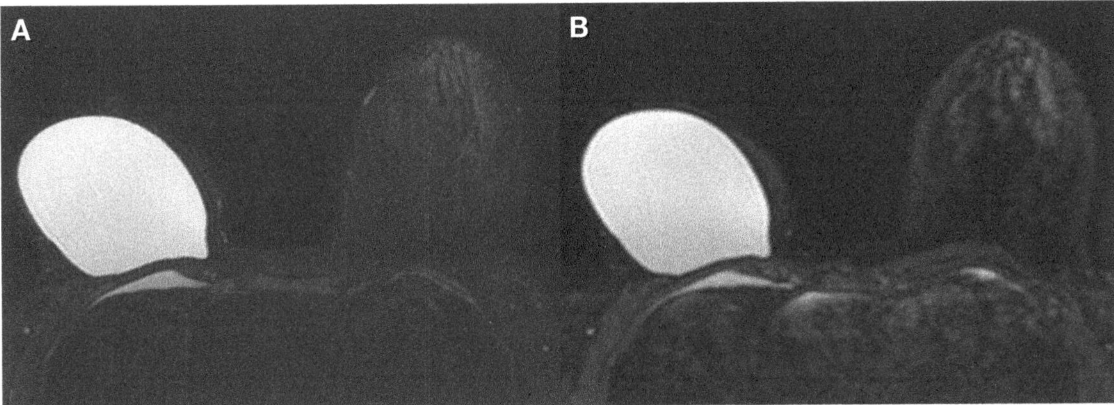

Figure 17.31.1

HISTORY: 49-year-old woman with a history of invasive right breast cancer with extensive ductal carcinoma in situ; she has undergone mastectomy and reconstruction with a saline implant

IMAGING FINDINGS: Axial water image (Figure 17.31.1A) from a T2-weighted FSE acquisition using a modified 3-point Dixon (IDEAL) method for fat suppression demonstrates water signal in a right breast implant. There is also a minimal amount of right pleural fluid. Axial FSE IR image with fat suppression and selective water suppression (silicone image) (Figure 17.31.1B) also demonstrates silicone signal in the right breast implant.

DIAGNOSIS: Incorrect selection of water peak

COMMENT: Since the Dixon water acquisition and the IR silicone acquisition appear essentially identical, it's easy to ignore the implications of the images and carry on with the examination (or with your interpretation). If you think about what the different series are showing, however, it should be obvious that a technical error has probably occurred. The IR sequence with water and fat suppression is essentially a silicone imaging acquisition (ie, silicone is bright and everything else is dark): While some implants do contain both silicone and saline, silicone is not soluble in water, and it would therefore be highly unlikely that 1) both silicone and water are uniformly distributed throughout the implant and 2) silicone has migrated to the right pleural space and has again uniformly mixed with normal pleural fluid.

Silicone imaging is usually performed using a 2D FSE IR sequence with the TI selected to suppress fat (about 100 ms) and with a spectral water suppression pulse whose success is dependent on excellent magnetic field homogeneity as well as on the ability to correctly identify the water peak for suppression. In this case, the technologist did not identify the correct peak to target for suppression, probably choosing instead the fat peak.

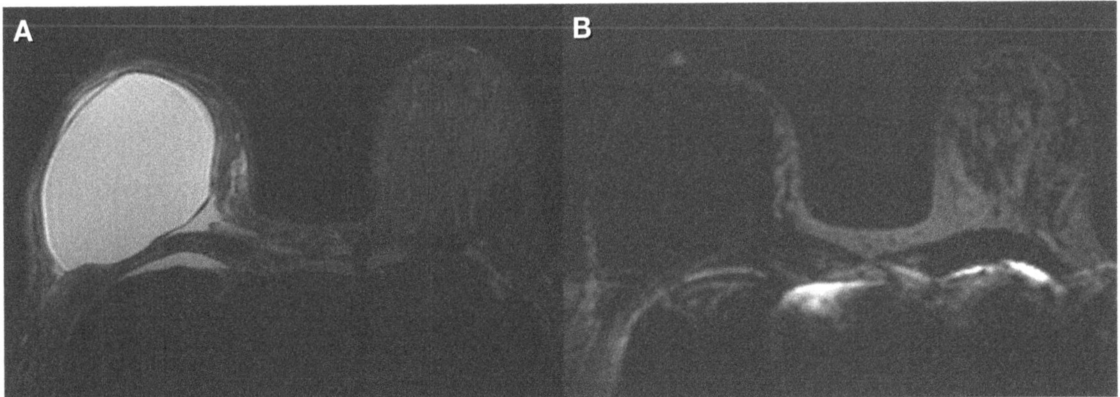

Figure 17.31.2

Figure 17.31.2 shows the same patient's breast MRI performed correctly 2 years earlier. Water image from a T2-weighted FSE 3-point Dixon (IDEAL) acquisition (Figure 17.31.2A) demonstrates the water signal from a saline implant as well as some peri-implant fluid (postoperative). There is again a small amount of physiologic right pleural effusion. The silicone image (Figure 17.31.2B) shows no silicone signal, certainly none in the saline implant, and fortunately none in the pleural fluid. The "silicone" signal along the pericardium is commonly seen and is related to the field inhomogeneities along the cardiac border.

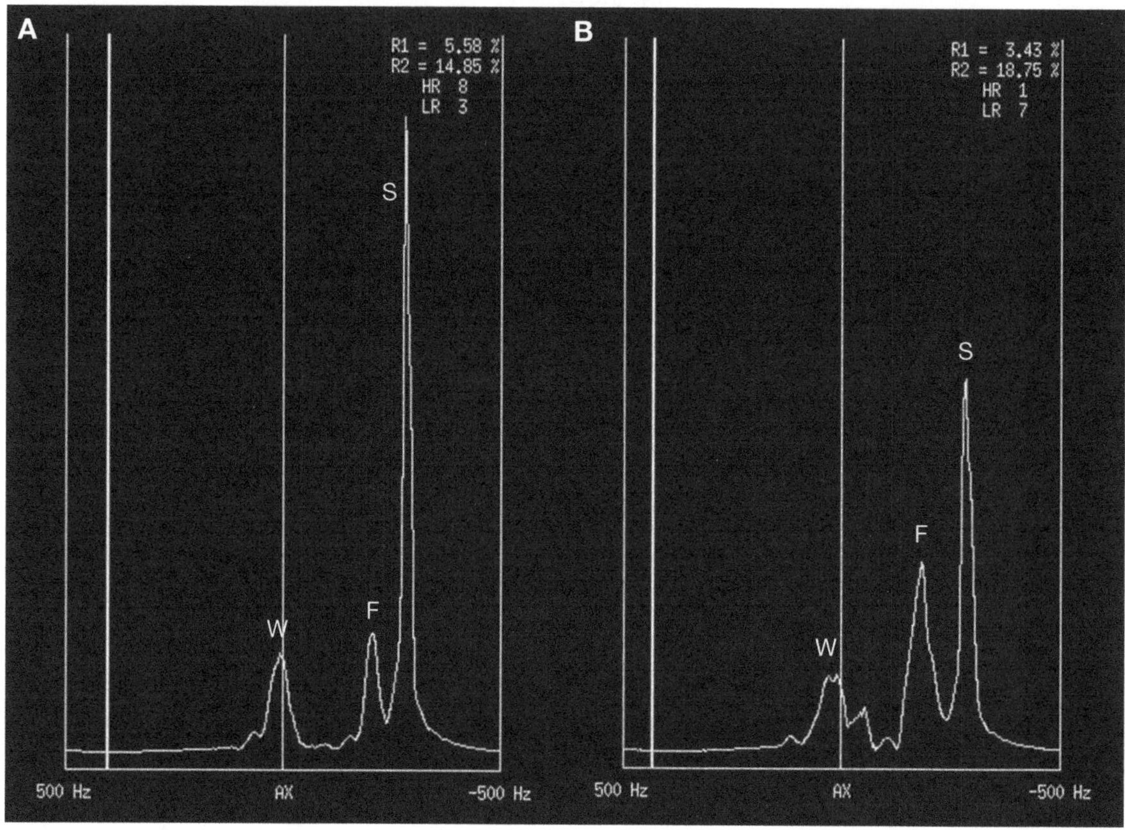

Figure 17.31.3

Even when your technologist knows which peak to suppress, this task is not always straightforward. Spectral peaks from 2 different patients with silicone implants are shown in Figure 17.31.3 (where *F* indicates fat; *S*, silicone; and *W*, water). When the peaks are narrowed, such as in Figure 17.31.3A, centering on the water peak is relatively straightforward. When the peaks are broader, as in Figure 17.31.3B, water suppression becomes a little more challenging, and a few additional adjustments may be necessary to optimize the acquisition, including increasing the amplitude of the suppression pulse and reshimming the volume to try to narrow the water peak. Since the fat peak is generally narrow, it's occasionally helpful to center on the fat peak and then add 220 Hz to find the water peak. In any case, it's always a good idea to turn on the suppression pulse while viewing the spectral peaks and make sure that the water peak disappears.

ABBREVIATIONS

ADC	apparent diffusion coefficient
ARC	autocalibrating reconstruction for Cartesian sampling
ASSET	array spatial and sensitivity encoding technique
CE	contrast-enhanced
CT	computed tomography
DWI	diffusion-weighted imaging
EPI	echo-planar imaging
ERCP	endoscopic retrograde cholangiopancreatography
ETL	echo train length
FOV	field of view
FRFSE	fast-recovery fast-spin echo
FSE	fast-spin echo
GRAPPA	generalized autocalibrating partially parallel acquisition
IDEAL	iterative decomposition of water and fat with echo asymmetric and least-squares estimation
IP	in-phase
IR	inversion-recovery
IVC	inferior vena cava
MAVRIC	multiacquisition variable resonance image combination
MIP	maximum intensity projection
MR	magnetic resonance
MRA	magnetic resonance angiography
MRCP	magnetic resonance cholangiopancreatography
MRI	magnetic resonance imaging
NPW	no-phase-wrap
OP	out-of-phase
RF	radiofrequency
ROI	region of interest
SEMAC	slice encoding for metal artifact correction
SENSE	sensitivity encoding
SMASH	simultaneous acquisition of spatial harmonics
SNR	signal to noise ratio
SPGR	spoiled gradient recalled
SSFP	steady-state free precession
SSFSE	single-shot fast-spin echo
STIR	short tau inversion recovery
TE	echo time
3D	3-dimensional
TI	inversion time
TOF	time-of-flight
TR	repetition time
2D	2-dimensional
US	ultrasonography
VR	volume-rendered

INDEX

B

D

E

R

Printed in the USA/Agawam, MA
February 21, 2023

806117.096